Veterinary Drug Handbook

3rd Edition

Donald C. Plumb, Pharm.D.

Hospital Director
Veterinary Teaching Hospitals, College of Veterinary Medicine
University of Minnesota
St. Paul, Minnesota

DISTRIBUTED BY
Iowa State University Press / Ames

Worldwide Print Distribution by:
   Iowa State University Press
   2121 South State Avenue
   Ames, Iowa 50014-8300
   Orders: 1-800-862-6657
   Office: 1-515-292-0140
   Fax: 1-515-292-3348
   Web site: www.isupress.edu

Pharma Vet Publishing
White Bear Lake, Minnesota

Printed in the United States of America
First edition, 1991
Second edition, 1995
Third edition, 1999

Library of Congress Cataloging-in-Publication Data

Plumb, Donald C.
   Veterinary drug handbook / Donald C. Plumb.—3rd ed.
      p.   cm.
   Includes bibliographical references (p.   ) and index.
   ISBN 0-8138-2444-3 (desk edition).—ISBN 0-8138-2353-6 (pocket edition)
   1. Veterinary drugs—Handbooks, manuals, etc.   I. Title.
   SF917.P58   1999
   636.089'51'03—dc21   98-53001

Desk edition ISBN: 0-8138-2444-3
Pocket edition ISBN: 0-8138-2353-6

Last digit is the print number: 9 8 7 6 5 4 3 2

This edition is dedicated to the veterinary profession
and to all the individuals who support it in the quest to better care for animals

* * *

Contributors to the 3rd Edition

Section on Ophthalmology Drugs
Dennis K. Olivero, DVM, DACVO
Veterinary Ophthalmology Spec.
St. Louis Park, MN 55416

Section on Dog and Cat Therapeutic Diets
C.A. Tony Buffington, DVM, PhD, DACVN
Professor of Veterinary Clinical Sciences

Cheryl Holloway, RVT
Nutrition Support Specialist
The Ohio State University Veterinary Hospital
Columbus, OH 43210-1089

Protocols for Chemotherapy
Carrie A. Wood, DVM,
Jeffrey S. Klausner, DVM, MS
Ford Watson Bell, DVM, MS
Chand Khanna, DVM, PhD
College of Veterinary Medicine
St. Paul, MN 55108

Preface to the Third Edition

The goal of the VDH remains the same as with the first two editions, namely to be a "...
quality, single-volume, veterinary drug reference, particularly one that included information on
not only those drugs approved for use in veterinary species, but also those non-approved
("human") drugs that are routinely used in veterinary practices today".

The major changes to this work are the addition of a new appendix on small animal therapeutic
diets, an additional 27+ drug monographs, an update of the older monographs, and a new
separate index that lists drugs by their classification or major indication. This last change should
allow a quick comparison of potential therapeutic options available for a given condition/species.
I hope the reader will find this new version a welcome addition to their reference
armamentarium.

Donald Plumb
October 1998

Acknowledgments-

I would like to thank my many colleagues in the Society of Veterinary Hospital Pharmacists for
their support and suggestions as well as the many readers of the first and second editions who
gave suggestions to improve this edition. Finally, I would like to thank my wife, Shirley for her
assistance in the preparation of the manuscript.

Abbreviations: OTC & Rx

In addition to the abbreviations used in writing prescriptions (*e.g.,* tid, q8h, etc.—see the abbreviation list in the appendix), the terms OTC or Rx are found in parentheses after a listed dosage form. If Rx, the drug is considered to be a prescription or legend product, and requires a prescription. OTC denotes that the item is available "over-the-counter" and does not require a prescription for purchase.

Caution!

While a sincere effort has been expounded to assure that the dosages and information included in this book are correct, errors may occur and it is suggested that the reader refer to the original reference or the approved labeling information of the product for additional information.

While this reference includes information on the use of non-approved drugs in food animals (extra-label use), this does not infer that the author or authors of the original references endorse the use of such drugs. Specific guidelines have been published with regard to the use of non-approved drugs in food animals and the reader should follow them before using any drug in those species. It is highly recommended to obtain the booklet: "**FDA and the Veterinarian**" [HHS publication No. (FDA) 89-6046] which discusses extra-label use and other related topics in an easily readable manner. It may be obtained from:

> U.S. Department of Health and Human Services
> Public Health Service
> Food and Drug Administration
> Center for Veterinary Medicine
> 5600 Fishers Lane,
> Rockville, MD 20857

The FDA's Center for Veterinary Medicine has an excellent web site. It is located at:
http://www.fda.gov/cvm/

DISCLAIMER

The author/publisher/distributor assume no responsibility for and make no warranty with respect to results that may be obtained from the uses, procedures, or dosages listed, and do not necessarily endorse such uses, procedures, or dosages. The author/publisher shall not be liable to any person whatsoever for any damages, or equivalencies, or by reason of any misstatement or error, negligent or otherwise obtained in this work. Should the purchaser not wish to be bound by the above, he/she may return the book to the distributor for a full refund.

Table of Contents

Drug Monographs

APPENDIX

ACEPROMAZINE MALEATE

Chemistry - Acepromazine maleate (formerly acetylpromazine) is a phenothiazine derivative which occurs as a yellow, odorless, bitter tasting powder. One gram is soluble in 27 ml of water, 13 ml of alcohol, and 3 ml of chloroform. Acepromazine is also known as "ACE", ACP, *Plegicil*®, *Notensil*®, & *Atravet*®.

Storage/Stability/Compatibility - Store protected from light. Tablets should be stored in tight containers. Acepromazine injection should be kept from freezing.

Although controlled studies have not documented the compatibility of these combinations, acepromazine has been mixed with atropine, buprenorphine, chloral hydrate, ketamine, meperidine, oxymorphone, and xylazine. Both glycopyrrolate and diazepam have been reported to be physically incompatible with phenothiazines. However, glycopyrrolate has been demonstrated to be compatible with promazine HCl for injection.

Pharmacology - Acepromazine is a phenothiazine neuroleptic agent. While the exact mechanisms of action are not fully understood, the phenothiazines block post-synaptic dopamine receptors in the CNS and may also inhibit the release of, and increase the turnover rate of dopamine. They are thought to depress portions of the reticular activating system which assists in the control of body temperature, basal metabolic rate, emesis, vasomotor tone, hormonal balance, and alertness. Additionally, phenothiazines have varying degrees of anticholinergic, antihistaminic, antispasmodic, and alpha-adrenergic blocking effects.

The primary desired effect for the use of acepromazine in veterinary medicine is its tranquilizing action. Additional pharmacologic actions that acepromazine possess, include antiemetic, antispasmodic, and hypothermic actions. Some researchers have reported that acepromazine has anticonvulsant activity, but in veterinary medicine it is generally felt that phenothiazines should not be used in epileptic animals or those susceptible to seizures (*e.g.*, post-myelography) as it may precipitate seizures.

Acepromazine may decrease respiratory rates, but studies have demonstrated that little or no effect occurs with regard to the blood gas picture, pH or oxyhemoglobin saturation. A dose dependent decrease in hematocrit is seen within 30 minutes after dosing in the horse and the dog. In horses, hematocrit values may decrease up to 50% of pre-dose values which is probably due to increased splenic sequestration of red cells.

Besides a lowering of arterial blood pressure in the dog, acepromazine causes an increase in central venous pressure, a vagally induced bradycardic effect and transient sinoatrial arrest. The bradycardia may be negated by a reflex tachycardic effect secondary to decreases in blood pressure. Acepromazine also has antidysrhythmic effects. Acepromazine has been demonstrated to inhibit the arrhythmias induced by the ultra-short acting barbiturates, and protect against the ventricular fibrillatory actions of halothane and epinephrine. Other pharmacologic actions are discussed in the adverse effects section below.

Uses/Indications - Acepromazine is approved for use in dogs, cats, and horses. Approved indications for dogs and cats include: "...as an aid in controlling intractable animals.....alleviate itching as a result of skin irritation; as an antiemetic to control vomiting associated with motion sickness" and as a preanesthetic agent. In horses, "...as an aid in controlling fractious animals", and in conjunction with local anesthesia for various procedures and treatments (Package Insert - *PromAce*®, Fort Dodge). It is also commonly used in horses as a pre-anesthetic agent, at very small doses to help control behavior.

Although not approved, it is used as a tranquilizer (see doses) in swine, cattle, rabbits, sheep and goats. Acepromazine has also been shown to reduce the incidence of halothane-induced malignant hyperthermia in susceptible pigs.

Pharmacokinetics - The pharmacokinetics of acepromazine has been studied in the horse (Ballard et al. 1982). The drug has a fairly high volume of distribution (6.6 L/kg), and is more than 99% protein bound. The onset of action is fairly slow, requiring up to 15 minutes following IV administration, with peak effects seen in 30-60 minutes. The elimination half-life in horses approximately 3 hours.

Acepromazine is metabolized in the liver with both conjugated and unconjugated metabolites eliminated in the urine. Metabolites may be found in equine urine for up to 96 hours after dosing. Do not administer to racing animals within 4 days of racing.

Contraindications/Precautions - Animals may require lower dosages of general anesthetics following acepromazine. Cautious use and smaller doses of acepromazine should be given to animals with hepatic dysfunction, cardiac disease, or general debilitation. Because of its hypotensive effects, acepromazine is relatively contraindicated in patients with hypovolemia or shock. Phenothiazines are relatively contraindicated in patients with tetanus or strychnine intoxication due to effects on the extrapyramidal system.

Intravenous injections should be made slowly. Do not administer intra-arterially in horses; may cause severe CNS excitement/depression, seizures and death. Because of its effects on thermoregulation, use cautiously in very young or debilitated animals.

Acepromazine has no analgesic effects; treat animals with appropriate analgesics to control pain. The tranquilization effects of acepromazine can be overridden and it cannot always be counted upon when used as a restraining agent. Do not administer to racing animals within 4 days of a race.

In dogs, acepromazine's effects may be individually variable and breed dependent. In geriatric patients, very low doses have been associated with prolonged effects of the drug. Giant breeds and greyhounds may be extremely sensitive to the drug, while terrier breeds are somewhat resistant to its effects. Boxers are reported to very sensitive to the hypotensive and bradycardic effects of acepromazine and should be used cautiously and in small doses in this breed. Atropine is often suggested to be given with acepromazine to help negate its bradycardic effects.

In addition to the legal aspects (not approved) of using acepromazine in cattle, the drug may cause regurgitation of ruminal contents when inducing general anesthesia.

Adverse Effects/Warnings - Acepromazine's effect on blood pressure (hypotension) is well described and an important consideration in therapy. This effect is thought to be mediated by both central mechanisms and also through the alpha-adrenergic actions of the drug. Cardiovascular collapse (secondary to bradycardia and hypotension) has been described in all major species. Dogs may be more sensitive to these effects than other animals.

In male large animals, acepromazine causes protrusion of the penis and corresponds to the sedative effects of the drug. In horses, this effect may last 2 hours. Stallions should be given acepromazine with caution as injury to the penis can occur with resultant swelling and permanent paralysis of the penis retractor muscle. Other symptoms that have been reported in horses include excitement, restlessness, sweating, trembling, tachypnea, tachycardia and, rarely, seizures and recumbency.

While acepromazine is a good tranquilizer, its effects of causing penis extension in horses and prolapse of the membrana nictitans in horses and dogs, may make its use unsuitable for show animals. There are also ethical considerations regarding the use of tranquilizers prior to showing an animal or having the animal examined before sale.

Occasionally an animal may develop the contradictory symptoms of aggressiveness and generalized CNS stimulation after receiving acepromazine. IM injections may cause transient pain at the injection site.

Overdosage - The LD$_{50}$ in mice is 61 mg/kg after IV dosage and 257 mg/kg after oral dose. Dogs receiving 20 - 40 mg/kg over 6 weeks apparently demonstrated no adverse effects. Dogs gradually receiving up to 220 mg/kg orally exhibited signs of pulmonary edema and hyperemia of internal organs, but no fatalities were noted.

Because of the apparent relative low toxicity of acepromazine, most overdoses can be handled by monitoring the animal and treating symptoms if they occur. Massive oral overdoses should definitely be treated by emptying the gut if possible. Hypotension should not be treated with epinephrine; use either phenylephrine or norepinephrine (levarterenol). Seizures may be controlled with barbiturates or diazepam. Doxapram has been suggested as an antagonist to the CNS depressant effects of acepromazine.

Drug Interactions - Acepromazine should not be given within one month of worming with an **organophosphate agent** as their effects may be potentiated. **Other CNS depressant agents (barbiturates, narcotics, anesthetics,** etc.) may cause additive CNS depression if used with acepromazine.

Quinidine when given with phenothiazines may cause additive cardiac depression.

Antidiarrheal mixtures (*e.g.,* Kaolin/pectin, bismuth subsalicylate mixtures) and **antacids** may cause reduced GI absorption of oral phenothiazines. Increased blood levels of both drugs may result if **propranolol** is administered with phenothiazines.

Phenothiazines block alpha-adrenergic receptors and if **epinephrine** is given, can lead to unopposed beta-activity causing vasodilation and increased cardiac rate. **Phenytoin** metabolism may be decreased if given concurrently with phenothiazines.

Procaine activity may be enhanced by phenothiazines.

Doses - Note: The manufacturer's dose of 0.5 - 2.2 mg/kg for dogs and cats is considered by many clinicians to be 10 times greater than is necessary for most indications. Give IV doses slowly; allow at least 15 minutes for onset of action.

Dogs:
    a) Premedication: 0.03 - 0.05 mg/kg IM or 1 - 3 mg/kg PO at least one hour prior to surgery (not as reliable). (Hall and Clarke 1983)
    b) Restraint/sedation: 0.025 - 0.2 mg/kg IV; maximum of 3 mg or 0.1 - 0.25 mg/kg IM.

Preanesthetic: 0.1 - 0.2mg/kg IV or IM; max. of 3 mg; 0.05 - 1 mg/kg IV, IM or SQ. (Morgan 1988)
c) 0.1 mg/kg IM or IV q8h (Davis 1985b)
d) 0.55 - 2.2 mg/kg PO or 0.55 - 1.1 mg/kg IV, IM or SQ (Package Insert, *PromAce*® - Fort Dodge)
e) 0.55 - 2.2 mg/kg PO or 0.055 - 0.11 mg/kg IV, IM or SQ (Kirk 1986)

Cats:
a) Restraint/sedation: 0.05 - 0.1 mg/kg IV, maximum of 1 mg (Morgan 1988)
b) 0.1 mg/kg IM or IV once daily (Davis 1985b)
c) 1.1 - 2.2 mg/kg PO, IV, IM or SQ (Package Insert, *PromAce*® - Fort Dodge)
d) 0.055 - 0.11 mg/kg IM or SQ or 1.1 - 2.2 mg/kg PO (Kirk 1986)
e) 0.11 mg/kg with atropine (0.045 - 0.067 mg/kg) 15-20 minutes prior to ketamine (22 mg/kg IM). (Booth 1988a)

Rabbits:
a) As a tranquilizer: 1 mg/kg IM, effect should begin in 10 minutes and last for 1-2 hours (Booth 1988a)

Cattle:
a) Sedation: 0.01 - 0.02 mg/kg IV or 0.03 - 0.1 mg/kg IM (Booth 1988a)
b) 0.05 - 0.1 mg/kg IV, IM or SQ (Howard 1986)
c) Sedative one hour prior to local anesthesia: 0.1 mg/kg IM (Hall and Clarke 1983)

Horses:
a) 0.04 - 0.1 mg/kg IV or IM (Robinson 1987)
b) 0.044 - 0.088 mg/kg (2 - 4 mg/100 lbs. body weight) IV, IM or SQ (Package Insert, *PromAce*® - Fort Dodge)
c) 0.02 - 0.05 mg/kg IM or IV as a preanesthetic (Booth 1988a)
d) Neuroleptanalgesia:0.02 mg/kg given with buprenorphine (0.004 mg/kg IV) or xylazine (0.6 mg/kg IV) (Thurmon and Benson 1987)

Swine:
a) 0.1 - 0.2 mg/kg IV, IM, or SQ (Howard 1986)
b) 0.03 - 0.1 mg/kg (Hall and Clarke 1983)
c) For brief periods of immobilization: acepromazine 0.5 mg/kg IM followed in 30 minutes by ketamine 15 mg/kg IM. Atropine (0.044 mg/kg IM) will reduce salivation and bronchial secretions. (Lumb and Jones 1984)

Sheep & Goats:
a) 0.05 - 0.1 mg/kg IM (Hall and Clarke 1983)

Monitoring Parameters -
1) Cardiac rate/rhythm/blood pressure if indicated and possible to measure
2) Degree of tranquilization
3) Male horses should be checked to make sure penis retracts and is not injured.
4) Body temperature (especially if ambient temperature is very hot or cold)

Client Information/FDA Approval Status - May discolor the urine to a pink or red-brown color; this is not abnormal.
Acepromazine is approved for use in dogs, cats, and horses not intended for food.

Dosage Forms/Preparations/FDA Approval Status/Withholding Times -
Veterinary-Approved Products:

Acepromazine Maleate for Injection 10 mg/ml for injection in 50 ml vials;*PromAce*® (Fort Dodge); generic; (Rx). Approved for use in dogs, cats and horses not intended for food.

Acepromazine Maleate Tablets 5, 10, & 25 mg in bottles of 100 and 500 tablets; *PromAce*® (Fort Dodge); generic; (Rx). Approved for use in dogs, cats and horses not intended for food.

Human-Approved Products: None

ACETAMINOPHEN

Chemistry - A synthetic non-opiate analgesic, acetaminophen (also known as paracetamol occurs as a crystalline, white powder with a slightly bitter taste. It is soluble in boiling water and freely soluble in alcohol. Acetaminophen is known in the U.K. as paracetamol.

Storage/Stability/Compatibility - Acetaminophen products should be stored at temperatures less than 40°C. Do not freeze the oral solution or suspension.

Pharmacology - Acetaminophen produces analgesia and antipyresis via mechanisms similar to the salicylates (inhibition of cyclooxygenase). Unlike aspirin, it does not possess significant anti-inflammatory activity.

Uses/Indications - Acetaminophen is occasionally used as an oral analgesic in dogs. In conditions of more severe pain, it may be used in combination with oral codeine phosphate.

Pharmacokinetics - Specific pharmacokinetic information in domestic animals was not located. In humans, acetaminophen is rapidly and nearly completely absorbed from the gut and is rapidly distributed into most tissues. Approximately 25% is plasma protein bound. Dogs apparently exhibit dose dependent metabolism (saturable).

Contraindications/Precautions/Reproductive Safety - Acetaminophen is contraindicated in cats at any dosage. Severe methemoglobinemia, hematuria, and icterus can be seen. Cats apparently are unable to significantly glucuronidate acetaminophen leading to toxic metabolites being formed and resultant toxicity. Dogs also do not metabolize acetaminophen as well as humans and its use must be judicious. In dogs, it is generally not recommended to use acetaminophen during the immediate post-operative phase (first 24 hours) due to an increased risk of hepatotoxicity developing.

  Absolute reproductive safety has not been established, but acetaminophen is apparently relatively safe for occasional use in pregnancy (no documented problems in humans). Animal data not located.

Adverse Effects/Warnings - Because acetaminophen is not routinely used in veterinary medicine, experience on its adverse effect profile is limited. At suggested dosages in dogs, there is a potential for renal, hepatic, GI and hematologic effects occurring.

Overdosage - Because of the potentially severe toxicity associated with acetaminophen, consultation with an animal poison center is recommended (see appendix). For overdosage in dogs or cats, standard gut emptying techniques and supportive care should be administered when applicable. Further treatment with acetylcysteine may be warranted (see acetylcysteine monograph for more information).

Drug Interactions - Large doses may potentiate the effects of **coumarin or inandione anticoagulants**. **Doxorubicin** may deplete hepatic glutathione, thereby leading to increased hepatic toxicity. Acetaminophen is not recommended to be used for post-operative analgesia in animals who received **halothane** anesthesia. Chronic use of acetaminophen in combination with **other analgesics** may lead to renal pathologies.

Laboratory Considerations - False positive results may occur for urinary **5-hydroxyindoleacetic acid**.

Doses -
  Dogs:
    As an analgesic:
      a) 15 mg/kg PO q8h (Dodman 1992)
      b) 10 mg/kg PO q12h (Kelly 1995)
      b) In the treatment of degenerative myelopathy (in German Shepherds): 5 mg/kg PO (not to exceed 20 mg/kg per day) (Clemmons 1991)

    In combination with codeine as an analgesic:
      a) Using a 60 mg codeine and 300 mg acetaminophen fixed-dose tablet (*e.g.*, *Tylenol®* *#4*), give 1 - 2 mg/kg (of the codeine) PO q6-8h. (Hansen 1994)

  Rabbits/Rodents:
    As an analgesic:
      a) Using Childrens Tylenol: 1 - 2 mg/ml in drinking water. Effective for controlling low-grade nociception. (Huerkamp 1995)

Monitoring Parameters - When used at recommended doses in otherwise healthy dogs for pain control, little monitoring should be necessary. However, with chronic therapy occasional liver, renal and hematologic monitoring may be warranted, particularly when symptoms occur.

Client Information - Follow directions carefully; do not exceed dosage or increase dosing frequency. Do not for any reasons administer to cats. Keep out of reach of children.

Dosage Forms/Preparations/FDA Approval Status/Withholding Times -
  Veterinary-Approved Products: None
  Human-Approved Products:
    There are many different trade names and products of acetaminophen available. The most commonly known trade name is *Tylenol®*. Acetaminophen is commonly available in 325 mg, 500 mg tablets; 650 mg tablets; 80 mg and 160 mg chewable tablets; 160 mg, 500 mg, 650 mg caplets; 500 mg gelcaps; 325 mg, 500 mg, capsules; 80 mg/2.5 ml, 80 mg/5 ml, 120 mg/5 ml, 160 mg/5 ml elixir; 16 mg/ml, 32 mg/ml, 80 mg/ml, 100 mg/ml and 160 mg/5 ml,

500 mg/15 ml, 80 mg/1.66 ml, oral solutions and suspensions. Combinations with other analgesics (aspirin, codeine phosphate, oxycodone or propoxyphene) are also available.

See the codeine monograph for more information on the use of acetaminophen-codeine combination preparations.

ACETAZOLAMIDE
ACETAZOLAMIDE SODIUM

Chemistry - A carbonic anhydrase inhibitor, acetazolamide occurs as a white to faintly yellowish-white, odorless, crystalline powder with pK_as of 7.4 and 9.1. It is very slightly soluble in water and sparingly soluble in hot water (90-100°C), and sparingly soluble in alcohol. Acetozolamide sodium occurs as a white lyophilized solid and is freely soluble in water. The injection has a pH of 9.2 after reconstitution with Sterile Water for Injection.

Storage/Stability/Compatibility - Acetazolamide products should be stored at room temperature. After reconstitution, the injection is stable for one week when refrigerated, but as it contains no preservatives, it should be used within 24 hours.

Acetazolamide sodium for injection is reportedly physically compatible with all commonly used IV solutions and cimetidine HCl for injection.

Pharmacology - The carbonic anhydrase inhibitors act by a noncompetitive, reversible inhibition of the enzyme carbonic anhydrase. This reduces the formation of hydrogen and bicarbonate ions from carbon dioxide and reduces the availability of these ions for active transport into body secretions.

Pharmacologic effects of the carbonic anhydrase inhibitors include decreased formation of aqueous humor, thereby reducing intraocular pressure; increased renal tubular secretion of sodium and potassium and, to a greater extent, bicarbonate, leading to increased urine alkalinity and volume; anticonvulsant activity, which is independent of its diuretic effects (mechanism not fully understood, but may be due to carbonic anhydrase or a metabolic acidosis effect).

Uses/Indications - Acetazolamide is used principally in veterinary medicine for its effects on aqueous humor production in the treatment of glaucoma. It has also been used for its diuretic action and in the treatment of metabolic alkalosis. In humans, the drug has been used as adjunctive therapy for epilepsy and for acute high-altitude sickness.

Pharmacokinetics - The pharmacokinetics of this agent have apparently not been studied in domestic animals. One report (Roberts 1985) states that after a dose of 22 mg/kg, the onset of action is 30 minutes; maximal effects occur in 2-4 hours; duration of action of 4-6 hours in small animals.

In humans, the drug is well absorbed after oral administration with peak levels occurring within 1 - 3 hours. It is distributed throughout the body with highest levels found in the kidneys, plasma and erythrocytes. Acetazolamide has been detected in the milk of lactating dogs and it crosses the placenta (unknown quantities). Within 24 hours of administration, an average of 90% of the drug is excreted unchanged into the urine by tubular secretion and passive reabsorption processes.

Contraindications/Precautions - Carbonic anhydrase inhibitors are contraindicated in patients with significant hepatic disease (may precipitate hepatic coma), renal or adrenocortical insufficiency, hyponatremia, hypokalemia, hyperchloremic acidosis or electrolyte imbalance. They should not be used in patients with severe pulmonary obstruction unable to increase alveolar ventilation or those who are hypersensitive to them. Long term use of carbonic anhydrase inhibitors are contraindicated in patients with chronic, noncongestive, angle-closure glaucoma as angle closure may occur and the drug may mask the condition by lowering intra-ocular pressures.

Acetazolamide should be used with caution in patients with severe respiratory acidosis or who have preexisting hematologic abnormalities. Cross sensitivity between acetazolamide and antibacterial sulfonamides may occur.

Adverse Effects/Warnings - Potential adverse effects that may be encountered include GI disturbances, CNS effects (sedation, depression, excitement, etc.), hematologic effects (bone marrow depression), renal effects (crystalluria, dysuria, renal colic, polyuria), hypokalemia, hyperglycemia, hyponatremia, hyperuricosemia, hepatic insufficiency, dermatologic effects (rash, etc.), and hypersensitivity reactions.

Overdosage - Information regarding overdosage of this drug is not readily available. It is suggested to monitor serum electrolytes, blood gases, volume status, and CNS status during an acute overdose. Treat symptomatically and supportively.

Drug Interactions - Oral acetozolamide can inhibit **primidone** absorption. **Primidone or phenytoin,** used with acetazolamide, may cause severe osteomalacia.

Because acetazolamide alkalinizes the urine, the excretion rates of many drugs (*e.g.,* **quinidine, procainamide, phenobarbital, methotrexate,** etc.) may be affected. It may also negate the effects of **methenamine** compounds in the urine.

Concomitant use with **corticosteroids, amphotericin B, corticotropin, or other diuretics** may exacerbate potassium depletion; this may be especially significant in patients receiving **digitalis preparations**.

Rarely, carbonic anhydrase inhibitors interfere with the hypoglycemic effects of **insulin**.

Laboratory Interactions - By alkalinizing the urine, carbonic anhydrase inhibitors may cause false positive results in determining **urine protein** using bromphenol blue reagent (*Albustix®, Albutest®, Labstix®*), sulfosalicylic acid (*Bumintest®, Exton's Test Reagent*), nitric acid ring test, or heat and acetic acid test methods.

Carbonic anhydrase inhibitors may **decrease iodine uptake** by the thyroid gland in hyperthyroid or euthyroid patients.

Doses - Directions for reconstitution of injection: Reconstitute 500 mg vial with at least 5 ml of Sterile Water for Injection; use within 24 hours after reconstitution.

Dogs:
For adjunctive treatment of metabolic alkalosis:
a) 10 mg/kg *qid* (may aggravate volume contraction and hypokalemia). (Hardy and Robinson 1986)
For adjunctive therapy of glaucoma:
a) 10 - 25 mg/kg divided 2-3 times daily (Brooks 1986)
b) 10 - 30 mg/kg divided *tid* (Wyman 1986)
c) 50 mg/kg IV one time; 7 mg/kg PO *tid* (Vestre 1985)

Cats:
For adjunctive therapy of glaucoma:
a) 50 mg/kg IV once; 7 mg/kg PO *tid* (Vestre 1985)

Ruminants:
a) 6 - 8 mg/kg IV, IM, or SQ (Howard 1986)

Swine:
a) 6 - 8 mg/kg IV, IM, or SQ (Howard 1986)

Monitoring Parameters - 1) Intraocular pressure/tonometry (if used for glaucoma); blood gases if used for alkalosis; 2) Serum electrolytes; 3) Baseline CBC with differential and periodic retests if using chronically; 4) Other adverse effects

Client Information - If using oral preparation and GI upset occurs, give with food. Notify veterinarian if abnormal bleeding or bruising occurs or if animal develops tremors or a rash.

Dosage Forms/Preparations/FDA Approval Status/Withholding Times -
Veterinary-Approved Products: None

Human-Approved Products:

Acetazolamide 125 mg, 250 mg Tablets; *Diamox®* (Lederle) (Rx); *.i.Dazamide®* (Major) (Rx); generic (Rx)

Acetazolamide Extended-release Capsules 500mg; *Diamox Sequels®* (Lederle); generic (Rx)

Acetazolamide Injection: 500 mg per vial; *Diamox®;* (Lederle);

Acetazolamide Powder 500 mg for Reconstitution; *Diamox®* (Lederle); Generic; (Rx)

To prepare parenteral solution: Reconstitute with at least 5 ml of Sterile Water for Injection. If refrigerated, potency will remain for 1 week, but it should be used within 24 hours as it contains no preservatives.

ACETIC ACID

Chemistry - Glacial acetic acid is $C_2H_4O_2$. Acetic acid has a distinctive odor and a sharp acid taste. It is miscible with water, alcohol or glycerin. Much confusion can occur with the percentages of $C_2H_4O_2$ contained in various acetic acid solutions. Acetic Acid USP is defined as having a concentration of 36-37% $C_2H_4O_2$. Diluted Acetic Acid NF contains 5.7 - 6.3% w/v of $C_2H_4O_2$. Solutions containing approximately 3-5% w/v of $C_2H_4O_2$ is commonly known as vinegar. Be certain of the concentration of the product you are using and your dilutions.

Storage/Stability/Compatibility - Acetic acid solutions should be stored in airtight containers.

Pharmacology/Indications - Via its acidifying qualities, acetic acid is used in ruminants to treat non-protein nitrogen-induced ammonia toxicosis. The acetic acid in the rumen lowers pH, thereby shifting ammonia to ammonium ions and reducing absorption. It is also used as a potential treatment to prevent enterolith formation in horses, supposedly by reducing colonic pH.

Pharmacokinetics - No information noted.

Contraindications/Precautions - Should not be administered to ruminants with potential lactic acidosis (grain overload, rumen acidosis) until ruled out.

Adverse Effects/Warnings - Because of the unpleasant taste and potential for causing mucous membrane irritation, acetic acid is generally recommended to be administered via stomach tube.

Overdosage/Acute Toxicity - When used for appropriate indications, there is little likelihood of serious toxicity occurring after minor overdoses. The greatest concern would occur if a concentrated form of acetic acid is mistakenly used due to its potential corrosiveness. However, one human patient who had glacial acetic acid used instead of 5% acetic acid during colposcopy (cervix), demonstrated no detectable harm.

Drug Interactions - There are no documented drug interactions with oral acetic acid, but because of its acidic qualities it could potentially affect the degradation of several drugs in the gut.

Doses -
   Cattle/Ruminants:
      For cattle with putrefaction of rumen associated with a high rumen pH:
         a)   4 - 10 liters of vinegar. (Constable 1993)

   Horses:
      For enterolith prevention:
         a)   Using vinegar: 250 ml/450 kg body weight PO once daily (Robinson 1992)

Dosage Forms/Preparations/FDA Approval Status/Withholding Times -
   Veterinary-Approved Products: None
   Human-Approved Products: None
      There are no systemic products commercially available. Acetic acid (in various concentrations) may be purchased from chemical supply houses.

ACETOHYDROXAMIC ACID

Chemistry - An inhibitor of urease, acetohydroxamic acid (also known as AHA, Acetic acid oxime, *N*-Acetylhydroxylamide, or *N*-Hydroxyacetamide) occurs as a white crystal having a pKa of 9.32-9.4 and a pH of about 9.4. In one ml of water, 850 mg is soluble and 400 mg is soluble in one ml of alcohol.

Storage/Stability/Compatibility - Tablets should be stored in tight containers.

Pharmacology - AHA inhibits urease, thereby reducing production of urea and subsequent urinary concentrations of ammonia, bicarbonate and carbonate. While the drug does not directly reduce urine pH, by reducing ammonia and bicarbonate production by urease-producing bacteria, it prevents increases in urine pH. The drug may act synergistically with several antimicrobial agents (*e.g.*, carbenicillin, gentamicin, clindamycin, trimethoprim/sulfa or chloramphenicol) in treating some urinary tract infections. The drug's effects on urinary pH and infection also indirectly inhibit the formation of urinary calculi (struvite, carbonate-apatite).

Uses/Indications - Acetohydroxamic acid is used as adjunctive therapy in some cases of recurrent canine urolithiasis (see pharmacology above) or in the treatment of persistent urinary tract infections caused by the following bacteria: *E. coli, Klebsiella spp., Morganella morganii, Staphylococci spp., Pseudomonas aeruginosa.*

Pharmacokinetics - No canine specific data was located. In humans, the drug is rapidly absorbed after PO administration. Absolute bioavailability "in animals" is reported to be 50-60%. AHA is well distributed throughout body fluids. It is partially metabolized to acetamide which is active. 36-65% of a dose is excreted in the urine unchanged, and 9-14% excreted in the urine as acetamide. The remainder is reportedly excreted as CO_2 via the respiratory tract. It is unknown if AHA is excreted into milk.

Contraindications/Precautions/Reproductive Safety - AHA is contraindicated in patients with poor renal function (*e.g.*, serum creatinine >2.5 mg/dl) or when it is not specifically indicated (see Indications).

   AHA use is considered contraindicated during pregnancy. In pregnant beagles, doses of 25 mg/kg/day caused cardiac, coccygeal, and abdominal wall abnormalities in puppies. At high doses (>750 mg/kg), leg deformities have been noted in test animals. Higher doses (1500 mg/kg) caused significant encephalopathologies.

Adverse Effects/Warnings - Potential adverse effects include CNS disturbances (anxiety, depression, tremulousness), GI effects (anorexia, vomiting), hematologic effects (reticulocytosis, Coombs negative hemolytic anemia, bone marrow depression), phlebitis, and skin rashes/alopecia. Effects on bilirubin metabolism have also been reported.

Overdosage/Acute Toxicity - In humans, mild overdoses have resulted in hemolysis particularly in patients with reduced renal function after several weeks of treatment. Acute overdoses would be expected to cause symptoms such as anorexia, tremors, lethargy, vomiting and anxiety. Laboratory findings that would be expected include increased reticulocyte counts, and a severe hemolytic reaction. Treatment for an acute overdose may include intensive hematologic monitoring with adjunctive supportive therapy, including possible transfusions.

Drug Interactions - AHA may chelate **iron** salts in the gut if given concomitantly. AHA may have a synergistic effect with **methenamine** in inhibiting the urine pH increases caused by urease-producing *Proteus* spp. AHA may also potentiate the antibacterial effect of methenamine against these bacteria. In humans, AHA taken with **alcohol** has resulted in a rash.

Laboratory Considerations - Although AHA is a true urease inhibitor, it apparently does not interfere with urea nitrogen determination using either the urease-Berthelot, urease-glutamate dehydrogenase or diacetyl monoxime methods.

Doses -
  Dogs:
    For adjunctive therapy of persistent struvite uroliths and persistent urease-producing bacteria after treating with antibiotics and calculolytic diets: 25 mg/kg/day in two divided doses PO. (Osborne, Lulich et al. 1993)

Monitoring Parameters - 1) CBC; 2) Renal/Hepatic (bilirubin) Function; 3) Efficacy

Client Information - Clients should be informed to monitor for symptoms associated with toxicity, particularly hematologic effects (*e.g.*, hematuria, etc.), as well as symptoms associated with urolithiasis or urinary tract infection.

Dosage Forms/Preparations/FDA Approval Status/Withholding Times -
  Veterinary-Approved Products: None
  Human-Approved Products:
    Acetohydroxamic Acid 250 mg scored Tablets; *Lithostat®* (Mission):

ACETYLCYSTEINE

Chemistry - The *N*-acetyl derivative of L-cysteine, acetylcysteine occurs as a white, crystalline powder with a slight acetic odor. It is freely soluble in water or alcohol. Acetylcysteine may also be known as N-acetylcysteine or N-Acetyl-L-cysteine.

Storage/Stability/Compatibility - When unopened, vials of sodium acetylcysteine should be stored at room temperature (15-30°C). After opening, vials should be kept refrigerated and used within 96 hours.

Acetylcysteine is incompatible with oxidizing agents and solutions can become discolored and liberate hydrogen sulfide when exposed to rubber, copper, iron, and during autoclaving. It does not react to aluminum, stainless steel, glass or plastic. If the solution becomes light purple in color, potency is not appreciably affected, but it is best to use non-reactive materials when giving the drug via nebulization. Acetylcysteine solutions are incompatible with amphotericin B, ampicillin sodium, erythromycin lactobionate, tetracycline, oxtetracycline, iodized oil, hydrogen peroxide and trypsin.

Pharmacology - When administered into the pulmonary tree, acetylcysteine reduces the viscosity of both purulent and nonpurulent secretions and expedites the removal of these secretions via coughing, suction, or postural drainage. The free sulfhydryl group on the drug is believed to reduce disulfide linkages in mucoproteins. This effect is most pronounced at a pH from 7-9. The drug has no effect on living tissue or fibrin.

Acetylcysteine also can reduce the extent of liver injury or methemoglobinemia after ingestion of acetaminophen, by providing an alternate substrate for conjugation with the reactive metabolite of acetaminophen, thus maintaining or restoring glutathione levels.

Uses/Indications - Acetylcysteine is used in veterinary medicine as both a mucolytic agent for pulmonary and ophthalmic use and a treatment for acetaminophen toxicity in small animals.

Pharmacokinetics - When given orally, acetylcysteine is absorbed from the GI tract. When administered via nebulization or intratracheally into the pulmonary tract, most of the drug is involved in the sulfhydryl-disulfide reaction and the remainder is absorbed. Absorbed drug is converted (deacetylated) into cysteine in the liver and then further metabolized.

Contraindications/Precautions/Reproductive Safety - Acetylcysteine is contraindicated (for pulmonary indications) in animals hypersensitive to it. There are no contraindications for its use as an antidote.

Because acetylcysteine may cause bronchospasm in some patients when used in the pulmonary system, animals with bronchospastic diseases should be monitored carefully when using this agent.

Reproduction studies in rabbits and rats have not demonstrated any evidence of teratogenic or embryotoxic effects when used in doses up to 17 times normal. It is unknown if acetylcysteine enters milk.

Adverse Effects/Warnings - When given orally for acetominophen toxicity, acetylcysteine can cause GI effects (nausea, vomiting) and rarely, urticaria. Because the taste of the solution is very bad, use of taste masking agents (*e.g.,* colas, juices) have been used. Because oral dosing of these drugs may be very difficult in animals, gastric or duodenal tubes may be necessary.

When administered into the pulmonary tract, acetylcysteine hypersensitivity has been reported rarely. Chest tightness, bronchoconstriction, and bronchial or tracheal irritation have also been reported, but these effects are also considered to occur rarely.

Overdosage/Acute Toxicity - The LD_{50} of acetylcysteine in dogs is 1 g/kg (PO) and 700 mg/kg (IV). It is believed that acetylcysteine is quite safe (with the exception of the adverse effects listed above) in most overdose situations.

Drug Interactions, Drug/Laboratory Interactions - The use of **activated charcoal** as a gut adsorbent of acetominophen is controversial, as charcoal may also adsorb acetylcysteine. In humans, at least 3 hours should pass between giving activated charcoal and the first dose of acetylcysteine. Because cats can develop methemoglobinemia very rapidly after ingestion of acetominophen, delay in treating with acetylcysteine cannot be recommended.

Doses -
  Dogs:
    For acetominophen toxicity:
      a) 150 mg/kg PO or IV initially, then 50 mg/kg q4h for 17 additional doses. (Bailey 1986a)
      b) Loading dose of 140 mg/kg PO or IV (as a 5% solution), then 70 mg/kg every 4 hours for 3-5 treatments. (Oehme 1986a)
      c) Loading dose of 140 mg/kg PO, then 70 mg/kg PO every 6 hours for 7 treatments. (Grauer and Hjelle 1988a)
    For respiratory use:
      a) 50 ml/hr for 30-60 minutes every 12 hours by nebulization. (Kirk 1986)
  Cats:
    For acetominophen toxicity:
      a) 140 mg/kg PO or IV (as a 5% solution) initially, then 70 mg/kg q4h PO or IV for 3-5 additional treatments. (Reid and Oehme 1989), (Oehme 1986a)
      b) 150 mg/kg PO or IV initially, then 50 mg/kg q4h for 17 additional doses. (Bailey 1986a)
      c) For methemoglobinemia secondary to acetominophen or other toxins: Using a 10% solution give 1.4 ml/kg (0.7 ml/kg if using 20% solution) PO q8h for a total of 3-7 treatments. (Maggio-Price 1988)
      d) Loading dose of 140 mg/kg PO, then 70 mg/kg PO every 6 hours for 7 treatments. (Grauer and Hjelle 1988a)
      e) 140 mg/kg PO initially (as a 5% solution in water (isotonic) or in 5-10% dextrose), then 70 mg/kg PO for 3-5 treatments. (Mount 1989)
    For respiratory use:
      a) 50 ml/hr for 30-60 minutes every 12 hours by nebulization. (Kirk 1986)

Monitoring Parameters -
  When used for acetominophen poisoning:
    1) Hepatic enzymes (particularly in dogs)
    2) Acetominophen level, if available (particularly in dogs)
    3) Hemogram, with methemoglobin value (particularly in cats)
    4) Serum electrolytes, hydration status

Client Information - This agent should be used in a clinically supervised setting only.

Dosage Forms/Preparations/FDA Approval Status/Withholding Times -
  Veterinary-Approved Products: None
  Human-Approved Products:
    Acetylcysteine (as sodium) 10% (100 mg/ml) and 20% (200 mg/ml) in 4 ml, 10 ml and 30 ml vials for oral inhalation, oral solution, or intratracheal instillation.; *Mucomyst*® (Apothecon); *Mucosil-10* ®(Dey Labs); *Mucosil-20* ®(Dey Labs); Generic. (Rx)

Acetylsalicylic Acid — See Aspirin

ACTH — See Corticotropin

Activated Charcoal — See Charcoal, Activated

ACYCLOVIR

Chemistry - An antiviral agent, acyclovir (also known as ACV or acycloguanosine), occurs as a white, crystalline powder. 1.3 mg is soluble in one ml of water. Acyclovir sodium has a solubility of greater than 100 mg/ml in water. However, at a pH of 7.4 at 37°C it is practically all unionized and has a solubility of only 2.5 mg/ml in water. There is 4.2 mEq of sodium in each gram of acyclovir sodium.

Storage/Stability/Compatibility - Acyclovir ointment should be stored in a dry place at room temperature. Acyclovir capsules and tablets should be stored in tight, light resistant containers at room temperature. Acyclovir suspension and sodium sterile powder should be stored at room temperature.

When reconstituting acyclovir sodium do not use bacteriostatic water with parabens as precipitation may occur. The manufacturer does not recommend using bacteriostatic water for injection with benzyl alcohol because of the potential toxicity in neonates. After reconstitution with 50-100 ml of a standard electrolyte or dextrose solution, the resulting solution is stable at 25°C for 24 hours. Acyclovir is reportedly incompatible with biologic or colloidial products (*e.g.*, blood products or protein containing solutions). It is also incompatible with dopamine HCl, dobutamine, fludarabine phosphate, foscarnet sodium, meperidine and morphine sulfate. Many other drugs have been shown to be compatible in specific situations. Compatibility is dependent upon factors such as pH, concentration, temperature and diluents used. It is suggested to consult specialized references (*e.g.*, *Handbook on Injectable Drugs* by Trissel; see bibliography) for more specific information.

Pharmacology - Acyclovir has antiviral activity against a variety of viruses including herpes simplex (types I and II), cytomegalovirus, Epstein-Barr, and varicella-Zoster. It is preferentially taken up by these viruses, converted into the active triphosphate form where it inhibits viral DNA replication.

Uses/Indications - Acyclovir may be useful in treating herpes infections in a variety of avian species and in cats with corneal and/or conjunctival herpes infections. Its use in veterinary medicine is not well established however, and it should be used with caution.

Pharmacokinetics - Acyclovir is poorly absorbed after oral administration (approx. 20%) and absorption is not significantly affected by the presence of food. It is widely distributed throughout body tissues and fluids, including the brain, semen, and CSF. It has low protein binding and crosses the placenta. Acyclovir is primarily hepatically metabolized and has a half life of about 3 hours in humans. Renal disease does not significantly alter half life unless anuria is present.

Contraindications/Precautions/Reproductive Safety - Acyclovir is potentially contraindicated (assess risk-benefit) during dehydrated states, pre-existing renal function impairment, hypersensitivity to it or other related antivirals, neurologic deficits, or previous neurologic reactions to other cytotoxic drugs.

Acyclovir crosses the placenta, but rodent studies have not demonstrated any teratogenic effects thus far. Acyclovir crosses into maternal milk, but associated adverse effects have not been noted.

Adverse Effects/Warnings - With parenteral therapy, potential adverse effects include thrombophlebitis, acute renal failure, and ecephalopathologic changes (rare). GI disturbances may occur with either oral or parenteral therapy.

Preliminary effects noted in cats, include leukopenia and anemias, that are apparently reversible with discontinuation of therapy.

Overdosage/Acute Toxicity - Oral overdose is unlikely to cause significant toxicity. It is recommended to contact a poison control center for further information should an overdose situation present itself.

Drug Interactions - Concomitant administration of IV acyclovir with **nephrotoxic medications** may increase the potential for nephrotoxicity occurring. Amphotericin B may potentiate the antiviral effects of acyclovir (but it also increases chances for development of nephrotoxicity).

Doses -
 Birds:
　　For treatment of Pacheco's Disease:
　　　a) 80 mg/kg PO q8h or 40 mg/kg q8h IM (do not use parenterally for greater than 72 hours as it can cause tissue necrosis at site of injection) (Oglesbee and Bishop 1994b)
　　　b) 80 mg/kg in oral suspension once daily PO; mix suspension with peanut butter or add to drinking water 50 mg in 4 oz of water for 7-14 days. (Jenkins 1993)
 Cats:
　　In cases of confirmed feline herpes virus infection (corneal and/or conjunctival) in which resolution is not achieved with time, time + antiviral topical agents: One 200 mg cap-

sule PO *qid*. Mixed results have been achieved. It is important to monitor the CBC of cats. Leukopenia and a mild non regenerative anemia which reversed with cessation of treatment have been noted in some cats. (Olivero 1994)

Monitoring Parameters - 1) Renal function tests (BUN, Serum Cr) with prolonged or IV therapy; 2) Cats: CBC

Dosage Forms/Preparations/FDA Approval Status/Withholding Times -
 Veterinary-Approved Products: None
 Human-Approved Products:

Acyclovir Tablets: 400 mg, 800 mg; *Zovirax* ®, (Glaxo Wellcome); generic (Rx)

Acyclovir Capsules 200 mg, 400 mg and 800 mg tablets; *Zovirax*® (Glaxo Wellcome); generic (Rx)

Acyclovir Suspension: 200 mg/5 ml; *Zovirax* ® (Glaxo Wellcome) (Rx)

Acyclovir Sodium Parenteral Injection (for IV infusion Only), 500 mg/vial (as sodium) in 10 ml vials; 1000 mg/vial (as sodium) in 20 ml vials; *Zovirax*®(Glaxo Wellcome); (Rx)

 Acyclovir is also available in a topical ointment.

ALBENDAZOLE

Chemistry - A benzimidazole anthelmintic structurally related to mebendazole, albendazole has a molecular weight of 265. It is insoluble in water and soluble in alcohol.

Storage/Stability/Compatibility - Albendazole suspension should be stored at room temperature(15-30°C); avoid freezing. Shake well before using.

Uses/Indications - Albendazole is approved for the following endoparasites of cattle: *Ostertagia ostertagi, Haemonchus spp., Trichostrongylus spp., Nematodius spp., Cooperia spp., Bunostomum phlebotomum, Oesphagostomum spp., Dictacaulus spp., Fasciola hepatica* (adults), and *Moniezia spp.* It is also used in sheep, goats and swine for endoparasite control.

 In cats, albendazole has been used to treat *Paragonimus kellicotti* infections. In dogs and cats, albendazole has been used to treat capillariasis. In dogs, albendazole has been used to treat *Filaroides* infections.

 Albendazole was implicated as being an oncogen in 1984, but subsequent studies were unable to demonstrate any oncogenic or carcinogenic activity of the drug.

Pharmacokinetics - Pharmacokinetic data for albendazole in cattle, dogs and cats were not located. The drug is thought to be better absorbed orally than other benzimidazoles. Approximately 47% of an oral dose was recovered (as metabolites) in the urine over a 9 day period.

 After oral dosing in sheep, the parent compound was either not detectable or only transiently detectable in the plasma due to a very rapid first-pass effect. The active metabolites, albendazole sulphoxide and albendazole sulfone reached peak plasma concentrations 20 hours after dosing.

Contraindications/Precautions - The drug is not approved for use in lactating dairy cattle. The manufacturer recommends not administering to female cattle during the first 45 days of pregnancy or for 45 days after removal of bulls. Albendazole has been associated with teratogenic and embryotoxic effects in rats, rabbits and sheep when given early in pregnancy.

 In humans, albendazole is recommended to be used with caution in patients with liver or hematologic diseases.

Adverse Effects/Warnings - Albendazole is tolerated without significant adverse effects when dosed in cattle at recommended dosages.

 Dogs treated at 50 mg/kg twice daily may develop anorexia.

 Cats may exhibit symptoms of mild lethargy, depression, anorexia, and resistance to taking the medication when albendazole is used to treat *Paragonimus.*

Overdosage/Toxicity - Doses of 300 mg/kg (30X recommended) and 200 mg/kg have caused death in cattle and sheep, respectively. Doses of 45 mg/kg (4.5X) those recommended did not cause any adverse effects in cattle tested. Cats receiving 100 mg/kg/day for 14-21 days showed signs of weight loss, neutropenia and mental dullness.

Drug Interactions - In humans, **dexamethasone** and **praziquantal** both have been demonstrated to increase albendazole serum levels. **Cimetidine** increased albendazole levels in bile and cystic fluid. Veterinary clinical relevance is unknown.

Doses -
 Dogs:
  For *Filaroides hirthi* infections:
   a) 50 mg/kg q12h PO for 5 days; repeat in 21 days. Symptoms may suddenly worsen during therapy, presumably due to a reaction to worm death. (Hawkins, Ettinger, and Suter 1989)

    b) 25 mg/kg PO q12h for 5 days; may repeat in 2 weeks (also for *Oslerus osleri)* (Reinemeyer 1995)

For *Filaroides osleri* (also known as *Oslerus osleri*) infections:
    a) 9.5 mg/kg for 55 days or 25 mg/kg PO *bid* for 5 days. Repeat therapy in 2 weeks. (Todd, Paul, and DiPietro 1985)

For *Capillaria plica*:
    a) 50 mg/kg q12h for 10-14 days. May cause anorexia. (Brown and Barsanti 1989)

For *Paragonimus kellicotti*:
    a) 50 mg/kg PO per day for 21 days. (Roberson 1988b)
    b) 30 mg/kg once daily for 12 days. (Todd, Paul, and DiPietro 1985)
    c) 25 mg/kg PO q12h for 14 days (Reinemeyer 1995)

For Giardia:
    a) 25 mg/kg PO q12h for 4 doses (Barr, Bowman et al.)
    b) 25 mg/kg PO bid for 5 days (Barr and Bowman 1994)

Cats:
For *Paragonimus kellicotti*:
    a) 50 mg/kg PO per day for 21 days. (Roberson 1988b)
    b) 25 mg/kg PO q12h for 10-21 days. (Hawkins, Ettinger, and Suter 1989)
    c) 30 mg/kg once a day for 6 days. (Todd, Paul, and DiPietro 1985)]
    d) 25 mg/kg PO q12h for 14 days (Reinemeyer 1995)

For Giardia:
    a) 25 mg/kg PO bid for 5 days (Barr and Bowman 1994)

Cattle:
For susceptible parasites:
    a) 10 mg/kg PO (Labeled directions; *Valbazen*®—SKB)
    b) 7.5 mg/kg PO; 15 mg/kg PO for adult liver flukes. (Roberson 1988b)
    c) For adult liver flukes: 10 mg/kg PO; best used in fall when the majority are adults (little or no efficacy against immature forms). A second treatment in winter may be beneficial. (Herd 1986b)
    d) For gastrointestinal cestodes: 10 mg/kg PO. (Herd 1986a)

Swine:
For susceptible parasites:
    a) 5 - 10 mg/kg PO. (Roberson 1988b)

Sheep & Goats:
For susceptible parasites:
    a) 7.5 mg/kg PO; 15 mg/kg PO for adult liver flukes. (Roberson 1988b)
    b) For adult liver flukes in sheep: 7.6 mg/kg (Paul 1986)

Monitoring Parameters -
    1) Efficacy
    2) Adverse effects if used in non-approved species or at dosages higher than recommended.

Client Information - Shake well before administering. Contact veterinarian if adverse effects occur.

Dosage Forms/Preparations/FDA Approval Status -
  Veterinary-Approved Products:
  Albendazole Suspension 113.6 mg/ml (11.36%) in 500 ml, 1 liter, 5 liter

  Albendazole Paste 205 g (7.2 oz); *Valbazen*® (Pfizer); (OTC) Approved for use in cattle (not female cattle of breeding age). Slaughter withdrawal=27 days.

  Human-Approved Products:
  Albendazole Tablets 200 mg *Albenza* ® (SmithKline Beecham), (Rx)

ALBUTEROL SULFATE

Chemistry - A synthetic sympathomimetic amine, albuterol sulfate occurs as a white, almost tasteless crystalline powder. It is soluble in water and slightly soluble in alcohol. One mg of albuterol is equivalent to 1.2 mg of albuterol sulfate. Albuterol is also known as salbutamol.

Storage/Stability/Compatibility - Oral albuterol sulfate products should be stored at 2-30°C. The capsules containing powder for inhalation should be left in the original packaging until just before use.

Pharmacology - Like other beta-agonists, albuterol is believed to act by stimulating production of cyclic AMP through activation of adenyl cyclase. Albuterol is considered to be predominantly a $beta_2$ agonist (relaxation of bronchial, uterine, and vascular smooth muscles). At usual doses, albuterol possesses minimal $beta_1$ agonist (heart) activity. beta adrenergics can promote a shift of potassium away from the serum and into the cell, perhaps via stimulation of $Na^+-K^+-ATPase$. Temporary decreases in either normal or high serum potassium levels are possible.

Uses/Indications - Albuterol is used principally in dogs and cats for its effects on bronchial smooth muscle to alleviate bronchospasm or cough. It potentially could also be used in horses as a bronchodilator.

Pharmacokinetics - The specific pharmacokinetics of this agent have apparently not been thoroughly studied in domestic animals. In general, albuterol is absorbed rapidly and well after oral administration. Effects occur within 5 minutes after oral inhalation, and 30 minutes after oral administration (*e.g.*, tablets). It does not cross the blood-brain barrier, but does cross the placenta. Duration of effect generally persists for 3-6 hours after inhalation and up to 12 hours (depending on dosage form) after oral administration. The drug is extensively metabolized in the liver, principally to the inactive metabolite, albuterol 4'-O-sulfate. After oral administration, the serum half life in humans has been reported as 2.7-5 hours.

Contraindications/Precautions/Reproductive Safety - Albuterol is contraindicated in patients hypersensitive to it. One veterinary school formulary (Schultz 1986) states that a related drug (**terbutaline**), is contraindicated in dogs and cats with heart disease, particularly when CHF or cardiomyopathy is present. It should be used with caution in patients with diabetes, hyperthyroidism, hypertension, seizure disorders, or cardiac disease (especially with concurrent arrhythmias).

In very large doses, albuterol is teratogenic in rodents. It should be used (particularly the oral dosage forms) during pregnancy only when the potential benefits outweigh the risks. Like some other beta agonists, it may delay pre-term labor after oral administration. It is unknown whether the drug crosses into maternal milk.

Adverse Effects/Warnings - Most adverse effects are dose-related and are those that would be expected with sympathomimetic agents including increased heart rate, tremors, CNS excitement (nervousness) and dizziness. These effects are generally transient and mild and usually do not require discontinuation of therapy. Decreased serum potassium values may be noted; rarely is potassium supplementation required.

Overdosage/Acute Toxicity - Symptoms of significant overdose after systemic administration may include arrhythmias (bradycardia, tachycardia, heart block, extrasystoles), hypertension, fever, vomiting, mydriasis, and CNS stimulation. Hypokalemia may also be noted. If recently ingested (orally), and if the animal does not have significant cardiac or CNS effects, it should be handled like other overdoses (empty gut, give activated charcoal and a cathartic). If cardiac arrhythmias require treatment, a beta-blocking agent (*e.g.,* propranolol) can be used, but may precipitate bronchoconstriction. The oral LD_{50} in rats is reported to be greater than 2 g/kg. Contact a poison control center for further information.

Drug Interactions - Use of albuterol with **other sympathomimetic amines** may increase the risk of developing adverse cardiovascular effects. **Beta-adrenergic blocking agents** (*e.g.,* propranolol) may antagonize the actions of albuterol. **Tricyclic antidepressants or monoamine oxidase inhibitors** may potentiate the vascular effects of albuterol. Use with inhalation anesthetics (*e.g.*, **halothane, isoflurane, methoxyflurane**), may predispose the patient to ventricular arrhythmias, particularly in patients with preexisting cardiac disease—use cautiously. Use with **digitalis** glycosides may increase the risk of cardiac arrhythmias.

Doses -
  Dogs:
    Warning:
      a) There are several sources that state that the oral dose is 50 <u>mg</u>/kg q8h. **This is an obvious overdose and should not be followed.** A more reasonable dose orally in dogs is: 0.05 mg/kg (50 <u>micrograms</u>/kg) PO q8h.
      b) For inhalation, based on a 60 lb dog: 0.5 ml of the 0.5% solution for nebulization in 4 ml of saline nebulized every 6 hours. (McConnell and Hughey 1992)
  Horses:
      a) 8 micrograms/kg PO q12h (Enos 1993)

Monitoring Parameters - 1) Clinical symptom improvement; auscultation, blood gases (if indicated); 2) Cardiac rate, rhythm (if warranted); 3) Serum potassium, early in therapy if animal susceptible to hypokalemia

Client Information - Contact veterinarian if animal's condition deteriorates or becomes acutely ill.

Dosage Forms/Preparations/FDA Approval Status/Withholding Times -
  Veterinary-Approved Products: None

Human-Approved Products:

Albuterol Tablets 2 mg, 4 mg tablets & 4 mg, 8 mg extended release tablets; *Proventil®* (Schering) *Proventil Repetabs* ®; *Ventolin®* (Glaxo Wellcome); *Volmax* (Muro); generic (Rx)

Albuterol Oral Syrup 2 mg (as sulfate)/5 ml; *Proventil®* (Schering); *Ventolin®* (Glaxo Wellcome); Generic; (Rx)

Albuterol Aerosol: Each actualization delivers 90 mcg albuterol in 17g & 6.7g canisters; *Proventil®* (Schering); *Proventil HFA®* (Key); *Ventolin®* (Glaxo Wellcome); generic. (Rx)

Albuterol for Inhalation: Solution for Inhalation 0.083% & 0.5% (as sulfate) in 3 ml or 20 ml; 200 micrograms capsules (powder) for inhalation; Airet® (Adams); *Albuterol* (Dey, Copley); *Proventil* ® (Schering);*Ventolin Nebules®* (Glaxo Wellcome); Ventolin Rotacaps® (Glaxo Wellcome); generic. (Rx)

ALLOPURINOL

Chemistry - A xanthine oxidase inhibitor, allopurinol occurs as a tasteless, fluffy white to off-white powder with a slight odor. It melts above 300° with decomposition and has an apparent pK_a of 9.4. Oxypurinol (*aka* oxipurinol, alloxanthine), its active metabolite, has a pK_a of 7.7. Allopurinol is only very slightly soluble in both water or alcohol.

Storage/Stability/Compatibility - Allopurinol tablets should be stored at room temperature in well-closed containers. The drug is stated to be stable in both light and air.

An extemporaneously prepared suspension containing 20 mg/ml allopurinol for oral use can be prepared from the commercially available tablets. Tablets are crushed and mixed with an amount of *Cologel®* suspending agent equal to 1/3 the final volume. A mixture of simple syrup and wild cherry syrup at a ratio of 2:1 is added to produce the final volume. This preparation has been reported to be stable for at least 14 days when stored in an amber bottle at either room temperature or refrigerated.

Pharmacology - Allopurinol and its metabolite, oxypurinol, inhibit the enzyme xanthine oxidase. Xanthine oxidase is responsible for the conversion of oxypurines (*e.g.,* hypoxanthine, xanthine) to uric acid. Hepatic microsomal enzymes may also be inhibited by allopurinol. It does not increase the renal excretion of uric acid nor does it possess any anti-inflammatory or analgesic activity.

Allopurinol, by inhibiting xanthine oxidase, can also inhibit the formation of superoxide anion radicals, thereby providing protection against hemorrhagic shock and myocardial ischemia in laboratory conditions. The clinical use of the drug for these indications requires further study.

Uses/Indications - The principle veterinary uses for allopurinol are for the prophylactic treatment of recurrent uric acid uroliths and hyperuricosuric calcium oxalate uroliths in small animals. It has also been used in an attempt to treat gout in pet birds.

Pharmacokinetics - No information was located on the pharmacokinetics of this agent in veterinary species. In humans, allopurinol is approximately 90% absorbed from the GI after oral dosing. Peak levels after oral allopurinol administration occur 1.5 and 4.5 hours later, for allopurinol and oxypurinol, respectively.

Allopurinol is distributed in total body tissue water, but levels in the CNS are only about 50% of those found elsewhere. Neither allopurinol or oxypurinol are bound to plasma proteins, but both drugs are excreted into milk.

Xanthine oxidase metabolizes allopurinol to oxypurinol. The serum half-life for allopurinol is 1 to 3 hours and for oxypurinol, 18-30 hours. Half-lives are increased in patients with diminished renal function. Both allopurinol and oxypurinol are dialyzable.

Contraindications/Precautions - Allopurinol is contraindicated in patients who are hypersensitive or have previously developed a severe reaction to it. It should be used cautiously and with intensified monitoring in patients with impaired hepatic or renal function. When used in patients with renal insufficiency, dosage reductions and increased monitoring are usually warranted.

While the safe use of allopurinol during pregnancy has not been established, dosages of up to 20 times normal in rodents have not demonstrated decreases in fertility. Infertility in males (humans) has been reported with the drug, but a causal effect has not been firmly established.

Adverse Effects/Warnings - Although adverse effects in dogs are apparently uncommon with allopurinol, several adverse effects have been reported in humans including GI distress, bone marrow suppression, skin rashes, hepatitis, and vasculitis. Human patients with renal dysfunction are at risk for further decreases in renal function and other severe adverse effects, unless dosages are reduced. Until further studies are performed in dogs with decreased renal function, the drug should be used with caution and at reduced dosages.

Prolonged use of allopurinol in dogs at dosages of 30 mg/kg/day may result in xanthine urolith formation. If the drug is required for chronic therapy, dosage reduction should be considered.

Overdosage - No reports of massive overdoses in either humans or veterinary species were located.

Drug Interactions - Increased bone marrow depression may occur in patients receiving both allopurinol and **cyclophosphamide**.

Urocosuric agents (e.g probenecid, sulfinpyrazone) may increase the renal excretion of oxypurinol and thereby reduce xanthine oxidase inhibition. In treating hyperuricemia however, the additive effects on blood uric acid may in fact be beneficial to the patient.

Urinary acidifiers (*e.g.,* **methionine, ammonium chloride**) may reduce the solubility of uric acid in the urine and induce urolithiasis.

In humans, concomitant use of allopurinol and **amoxicillin, hetacillin or ampicillin** has been implicated in increased occurrences of skin rashes. The veterinary significance of this interaction is unknown.

Allopurinol may inhibit the metabolism of **azathioprine or mercaptopurine** and increase their toxicity. If concurrent use is necessary, dosages of the antineoplastic/immunosuppressive agent should be reduced initially to 25-33% of their usual dose and then adjusted, dependent upon patient's response.

Most **diuretics (furosemide, thiazides), diazoxide, and alcohol** can increase uric acid levels.

In a few human patients, allopurinol used with **trimethoprim/sulfamethoxazole** has been associated with thrombocytopenia.

Allopurinol may reduce the metabolism of **oral anticoagulants** (*e.g.,* **warfarin**), thereby increasing their effect.

Large doses of allopurinol may decrease the metabolism of **aminophylline or theophylline**, thereby increasing their serum levels.

Doses -
  Dogs:
    For urate uroliths:
      a) 7 - 10 mg/kg PO *tid* for both dissolution or prevention. Goal is to reduce urine urate:creatinine ratio by 50%. (Senior 1989)
      b) For dissolution: 30 mg/kg/day PO divided into 2-3 doses per day. For prevention: 10 - 20 mg/kg/day. (Osborne et al. 1989)
      c) Alkalinize urine to a pH of 6.5 - 7 (see sodium bicarbonate monograph), give low purine diet and eliminate any UTI. Allopurinol at 10 mg/kg *tid* for the first month, then 10 mg/kg once daily thereafter. Reduce dose in patients with renal failure. (Polzin and Osborne 1985), (Lage, Polzin, and Zenoble 1988)
    Prior to surgery:
      a) 5 mg/kg PO 2 hours before surgery (McConnell and Hughey 1987)
  Cats:
    For urate uroliths:
      a) 9 mg/kg PO per day (Schultz 1986)
  Birds:
    For gout:
      a) In budgies and cockatiels: Crush one 100 mg tablet into 10 ml of water. Add 20 drops of this solution to one ounce of drinking water. (McDonald 1989)
      b) For parakeets: Crush one 100 mg tablet into 10 ml of water. Add 20 drops of this solution to one ounce of drinking water or give 1 drop 4 times daily. (Clubb 1986)

Monitoring Parameters -
  1) Urine uric acid (for urolithiasis)
  2) Adverse effects
  3) Periodic CBC, liver & renal function tests (*e.g.,* BUN, Creatinine, liver enzymes); especially early in therapy.

Client Information - Unless otherwise directed, administer after meals. Notify veterinarian if animal develops a rash, becomes lethargic or ill.

Dosage Forms/Preparations/FDA Approval Status/Withholding Times -
  Veterinary-Approved Products: None
  Human-Approved Products:
    Allopurinol Tablets 100 mg, 300 mg; *Zyloprim*® (Glaxo Wellcome); *Purinol* ® (Horner); Generic. (Rx)

ALTRENOGEST

Chemistry - An orally administered synthetic progestational agent, altrenogest has a chemical name of 17 alpha-Allyl-17β-hydroxyestra-4,9,11-trien-3-one. It may also be known as allyl trenbolone.

Storage/Stability/Compatibility - Altrenogest oral solution should be stored at room temperature.

Pharmacology - Progestins are primarily produced endogenously by the corpus luteum. They transform proliferative endometrium to secretory endometrium, enhance myometrium hypertrophy and inhibit spontaneous uterine contraction. Progestins have a dose-dependent inhibitory effect on the secretion of pituitary gonadotropins and also have some degree of estrogenic, anabolic and androgenic activity.

Uses/Indications - Altrenogest is indicated (labeled) to suppress estrus in mares to allow a more predictable occurrence of estrus following withdrawal of the drug. It is used clinically to assist mares to establish normal cycles during the transitional period from anestrus to the normal breeding season often in conjunction with an artificial photoperiod. It is more effective in assisting in pregnancy attainment later in the transition period. One group of authors (Squires et al. 1983) suggest selecting mares with considerable follicular activity (mares with one or more follicles 20 mm or greater in size) for treatment during the transitional phase. Mares that have been in estrus for 10 days or more and have active ovaries are also considered to be excellent candidates for progestin treatment.

Altrenogest is effective in normally cycling mares for minimizing the necessity for estrus detection, for the synchronization of estrus and permitting scheduled breeding. Estrus will ensue 2-5 days after treatment is completed and most mares ovulate between 8-15 days after withdrawal. Altrenogest is also effective in suppressing estrus expression in show mares or mares to be raced. Although the drug is labeled as contraindicated during pregnancy, it has been demonstrated to maintain pregnancy in oophorectomized mares and may be of benefit in mares who abort due to sub-therapeutic progestin levels.

Pharmacokinetics - The pharmacokinetic parameters of altrenogest were not found. Other progestin agents are rapidly metabolized by the liver.

Contraindications/Precautions - The manufacturer (*Regu-Mate*® — Hoechst) lists pregnancy as a contraindication to the use of altrenogest, however it has been used clinically to maintain pregnancy in certain mares (see Dosages below). Altrenogest should also not be used in horses intended for food purposes.

Adverse Effects/Warnings - Adverse effects of altrenogest appear to be minimal when used at labeled dosages. One study (Shideler et al. 1983) found negligible changes in hematologic and most "standard" laboratory tests after administering altrenogest to 4 groups of horses (3 dosages, 1 control) over 86 days. Occasionally, slight changes in Ca^{++}, K^+, alkaline phosphatase and AST were noted in the treatment group, but values were only slightly elevated and only noted sporadically. No pattern or definite changes could be attributed to altrenogest. No outward adverse effects were noted in the treatment group during the trial.

Use of progestational agents in mare's with chronic uterine infections should be avoided as the infection process may be enhanced.

The manufacturer (*Regu-Mate*® — Hoechst) lists the following people as those who should not handle the product:

1. Women who are or suspect that they are pregnant
2. Anyone with thrombophlebitis or thromboembolic disorders or with a history of these events
3. Anyone having cerebrovascular or coronary artery disease
4. Women with known or suspected carcinoma of the breast
5. People with known or suspected estrogen-dependent neoplasia
6. Women with undiagnosed vaginal bleeding
7. People with benign or malignant tumor which developed during the use of oral contraceptives or other estrogen containing products

Altrenogest can be absorbed after skin contact and absorption can be enhanced if the drug is covered by occlusive materials (*e.g.,* under latex gloves, etc.). If exposed to the skin, wash off immediately with soap and water. If the eyes are exposed, flush with water for 15 minutes and get medical attention. If the product is swallowed, do not induce vomiting and contact a physician or poison control center.

Overdosage - The LD_{50} of altrenogest in is 175-177 mg/kg in rats. No information was located regarding the effects of an accidental acute overdose in horses.

Drug Interactions - **Rifampin** may decrease progestin activity if administered concomitantly. This is presumably due to microsomal enzyme induction with resultant increase in progestin metabolism. The clinical significance of this potential interaction is unknown.

Doses -
Horses:
To suppress estrus for synchronization:
a) Administer 1 ml per 110 pounds body weight (0.044 mg/kg) PO once daily for 15 consecutive days. May administer directly on tongue using a dose syringe or on the usual grain ration. (Package insert; *Regu-Mate*® — Hoechst)
b) 0.044 mg/kg PO for 8-12 days (Bristol 1987)

To maintain pregnancy in mares with deficient progesterone levels:
a) 22 - 44 mg daily PO (Squires et al. 1983)

To suppress estrus (long-term):
a) 0.044 mg/kg PO daily (Squires et al. 1983)

Client Information - See the Adverse Effects/Warnings section for specific recommendations on handling, etc.

Dosage Forms/Preparations/FDA Approval Status/Withholding Times -
Veterinary-Approved Products:
Altrenogest 0.22% (2.2 mg/ml) in oil solution in 150 ml & 1000 ml bottles; *Regu-Mate*® (Hoechst); (Rx) Approved for use in horses not intended for food.

Human-Approved Products: None

AMIKACIN SULFATE

Chemistry - A semi-synthetic aminoglycoside derived from kanamycin, amikacin occurs as a white, crystalline powder that is sparingly soluble in water. The sulfate salt is formed during the manufacturing process. 1.3 grams of amikacin sulfate is equivalent to 1 gram of amikacin. Amikacin may also be expressed in terms of units. 50,600 Units are equal to 50.9 mg of base. The commercial injection is a clear to straw-colored solution and the pH is adjusted to 3.5 - 5.5 with sulfuric acid.

Storage/Stability/Compatibility - Amikacin sulfate for injection should be stored at room temperature (15-30°C); freezing or temperatures above 40°C should be avoided. Solutions may become very pale yellow with time, but this does not indicate a loss of potency.

Amikacin is stable for at least 2 years at room temperature. Autoclaving commercially available solutions at 15 pounds of pressure at 120°C for 60 minutes did not result in any loss of potency.

Amikacin sulfate is reportedly **compatible** and stable in all commonly used intravenous solutions and with the following drugs: amobarbital sodium, ascorbic acid injection, bleomycin sulfate, calcium chloride/gluconate, cefoxitin sodium, chloramphenicol sodium succinate, chlorpheniramine maleate, cimetidine HCl, clindamycin phosphate, colistimethate sodium, dimenhydrinate, diphenhydramine HCl, epinephrine HCl, ergonovine maleate, hyaluronidase, hydrocortisone sodium phosphate/succinate, lincomycin HCl, metaraminol bitartrate, metronidazole (with or without sodium bicarbonate), norepinephrine bitartrate, pentobarbital sodium, phenobarbital sodium, phytonadione, polymyxin B sulfate, prochlorperazine edisylate, promethazine HCl, secobarbital sodium, sodium bicarbonate, succinylcholine chloride, vancomycin HCl and verapamil HCl.

The following drugs or solutions are reportedly **incompatible** or only compatible in specific situations with amikacin: aminophylline, amphotericin B, ampicillin sodium, carbenicillin disodium, cefazolin sodium, cephalothin sodium, cephapirin sodium, chlorothiazide sodium, dexamethasone sodium phosphate, erythromycin gluceptate, heparin sodium, methicillin sodium, nitrofurantoin sodium, oxacillin sodium, oxytetracycline HCl, penicillin G potassium, phenytoin sodium, potassium chloride (in dextran 6% in sodium chloride 0.9%; stable with potassium chloride in "standard" solutions), tetracycline HCl, thiopental sodium, vitamin B-complex with C and warfarin sodium. Compatibility is dependent upon factors such as pH, concentration, temperature and diluents used. It is suggested to consult specialized references for more specific information (*e.g., Handbook on Injectable Drugs* by Trissel; see bibliography).

In vitro inactivation of aminoglycoside antibiotics by beta-lactam antibiotics is well documented. While amikacin is less susceptible to this effect, it is usually recommended to avoid mixing these compounds together in the same syringe or IV bag, unless administration occurs promptly. See also the information in the Drug Interaction and Drug/Lab Interaction sections.

Pharmacology - Amikacin, like the other aminoglycoside antibiotics, act on susceptible bacteria presumably by irreversibly binding to the 30S ribosomal subunit thereby inhibiting protein synthesis. It is considered to be an bactericidal antibiotic.

Amikacin's spectrum of activity include coverage against many aerobic gram negative and some aerobic gram positive bacteria, including most species of *E. coli, Klebsiella, Proteus, Pseudomonas, Salmonella, Enterobacter, Serratia*, and *Shigella, Mycoplasma*, and *Staphylococcus*. Several strains of *Pseudomonas aeruginosa, Proteus*, and *Serratia* that are resistant to gentamicin will still be killed by amikacin.

Antimicrobial activity of the aminoglycosides are enhanced in an alkaline environment.

The aminoglycoside antibiotics are inactive against fungi, viruses and most anaerobic bacteria.

Uses/Indications - While parenteral use is only approved in dogs, amikacin is used clinically to treat serious gram negative infections in most species. It is often used in settings where gentamicin-resistant bacteria are a clinical problem. The inherent toxicity of the aminoglycosides limit their systemic use to serious infections when there is either a documented lack of susceptibility to other less toxic antibiotics or when the clinical situation dictates immediate treatment of a presumed gram negative infection before culture and susceptibility results are reported.

Amikacin is also approved for intrauterine infusion in mares.

Pharmacokinetics - Amikacin, like the other aminoglycosides is not appreciably absorbed after oral or intrauterine administration, but it is absorbed from topical administration (not skin or urinary bladder) when used in irrigations during surgical procedures. Patients receiving oral aminoglycosides with hemorrhagic or necrotic enteritises may absorb appreciable quantities of the drug. After IM administration to dogs and cats, peak levels occur from 1/2 to 1 hour later. Subcutaneous injection results in slightly delayed peak levels and with more variability than after IM injection. Bioavailability from extravascular injection (IM or SQ) is greater than 90%.

After absorption, aminoglycosides are distributed primarily in the extracellular fluid. They are found in ascitic, pleural, pericardial, peritoneal, synovial and abscess fluids, and high levels are found in sputum, bronchial secretions and bile. Aminoglycosides are minimally protein bound (<20%, streptomycin 35%) to plasma proteins. Aminoglycosides do not readily cross the blood-brain barrier nor penetrate ocular tissue. CSF levels are unpredictable and range from 0-50% of those found in the serum. Therapeutic levels are found in bone, heart, gallbladder and lung tissues after parenteral dosing. Aminoglycosides tend to accumulate in certain tissues such as the inner ear and kidneys, that may help explain their toxicity. Volumes of distribution have been reported to be 0.15-0.3 L/kg in adult cats and dogs, and 0.26-0.58 L/kg in horses. Volumes of distribution may be significantly larger in neonates and juvenile animals due to their higher extracellular fluid fractions. Aminoglycosides cross the placenta and fetal concentrations range from 15-50% of those found in maternal serum.

Elimination of aminoglycosides after parenteral administration occurs almost entirely by glomerular filtration. The elimination half-lives for amikacin have been reported to be 1.14-2.3 hours in horses, 2.2-2.7 hours in calves, and 0.5-1.5 hours in dogs and cats. Patients with decreased renal function can have significantly prolonged half-lives. In humans with normal renal function, elimination rates can be highly variable with the aminoglycoside antibiotics.

Contraindications/Precautions/Reproductive Safety - Aminoglycosides are contraindicated in patients who are hypersensitive to them. Because these drugs are often the only effective agents in severe gram-negative infections there are no other absolute contraindications to their use. However, they should be used with extreme caution in patients with preexisting renal disease with concomitant monitoring and dosage interval adjustments made. Other risk factors for the development of toxicity include age (both neonatal and geriatric patients), fever, sepsis and dehydration.

Because aminoglycosides can cause irreversible ototoxicity, they should be used with caution in "working" dogs (*e.g.,* "seeing-eye", herding, dogs for the hearing impaired, etc.).

Aminoglycosides should be used with caution in patients with neuromuscular disorders (*e.g.,* myasthenia gravis) due to their neuromuscular blocking activity.

Because aminoglycosides are eliminated primarily through renal mechanisms, they should be used cautiously, preferably with serum monitoring and dosage adjustment in neonatal or geriatric animals.

Aminoglycosides are generally considered contraindicated in rabbits/hares as they adversely affect the GI flora balance in these animals.

Aminoglycosides can cross the placenta and while rare, may cause 8th cranial nerve toxicity or nephrotoxicity in fetuses. Because the drug should only be used in serious infections, the benefits of therapy may exceed the potential risks.

Adverse Effects/Warnings - The aminoglycosides are infamous for their nephrotoxic and ototoxic effects. The nephrotoxic (tubular necrosis) mechanisms of these drugs are not completely understood, but are probably related to interference with phospholipid metabolism in the lysosomes of proximal renal tubular cells, resulting in leakage of proteolytic enzymes into the cytoplasm. Nephrotoxicity is usually manifested by increases in BUN, creatinine, nonprotein nitrogen in the serum and decreases in urine specific gravity and creatinine clearance. Proteinuria and cells or casts may also be seen in the urine. Nephrotoxicity is usually reversible once the drug is discontinued. While gentamicin may be more nephrotoxic than the other aminoglycosides, the incidences of nephrotoxicity with all of these agents require equal caution and monitoring.

Ototoxicity (8th cranial nerve toxicity) of the aminoglycosides can be manifested by either auditory and/or vestibular symptoms and may be irreversible. Vestibular symptoms are more frequent with streptomycin, gentamicin, or tobramycin. Auditory symptoms are more frequent with amikacin, neomycin, or kanamycin, but either forms can occur with any of the drugs. Cats are apparently very sensitive to the vestibular effects of the aminoglycosides.

The aminoglycosides can also cause neuromuscular blockade, facial edema, pain/inflammation at injection site, peripheral neuropathy and hypersensitivity reactions. Rarely, GI symptoms, hematologic and hepatic effects have been reported.

Overdosage/Acute Toxicity - Should an inadvertant overdosage be administered, three treatments have been recommended. Hemodialysis is very effective in reducing serum levels of the drug, but is not a viable option for most veterinary patients. Peritoneal dialysis also will reduce serum levels, but is much less efficacious. Complexation of drug with either carbenicillin or ticarcillin (12-20 g/day in humans) is reportedly nearly as effective as hemodialysis. Since amikacin is less affected by this effect than either tobramycin or gentamicin, it is assumed that reduction in serum levels will also be minimized using this procedure.

Drug Interactions - Aminoglycosides should be used with caution with other nephrotoxic, ototoxic, and neurotoxic drugs. These include **amphotericin B**, **other aminoglycosides**, **acyclovir**, **bacitracin** (parenteral use), **cisplatin**, **methoxyflurane**, **polymyxin B**, or **vancomycin**.

The concurrent use of aminoglycosides with **cephalosporins** is controversial. Potentially, cephalosporins could cause additive nephrotoxicity when used with aminoglycosides, but this interaction has only been well documented with cephaloridine (no longer marketed) and cephalothin.

Concurrent use with loop (**furosemide**, **ethacrynic acid**) or osmotic diuretics (**mannitol**, **urea**) may increase the nephrotoxic or ototoxic potential of the aminoglycosides.

Concomitant use with **general anesthetics** or **neuromuscular blocking agents** could potentiate neuromuscular blockade.

Synergism against *Pseudomonas aeruginosa* and *enterococci* may occur with beta-**lactam antibiotics** and the aminoglycosides. This effect is apparently not predictable and its clinical usefulness is in question.

Drug/Laboratory Interactions - Amikacin **serum concentrations** may be falsely decreased if the patient is also receiving beta-lactam antibiotics and the serum is stored prior analysis. It is recommended that if assay is delayed, samples be frozen and if possible, drawn at times when the beta-lactam antibiotic is at a trough.

Doses - Note: There is significant interpatient variability with regards to aminoglycoside pharmacokinetic parameters. To insure therapeutic levels and to minimize the risks for toxicity development, it is recommended to consider monitoring serum levels for this drug.

For small animals, one pair of authors (Aronson and Aucoin 1989) make the following recommendations with regard to minimizing risks of toxicity yet maximizing efficacy:

1) Dose according to animal size. The larger the animal, the smaller the dose (on a mg/kg basis).
2) The more risk factors (age, fever, sepsis, renal disease, dehydration) the smaller the dose.
3) In old patients or those suspected of renal disease, increase dosing interval from q8h to q16-24h.
4) Determine serum creatinine prior to therapy and adjust by changes in level even if it remains in "normal range".
5) Monitor urine for changes in sediment (*e.g.,* casts) or concentrating ability. Not very useful in patients with UTI.
6) Therapeutic drug monitoring is recommended when possible.

Dogs:
For susceptible infections:
  a) 11 mg/kg IM or SQ q12h (Kirk 1989)
  b) 5 - 10 mg/kg IV, IM or SubQ q8h (avoid use or reduce dosage in patients with renal failure; recommend therapeutic drug monitoring, particularly in young animals) (Vaden and Papich 1995)
  c) 5 mg/kg IV, or IM *tid* (Morgan 1988)
  d) 10 mg/kg IM or SQ *tid*; soft tissue or skin infections should be treated for a minimum of 7 days and genitourinary infections treated for 7-21 days or until culture negative and asymptomatic. Do not exceed 30 days of treatment. (Package insert; *Amiglyde-V*®—Fort Dodge)

    e) In dogs with normal renal function: 10 mg/kg IM or SQ q8h for systemic infections, and q12h for UTI. (Baggot, Ling, and Chatfield 1985)

    f) 8.8 - 17.6 mg/kg IV (only if acute sepsis), IM q8h (see adjustment guidelines above). (Aronson and Aucoin 1989)

Cats:
For susceptible infections:

    a) 5 - 10 mg/kg IV, IM or SubQ q8h (avoid use or reduce dosage in patients with renal failure; recommend therapeutic drug monitoring, particularly in young animals) (Vaden and Papich 1995)

    b) 10 mg/kg SQ q8h (Jernigan, Wilson, and Hatch 1988)

    c) 8.8 - 17.6 mg/kg IV (only if acute sepsis), IM q8h (see adjustment guidelines above). (Aronson and Aucoin 1989)

Cattle:
For susceptible infections:

    a) 10 mg/kg IM q8h or 25 mg/kg q12h. (Beech 1987b)

    b) 22 mg/kg/day IM divided *tid* (Upson 1988)

Horses:
For susceptible infections:

    a) 6.6 mg/kg IM or IV *tid* (Robinson 1987)

    b) For gram negative respiratory infections: 6.6 mg/kg IM or IV q4-6 h; IV use is recommended for bronchopneumonia. (Beech 1987a)

    c) In foals: 7.5 mg/kg IV q12h; monitor serum levels if possible. (Caprile and Short 1987)

    d) 4.4 - 6.6 mg/kg IV or IM *bid - tid*, *tid* if severe infection (serious life-threatening). (Orsini et al. 1985)

    e) 4 - 8 mg/kg q8-12h IM (Baggot and Prescott 1987)

For uterine infusion:

    a) 2 grams mixed with 200 ml sterile normal saline (0.9% sodium chloride for injection) and aseptically infused into uterus daily for 3 consecutive days. (Package insert; *Amiglyde-V®*—Fort Dodge)

Birds:
For susceptible infections:

    a) For sunken eyes/sinusitis in macaws caused by susceptible bacteria: 40 mg/kg IM once daily or *bid*. Must also flush sinuses with saline mixed with appropriate antibiotic (10-30 ml per nostril). May require 2 weeks of treatment. (Karpinski and Clubb 1986)

    b) 15 mg/kg IM or SubQ q12h (Hoeffer 1995)

    c) For gram negative infections resistant to gentamicin: Dilute commercial solution and administer 15-20 mg/kg (0.015 mg/g) IM once a day or twice a day. (Clubb 1986)

Reptiles:
For susceptible infections:

    a) For snakes: 5 mg/kg IM (forebody) loading dose, then 2.5 mg/kg q72h for 7 - 9 treatments. Commonly used in respiratory infections. Use a lower dose for *Python curtus*. (Gauvin 1993)

    b) Study done in gopher snakes: 5 mg/kg IM loading dose, then 2.5 mg/kg q72h. House snakes at high end of their preferred optimum ambient temperature. (Mader, Conzelman, and Baggot 1985)

    c) For bacterial shell diseases in turtles: 10 mg/kg daily in water turtles, every other day in land turtles and tortoises for 7-10 days. Used commonly with a beta-lactam antibiotic. Recommended to begin therapy with 20 ml/kg fluid injection. Maintain hydration and monitor uric acid levels when possible. (Rosskopf 1986)

Monitoring Parameters -

    1) Efficacy (cultures, clinical signs and symptoms associated with infection)

    2) Renal toxicity; baseline urinalysis, serum creatinine/BUN. Casts in the urine are often the initial sign of impending nephrotoxicity. Frequency of monitoring during therapy is controversial. It can be said that monitoring daily urinalyses early in the course of treatment or daily creatinines once casts are seen or increases are noted in serum creatinine levels are not too frequent .

    3) Gross monitoring of vestibular or auditory toxicity is recommended

    4) Serum levels if possible; see the reference by Aronson and Aucoin in Ettinger (Aronson and Aucoin 1989) for more information.

Client Information - With appropriate training, owners may give subcutaneous injections at home, but routine monitoring of therapy for efficacy and toxicity must still be done. Clients should also understand that the potential exists for severe toxicity (nephrotoxicity, ototoxicity) developing from this medication.

Dosage Forms/Preparations/FDA Approval Status -
   Veterinary-Approved Products:
   Amikacin Sulfate Injection 50 mg (of amikacin base) per ml in 50 ml vials; *Amiglyde-V®* (Fort Dodge); Generic; (Rx) Approved for use in dogs.

   Amikacin Sulfate Intrauterine Solution 250 mg (of amikacin base) per ml in 48 ml vials; *Amiglyde-V®* (Fort Dodge); (Rx) Approved for use in horses.

   Human-Approved Products:
   Amikacin Injection 50 mg (of amikacin base) and 250 mg (of amikacin base) per ml; *Amikin®* (Apothecon); Generic (Rx)

AMINOCAPROIC ACID

Chemistry - An inhibitor of fibrinolysis, aminocaproic acid is a synthetic monamino carboxylic acid occurring as a fine, white crystalline powder. It is slightly soluble in alcohol and freely soluble in water and has pKa's of 4.43 and 10.75. The injectable product has its pH adjusted to approximately 6.8. Aminocaproic acid may also be known by the acronym EACA.

Storage/Stability/Compatibility - Products should be stored at room temperature. Avoid freezing liquid preparations. Discoloration will occur if aldehydes or aldehydic sugars are present. When given as an intravenous infusion, normal saline, D5W and Ringer's Injection have been recommended to be used as the infusion diluent.

Pharmacology - Aminocaproic acid inhibits fibrinolysis via its inhibitory effects on plasminogen activator substances and also via some antiplasmin action.
Aminocaproic acid is thought to affect degenerative myelopathy by its antiprotease activity, thereby reducing the activation of inflammatory enzymes that damage myelin.

Uses/Indications - Aminocaproic acid has been used as a treatment to degenerative myelopathy (seen primarily in German shepherds). In humans, it is primarily used for treating hyperfibrinolysis-induced hemorrhage.

Pharmacokinetics - In humans, the drug is rapidly and completely absorbed after oral administration. The drug is well distributed in both intravascular and extravascular compartments and penetrates cells (including red blood cells). It unknown if the drug enters maternal milk. It does not bind to plasma proteins. Terminal half life is about 2 hours in humans and the drug is primarily renally excreted as unchanged drug.

Contraindications/Precautions/Reproductive Safety - Aminocaproic acid is contraindicated in patients with active intravascular clotting. It should be used when the benefits outweigh the risks in patients with preexisting cardiac, renal or hepatic disease. Some, but not all, animal studies have demonstrated teratogenicity; use when risk to benefit ratio merits.

Adverse Effects/Warnings - In dogs treated, about 1% exhibit symptoms of GI irritation.

Overdosage/Acute Toxicity - There is very limited information on overdoses with aminocaproic acid. The IV lethal dose in dogs is reportedly 2.3 g/kg. At lower IV overdosages, tonic-clonic seizures were noted in some dogs. There is no known antidote, but the drug is dialyzable.

Drug Interactions - Hypercoagulation states may occur in patients receiving **estrogens**.

Laboratory Considerations - Serum **potassium** may be elevated by aminocaproic acid especially in patients with preexisting renal failure.

Doses -
   Dogs:
   For adjunctive treatment of degenerative myelopathy (seen primarily in German shepherds):
   a) In combination with exercise, vitamin support (vitamin B-complex, vitamin E), and analgesia (if required; using acetaminophen): Aminocaproic acid: 500 mg (regardless of size of animal, approximate dose is 15 mg/kg) PO q8h. Mix 192 ml of the 250 mg/ml injection with 96 ml of hematinic compound (*e.g. Lixotinic®*) producing a 288 ml final volume. Give 3 ml per dose (500 mg). Store solution in refrigerator. Clinical improvement seen within 8 weeks. (Clemmons 1991)

Client Information - Drug costs to treat a German shepherd-sized dog can be substantial.

Dosage Forms/Preparations/FDA Approval Status/Withholding Times -
   Veterinary-Approved Products: None
   Human-Approved Products:
   Aminocaproic Acid Tablets 500 mg; Aminocaproic Oral Solution 250 mg/ml; *Amicar®* (Immunex); (Rx)

Aminocaproic Acid Injection for Intravenous Infusion 250 mg/ml (5 gram); *Amicar*®
Intravenous (Immunex); Generic; (Rx)

AMINOPENTAMIDE HYDROGEN SULFATE

Chemistry - An antispamodic, anticholinergic agent, aminopentamide hydrogen sulfate has a
chemical name of 4-(dimethylamino)-2,2-diphenylvaleramide.

Storage/Stability/Compatibility - No information located.

Pharmacology - Aminopentamide is an anticholinergic agent that has been described when
compared to atropine as having a greater effect on reducing colonic contractions and less mydriatic and salivary effects. It reportedly also may reduce gastric acid secretion.

Uses/Indications - The manufacturer states that the drug is indicated "in the treatment of acute
abdominal visceral spasm, pylorospasm or hypertrophic gastritis and associated nausea, vomiting
and/or diarrhea" for use in dogs and cats.

Pharmacokinetics - No information located.

Contraindications/Precautions - The manufacturer lists glaucoma as an absolute contraindication to therapy and to use the drug cautiously, if at all, in patients with pyloric obstruction.
Additionally, aminopentamide should not be used if the patient has a history of hypersensitivity
to anticholinergic drugs, tachycardias secondary to thyrotoxicosis or cardiac insufficiency, myocardial ischemia, unstable cardiac status during acute hemorrhage, GI obstructive disease, paralytic ileus, severe ulcerative colitis, obstructive uropathy or myasthenia gravis (unless used to reverse adverse muscarinic effects secondary to therapy).

Antimuscarinic agents should be used with extreme caution in patients with known or suspected
GI infections. Atropine or other antimuscarinic agents can decrease GI motility and prolong retention of the causative agent(s) or toxin(s) resulting in prolonged symptoms. Antimuscarinic
agents must also be used with extreme caution in patients with autonomic neuropathy.

Antimuscarinic agents should be used with caution in patients with hepatic disease, renal disease, hyperthyroidism, hypertension, CHF, tachyarrhythmias, prostatic hypertrophy, esophogeal
reflux, and geriatric or pediatric patients.

Adverse Effects/Warnings - Adverse effects resulting from aminopentamide therapy may include dry mouth, dry eyes, blurred vision, and urinary hesitancy.Urinary retention is a symptom
of too high a dose and the drug should be withdrawn until resolved.

Overdosage - No specific information was located regarding acute overdosage symptoms or
treatment for this agent. The following discussion is from the Atropine monograph which could
be used as a guideline for treating overdoses:

If a recent oral ingestion, emptying of gut contents and administration of activated charcoal and
saline cathartics may be warranted. Treat symptoms supportively and symptomatically. Do not
use phenothiazines as they may contribute to the anticholinergic effects. Fluid therapy and standard treatments for shock may be instituted.

The use of physostigmine is controversial and should probably be reserved for cases where the
patient exhibits either extreme agitation and is at risk for injuring themselves or others, or for
cases where supraventricular tachycardias and sinus tachycardias are severe or life-threatening.
The usual dose for physostigmine (human) is: 2 mg IV slowly (for average sized adult), if no response may repeat every 20 minutes until reversal of toxic antimuscarinic effects or cholinergic
effects takes place. The human pediatric dose is 0.02 mg/kg slow IV (repeat q10 minutes as
above) and may be a reasonable choice for treatment of small animals. Physostigmine adverse effects (bronchoconstriction, bradycardia, seizures) may be treated with small doses of IV atropine.

Drug Interactions - No specific interactions were noted for this product. The following are
listed in the Atropine monograph and may also apply to aminopentamide: The following drugs
may enhance the activity of atropine and its derivatives: **antihistamines, procainamide, quinidine, meperidine, benzodiazepines, phenothiazines**.

The following drugs may potentiate the adverse effects of atropine and its derivatives: **primidone, disopyramide, nitrates, long-term corticosteroid use** (may increase intraocular pressure).

Atropine and its derivatives may enhance the actions of **nitrofurantoin, thiazide diuretics,
sympathomimetics**.

Atropine and its derivatives may antagonize the actions of **metoclopramide**.

Doses -
  Dogs:
   a) May be administered every 8-12 hours via IM, SQ or oral routes. If the desired effect
      is not attained, the dosage may be gradually increased up to 5 times those listed be-
      low: Animals weighing: 10 lbs or less: 0.1 mg; 1-20 lbs: 0.2 mg; 21-50 lbs: 0.3 mg;
      51-100 lbs: 0.4 mg; over 100 lbs: 0.5 mg. (Package Insert; *Centrine*® - Fort Dodge)

    b) To decrease tenesmus in malabsorption/maldigestion syndromes: 0.1 - 0.4 mg SQ, or IM *bid - tid* (Chiapella 1988)
    c) As an antiemetic: 0.1 - 0.4 mg SQ, or IM *bid - tid* (Johnson 1984)

Cats:
    a) as above for dogs under "a"
    b) As an antiemetic: 0.1 - 0.4 mg SQ, or IM *bid - tid* (Johnson 1984)

Monitoring Parameters -
    1) Clinical efficacy
    2) Adverse effects (see above)

Client Information - Contact veterinarian if animal has difficulty urinating or if animal is bothered by dry eyes or mouth.

Dosage Forms/Preparations/FDA Approval Status/Withholding Times -
Veterinary-Approved Products:

Aminopentamide Hydrogen Sulfate Tablets 0.2 mg; *Centrine*® (Fort Dodge); (Rx) Approved for use in dogs and cats only.

Aminopentamide Hydrogen Sulfate Injection 0.5 mg/ml, 10 ml vials; *Centrine*® (Fort Dodge); (Rx) Approved for use in dogs and cats only.

Human-Approved Products: None

AMINOPHYLLINE
THEOPHYLLINE

Chemistry - Xanthine derivatives, aminophylline and theophylline are considered to be respiratory smooth muscle relaxants, but also have other pharmacologic actions. Aminophylline differs from theophylline only by the addition of ethylenediamine to its structure and may have different amounts of molecules of water of hydration. 100 mg of aminophylline (hydrous) contains approximately 79 mg of theophylline (anhydrous) and 100 mg of aminophylline (anhydrous) contains approximately 86 mg theophylline (anhydrous). Conversely, 100 mg of theophylline (anhydrous) is equivalent to 116 mg of aminophylline (anhydrous) and 127 mg aminophylline (hydrous).

Aminophylline occurs as bitter-tasting, white or slightly yellow granules or powder with a slight ammoniacal odor and a pK_a of 5. Aminophylline is soluble in water and insoluble in alcohol.

Theophylline occurs as bitter-tasting, odorless, white, crystalline powder with a melting point between 270-274°C. It is sparingly soluble in alcohol and only slightly soluble in water at a pH of 7, but solubility increases with increasing pH.

Storage/Stability/Compatibility - Aminophylline for injection should be stored in single-use containers in which carbon dioxide has been removed. It should also be stored at temperatures below 30°C and protected from freezing and light. Upon exposure to air (carbon dioxide), aminophylline will absorb carbon dioxide, lose ethylenediamine and liberate free theophylline which can precipitate out of solution. Do not inject aminophylline solutions that contain a precipitate or visible crystals.

Aminophylline for injection is reportedly **compatible** when mixed with all commonly used IV solutions, but may be **incompatible** with 10% fructose or invert sugar solutions.

Aminophylline is reportedly **compatible** when mixed with the following drugs: amobarbital sodium, bretylium tosylate, calcium gluconate, chloramphenicol sodium succinate, dexamethasone sodium phosphate, dopamine HCl, erythromycin lactobionate, heparin sodium, hydrocortisone sodium succinate, lidocaine HCl, mephentermine sulfate, methicillin sodium, methyldopate HCl, metronidazole with sodium bicarbonate, pentobarbital sodium, phenobarbital sodium, potassium chloride, secobarbital sodium, sodium bicarbonate, sodium iodide, terbutaline sulfate, thiopental sodium, and verapamil HCl.

Aminophylline is reportedly **incompatible** (or data conflicts) with the following drugs: amikacin sulfate, ascorbic acid injection, bleomycin sulfate, cephalothin sodium, cephapirin sodium, clindamycin phosphate, codeine phosphate, corticotropin, dimenhydrinate, dobutamine HCl, doxorubicin HCl, epinephrine HCl, erythromycin gluceptate, hydralazine HCl, hydroxyzine HCl, insulin (regular), isoproterenol HCl, levorphanol bitartrate, meperidine HCl, methadone HCl, methylprednisolone sodium succinate, morphine sulfate, nafcillin sodium, norepinephrine bitartrate, oxytetracycline, penicillin G potassium, pentazocine lactate, procaine HCl, prochlorperazine edisylate or mesylate, promazine HCl, promethazine HCl, sulfisoxasole diolamine, tetracycline HCl, vancomycin HCl, and vitamin B complex w/C. Compatibility is dependent upon factors such as pH, concentration, temperature, and diluents used and it is suggested to consult specialized references for more specific information.

Pharmacology - The theophyllines competitively inhibit phosphodiesterase, thereby increasing amounts of cyclic AMP which increases the release of endogenous epinephrine. The increased levels of cAMP may also inhibit the release of histamine and slow reacting substance of anaphylaxis (SRS-A). The myocardial and neuromuscular transmission effects that the theophyllines posses may be a result of translocating intracellular ionized calcium.

The theophyllines directly relax smooth muscles in the bronchi and pulmonary vasculature, induce diuresis, increase gastric acid secretion and inhibit uterine contractions. They also have weak chronotropic and inotropic action, stimulate the CNS and can cause respiratory stimulation (centrally-mediated).

Uses/Indications - The theophyllines are used primarily for their bronchodilitory effects, often in patients with myocardial failure and/or pulmonary edema.

Pharmacokinetics - The pharmacokinetics of theophylline have been studied in several domestic species. After oral administration, the rate of absorption of the theophyllines is limited primarily by the dissolution of the dosage form in the gut. In studies in cats, dogs, and horses, bioavailabilities after oral administration are nearly 100% when non-sustained release products are used. One study in dogs that compared various sustained-release products (Koritz, Neff-Davis, and Munsiff 1986), found bioavailabilities to range from approximately 30 - 76%, depending on the product used.

Theophylline is distributed throughout the extracellular fluids and body tissues. It crosses the placenta and is distributed into milk (70% of serum levels). In dogs, at therapeutic serum levels, only about 7-14% is bound to plasma proteins. The volume of distribution of theophylline for dogs has been reported to be 0.82 L/kg. The volume of distribution in cats is reported to be 0.46 L/kg, and in horses, 0.85 - 1.02 L/kg. Because of the low volumes of distribution and theophylline's low lipid solubility, obese patients should be dosed on a lean body weight basis.

Theophylline is metabolized primarily in the liver (in humans) to 3-methylxanthine, which has weak bronchodilitory activity. Renal clearance contributes only about 10% to the overall plasma clearance of theophylline. The reported elimination half-lives (mean values) in various species are: dogs ≈ 5.7 hours; cats ≈ 7.8 hours, pigs ≈ 11 hours; and horses ≈ 11.9 to 17 hours. In humans, there are very wide interpatient variations in serum half lives and resultant serum levels. It could be expected that similar variability exists in veterinary patients, particularly those with concurrent illnesses.

Contraindications/Precautions - The theophyllines are contraindicated in patients who are hypersensitive to any of the xanthines, including theobromine or caffeine. Patients who are hypersensitive to ethylenediamine should not take aminophylline.

The theophyllines should be administered with caution in patients with severe cardiac disease, gastric ulcers, hyperthyroidism, renal or hepatic disease, severe hypoxia, or severe hypertension. Becuase it may cause or worsen preexisting arrhythmias, patients with cardiac arrhythmias should receive theophylline only with caution and enhanced monitoring. Neonatal and geriatric patients may have decreased clearances of theophylline and be more sensitive to its toxic effects. Patients with CHF may have prolonged serum half-lifes of theophylline.

Adverse Effects/Warnings - The theophyllines can produce CNS stimulation and gastrointestinal irritation after administration by any route. Most adverse effects are related to the serum level of the drug and may be symptomatic of toxic blood levels. Some mild CNS excitement and GI disturbances are not uncommon when starting therapy and generally resolve with chronic administration in conjunction with monitoring and dosage adjustments.

Dogs and cats can exhibit symptoms of nausea and vomiting, insomnia, increased gastric acid secretion, diarrhea, polyphagia, polydipsia, and polyuria. Side effects in horses are generally dose related and may include: nervousness, excitability (auditory, tactile, and visual), tremors, diaphoresis, tachycardia, and ataxia. Seizures or cardiac dysrhythmias may occur in severe intoxications.

Overdosage - Symptoms of toxicity (see above) are usually associated with levels greater than 20 micrograms/ml in humans and become more severe as the serum level exceeds that value. Tachycardias, arrhythmias, and CNS effects (seizures, hyperthermia) are considered to be the most life-threatening aspects of toxicity.

Treatment of theophylline toxicity is basically supportive. The gut should be emptied, charcoal and a cathartic administered after an oral ingestion, using the standardized methods and cautions associated with these practices. Patients suffering from seizures should have an adequate airway maintained and treated with IV diazepam. The patient should be constantly monitored for cardiac arrhythmias and tachycardia. Fluid and electrolytes should be monitored and corrected as necessary. Hyperthermia may be treated with phenothiazines and tachycardia treated with propranolol if either condition is considered life-threatening.

Drug Interactions - **Phenobarbital or Phenytoin** may decrease the effect of theophylline by increasing its clearance.

Agents which may increase theophylline effects, include **cimetidine, erythromycin, allopurinol, thiabendazole, clindamycin, lincomycin.**

Theophylline may decrease the effects of **phenytoin, lithium carbonate, or pancuronium.**

Theophylline and beta-**adrenergic blockers (propranolol, etc.)** may antagonize each other's effect.

Toxic synergism (arrhythmias) can occur if theophylline is used concurrently with sympathomimetics (especially **ephedrine**) or possibly **isoproterenol.** Theophylline with **halothane** may cause increased incidence of cardiac dysrhythmias.

Theophylline with **ketamine** can cause an increased incidence of seizures.

Laboratory Interactions - Theophylline can cause falsely elevated values of serum **uric acid** if measured by the Bittner or colorimetric methods. Values are not affected if using the uricase method.

Theophylline serum levels can be falsely elevated by **furosemide, phenylbutazone, probenecid, theobromine, caffeine, sulfathiazole, chocolate, or acetominophen** if using a spectrophotometric method of assay.

Doses - Note: Theophyllines have a low therapeutic index; determine dosage carefully. Because of aminophylline/theophylline's pharmacokinetic characteristics, it should be dosed on a lean body weight basis in obese patients. Dosage conversions between aminophylline and theophylline can be easily performed by using the information found in the Chemistry section above. Aminophylline causes intense local pain when administered IM and is rarely used or recommended via this route.

Dogs:
- a) 10 mg/kg PO, IM, or IV q8h (Kirk 1986)
- b) 10 mg/kg PO (aminophylline) q8h; 5-7 mg/kg (theophylline) q8h PO (Roudebush 1985)
- c) 6 - 11 mg/kg PO, IM or IV *tid* (Morgan 1988)
- d) 20 mg/kg PO using sustained-release theophylline tablets (*Theo-Dur*®; Key Pharmaceuticals) q12h (Koritz, Neff-Davis, and Munsiff 1986)

Cats:
- a) 4.25 mg/kg theophylline (5 mg/kg aminophylline) PO q8-12h (McKiernan et al. 1983)
- b) 4 mg/kg IM, PO *bid* (Morgan 1988)
- c) 25 mg aminophylline PO (1/4 or one 100 mg tablet) *bid-tid* (Noone 1986)

Horses:
Note: Intravenous aminophylline should be diluted in at least 100 ml of D_5W or normal saline and administered slowly (not > than 25 mg/min).
- a) 4 - 7 mg/kg PO *tid* (Robinson 1987)
- b) 10 - 15 mg/kg PO theophylline *bid*; or up to 15 mg/kg given slowly IV. Monitor serum levels; do not exceed 15 micrograms/ml. (Beech 1987)
- c) Loading dose of 12 mg/kg PO (theophylline), followed by maintenance doses of 5 mg/kg PO *bid* (Button, Errecalde, and Mulders 1985)

Monitoring Parameters -
1) Therapeutic efficacy and symptoms of toxicity
2) Serum levels at steady state.The therapeutic serum levels of theophylline in humans are generally described to be between 10 - 20 micrograms/ml. Therapeutic and toxic levels have not been firmly established in veterinary species, so the human values should be used as a guide (Note: Some recommend not exceeding 15 micrograms/ml in horses).

Client Information - Give dosage as prescribed by veterinarian to maximize the drug's benefit.

Dosage Forms/Preparations/FDA Approval Status/Withholding Times -
Veterinary-Approved Products: None
Human-Approved Products: The listing below is a sampling of products and sizes available; consult specialized references for a more complete listing.

Aminophylline Tablets 100 mg (78.9 mg theophylline), 200 mg (158 mg theophylline); (Rx); 225 mg (178 mg theophylline) controlled release tablets (Rx)

Aminophylline Injection 25 mg/ml (19.7 mg/ml theophylline) in 10 ml, & 20 ml vials amps and vials); (Rx)

Aminophylline oral liquid 105 mg/5 ml (90 mg theophylline); generic; (Rx)

Aminophylline suppositories 250mg (197.5 mg theophylline) & 500 mg (395 mg theophylline); (Rx)

Theophylline Time Released Capsules and Tablets; 50 mg, 60 mg, 65 mg, 75 mg, 100 mg, 125 mg, 130 mg, 200 mg, 250 mg, 260 mg, & 300 mg, 450 mg, 500 mg, 600 mg are available (Note: Different products have different claimed release rates which may or may not correspond to actual times in veterinary patients; (Rx)

Theophylline Tablets and Capsules: 100 mg, 125 mg, 200 mg, 250 mg, 300 mg (Rx)

Theophylline Syrup; 80 mg/15 ml (26.7 mg/5 ml), 150 mg/15 ml (50 mg/5 ml) (Rx)

Theophylline Elixir/Solution 80 mg/15 ml (26.7 mg/5 ml) (Rx)

AMINOPROPAZINE FUMARATE

Chemistry - A phenothiazine derivative, aminopropazine fumarate occurs as a white powder with a melting point of 168°C. One gram is soluble in 11 ml of water; 200 ml of alcohol. 118 mg of the fumarate salt is equivalent to 100 mg of the base.

Storage/Stability/Compatibility - Protect from light and excessive heat.

The injectable solution is colorless to light amber in color. Should marked deviation occur from the above color, do not use.

Pharmacology - Reportedly, aminopropazine causes smooth muscle relaxation by direct action on the muscle rather than a neurotropic mechanism. It primarily reduces muscle contractions in the GI, GU, and respiratory systems. It has little CNS effect (sedation) and does not affect biliary secretion, or exhibit histaminic, sympatholytic or ganglionic blocking actions.

Uses/Indications - Aminopropazine is indicated for: "reducing excessive smooth muscle contractions, such as occur in urethral spasms associated with urolithiasis in cats and dogs, and colic spasms in horses." (Package insert, *Jenotone®*—Coopers)

Pharmacokinetics - No pharmacokinetic information was located for this agent.

Contraindications/Precautions - The intravenous route is not recommended in patients with history of severe cardiac, renal or hepatic disease and the oral form of the drug should be used very cautiously in these patients.

The parenteral preparation should be given IV slowly or into a large muscle mass IM (avoid IM injections near nerves). Avoid extravascular injections and do not give subcutaneously. See Drug Interactions for more information.

Adverse Effects/Warnings - Mild tranquilization or hyperexcitability are listed as possible side effects by the manufacturer.

Overdosage - No specific information was located for this agent. It is suggested that standard overdose procedures be followed, including emptying the gut after oral ingestion if possible and treating supportively. Do not give epinephrine for hypotension (use either phenylephrine or norepinephrine if sympathomimetic pressor agents are indicated).

Drug Interactions - Aminopropazine should not be given within one month of worming with an **organophosphate agent** as their effects may be potentiated. **Other CNS depressant agents (barbiturates, narcotics, anesthetics,** etc.) may cause additive CNS depression if used with aminopropazine.

Quinidine when given with phenothiazines may cause additive cardiac depression.

Antidiarrheal mixtures (*e.g.,* Kaolin/pectin, bismuth subsalicylate mixtures) and **antacids** may cause reduced GI absorption of oral phenothiazines. Increased blood levels of both drugs may occur if **propranolol** is administered with phenothiazines.

Phenothiazines block alpha-adrenergic receptors, if **epinephrine** is then given, unopposed beta activity causing vasodilation and increased cardiac rate can occur. The manufacturer lists epinephrine as being contraindicated with aminopropazine.

Phenytoin metabolism may be decreased if given concurrently with phenothiazines.

Procaine activity may be enhanced by phenothiazines.

Doses - The parenteral preparation should be given slowly IV or IM into a large muscle mass.

Dogs:

    a) 2.2 - 4.4 mg/kg IM or IV; or 1 - 2 tablets (25 mg tablets) per 25 lbs of body weight q12h. (Package insert; *Jenotone®* — Coopers)

    b) For urge incontinence: 2 mg/kg PO *bid* (Chew, DiBartola, and Fenner 1986)

Cats:

    a) 2.2 - 4.4 mg/kg IM or IV; or 1/4 - 1/2 tablet (25 mg tablets) per 6 lbs of body weight q12h. (Package insert; *Jenotone®* — Coopers)

    b) For urge incontinence: 2 mg/kg PO *bid* (Chew, DiBartola, and Fenner 1986)

Horses:

    a) 0.55 mg/kg (1 ml/100 lbs body weight) IM or IV q12h (Package insert; *Jenotone®* - Coopers)

Monitoring Parameters - Dependent on reason for use; monitor for efficacy.

Dosage Forms/Preparations/FDA Approval Status/Withholding Times -
Veterinary-Approved Products:

Aminopropazine Fumarate for Injection 25 mg/ml, (as base) 50 ml vials; *Jenotone®* (Schering-Plough); (Rx)

Aminopropazine Fumarate Tablets 25 mg, bottles of 100; *Jenotone®* (Schering-Plough); (Rx)

Human-Approved Products: None

Aminopropazine Fumarate may also be known as proquamezine fumarate, tetrameprozine fumarate, or *Myspamol®* (May & Baker, U.K.).

AMIODARONE HCL

Chemistry - An iodinated benzofuran, amiodarone is unique structurally and pharmacologically from other antiarrhythmic agents. It occurs as a white to cream colored lipophilic powder having a pKa of approximately 6.6. Amiodarone 200 mg tablets each contain approximately 75 mg of iodine.

Storage/Stability/Compatibility - Tablets should be stored in tight containers, at room temperature and protected from light. A 3 year expiration date is assigned from the date of manufacture.

Pharmacology - Amiodarone's mechanism of action is not fully understood, but it is believed that it possesses unique pharmacology from other antiarrhythmic agents. It can be best classified as a class III antiarrhythmic agent. Major properties include prolongation of myocardial cell-action potential duration and refractory period, and non-competitive alpha- and beta-adrenergic inhibition.

Uses/Indications - Because of its toxicity, amiodarone should only be considered for use in dogs with recurrent ventricular tachycardias that are not controlled with other therapies. As the risk of sudden death is high in Doberman pinschers exhibiting rapid, wide-complex ventricular tachycardia or syncope with recurrent VPC's, amiodarone may be useful when other drug therapies are ineffective.

Pharmacokinetics - Amiodarone may be administered parenterally or orally. In humans, the oral absorption is slow and variable, with bioavailabilities ranging from 22-86%. Amiodarone is widely distributed throughout the body and can accumulate in adipose tissue. Amiodarone is metabolized by the liver into the active metabolite desethylamiodarone. After oral administration of a single dose in normal dogs, amiodarone's plasma half-life averaged 7.5 hours, but repeated dosing increased its half-life to 3.2 days.

Contraindications/Precautions/Reproductive Safety - Amiodarone is considered contraindicated in patients (people) hypersensitive to it; have severe sinus-node dysfunction with severe sinus bradycardia, 2nd or 3rd degree heart block or bradycardial syncope.

Clinical experience in veterinary patients is limited. Use only when other less toxic and more commonly used (and understood) drugs are ineffective.

In laboratory animals, amiodarone has been embryotoxic at high doses and congenital thyroid abnormalities have been detected in offspring. Use during pregnancy only when the potential benefits outweigh the risks of the drug.

Adverse Effects/Warnings - Gastrointestinal effects (*e.g.*, anorexia, vomiting) are apparently the most likely adverse effects seen in the limited number of canine patients treated. However, in people, adverse effects are very common while on amiodarone therapy. Those that most commonly cause discontinuation of the drug include: pulmonary infiltrates or pulmonary fibrosis (sometimes fatal), liver enzyme elevations, congestive heart failure, paroxysmal ventricular tachycardia and thyroid dysfunction (hypo- or hyperthyroidism). An odd effect seen in some individuals is a bluish cast to their skin.

Clinical experience in dogs is limited and the adverse effect profile of this drug in people warrants its use only when other less toxic agents are ineffective and treatment is deemed necessary.

Overdosage - Clinical overdosage experience is limited; most likely adverse effects seen are hypotension, bradycardia, cardiogenic shock, AV block, and hepatotoxicity. Treatment is supportive. Bradycardia may be managed with a pacemaker or $beta_1$ agonists (*e.g.*, isoproterenol); hypotension managed with positive inotropic agents or vasopressors. Neither amiodarone or its active metabolite are dialyzable.

Drug/Drug Interactions - There are several potentially significant interactions that may occur with amiodarone. The following is partial list of interactions that are most likely seen in veterinary patients: amiodarone may significantly increase the serum levels and/or pharmacologic effects of **anticoagulants, beta blockers, calcium channel blockers (e.g. diltiazem, verapamil), cyclosporin, digoxin, lidocaine, methotrexate, procainamide, quinidine and theophylline**. **Cimetidine** may increase the serum levels of amiodarone.

Drug/Lab Interactions - While most human patients remain euthyroid while receiving amiodarone, it may cause an increase in serum T_4 and serum reverse T_3 levels, and a reduction in serum T_3 levels.

Doses -
  Dogs:
      For recurrent ventricular tachycardia not controlled with other less toxic drugs:
      a) 10 - 25 mg/kg PO twice daily for 7 days, followed by 5 - 7.5 mg/kg PO twice daily for 14 days, followed by 7.5 mg/kg PO once daily. (Calvert 1995)
      Note: Some human references state that because of the potential for drug interactions with previous drug therapies, the life-threatening nature of the arrhythmias being treated, and the unpredictability of response from amiodarone, the drug should be initially given (loaded) over several days in an inpatient setting where adequate monitoring can occur.

Monitoring Parameters -
      1) Efficacy (ECG)
      2) Toxicity (GI effects; liver enzymes; thyroid function tests; blood pressure; pulmonary radiographs if symptoms such as dyspnea/cough occur)

Client Information - Because of the "experimental" nature (relatively few canine patients have received this agent) and the toxicity dangers associated with its use, clients should give informed consent before the drug is prescribed.

Dosage Forms/Preparations/FDA Approval Status -
  Veterinary-Approved Products: None
  Human-Approved Products:
      Amiodarone Oral Tablets 200 mg; Amiodarone Concentrate for Injection for IV Infusion 50 mg/ml in 3 ml ampules;*Cordarone*® (Wyeth-Ayerst); (Rx)

AMITRAZ

Chemistry - A diamide topical antiparasitic agent, amitraz is pale yellow with a melting point of 86°-87°C. It is sparingly soluble in water, but soluble in most organic solvents. It is non-hygroscopic and relatively stable to heat.

Storage/Stability/Compatibility - Compatibility with other agents have apparently not been determined. Do not mix with other antiparasiticides.

Pharmacology - The pharmacologic action of amitraz is not well understood. It may have effects on the CNS of susceptible organisms. It apparently also possess alpha-2 adrenergic activity. Amitraz can cause a significant increase in plasma glucose levels, presumably by inhibiting insulin release via its alpha 2-adrenergic activity. Yohimbine (alpha 2 blocker) can antagonize this effect).

Uses/Indications - In dogs, amitraz is used topically primarily in the treatment of generalized demodicosis. It is also used as a general insecticidal/miticidal agent in several other species (see label information).

Pharmacokinetics - No information located.

Contraindications/Precautions/Reproductive Safety - Safety has not been demonstrated in dogs less than 4 months of age. The manufacturer of *Mitaban*® does not recommend use in these animals. Toy breeds may be more susceptible to CNS effects (transient sedation); lower dose rates (1/2 of recommended) has been recommended in these breeds. Because of the drug's effects on plasma glucose, use with caution in brittle diabetic patients.
  Reproductive safety has not been established. Use only when benefits outweigh potential risks of therapy.

Adverse Effects/Warnings - The most commonly reported adverse effect after amitraz topical administration is transient sedation that may persist for up to 72 hours (24 hours is usual). If treating around eyes, use an ophthalmic protectant (*e.g.*, petrolatum ophthalmic ointment) before treating. Do not use if dog has deep pyodermas with drainage tracts; postpone application until lesions improve after treating with antibiotic and shampoo therapy.
  Amitraz can be toxic to cats and rabbits and it is probably best to avoid its use in these species.

Overdosage/Acute Toxicity - Amitraz may be toxic if swallowed (by either animals or humans). Beagles receiving 4 mg/kg PO daily for 90 days, demonstrated transient ataxia, CNS depression, hyperglycemia, decreased pulse rates and lowered body temperature. No animals died.
  Amitraz toxicity can be significant if amitraz-containing insecticide collars are ingested. Treatment should consist of emesis, retrieval of the collar using endoscopy if possible and administration of activated charcoal and a cathartic to remove any remaining collar fragments. Because of the risk of an increased chance of gastric dilatation, gastrotomy may not be a viable

option. Yohimbine at a dose of 0.11- 0.2 mg/kg IV (start with low dosage) may be of benefit for overdose effects. Because yohimbine has a short half-life it may need to be repeated, particularly if the animal has ingested an amitraz-containing collar that has not been retrieved from the GI tract. Atipamezole has also been used to treat amitraz toxicity; refer to that monograph for more information. Contact a poison center for more information, if necessary.

Drug Interactions - Because of their immunosuppressive effects, **corticosteroids** and **other immunosuppressant drugs** (*e.g.*, azathioprine, cyclophosphamide, etc) should not be used in animals with demodicosis.

Doses -
 Dogs:
  For treatment of generalized demodicosis:
  a) Long and medium haired dogs should be clipped closely and given a shampoo with mild soap and water prior to first treatment. Topically treat at a concentration of 250 ppm (one 10.6 ml bottle of Mitaban® in 2 gallons of warm water, by applying to entire animal and allowing to air dry. DO not rinse or towel dry. Use a freshly prepared dilution for additional dogs or additional treatments. Repeat every 14 days for 3 - 6 treatments (continue until six treatments done or two successive skin scrapings demonstrate no live mites. Chronic cases may require additional courses of therapy. (Package Insert - *Mitaban*®—Upjohn)
  b) For dogs who are only controlled with chronic therapy (as above) and whose owners accept the risk of using the drug in an "unlicensed" manner in an attempt for cure: Owners should be made aware of the risks of therapy and accept them. First, try the 250 ppm solution (as above once weekly for 4 weeks. If positive response is seen, continue until all mites eradicated (using skin scrapings) and then for an additional 30 days. If weekly 250 ppm application fails, a 500 ppm solution may be tried (1 bottle in 1 gallon of water) weekly as above. In dogs failing 500 ppm, 1000 ppm may also be attempted, but likelihood of toxicity increases and the author has no experience using it. If these methods fail, the dog is unlikely to be cured using amitraz. (Miller 1992)
  c) For dogs not responding to conventional (labeled) therapy: Prepare a 0.125% solution by diluting 1 ml of the 12.5% commercially available large animal product (*Taktic*®) in 100 ml of water. Clip and bathe with appropriate shampoos once weekly if required. Using a sponge rub the diluted solution (0.125%) daily onto one-half of the dog's body and alternate sides on a daily basis. Air dry. During first week of therapy, keep dog hospitalized and observe for adverse effects. Continue therapy for 2 weeks after multiple skin scrapings are negative for mites. Dogs also receive otic therapy with a diluted solution of amitraz (1 ml of *Tactic* in 8.5 ml of mineral oil) every 3 - 7 days unless irritation develops and one researcher also treats dogs with pododermatitis with daily foot soaks of the 0.125% solution. Preliminary results look promising and reported adverse effects in dogs are low in frequency and mild. Owners accepting this un-approved therapy, must be carefully screened and trained to carefully handle the amitraz solutions. (Mundell 1994)

  For scabies in older puppies and adult dogs:
  a) Dilute and treat per label recommendation (see "a" above for demodicosis) for 3 treatments. (Moriello 1992)

 Goats:
 For demodectic mange:
  a) 10.6 ml of amitraz solution (19.9%—*Mitaban*®) in 2 gallons of water. Use as a whole body dip; repeat every 14 days for 2-3 treatments. (Rosser 1993)

Client Information - Amitraz liquid (Mitaban®) is flammable until diluted with water. Do not stress animals for at least 24 hours after application of *Mitaban*®. When mixing with water, protect exposed skin with rubber gloves, etc. Wash hands and arms well after application to animal. Dispose of unused diluted solution by flushing down the drain. Rinse Mitaban container with water and dispose; do not re-use. Do not re-use collar or container, wrap in newspaper and throw in trash. Avoid inhalation of vapors. Animals treated may exhibit signs of sedation; if animal is un-arousable or sedation persists for longer than 72 hours, contact your veterinarian.
 Because of amitraz's effects on glucose, human diabetics should use these products with extreme caution.

Dosage Forms/Preparations/FDA Approval Status/Withholding Times -
 Veterinary-Approved Products:
  Amitraz 19.9% Topical Solution for Dilution in 10.6 ml bottles; *Mitaban*®(Upjohn); (Rx)

  Amitraz 9% Tick Collar for dogs - 25 inch; *Preventic*® (Allerderm/Virbac); OTC

Amitraz 10% Collar for Dairy Cattle - 7 collars/tray; *Taktic Dairy Collar*® (Hoechst/Roussel) (OTC); Approved for use in all breeds, all ages, lactating or non-lactating. There are no withdrawal times required for milk or meat.

Amitraz 12.5% Concentrated Solution for dilution and topical application to swine, dairy or beef cattle in 760 ml cans. *Taktic EC*®; (Hoechst/Roussel) (OTC)

Human-Approved Products: None

AMITRIPTYLINE HCL

Chemistry - A tricyclic dibenzocycloheptene-derivative antidepressant, amitriptyline HCl occurs as a white or practically white, odorless or practically odorless crystalline powder that is freely soluble in water or alcohol. It has a bitter, burning taste and a pK_a of 9.4.

Storage/Stability/Compatibility - Amitriptyline tablets should be stored at room temperature. The injection should be kept from freezing and protected from light.

Pharmacology - Amitriptyline (and its active metabolite, nortriptyline) has a complicated pharmacologic profile. From a slightly oversimplified viewpoint, it has 3 main characteristics: blockage of the amine pump, thereby increasing neurotransmitter levels (principally serotonin, but also norepinephrine), sedation, and central and peripheral anticholinergic activity. In animals, tricyclic antidepressants are similar to the actions of phenothiazines in altering avoidance behaviors.

Uses/Indications - Amitriptyline has been used for separation anxiety in dogs, and excessive grooming, spraying and anxiety in cats.

Pharmacokinetics - Amitriptyline is rapidly absorbed from both the GI tract and from parenteral injection sites. Peak levels occur within 2-12 hours. Amitriptyline is highly bound to plasma proteins, enters the CNS, and enters maternal milk in levels at or greater than that found in maternal serum. The drug is metabolized in the liver to several metabolites, including nortriptyline, which is active. In humans the terminal half life is approximately 30 hours. Half life in dogs has been reported to be 6-8 hours.

Contraindications/Precautions/Reproductive Safety - These agents are contraindicated if prior sensitivity has been noted with any other tricyclic. Concomitant use with monoamine oxidase inhibitors is generally contraindicated. Isolated reports of limb reduction abnormalities have been noted; restrict use to pregnant animals only when the benefits clearly outweigh the risks.

Adverse Effects/Warnings - The most predominant adverse effects seen with the tricyclics are related to their sedating and anticholinergic properties. Occasionally, dogs exhibit hyperexcitability. However, adverse effects can run the entire gamut of systems, including hematologic effects (bone marrow suppression), GI effects (diarrhea, vomiting), endocrine effects, etc. Refer to other references for additional information.

Overdosage/Acute Toxicity - Overdosage with tricyclics can be life-threatening (arrhythmias, cardiorespiratory collapse). Because the toxicities and therapies for treatment are complicated and controversial, it is recommended to contact a poison control center for further information in any potential overdose situation.

Drug Interactions - Because of additive effects, use amitriptyline cautiously with other agents with **anticholinergic** or **CNS depressant** effects. Tricyclic antidepressants used with antithyroid agents may increase the potential risk of agranulocytosis. **Cimetidine** may inhibit tricyclic antidepressant metabolism and increase the risk of toxicity. Use in combination with **sympathomimetic agents** may increase the risk of cardiac effects (arrhythmias, hypertension, hyperpyrexia). Concomitant use with **monoamine oxidase inhibitors** is generally contraindicated.

Laboratory Considerations - Tricyclics can widen QRS complexes, prolong PR intervals and invert or flatten T-waves on **ECG**. The response to **metapyrone** may be decreased by amitriptyline. Tricyclics may alter (increase or decrease) **blood glucose** levels.

Doses -
 Dogs:
   For adjunctive treatment of pruritus:
     a) 1 - 2 mg/kg PO q12h (Paradis and Scott 1992)
     b) For acral pruritic dermatitis: 2.2 mg/kg PO *bid*; only occasionally effective. A 2-4 week trial is recommended. (Rosychuck 1991)

   For self-mutilation behaviors:
     a) 1 - 2 mg/kg PO q12h; with behavior modification. (Shanley and Overall 1992)

   For adjunctive treatment of separation anxiety or other tricyclic antidepressant-responsive behavior disorders:
     a) 2.2 - 4.4 mg/kg PO once daily. (Marder 1991)

Cats:
For adjunctive treatment of behavior disorders:
a) 5 -10 mg per cat PO once daily (Miller 1989), (Marder 1991)
b) For spraying: 5 mg PO daily (McConnell and Hughey 1992)

For self-mutilation behaviors:
a) 5 -10 mg per cat PO once to twice daily; with behavior modification. (Shanley and Overall 1992)

Monitoring Parameters - 1) Efficacy; 2) Adverse Effects

Client Information - All tricyclics should be dispensed in child-resistant packaging and kept well away from children or pets. Inform clients that several weeks may be required before efficacy is noted and to continue dosing as prescribed.

Dosage Forms/Preparations/FDA Approval Status/Withholding Times -
Veterinary-Approved Products: None
Human-Approved Products:
Amitriptyline HCl tablets 10, 25, 50, 75, 100, 150 mg; *Elavil*® (Zeneca) (Rx); generic; (Rx)

Amitriptyline HCl for Injection 10 mg/ml; *Elavil*® (Zeneca); (Rx)

There are also fixed dose oral combination products containing amitriptyline and chlordiazepoxide, and amitriptyline and perphenazine.

AMLODIPINE BESYLATE

Chemistry - Amlodipine besylate, a dihydropyridine calcium channel blocking agent, occurs as a white crystalline powder that is slightly soluble in water and sparingly soluble in alcohol.

Storage/Stability/Compatibility - Store amlodipine at room temperature, in tight, light resistant containers.

Pharmacology - Amlodipine inhibits calcium influx across cell membranes in both cardiac and vascular smooth muscle. It has a greater effect on vascular smooth muscle, thereby acting as a peripheral arteriolar vasodilator and reducing afterload. Amlodipine also depresses impulse formation (automaticity) and conduction velocity in cardiac muscle.

Uses/Indications - Oral amlodipine appears to be a useful agent in the treatment of hypertension in cats. The drug potentially could be useful in other veterinary species as well, but safety and efficacy data are lacking.

Hypertension in cats is usually secondary to other diseases (often renal failure or cardiac causes such as thyrotoxic cardiomyopathy or primary hypertrophic cardiomyopathy, etc.) and is most often seen in middle-aged or geriatric cats. These animals often present with acute symptoms such as blindness, seizures, collapse or paresis. A cat is generally considered hypertensive if systolic blood pressure is >160mmHg. Early reports indicate that if antihypertensive therapy is begun acutely, some vision may be restored in about 50% of cases with blindness secondary to hypertension.

Pharmacokinetics - No feline-specific data on the drug's pharmacokinetics was located. In humans amlodipine's bioavailability does not appear to be altered by the presence of food in the gut. The drug is slowly but almost completely absorbed after oral administration. Peak plasma concentrations occur between 6-9 hours post-dose and effects on blood pressure are correspondingly delayed. The drug has very high plasma protein binding characteristics (approximately 93%). However, drug interactions associated with potential displacement from these sites have not been elucidated. Amlodipine is slowly, but extensively metabolized to inactive compounds in the liver. Terminal plasma half-life is approximately 35 hours in healthy humans, but is prolonged in the elderly and in those patients with hypertension or hepatic dysfunction.

Contraindications/Precautions/Reproductive Safety - Because amlodipine may have slight negative inotropic effects, it should be used cautiously in patients with heart failure or cardiogenic shock. It should also be used cautiously in patients with hepatic disease or at risk for developing hypotension. A relative contraindication for amlodipine exists for humans with advanced aortic stenosis.

Amlodipine is classified as a pregnancy category C drug for humans. While no evidence of impaired fertility was noted in rats given 8X overdoses, amlodipine has been shown to be fetotoxic (intrauterine death rates increased 5 fold) in laboratory animals (rats, rabbits) at very high dosages. No evidence of teratogenicity or mutagenicity were observed in lab animal studies. In rats, amlodipine prolonged labor. It is unknown whether amlodipine enters maternal milk.

Adverse Effects/Warnings - Adverse effect profile is not well determined for cats at this time. In the limited number of cats treated, amlodipine appears to have minimal adverse effects. In humans taking amlodipine, headache (7.3%) is the most frequent problem reported.

Overdosage - Little information is available. Limited experience with other calcium channel blockers in humans have shown that profound hypotension and bradycardia may result. When possible, massive overdoses should be managed with gut emptying and supportive treatment. Beta-agonists and intravenous calcium may be beneficial.

Drug Interactions - No clinically significant drug-drug interactions have been noted specifically with amlodipine at this time. However, concomitant use of **diuretics**, **beta blockers**, other **vasodilators or other agents that may reduce blood pressure** (e.g. fentanyl) may cause hypotension if used with amlodipine.

Doses -

Cats:
> For treatment of systemic hypertension:
> a) 0.625 mg (1/4 of a 2.5 mg tab) once daily PO (Snyder 1998), (Henik et al. 1997)

Dogs:
> For adjunctive treatment of systemic hypertension:
> a) 0.5 - 1 mg/kg PO once daily (Brown 1997) (**NOTE**: Although the aforementioned reference is cited correctly, recently obtained information suggests that the actual dose may be 0.05 - 0.1 mg/kg PO once daily—Plumb; March 1999)
> b) 0.132 - 0.22 mg/kg PO once daily (anecdotal communication to the author)

Monitoring Parameters - 1) Blood pressure; 2) Ophthalmic exam

Client Information- May give with food. Clients should understand that missing dosages may cause rapid redevelopment of symptoms and damage secondary to hypertension.

Dosage Forms/Preparations/FDA Approval Status -
Veterinary-Approved Products: None
Human-Approved Products:
> Amlodipine Oral Tablets 2.5 mg, 5 mg, 10 mg; *Norvasc®* (Pfizer); (Rx)

AMMONIUM CHLORIDE

Chemistry - An acid-forming salt, ammonium chloride occurs as colorless crystals or as white, fine or course, crystalline powder. It is somewhat hygroscopic, and has a cool, saline taste. When dissolved in water, the temperature of the solution is decreased. One gram is soluble in approximately 3 ml of water at room temperature; 1.4 ml at 100°C. One gram is soluble in approximately 100 ml of alcohol.

One gram of ammonium chloride contains 18.7 mEq of ammonium and chloride ions. The commercially available concentrate for injection (26.75%) contains 5 mEq of each ion per ml and contains disodium edetate as a stabilizing agent. The pH of the concentrate for injection is approximately 5. Synonyms for ammonium chloride include muriate of ammonia and sal ammoniac.

Storage/Stability/Compatibility - Ammonium chloride for injection should be stored at room temperature; avoid freezing. At low temperatures, crystallization may occur; it may be resolubolized by warming to room temperature in a water bath.

Ammonium chloride should not be titrated with strong oxidizing agents (*e.g.*, potassium chlorate) as explosive compounds may result.

Ammonium chloride is reported to be physically **compatible** with all commonly used IV replacement fluids and potassium chloride.

It is **incompatible** with: codeine phosphate, dimenhydrinate, methadone HCl, nitrofurantoin sodium, sulfisoxazole diolamine, and warfarin sodium. It is also reportedly incompatible with alkalis and their hydroxides.

Pharmacology - The acidification properties of ammonium chloride are caused by its dissociation into chloride and ammonium ions *in vivo*. The ammonium cation is converted by the liver to urea with the release of a hydrogen ion. This ion combines with bicarbonate to form water and carbon dioxide. In the extracellular fluid, chloride ions combine with fixed bases and decrease the alkaline reserves in the body. The net effects are decreased serum bicarbonate levels and a decrease in blood and urine pH.

The excess chloride ions presented to the kidney, are not completely reabsorbed by the tubules and are excreted with cations (principally sodium) and water. This diuretic effect is usually compensated for by the kidneys after a few days of therapy.

Uses/Indications - The veterinary indications for ammonium chloride are as a urinary acidifying agent to help prevent and dissolve certain types of uroliths (*e.g.*, struvite), to enhance renal excretion of some types of toxins (*e.g.*, strontium) or drugs (*e.g.*, quinidine), or to enhance the efficacy of certain antimicrobials (*e.g.*, chlortetracycline, methenamine mandelate, nitrofurantoin, oxytetracycline, penicillin G or tetracycline) when treating urinary tract infections. Ammonium chloride has also been used intravenously for the rapid correction of metabolic alkalosis.

Pharmacokinetics - No information was located on the pharmacokinetics of this agent in veterinary species. In humans, ammonium chloride is rapidly absorbed from the GI.

Contraindications/Precautions - Ammonium chloride is contraindicated in patients with severe hepatic disease as ammonia may accumulate and cause toxicity. In general, ammonium chloride should not be administered to uremic patients as it may intensify the metabolic acidosis already existing in some of these patients. Ammonium chloride should not be used alone in patients with severe renal insufficiency and metabolic alkalosis secondary to vomiting hydrochloric acid as sodium depletion can occur. In these cases, sodium chloride repletion with or without ammonium chloride administration should be performed to correct both sodium and chloride deficits. Ammonium chloride is contraindicated in patients with urate calculi or respiratory acidosis and high total CO_2 and buffer base. Ammonium chloride cannot alone correct hypochloremia with secondary metabolic alkalosis due to intracellular potassium chloride depletion. Potassium chloride must be administered to these patients.

Do not administer subcutaneously, rectally or intraperitoneally.

Use ammonium chloride with caution in patients with pulmonary insufficiency or cardiac edema.

Adverse Effects/Warnings - Development of metabolic acidosis (sometimes severe) can occur unless adequate monitoring is performed. When used intravenously, pain at the injection site can develop; slow administration lessens this effect. Gastric irritation, nausea and vomiting can be associated with oral dosing of the drug.

Overdosage - Symptoms of overdosage may include: nausea, vomiting, excessive thirst, hyperventilation, bradycardias or other arrhythmias, and progressive CNS depression. Profound acidosis and hypokalemia may be noted on laboratory results.

Treatment should consist of correcting the acidosis by administering sodium bicarbonate or sodium acetate intravenously. Hypokalemia should be treated by using a suitable oral (if possible) potassium product. Intense acid-base and electrolyte monitoring should be performed on an ongoing basis until the patient is stable.

Drug Interactions - Urine acidification may increase the renal excretion of **quinidine**.

The **aminoglycosides** (*e.g.,* gentamicin) and **erythromycin** are more effective in an alkaline medium; urine acidification may diminish these drugs effectiveness in treating bacterial urinary tract infections.

Doses -
  Dogs:
    For urine acidification:
     a) In struvite dissolution therapy if diet and antimicrobials do not result in acid urine: 200 mg/kg/day PO divided *tid* (Lage, Polzin, and Zenoble 1988)
     b) To enhance the renal elimination of certain toxins/drugs: 200 mg/kg/day divided *qid* (Grauer and Hjelle 1988)
     c) To enhance elimination of strontium: 0.2 - 0.5 grams PO 3-4 times a day (used with calcium salts) (Bailey 1986)

  Cats:
    For urine acidification:
     a) In struvite dissolution therapy if diet and antimicrobials do not result in acid urine or to help prevent idiopathic FUS in a non-obstructed cat: 20 mg/kg PO *bid* (Lage, Polzin, and Zenoble 1988)
     b) 800 mg per day given in the food once daily (if diet and antimicrobials do not reduce pH) (Lewis, Morris, and Hand 1987)

  Horses:
     a) 4 - 15 grams PO (Swinyard 1975)

  Cattle:
     a) For urolithiasis prevention: 200 mg/kg PO (Howard 1986)
     b) 15 - 30 grams PO (Swinyard 1975)

  Sheep & Goats:
     a) For urolithiasis prevention: 200 mg/kg PO (Howard 1986)
     b) 1 - 2 grams PO (Swinyard 1975)

Monitoring Parameters -
  1) Urine pH (Urine pH's of ≤6.5 have been recommended as goals of therapy)
  2) Blood pH if there are symptoms of toxicity or treating metabolic alkalosis
  3) Serum electrolytes, if using chronically or if treating metabolic acidosis
  4) Prior to IV use it is recommended that the carbon dioxide combining power of the patient's serum be measured to insure that serious acidosis is prevented

Client Information - Contact veterinarian if animal exhibits signs of nausea, vomiting, excessive thirst, hyperventilation or progressive lethargy.

Dosage Forms/Preparations/FDA Approval Status/Withholding Times -

Veterinary-Approved Products:

Ammonium Chloride Tablets: 357 mg (6.7 mEq/tablet) 50 & 500 tabs/bottle *MEq-AC* ® (Vet-A-Mix); 200 mg tablets in btls of 100 and 500 *Uroeze-200*® (Daniels) Approved for use in cats and dogs. (Rx)

Ammonium Chloride Granules:*MEq-5AC*® (Vet-A-Mix) Each teaspoonsful (3.35 grams) contains 535 mg (10mEq) in 4 oz and 1 lb bottles; *Uroeze*® (Daniels) each 1/4 teaspoonsful contains 200 mg of ammonium chloride. Approved for cats and dogs (Rx)

Human-Approved Products:

Ammonium Chloride Tablets 500 mg (enteric-coated & plain) Note: enteric-coated tablets may be excreted unchanged into the feces and are not recommended.
  Generic; (OTC)

Ammonium Chloride Concentrate for Injection 26.75% (5 mEq/ml) in 20 ml (100 mEq) vials. Must be diluted before infusion.
  Generically labeled (Abbott); (Rx).

Preparation of solution for IV administration: Dilute 1 or 2 vials (100 - 200 mEq) in either 500 or 1000 ml of sodium chloride 0.9% for Injection. Do not administer at a rate greater than 5 ml/min (human adult).

AMMONIUM MOLYBDATE

Uses/Indications - Ammonium molybdate is used for the investigational or compassionate treatment of copper poisoning in sheep.

Doses -

Sheep:

For treatment of copper poisoning:
  a) 100 mg with 1 gram sodium sulfate by mouth daily. (Debuf 1991)
  b) 50 - 500 mg ammonium (or sodium) molybdate with 0.3 - 1 gm thiosulfate per day for up to 3 weeks. Whole blood transfusions may be required in some situations. (Buck 1986)
  c) 100 mg/head/day and sodium sulfate 1 gram/head/day for 30 days. Mix each with 2 ml of water and give orally. (McConnell and Hughey 1992)
  d) 200 mg ammonium or sodium molybdate plus 500 mg of sodium thiosulfate given daily PO for up to 3 weeks. (Thompson and Buck 1993a)

Dosage Forms/Preparations/FDA Approval Status/Withholding Times -

Veterinary-Approved Products: None.

Note: Ammonium Molybdate can be obtained from various chemical supply houses, but there has been some concern raised that the FDA will not allow molybdate salts to be used in food animals. It is recommended to contact the FDA before treating for guidance when contemplating using molybdate.

Human-Approved Products:

Ammonium Molybdate Injection 25 mcg/ml (as 46 mcg/ml ammonium molybdate tetrahydrate in 10 ml vials) .i.*Molypen* ® (Lyphomed); Generic, (Rx)

AMOXICILLIN

For general information on the penicillins, including adverse effects, contraindications, overdosage, drug interactions and monitoring parameters, refer to the monograph: Penicillins, General Information.

Chemistry - An aminopenicillin, amoxicillin is commercially available as the trihydrate. It occurs as a practically odorless, white, crystalline powder that is sparingly soluble in water. Amoxicillin differs structurally from ampicillin only by having an additional hydroxyl group on the phenyl ring. Amoxicillin may also be known as amoxycillin, *p*-hydroxyampicillin, or BRL 2333.

Storage/Stability/Compatibility - Amoxicillin capsules, tablets, and powder for oral suspension should be stored at room temperature (15-30°C) in tight containers. After reconstitution, the oral suspension should preferably be refrigerated (refrigeration not absolutely necessary) and any unused product discarded after 14 days. After reconstitution, the injectable veterinary suspension is stable for 3 months at room temperature and 12 months when refrigerated.

Pharmacology/Uses/Indications - Although there may be some slight differences in activity against certain organisms, amoxicillin generally shares the same spectrum of activity and uses as ampicillin. Because it is better absorbed orally (in non-ruminants), higher serum levels may be attained than with ampicillin. Refer to the ampicillin monograph or the general penicillin statement for more information.

Pharmacokinetics (specific) - Amoxicillin trihydrate is relatively stable in the presence of gastric acid. After oral administration, it is about 74-92% absorbed in humans and animals (monogastric). Food will decrease the rate, but not the extent of oral absorption and many clinicians suggest giving the drug with food, particularly if there is concomitant associated GI distress. Amoxicillin serum levels will generally be 1.5-3 times greater than those of ampicillin after equivalent oral doses.

After absorption the volume of distribution for amoxicillin is approximately 0.3 L/kg in humans and 0.2 L/kg in dogs. The drug is widely distributed to many tissues, including liver, lungs, prostate (human), muscle, bile, and ascitic, pleural and synovial fluids. Amoxicillin will cross into the CSF when meninges are inflamed in concentrations that may range from 10-60% of those found in serum. Very low levels of the drug are found in the aqueous humor, and low levels found in tears, sweat and saliva. Amoxicillin crosses the placenta, but it is thought to be relatively safe to use during pregnancy. It is approximately 17-20% bound to human plasma proteins, primarily albumin. Protein binding in dogs is approximately 13%. Milk levels of amoxicillin are considered to be low.

Amoxicillin is eliminated primarily through renal mechanisms, principally by tubular secretion, but some of the drug is metabolized by hydrolysis to penicilloic acids (inactive) and then excreted in the urine. Elimination half-lives of amoxicillin have been reported as 45-90 minutes in dogs and cats, and 90 minutes in cattle. Clearance is reportedly 1.9 ml/kg/min in dogs.

Doses -

Dogs:
    For susceptible infections:
- a) 10 - 22 mg/kg PO or SubQ q8h (Vaden and Papich 1995)
- b) Trihydrate injectable (*Amoxi-Inject®*): 5.5 - 11 mg/kg IM or SQ q8h
  Oral Forms: 11 - 22 mg/kg PO q8-12h (Aronson and Aucoin 1989)
- c) For routine infections: 10 mg/kg PO, SQ *bid*
  For chlolangiohepatitis: 20 mg/kg PO, SQ *bid* (Morgan 1988)
- d) 22 mg/kg PO q12h (Kirk 1989)
- e) 10 - 55 mg/kg q6-12h PO; 5 - 11 mg/kg IV, IM, or SQ q6-12h (Greene 1984)
- f) For Lyme Disease: 22 mg/kg PO q12h for 21-28 days (Appel and Jacobson 1995)

Cats:
    For susceptible infections:
- a) 10 - 22 mg/kg PO or SubQ q8h (Vaden and Papich 1995)
- b) Trihydrate injectable (*Amoxi-Inject®*): 5.5 - 11 mg/kg IM or SQ q8h
  Oral Forms: 11 - 22 mg/kg PO q8-12h (Aronson and Aucoin 1989)
- c) 11 - 22 mg/kg PO q8-12h (Ford and Aronson 1985)
- d) For bacterial respiratory infections: 10 mg/kg PO or parenterally q12-24h (Roudebush 1985)
- e) 22 mg/kg PO q12h (Kirk 1989)

Cattle:
    For susceptible infections:
- a) 6 -10 mg/kg SQ or IM q24h (Withdrawal time = 30 days). (Jenkins 1986)
- b) For respiratory infections: 11 mg/kg IM or SQ q12h. (Hjerpe 1986)
- c) For respiratory infections: 11 mg/kg IM or SQ q12h (Beech 1987b)
- d) Calves: Amoxicillin trihydrate: 7 mg/kg PO q8-12h (Baggot 1983)
- e) 13.2 - 15.4 mg/kg IM or SQ once daily (Upson 1988)

Horses:
    For susceptible infections:
- a) For respiratory infections: 20 - 30 mg/kg PO q6h (Beech 1987b)
- b) Amoxicillin trihydrate: 20 mg/kg q12h IM. (Upson 1988)

Birds:
    For susceptible infections:

    a) For most species: 150 - 175 mg/kg PO once to twice daily (using 50 mg/ml suspension) (Clubb 1986)

    b) 100 mg/kg q8h PO (Bauck and Hoefer 1993)

    c) 100mg/kg q8h, IM, SubQ, PO (Hoeffer 1995)

Reptiles:

For susceptible infections:

    a) For all species: 22 mg/kg PO q12-24h; not very useful unless used in combination with aminoglycosides. (Gauvin 1993)

Client Information - The oral suspension should preferably be refrigerated, but refrigeration is not absolutely necessary; any unused oral suspension should be discarded after 14 days. Amoxicillin may be administered orally without regard to feeding status. If the animal develops gastrointestinal symptoms (*e.g.,* vomiting, anorexia), giving with food may be of benefit.

Dosage Forms/Preparations/FDA Approval Status/Withholding Times -
Veterinary-Approved Products:

Amoxicillin Oral Tablets 50 mg, 100 mg, 150 mg, 200 mg, , 400 mg; *Amoxi-Tabs*® (Pfizer), (Rx) Approved for use in dogs and cats. *Robamox-V*® (Fort Dodge); (Rx) Approved for use in dogs only.

Amoxicillin Powder for Oral Suspension 50 mg/ml (after reconstitution) in 15 ml or 30 ml bottles; *Amoxi-Drop*® (Pfizer); (Rx); Approved for use in dogs and cats.*Robamox-V*® (Fort Dodge) (Rx); Approved for use in dogs.

Amoxicillin Oral Bolus 400 mg; *Amoxi-Bol*® (Pfizer); (Rx) Approved for use in non-ruminating calves, including veal calves. Slaughter withdrawal = 20 days.

Amoxicillin Powder for Suspension (Injection): 3 gram vial (Dogs, Cats) and 25 g vial (non-lactating cattle); *Amoxi-Inject*® (Pfizer); (Rx) Approved for use in dogs and cats (3 g vial), Slaughter withdrawal (cattle) = 25 days. Milk withdrawal = 96 hours.

Amoxicillin Intramammary Infusion 62.5 mg/syringe in 10 ml syringes; *Amoxi-Mast*® (Pfizer); (Rx) Approved for use in lactating dairy cattle. Slaughter withdrawal = 12 days; Milk withdrawal = 60 hours.

Human-Approved Products:

Amoxicillin Tablets (chewable) 125 mg (As trihydrate) & 250 mg (as trihydrate);*Amoxil*®(SK Beecham); generic, (Rx)

Amoxicillin Capsules (as trihydrate) 250 mg, 500 mg; *Polymox*® (Apothecon); *Wymox*® (Wyeth-Ayerst); generic (Rx)

Amoxicillin (as the trihydrate) Powder for Oral Suspension 50 mg/ml (as trihydrate) (in 15 and 30 ml bottles), 125 mg/5 ml (as trihydrate) and 250 mg/5 ml (as trihydrate) 80 ml, 100 ml, 150 ml, and 200 ml bottles. *(Rx)*

AMOXICILLIN/CLAVULANATE POTASSIUM
AMOXICILLIN/CLAVULANIC ACID

For general information on the penicillins, including adverse effects, contraindications, overdosage, drug interactions and monitoring parameters, refer to the monograph: Penicillins, General Information. A separate monograph for amoxicillin is found earlier in this section. Refer to it for more information on amoxicillin chemistry, storage, stability, doses, etc..

Chemistry - A beta-lactamase inhibitor, clavulanate potassium occurs as an off-white, crystalline powder that has a pK_a of 2.7 (as the acid) and is very soluble in water and slightly soluble in alcohol at room temperatures. Although available in commercially available preparations as the potassium salt, potency is expressed in terms of clavulanic acid. Synonyms include: clavulanic acid and potassium clavulanate.

Storage/Stability/Compatibility - All commercially available amoxicillin/potassium clavulanate products should be stored at temperatures less than 24°C (75°F) in tight containers. Potassium clavulanate is reportedly very susceptible to moisture and should be protected from excessive humidity.

  After reconstitution, oral suspensions are stable for 10 days when refrigerated. Unused portions should be discarded after that time.

Pharmacology - Clavulanic acid has only weak antibacterial activity when used alone and presently it is only available in fixed-dose combination with either amoxicillin (oral) or ticarcillin (parenteral). Clavulanic acid acts by competitively and irreversibly binding to beta-lactamases, including types II, III, IV, and V, and penicillinases produced by Staphylococcus. Staphylococci that are resistant to penicillinase-resistant penicillins (*e.g.,* oxacillin) are considered to be resistant to amoxicillin/potassium clavulanate, although susceptibility testing may indicate otherwise.

Amoxicillin/potassium clavulanate is usually ineffective against type I cephalosporinases. These plasmid-mediated cephalosporinases are often produced by members of the family Enterobacteriaceae, particularly *Pseudomonas aeruginosa*. When combined with amoxicillin, there is little if any synergistic activity against organisms already susceptible to amoxicillin, but amoxicillin-resistant strains (due to beta-lactamase inactivation) may be covered.

When performing Kirby-Bauer susceptibility testing, the *Augmentin*® (human-product trade name) disk is used. Because the amoxicillin:clavulanic acid ratio of 2:1 in the susceptibility tests may not correspond to *in vivo* drug levels, susceptibility testing may not always accurately predict efficacy for this combination.

Uses/Indications - Amoxicillin/potassium clavulanate tablets and oral suspension products are approved for use in dogs and cats for the treatment of urinary tract, and skin and soft tissue infections caused by susceptible organisms. It is also indicated for canine periodontal disease due to susceptible strains of bacteria.

Pharmacokinetics (specific) - The pharmacokinetics of amoxicillin are presented in that drug's monograph. There is no evidence to suggest that the addition of clavulanic acid alters amoxicillin pharmacokinetics.

Clavulanate potassium is relatively stable in the presence of gastric acid and is readily absorbed. In dogs, the absorption half-life is reportedly 0.39 hours with peak levels occurring about 1 hour after dosing. Bioavailability data for dogs or cats was not located.

Clavulanic acid has an apparent volume of distribution of 0.32 L/kg in dogs and is distributed (with amoxicillin) into the lungs, pleural fluid and peritoneal fluid. Low concentrations of both drugs are found in the saliva, sputum and CSF (uninflamed meninges). Higher concentrations in the CSF are expected when meninges are inflamed, but it is questionable whether therapeutic levels are attainable. Clavulanic acid is 13% bound to proteins in dog serum. The drug readily crosses the placenta, but is not believed to cause any teratogenic problems. Clavulanic acid and amoxicillin are both found in milk in low concentrations.

Clavulanic acid is apparently extensively metabolized in the dog (and rats) primarily to 1-amino-4-hydroxybutan-2-one. It is not known if this compound possess any beta-lactamase inhibiting activity. The drug is also excreted unchanged in the urine via glomerular filtration. In dogs, 34-52% of a dose is excreted in the urine as unchanged drug and metabolites, 25-27% excreted in the feces, and 16-33% into respired air. Urine levels of active drug are considered to be high, but may be only 1/5th of those of amoxicillin.

Doses - All doses are for combined quantities of both drugs (unless noted otherwise).
  Dogs:
    For susceptible infections:
      a) 13.75 mg/kg PO *bid*; do not exceed 30 days of therapy. (Package insert; *Clavamox*®—Beecham)
      b) 10 - 20 mg/kg (amoxicillin) PO *bid* (Morgan 1988)
      c) 11 - 22 mg/kg PO q8-12h (Aronson and Aucoin 1989)
      d) 12.5 - 25 mg/kg PO q8-12h (Vaden and Papich 1995)
  Cats:
    For susceptible infections:
      a) 62.5 mg PO *bid*; do not exceed 30 days of therapy. (Package insert; *Clavamox*®—Beecham)
      b) 62.5 mg PO q8-12h (Vaden and Papich 1995)
      c) 11 - 22 mg/kg PO q8-12h (Aronson and Aucoin 1989)
  Birds:
    For susceptible infections:
      a) 50 - 100 mg/kg PO q6-8h (Hoeffer 1995)

Dosage Forms/Preparations/FDA Approval Status/Withholding Times -
Veterinary-Approved Products:
  Oral Tablets:
    62.5 mg: Amoxicillin 50 mg/12.5 mg clavulanic acid (as the potassium salt),
    125 mg: Amoxicillin 100 mg/25 mg clavulanic acid (as the potassium salt),
    250 mg: Amoxicillin 200 mg/50 mg clavulanic acid (as the potassium salt),
    375 mg: Amoxicillin 300 mg/75 mg clavulanic acid (as the potassium salt)
    Clavamox Tablets® (Pfizer); (Rx) Approved for use in dogs and cats.

  Powder for Oral Suspension:
    Amoxicillin 50 mg/12.5 mg clavulanic acid (as the potassium salt) per ml in 15 ml dropper bottles. Add 14 ml of water and shake vigorously; refrigerate and discard any unused portion after 10 days.
    Clavamox® *Drops* (Pfizer); (Rx) Approved for use in dogs and cats.

Human-Approved Products:
Oral Tablets:
Amoxicillin 250 mg/125 mg clavulanic acid (as the potassium salt,; Amoxicillin 500 mg/125 mg clavulanic acid (as the potassium salt); Amoxicillin 875 mg/125 mg clavulanic acid (as the potassium salt); Amoxicillin 125 mg/31.25 mg clavulanic acid (as the potassium salt) (Chewable); Amoxicillin 200 mg/28.5 mg clavulanic acid (Chewable); Amoxicillin 250 mg/62.5 mg clavulanic acid (as the potassium salt) (Chewable); Amoxicillin 400 mg/57 mg clavulanic acid (Chewable)
Augmentin® (SK-Beecham); (Rx)

Powder for Oral Suspension:
Amoxicillin 125 mg/31.25 mg clavulanic acid (as the potassium salt) per 5 ml in 75, 100 & 150 ml; Amoxicillin 200 mg/28.5 mg clavulanic acid (as the potassium salt) per 5 ml in 50, 75, & 100 ml; Amoxicillin 250 mg/62.5 mg clavulanic acid (as the potassium salt) per 5 ml in 75, 100 & 150 ml; Amoxicillin 400 mg/57 mg clavulanic acid (as the potassium salt) per 5 ml in 50, 75, & 100 ml
Augmentin® (SK-Beecham); (Rx)

AMPHOTERICIN B

Chemistry - A polyene macrolide antifungal agent produced by *Streptomyces nodosus*, amphotericin B occurs as a yellow to orange, odorless or practically odorless powder. It is insoluble in water and anhydrous alcohol. Amphotericin B is amphoteric and can form salts in acidic or basic media. These salts are more water soluble, but possess less antifungal activity than the parent compound. Each mg of amphotericin B must contain not less than 750 micrograms of anhydrous drug. Amphotericin A may be found as a contaminant in concentrations not exceeding 5%. The commercially available powder for injection contains sodium desoxycholate as a solubolizing agent.

Storage/Stability/Compatibility - Vials of amphotericin B powder for injection should be stored in the refrigerator (2-8°C), protected from light and moisture. Reconstitution of the powder must be done with sterile water for injection (no preservatives—see directions for preparation in the Dosage Form section below).

After reconstitution, if protected from light, the solution is stable for 24 hours at room temperature and for 1 week if kept refrigerated. After diluting with D5W (must have pH >4.3) for IV use, the manufacturer recommends protecting the solution during administration. Additional studies however, have shown that potency remains largely unaffected if the solution is exposed to light for 8-24 hours.

Amphotericin B is reportedly **compatible** with the following solutions and drugs: D5W, D5W in sodium chloride 0.2%, heparin sodium, heparin sodium with hydrocortisone sodium phosphate, hydrocortisone sodium phosphate/succinate and sodium bicarbonate.

Amphotericin B is reportedly **incompatible** with the following solutions and drugs: normal saline, lactated Ringer's, D5-normal saline, D5-lactated Ringer's, amino acids 4.25% - dextrose 25%, amikacin, calcium chloride/gluconate, carbenicillin disodium, chlorpromazine HCl, cimetidine HCl, diphenhydramine HCl, dopamine HCl, edetate calcium disodium (Ca EDTA), gentamicin sulfate, kanamycin sulfate, lidocaine HCl, metaraminol bitartrate, methyldopate HCl, nitrofurantoin sodium, oxytetracycline HCl, penicillin G potassium/sodium, polymyxin B sulfate, potassium chloride, prochlorperazine mesylate, streptomycin sulfate, tetracycline HCl, and verapamil HCl. Compatibility is dependent upon factors such as pH, concentration, temperature and diluents used. It is suggested to consult specialized references for more specific information (*e.g.*, *Handbook on Injectable Drugs* by Trissel; see bibliography).

Pharmacology - Amphotericin B is usually fungistatic, but can be fungicidal against some organisms depending on drug concentration. It acts by binding to sterols (primarily ergosterol) in the cell membrane and alters the permeability of the membrane allowing intracellular potassium and other cellular constituents to "leak out". Because bacteria and rickettsia do not contain sterols, amphotericin B has no activity against those organisms. Mammalian cell membranes do contain sterols (primarily cholesterol) and the drug's toxicity may be a result of a similar mechanism of action, although amphotericin binds less strongly to cholesterol than ergosterol.

Amphotericin B has *in vitro* activity against a variety of fungal organisms, including *Blastomyces, Aspergillus, Paracoccidiodes, Coccidiodes, Histoplasma, Cryptococcus, Mucor*, and *Sporothrix. Zygomycetes* is reportedly variable in its response to amphotericin. Aspergillosis in dogs and cats does not tend to respond satisfactorily to amphotericin therapy. Additionally, amphotericin B has *in vivo* activity against some protozoa species, including *Leishmania spp.* and *Naegleria spp.*.

It has been reported that amphotericin B has immunoadjuvant properties, but further work is necessary to confirm the clinical significance of this effect.

Uses/Indications - Because the potential exists for severe toxicity associated with this drug, it should only be used for progressive, potentially fatal fungal infections. Veterinary use of amphotericin has been primarily in dogs, but other species have been treated successfully. For further information on fungal diseases treated, see the Pharmacology and Dosage sections.

Pharmacokinetics - Pharmacokinetic data on veterinary species is apparently unavailable. In humans (and presumably animals), amphotericin B is poorly absorbed from the GI tract and must be given parenterally to achieve sufficient concentrations to treat systemic fungal infections. After intravenous injection, the drug reportedly penetrates well into most tissues, but does not penetrate well into the pancreas, muscle, bone, aqueous humor, pleural, pericardial, synovial, or peritoneal fluids. The drug does enter the pleural cavity and joints when inflamed. CSF levels are approximately 3% of those found in the serum. Approximately 90-95% of amphotericin in the vascular compartment is bound to serum proteins.

The metabolic pathways of amphotericin are not known, but it exhibits biphasic elimination. An initial serum half-life of 24-48 hours, and a longer terminal half-life of about 15 days have been described. Seven weeks after therapy has stopped, amphotericin can still be detected in the urine. Approximately 2-5% of the drug is recovered in the urine in unchanged (biologically active) form.

Contraindications/Precautions/Reproductive Safety - Amphotericin is contraindicated in patients who are hypersensitive to it, unless the infection is life-threatening and no other alternative therapies are available.

Because of the serious nature of the diseases treated with systemic amphotericin, it is not contraindicated in patients with renal disease, but should be used cautiously with adequate monitoring.

The safety of amphotericin B during pregnancy has not been established, but there are apparently no reports of teratogenicity associated with the drug. The risks of therapy should be weighed against the potential benefits.

Adverse Effects/Warnings - Amphotericin B is notorious for its nephrotoxic effects and most canine patients will show some degree of renal toxicity after receiving the drug. The proposed mechanism of nephrotoxicity is via renal vasoconstriction with a subsequent reduction in glomerular filtration rate. The drug may also directly act as a toxin to renal epithelial cells. Renal damage may be more common and severe in patients who receive higher individual doses.

The patient's renal function should be aggressively monitored during therapy. A pre-treatment serum creatinine, BUN (serum urea nitrogen/SUN), serum electrolytes (including magnesium if possible), total plasma protein (TPP), packed cell volume (PCV), body weight, and urinalysis should be done prior to starting therapy. BUN, creatinine, PCV, TPP, and body weight are rechecked before each dose is administered. Electrolytes and urinalysis should be monitored at least weekly during the course of treatment. Several different recommendations regarding stopping therapy when a certain BUN is reached have been made. Most clinicians recommend stopping, at least temporarily, amphotericin treatment if the BUN reaches 30-40 mg/dl, serum creatinine >3 mg/dl or if other symptoms of systemic toxicity develop such as serious depression or vomiting.

At least two regimens have been used in the attempt to reduce nephrotoxicity in dogs treated with amphotericin. Mannitol (12.5 grams or 0.5 - 1 g/kg) given concurrently with amphotericin B (slow IV infusion) to dogs may reduce nephrotoxicity, but may also reduce the efficacy of the therapy, particularly in blastomycosis. Mannitol treatment also increases the total cost of therapy by approximately two times.

Sodium loading prior to treating has garnered considerable support in recent years. A tubuloglomerular feedback mechanism that induces vasoconstriction and decreased GFR has been postulated for amphotericin B toxicity; increased sodium load at the glomerulus may help prevent that feedback. One clinician (Foil 1986), uses 5 ml/kg of normal saline given in two portions, before and after amphotericin B dosing and states that is has been "... helpful in averting renal insufficiency... ".

Cats are apparently more sensitive to the nephrotoxic aspects of amphotericin B, and many clinicians recommend using reduced dosages in this species (see Dosage section).

Other adverse effects that have been reported with amphotericin B include anorexia, vomiting, hypokalemia, phlebitis and fever.

Overdosage/Acute Toxicity - No case reports were located regarding acute intravenous overdose of amphotericin B. Because of the toxicity of the drug, dosage calculations and solution preparation procedures should be double-checked. If an accidental overdose is administered, renal toxicity may be minimized by administering fluids and mannitol as outlined above in the Adverse effects section.

Drug Interactions - Since the renal effects of other nephrotoxic drugs may be additive with amphotericin B, avoid, if possible the concurrent or sequential use of **aminoglycosides**

(gentamicin, amikacin, kanamycin, etc), polymyxin B, colistin, cisplatin, methoxyflurane or vancomycin.

Amphotericin B therapy may cause potassium-loss or hypokalemia. This may be of particular concern in patients receiving **cardiac glycosides** (*e.g.,* **digoxin**), **skeletal muscle relaxants, or other potassium-depleting drugs** (*e.g.,* **thiazide or loop diuretics**). **Corticosteroids** may exacerbate the potassium-losing effects of amphotericin.

Synergy between amphotericin and **flucytosine** can occur against strains of *Cryptococcus* and *Candida spp.*, but increased flucytosine toxicity may also occur. Synergism with **rifampin** (against *Candida*, *Histoplasma*, and *Aspergillus*) and **tetracycline** (*Cryptococcus* and *Candida spp.*) have also been reported against fungi susceptible to amphotericin B. Antagonism of activity has been suggested between amphotericin B and **miconazole**. Further studies need to confirm this, however.

Reconstitution with **saline solutions** or with **solutions containing a preservative** may cause precipitation.

Doses -

Note: Some clinicians have recommended administering a 1 mg test dose (less in small dogs or cats) IV over anywhere from 20 minutes to 4 hours and monitoring pulse, respiration rates, temperature, and if possible, blood pressure. If a febrile reaction occurs some clinicians recommend adding a glucocorticoid to the IV infusion solution or using an antipyretic prior to treating, but these practices are controversial.

A recently published study (Rubin et al. 1989) demonstrated less renal impairment and systemic adverse effects in dogs who received amphotericin B IV slowly over 5 hours in 1 L of D5W than in dogs who received the drug IV in 25 ml of D5W over 3 minutes.

Dogs:

For treatment of susceptible systemic fungal infections:
- a) Two regimens can be used; after diluting vial (as outlined below in preparation of solution section), either:
    1) Rapid-Infusion Technique:
    Dilute quantity of stock solution to equal 0.25 mg/kg in 30 ml of 5% dextrose. Using butterfly catheter, flush with 10 ml of D5W. Infuse amphotericin B solution IV over 5 minutes. Flush catheter with 10 ml of D5W and remove catheter. Repeat above steps using 0.5 mg/kg 3 times a week until 9-12 mg/kg accumulated dosage is given.
    2) Slow IV Infusion Technique:
    Dilute quantity of stock solution to equal 0.25 mg/kg in 250 - 500 ml of D5W. Place indwelling catheter in peripheral vein and give total volume over 4-6 hours. Flush catheter with 10 ml of D5W and remove catheter. Repeat above steps using 0.5 mg/kg 3 times a week until 9-12 mg/kg accumulated dosage is given. (Noxon 1989)
- b) In dehydrated, sodium-depleted animals, must rehydrate before administration. Dosage is 0.5 mg/kg diluted in D5W. In dogs with normal renal function, may dilute in 60-120 ml of D5W and give by slow IV over 15 minutes. In dogs with compromised renal function, dilute in 500 ml or 1 l of D5W and give over slowly IV over 3-6 hours. Readminister every other day if BUN remains below 50 mg/dl. If BUN exceeds 50 mg/dl, discontinue until BUN decreases to at least 35 mg/dl. Cumulative dose of 8-10 mg/kg is required to cure blastomycosis or histoplasmosis. Coccidioidomycosis, aspergillosis and other fungal diseases require a greater cululative dosage. (Legendre 1995)

For blastomycosis (see general dosage guidelines above) :
- a) Amphotericin B 0.5 mg/kg 3 times weekly until a total dose of 6 mg/kg is given, with ketoconazole at 10 - 20 mg/kg (30 mg/kg for CNS, bone or eye involvement) divided for 3-6 months. (Foil 1986)
- b) Amphotericin B 0.15 - 0.5 mg/kg IV 3 times a week with ketoconazole 20 mg/day PO once daily or divided *bid*; 40 mg/kg divided *bid* for ocular or CNS involvement (for at least 2-3 months or until remission then start maintenance). When a total dose of amphotericin B reaches 4 - 6 mg/kg start maintenance dosage of amphotericin B at 0.15 - 0.25 mg/kg IV once a month or use ketoconazole at 10 mg/kg PO either once daily, divided *bid* or ketoconazole at 2.5 - 5 mg/kg PO once daily. If CNS/ocular involvement use ketoconazole at 20 - 40 mg/kg PO divided *bid*. (Greene, O'Neal, and Barsanti 1984)

For cryptococcosis (see general dosage guidelines above):
- a) Amphotericin B 0.15 - 0.4 mg/kg IV 3 times a week with flucytosine 150 - 175 mg/kg PO divided *tid-qid*. When a total dose of amphotericin B reaches 4 - 6 mg/kg start maintenance dosage of amphotericin B at 0.15 - 0.25 mg/kg IV once a month with

flucytosine at dosage above or with ketoconazole at 10 mg/kg PO once daily or divided *bid*. (Greene, O'Neal, and Barsanti 1984)

For histoplasmosis (see general dosage guidelines above):
a) Amphotericin B 0.15 - 0.5 mg/kg IV 3 times a week with ketoconazole 10 - 20 mg/day PO once daily or divided *bid* (for at least 2-3 months or until remission then start maintenance). When a total dose of amphotericin B reaches 2 - 4 mg/kg start maintenance dosage of amphotericin B at 0.15 - 0.25 mg/kg IV once a month or use ketoconazole at 10 mg/kg PO either once daily, divided *bid* or at 2.5 - 5 mg/kg PO once daily. (Greene, O'Neal, and Barsanti 1984)
b) As an alternative to ketoconazole treatment: 0.5 mg/kg IV given over 6-8 hours. If dose is tolerated, increase to 1 mg/kg given on alternate day until total dose of 7.5-8.5 mg/kg cumulative dose is achieved. (Macy 1987)

Cats:

For treatment of susceptible systemic fungal infections:
a) Rapid-Infusion Technique: After diluting vial (as outlined below in preparation of solution section), dilute quantity of stock solution to equal 0.25 mg/kg in 30 ml of 5% dextrose. Using butterfly catheter, flush with 10 ml of D5W. Infuse amphotericin B solution IV over 5 minutes. Flush catheter with 10 ml of D5W and remove catheter. Repeat above steps using 0.25 mg/kg 3 times a week until 9-12 mg/kg accumulated dosage is given. (Noxon 1989)

For cryptococcosis (see general dosage guidelines above):
a) As an alternative therapy to ketoconazole: Amphotericin B: 0.25 mg/kg in 30 ml D5W IV over 15 minutes q48h with flucytosine: 200 mg/kg/day divided q6h PO. Continue therapy for 3-4 weeks after clinical signs have resolved or until BUN > 50 mg/dl. (Legendre 1989)
b) Amphotericin B 0.15 - 0.4 mg/kg IV 3 times a week with flucytosine 125 - 250 mg/day PO divided *bid-qid*. When a total dose of amphotericin B reaches 4 - 6 mg/kg start maintenance dosage of amphotericin B at 0.15 - 0.25 mg/kg IV once a month with flucytosine at dosage above or with ketoconazole at 10 mg/kg PO once daily or divided *bid*. (Greene, O'Neal, and Barsanti 1984)

For histoplasmosis (see general dosage guidelines above):
a) Amphotericin B: 0.25 mg/kg in 30 ml D5W IV over 15 minutes q48h with ketoconazole: 10 mg/kg q12h PO. Continue therapy for 4-8 weeks or until BUN > 50 mg/dl. If BUN increases greater than 50 mg/dl, continue ketoconazole alone. Ketoconazole is used long-term (at least 6 months of duration. (Legendre 1989)
b) Amphotericin B 0.15 - 0.5 mg/kg IV 3 times a week with ketoconazole 10 mg/day PO once daily or divided *bid* (for at least 2-3 months or until remission, then start maintenance). When a total dose of amphotericin B reaches 2 - 4 mg/kg start maintenance dosage of amphotericin B at 0.15 - 0.25 mg/kg IV once a month or use ketoconazole at 10 mg/kg PO either once daily, divided *bid* or at 2.5 - 5 mg/kg PO once daily. (Greene, O'Neal, and Barsanti 1984)

For blastomycosis (see general dosage guidelines above):
a) Amphotericin B: 0.25 mg/kg in 30 ml D5W IV over 15 minutes q48h with ketoconazole: 10 mg/kg q12h PO (for at least 60 days). Continue amphotericin B therapy until a cumulative dose of 4 mg/kg is given or until BUN > 50 mg/dl. If renal toxicity does not develop, may increase dose to 0.5 mg/kg of amphotericin B. (Legendre 1989)
b) Amphotericin B 0.15 - 0.5 mg/kg IV 3 times a week with ketoconazole 10 mg/day PO once daily or divided *bid* (for at least 2-3 months or until remission then start maintenance). When a total dose of amphotericin B reaches 4 - 6 mg/kg start maintenance dosage of amphotericin B at 0.15 - 0.25 mg/kg IV once a month or use ketoconazole at 10 mg/kg PO either once daily, divided *bid* or ketoconazole at 2.5 - 5 mg/kg PO once daily. If CNS/ocular involvement, use ketoconazole at 20 - 40 mg/kg PO divided *bid*. (Greene, O'Neal, and Barsanti 1984)

Horses:

For treatment of susceptible systemic fungal infections:
a) 0.3 mg/kg in D5W IV (Robinson 1987)
b) For phycomycoses and pulmonary mycoses: After reconstitution (see below) transfer appropriate amount of drug to 1L of D5W and administer using a 16 g needle IV at a rate of 1 L/hr. Dosage schedule follows:
Day 1: 0.3 mg/kg IV
Day 2: 0.45 mg/kg IV
Day 3: 0.6 mg/kg IV; then every other day for 3 days per week (MWF or TTHSa) until clinical signs of improvement or toxicity takes place. It toxicity occurs, a dose

may be skipped, dose reduced or dosage interval lengthened. Administration may extend from 10-80 days. (Brumbaugh 1987)

Llamas:
For treatment of susceptible systemic fungal infections:
   a) A single case report. Llama received 1 mg test dose, then initially at 0.3 mg/kg IV over 4 hours, followed by 3 L of LRS with 1.5 ml of B-Complex and 20 mEq of KCl added. Subsequent doses were increased by 10 mg and given every 48 hours until reaching 1 mg/kg q48h IV for 6 weeks. Animal tolerated therapy well, but treatment was ultimately unsuccessful (Coccidiodomycoses). (Fowler 1989)

Birds:
For treatment of susceptible systemic fungal infections:
   a) For raptors and psittacines with aspergillosis: 1.5 mg/kg IV *tid* for 3 days with flucytosine or follow with flucytosine.
      May also use intratracheally at 1 mg/kg diluted in sterile water once to 3 times daily for 3 days in conjunction with flucytosine or nebulized (1 mg/ml of saline) for 15 minutes *bid*.
      Potentially nephrotoxic and may cause bone marrow suppression. (Clubb 1986)

Reptiles:
For susceptible fungal respiratory infections:
   a) For most species: 1 mg/kg diluted in saline and given intra tracheally once daily for 14-28 treatments (Gauvin 1993)

Monitoring Parameters - Also see Adverse effects section
   1) BUN and serum creatinine every other day while dosage is being increased, and at least weekly thereafter during therapy
   2) Serum electrolytes (sodium, potassium and magnesium) weekly
   3) Liver function tests weekly
   4) CBC weekly
   5) Urinalysis weekly
   6) TPP at least weekly
   7) Animal's weight

Client Information - Clients should be informed of the potential seriousness of toxic effects that can occur with amphotericin B therapy, as well as the costs associated with therapy.

Dosage Forms/Preparations/FDA Approval Status/Solution Preparation -
   Veterinary-Approved Products: None
   Human-Approved Products:

Amphotericin B for Powder for Injection 50 mg/vial (as deoxycholate); *Fungizone*® *Intravenous* (Bristol-Myers Squibb); (Rx);*Amphotericin B*® (Pharma-Tek); (Rx)
   Directions for reconstitution/administration: Using strict aseptic technique and a 20 gauge or larger needle, rapidly inject 10 ml of sterile water for injection (without a bacteriostatic agent) directly into the lyophylized cake; immediately shake well until solution is clear. A 5 mg/ml colloidal solution results. Further dilute (1:50) for administration to a concentration of 0.1 mg/ml with 5% dextrose in water (pH >4.2). An in-line filter may be used during administration, but must have a pore diameter >1 micron.

Amphotericin B Suspension for Injection: 100 mg/20 ml (as lipid complex) in single use vials with 5 micron filter needles:*Abelcet*® (Liposome Co.) (Rx)

Amphotericin B for Powder for Injection 50 mg/vial (as cholesteryl) in 20 ml vials with 52.8 mg sodium cholesteryl sulfate & 100 mg (as cholesteryl) in 50 ml vials with 52.8 mg sodium cholesteryl sulfate; *Amphotec*® (Sequus Pharmaceuticals) (Rx)

Amphotericin B for Powder for Injection 50 mg/vial (as liposomal) in single use vials with 5 micron filter needles:*AmBisome*® (Fujisawa) (Rx)

Amphotericin B is also available in a topical formulation.

AMPICILLIN
AMPICILLIN SODIUM
AMPICILLIN TRIHYDRATE

For general information on the penicillins, including adverse effects, contraindications, overdosage, drug interactions and monitoring parameters, refer to the monograph: Penicillins, General Information.

Chemistry - A semi-synthetic aminopenicillin, ampicillin anhydrous and trihydrate occur as practically odorless, white, crystalline powders that are slightly soluble in water. At usual temperatures (<42°C), ampicillin anhydrous is more soluble in water than is the trihydrate (13 mg/ml vs. 6 mg/ml at 20°C). Ampicillin anhydrous or trihydrate oral suspensions have a pH of 5-7.5 after reconstitution with water.

Ampicillin sodium occurs as an odorless or practically odorless, white to off-white, crystalline hygroscopic powder. It is very soluble in water or other aqueous solutions. After reconstitution, ampicillin sodium has a pH of 8-10 at a concentration of 10 mg/ml. Commercially available ampicillin sodium for injection has approximately 3 mEq of sodium per gram of ampicillin.

Potency of the ampicillin salts are expressed in terms of ampicillin anhydrous. Ampicillin may also be known as aminobenzylpenicillin, AY-6108, or BRL 1341.

Storage/Stability/Compatibility - Ampicillin anhydrous or trihydrate capsules and powder for oral suspension should be stored at room temperature (15-30°C). After reconstitution, the oral suspension is stable for 14 days if refrigerated (2-8°C) and is stable for 7 days when kept at room temperature.

Ampicillin trihydrate for injection (*Polyflex®*) is stable for 12 months if refrigerated (2-8°C) and is stable for 3 months when kept at room temperature.

Ampicillin sodium for injection is relatively unstable after reconstitution and should generally be used within 1 hour of reconstitution. As the concentration of the drug in solution increases, the stability of the drug decreases. Dextrose may also speed the destruction of the drug by acting as a catalyst in the hydrolysis of ampicillin.

While most sources recommend using solutions of ampicillin sodium immediately, studies have demonstrated that at concentrations of 30 mg/ml, ampicillin sodium solutions are stable in sterile water for injection or 0.9% sodium chloride for up to 48 hours (72 hours if concentrations are 20 mg/ml or less) if kept at 4°C. Solutions with a concentration of 30 mg/ml or less have also been shown to be stable for up to 24 hours in solutions of lactated Ringer's solution if kept at 4°C. Solutions of 20 mg/ml or less are reportedly stable for up to 4 hours in D5W if refrigerated.

Ampicillin sodium is reportedly **compatible** with the following additives (see the above paragraph for more information): heparin sodium, chloramphenicol sodium succinate, procaine HCl and verapamil HCl.

Ampicillin sodium is reportedly **incompatible** with the following additives: amikacin sulfate, chlorpromazine HCl, dopamine HCl, erythromycin lactobionate, gentamicin HCl, hydralazine HCl, hydrocortisone sodium succinate, kanamycin sulfate, lincomycin HCl, oxytetracycline HCl, polymyxin B sulfate, prochlorperazine edisylate, sodium bicarbonate and tetracycline HCl. Compatibility is dependent upon factors such as pH, concentration, temperature and diluents used. It is suggested to consult specialized references for more specific information (*e.g.,* *Handbook on Injectable Drugs* by Trissel; see bibliography).

Pharmacology - Ampicillin and the other aminopenicillins have increased activity against many strains of gram negative aerobes not covered by either the natural penicillins or penicillinase-resistant penicillins, including some strains of *E. coli, Klebsiella* and *Haemophilus.* Like the natural penicillins they are susceptible to inactivation by beta-lactamase-producing bacteria (*e.g.,* *Staph aureus*). Although not as active as the natural penicillins, they do have activity against many anaerobic bacteria, including *Clostridial* organisms. Organisms that are generally not susceptible include *Pseudomonas aeruginosa, Serratia,* Indole-positive *Proteus* (*Proteus mirabilis* is susceptible), *Enterobacter, Citrobacter,* and *Acinetobacter.* The aminopenicillins also are inactive against *Rickettsia,* mycobacteria, fungi, *Mycoplasma,* and viruses.

Uses/Indications - In dogs and cats, ampicillin is not as well absorbed after oral administration as is amoxicillin and its oral use has largely been supplanted by amoxicillin. It is used commonly in parenteral dosage forms when an aminopenicillin is indicated in all species.

Pharmacokinetics (specific) - Ampicillin anhydrous and trihydrate is relatively stable in the presence of gastric acid. After oral administration, it is about 30-55% absorbed in humans (empty stomach) and animals (monogastric). Food will decrease the rate and extent of oral absorption.

When administered parenterally (IM, SQ) the trihydrate salt will achieve serum levels of approximately 1/2 of those of a comparable dose of the sodium salt. The trihydrate parenteral dosage form should not be used where higher MIC's are required for treating systemic infections.

After absorption the volume of distribution for ampicillin is approximately 0.3 L/kg in humans and dogs, and 0.167 L/kg in cats. The drug is widely distributed to many tissues, including liver, lungs, prostate (human), muscle, bile, and ascitic, pleural and synovial fluids. Ampicillin will cross into the CSF when meninges are inflamed in concentrations that may range from 10-60% of those found in serum. Very low levels of the drug are found in the aqueous humor and low levels are found in tears, sweat and saliva. Ampicillin crosses the placenta, but is thought to be relatively safe to use during pregnancy. Ampicillin is approximately 20% bound to plasma proteins, primarily albumin. Milk levels of ampicillin are considered to be low.

Ampicillin is eliminated primarily through renal mechanisms, principally by tubular secretion, but some of the drug is metabolized by hydrolysis to penicilloic acids (inactive) and then excreted in the urine. Elimination half-lives of ampicillin have been reported as 45-80 minutes in dogs and cats, and 60 minutes in swine.

Doses -
 Dogs:
   For susceptible infections:
   a) 10 - 20 mg/kg IV, IM, or SQ q6-8h (Vaden and Papich 1995)
   b) Trihydrate injectable (*Polyflex®*): 5.5 - 11 mg/kg IM or SQ q8h
       Sodium salt: 5.5 - 11 mg/kg IV or SQ q8h
       Oral Forms: 22 - 33 mg/kg PO q8h (Aronson and Aucoin 1989)
   c) For routine infections: 22 mg/kg PO *tid*, or 11 - 22 mg/kg IM, IV, or SQ *tid-qid* (Morgan 1988)
   d) For susceptible UTI's: 77 mg/kg/day PO divided *tid* (Rogers and Lees 1989)
   e) 10 - 20 mg/kg PO q6h; 5 - 10 mg/kg q6h IV, IM or SQ (Kirk 1989)
   f) 10 - 55 mg/kg q6-12h PO; 5 - 11 mg/kg IV, IM, or SQ q6-12h (Greene 1984)
   g) Trihydrate injectable (*Polyflex®*): 10 - 50 mg/kg IM or SQ q6-8h;
       For beta-hemolytic *Streptococcus* osteomyelitis: 20 mg/kg PO q6h (Ford and Aronson 1985)

 Cats:
   For susceptible infections:
   a) 10 - 20 mg/kg IV, IM, or SQ q6-8h (Vaden and Papich 1995)
   b) Trihydrate injectable (*Polyflex®*): 5.5 - 11 mg/kg IM or SQ q8h
       Sodium salt: 5.5 - 11 mg/kg IV or SQ q8h
       Oral Forms: 22 - 33 mg/kg PO q8h (Aronson and Aucoin 1989)
   c) Oral: 10 - 20 mg/kg PO q8-12h (Ford and Aronson 1985)
   d) For bacterial respiratory infections: 10 - 20 mg/kg PO or parenterally q8-12h (Roudebush 1985)
   e) 10 - 20 mg/kg PO q6h; 5 - 10 mg/kg q6h IV, IM or SQ (Kirk 1989)
   f) For routine infections: 22 mg/kg PO *tid*, or 11 - 22 mg/kg IM, IV, or SQ *tid-qid* (Morgan 1988)
   g) 10 - 60 mg/kg q6-12h PO; 5 - 11 mg/kg IV, IM, or SQ q6-12h (Greene 1984)

 Cattle:
   For susceptible infections:
   a) 4 - 10 mg/kg IM q24h (salt not indicated); 4 - 10 mg/kg PO q12-24h. (Jenkins 1986)
   b) For respiratory infections: Ampicillin trihydrate (*Polyflex®*): 22 mg/kg SQ q12h (60 day slaughter withdrawal suggested). (Hjerpe 1986)
   c) For respiratory infections: ampicillin sodium 22 mg/kg SQ q12h;
       Ampicillin trihydrate: 11 mg/kg IM q24h (Beech 1987b)
   d) Ampicillin trihydrate: 15 - 22 mg/kg SQ or IM *tid* (Upson 1988)

 Horses:
   For susceptible infections:
   a) Ampicillin sodium: 10 - 50 mg/kg IV or IM *tid*
       Ampicillin trihydrate: 5 - 20 mg/kg IM *bid* (Robinson 1987)
   b) Ampicillin sodium: 11 - 15 mg/IM or IV *tid-qid* (Beech 1987a)
   c) Foals: Ampicillin sodium 20 mg/kg IV q6-8h (dose extrapolated from adult horses; use longer dosage interval in premature foals or those less than 7 days of age) (Caprile and Short 1987)
   d) Ampicillin trihydrate: 11 mg/kg IM q6h
       Ampicillin sodium: 22 mg/kg IM q12h (Upson 1988)
   e) Ampicillin sodium 22 mg/kg IM q6-12h or 25 - 100 mg/kg IV q6h.
       Ampicillin trihydrate: 11 - 22 mg/kg IM q12h (Brumbaugh 1987)

 Swine:
   For susceptible infections:
   a) Ampicillin sodium: 6 - 8 mg/kg SQ or IM q8h (Baggot 1983)

 Rabbits:
   For susceptible infections:
   a) 10 - 25 mg/kg IM or SQ q6-12h (Warning: Do not give orally to rabbits) (McConnell and Hughey 1987)

 Birds:
   For susceptible infections:
   a) Amazon parrots: 150 - 200 mg/kg PO *bid - tid* (poorly absorbed PO); 100 mg/kg IM (as the trihydrate/*Polyflex®*) q4h.
       Pet birds: 250 mg capsule in 8 oz. of drinking water (poorly absorbed; rapidly excreted)
       Chickens: 1.65 g/L drinking water (see above)

Most birds: 250 mg/kg via feed for 5-10 days. Sprinkle on favorite food or add to mash or corn mix. (Clubb 1986)
  b) 100 mg/kgIM or IM q8h (Hoeffer 1995)

Reptiles:
For susceptible infections:
  a) Snakes: 3 - 6 mg/kg IM or SQ daily (McConnell and Hughey 1987)]
  b) All species: 3 - 6 mg/kg PO, SubQ or IM every 12-24 hours for 2 weeks; not very useful unless used in combination with aminoglycosides. (Gauvin 1993)

Client Information - Unless otherwise instructed by the veterinarian, this drug should be given orally on an empty stomach, at least 1 hour before feeding or 2 hours after. Keep oral suspension in the refrigerator and discard any unused suspension after 14 days. If stored at room temperature, discard unused suspension after 7 days.

Dosage Forms/Preparations/FDA Approval Status/Withholding Times -
Veterinary-Approved Products:
Ampicillin Trihydrate Injection Powder for Suspension 10 g & 25 g (of ampicillin) vials.
  Polyflex® (Fort Dodge); (Rx) Approved for use in dogs, cats, and cattle. Withdrawal times (cattle; do not treat for more than 7 days): Milk = 48 hours; Slaughter = 6 days.
Ampicillin Sodium for Injection 1 gram & 3 gram vials (of ampicillin)
  Amp-Equine® (Pfizer); (Rx) Approved for use in horses not intended for food.

Human-Approved Products:
Ampicillin Sodium Powder for Injection Vials 125 mg, 250 mg, 500 mg, 1 g, 2 g, 10 g; 500 mg, 1 g, and 2 gram piggyback units; *Omnipen-N*® (Wyeth-Ayerst) (Rx);*Polycillin-N*® (Apothecon) (Rx);*Totacillin-N*® (SK-Beecham) (Rx); generic (Rx)
Ampicillin Capsules (as either trihydrate or anhydrous) 250 mg, 500 mg; Many tradenames and generics; (Rx)
Ampicillin (as the trihydrate) Powder for Oral Suspension 25 mg/ml, 50 mg/ ml, 100 mg/ml in 20 ml, 80 ml, 100 ml, 150 ml, and 200 ml bottles; Many tradenames; (Rx)
Also available in fixed dose combinations with:
Probenecid: Powder for Oral Suspension: 3.5 g ampicillin (as trihydrate) & 1g probenecid/probenecid (oral): *Polycillin-PRB*® (Apothecon); *Probampacin*®, generic (Rx)
Sulbactam Sodium (injection): 1.5 g (1 g ampicillin sodium/.05 g sulbactam sodium) & 3 g (2 g ampicillin sodium/1 g sulbactam sodium);*Unasyn*® (Roerig) (Rx)

AMPROLIUM HYDROCHLORIDE

Chemistry - A structural analogue of thiamine (vitamin B$_1$), amprolium hydrochloride occurs as a white or almost white, odorless or nearly odorless powder. One gram is soluble in 2 ml of water and is slightly soluble in alcohol.

Storage/Stability/Compatibility - Unless otherwise instructed by the manufacturer, amprolium products should be stored at room temperature (15-30°C).

Pharmacology - By mimicking its structure, amprolium competitively inhibits thiamine utilization by the parasite. Prolonged high dosages can cause thiamine deficiency in the host and excessive thiamine in the diet can reduce or reverse the anticoccidial activity of the drug.
  Amprolium reportedly acts primarily upon the first generation schizont in the cells of the intestinal wall, preventing differentiation of the metrozoites. It may also suppress the sexual stages and sporulation of the oocysts.

Uses/Indications - Amprolium has good activity against *Eimeria tenella, E. acervulina* in poultry and can be used as a therapeutic agent for these organisms. It only has marginal activity or weak activity against *E. maxima, E. mivati, E. necatrix,* or *E. brunetti*. It is often used in combination with other agents (*e.g.,* ethopabate) to improve control against those organisms.
  In cattle, amprolium has approval for the treatment and prevention of *E. bovis* and *E. zurnii* in cattle and calves. Amprolium has been used in dogs, swine, sheep, and goats for the control of coccidiosis, although there are no approved products in the U.S.A. for these species.

Pharmacokinetics - No information was located for this agent.

Contraindications/Precautions/Reproductive Safety - Not recommended to be used for over 12 days in puppies.

Adverse Effects/Warnings - In dogs, neural disturbances, depression, anorexia, and diarrhea have been reported but are rare and are probably dose-related. See Overdosage section below for treatment recommendations.

Overdosage/Acute Toxicity - Amprolium has induced polioencephalomalacia (PEM) in sheep when administered at 880 mg/kg PO for 4-6 weeks and at 1 gram/kg for 3-5 weeks. Erythrocyte production in lambs receiving these high dosages of amprolium also ceased.

It is reported that overdoses of amprolium will produce neurologic symptoms in dogs. Treatment should consist of stopping amprolium therapy and administering parenteral thiamine (1 - 10 mg/day IM or IV).

Drug Interactions - Exogenously administered **thiamine** in high doses may reverse or reduce the efficacy of amprolium.

Doses -
  Dogs:
    For coccidiosis:
      a) 100 - 200 mg/kg PO in food or water for 7-10 days. (Morgan 1988), (Kirk 1989), (Greene 1984)
      b) Prophylaxis: 30 ml of 9.6% solution in one gallon (3.8 L) of drinking water or (not both) 1.25 grams of 20% powder in food to feed 4 pups daily. Give as sole source of food or water for 7 days prior to shipping. Bitches may be given medicated water (as above) as the sole source of water for 10 days prior to whelping. (USPC 1989)
      c) Prophylaxis: 0.075% solution as drinking water (Matz 1995)
  Cattle:
    For coccidiosis:
      a) Treatment: 10 mg/kg PO for 5 days; 5 mg/kg for 21 days for prophylaxis. (Todd, Dipietro, and Guterbock 1986)
  Swine:
    For coccidiosis:
      a) Treatment: 25 - 65 mg/kg PO once or twice daily for 3-4 days. (Todd, Dipietro, and Guterbock 1986)
      b) 100 mg/kg/day in food or water. (Howard 1986)
  Sheep & Goats:
    For coccidiosis:
      a) Lambs: 55 mg/kg daily PO for 19 days. (Todd, Dipietro, and Guterbock 1986)
  Birds:
      a) For coccidiosis in pet birds: 2 ml (using the 9.6% solution)/gallon of water for 5 days or longer. Cages should be steam cleaned to prevent reinfection. Supplement diet with B vitamins. Some strains resistant in Toucans and Mynahs. (Clubb 1986)
      For chickens (broilers or layers), turkeys, and pheasants: Refer to individual product instructions.

Monitoring Parameters -
  1) Clinical efficacy

Dosage Forms/Preparations/FDA Approval Status/Withholding Times -
  Veterinary-Approved Products:
    Amprolium 1.25% Medicated Crumbles for Top Dressing in 50 lb bags.; *Corid® 1.25% Crumbles* (MSD-AgVet); (OTC) Approved for use in calves. Slaughter withdrawal = 24 hours.

    Amprolium 9.6% (96 mg/ml) Oral Solution; *Corid® 9.6% Oral Solution* (MSD-AgVet); (OTC) Approved for use in calves. Slaughter withdrawal = 24 hours

    Amprolium 20 % Soluble Powder; *Corid® 20% Soluble Powder* (MSD-AgVet); (OTC) Approved for use in calves. Slaughter withdrawal = 24 hours

There are many combination products (medicated feeds, feed additives) containing amprolium with other therapeutic agents. These products are approved for chickens (broilers only) and/or turkeys. There are some products containing amprolium alone for use in laying hens.

  Human-Approved Products: None

AMRINONE LACTATE

Chemistry - Unrelated structurally to cardiac glycosides or catecholamines, amrinone is a bipyrdine cardiac inotropic agent. It occurs as a pale yellow, crystalline powder and is insoluble in water and slightly soluble in alcohol. The commercially available injection has a pH adjusted to 3.2-4 and an osmolality of 101 mOsm/L.

Storage/Stability/Compatibility - The commercially available injection should be stored at room temperature and protected from light. It is stable for 2 years after manufacture.

Amrinone lactate for injection is reportedly **compatible** with 0.45% or 0.9% sodium chloride injection, propranolol HCl, verapamil HCl. It is reportedly **incompatible** with solutions containing dextrose or sodium bicarbonate. Compatibility is dependent upon factors such as pH, concentration, temperature and diluents used. It is suggested to consult specialized references (*e.g., Handbook on Injectable Drugs* by Trissel; see bibliography) for more specific information.

Pharmacology - The exact mechanisms of amrinone's cardiac effects are not well understood. It is thought the primary effects are due to its vasodilatory effects, thereby reducing both preload and afterload. Because it inhibits phosphodiesterase, it may also directly stimulate cardiac contractility.

Uses/Indications - Amrinone is considered to be a second line agent for the short term management of CHF.

Pharmacokinetics - Although no commercial dosage forms are available, amrinone is rapidly absorbed after oral administration. After initial intravenous injection, effects begin within 2-3 minutes and peak effects occur within 10 minutes. Cardiac effects generally correlate with the drug's serum level. Amrinone's distribution characteristics are not well described. In humans, it has an apparent volume of distribution of 1.2 L/kg. It exhibits low to moderate protein binding (10-49%). It is unknown if it crosses the placenta, blood-brain barrier or enters into maternal milk. Amrinone is eliminated primarily via the kidneys. About 63% of a dose is excreted (10-40% unchanged) into the urine. The duration of effect (in humans) is dose related with a single dose lasting from 30 minuets after a 0.75 mg/kg IV dose to 2 hours after a 3 mg/kg dose. Plasma half lives may be prolonged in patients with CHF.

Contraindications/Precautions/Reproductive Safety - Amrinone is considered contraindicated when severe aortic or pulmonic valve disease is present or in patients hypersensitive to it or bisulfites. The potential risks versus benefits of therapy with amrinone should be carefully considered in patients with hypertrophic cardiomyopathy. Reproductive safety data are conflicting; use only when benefits outweigh risks.

Adverse Effects/Warnings - Use in domestic animals is limited. Adverse effects that potentially could be seen include arrhythmias (drug is not inherently arrhythmogenic, but CHF patients are more susceptible to arrhythmias secondary to any drug), hypotension, GI effects (vomiting, diarrhea), thrombocytopenia (particularly with prolonged therapy), hepatotoxicity, and hypersensitivity reactions (variable symptomatology: pericarditis to myositis, etc.). Amrinone should only be used in settings where appropriate monitoring may be employed.

Overdosage/Acute Toxicity - Only one case (human) of accidental massive overdose resulting in death has been reported (causal relationship not unequivocally established). Because hypotension is the primary problem that would generally be seen, circulatory support should be instituted.

Drug Interactions - **Digoxin** and other inotropic cardiac glycosides have an additive effect with amrinone. This is generally considered to be a positive drug interaction. **Disopyramide** may cause excessive hypotension when used with amrinone.

Doses -
  Dogs:
    As a positive inotropic agent:
      a) In cardiogenic shock: Slow IV bolus (over 2-3 minutes) of 0.75 mg/kg, then a constant infusion of 5 -10 micrograms/kg/min. (Keene 1989)
      b) 1 - 3 mg/kg IV followed by 30 - 100 micrograms/kg/min IV infusion (Muir and Bonagura 1994)

  Cats:
      a) 1 - 3 mg/kg IV followed by 30 - 100 micrograms/kg/min IV infusion (Muir and Bonagura 1994)

Monitoring Parameters -
  1) Blood pressure; 2) Heart rate/rhythm; 3) Body weight; 4) Platelet counts

Client Information - Clients should be made aware of the "investigational nature" of the use of this drug in dogs or cats prior to its usage.

Dosage Forms/Preparations/FDA Approval Status/Withholding Times -
  Veterinary-Approved Products: None

  Human-Approved Products:
Amrinone Lactate for Injection 5 mg/ml (as lactate); *Inocor*® (Sanofi Winthrop) (Rx)

Antacids, Oral

Pharmacology - Oral antacids used in veterinary medicine are generally relatively non-absorbable salts of aluminum, calcium or magnesium. Up to 20% of an oral dose of magnesium can be absorbed, however. Antacids decrease HCl concentrations in the GI. One gram of these compounds generally neutralize 20-35 mEq of acid (*in vitro*). Although the pH of the gastric fluid can rarely be brought to near-neutral conditions, at a pH of 3.3, 99% of all gastric acid is neutralized, thereby reducing gastric acid back-diffusion through the gastric mucosa and reducing the amount of acid presented to the duodenum. Pepsin proteolytic activity is also reduced by raising the pH and can be minimized if the pH of the gastric contents can be increased to >4.

Uses/Indications - Antacids have been used in veterinary medicine for the adjunctive treatment of esophagitis, gastric hyperacidity, peptic ulcer and gastritis. Because of difficulty in administration and the frequent dosing that is often required, and with the advent of the histamine-2 blocking agents (cimetidine, ranitidine, *et al*) and/or sucralfate, antacids have largely been relegated to adjunctive roles in therapy for these indications in foals and small animals. They still remain important in reducing hyperphosphatemia in patients with renal failure.

In ruminants, magnesium hydroxide is used to increase rumen pH and as a laxative in the treatment of rumen overload syndrome (*aka* acute rumen engorgement, rumen acidosis, grain overload, engorgement toxemia, rumen impaction).

Contraindications/Precautions - Magnesium-containing antacids are contraindicated in patients with renal disease. Some products have significant quantities of sodium or potassium and should be used cautiously in patients who should have these electrolytes restricted in their diet. Aluminum-containing antacids may inhibit gastric emptying; use cautiously in patients with gastric outlet obstruction.

Adverse Effects/Warnings - In monogastric animals, the most common side effects of antacid therapy are constipation with aluminum- and calcium-containing antacids, and diarrhea or frequent loose stools with magnesium containing antacids. Many products contain both aluminum and magnesium salts in the attempt to balance the constipating and laxative actions of the other.

If the patient is receiving a low phosphate diet, hypophosphatemia can develop if the patient chronically receives aluminum antacids. Magnesium-containing antacids can cause hypermagnesemia in patients with severe renal insufficiency.

If administering calcium carbonate in high doses or chronically, significant quantities of calcium can be absorbed from the gut resulting in hypercalcemia in susceptible patients. Calcium carbonate has also been implicated in causing a gastric acid rebound phenomena. Patients with significant renal impairment or dehydration and electrolyte imbalance can develop the milk-alkali syndrome. If the patient is receiving a low phosphate diet, hypophosphatemia can develop if the patient chronically receives calcium carbonate antacids.

In ruminants, alkalinization of the rumen may enhance the absorption of ammonia, histamine or other basic compounds.

Overdosage - See the Adverse Effects section above. If necessary, GI and electrolyte imbalances that can occur with chronic or acute overdose should be treated symptomatically.

Drug Interactions - By altering GI transit time, stomach pH, or by chelation, all orally administered non-absorbable antacids can affect the rate and potentially the extent of absorption of other drugs. The reader is referred to specific references (see bibliography) for more information on the clinical significance and the individual salt(s) that have been implicated in the listing below. As a general guideline, it is best not to give antacids within 1-2 hours of other oral medications.

Orally administered **tetracycline** products can be chelated and prevented from being absorbed by antacids. Antacids should not be administered within 1-2 hours of tetracycline dosing. Antacids can decrease the amount absorbed or the pharmacologic effect of: **chlordiazepoxide, captopril, chloroquine, cimetidine, corticosteroids, digoxin, iron salts, indomethicin, isoniazid** (aluminum antacids only), **ketoconazole, nitrofurantoin, pancrelipase, penicillamine, phenothiazines, phenytoin, ranitidine, and valproic acid**.

Increased absorption or pharmacologic effect may occur when antacids are administered with the following: **dicumarol, flecainide, quinidine, and sympathomimetics. Aspirin** absorption and also excretion can be enhanced when concomitantly administered with antacids.

Use of **sodium polystyrene sulfonate** (*Kayexalate®*) with antacids, may decrease the potassium lowering effectiveness of the drug and in patients in renal failure may cause metabolic alkalosis.

Doses -
  Dogs:
    For hyperphosphatemia:
      a) Aluminum hydroxide: Initially at 30 - 90 mg/kg per day. Dosage must be individualized. Prefer capsules or suspension as they are more easily mixed with food and dis-

persed throughout ingesta. Evaluate serum phosphate levels at 10-14 days intervals to determine optimum dosage. (Polzin and Osborne 1985)
b) Aluminum hydroxide: 30 - 90 mg/kg PO once a day to three times a day with meals (Morgan 1988)

For adjunctive therapy for gastric ulcers:
a) Aluminum hydroxide suspension or aluminum hydroxide/magnesium hydroxide suspension: 2 - 10 ml PO q2-4h (Hall and Twedt 1988)
b) Aluminum hydroxide tablets: 0.5 - 1 tablet PO q6h (Matz 1995)

As an antacid:
a) Magnesium hydroxide (Milk of Magnesia): 5 - 30 ml PO once to twice daily (Morgan 1988)

Cats:
For hyperphosphatemia:
a) Aluminum hydroxide: Initially at 30 - 90 mg/kg per day. Dosage must be individualized. Prefer capsules or suspension as they are more easily mixed with food and dispersed throughout ingesta. Evaluate serum phosphate levels at 10-14 days intervals to determine optimum dosage. (Polzin and Osborne 1985)

As an antacid:
a) Magnesium hydroxide (Milk of Magnesia): 5 - 15 ml PO once to twice daily (Morgan 1988)
b) Aluminum hydroxide tablets: 0.25 tablets PO q6h (Matz 1995)

Cattle:
For rumen overload syndrome:
a) For adult animals: Up to 1 gm/kg (MgOH) mixed in 2-3 gallons of warm water and given PO per tube. May repeat (use smaller doses) at 6-12 hour intervals. If the rumen has been evacuated, do not exceed 225 grams initially. Dehydration and systemic acidosis must be concomitantly corrected.
Calves: As above but use 1/8th-1/4th the amount. (Wass et al. 1986a)

As an antacid:
a) Aluminum hydroxide: 30 grams;
Calcium carbonate: 60 - 360 grams (Jenkins 1988)

Horses:
For adjunctive gastroduodenal ulcer therapy in foals:
a) Aluminum/magnesium hydroxide suspension: 15 ml 4 times a day (Clark and Becht 1987)

Sheep & Goats:
For rumen overload syndrome:
a) As above for cattle, but use 1/8th-1/4th the amount. (Wass et al. 1986a)

Monitoring Parameters - Monitoring parameters are dependent upon the indication for the product and the salt used. Patients receiving high dose or chronic therapy should be monitored for electrolyte imbalances outlined above.

Client Information/FDA Approval Status - Oral antacids are available without prescription (OTC). Most products are labeled for use in humans. There are veterinary approved products for use in food animals.

Dosage Forms/Preparations-
Veterinary-Approved Products:
Magnesium Hydroxide
Oral Boluses 27 grams of magnesium hydroxide, ginger 200 mg, capsicum 100 mg, methyl salicylate 56 mg
Magnalax® (OTC)
Oral Powder, each pound of powder contains: 350 grams of magnesium hydroxide, ginger 2.6 grams, capsicum 1.3 grams, methyl salicylate 56 mg
Rulax II® (OTC)

Human-Approved Products: The following is a list of some antacids available, it is not meant to be all inclusive.

Aluminum Carbonate, basic
Capsules, equivalent to dried aluminum hydroxide gel 608 mg or aluminum hydroxide 500 mg
Basalgel® (Wyeth)

Suspension, equivalent to aluminum hydroxide 400 mg/5ml
Basalgel® (Wyeth)

Aluminum Hydroxide
  Capsules,
     475 mg; *Alu-Cap®* (Riker)
     500 mg; *Dialume®* (Armour)
  Suspension
     320 mg/5 ml; *Amphogel®* (Wyeth-Ayerst)
     400 mg/5 ml; *Aluminum Hydroxide Gel®* (Roxane)
     600 mg/5 ml; *Alternagel®* (Stuart), *Aluminum Hydroxide Concentrated®* (Roxane)
Magnesium Hydroxide
  Powder
  Oral Suspension (Milk of Magnesia) ≈77.5 mg/gram
Aluminum Hydroxide and Magnesium Hydroxide
  Suspension (Note: there are too many products and concentrations to list in this reference; a representative product is *Maalox®* Suspension (Rorer) which contains 225 mg aluminum hydroxide and 200 mg magnesium hydroxide per 5 ml.)

Other dosage forms that are available commercially include: tablets, chewable tablets, and aerosol foam suspension.

ANTIVENIN (CROTALIDAE) POLYVALENT
ANTIVENIN (MICRURUS FULVIAS) CORAL SNAKE

NOTE: The location of antivenins for rare species and the telephone numbers for envenomation experts is available from the Arizona Poison Control Center: (602) 626-6061.

Chemistry - These products are concentrated serum globulins obtained from horses immunized with the venoms of several types of snakes. They are provided as refined, lyophilized product with a suitable diluent.

Storage/Stability/Compatibility - Do not store above 98°F (37°C). The coral snake product should be stored in the refrigerator.

Pharmacology - Antivenins act by neutralizing the venoms (complex proteins) in patients via passive immunization of globulins obtained from horses immunized with the venom.

Uses/Indications - These products are indicated for the treatment of envenomation from most venomous snakes found in North America (not Sonoran or Arizona Coral Snake) causing serious systemic toxicity or potential serious toxicity in domestic animals. There is a fair amount of controversy with regard to these products' use in domestic animals. The risks of administration (*e.g.*, anaphylaxis—see below) may outweigh their potential benefits in certain circumstances. However, these agents can be life-saving when given early in select situations. Many factors contribute to the potential for toxicity (victim's size and general health, bite site(s), number of bites, age, species and size of snake, etc.).

  Antivenin can be very expensive. One 10 ml vial of Crotalidae antivenin approved for use in dogs costs approximately $100. The coral snake product (for human use) cost is >$150 per vial and to treat a coral snake bite may require 5 or more vials. Because of the high cost, not being returnable for credit, and potential adverse effects, veterinary practices need to assess all factors before stocking and using these products.

Contraindications/Precautions - The coral snake antivenin will not neutralize *M euryxanthus* (Sonoran or Arizona Coral Snake) venom. Because there is a risk of anaphylaxis occurring secondary to the horse serum, many recommend perform sensitivity testing before administration.

Adverse Effects/Warnings - The most significant adverse effect associated with the use of these products is anaphylaxis secondary to the equine serum source of this product. A 1:10 dilution of the antivenin given intracutaneously at a dose of 0.02 - 0.03 ml may be useful as a test for hypersensitivity. Wheal formation and erythema indicate a positive reaction and are generally seen within 30 minutes of administration. A negative response does not insure that anaphylaxis will not occur however.

Drug Interactions - Although reducing excessive movement and other supportive therapy are important parts of treating envenomation, drugs that can mask the clinical signs associated with the venom (*e.g.*, analgesics and sedatives) should be used with discretion. It has also been stated that antihistamines (Controversial: See equine dose below) and tranquilizers are contraindicated as they may potentiate the venom.

Doses -
  Dogs:
     Crotilidae Antivenin: Administer 1-5 rehydrated vials (10-50 ml) IV depending on severity of symptoms, duration of time after the bite, snake size, patient size (smaller the

victim, the larger the dose). Additional doses may be given every 2 hours as required. If unable to give IV, may administer IM as close to bite as practical. Give supportive therapy (*e.g.*, corticosteroids, antibiotics, fluid therapy, blood products, and tetanus prophylaxis) as required. (Package Insert; *Antivenin*®—Fort Dodge)

Coral Snake antivenin (not Sonoran or Arizona variety): After testing for hypersensitivity (see above) give 1-2 vials initially, and more in 4-6 hours if necessary. Therapy is best started within 4 hours after envenomation. Supportive care includes broad spectrum antibiotics, fluid therapy and mechanical ventilation if necessary. Corticosteroids are not recommended. (Marks, Mannella et al. 1990)

Horses:

Crotilidae Antivenin: Use only if necessary to treat systemic effects otherwise avoid use. Administer 1-2 vials slowly IV diluted in 250-500 ml saline or lactated Ringer's. Administer antihistamines; corticosteroids are contraindicated.

Coral Snake (not Sonoran or Arizona variety): As above; same cautions. May be used with Crotilidae antivenin. (Bailey and Garland 1992b)

Species Not Identified:

Crotilidae Antivenin: 1 - 10 vials IV depending on severity of symptoms, time after envenomation, size of animal and snake (5-10 vials usually needed for Eastern Diamondback Rattlesnake envenomation). Best effects when given within 4 hours of envenomation.

Coral Snake: 1 - 10 vials IV given as soon as possible after envenomation. (Thompson 1992)

Client Information - Clients must be made aware of the potential for anaphylaxis as well as the expenses associated with treatment and associated monitoring and hospitalization.

Dosage Forms/Preparations/FDA Approval Status -

Veterinary-Approved Products:

Antivenin (*Crotalidae*) Polyvalent Equine Origin single dose vial lyophilized; 10 ml diluent. *Antivenin*® (Fort Dodge); (Rx) Approved for use in dogs.

Human-Approved Products:

Antivenin (*Crotalidae*) Polyvalent Equine Origin single dose vial lyophilized; 10 ml diluent. Includes 1 ml of normal horse serum diluted 1:10 for use for sensitivity testing; *Antivenin (Crotalidae) Polyvalent* (Wyeth-Ayerst); (Rx)

Antivenin (*Micrucus fulvius*) single dose vial lyophilized; 10 ml diluent; *Antivenin (Micrucus fulvius)* (Wyeth-Ayerst); (Rx)

APOMORPHINE HCL

Chemistry - A centrally-acting emetic, apomorphine occurs as a white powder or minute, white or grayish-white crystals and is sparingly soluble in water or alcohol.

Storage/Stability/Compatibility - Apomorphine soluble tablets should be stored in tight containers at room temperature (15-30°C) and be protected from light.

Upon exposure to light and air, apomorphine gradually darkens in color. Discolored tablets should not be used. Apomorphine solutions are more stable in acidic than alkaline solutions. A 0.3% solution of apomorphine has a pH of about 3-4.

Solutions of apomorphine can be made by solubilizing tablets in at least 1 - 2 ml of either sterile water for injection or 0.9% sodium chloride for injection. After being sterilized by filtration, the solution is stable for 2 days if protected from light and air and stored in the refrigerator. Do not use solutions that are discolored or form a precipitate after filtering.

Pharmacology - Apomorphine stimulates dopamine receptors in the chemoreceptor trigger zone, thus inducing vomiting. It can cause both CNS depression and stimulation, but tends to cause more stimulatory effects. Medullary centers can be depressed with resultant respiratory depression.

Uses/Indications - Apomorphine is used primarily as an emetic in dogs, and is considered to be the emetic of choice in dogs by many clinicians.

Pharmacokinetics - Apomorphine is slowly absorbed after oral administration and has unpredictable efficacy when given by this route and, therefore, is usually administered parenterally or topically to the eye. When given intravenously in dogs, emesis occurs very rapidly; after IM use, vomiting occurs generally within 5 minutes but may be more prolonged. Topical administration to the conjunctival sac is usually effective, but less so than either IV or IM administration.

Apomorphine is primarily conjugated in the liver and then excreted in the urine.

Contraindications/Precautions/Reproductive Safety - Emetics can be an important aspect in the treatment of orally ingested toxins, but must not be used injudiciously. Emetics should not be used in rodents or rabbits, because they are either unable to vomit or do not have stomach walls strong enough to tolerate the act of emesis. Emetics are also contraindicated in patients that are: hypoxic, dyspneic, in shock, lack normal pharyngeal reflexes, seizuring, comatose, severely CNS depressed or where CNS function is deteriorating, or extremely physically weak. Emetics should also be withheld in patients who have previously vomited repeatedly. Emetics are contraindicated in patients who have ingested strong acids, alkalies, other caustic agents because of the risks of additional esophogeal or gastric injury with emesis. Because of the risks of aspiration, emetics are usually contraindicated after petroleum distillate ingestion, but may be employed when the risks of toxicity of the compound are greater than the risks of aspiration. Use of emetics after ingestion of strychnine or other CNS stimulants may precipitate seizures.

Emetics generally do not remove more than 80% of the material in the stomach (usually 40-60%) and successful induction of emesis does not signal the end of appropriate monitoring or therapy. In addition to the contraindications outlined in the general statement, apomorphine should not be used in cases of oral opiate or other CNS depressant (*e.g.,* barbiturates) toxicity, or in patients hypersensitive to morphine.

The use of apomorphine in cats is controversial, and several clinicians state that it should not be used in this species as it is much less effective than either xylazine or ipecac syrup and possibly less safe.

If vomiting does not occur within the expected time after apomorphine administration, repeated doses are also unlikely to induce emesis and may cause symptoms of toxicity.

The reproductive safety of this drug has not been established; weigh the risks of use versus the potential benefits.

Adverse Effects/Warnings - At usual doses, the principal adverse effect that may be seen with apomorphine, is protracted vomiting. Protracted vomiting after ophthalmic administration may be averted by washing the conjunctival sac with sterile saline or ophthalmic rinsing solution. Excitement, restlessness, CNS depression or respiratory depression are usually only associated with overdoses of the drug.

Overdosage/Acute Toxicity - Excessive doses of apomorphine may result in respiratory and/or cardiac depression, CNS stimulation (excitement, seizures) or depression and protracted vomiting. Naloxone may reverse the CNS and respiratory effects of the drug, but cannot be expected to halt the vomiting. Atropine has been suggested to treat severe bradycardias.

Drug Interactions - Antiemetic drugs, particularly **antidopaminergic drugs** (*e.g.,* **phenothiazines**) may negate the emetic effects of apomorphine.

Additive CNS, or respiratory depression may occur when apomorphine is used with **opiates or other CNS or respiratory depressants** (*e.g.,* **barbiturates**).

Doses -
 Dogs:
   For induction of emesis:
    a) 0.03 mg/kg IV or 0.04 mg/kg IM (IV route preferred); alternatively a portion of tablet may be crushed in a syringe and dissolved with few drops of water, and administered into the conjunctival sac. After sufficient vomiting occurs, rinse conjunctival sac free of unabsorbed apomorphine. (Beasley and Dorman 1990)
    b) 0.04 mg/kg IV or 0.08 mg/kg IM or SQ (Bailey 1989), (Riviere 1985), (Mount 1989)
    c) 0.04 mg/kg IV, 0.07 mg/kg IM, or 0.25 mg/kg into the conjunctival sac. (Jenkins 1988)
 Cats:
   For induction of emesis:
    a) 0.04 mg/kg IV or 0.08 mg/kg IM or SQ (Bailey 1989), (Reid & Oehme 1989)

Monitoring Parameters -
 1) CNS, respiratory, and cardiac systems should monitored
 2) Vomitus should be quantitated, examined for contents and saved for possible later analysis

Client Information - This agent must be used in a professionally supervised setting only.

Dosage Forms/Preparations/FDA Approval Status/Withholding Times -
 Veterinary-Approved Products: None, but the product may be available from "compounding" pharmacies
 Human-Approved Products: An orphan product is available

APRAMYCIN SULFATE

Chemistry - An aminocyclitol antibiotic produced from *Streptomyces tenebrarius*, apramycin is water soluble.

Storage/Stability/Compatibility - Apramycin powder should be stored in a cool dry place, in tightly closed containers; protect from moisture. If exposed to rust, as in a rusty waterer, the drug can be inactivated. The manufacturer recommends preparing fresh water daily.

Pharmacology - Apramycin is bactericidal against many gram negative bacteria (*E. coli, Pseudomonas, Salmonella, Klebsiella, Proteus, Pasturella, Treponema hyodysenteriae, Bordetella bronchiseptica*), Staphylococcus and Mycoplasma. Its mechanism of action is by preventing protein synthesis by susceptible bacteria, presumably by binding to the 30S ribosomal subunit.

Uses/Indications - Apramycin is approved for the treatment of porcine colibacillosis secondary to *E. coli* sensitive to the drug. Although not approved, it has also been used for the same indication in calves. The injectable form of the drug, which is not available in the United States, has also been used to treat gram negative infections in various species.

Pharmacokinetics - After oral administration, apramycin is partially absorbed, particularly in neonates. Absorption is dose related and decreases substantially with the age of the animal. Absorbed drug is eliminated via the kidneys unchanged.

Contraindications/Precautions/Reproductive Safety - When used as labeled, the manufacturer does not list any contraindications. The drug apparently has a wide margin of safety when used orally and is safe to use in breeding swine.

Adverse Effects/Warnings - When used as labeled, the manufacturer does not list any adverse reactions. Should substantial amounts of the drug be absorbed, both ototoxicity and nephrotoxicity are a distinct possibility.

Drug Interactions, Drug/Laboratory Interactions - None listed. May have similar interaction potential as neomycin; refer to that monograph for more information.

Doses -
  Swine:
    For bacterial enteritis caused by susceptible organisms:
      a) Treated pigs should consume enough water to receive 12.5 mg/kg body weight per day for 7 days. Add to drinking water at a rate of 375 mg per gallon. After adding to water, stir and allow to stand for 15 minutes, then stir again. (Label directions; *Apralan*® *Soluble Powder*—SKB)
      b) 20 - 40 mg/kg PO daily in drinking water. (Huber 1988a)

  Cattle:
    For bacterial enteritis caused by susceptible organisms:
      a) 20 - 40 mg/kg PO daily in drinking water. (Huber 1988a)

Monitoring Parameters -
  1) Clinical efficacy

Dosage Forms/Preparations/FDA Approval Status/Withholding Times -
  Veterinary-Approved Products:

  Apramycin Sulfate Soluble Powder 37.5 g (base) bottle; *Apralan*® (Elanco); (OTC) Approved for use in swine. Withdrawal time = 28 days.

  Apramycin Sulfate Type A medicated feed articles containing 75 g/lb.; *Apralan*® *75* (Elanco); (OTC) Approved for use in swine. Withdrawal time = 28 days.

An injectable product is available in some European countries.

  Human-Approved Products: None

ASA - see Aspirin

ASCORBIC ACID
VITAMIN C

Chemistry - A water soluble vitamin, ascorbic acid occurs as white to slightly yellow crystal or powder. It is freely soluble in water and sparingly soluble in alcohol. The parenteral solution has a pH of 5.5-7.

Storage/Stability/Compatibility - Protect from air and light. Ascorbic acid will slowly darken upon light exposure. Slight discoloration does not affect potency. Because with time ascorbic acid will decompose with the production of CO_2, open ampules and multidose vials carefully. To reduce the potential for excessive pressure within ampules, store in refrigerator and open while still cold.

Ascorbic acid for injection is **compatible** with most commonly used IV solutions, but is **incompatible** with many drugs when mixed in syringes or IV bags. Compatibility is dependent upon factors such as pH, concentration, temperature and diluents used. It is suggested to consult specialized references (*e.g., Handbook on Injectable Drugs* by Trissel; see bibliography) for more specific information.

Pharmacology - Exogenously supplied ascorbic acid is a dietary requirement in some exotic species (including rainbow trout, Coho salmon), guinea pigs, and in primates. The other domestic species are able to synthesize *in vivo* enough Vitamin C to meet their nutritional needs. Vitamin C is used for tissue repair and collagen formation. It may also be involved with some oxidation-reduction reactions, and is involved with the metabolism of many substances (iron, folic acid, norepinephrine, histamine, phenylalanine, tyrosine, some drug enzyme systems). Vitamin C is believed to play a role in protein, lipid and carnitine synthesis, maintaining blood vessel integrity, and immune function.

Uses/Indications - Ascorbic acid may be used as a urinary acidifier, but its efficacy is in question. Sodium ascorbate does not acidify the urine. It is also used to treat copper-induced hepatopathy in dogs.

Pharmacokinetics - Vitamin C is generally well absorbed in the jejunum (human data) after oral administration, but absorption may be reduced with high doses as an active process is involved with absorption. Ascorbic acid is widely distributed and only about 25% is bound to plasma proteins. Vitamin C is biotransformed in the liver. When the body is saturated with vitamin C and the blood concentrations exceed the renal threshold the drug is more readily excreted unchanged into the urine.

Contraindications/Precautions/Reproductive Safety - Vitamin C (high doses) should be used with caution in patients with diabetes mellitus due to the laboratory interactions (see below) or in patients susceptible to urolithiasis. The reproductive safety of vitamin C has not been studied, but it is generally considered to be safe at moderate dosages.

Adverse Effects/Warnings - At usual doses vitamin C has minimal adverse effects. Occasionally GI disturbances have been noted in humans. At higher dosages, there is an increased potential for urate, oxalate or cystine stone formation, particularly in susceptible patients.

Overdosage/Acute Toxicity - Very large doses may result in diarrhea and potentially urolithiasis. Generally, treatment should consist of monitoring and keeping the patient well hydrated.

Drug Interactions - Large doses causing acidification of urine may increase the renal excretion of some drugs (*e.g.*, **mexiletine, quinidine**) and reduce the efficacy of some antimicrobials in the urine (*e.g.*, **aminoglycosides, erythromycin**). Vitamin C may be synergistic with **deferoxamine** in removing iron, but may in fact, lead to increased iron tissue toxicity especially in cardiac muscle. It should be used with caution, particularly in patients with preexisting cardiac disease.

Laboratory Considerations - Large doses may cause false-negative **urine glucose** values. False-negative results may occur if vitamin C is administered within 48-72 hours of an amine-dependent **stool occult blood** test. Vitamin C may decrease **serum bilirubin** concentrations.

Doses -
  Dogs:
      To decrease intestinal copper absorption: 500 - 1000 mg per day given with meals. Note: efficacy not proven. (Johnson and Sherding 1994)
  Cats:
      For adjunctive treatment of FIP: 125 mg PO q12h (Weiss 1994)
  Guinea Pigs:
      For treatment of scurvy during pregnancy: 30 mg/kg either parenterally or PO (in feed or water) (Fish and Besch-Williford 1992)
      For prevention of scurvy: Add 200 mg vitamin C to one liter of dechlorinated water and add to water bottle. For treatment of scurvy: 20 - 200 mg/kg IM or SubQ (Anderson 1994)
  Horses:
      For replacement therapy after stress (*e.g.* strenuous exercise): 20 grams PO daily (Ferrante and Kronfeld 1992)
  Cattle:
      For vitamin C-responsive dermatitis in calves: 3 grams SubQ once or twice. (Miller 1993)

Dosage Forms/Preparations/FDA Approval Status/Withholding Times -
Veterinary-Approved Products:
Parenteral Injection 250 mg/ml in 100 and 250 ml vials; Generic (Rx or OTC depending on labeling)

Human-Approved Products:
As ascorbic acid or sodium ascorbate: Oral tablets 25 mg, 50 mg, 100 mg, 250 mg, 500 mg, 1000 mg; chewable tablets: 60 mg, 100 mg, 250 mg, 500 mg,; (various); (OTC)

Oral extended release capsules and tablets 500 mg; 1000 mg, 1500 mg; (various); (OTC)

Crystals/Powder: 4 g/tsp (in 100 & 500g); 5 g/tsp (in 180 g); (OTC)

Liquid/Syrup: 35 mg/0.6ml, 100 mg/ml, (OTC)

Parenteral Injection 250 mg/ml in 2 ml ampules and 30 & 50 ml multidose vials; various & generic; (Rx)

ASPARAGINASE

Chemistry - Asparaginase is an enzyme derived from *E. coli* and occurs as a white or almost white, slightly hygroscopic powder that is soluble in water. The commercially available product is a lyophilized powder that also contains mannitol which after reconstituting has a pH of about 7.4. Activity of asparaginase is expressed in terms of International Units ((I.U.). Asparaginase may also be known by the following monikers: L-asparaginase, L-asparagine amidohydrolase, Coloaspase, A-ase, or ASN-ase.

Storage/Stability/Compatibility - Asparaginase powder for injection should be stored at temperatures less than 8°C, but it is stable for at least 48 hours at room temperature. After reconstituting, the manufacturer states that the drug is stable when refrigerated for up to 8 hours, but other sources state that it is stable for up to 14 days.

Solutions should be used only if clear; turbid solutions should be discarded. Upon standing, gelatinous fibers may be noted in the solution occasionally. These may be removed without loss of potency with a 5 micron filter. Some loss of potency may occur if a 0.2 micron filter is used.

The solution may be shaken while reconstituting, but vigorous shaking should be avoided as the solution may become foamy and difficult to withdraw from the vial, and some loss of potency can also occur. Recommended intravenous diluents for asparaginase include D5W and sodium chloride 0.9%.

Pharmacology - Some malignant cells are unable to synthesize asparagine and are dependent on exogenous asparagine for DNA and protein synthesis. Asparaginase catalyzes asparagine into ammonia and aspartic acid. The antineoplastic activity of asparaginase is greatest during the postmitotic (G_1) cell phase. While normal cells are able to synthesize asparagine intracellularly, some normal cells having a high rate of protein synthesis require some exogenous asparagine and may be adversely affected by asparaginase.

Resistance to asparaginase can develop rapidly, but apparently there is no cross-resistance between asparaginase and other antineoplastic agents.

Asparaginase possesses antiviral activity, but its toxicity prevents it from being clinically useful in this regard.

Uses/Indications - Asparaginase has been useful in combination with other agents in the treatment of lymphosarcoma in dogs. The drug is most useful in inducing remission of disease, but is occasionally used in some maintenance protocols.

Pharmacokinetics - Asparaginase is not absorbed from the GI tract and must be given either IV or IM. After IM injection, serum levels of asparaginase are approximately 1/2 of those after IV injection. Because of its high molecular weight, asparaginase does not diffuse readily out of the capillaries and about 80% of the drug remains within the intravascular space.

In humans after IV dosing, serum levels of asparagine fall almost immediately to zero and remain that way as long as therapy continues. Once therapy is halted, serum levels of asparagine do not recover for at least 23 days.

The metabolic fate of asparaginase is not known. In humans, the plasma half-life is highly variable and ranges from 8-30 hours.

Contraindications/Precautions/Reproductive Safety - Asparaginase is contraindicated in patients who have exhibited anaphylaxis to it, or in patients with pancreatitis or a history of pancreatitis. Asparaginase should be used with caution in patients with preexisting hepatic, renal, hematologic, gastrointestinal, or CNS dysfunction.

No special precautions are required for handling asparaginase, but any inadvertent skin contact should be washed off as the drug can be a contact irritant.

Adverse Effects/Warnings - Asparaginase adverse reactions are classified in two main categories, hypersensitivity reactions and its effects on protein synthesis. Hypersensitivity reactions can occur with symptoms of vomiting, diarrhea, urticaria, pruritis, dyspnea, restlessness, hypotension and collapse. The likelihood of hypersensitivity reactions occurring increases with subsequent doses and intravenous administration. Some clinicians recommend giving a test dose before the full dose to test for local hypersensitivity and/or administering antihistamines (*e.g.,* diphenhydramine) prior to dosing. If a hypersensitivity reaction occurs, diphenhydramine (0.2 - 0.5 mg/kg slow IV), dexamethasone sodium phosphate (1 - 2 mg/kg IV), intravenous fluids and, if severe, epinephrine (0.1 - 0.3 ml of a 1:1000 solution IV) have been suggested (O'Keefe and Harris 1990).

The other broad category of toxicity is associated with asparaginase's effects on protein synthesis. Hemorrhagic pancreatitis or other gastrointestinal disturbances, hepatotoxicity and coagulation defects may be noted. Large doses may be associated with hyperglycemia secondary to altered insulin synthesis. Bone marrow depression is an uncommon consequence of asparaginase therapy, but leukopenia has been reported.

Overdosage/Acute Toxicity - Little information was located regarding overdosages with this agent. It would be expected that toxicity secondary to the protein synthesis altering effects of the drug would be encountered. In dogs it has been reported that the maximally tolerated dose of asparaginase is 10,000 IU/kg and the lethal dose is 50,000 IU/kg.

It is recommended to treat supportively if an overdose occurs.

Drug Interactions - Asparaginase may reduce **methotrexate** effectiveness against tumor cells until serum asparagine levels return to normal.

In humans, increased toxicity may occur when asparaginase (IV) is given concurrently with or before **prednisone and vincristine**.

Drug/Laboratory Interactions - **Serum ammonia and urea nitrogen** levels may be increased by the action of the drug.

Asparaginase may cause rapid (within 2 days) and profound decreases in circulating **thyroxine-binding globulin**, which may alter interpretation of thyroid function studies. Values may return to normal after approximately 4 weeks.

Doses - For more information, refer to the protocol references found in the appendix or other protocols found in other references, including: *Current Veterinary Therapy X: Small Animal Practice* (Matus 1989) and *Handbook of Small Animal Practice* (Cotter 1988).

Dogs:
For neoplastic diseases (usually used in combination protocols with other drugs; rarely used alone):
a)   20,000 IU/m^2 IM or IP weekly. (MacEwen and Rosenthal 1989)
b)   400 IU/kg IV, IP, or IM weekly. (Macy 1986)
c)   Large dogs: 30,000 IU/m^2 IV, or intraperitoneally once weekly.
      Small dogs: 10,000 IU/m^2 IV, or intraperitoneally once weekly. (Coppoc 1988)

Cats:
For neoplastic diseases (usually used in combination protocols with other drugs; rarely used alone):
a)   10,000 IU/m^2 SQ, intraperitoneally, or IM every 1-3 weeks. (Couto 1989b)
b)   10,000 IU/m^2 IV, or intraperitoneally once weekly. (Coppoc 1988)

Monitoring Parameters - Animals should have hepatic, renal, pancreatic (blood glucose, amylase), hematopoietic, function determined prior to initiating therapy and regularly monitored during therapy.

Client Information - Clients must be briefed on the possibilities of severe toxicity developing from this drug, including drug-related mortality. Clients should contact the veterinarian if the patient exhibita any symptoms of profound depression, severe diarrhea, abnormal bleeding (including bloody diarrhea) and/or bruising.

Dosage Forms/Preparations/FDA Approval Status/Withholding Times -
Veterinary-Approved Products: None
Human-Approved Products:
Asparaginase 10,000 IU Powder for Injection in 10 ml vials (with 80 mg mannitol); Reconstitute vial with 5 ml Sodium Chloride Injection or Sterile Water for Injection for IV use. For IM use, add 2 ml Sodium Chloride Injection. See Storage/Stability section above for more information.
Elspar® (Merck); (Rx)

ASPIRIN

Chemistry - Aspirin, sometimes known as acetylsalicylic acid or ASA, is the salicylate ester of acetic acid. The compound occurs as a white, crystalline powder or tabular or needle-like crystals. It is a weak acid with a pK_a of 3.5. Aspirin is slightly soluble in water and is freely soluble in alcohol. Each gram of aspirin contains approximately 760 mg of salicylate.

Storage/Stability/Compatibility - Aspirin tablets should be stored in tight, moisture resistant containers. Do not use products past the expiration date or if a strong vinegar-like odor is noted emitting from the bottle.

Aspirin is stable in dry air, but readily hydrolyzes to acetate and salicylate when exposed to water or moist air. It will then exude a strong vinegar-like odor. The addition of heat will speed the rate of hydrolysis. In aqueous solutions, aspirin is most stable at pH's of 2-3 and least stable at pH's below 2 or greater than 8. Should an aqueous solution be desirable as a dosage form, the commercial product *Alka-Seltzer*® will remain stable for 10 hours at room temperature in solution.

Pharmacology - Aspirin inhibits cyclooxygenase (prostaglandin synthetase) thereby reducing the synthesis of prostaglandins and thromboxanes. These effects are thought to be how aspirin produces analgesia, antipyrexia, and reduces platelet aggregation and inflammation. Most cells can synthesize new cyclooxygenase, but platelets cannot. Therefore, aspirin causes an irreversible effect on platelet aggregation. Aspirin has been shown to decrease the clinical symptoms of experimentally induced anaphylaxis in calves and ponies.

Pharmacokinetics - Aspirin is rapidly absorbed from the stomach and proximal small intestine in monogastric animals. The rate of absorption is dependent upon factors as stomach content, gastric emptying times, tablet disintegration rates and gastric pH. Absorption is slow from the GI tract in cattle, but approximately 70% of an oral dose will be absorbed.

During absorption, aspirin is partially hydrolyzed to salicylic acid where it is distributed widely throughout the body. Highest levels may be found in the liver, heart, lungs, renal cortex, and plasma. The amount of plasma protein binding is variable, depending on species, serum salicylate and albumin concentrations. At lower salicylate concentrations, it is 90% protein bound, but only 70% protein bound at higher concentrations. Salicylate is excreted into milk, but levels appear to be very low. Salicylate will cross the placenta, and fetal levels may actually exceed those found in the mother.

Salicylate is metabolized in the liver primarily by conjugation with glycine and glucuronic acid via glucuronyl transferase. Because cats are deficient in this enzymatic pathway, they have prolonged half-lives and are susceptible to accumulating the drug. Minor metabolites formed include gentisic acid and 2,3-dihydroxybenzoic acid, and 2,3,5-trihydroxybenzoic acid. Gentisic acid appears to be the only active metabolite, but because of its small concentrations, it appears to play an insignificant role therapeutically. The rate of metabolism is determined by both first order kinetics and dose-dependent kinetics depending on which metabolic pathway is looked at. Generally, steady-state serum levels will increase to levels higher (proportionally) than expected with dosage increases. These effects have not been well studied in domestic animals, however.

Salicylate and its metabolites are rapidly excreted by the kidneys by both filtration and renal tubular secretion. Significant tubular reabsorption occurs which is highly pH dependent. Salicylate excretion can be significantly increased by raising urine pH to 5-8. Salicylate and metabolites may be removed using peritoneal dialysis or more rapidly using hemodialysis.

Uses/Indications - Aspirin is used in all species for its analgesic and antipyretic effects. It is the one nonsteroidal anti-inflammatory agent that is relatively safe to use in both dogs and cats. Besides its analgesic, anti-inflammatory and antipyretic effects, aspirin is used therapeutically for its effects on platelet aggregation in the treatment of DIC and pulmonary artery disease secondary to heartworm infestation in dogs. It is also used in cats with cardiomyopathy.

Contraindications/Precautions - Aspirin is contraindicated in patients demonstrating previous hypersensitivity reactions to it. It is also contraindicated in patients with bleeding ulcers. It is relatively contraindicated in patients with hemorrhagic disorders, asthma, or renal insufficiency.

Because aspirin is highly protein bound to plasma albumin, patients with hypoalbuminemia may require lower dosages to prevent symptoms of toxicity. Aspirin should be used cautiously, with enhanced monitoring, in patients with severe hepatic failure or diminished renal function. Because of its effects on platelets, aspirin therapy should be halted, if possible, one week prior to surgical procedures. Aspirin has been shown to delay parturition and therefore should be avoided during the last stages of pregnancy.

Aspirin must be used cautiously in cats because of their inability to rapidly metabolize and excrete salicylates. Symptoms of toxicity may occur if dosed recklessly or without stringent monitoring. Aspirin should be used cautiously in neonatal animals; adult doses may lead to toxicity.

Adverse Effects/Warnings - The most common adverse effect of aspirin at therapeutic doses is gastric or intestinal irritation with varying degrees of occult GI blood loss occurring. The resultant irritation may result in vomiting and/or anorexia. Severe blood loss may result in a secondary anemia or hypoproteinemia. In dogs, plain uncoated aspirin may be more irritating to the gastric mucosa   n either buffered aspirin or enteric coated tablets. Hypersensitivity reactions have been reported in dogs, although they are thought to occur rarely.

Salicylates are possible teratogens and their use should be avoided during pregnancy, particularly during the later stages.

Overdosage - Symptoms of acute overdosage in dogs and cats include: depression, vomiting (may be blood tinged), anorexia, hyperthermia, and increased respiratory rate. Initially, a respiratory alkalosis occurs with a compensatory hyperventilation response. A profound metabolic acidosis follows. If treatment is not provided, muscular weakness, pulmonary and cerebral edema, hypernatremia, hypokalemia, ataxia and seizures, may all develop with eventual coma and death.

Treatment of acute overdosage initially consists of emptying the gut if ingestion has occurred within 12 hours, giving activated charcoal and an oral cathartic, placing an intravenous line, beginning fluids and drawing appropriate lab work (*e.g.,* blood gases). Some clinicians suggest performing gastric lavage with a 3-5% solution of sodium bicarbonate to delay the absorption of aspirin. A reasonable choice for an intravenous solution to correct dehydration would be dextrose 5% in water. Acidosis treatment and forced alkaline diuresis with sodium bicarbonate should be performed for serious ingestions. Diuresis may be enhanced by the administration of mannitol (1-2 gm/kg/hr). Seizures may be controlled with IV diazepam. Treatment of hypoprothrombinemia may be attempted by using phytonadione (2.5 mg/kg divided q8-12h) and ascorbic acid (25 mg parenterally), but ascorbic acid may negate some of the urinary alkalinization effects of bicarbonate. Peritoneal dialysis or exchange transfusions may be attempted in very severe ingestions when heroic measures are desired.

Drug Interactions - Drugs that alkalinize the urine (*e.g.,* **acetazolamide, sodium bicarbonate**) significantly increase the renal excretion of salicylates. Because carbonic anhydrase inhibitors (*e.g.,* acetazolamide, dichlorphenamide) may cause systemic acidosis and increase CNS levels of salicylates, toxicity may occur.

Urinary acidifying drugs (**methionine, ammonium chloride, ascorbic acid**) will decrease the urinary excretion of salicylates.

Furosemide may compete with the renal excretion of aspirin and delay its excretion. This may cause symptoms of toxicity in animals receiving high aspirin doses.

Phenobarbital may increase the rate of metabolism of aspirin by inducing hepatic enzymes.

Corticosteroids may increase the clearance of salicylates and decrease serum levels.

Increased chances of developing GI ulceration exist if administering aspirin with **corticosteroids** or **phenylbutazone or other non-steroidal agents** concurrently. Aspirin may increase the risks of bleeding associated with **heparin** or **oral anticoagulant** therapy.

At usual doses, aspirin may antagonize the uricosuric effects of **probenicid** or **sulfinpyrazone**.

Aspirin may inhibit the diuretic activity of **spironolactone**.

Aspirin may displace highly protein bound drugs from plasma proteins thus increasing free drug levels and pharmacologic effect. The following drugs may be affected by this mechanism (clinical significance is unknown, but increased monitoring should be performed if adding aspirin): **methotrexate, valproic acid, phenytoin, oral anticoagulants, penicillins**, and **sulfonamides**.

The antacids in buffered aspirin may chelate **tetracycline** products if given simultaneously, space doses apart by at least one hour.

In dogs, aspirin has been demonstrated to increase the plasma levels of **digoxin** by decreasing the clearance of the drug.

Some clinicians feel that aspirin should not be given concomitantly with **aminoglycoside antibiotics** because of an increased likelihood of nephrotoxicity developing. The actual clinical significance of this interaction is not entirely clear, and the risk versus benefits should be weighed when contemplating therapy.

Laboratory Test Interference - At high doses, aspirin may cause false-positive results for **urinary glucose** if using the cupric sulfate method (*Clinitest*® , Benedict's solution) and false-negative results if using the glucose oxidase method (*Clinistix*® or *Tes-Tape*®).

Urinary ketones measured by the ferric chloride method (Gerhardt) may be affected if salicylates are in the urine (reddish-color produced). **5-HIAA** determinations by the fluorometric method may be interfered by salicylates in the urine. Falsely elevated **VMA** (vanillylmandelic acid) may be seen with most methods used if salicylates are in the urine. Falsely lowered **VMA** levels may be seen if using the Pisano method.

Urinary excretion of **xylose** may be decreased if aspirin is given concurrently. Falsely elevated **serum uric acid** values may be measured if using colorimetric methods.

Doses -
Dogs:
For analgesia:
a) 10 - 25 mg/kg PO *bid-tid* (Morgan 1988)

    b) 10 - 20 mg/kg PO q12h (Jenkins 1987), (Holland and Chastain 1995)

    c) 11 mg/kg PO *bid* (Chastain 1987)

    d) 11 - 26 mg/kg PO q12h (Kelly 1995)

As an antiinflammatory/antirheumatic:
    a) 25 - 35 mg/kg PO q8h (Chastain 1987)
    b) 25 mg/kg PO q8h (Holland and Chastain 1995)
    c) Higher doses of up to 50 mg/kg q8-12h have been suggested for antirheumatic indications (Handagama 1986)

For antipyrexia:
    a) 10 mg/kg PO *bid* (Morgan 1988); (Holland and Chastain 1995)
    b) 11 mg/kg PO *bid* (Chastain 1987)

Post-Adulticide therapy for heartworm disease:
    a) 5 - 10 mg/kg PO once a day (Morgan 1988)
    b) 7 - 10 mg/kg PO once a day (Calvert 1987)

To decrease platelet aggregation/antithrombotic:
    a) 0.5 mg/kg PO *bid* (Rackear et al. 1988); (Holland and Chastain 1995)

For Disseminated Intravascular Coagulation (DIC):
    a) 150 - 300 mg/20kg animal PO once a day to once every other day for 10 days (Morgan 1988)

As an analgesic/antiinflammatory prior to elective intraocular surgery:
    a) 6.5 mg/kg *bid-tid* (Wyman 1986)

Cats:
For analgesia:
    a) 10 mg/kg PO every other day (Jenkins 1987); (Holland and Chastain 1995)
    b) 10 mg/kg PO daily (Handagama 1986) ; (Davis 1985a)
    c) 11 - 22 mg/kg PO q48h (every other day) (Kelly 1995)

For the treatment of arthritis/antirheumatic/antiinflammatory:
    a) one 81 mg tablet ("baby" aspirin) PO in an average sized cat, on Monday, Wednesday, and Friday of each week. (Davis 1985a)
    b) 25 mg/kg PO once daily (Chastain 1987); (Holland and Chastain 1995)

For antipyrexia:
    a) 10 mg/kg PO q48h (every other day) (Holland and Chastain 1995)

For adjunctive treatment of hypertropic feline cardiomyopathy or intermediate (restrictive) feline cardiomyopathy (as an anti-thrombogenic agent):
    a) 162 mg (two 81 mg "baby" aspirin or one-half 5 grain tablet) PO twice weekly (Harpster 1986)
    b) 11 mg/kg PO every other day (q48h) (Chastain 1987)
    c) As an anti-thrombotic: 25 mg/kg PO q56-84h (Holland and Chastain 1995)

As an analgesic/antiinflammatory prior to elective intraocular surgery:
    a) 6.5 mg/kg *bid-tid* (Wyman 1986)

Cattle:
For analgesia/antipyrexia:
    a) 50 - 100 mg/kg PO q12h (Jenkins 1987)
    b) 100 mg/kg PO q12h (Koritz 1986)
    c) Mature Cattle: two to four 240 grain boluses PO; Calves: one to two 240 grain boluses, allow animals to drink water after administration. (Label directions - Vedco Brand)

Horses:
For analgesia:
    a) Mature Horses: two to four 240 grain boluses PO;
    Foals: one to two 240 grain boluses, allow animals to drink water after administration. (Label directions - Vedco Brand)
    b) 25 mg/kg PO q12h initially, then 10 mg/kg once daily (Jenkins 1987)
    c) 15 - 100 mg/kg PO once daily (Robinson 1987)

Swine:
For analgesia:
    a) 10 mg/kg q4h PO (Jenkins 1987), (Koritz 1986)
    b) 10 mg/kg q6h PO (Davis 1979)

Avian:
    a) 5 grams in 250 ml of water as sole water source (Clubb 1986)

Note: Because of the significant hydrolysis that will occur, this solution should be freshly prepared every 12 hours if stored at room temperature or every 4 days if kept refrigerated at 5° C.

Monitoring Parameters -
1) Analgesic effect &/or antipyrexic effect
2) Bleeding times if indicated
3) PCV & stool guiaic tests if indicated

Client Information - Contact veterinarian if symptoms of GI bleeding or distress occur (black, tarry feces; anorexia or vomiting, etc).

Because aspirin is a very old drug, formal approvals from the FDA for its use in animals have not been required (so-called "grandfather" drug). There is no listed meat or milk withdrawal times listed for food-producing animals, but because there are salicylate-sensitive people, in the interest of public health this author suggests a minimum of 1 day withdrawal time for either milk or meat.

Dosage Forms/Preparations - Note: Many dosage forms and brand names are commercially available; the following is an abbreviated list of some products that have been used for veterinary indications:

Aspirin, Tablets, Children's; 65 mg (1 grain) and 81 mg (1.25 grains) in bottles of 36, 100, & 1000 tabs (Note: some varieties are chewable; orange flavor)

Aspirin, Tablets; plain uncoated;325 mg (5 grain), or 500 mg (7.8 grain) in bottles of 12 - 1000 tablets

Aspirin, Tablets; buffered uncoated; 325 mg (5 grain), or 500 mg (7.8 grain) with aluminum &/or magnesium salts in bottles of 12 - 1000 tablets

Aspirin Tablets (veterinary) 60 grain (3.89 grams) in 100's

Aspirin Boluses (veterinary) 240 grain (15.55 gram) in boxes/bottles of 50

Rectal suppositories, and enteric coated or sustained-release oral dosage forms are also available commercially for human use. A combination veterinary product, *Cortaba*® (Upjohn), containing 300 mg of aspirin and 0.5 mg methylprednisolone per tablet is also available commercially.

ATENOLOL

Chemistry - A beta$_1$ adrenergic blocking agent, atenolol occurs as a white, crystalline powder. At 37°C, 26.5 mg are soluble in 1 ml of water. The pH of the commercially available injection is adjusted to 5.5-6.5.

Storage/Stability/Compatibility - Tablets should be stored at room temperature and protected from heat, light and moisture. The injection solution should be stored at room temperature and protected from light.

Atenolol injection is reported to be physically compatible with morphine sulfate injection and meperidine HCl for at least 4 hours. Dextrose injections, sodium chloride injections and combinations of the two are recommended to be used as diluents when given parenterally.

Pharmacology - Atenolol is a relatively specific beta 1 blocker. At higher dosages this specificity may be lost and beta 2 blockade can occur. Atenolol does not possess any intrinsic sympathomimetic activity like pindolol nor does it possess membrane stabilizing activity like pindolol or propranolol. Cardiovascular effects secondary to atenolol's negative inotropic and chronotropic actions include: decreased sinus heart rate, slowed AV conduction, diminished cardiac output at rest and during exercise, decreased myocardial oxygen demand, reduced blood pressure, and inhibition of isoproterenol-induced tachycardia.

Uses/Indications - Because atenolol is relatively safe to use in animals with bronchospastic disease, it is often chosen over propranolol. It may be effective in supraventricular tachyarrhythmias, premature ventricular contractions (PVC's, VPC's), systemic hypertension and in treating cats with hypertrophic cardiomyopathy.

Pharmacokinetics - Only about 50-60% of an oral dose is absorbed in humans, but it is rapidly absorbed. The drug has very low protein binding characteristics (5-15%) and is distributed well into most tissues. Atenolol has low lipid solubility and unlike propranolol, only small amounts of atenolol are distributed into the CNS. Atenolol crosses the placenta and levels in milk are higher than those found in plasma. Atenolol is minimally biotransformed in the liver; 40-50% is excreted unchanged in the urine and the bulk of the remainder is excreted in the feces unchanged (unabsorbed drug). Reported half life in dogs is 3.2 hours; 6-7 hours in humans.

Contraindications/Precautions/Reproductive Safety - Atenolol is contraindicated in patients with overt heart failure, hypersensitivity to this class of agents, greater than first degree heart block, or sinus bradycardia. Non-specific beta-blockers are generally contraindicated in patients with CHF unless secondary to a tachyarrhythmia responsive to beta-blocker therapy. They are also relatively contraindicated in patients with bronchospastic lung disease.

Atenolol should be used cautiously in patients with significant renal insufficiency. It should also be used cautiously in patients with sinus node dysfunction.

Atenolol (at high dosages) can mask the symptoms associated with hypoglycemia. It can also cause hypoglycemia or hyperglycemia and, therefore, should be used cautiously in labile diabetic patients.

Atenolol can mask the symptoms associated with thyrotoxicosis, but it may be used clinically to treat the symptoms associated with this condition.

Adverse Effects/Warnings - It is reported that adverse effects most commonly occur in geriatric animals or those that have acute decompensating heart disease. Adverse effects considered to be clinically relevant include: bradycardia, lethargy and depression, impaired AV conduction, CHF or worsening of heart failure, hypotension, hypoglycemia, and bronchoconstriction (less so with beta 1 specific drugs like atenolol). Syncope and diarrhea have also been reported in canine patients with beta blockers.

Exacerbation of symptoms have been reported following abrupt cessation of beta-blockers in humans. It is recommended to withdraw therapy gradually in patients who have been receiving the drug chronically.

Overdosage - There is limited information available on atenolol overdosage. Humans have apparently survived dosages of up to 5 grams. The most predominant symptoms expected would be extensions of the drug's pharmacologic effects: hypotension, bradycardia, bronchospasm, cardiac failure and hypoglycemia.

If overdose is secondary to a recent oral ingestion, emptying the gut and charcoal administration may be considered. Monitor ECG, blood glucose, potassium and, if possible, blood pressure. Treatment of the cardiovascular effects are symptomatic. Use fluids and pressor agents to treat hypotension. Bradycardia may be treated with atropine. If atropine fails, isoproterenol given cautiously has been recommended. Use of a transvenous pacemaker may be necessary. Cardiac failure can be treated with a digitalis glycosides, diuretics and oxygen. Glucagon (5-10 mg IV - Human dose) may increase heart rate and blood pressure and reduce the cardiodepressant effects of atenolol.

Drug Interactions - Sympathomimetics (metaproterenol, terbutaline, beta effects of epinephrine, phenylpropanolamine, etc.) may have their actions blocked by atenolol and they may, in turn, reduce the efficacy of atenolol. Additive myocardial depression may occur with the concurrent use of atenolol and myocardial depressant **anesthetic agents**. **Phenothiazines** given with atenolol may exhibit enhanced hypotensive effects. **Furosemide and hydralazine** or other hypotensive producing drugs may increase the hypotensive effects of atenolol. Atenolol may prolong the hypoglycemic effects of **insulin** therapy. Concurrent use of beta blockers with **calcium channel blockers** (or other negative inotropics) should be done with caution, particularly in patients with preexisting cardiomyopathy or CHF.

Doses -
Dogs:
    For indications where beta blockade may be indicated (cardiac arrhythmias, obstructive heart disease, hypertension, myocardial infarction, etc.):
        a) 12.5 - 50 mg once or twice daily. Start at a low dose and titrate upwards as necessary. (Ware 1992)
        b) 0.25 - 1 mg/kg PO q12-24h (Miller, Tilley et al. 1994)
        c) 6.25 - 25 mg (total dose) q12h (Muir and Bonagura 1994)
    For treatment of hypertension:
        a) 2 mg/kg once daily (Littman 1992)

Cats:
    For treatment of hypertension:
        a) 2 mg/kg once daily; hyperthyroid cats being started on methimazole are treated usually for 2 weeks with atenolol. It is important to closely monitor geriatric cats as renal disease may be a concurrent problem with hyperthyroidism or hypertension. (Littman 1992)

    For indications where beta blockade may be indicated (cardiac arrhythmias, obstructive heart disease, hypertension, myocardial infarction, etc.):
        a) 6.25 - 12.5 mg total dose PO once daily (q24h) (Miller, Tilley et al. 1994), (Muir and Bonagura 1994)

Monitoring Parameters -
        1) Cardiac function, pulse rate, ECG if necessary, BP if indicated; 2) Toxicity (see Adverse Effects/Overdosage)

Client Information - To be effective, the animal must receive all doses as prescribed. Notify veterinarian if animal becomes lethargic or becomes exercise intolerant, develops shortness of breath or cough, or develops a change in behavior or attitude. Do not stop therapy without first conferring with veterinarian.

Dosage Forms/Preparations/FDA Approval Status/Withholding Times -
  Veterinary-Approved Products: None
  Human-Approved Products:
    Atenolol Tablets 25, 50, & 100 mg; *Tenormin*® (ICI), Generic; (Rx)

    Atenolol Injection 5 mg/ml in 10 ml amps; *Tenormin*® (ICI); (Rx)

    Also available in an oral fixed dose combination product with chlorthalidone.

ATIPAMEZOLE HCL

Chemistry/Storage/Stability/Compatibility - An alpha2-adrenergic antagonist, atipamezole HCl injection should be stored at room temperature (15°-30°C) and protected from light.

Pharmacology - Atipamezole competitively inhibits alpha2-adrenergic receptors, thereby acting as a reversal agent for alpha2-adrenergic agonists (*e.g.*, medetomidine). Net pharmacologic effects are to reduce sedation, decrease blood pressure, increase heart and respiratory rates, and reduce the analgesic effects of alpha2-adrenergic agonists.

Uses/Indications - Atipamezole is labeled for use as a reversal agent for medetomidine. It potentially could be useful for reversal of other alpha2-adrenergic agonists as well (*e.g.*, amitraz, xylazine).

Pharmacokinetics - After IM administration in the dog, peak plasma levels occur in about 10 minutes. Atipamezole is apparently metabolized in the liver to compounds that are eliminated in the urine. The drug has an average plasma elimination half life of about 2-3 hours.

Contraindications/Precautions/Reproductive Safety - While the manufacturer lists no absolute contraindications to the use of atipamezole, it states that the drug is not recommended in pregnant or lactating animals due to lack of data establishing safety in these animals. Caution should be used in administration of anesthetic agents to elderly or debilitated animals.

Adverse Effects/Warnings - Potential adverse effects include occasional vomiting, diarrhea, hypersalivation, tremors, and brief excitation/apprehensiveness.
  Because reversal can occur rapidly, care should be exercised as animals emerging from sedation and analgesia may exhibit apprehensive or aggressive behaviors. After reversal, animals should be protected from falling. Additional analgesia (*e.g.,* butorphanol) should be considered, particularly after painful procedures.

Overdosage - Dogs receiving up to 10X the listed dosage apparently tolerated the drug without major effects. When overdosed, dose related effects seen included panting, excitement, trembling, vomiting, soft or liquid feces, vasodilatation of sclera and some muscle injury at the IM injection site. Specific overdose therapy should generally not be necessary.

Drug Interactions - The manufacturer states that information on the use of atipamezole with other drugs is lacking, therefore, caution should be taken when using with other drugs (other than medetomidine).

Doses -
  Dogs:
       For reversal of medetomidine:
          a) Give IM an equal volume of Antisedan® as Domitor® is administered (ml per ml). The actual concentration of Antisedan® will be 5X that of Domitor®, as Antisedan® is 5 mg/ml versus Domitor®'s 1 mg/ml. (Package Insert; Antisedan®—Pfizer)
          b) As above, but may give IV as well as IM. If it has been at least 45 minutes since medetomidine was given, may give atipamezole at half the volume of medetomidine if administered IV. If after 10-15 minutes an IM dose of atipamezole has not seemed to reverse the effects of medetomidine, an additional dose of atipamezole at 1/2 the volume of the medetomidine dose may be given. (McGrath and Ko 1997b)

       For treatment of amitraz toxicity:
          a) 50 mcg/kg IM (Hugnet, Buronrosse et al. 1996)

Monitoring Parameters - Level of sedation and analgesia; heart rate; body temperature

Client Information - Atipamezole should be administered by veterinary professionals only. Clients should be informed that occasionally vomiting, diarrhea, hypersalivation, excitation and tremors may be seen after atipamezole administration. Should these be severe or persist after leaving the clinic, clients should contact the veterinarian.

Dosage Forms/Preparations/FDA Approval Status -

Veterinary-Approved Products:

Atipamezole HCl for Injection 5 mg/ml in 10 ml multidose vials; *Antisedan®*; (Pfizer); (Rx) Approved for use in dogs.

Human-Approved Products: None

ATRACURIUM BESYLATE

Chemistry - A synthetic, non-depolarizing neuromuscular blocking agent, atracurium, is a bisquaternary, non-choline diester structurally similar to metocurine and tubocurarine. It occurs as white to pale yellow powder. 50 mg is soluble in 1 ml of water, 200 mg is soluble in 1 ml of alcohol, and 35 mg is soluble in 1 ml of normal saline.

The commercially available injection occurs as clear, colorless solution and is a sterile solution of the drug in sterile water for injection. The pH of this solution is 3.25 - 3.65. Atracurium besylate may also be known as: atracurium besilate.

Storage/Stability/Compatibility - Atracurium injection should be stored in the refrigerator and protected against freezing. At room temperature, approximately 5% potency loss occurs each month; when refrigerated, a 6% potency loss occurs over a years time.

Atracurium is compatible with the standard IV solutions, but while stable in lactated Ringer's for 8 hours, degradation occurs more rapidly. It should not be mixed in the same IV bag or syringe, or given through the same needle with alkaline drugs (*e.g.,* barbiturates) or solutions (sodium bicarbonate) as precipitation may occur.

Pharmacology - Atracurium is a nondepolarizing neuromuscular blocking agent and acts by competitively binding at cholinergic receptor sites at the motor end-plate, thereby inhibiting the effects of acetylcholine. Atracurium is considered to be 1/4 to 1/3 as potent as pancuronium. In horses, atracurium is more potent than in other species tested and more potent than other nondepolarizing muscle relaxants studied.

At usual doses, atracurium exhibits minimal cardiovascular effects, unlike most other nondepolarizing neuromuscular blockers. While atracurium can stimulate histamine release, it is considered to cause less histamine release than either tubocurarine or metocurine. In humans, less than one percent of patients receiving atracurium exhibit clinically significant adverse reactions or histamine release.

Uses/Indications - Atracurium is indicated as an adjunct to general anesthesia to produce muscle relaxation during surgical procedures or mechanical ventilation and also to facilitate endotracheal intubation. Atracurium can be used in patients with significant renal or hepatic disease.

Pharmacokinetics - After IV injection, maximal neuromuscular blockade generally occurs within 3-5 minutes. The duration of maximal blockade increases as the dosage increases. Systemic alkalosis may diminish the degree and duration of blockade; acidosis potentiates it. In conjunction with balanced anesthesia, the duration of blockade generally persists for 20-35 minutes. Recovery times do not change after maintenance doses are given, so predictable blocking effects can be attained when the drug is administered at regular intervals.

Atracurium is metabolized by ester hydrolysis and Hofmann elimination which occurs independently of renal or hepatic function.

Contraindications/Precautions - Atracurium is contraindicated in patients who are hypersensitive to it. Because it may rarely cause significant release of histamine it should be used with caution in patients where this would be hazardous (severe cardiovascular disease, asthma, etc.). Atracurium has minimal cardiac effects and will not counteract the bradycardia or vagal stimulation induced by other agents. Use of neuromuscular blocking agents must be done with extreme caution, or not at all, in patients suffering from myasthenia gravis. Atracurium has no analgesic or sedative/anesthetic actions.

Adverse Effects/Warnings - Clinically significant adverse effects are apparently quite rare in patients (<1% in humans) receiving recommended doses of atracurium and usually are secondary to histamine release. They can include: allergic reactions, inadequate or prolonged block, hypotension vasodilatation, bradycardia, tachycardia, dyspnea, broncho-, laryngo- spasm, rash, urticaria, and a reaction at the injection site. Patients developing hypotension usually have preexisting severe cardiovascular disease.

Overdosage - Overdosage possibilities can be minimized by monitoring muscle twitch response to peripheral nerve stimulation. Increased risks of hypotension and histamine release occur with overdoses, as well as prolonged duration of muscle blockade.

Besides treating conservatively (mechanical ventilation, O_2, fluids, etc.), reversal of blockade may be accomplished by administering an anticholinesterase agent (edrophomium, physostigmine, or neostigmine) with an anticholinergic (atropine or glycopyrrolate). Reversal is usually attempted (in humans) approximately 20-35 minutes after the initial dose, or 10-30 minutes after the last maintenance dose. Reversal is usually complete within 8-10 minutes.

Drug Interactions - The following agents may enhance the neuromuscular blocking activity of atracurium: **procainamide, quinidine, verapamil, aminoglycoside antibiotics (gentamicin**, etc), **lincomycin, clindamycin, bacitracin, polymyxin B, lithium, magnesium sulfate, thiazide diuretics, enflurane, isoflurane,** and **halothane**.

Loop diuretics (*e.g., furosemide*) have been reported to both decrease and increase the effects of nondepolarizing neuromuscular blockers.

Other muscle relaxant drugs may cause a synergistic or antagonistic effect. **Succinylcholine** may speed the onset of action and enhance the neuromuscular blocking actions of atracurium. Do not give atracurium until succinylcholine effects have diminished.

Theophylline or **phenytoin** may inhibit or reverse the neuromuscular blocking action of atracurium.

Doses -
Dogs:
    a) Induction dose: 0.22 mg/kg IV, give 1/10th to 1/6th of this dose initially as a "priming" dose, followed 4-6 minutes later with the remainder and a sedative/hypnotic agent.
    Intraoperative dose: 0.11 mg/kg IV (Mandsager 1988)
    b) After acepromazine and/or meperidine premedication, give 0.5 mg/kg IV initially. Induce anesthesia with thiopental or methohexital; after intratracheal intubation maintain anesthesia with nitrous oxide:oxygen (2:1) and halothane (0.5%), using controlled ventilation. Additional doses of atracurium may be administered at 0.2 mg/kg IV. (Jones 1985b)

Cats:
    a) Induction dose: 0.22 mg/kg IV, give 1/10th to 1/6th of this dose initially as a "priming" dose, followed 4-6 minutes later with the remainder and a sedative/hypnotic agent.
    Intraoperative dose: 0.11 mg/kg IV (Mandsager 1988)

Horses:
    a) Intraoperative dose: 0.055 mg/kg IV (Mandsager 1988)

Monitoring Parameters -
    1) Level of neuromuscular blockade; cardiac rate

Client Information - This drug should only be used by professionals familiar with its use.

Dosage Forms/Preparations/FDA Approval Status/Withholding Times -
Veterinary-Approved Products: None
Human-Approved Products:
    Atracurium Besylate Injection 10 mg/ml in 5 ml amps and 10 ml vials; *Tracrium*® (Glaxo Wellcome); (Rx)

ATROPINE SULFATE

Chemistry - The prototype tertiary amine antimuscarinic agent, atropine sulfate is derived from the naturally occurring atropine. It is a racemic mixture of *d*-hyoscyamine and *l*-hyoscyamine. The *l*- form of the drug is active, while the *d*- form has practically no antimuscarinic activity. Atropine sulfate occurs as colorless and odorless crystals, or white, crystalline powder. One gram of atropine sulfate is soluble in approximately 0.5 ml of water, 5 ml of alcohol, or 2.5 ml of glycerin. Aqueous solutions are practically neutral or only slightly acidic. Commercially available injections may have the pH adjusted to 3.0 - 6.5. Atropine may also be known as *dl*-hyoscyamine.

Storage/Stability/Compatibility - Atropine sulfate tablets or soluble tablets should be stored in well-closed containers at room temperature (15-30°C). Atropine sulfate for injection should be stored at room temperature; avoid freezing.

Atropine sulfate for injection is reportedly **compatible** with the following agents: benzquinamide HCl, butorphanol tartrate, chlorpromazine HCl, cimetidine HCl (not with pentobarbital), dimenhydrinate, diphenhydramine HCl, dobutamine HCl, droperidol, fentanyl citrate, glycopyrrolate, hydromorphone HCl, hydroxyzine HCl (also w/meperidine), meperidine HCl, morphine sulfate, nalbuphine HCl, pentazocine lactate, pentobarbital sodium (OK for 5 minutes, not 24 hours), perphenazine, prochlorperazine edisylate, promazine HCl, promethazine HCl (also w/meperidine), and scopolamine HBr. Atropine sulfate is reported physically **incompatible** with norepinephrine bitartrate, metaraminol bitartrate, methohexital sodium, and sodium bicarbonate. Compatibility is dependent upon factors such as pH, concentration, temperature, and diluents used and it is suggested to consult specialized references for more specific information.

Pharmacology - Atropine, like other antimuscarinic agents, competitively inhibits acetylcholine or other cholinergic stimulants at postganglionic parasympathetic neuroeffector sites. High doses may block nicotinic receptors at the autonomic ganglia and at the neuromuscular junction. Pharmacologic effects are dose related. At low doses salivation, bronchial secretions, and sweating (not horses) are inhibited. At moderate systemic doses, atropine dilates and inhibits accommodation of the pupil, and increases heart rate. High doses will decrease GI and urinary tract motility. Very high doses will inhibit gastric secretion.

Uses/Indications - The principal veterinary indications for systemic atropine include:
1) Preanesthetic to prevent or reduce secretions of the respiratory tract
2) Treat sinus bradycardia, sinoatrial arrest, incomplete AV block
3) As an antidote for overdoses of cholinergic agents (*e.g.,* physostigmine, etc.)
4) As an antidote for organophosphate or muscarinic mushroom intoxication
5) Hypersialism
6) Treatment of bronchoconstrictive disease

Pharmacokinetics - Atropine sulfate is well absorbed after oral administration, IM injection, inhalation, or endotracheal administration. After IV administration, peak effects in heart rates occur within 3-4 minutes.

Atropine is well distributed throughout the body and crosses into the CNS, across the placenta, and can distribute into the milk in small quantities.

Atropine is metabolized in the liver and excreted into the urine. Approximately 30-50% of a dose is excreted unchanged into the urine. The plasma half-life in humans has been reported to be between 2-3 hours.

Contraindications/Precautions - Atropine is contraindicated in patients with narrow-angle glaucoma, synchiae (adhesions) between the iris and lens, hypersensitivity to anticholinergic drugs, tachycardias secondary to thyrotoxicosis or cardiac insufficiency, myocardial ischemia, unstable cardiac status during acute hemorrhage, GI obstructive disease, paralytic ileus, severe ulcerative colitis, obstructive uropathy, and myasthenia gravis (unless used to reverse adverse muscarinic effects secondary to therapy).

Antimuscarinic agents should be used with extreme caution in patients with known or suspected GI infections. Atropine or other antimuscarinic agents can decrease GI motility and prolong retention of the causative agent(s) or toxin(s) resulting in prolonged symptoms. Antimuscarinic agents must also be used with extreme caution in patients with autonomic neuropathy.

Antimuscarinic agents should be used with caution in patients with hepatic or renal disease, geriatric or pediatric patients, hyperthyroidism, hypertension, CHF, tachyarrhythmias, prostatic hypertrophy, or esophogeal reflux. Systemic atropine should be used cautiously in horses as it may decrease gut motility and induce colic in susceptible animals. It may also reduce the arrhythmogenic doses of epinephrine. Use of atropine in cattle may result in inappetance and rumen stasis which may persist for several days.

Adverse Effects/Warnings - Adverse effects are basically extensions of the drug's pharmacologic effects and are generally dose related. At usual doses effects tend to mild in relatively healthy patients. The more severe effects listed tend to occur with high or toxic doses. GI effects can include dry mouth (xerostomia), dysphagia, constipation, vomiting, and thirst. GU effects may include urinary retention or hesitancy. CNS effects may include stimulation, drowsiness, ataxia, seizures, respiratory depression, etc. Ophthalmic effects include blurred vision, pupil dilation, cycloplegia, and photophobia. Cardiovascular effects include sinus tachycardia (at higher doses), bradycardia (initially or at very low doses), hypertension, hypotension, arrhythmias (ectopic complexes), and circulatory failure.

Overdosage - For signs and symptoms of atropine toxicity see adverse effects above. If a recent oral ingestion, emptying of gut contents and administration of activated charcoal and saline cathartics may be warranted. Treat symptoms supportively and symptomatically. Do not use phenothiazines as they may contribute to the anticholinergic effects. Fluid therapy and standard treatments for shock may be instituted.

The use of physostigmine is controversial and should probably be reserved for cases where the patient exhibits either extreme agitation and is at risk for injuring themselves or others, or for cases where supraventricular tachycardias and sinus tachycardias are severe or life-threatening. The usual dose for physostigmine (human) is: 2 mg IV slowly (for average sized adult) If no response, may repeat every 20 minutes until reversal of toxic antimuscarinic effects or cholinergic effects takes place. The human pediatric dose is 0.02 mg/kg slow IV (repeat q10 minutes as above) and may be a reasonable choice for initial treatment of small animals. Physostigmine adverse effects (bronchoconstriction, bradycardia, seizures) may be treated with small doses of IV atropine.

Drug Interactions - The following drugs may enhance the activity of atropine and its derivatives: **antihistamines, procainamide, quinidine, meperidine, benzodiazepines, phenothiazines**.

The following drugs may potentiate the adverse effects of atropine and its derivatives: **Primidone, disopyramide, nitrates, long-term corticosteroid use** (may increase intraocular pressure).

Atropine and its derivatives may enhance the actions of **nitrofurantoin, thiazide diuretics, sympathomimetics**.

Atropine and its derivatives may antagonize the actions of **metoclopramide**.

Doses -

Dogs:

As a preanesthetic adjuvant:
a) 0.022 - 0.044 mg/kg IM or SQ (Muir)
b) 0.074 mg/kg IV, IM or SQ (Package Insert; Atropine Injectable, S.A. - Fort Dodge)
c) 0.02 - 0.04 mg/kg SQ, IM or IV (Morgan 1988)

For adjunctive treatment of bradycardias, Incomplete AV block, etc:
a) 0.022 - 0.044 mg/kg IM, SQ, or IV *prn*; or 0.04 mg/kg PO *tid-qid* (Morgan 1988)
b) 0.02 - 0.04 mg/kg IV or IM (Russell and Rush 1995)

For treatment of cholinergic toxicity:
a) 0.2 - 2.0 mg/kg ; give 1/4th of the dose IV and the remainder SQ or IM (Morgan 1988)

For treatment of bronchoconstriction:
a) 0.02 - 0.04 mg/kg for a duration of effect of 1 - 1.5 hours (Papich 1986)

Cats:

As a preanesthetic adjuvant:
a) 0.022 - 0.044 mg/kg IM or SQ (Muir))
b) 0.074 mg/kg IV, IM or SQ (Package Insert; Atropine Injectable, S.A. - Fort Dodge)
c) 0.02 - 0.04 mg/kg SQ, IM or IV (Morgan 1988)

For treatment of bradycardias:
a) 0.022 - 0.044 mg/kg IM, SQ, or IV *prn*; or 0.04 mg/kg PO *tid-qid* (Morgan 1988)
b) 0.02 - 0.04 mg/kg SQ, IM or IV q4-6h (Miller 1985)

For treatment of cholinergic toxicity:
a) 0.2 - 2.0 mg/kg ; give 1/4th of the dose IV and the remainder SQ or IM (Morgan 1988)

Cattle:

As a preanesthetic:
a) Because of a lack of extended efficacy and potential adverse reactions, atropine is not used routinely as a preoperative agent in ruminants. If it is desired for use, a dose of 0.06 - 0.12 mg/kg IM has been suggested. (Thurmon and Benson 1986)

For adjunctive treatment of bovine hypersensitivity disease:
a) 1 gram per cow once daily followed by 0.5 gram/cow in 2 - 3 days (method of administration not specified) (Manning and Scheidt 1986)

For treatment of cholinergic toxicity (organophosphates):
a) 0.5 mg/kg (average dose); give 1/4th of the dose IV and the remainder SQ or IM; may repeat q3-4h for 1-2 days (Bailey 1986)

Horses:

For treatment of bradyarrhythmias due to increased parasympathetic tone:
a) 0.02 mg/kg IV (Muir and McGuirk 1987a)
b) 0.045 mg/kg parenterally (Hilwig 1987)

As a bronchodilator:
a) 5 mg IV for a 400-500 kg animal (Beech 1987)

For organophosphate poisoning:
a) Approximately 1 mg/kg given to effect IV (use mydriasis and absence of salivation as therapy endpoints), may repeat every 1.5 - 2 hours as required subcutaneously (Oehme 1987)
b) 0.22 mg/kg, 1/4th of the dose administered IV and the remainder SQ or IM (Package Insert; Atropine Injectable, L.A. - Fort Dodge)

Swine: The equine dose (above) may be used to initially treat organophosphate toxicity in swine.

As an adjunctive preanesthetic agent:
a) 0.04 mg/kg IM (Thurmon and Benson 1986)

Sheep, Goats:
  As a preanesthetic:
    a) Because of a lack of extended efficacy and potential adverse reactions, atropine is not used routinely as a preoperative agent in ruminants. If it is desired for use, a dose of 0.15 - 0.3 mg/kg IM has been suggested. (Thurmon and Benson 1986)
  For treating organophosphate toxicity: Use the dose for cattle (above).

Birds:
  For organophosphate poisoning:
    a) 0.1 - 0.2 mg/kg IM or SQ *prn* (Clubb 1986)
  As a preanesthetic:
    a) 0.04 - 0.1 mg/kg IM or SQ once (Clubb 1986)

Reptiles:
    a) For organophosphate toxicity in most species: 0.1 - 0.2 mg/kg subQ or IM as needed.

    For ptyalism in tortoises: 0.05 mg/kg (50 µg/kg) Sub Q or IM once daily. (Gauvin 1993)

Monitoring Parameters - Dependent on dose and indication
  1) Heart rate and rhythm
  2) Thirst/appetite; urination/defecation capability
  3) Mouth/secretions dryness

Client Information - Parenteral atropine administration is best performed by professional staff and where adequate cardiac monitoring is available. If animal is receiving atropine tablets, allow animal free access to water and encourage drinking if dry mouth is a problem.

Dosage Forms/Preparations/FDA Approval Status/Withholding Times -
  Veterinary-Approved Products: Atropine is approved for use in dogs, cats, horses, cattle, sheep, and swine. No information is available regarding meat or milk withdrawal. Atropine products are available by prescription only.
  Atropine Sulfate for Injection
    0.5 mg/ml 30 ml, 100 ml vials
    2 mg/ml 100 ml vial
    15 mg/ml (Organophosphate Tx) 100 ml vial
  Human-Approved Products:
  Atropine Sulfate for Injection
    0.05 mg/ml in 5 ml syringes
    0.1 mg/ml in 5 and 10 ml syringes
    0.3 mg/ml in 1 ml and 30 ml vials
    0.4 mg/ml in 1 ml amps and 1, 20, and 30 ml vials
    0.5mg/ml in 1 & 30 ml vials and 5 ml syringes
    0.8 mg/ml in 0.5 & 1 ml amps and 0.5 ml syringes
    1 mg/ml in 1 ml amps & vials and 10 ml syringes
  Atropine Sulfate Tablets
    0.4 mg in 100's
  Also see the monograph for atropine sulfate for ophthalmic use in the appendix.

AURANOFIN

Chemistry - An orally administered gold compound, auranofin occurs as a white, odorless, crystalline powder. It is very slightly soluble in water and soluble in alcohol. Auranofin contains 29% gold.

Storage/Stability/Compatibility - Store capsules in tight, light resistant containers at room temperature. After manufacture, expiration dates of 4 years are assigned to the capsules.

Pharmacology - Auranofin is an orally available gold salt. Gold has anti-inflammatory, antirheumatic, immunomodulating, and antimicrobial (*in vitro*) effects. The exact mechanisms for these actions are not well understood. Gold is taken up by macrophages where it inhibits phagocytosis and may inhibit lysosomal enzyme activity. Gold also inhibits the release of histamine, and the production of prostaglandins. While gold does have antimicrobial effects *in vitro*, it is not clinically useful for this purpose. Auranofin suppresses helper T-cells, without affecting suppressor T-cell populations.

Uses/Indications - Auranofin has been used to treat idiopathic polyarthritis and pemphigus foliaceus in dogs. Several clinicians report that while auranofin may be less toxic, it also less efficacious than injectable gold (aurothioglucose).

Pharmacokinetics - Unlike other available gold salts, auranofin is absorbed when given by mouth (20-25% of the gold) primarily in the small and large intestines. In contrast to the other gold salts, auranofin is only moderately bound to plasma proteins (the others are highly bound). Auranofin crosses the placenta and is distributed into maternal milk. Tissues with the highest levels of gold are kidneys, spleen, lungs, adrenals and liver. Accumulation of gold does not appear to occur, unlike the parenteral gold salts. About 15% of an administered dose (60% of the absorbed dose) is excreted by the kidneys and remainder in the feces.

Contraindications/Precautions/Reproductive Safety - Auranofin should only be administered to dogs where other less expensive and toxic therapies are ineffective and the veterinarian and owner are aware of the potential pitfalls of auranofin therapy and are willing to accept the associated risks and expenses. Auranofin has been demonstrated to be teratogenic and maternotoxic in laboratory animals; it should not be used during pregnancy unless the owner accepts the potential risks of use.

Adverse Effects/Warnings - A dose dependent immune-mediated thrombocytopenia, hemolytic anemia or leukopenias have been noted in dogs. Discontinuation of the drug and administration of steroids have been recommended. Auranofin has a higher incidence of dose dependent GI disturbances (particularly diarrhea) in dogs than with the injectable products. Discontinuation of the drug or a lowered dose will generally resolve the problem. Renal toxicity manifested by proteinuria is possible as is hepatotoxicity (increased liver enzymes). These effects are less likely than either the GI or hematologic effects.

Overdosage/Acute Toxicity - Very limited data is available. The minimum lethal oral dose in rats is 30 mg/kg It is recommended that gut emptying protocols be employed after an acute overdose when applicable. Use of chelating agents (*e.g.*, penicillamine, dimercaprol) for severe toxicities have been used, but are controversial. One human patient who took an overdose over 10 days developed various neurologic sequelae, but eventually (after 3 months) recovered completely after discontinuation of the drug and chelation therapy.

Drug Interactions - There is one report of a human patient who had increased blood **phenytoin** levels after receiving auranofin. The veterinary significance of this potential interaction is minimal. Use of **penicillamine** or **antimalarial drugs** with gold salts is not recommended due to the increased potential for hematologic or renal toxicity. Auranofin's safety when used with other **cytotoxic agents**, including high dose **steroids**, has not been established; use with caution.

Laboratory Considerations - In humans, response to **tuberculin skin** tests may be enhanced; veterinary significance is unclear.

Doses -
  Dogs:
      For treatment of gold-responsive dermatoses:
          a) 0.1 - 0.2 mg/kg PO daily (note: preliminary dosage) (Rosenkrantz 1989)

      For immune-mediated arthropathies and dermatopathies:
          a) 0.05 - 0.2 mg/kg (up to 9 mg/day total dose) PO q12h (Vaden and Cohn 1994)

Monitoring Parameters - 1) Hepatic and renal function tests (prior to initiation of therapy and at regular intervals—at least every 6 months); 2) CBC, platelet counts, and urinalyses (twice a month initially, then monthly for at least 3 months, then at least every 3-4 months)

Client Information - Clients must understand that several months may be required before a positive response may be seen. Commitment to the dosing schedule (*bid*), the costs associated with therapy, and the potential adverse effects should be discussed before initiating therapy.

Dosage Forms/Preparations/FDA Approval Status/Withholding Times -
  Veterinary-Approved Products: None
  Human-Approved Products:
    Auranofin 3 mg Capsules; *Ridaura*® (SKBeecham); (Rx)

AUROTHIOGLUCOSE

Chemistry - A water soluble gold salt, aurothioglucose contains approximately 50% gold. It is practically insoluble in alcohol and insoluble in vegetable oils. The commercial product is a 5% (50 mg/ml) suspension in sesame oil, 2% aluminum monostearate, and propylparaben is added as a preservative.

Storage/Stability/Compatibility - Protect from light and store between 15-30° C; avoid freezing. A five year expiration date is assigned after manufacture. Do not mix with any other compound when injecting.

Pharmacology - Aurothioglucose has anti-inflammatory, antirheumatic, immunomodulating, and antimicrobial (*in vitro*) effects. The exact mechanisms for these actions are not well understood. Gold is taken up by macrophages where it inhibits phagocytosis and may inhibit lysosomal enzyme activity. Gold also inhibits the release of histamine, and the production of prostaglandins. While gold does have antimicrobial effects *in vitro*, it is not clinically useful for this purpose.

Uses/Indications - In human medicine, gold compounds are used primarily as a treatment for rheumatoid arthritis that has not adequately responded to less toxic treatment modalities. In veterinary medicine (primarily small animal medicine), it use has been generally used for treating immune-mediated serious skin disorders such as pemphigus complex.

Pharmacokinetics - After IM injection, aurothioglucose is quite rapidly absorbed and peak serum concentrations are reached in 4-6 hours. It is distributed to several tissues (liver, kidney, spleen, bone marrow, adrenals, and lymph nodes), but highest levels are found in the synovium. In the plasma, 95% is bound to plasma proteins. Gold salts may be found in the epithelial cells in the renal tubules years after dosing has ended. Plasma half-lives increase in length after multiple doses have been given. These values have ranged from 21 - 168 hours in humans. Approximately 70% of a dose is excreted by the kidneys, while the remaining 30% is excreted in the feces.

There appears to be no correlation with serum levels and efficacy. It usually takes from 6-12 weeks for a beneficial effect to be noted after beginning therapy.

Contraindications/Precautions - Contraindications for chrysotherapy (gold therapy) include patients with renal or hepatic disease, SLE (lupus erythematosus, diabetes mellitus (uncontrolled), severe debilitation, and preexisting hematologic disorders.

The safety of aurothioglucose has not been established during pregnancy, it should only be used when the potential benefits outweigh the risks involved. Gold salts are distributed into milk and there have been reports of human infants developing rashes after nursing from mothers taking gold.

Adverse Effects/Warnings - Veterinary experience with aurothioglucose is limited. Pain at the injection site is common and some animals may develop thrombocytopenia with petechia and echymoses. One author (Kummel 1995) reports that four pemphigus canine cases treated with aurothioglucose that was given immediately after cessation of azathioprine, developed a fatal toxic epidermal necrolysis.

Adverse reactions seen in people include, mucocutaneous reactions which are fairly common (15-20%) and are characterized by rashes, (with or preceded by pruritis), and mucosal lesions (usually seen as a stomatitis). Hematologic reactions (thrombocytopenia, leukopenia, aplastic anemias), although rare in humans, can be life-threatening. Renal effects are generally mild and reversible with cessation of therapy if noted early. Proteinuria is an early sign associated with the proximal tubule damage that gold can cause. Reversible pulmonary infiltrates have been noted, but are reversible when therapy is discontinued. Enterocolitis, which may be fatal, has been reported in rare instances.

Because of the serious nature of these adverse reactions, adequate patient monitoring is essential.

Overdosage - Overdosages resulting from a too rapid increase in dosages are exhibited by rapid development of toxic signs, primarily renal (hematuria, proteinuria) and hematologic (thrombocytopenia, granulocytopenia) effects. Other symptoms include: nausea, vomiting, diarrhea, skin lesions, and fever.

Treat with dimercaprol (BAL) to chelate the gold and treat the hematologic and renal effects supportively.

Drug Interactions - Patients receiving aurothioglucose should generally not receive **penicillamine**, **antimalarials**, **hydroxychloroquin**, **immunosuppresive** or **cytotoxic drugs** (*e.g.*, **cyclophosphamide**, **methotrexate**, **azathioprine**) other than corticosteroids, because of similar toxicity profiles.

Doses -
  Dogs:
       For canine pemphigus foliaceus/vulgaris:
       a) For those cases where corticosteroids and/or azathioprine are ineffective or causing unacceptable adverse effects: Discontinue azathioprine for one month and then give 1 mg/5kg of body weight IM weekly for 10 weeks and then monthly thereafter. Note: Before treating, the reader is advised to refer to the full reference for additional information. (Kummel 1995)
       b) Test dose of 1 - 5 mg IM, then 1 mg/kg IM weekly until remission, then monthly (Morgan 1988)

  Cats:
       a) Give animal test dose of 1 mg IM the first week and 2 mg the second week. If no adverse reactions seen (see adverse effects), give 1 mg/kg IM once weekly until either clinical improvement, toxic reactions occur, or weekly dosing has gone on for 20

weeks. Once remission is achieved, attempt to reduce dose and/or increase dosing interval to denote animals that have gone into remission. (Long 1986)
b) Test dose of 1 - 5 mg IM, then 1 mg/kg IM weekly until remission, then monthly (Morgan 1988)
c) First week 1 mg IM, 2nd week 2 mg IM; then 1 mg/kg once weekly IM decreasing to once per month (Kirk 1986)

Horses:
a) 1 mg/kg IM once a week decreasing to once a month (Schultz 1986)

Monitoring Parameters -
1) Urinalysis—baseline, then weekly
2) CBC - baseline, then every 2 weeks
After the patient is on maintenance therapy, hemograms and urinalyses may be done every month or two.

Client Information - Clients should be instructed to notify the veterinarian if pruritis, rash, or diarrhea develops, or if the animal becomes ill or depressed.

Dosage Forms/Preparations/FDA Approval Status/Withholding Times -
Veterinary-Approved Products: None
Human-Approved Products:
Aurothioglucose Injection 50 mg/ml suspension (contains approximately 50% gold); in 10 ml vials; *Solganal*® (Schering); (Rx)

AZAPERONE

Chemistry - A butyrephone neuroleptic, azaperone occurs as a white to yellowish-white macro-crystalline powder with a melting point between 90 - 95°C. It is practically insoluble in water and 1 gram is soluble in 29 ml of alcohol.

Storage/Stability/Compatibility - Azaperone should be stored at room temperature (15-30°C) and away from light. No information was located regarding mixing azaperone with other compounds.

Pharmacology - The butyrephenones as a class cause tranquilization and sedation (sedation may be less so than with the phenothiazines), anti-emetic activity, reduced motor activity, and inhibition of CNS catecholamines (dopamine, norepinephrine). Azaperone appears to have minimal effects on respiration and may inhibit some of the respiratory depressant actions of general anesthetics. A slight reduction of arterial blood pressure has been measured in pigs after IM injections of azaperone, which is apparently due to slight alpha-adrenergic blockade. Azaperone has been demonstrated to prevent the development of halothane-induced malignant hyperthermia in susceptible pigs. Preliminary studies have suggested that the effects of butyrephenones may be antagonized by 4-aminopyridine.

Uses/Indications - Azaperone is officially indicated for the "control of aggressiveness when mixing or regrouping weanling or feeder pigs weighing up to 36.4 kg" (Package Insert, *Stresnil*® - P/M; Mallinckrodt). It is also used clinically as a general tranquilizer for swine, in aggressive sows to allow piglets to be accepted, and as a preoperative agent prior to general anesthesia or cesarian section with local anesthesia.

Azaperone has also been used as a neuroleptic in horses, but some horses develop adverse reactions (sweating, muscle tremors, panic reaction, CNS excitement) and IV administration has resulted in significant arterial hypotension in the horse. Because of these effects, most clinicians avoid the use of this drug in equines.

Pharmacokinetics - Minimal information was located regarding actual pharmacokinetic parameters, but the drug is considered to have a fairly rapid onset of action following IM injections in pigs (5-10 minutes) with a peak effect at approximately 30 minutes post injection. It has a duration of action of 2-3 hours in young pigs and 3-4 hours in older swine. The drug is metabolized in the liver with 13% of it excreted in the feces. At 16 hours post-dose, practically all of the drug is eliminated from the body.

Contraindications/Precautions - When used as directed, the manufacturer reports no contraindications for the drug. It should not be given IV as a significant excitatory phase may be seen in pigs.

Adverse Effects/Warnings - Transient salivation, piling, and shivering have been reported in pigs. Pigs should be left undisturbed after injection (for approximately 20 minutes) until the drug's full effects have been expressed, as disturbances during this period may trigger excitement.

Azaperone has minimal analgesic effects and is not a substitute for appropriate anesthesia or analgesia. It is recommended that in large boars dosage not exceed 2 mg/kg IM.

Overdosage - No specific information was discovered regarding overdoses of azaperone, but it would be expected that symptoms would be an extension of its pharmacologic effects. It is suggested that treatment be supportive. Do not use epinephrine to treat cardiovascular symptoms. More work needs to done before 4-aminopyridine can be recommended as a reversal agent for azaperone.

Drug Interactions - No specific drug interactions have been reported for azaperone. The following interactions have been reported for the closely related compounds, haloperidol or droperidol: **CNS depressant agents (barbiturates, narcotics, anesthetics**, etc.) may cause additive CNS depression if used with butyrephenones.

Doses -
  Swine:
  a) For approved indication of mixing feeder or weanling pigs: 2.2 mg/kg deeply IM (see client information below) (Package Insert; *Stresnil*® — P/M; Mallinckrodt)
  b) Preanesthetic: 2 - 4 mg/kg IM; Immobilizing agent: 5.3 - 8 mg/kg IM (Swindle 1985)
  c) Sedation: 1 mg/kg IM
      Reduction of aggressiveness: 2.5 mg/kg IM
      Knock-down or immobilant: 5 - 10 mg/kg IM (Booth 1988a)

Monitoring Parameters -
  1) Level of sedation

Client Information - Must be injected IM deeply, either behind the ear and perpendicular to the skin or in the back of the ham. All animals in groups to be mixed must be treated.

Dosage Forms/Preparations -
  Veterinary-Approved Products: May not be currently marketed in the USA

  Azaperone 40 mg/ml for Injection in 20 ml vials (6 vials/box); *Stresnil*®; (Schering-Plough) (Rx). Approved for use in pigs. There is no specific tolerance for residues published and there is no specified withdrawal time before slaughter.

  Also known by the trade name *Suicalm*® in the United Kingdom.
  Human-Approved Products: None

AZATHIOPRINE
AZATHIOPRINE SODIUM

Chemistry - Related structurally to adenine, guanine and hypoxanthine, azathioprine is a purine antagonist antimetabolite that is used primarily for its immunosuppressive properties. Azathioprine occurs as an odorless, pale yellow powder that is insoluble in water and slightly soluble in alcohol. Azathioprine sodium powder for injection occurs as a bright yellow, amorphous mass. After reconstituting with sterile water for injection to a concentration of 10 mg/ml it has an approximate pH of 9.6.

Storage/Stability/Compatibility - Azathioprine tablets should be stored at room temperature in well-closed containers and protected from light.
  The sodium powder for injection should be stored at room temperature and protected from light. It is reportedly stable at neutral or acidic pH, but will hydrolyze to mercaptopurine in alkaline solutions. This conversion is enhanced upon warming or in the presence of sulfhydryl-containing compounds (*e.g.,* cysteine). After reconstituting, the injection should be used within 24 hours as no preservative is present.
  Azathioprine sodium is reportedly **compatible** with the following intravenous solutions: dextrose 5% in water, and sodium chloride 0.45% or 0.9%. Compatibility is dependent upon factors such as pH, concentration, temperature and diluents used. It is suggested to consult specialized references for more specific information (*e.g., Handbook on Injectable Drugs* by Trissel; see bibliography).

Pharmacology - While the exact mechanism how azathioprine exerts its immunosuppressive action has not been determined, it is probably dependent on several factors. Azathioprine antagonizes purine metabolism thereby inhibiting RNA, DNA synthesis and mitosis. It also may cause chromosome breaks secondary to incorporation into nucleic acids and cellular metabolism may become disrupted by the drug's ability to inhibit coenzyme formation. Azathioprine has greater activity on delayed hypersensitivity and cellular immunity than on humoral antibody responses. Clinical response to azathioprine may require up to 6 weeks.

Uses/Indications - In veterinary medicine, azathioprine is used primarily as a second or third line immunosuppressive agent in the treatment of immune-mediated diseases in dogs. See *Doses* below for more information.

Pharmacokinetics - Azathioprine is absorbed from the GI tract and is rapidly metabolized to mercaptopurine which is then further metabolized to several other compounds. These metabolites are excreted by the kidneys. Only minimal amounts of either azathioprine or mercaptopurine are excreted unchanged.

Contraindications/Precautions/Reproductive Safety - Azathioprine is contraindicated in patients hypersensitive to it. The drug should be used cautiously in patients with hepatic dysfunction.

Azathioprine is mutagentic and teratogenic (in lab animals).

Adverse Effects/Warnings - The principal adverse effect associated with azathioprine is bone marrow suppression. Cats are more prone to develop these effects and the drug is generally not recommended to be used in that species. Leukopenia is the prevalent consequence, but anemias and thrombocytopenia may also be seen. Acute pancreatitis and hepatotoxicity have also been associated with azathioprine therapy in dogs.

Because azathioprine depresses the immune system, animals may be susceptible to infections or neoplastic illnesses (long-term use).

In recovering dogs with immune-mediated hemolytic anemia, taper the withdrawal of the drug slowly over several months and monitor for early signs of relapse. Rapid withdrawal can lead to a rebound hyperimmune response.

Overdosage/Acute Toxicity - No specific information was located regarding acute overdose of azathioprine. It is suggested to use standard protocols to empty the GI tract if ingestion was recent and to treat supportively.

Drug Interactions - The hepatic metabolism of azathioprine may be decreased by concomitant administration of **allopurinol**. In humans, it is recommended to reduce the azathioprine dose to 1/4-1/3 usual if both drugs are to used together.

The neuromuscular blocking activity of **non-depolarizing muscle relaxants** (*e.g.,* **pancuronium, tubocurarine**) may be inhibited or reversed by azathioprine.

Doses -
  Dogs:
    As an immunosuppressive:
      a) For adjunctive therapy for immune-mediated hemolytic anemia (probably should be reserved for dogs w/fulminant intravascular hemolysis, autoagglutination or those that require repeated transfusion or have persistant reticulocytopenia): Initially at 2 mg/kg/day PO. Reduce to 1 mg/kg/day after the first 7-10 days. (Bucheler and Cotter 1995)
      b) For adjunctive therapy of immune-mediated glomerulopathy: 2 mg/kg PO once daily initially. When remission is achieved, give at same dose every other day. Prednisolone and azathioprine should be given on alternate days at this time. (Polzin and Osborne 1985)
      c) For adjunctive therapy in myasthenia gravis in non-responsive patients: 2 mg/kg PO once a day to every other day; may decrease dose if response is seen. (LeCouteur 1988)
      d) For adjunctive therapy of chronic atrophic gastritis: 0.5 mg/kg PO once a day to every other day (with corticosteroids). (Hall and Twedt 1988)
      e) For adjunctive therapy in chronic active hepatitis: If no improvement seen with corticosteroids, add azathioprine at 2 - 2.5 mg/kg PO once daily; recheck in 10-14 days. If improved, continue for additional 2-3 months; if no improvement, reconsider diagnosis. (Cornelius and Bjorling 1988)
      f) For adjunctive therapy in immune-mediated hemolytic anemia:
        2 mg/kg PO once daily (in combination with corticosteroids ± cyclophosphamide; *see reference or individual monographs*). (Maggio-Price 1988)
      g) For adjunctive therapy in immune-mediated thrombocytopenia: If corticosteroids ineffective, may add azathioprine at 2 mg/kg PO; taper to 0.5 - 1.0 mg/kg PO every other day. Alternatively, may use vincristine or cyclophosphamide. (Young 1988)
      h) For adjunctive therapy in autoimmune skin diseases: 2.2 mg/kg PO once a day to every other day. May require 2-3 weeks before benefits are seen; may allow reduction or withdrawal of prednisone. (Giger and Werner 1988)
      i) For adjunctive therapy of SLE or other multisystemic immune-mediated diseases: 2.2 mg/kg PO once a day to every other day;. used alone or in combination with other immunosuppressants. Once remission is achieved, may reduce dose to 1 - 2 mg/kg every other day. (Giger and Werner 1988)
      j) For immune-mediated chronic inflammatory bowel disease: 50 mg/m^2 once daily for 2 weeks, then every other day. Used rarely, but is helpful in a few cases. (Richter 1989)
      i) For rheumatoid arthritis: In conjunction with a glucocorticoid (predniso(lo)ne); give azathioprine 2 mg/kg PO once daily for 14-21 days; then give every other day

(usually alternating with corticosteroids) until 1 month after remission of synovial inflammation. (Tangner and Hulse 1988)

For adjunctive treatment of ocular fibrous histiocytomas:

    a) 2 mg/kg PO daily for 2 weeks, reevaluate, and reduce to 1 mg/kg every other day for 2 weeks, then 1 mg/kg once weekly for 1 month. (Riis 1986)

Cats: Note: Several authors do not recommend azathioprine for use in cats because of the potential for development of fatal toxicity and the difficulty in accurately dosing.

As an immunosuppressive:

    a) For immune-mediated dermatologic diseases: Cats are prone to develop bone marrow toxicity from azathioprine and the drug is generally recommended not to be used in that species. However, if the drug is to be used, the dose is 1.1 mg/kg PO every other day. (Rosenkrantz 1989)

Monitoring Parameters -

    1) Hemograms (including platelets) should be monitored closely; initially every 1-2 weeks and every 1-2 months once on maintenance therapy. It is recommended by some clinicians that if the WBC count drops to between 5,000-7,000 cells/mm^3 the dose be reduced by 25%. If WBC count drops below 5,000 cells/mm^3 treatment should be discontinued until leukopenia resolves.

    2) Liver function tests; serum amylase, if indicated

    4) Efficacy

Client Information - Clients must be briefed on the possibilities of severe toxicity developing from this drug, including drug-related neoplasms or mortality. Clients should contact veterinarian should the animal exhibit symptoms of abnormal bleeding, bruising, anorexia, vomiting or infection.

Although, no special precautions are necessary with handling intact tablets, it is recommended to wash hands after administering the drug.

Dosage Forms/Preparations/FDA Approval Status/Withholding Times -

  Veterinary-Approved Products: None

  Human-Approved Products:

Azathioprine Tablets 50 mg; *Imuran*® (Glaxo Wellcome) (Rx)

Azathioprine Sodium Injection 100 mg per vial in 20 ml vials; *Imuran*® (Glaxo Wellcome) ; (Rx); generic, (Rx)

BAL in Oil — see Dimercaprol

BARBITURATE PHARMACOLOGY

Also see the monographs for Phenobarbital, Pentobarbital, Thiamylal, & Thiopental

While barbiturates are generally considered to be CNS depressants, they can invoke all levels of CNS mood alteration from paradoxical excitement to deep coma and death. While the exact mechanisms for the CNS effects caused by barbiturates are unknown, they have been shown to inhibit the release of acetylcholine, norepinephrine, and glutamate. The barbiturates also have effects on GABA and pentobarbital has been shown to be GABA-mimetic. At high anesthetic doses, barbiturates have been demonstrated to inhibit the uptake of calcium at nerve endings.

The degree of depression produced is dependent on the dosage, route of administration, pharmacokinetics of the drug, and species treated. Additionally, effects may be altered by the age or physical condition of the patient, or the concurrent use of other drugs. The barbiturates depress the sensory cortex, lessen motor activity, and produce sedation at low dosages. Some barbiturates such as phenobarbital are useful as anticonvulsants because they tend to have sufficient motor activity depression, without causing excessive sedation. In humans, it has been shown that barbiturates reduce the rapid-eye movement (REM) stage of sleep. Barbiturates have no true intrinsic analgesic activity.

In most species, barbiturates cause a dose-dependent respiratory depression, but in some species they can cause slight respiratory stimulation. At sedative/hypnotic doses respiratory depression is similar to that during normal physiologic sleep. As doses increase, the medullary respiratory center is progressively depressed with resultant decreases in rate, depth, and volume. Respiratory arrest may occur at 4 times lower the dose that will cause cardiac arrest. These drugs must be used very cautiously in cats as they are particularly sensitive to the respiratory depressant effects of barbiturates.

Besides the cardiac arresting effects of the barbiturates at euthanatizing dosages, the barbiturates have other cardiovascular effects. In the dog, pentobarbital has been demonstrated to cause tachycardia, decreased myocardial contractility and stroke volume, and decreased mean arterial pressure and total peripheral resistance.

The barbiturates cause reduced tone and motility of the intestinal musculature, probably secondary to its central depressant action. The thiobarbiturates (thiamylal, thiopental) may, after initial depression, cause an increase in both tone and motility of the intestinal musculature. However, these effects do not appear to have much clinical significance. Administration of barbiturates reduces the sensitivity of the motor end-plate to acetylcholine, thereby slightly relaxing skeletal muscle. Because the musculature is not completely relaxed, other skeletal muscle relaxants may be necessary for surgical procedures.

There is no direct effect on the kidney by the barbiturates, but severe renal impairment may occur secondary to hypotensive effects in overdose situations. Liver function is not directly affected when used acutely, but hepatic microsomal enzyme induction is well documented with extended barbiturate (especially phenobarbital) administration. Although barbiturates reduce oxygen consumption of all tissues, no change in metabolic rate is measurable when given at sedative dosages. Basal metabolic rates may be reduced with resultant decreases in body temperature when barbiturates are given at anesthetic doses.

BENAZEPRIL HCL

Chemistry - Benazepril HCl, an angiotensin converting enzyme inhibitor, occurs as white to off-white crystalline powder. It is soluble in water and ethanol. Benazepril does not contain a sulfhydryl group in its structure.

Storage/Stability/Compatibility - Benazepril (and combination products) tablets should be stored at temperatures less than 86°F (30°C) and protected from moisture. They should be dispensed in tight containers.

Pharmacology - Benazepril is a prodrug, and has little pharmacologic activity of its own. After being hydrolyzed in the liver to benazeprilat, the drug inhibits the conversion of angiotensin I to angiotensin II by inhibiting angiotensin-converting enzyme (ACE). Angiotensin II acts both as a vasoconstrictor and stimulates production of aldosterone in the adrenal cortex. By blocking angiotensin II formation, ACE inhibitors generally reduce blood pressure in hypertensive patients and vascular resistance in patients with congestive heart failure.

Like enalapril and lisinopril, but not captopril, benazepril does not contain a sulfhydryl group. ACE inhibitors containing sulfhydryl groups (e.g., captopril) may have a greater tendency towards causing immune-mediated reactions.

Uses/Indications - Benazepril may be useful as a vasodilator in the treatment of heart failure and as a an antihypertensive agent. It may also be of benefit in treating the effects associated with valvular heart disease and left to right shunts. ACE inhibitors may also be of benefit in the adjunctive treatment of chronic renal failure and for protein losing nephropathies.

Pharmacokinetics - In healthy dogs, benazepril after oral dosing is rapidly absorbed and converted into the active metabolite benazeprilat with peak levels of benazeprilat occurring approximately 75 minutes after dosing. The elimination half-life of benazeprilat is approximately 3.5 hours in healthy dogs.

In humans, approximately 37% of an oral dose is absorbed after oral dosing and food apparently does not affect the extent of absorption. About 95% of the parent drug and active metabolite are bound to serum proteins. Benazepril and benazeprilat are primarily eliminated via the kidneys and mild to moderate renal dysfunction apparently does not significantly alter elimination as biliary clearance may compensate somewhat for reductions in renal clearances. Hepatic dysfunction or age does not appreciably alter benazeprilat levels.

Contraindications/Precautions /Reproductive Safety - Benazepril is contraindicated in patients who have demonstrated hypersensitivity to the ACE inhibitors.

ACE inhibitors should be used with caution in patients with hyponatremia or sodium depletion, coronary or cerebrovascular insufficiency, preexisting hematologic abnormalities or a collagen vascular disease (*e.g.,* SLE). Patients with severe CHF should be monitored very closely upon initiation of therapy.

Benazepril apparently crosses the placenta. High doses of ACE inhibitors in rodents have caused decreased fetal weights and increases in fetal and maternal death rates; no teratogenic effects have been reported to date, but use during pregnancy should occur only when the potential benefits of therapy outweigh the risks to the offspring.

Minimal amounts of benazepril and benazeprilat enter maternal milk and do not apparently convey much risk to nursing offspring.

Adverse Effects/Warnings - Benazepril's adverse effect profile in dogs is not well described, but other ACE inhibitors effects in dogs usually center around GI distress (anorexia, vomiting, diarrhea). Potentially, hypotension, renal dysfunction and hyperkalemia could occur. Because it lacks a sulfhydryl group (unlike captopril), there is less likelihood that immune-mediated reactions will occur, but rashes, neutropenia and agranulocytosis have been reported in humans.

Overdosage - In overdose situations, the primary concern is hypotension; supportive treatment with volume expansion with normal saline is recommended to correct blood pressure. Because of the drug's long duration of action, prolonged monitoring and treatment may be required. Recent massive overdoses should be managed using gut emptying protocols as appropriate.

Drug Interactions - Concomitant **diuretics** or other **vasodilators** may cause hypotension if used with benazepril; titrate dosages carefully. Some clinicians recommend reducing **furosemide** doses (by 25 - 50%) when adding enalapril to therapy in CHF.

Hyperkalemia may develop if given with **potassium** or **potassium sparing diuretics** (*e.g.,* **spironolactone**).

Non-steroidal anti-inflammatory agents (NSAIDs) may reduce the clinical efficacy of ACE inhibitors when they are being used as an antihypertensive agent. Indomethacin appears to be most likely to evoke this problem.

Laboratory Considerations - When using **iodohippurate sodium I^{123}/I^{134} or Technetium Tc^{99} pententate renal imaging** in patients with renal artery stenosis, ACE inhibitors may cause a reversible decrease in localization and excretion of these agents in the affected kidney which may lead to confusion in test interpretation.

Doses -

Dogs:
For adjunctive treatment of heart failure:
a) 0.25 - 0.5 mg/kg PO once daily (Miller and Tilley 1995)
b) 0.25 - 0.5 mg/kg PO once to twice daily (Ware 1997)

For adjunctive treatment of renal failure (progressive renal disease) or hypertension:
a) 0.25 mg/kg PO once to twice daily (Brown 1997)

Monitoring Parameters - 1) Clinical symptoms of CHF; 2) Serum electrolytes, creatinine, BUN, urine protein; 3) Blood pressure (if treating hypertension or symptoms associated with hypotension arise)

Client Information - Do not abruptly stop or reduce therapy without veterinarian's approval. Contact veterinarian if vomiting or diarrhea persist or is severe or if animal's condition deteriorates.

Dosage Forms/FDA Approval Status -
Veterinary-Approved Products: None
Human-Approved Products:
Benazepril HCl Oral Film-coated Tablets 5 mg, 10 mg, 20 mg, & 40 mg; *Lotensin®*; (Novartis); (Rx)
Also available in fixed dose combination products containing amlodipine (*Lotrel®*) or hydrochlorothiazide (*Lotensin HCT®*)

BETAMETHASONE
BETAMETHASONE DIPROPIONATE
BETAMETHASONE SODIUM PHOSPHATE

Note: For more information refer to the monograph: Glucocorticoids, General information .

Chemistry - A synthetic glucocorticoid, betamethasone is available as the base and as the dipropionate, acetate and sodium phosphate salts. The base is used for oral dosage forms. The sodium phosphate and acetate salts are used in injectable preparations. The dipropionate salt is used in topical formulations and in combination with the sodium phosphate salt in a veterinary-approved injectable preparation. Betamethasone may also be known as flubenisolone.

Betamethasone occurs as an odorless, white to practically white, crystalline powder. It is insoluble in water and practically insoluble in alcohol. The dipropionate salt occurs as a white or creamy-white, odorless powder. It is practically insoluble in water and sparingly soluble in alcohol. The sodium phosphate salt occurs as an odorless, white to practically white, hygroscopic powder. It is freely soluble in water and slightly soluble in alcohol.

Storage/Stability/Compatibility - Betamethasone tablets should be stored in well-closed containers at 2-30°C. The oral solution should be stored in well-closed containers, protected from light and kept at temperatures less than 40°C. The sodium phosphate injection should be protected from light and stored at room temperature (15-30°C); protect from freezing. The combination veterinary injectable product (*Betasone®*) should be stored between 2 - 30°C and protected from light or freezing.

When betamethasone sodium phosphate was mixed with heparin sodium, hydrocortisone sodium succinate, potassium chloride, vitamin B-complex with C, dextrose 5% in water (D5W),

D5 in Ringer's, D5 in lactated Ringer's, Ringer's lactate injection or normal saline, no physical incompatibility was noted immediately or after 4 hours.

Contraindications/Precautions/Adverse effects - For the product *Betasone*® (Schering), the manufacturer states that the drug is "contraindicated in animals with acute or chronic bacterial infections unless therapeutic doses of an effective antimicrobial agent are used." See the monograph: Glucocorticoids, General Information for additional information.

In addition to the contraindications, precautions and adverse effects outlined in the opening section of glucocorticoids, betamethasone has been demonstrated to cause decreased sperm output and semen volume and increased percentages of abnormal sperm in dogs.

Doses -
Dogs:
For the control of pruritis:
 a) *Betasone*® aqueous suspension: 0.25 - 0.5 ml per 20 pounds body weight IM. Dose dependent on severity of condition. May repeat when necessary. Relief averages 3 weeks in duration. Do not exceed more than 4 injections. (Package Insert; *Betasone*®- Schering)

Dosage Forms/Preparations/Approval Status/Withdrawal Times -
Veterinary-Approved Products:
Betamethasone diproprionate equivalent to 5 mg/ml of betamethasone and betamethasone sodium phosphate equivalent to 2 mg/ml betamethasone in 5 ml vials; *Betasone*® (Schering); (Rx) Approved for use in dogs.

Betamethasone valerate is also found in *Gentocin*® *Otic, Gentocin*® *Topical Spray* and *Topagen*® *Ointment,* all from Schering Animal Health.

Human-Approved Products:
Betamethasone sodium phosphate Injection 4 mg/ml (equivalent to 3 mg/ml betamethasone) in 5 ml vials; *Celestone Phosphate*® (Schering) (Rx); *Cel-U-Jec*® (Hauck); generic; (Rx)

Betamethasone sodium phosphate Injection 3 mg/ml and betamethasone acetate 3 mg/ml in 5 ml vials; *Celestone Soluspan*® (Schering); Generic (Rx)

Betamethasone oral solution 0.6 mg/5 ml andBetamethasone tablets 0.6 mg; *Celestone*® (Schering); (Rx)

Also many topical formulations available.

BETHANECHOL CHLORIDE

Chemistry - A synthetic cholinergic ester, bethanechol occurs as a slightly hygroscopic, white or colorless crystalline powder with a slight, amine-like or "fishy" odor. It exhibits polymorphism, with one form melting at 211° and the other form at 219°. One gram of the drug is soluble in approximately 1 ml of water or 10 ml of alcohol. The commercially available injection has a pH from 5.5 - 7.5.

Storage/Stability/Compatibility - Bethanechol tablets should be stored at room temperature in tight containers. The injectable form should be stored at room temperature; avoid freezing. It may be autoclaved at 120°C for 20 minutes without any loss of potency.

Pharmacology - Bethanechol directly stimulates cholinergic receptors. Its effects are principally muscarinic and at usual doses has negligible nicotinic activity. It is more resistant to hydrolysis than acetylcholine by cholinesterase and, therefore, has an increased duration of activity.

Pharmacologic effects include increased esophageal peristalsis and lower esophageal sphincter tone, increased tone and peristaltic activity of the stomach and intestines, increased gastric and pancreatic secretions, increased tone of the detrusor muscle of the bladder, and decreased bladder capacity. At high doses after parenteral administration, effects such as increased bronchial secretions and constriction, miosis, lacrimation, and salivation can be seen. When administered SQ or orally, effects are predominantly on the GI and urinary tracts.

Uses/Indications - In veterinary medicine, bethanechol is used primarily to stimulate bladder contractions in small animals. It also can be used as an esophageal or general GI stimulant, but metoclopramide and/or neostigmine have largely supplanted it for these uses.

Pharmacokinetics - No information was located on the pharmacokinetics of this agent in veterinary species. In humans, bethanechol is poorly absorbed from the GI tract, and the onset of action is usually within 30-90 minutes after oral dosing. After subcutaneous administration, effects begin within 5-15 minutes and usually peak within 30 minutes. The duration of action after oral dosing may persist for up to 6 hours after large doses and 2 hours after SQ dosing. Subcutaneous administration yields a more enhanced effect on urinary tract stimulation than does oral administration.

Bethanechol does not enter the CNS after usual doses; other distribution aspects of the drug are not known. The metabolic or excretory fate of bethanechol have not been described.

Contraindications/Precautions - Contraindications to bethanechol therapy include: bladder neck or other urinary outflow obstruction, when the integrity of the bladder wall is in question (*e.g.,* as after recent bladder surgery), hyperthyroidism, peptic ulcer disease or when other inflammatory GI lesions are present, recent GI surgery with resections/anastomoses, GI obstruction or peritonitis, hypersensitivity to the drug, epilepsy, asthma, coronary artery disease or occlusion, hypotension, severe bradycardia or vagotonia or vasomotor instability. If urinary outflow resistance is increased due to enhanced urethral tone (not mechanical obstruction!), bethanechol should only be used in conjunction with another agent that will sufficiently reduce outflow resistance (*e.g.,* diazepam, dantrolene (striated muscle) or phenoxybenzamine (smooth muscle)).

Adverse Effects/Warnings - When administered orally to small animals, adverse effects are usually mild, with vomiting, diarrhea, salivation, and anorexia being the most likely to occur. Cardiovascular (arrhythmias, hypotension) and respiratory effects (asthma) are most likely only seen after overdosage situations or with high dose SQ therapy.

IM or IV use is not recommended, except in emergency situations when the IV route may be used. Severe cholinergic reactions are likely if given IV. If injecting the drug (SQ or IV), it is recommended that atropine be immediately available.

Overdosage - Symptoms of overdosage are basically cholinergic in nature. Muscarinic effects (salivation, urination, defecation, etc.) are usually seen with oral or SQ administration. If given IM or IV, a full-blown cholinergic crisis can occur with circulatory collapse, bloody diarrhea, shock and cardiac arrest possible.

Treatment for bethanechol toxicity is atropine. Refer to the atropine monograph for more information on its use. Epinephrine may also be employed to treat symptoms of bronchospasm.

Drug Interactions - Bethanechol should not be used concomitantly with other **cholinergic** (*e.g.,* **carbachol**) **or anticholinesterase** (*e.g.,* **neostigmine**) **agents** because of additive effects and increased likelihood of toxicity developing.

Quinidine, procainamide, epinephrine (or sympathomimetic amines) or atropine can antagonize the effects of bethanechol.

Bethanechol used in combination with **ganglionic blocking drugs** (*e.g.,* mecamylamine) can produce severe GI and hypotensive effects.

Doses -
   Dogs:
      For urinary indications:
         a) 2.5 - 10 mg SQ q8h; or 5 - 25 mg q8h PO (Polzin and Osborne 1985), (Labato 1988)
         b) 5 - 15 mg PO *tid*; often used with phenoxybenzamine (Chew, DiBartola, and Fenner 1986)

      For increased esophageal sphincter tone: 0.5 - 1.0 mg/kg PO q8h (Jones 1985)

   Cats:
      For urinary indications:
         a) 2.5 - 5 mg q8-12h PO (Polzin and Osborne 1985), (Labato 1988)
         b) 1.25 - 5 mg PO *tid*; often used with phenoxybenzamine (Chew, DiBartola, and Fenner 1986)

   Horses:
         a) 0.05 mg/kg SQ; 0.11 - 0.22 mg/kg IV; Start at lower dose first and use cautiously (McConnell and Hughey 1987)

   Reptiles:
         a) 2.5 mg/kg SQ (McConnell and Hughey 1987)

Monitoring Parameters -Clinical efficacy; urination frequency, amount voided, bladder palpation; Adverse effects (see above section)

Client Information - Give medication on an empty stomach unless otherwise instructed by veterinarian. Contact veterinarian if salivation or GI (vomiting, diarrhea, or anorexia) effects are pronounced or persist.

Dosage Forms/Preparations/FDA Approval Status/Withholding Times -
   Veterinary-Approved Products: None
   Human-Approved Products:

      Bethanechol Chloride Tablets 5 mg, 10 mg, 25 mg, 50 mg; *Urecholine*® ((Merck, Frosst); *Duvoid*® (Roberts); *Myotonachol*® (Glenwood); *PMS-Bethanechol Chloride*® (Glenwood); Generic; (Rx)

      Bethanechol Chloride for Injection 5 mg/ml in 1 ml vials and amps; *Urecholine*® (Frosst); (Rx)

Bicarbonate — see Sodium Bicarbonate

BISACODYL

Chemistry - A diphenylmethane laxative, bisacodyl occurs as white to off-white crystalline powder. It is practically insoluble in water and sparingly soluble in alcohol.

Storage/Stability/Compatibility - Bisacodyl suppositories and enteric-coated tablets should be stored at temperatures less than 30°C.

Pharmacology - A stimulant laxative, bisacodyl's exact mechanism is unknown. It is thought to produce catharsis by increasing peristalsis by direct stimulation on the intramural nerve plexuses of intestinal smooth muscle. Another effect is it has been shown to increase fluid and ion accumulation in the large intestine thereby enhancing catharsis.

Uses/Indications - Bisacodyl oral and rectal products are used as stimulant cathartics in dogs and cats.

Pharmacokinetics - Bisacodyl is minimally absorbed after either oral or rectal administration. Onset of action after oral administration is generally 6-10 hours and 15 minutes to an hour after rectal administration.

Contraindications/Precautions/Reproductive Safety - Stimulant cathartics are contraindicated in the following conditions: intestinal obstruction (not constipation), undiagnosed rectal bleeding, or when the patient is susceptible to intestinal perforation.

Adverse Effects/Warnings - Bisacodyl has relatively few side effects; occasional cramping, nausea, or diarrhea may be noted after use.

Overdosage/Acute Toxicity - Overdoses may result in severe cramping, diarrhea, vomiting and potentially, fluid and electrolyte imbalances. Animals should be monitored and given replacement parenteral fluids and electrolytes as necessary.

Drug Interactions - Do not give **milk or antacids** within an hour of bisacodyl tablets as it may cause premature disintegration of the enteric coating. Stimulant laxatives may potentially decrease GI transit time thereby affecting absorption of other **oral drugs**. Separate doses by two hours if possible.

Doses -
  Dogs:
    As a cathartic:
      a)   One 5 mg tablet PO (Papich 1992)
      b)   5 - 20 mg (1- 4 tablets) PO once daily, 1 - 2 ml of the enema (as an enema), or 1 - 3 pediatric suppositories (Sherding 1994)

  Cats:
    As a cathartic:
      a)   One 5 mg tablet PO; or 1-3 pediatric rectal suppositories; or 1 ml/kg of the bisacodyl enema (DeNovo and Bright 1992)
      b)   5 mg (1 tablet) PO once daily, 1 - 2 ml of the enema (as an enema), or 1 - 3 pediatric suppositories (Sherding 1994)
      c)   1 - 2 tablets daily PO; requires 6-12 hours for action. (Ford 1991)

Client Information - 1) If using oral tablets do not crush or allow animal to chew or intense cramping may occur. 2) Unless otherwise directed by veterinarian, bisacodyl should be used on an "occasional" basis only. Chronic use has led to laxative dependence in humans.

Dosage Forms/Preparations/FDA Approval Status/Withholding Times -
  Veterinary-Approved Products: None
  Human-Approved Products:
    Bisacodyl 5 mg Oral Enteric-coated Tablets; *Dulcolax*® (Ciba), *Bisco-Lax*® (Schein), *Fleet*® *Bisacodyl* (Fleet), *Carter's Little Pills*® (Carter), generic; (OTC)

    Bisacodyl 5 mg (Pediatric) and 10 mg Rectal Suppositories; *Dulcolax*® (Ciba), *Bisco-Lax*® (Schein), *Fleet*® *Bisacodyl* (Fleet), generic; (OTC)

    Bisacodyl Enema: 10 mg/30 ml in 37 ml disposable bottles; *Fleet*® *Bisacodyl* (Fleet); (OTC)

BISMUTH SUBSALICYLATE

Chemistry - Bismuth subsalicylate occurs as white or nearly white, tasteless, odorless powder and contains about 58% bismuth. It is insoluble in water, glycerin and alcohol. It may also be known as bismuth salicylate, or bismuth oxysalicylate.

Storage/Stability/Compatibility - Bismuth subsalicylate should be stored protected from light. It is incompatible with mineral acids and iron salts. When exposed to alkali bicarbonates, bismuth subsalicylate decomposes with effervescence.

Pharmacology - Bismuth subsalicylate is thought to posses protectant, anti-endotoxic and weak antibacterial properties. It is believed that the parent compound is cleaved in the small intestine into bismuth carbonate and salicylate. The protectant, anti-endotoxic and weak antibacterial properties are thought to be as a result of the bismuth. The salicylate component has antiprostaglandin activity which may contribute to its effectiveness and reduce symptoms associated with secretory diarrheas.

Uses/Indications - In veterinary medicine, bismuth subsalicylate products are used to treat diarrhea. The drug is also used in humans for other GI symptoms (indigestion, cramps, gas pains) and in the treatment and prophylaxis of traveler's diarrhea.

Pharmacokinetics - No specific veterinary information was located. In humans, the amount of bismuth absorbed is negligible while the salicylate component is rapidly and completely absorbed. Salicylates are highly bound to plasma proteins and are metabolized in the liver to salicylic acid. Salicylic acid, conjugated salicylate metabolites and any absorbed bismuth are all excreted renally.

Contraindications/Precautions - Salicylate absorption may occur; use with caution in patients with preexisting bleeding disorders. Because of the potential for adverse effects caused by the salicylate component, this drug should be used cautiously, if at all, in cats.

Adverse Effects/Warnings - Antidiarrheal products are not a substitute for adequate fluid and electrolyte therapy when required. May change stool color to a gray-black or greenish-black; do not confuse with melena. In human infants and debilitated individuals, use of this product may cause impactions to occur.

As bismuth is radiopaque, it may interfere with GI tract radiologic examinations.

Overdosage - No specific information located, but theoretically may cause salicylism. See the Aspirin monograph for more information.

Drug Interactions - Bismuth containing products can decrease the absorption or orally administered **tetracycline** products. If both agents are to be used, separate drugs by at least 2 hours and administer tetracycline first.

Because bismuth subsalicylate contains salicylate, concomitant administration with **aspirin** may increase salicylate serum levels; monitor appropriately.

Laboratory Test Interference - At high doses, salicylates may cause false-positive results for **urinary glucose** if using the cupric sulfate method (Clinitest®, Benedict's solution) and false-negative results if using the glucose oxidase method (Clinistix® or Tes-Tape®). **Urinary ketones** measured by the ferric chloride method (Gerhardt) may be affected if salicylates are in the urine (reddish-color produced). **5-HIAA** determinations by the fluoremetric method may be interfered by salicylates in the urine. Falsely elevated **VMA** (vanillylmandelic acid) may be seen with most methods used if salicylates are in the urine. Falsely lowered **VMA** levels may be seen if using the Pisano method. Urinary excretion of **xylose** may be decreased if salicylates are given concurrently. Falsely elevated **serum uric acid** values may be measured if using colorimetric methods.

Doses -
  Dogs:
        a) Pepto-Bismol: 1 ml/kg PO initially, then decrease dosage (Jergens 1995)
        b) Pepto-Bismol: 2 ml/kg PO *tid-qid* (Chiapella 1988)
        c) Pepto-Bismol: 0.25 ml/kg PO *qid*
          Corrective Mixture w/Paregoric: 0.25 ml/kg initially, then 0.125 ml/kg PO *qid* (DeNovo 1988)

  Cattle:
        a) For calves: 60 ml *bid-qid* for two days (Label Directions - *Corrective Mixture*® (Beecham))
        b) 2 - 3 ounces PO 2-4 times a day (Braun 1986)

  Horses:
    For diarrhea:
        a) For foals: 0.5 ml per kg PO q4-6h, response usually within 48 hours. After diarrhea resolves, taper off drug. (Wilson 1987)
        b) For foals or adults:1 ounce per 8 kg of body weight PO *tid-qid* (Clark and Becht 1987)
        c) For foals: 3 - 4 oz. PO q6-8h (Martens and Scrutchfield 1982)

    d) For foals: 60 ml *bid-qid* for two days (Label Directions - *Corrective Mixture*® (Beecham))

Swine:
  For diarrhea in baby pigs:
    a) 2 - 5 ml PO *bid-qid* for 2 days (Label Directions - *Corrective Mixture*® (Beecham))

Monitoring Parameters -
  1) Clinical efficacy
  2) Fluid & electrolyte status in severe diarrhea

Client Information - Shake well before using. If diarrhea persists, contact veterinarian. May change stool color to a gray-black or greenish-black; contact veterinarian if stool becomes "tarry" black. Refrigeration of the suspension may improve palatability. Do not mix with milk before administering.

Dosage Forms/Preparations/FDA Approval Status/Withholding Times -
  Veterinary-Approved Products:
    Corrective Suspension® (Phoenix): Bismuth subsalicylate 17.5 mg/ml. Available in gallons.; (OTC) Labeled for use in cattle, horses, calves, folas, dogs and cats.

  Human-Approved Products:
    Bismuth Subsalicylate Suspension 262 mg/15 ml & 524 mg/15 ml in 120 ml, 240 ml, 360 ml bottles.; *Pepto-Bismol*® (Procter & Gamble); *Bismatrol Extra Strength*® (Major); *Pepto-Bismol Extra Strength*® (Procter & Gamble); Generic (OTC)

    Bismuth Subsalicylate Tablets & Caplets (Chewable) 262 mg;*Pepto-Bismol*® (Procter & Gamble); (OTC);*Bismatrol*® (Major); (OTC)

BLEOMYCIN SULFATE

Chemistry - An antibiotic antineoplastic agent, bleomycin sulfate is obtained from *Streptomyces verticullis*. It occurs as a cream colored, amorphous powder that is very soluble in water and sparingly soluble in alcohol. After reconstitution, the pH of the solution ranges from 4.5-6. Bleomycin is assayed microbiologically. One unit of bleomycin is equivalent to one mg of the reference Bleomycin A_2 standard.

Storage/Stability/Compatibility - Powder for injection should be kept refrigerated. After re-constituting with (sterile saline, water, or dextrose) the resulting solution is stable for 24 hours. Bleomycin is less stable in dextrose solutions than in saline. After reconstituting with normal saline, bleomycin is reportedly stable for at least two weeks at room temperature and for 4 weeks when refrigerated. However, since there are no preservatives in the resulting solution, the product is recommended to be used with 24 hours.

  Bleomycin sulfate is reported to be compatible with the following drugs: amikacin sulfate, cis-platin, cyclophosphamide, dexamethasone sodium phosphate, diphenhydramine HCl, doxoru-bicin, heparin sodium, metoclopramide HCl, vinblastine sulfate, and vincristine sulfate. Compatibility is dependent upon factors such as pH, concentration, temperature and diluents used. It is suggested to consult specialized references (*e.g., Handbook on Injectable Drugs* by Trissel; see bibliography) for more specific information.

Pharmacology - Bleomycin is an antibiotic that has activity against a variety of gram-negative and gram-positive bacteria as well as some fungi. While its cytotoxicity prevents it from being clinically useful as an antimicrobial, it is useful against a variety of tumors in small animals. Its exact mechanism of action is unknown, but it is possible it inhibits the incorporation of thymi-dine into DNA. Bleomycin also appears to labilize DNA, thereby splitting both single stranded and double stranded DNA.

Uses/Indications - Bleomycin has been used as adjunctive treatment of lymphomas, squamous cell carcinomas, teratomas, and nonfunctional thyroid tumors in both dogs and cats.

Pharmacokinetics - Bleomycin is not appreciably absorbed from the gut and thus must be ad-ministered parenterally. It is mainly distributed to the lungs, kidneys, skin, lymphatics and peri-toneum. In patients with normal renal function, terminal half life is about 2 hours. In humans, 60-70% of a dose is excreted as active drug in the urine.

Contraindications/Precautions/Reproductive Safety - Because bleomycin is a toxic drug with a low therapeutic index, it should be used only by those with the facilities to actively monitor the patient and deal with potential complications. The drug should be used very cautiously in pa-tients with significant renal insufficiency or pulmonary disease (not due to tumor). Bleomycin can be teratogenic, it should only be used in pregnant animals when the owners accept the asso-ciated risks.

Adverse Effects/Warnings - Toxicity falls into two broad categories: acute and delayed. Acute toxicities include fever, anorexia, vomiting, and allergic reactions (including anaphylaxis). Delayed toxic effects include dermatologic effects (*e.g.*, alopecia, rashes, etc.), stomatitis, pneumonitis and pulmonary fibrosis. These latter two effects have been associated with drug induced fatalities. Unlike many other antineoplastics, bleomycin does not usually cause bone marrow toxicity, but thrombocytopenia, leukopenia and slight decreases in hemoglobin levels are possible. Renal and hepatotoxicity are also potentially possible.

Overdosage/Acute Toxicity - No specific information located. Because of the toxicity of the drug, it is important to determine dosages carefully.

Drug Interactions - Use of **general anesthetics** in patients treated previously with bleomycin should be exercised with caution. Bleomycin sensitizes lung tissue to oxygen (even to concentrations of inspired oxygen considered to be safe) and rapid deterioration of pulmonary function with post-operative pulmonary fibrosis can occur. **Prior chemotherapy** with other agents **or radiation therapy** can lead to increased hematologic, mucosal and pulmonary toxicities with bleomycin therapy. There are some reports that **digoxin** or **phenytoin** serum levels may be decreased by combination chemotherapy; the significance of these interactions are in question.

Doses - (Note: Refer to specific treatment protocols for more information)
Small Animals:

> For squamous cell carcinomas, lymphomas and other carcinomas: 10 U/m^2 IV or SubQ once daily for 3-4 doses, then 10 U/m^2 every 7 days. Maximum accumulative dose: 200 U/m^2. (Jacobs, Lumsden et al. 1992)

Monitoring Parameters - 1) Efficacy; 2) Pulmonary Toxicity: Obtain chest films, (baseline and on a regular basis—in humans they are recommended q1-2 weeks); lung auscultation (dyspnea and fine rales are early signs of toxicity). Other pulmonary function tests are recommended in humans, but are unlikely to be available in veterinary medicine. 3) Blood chemistry (encompassing renal and hepatic function markers) and hematologic profiles (CBC) may be useful to monitor potential renal, hepatic and hematologic toxicities.

Client Information - Clients must be informed of the potential toxicities associated with therapy and urged to report any change in pulmonary function (*e.g.*, shortness of breath, wheezing) immediately.

Dosage Forms/Preparations/FDA Approval Status/Withholding Times -
Veterinary-Approved Products: None
Human-Approved Products:

Bleomycin Powder for Injection 15 & 30 units per vial; *Blenoxane* ®(MSD) (Rx)

BOLDENONE UNDECYLENATE

Chemistry - An injectable anabolic steroid derived from testosterone, boldenone undecylenate has a chemical name of 17 beta-hydroxyandrosta-1,4-dien-3-one. The commercially available product is in a sesame oil vehicle. It may also be known by the name boldenone undecenoate or in the U.K. by the trade name, *Vebonol*® (Ciba-Geigy).

Storage/Stability/Compatibility - Boldenone injection should be stored at room temperature; avoid freezing. Because it is in an oil vehicle, it should not be physically mixed with any other medications.

Pharmacology - In the presence of adequate protein and calories, anabolic steroids promote body tissue building processes and can reverse catabolism. As these agents are either derived from or are closely related to testosterone, the anabolics have varying degrees of androgenic effects. Endogenous testosterone release may be suppressed by inhibiting lutenizing hormone (LH). Large doses can impede spermatogenesis by negative feedback inhibition of FSH.

Anabolic steroids can also stimulate erythropoiesis. The mechanism for this effect may occur by stimulating erythropoeitic stimulating factor. Anabolics can cause nitrogen, sodium, potassium and phosphorus retention and decrease the urinary excretion of calcium.

Uses/Indications - Boldenone is labeled for use as adjunctive therapy "... as an aid for treating debilitated horses when an improvement in weight, haircoat, or general physical condition is desired" (*Equipoise*® package insert—Solvay).

Pharmacokinetics - No specific information was located for this agent. It is considered to be a long-acting anabolic, with effects persisting for up to 8 weeks. It is unknown if the anabolic agents cross into milk.

Contraindications/Precautions - The manufacturer (Solvay) recommends not using the drug on stallions or pregnant mares. Other clinicians state the that anabolic steroids should not be used in either stallions or non-pregnant mares intended for reproduction. Boldenone should not be administered to horses intended for food purposes.

In humans, anabolic agents are also contraindicated in patients with hepatic dysfunction, hypercalcemia, patients with a history of myocardial infarction (can cause hypercholesterolemia), pituitary insufficiency, prostate carcinoma, in selected patients with breast carcinoma, benign prostatic hypertrophy and during the nephrotic stage of nephritis.

The anabolic agents are category X (risk of use outweighs any possible benefit) agents for use in pregnancy and are contraindicated because of possible fetal masculinization.

Adverse Effects/Warnings - In the manufacturer's (*Equipoise*®—Solvay) package insert, only androgenic (overaggressiveness) effects are listed. However, in work reported in both stallions and mares (Squires and McKinnon 1987), boldenone caused a detrimental effect in testis size, sperm production and quality in stallions. In mares, the drug caused fewer total and large follicles, smaller ovaries, increased clitoral size, shortened estrus duration, reduced pregnancy rates and severely altered sexual behavior.

Although not reported in horses, anabolic steroids have the potential to cause hepatic toxicity.

Overdosage - No information was located for this specific agent. In humans, sodium and water retention can occur after overdosage of anabolic steroids. It is suggested to treat supportively and monitor liver function should an inadvertent overdose be administered.

Drug Interactions - No drug interactions were located for boldenone specifically. Anabolic agents as a class may potentiate the effects of **anticoagulants**. Monitoring of PT's and dosage adjustment, if necessary, of the anticoagulant are recommended.

Diabetic patients receiving **insulin**, may need dosage adjustments if anabolic therapy is added or discontinued. Anabolics may decrease blood glucose and decrease insulin requirements.

Anabolics may enhance the edema that can be associated with **ACTH** or **adrenal steroid** therapy.

Drug/Laboratory Interactions - Concentrations of **protein bound iodine (PBI)** can be decreased in patients receiving androgen/anabolic therapy, but the clinical significance of this is probably not important. Androgen/anabolic agents can decrease amounts of **thyroxine-binding globulin** and decrease **total T4** concentrations and increase **resin uptake of T3 and T4**. Free thyroid hormones are unaltered and clinically, there is no evidence of dysfunction.

Both **creatinine** and **creatine excretion** can be decreased by anabolic steroids. Anabolic steroids can increase the urinary excretion of **17-ketosteroids**.

Androgenic/anabolic steroids may alter **blood glucose** levels. Androgenic/anabolic steroids may suppress **clotting factors II, V, VII, and X**. Anabolic agents can affect **liver function tests** (BSP retention, SGOT, SGPT, bilirubin, and alkaline phosphatase).

Doses -
  Horses:
        a) 1.1 mg/kg IM; may repeat in 3 week intervals (most horses will respond with one or two treatments) (Package Insert; *Equipoise*®—Solvay)
        b) 1 mg/kg IM; repeated at 3 week intervals (Robinson 1987)

Monitoring Parameters -
    1) Androgenic side effects
    2) Fluid and electrolyte status, if indicated
    3) Liver function tests if indicated
    4) Red blood cell count, indices, if indicated
    5) Weight, appetite

Client Information - Because of the potential for abuse of anabolic steroids by humans, many states have included, or are considering including this agent as a controlled drug. It should be kept in a secure area and out of the reach of children.

Dosage Forms/Preparations/FDA Approval Status/Withholding Times -
  Veterinary-Approved Products:
    Boldenone Undecylenate for Injection 25 mg/ml in 10 ml vials; 50 mg/ml in 10 ml & 50 ml vials; *Equipoise*® (Fort Dodge); (Rx) Approved for use in horses not to be used for food.

  Human-Approved Products: None

BROMIDES
POTASSIUM BROMIDE
SODIUM BROMIDE

Chemistry - Potassium bromide occurs as white, odorless, cubical crystals or crystalline powder. One gram will dissolve in 1.5 ml of water. Potassium bromide contains 67.2% bromide. Each gram contains 8.4 mEq (mmol) of potassium and bromide.

Sodium bromide occurs as white, odorless, cubic crystals or granular powder. One gram will dissolve in 1.2 ml of water. Sodium bromide contains 77.7% bromide.

Storage/Stability/Compatibility - Store in tight containers. Bromides can precipitate out alkaloids in solution. Mixing with strong oxidizing agents can liberate bromine. Metal salts can precipitate solutions containing bromides. Sodium bromide is hygroscopic; potassium bromide is not.

Pharmacology - Bromide's anti-seizure activity is thought to be the result of its generalized depressant effects on neuronal excitability and activity. Bromide ions compete with chloride transport across cell membranes resulting in membrane hyperpolarization, thereby raising seizure threshold and limiting the spread of epileptic discharges.

Uses/Indications - Bromides are used as adjunctive therapy to control seizures in dogs who are not adequately controlled by phenobarbital (or primidone) alone. In patients suffering from phenobarbital (or primidone) hepatotoxicity, bromides may be used alone (renally excreted). Early indications are that approximately 50% of dogs show improvement in seizure control after the addition of bromides.

Pharmacokinetics - Bromides are well absorbed after oral administration, primarily in the small intestine. Bromide is distributed in the extracellular fluid and mimics the volume of distribution of chloride (0.2-0.4 L/Kg). It is not bound to plasma proteins and readily enters the CSF (in dogs: 87% of serum concentration; in humans: 37%). Bromides enter maternal milk (see reproductive safety below). Bromides are principally excreted by the kidneys. The half life in dogs has been reported to be about 25 days; in humans, 12 days.

Contraindications/Precautions/Reproductive Safety - Older animals and those with additional diseases, may be prone to intolerance (see side effects below) at blood levels that are easily tolerable by younger, more healthy dogs.

Reproductive safety has not been established. Human infants have suffered bromide intoxication and growth retardation after maternal ingestion of bromides during pregnancy. Bromide intoxication has also been reported in human infants breast feeding from mothers taking bromides.

Adverse Effects/Warnings - A transient sedation (lasting up to 3 weeks) is commonly seen in dogs receiving bromides in addition to phenobarbital. Toxicity generally presents as profound sedation to stupor, ataxia, tremors, or other CNS manifestations. Pancreatitis has been reported in dogs receiving combination therapy of bromides with either primidone or phenobarbital. However, since this effect has been reported with both primidone and phenobarbital, its relationship with bromide is unknown. Additional potential adverse effects reported include, anorexia, vomiting, and constipation. Rashes have been reported in humans taking bromides.

If administering an oral loading dose of potassium bromide, acute GI upset may occur if given too rapidly. Potentially, large loading doses could affect serum potassium levels in patients receiving potassium bromide.

Overdosage/Acute Toxicity - Toxicity is more likely with chronic overdoses, but acute overdoses are a possibility. In addition to the adverse effects noted above, animals who have developed bromism (whether acute or chronic) may develop signs of muscle pain, conscious proprioceptive deficits, anisocoria, and hyporeflexia.

Standard gut removal techniques should be employed after a known acute overdose. Death after an acute oral ingestion is apparently rare, as vomition generally occurs spontaneously. Administration of parenteral or oral sodium chloride, parenteral glucose and diuretics (*e.g.*, furosemide) may be helpful in reducing bromide loads in either acutely or chronically intoxicated individuals.

Drug Interactions - Bromide toxicity can occur if chloride ion ingestion is markedly reduced. Patients put on low **salt** diets may be at risk. Conversely, additional sodium chloride in the diet could reduce serum bromide levels, affecting seizure control. Because bromides can cause sedation, other **CNS sedating drugs** may cause additive sedation. **Diuretics** may enhance the excretion of bromides thereby affecting dosage requirements.

Laboratory Considerations - See drug interactions above regarding chloride.

Doses - Because of the extraordinarily long serum half life in dogs (it may take up to 4-5 months for blood levels to reach steady state), some dosing regimens include an initial oral bolus loading dose to reduce this time period. Whether to load or not is still a controversial issue. Apparently the majority of clinicians using bromides at this time do not routinely load and achieve efficacy in many dogs long before serum steady-state is reached. If, however, reaching a sustainable "therapeutic" level with rapidity is important, loading should be considered.

  Dogs:
    a) For adjunctive therapy (with either phenobarbital or primidone) of refractory seizures: 30 - 40 mg/kg PO daily of potassium bromide (either as capsules or dissolved in water). Elevated plasma concentrations may be obtained earlier by giving double or

triple the above dose the first day of therapy. Adjust dosage by monitoring adverse effects, efficacy and serum levels. (Schwartz-Porsche 1992)

b) For seizures: Loading dose: 400 mg/kg/day divided *bid* for 2-3 days, the go to maintenance dose. Maintenance dose: 22 - 30 mg/kg/day if concurrently using phenobarbital; 70-80 mg/kg/day as a single agent. Suggested therapeutic blood levels: 1 - 1.5 mg/ml. May take several weeks to attain therapeutic levels. (Neer 1994)

Monitoring Parameters - 1) Efficacy/Toxicity; 2) Serum Levels; "Normal" therapeutic levels in dogs probably range from 0.5 - 2.0 mg/ml. Most dogs can tolerate levels of at least 1.5 mg/ml and some younger, otherwise healthy dogs can tolerate levels of up to 2.5 mg/ml.

Client Information - Clients must be committed to administering doses of anticonvulsant medications on a regular basis. Lack of good compliance with dosing regimens is a major cause of therapeutic failures with anti-seizure medications. Clients should also understand and accept that this treatment involves using a non-approved "drug" Dose measurements of bromide solutions should be done with a needle-less syringe or other accurate measuring device. The dose may either be sprinkled on the dog's food (assuming he/she consumes it entirely) or squirted in the side of the mouth. Toxic effects (*e.g.*, profound sedation, ataxia, stupor, GI effects) should be explained to the owner and if they occur, owners should report them.

Dosage Forms/Preparations/FDA Approval Status/Withholding Times -
 Veterinary-Labeled or Human-Approved Products: None.
Neither potassium or sodium bromide are available in approved dosage forms in North America. Reagent grade or USP grade may be obtained from various chemical supply houses to compound an acceptable oral product. If purchasing a reagent grade, specify American Chemical Society (ACS) grade. At a concentration of 250 mg/ml (25 grams of potassium/sodium bromide *qs ad* to 100 ml distilled water), both sodium and potassium bromide dissolve easily in water. Flavoring agents are not usually necessary for patient acceptance.

BROMOCRIPTINE MESYLATE

Chemistry - A dopamine agonist and prolactin inhibitor, bromocriptine mesylate is a semisynthetic ergot alkaloid derivative. It occurs as a yellowish-white powder and is slightly soluble in water and sparingly soluble in alcohol. Bromocriptine mesylate may also be known as bromocryptine, Brom-ergocryptine, or 2-Bromergocryptine.

Storage/Stability/Compatibility - Tablets and capsules should be protected from light and stored in tight containers at temperatures less than 25°C.

Pharmacology - Bromocriptine exhibits multiple pharmacologic actions. It inhibits prolactin release from the anterior pituitary thereby reducing serum prolactin. The mechanism for this action is by a direct effect on the pituitary and/or stimulating postsynaptic dopamine receptors in the hypothalamus to cause release of prolactin-inhibitory factor. Bromocriptine also activates dopaminergic receptors in the neostriatum of the brain.

Uses/Indications - Bromocriptine may potentially be of benefit in treating acromegaly/pituitary adenomas or pseudopregnancy in a variety of species. However, because of adverse effects, its potential value for treating hyperadrenocorticism in dogs is low.

Pharmacokinetics - In humans, only about 28% of a bromocriptine dose is absorbed from the gut and due to a high first-pass effect only about 6% reaches the systemic circulation. Distribution characteristics are not well described, but in humans it is highly protein bound (90-96%) to serum albumin. Bromocriptine is metabolized by the liver to inactive and non-toxic metabolites. It has a biphasic half life; the alpha phase is about 4 hours and the terminal phase is about 15 hours (Note: one source says 45-50 hours).

Contraindications/Precautions/Reproductive Safety - Bromocriptine is generally contraindicated in patients with hypertension. It should be used with caution in patients with hepatic disease as metabolism of the drug may be reduced. Usage during pregnancy is contraindicated, although documented teratogenicity has not been established. Because bromocriptine interferes with lactation, it should not be used in animals who are nursing.

Adverse Effects/Warnings - Bromocriptine may cause a plethora of adverse effects which are usually dose related and minimized with dosage reduction. Some more likely possibilities include: gastrointestinal effects (nausea, vomiting), nervous system effects (sedation, fatigue, etc.), and hypotension (particularly with the first dose, but it may persist).

Overdosage/Acute Toxicity - Overdosage may cause vomiting, severe nausea, and profound hypotension. Standardized gut removal techniques should be employed when applicable and cardiovascular support instituted as needed.

Drug Interactions - If using bromocriptine for serum prolactin reduction: **butyrophenones** (*e.g.*, haloperidol, azaperone), **amitriptyline, phenothiazines, & reserpine** may increase prolactin concentrations and bromocriptine doses may need to be increased. **Estrogens** or **progestins** may interfere with the effects of bromocriptine. When used with other **antihypertensive drugs**, hypotensive effects may be additive. Although no conclusive evidence exists, use of bromocriptine and **ergot alkaloids** is not recommended. Some human patients receiving both have developed severe hypertension and myocardial infarction. Use with **alcohol** may cause a disulfiram-type reaction.

Doses -
  Dogs:
    For treatment of pseudopregnancy:
      a) 10 micrograms/kg PO for 10 days or 30 micrograms/kg for 16 days. If vomiting is a problem, may treat with metoclopramide. (Janssens 1986)

  Horses:
    For treatment of pituitary adenoma:
      a) 5 mg IM q12h. To prepare an injectable formulation for IM use from oral dosage forms: Bromocriptine mesylate 70 mg is added to 7 ml of a solution of 80% normal saline and 20% absolute alcohol (v/v). Final concentration is 1% (10 mg/ml). (Beck 1992)

Monitoring Parameters - Monitoring is dependent upon the reason for use to evaluate efficacy. However, blood pressures should be evaluated if patients have symptoms associated with hypotension.

Client Information - Have client administer drug with food to reduce GI adverse effects.

Dosage Forms/Preparations/FDA Approval Status/Withholding Times -
  Veterinary-Approved Products: None
  Human-Approved Products:

    Bromocriptine mesylate 5 mg (of bromocriptine) Capsules; *Parlodel*® (Sandoz); Rx

    Bromocriptine mesylate 2.5 mg (of bromocriptine) Tablets; *Parlodel*® *Snaptabs* (Sandoz); Rx

BUPRENORPHINE HCL

Chemistry - A thebaine derivative, buprenorphine is a synthetic partial opiate agonist. It occurs as a white, crystalline powder with a solubility of 17 mg/ml in water and 42 mg/ml in alcohol. The commercially available injectable product (*Buprenex*® - Norwich Eaton) has a pH of 3.5-5 and is a sterile solution of the drug dissolved in D5W. Terms of potency are expressed in terms of buprenorphine. The commercial product contains 0.324 mg/ml of buprenorphine HCl, which is equivalent to 0.3 mg/ml of buprenorphine.

Storage/Stability/Compatibility - Buprenorphine should be stored at room temperature (15-30° C). Temperatures above 40° C or below freezing should be avoided. Buprenorphine products should be stored away from bright light. Autoclaving may decrease drug potency considerably. The drug is stable between a pH of 3.5-5.

Buprenorphine is reported to be **compatible** with the following IV solutions and drugs: acepromazine, atropine, diphenhydramine, D5W, D5W & normal saline, droperidol, glycopyrrolate, hydroxyzine, lactated Ringer's, normal saline, scopolamine, and xylazine. Buprenorphine is reportedly **incompatible** with diazepam and lorazepam.

Pharmacology - Buprenorphine has partial agonist activity at the *mu* receptor. This is in contrast to pentazocine which acts as an antagonist at the *mu* receptor. Buprenorphine is considered to be 30 times as potent as morphine and exhibits many of the same actions as the opiate agonists; it produces a dose-related analgesia. It appears to have a high affinity for *mu* receptors in the CNS, which may explain its relatively long duration of action.

The cardiovascular effects of buprenorphine may cause a decrease in both blood pressure and cardiac rate. Rarely, human patients may exhibit increases in blood pressure and cardiac rate. Respiratory depression is a possibility, and decreased respiratory rates have been noted in horses treated with buprenorphine. Gastrointestinal effects appear to be minimal with buprenorphine, but further studies are needed to clarify this.

Pharmacokinetics - Buprenorphine is rapidly absorbed following IM injection, with 40-90% absorbed systemically when tested in humans. The drug is also absorbed sublingually (bioavailability≈55%) in people. Oral doses appear to undergo a high first-pass effect with metabolism occurring in the GI mucosa and liver.

The distribution of the drug has not been well studied. Data from work done in rats reflects that buprenorphine concentrates in the liver, but is also found in the brain, GI tract, and placenta. It is highly bound (96%) to plasma proteins (not albumin), crosses the placenta, and it (and metabolites) are found in maternal milk at concentrations equal to or greater than those found in plasma.

Buprenorphine is metabolized in the liver by N-dealkylation and glucuronidation. These metabolites are then eliminated by biliary excretion into the feces ($\approx$70%) and urinary excretion ($\approx$27%).

In the horse, onset of action is approximately 15 minutes after IV dosing. The peak effect occurs in 30-45 minutes and the duration of action may last up to 8 hours. Because acepromazine exhibits a similar onset and duration of action, many clinicians favor using this drug in combination with buprenorphine in the horse.

Uses/Indications - Because buprenorphine is a relatively new addition to the pharmacologic armamentarium, present indications appear to be limited to its use in horses as a neuroleptanalgesic (when used in combination with either acepromazine or xylazine) and as an analgesic in dogs and cats.

Contraindications/Precautions - All opiates should be used with caution in patients with hypothyroidism, severe renal insufficiency, adrenocortical insufficiency (Addison's), and in geriatric or severely debilitated patients.

Rarely, patients may develop respiratory depression from buprenorphine, it therefore should be used cautiously in patients with compromised cardiopulmonary function. Like other opiates, buprenorphine must be used with extereme caution in patients with head trauma, increased CSF pressure or other CNS dysfunction (*e.g.,* coma).

Patients with severe hepatic dysfunction may eliminate the drug more slowly than normal patients. Buprenorphine may increase bile duct pressure and should be used cautiously in patients with biliary tract disease.

Although no controlled studies have been performed in domestic animals or humans, the drug has exhibited no evidence of teratogenicity or of causing impaired fertility in laboratory animals.

The drug is contraindicated in patients having known hypersensitivity to it.

Adverse Effects/Warnings - Although rare, respiratory depression appears to be the major adverse effect to monitor with this agent, but because it has only recently been used in veterinary medicine, other adverse effects may be noted. The primary side effect seen in humans is sedation with an incidence of approximately 66%.

Overdosage - The intraperitoneal LD$_{50}$ of buprenorphine has been reported to be 243 mg/kg in rats. The ratio of lethal dose to effective dose is at least 1000:1 in rodents. Because of the apparent high index of safety, acute overdoses should be a rare event in veterinary medicine. In such a case however, treatment with naloxone and doxapram has been suggested in cases with respiratory or cardiac effects. High doses of nalaxone may be required to treat respiratory depression should it occur.

Drug Interactions - Other **CNS depressants** (*e.g.,* anesthetic agents, antihistamines, phenothiazines, barbiturates, tranquilizers, alcohol, etc.) may cause increased CNS or respiratory depression when used with buprenorphine. Buprenorphine may decrease the analgesic effects of the **opiate agonists** (morphine, etc.).

Pancuronium if used with buprenorphine may cause increased conjunctival changes.

Buprenorphine is contraindicated in human patients receiving **monamine oxidase (MOA) inhibitors** (rarely used in veterinary medicine) for at least 14 days after receiving MOA inhibitors in humans. One study done in rabbits did not demonstrate any appreciable interaction, however.

Local anesthetics (mepivicaine, bupivicaine) may be potentiated by concomitant use of buprenorphine.

Doses -
Horses:
    For neuroleptanalgesia:
        a) 0.004 mg/kg IV (given with acepromazine 0.02 mg/kg) (Thurmon and Benson 1987)
        b) 0.006 mg/kg IV (given with xylazine 0.07 mg/kg) (Thurmon and Benson 1987)
Rabbits/Rodents:
    As an analgesic (for control of acute or chronic visceral pain):
        a) Rabbits: 0.02 - 0.05 mg/kg SubQ or IM q6-12h; 0.5 mg/kg per rectum q12h
            Rodents: 0.1 - 3 mg/kg IM or SubQ q6-12h (Huerkamp 1995)

Monitoring Parameters -
    1) Analgesic efficacy
    2) Respiratory status
    3) Cardiac status

Client Information - This agent should be used in an inpatient setting or with direct professional supervision.

Dosage Forms/Preparations/FDA Approval Status/Withholding Times -
  Veterinary-Approved Products: None
  Human-Approved Products:
    Buprenorphine HCl for Injection: 0.324 mg/ml (equivalent to 0.3 mg/ml buprenorphine); 1 ml ampules; *Buprenex®* (Reckitt & Colman); (Rx)

BUSPIRONE HCL

Chemistry - An arylpiperazine derivative anxiolytic agent, buspirone HCl differs structurally from the benzodiazepines. It occurs as a white, crystalline powder with solubilities at 25°C of 865 mg/ml in water and about 20 mg/ml in alcohol.

Storage/Stability/Compatibility - Buspirone HCl tablets should be stored in tight, light-resistant containers at room temperature. After manufacture, buspirone tablets have an expiration date of 36 months.

Pharmacology - Buspirone is an anxioselective agent. Unlike the benzodiazepines, buspirone does not possess any anticonvulsant or muscle relaxant activity and little sedative or psychomotor impairment activity. The mechanism for buspirone's anxiolytic action is not well understood, but it does not appear to share the same mechanisms as the benzodiazepines (does not have significant affinity for benzodiazepine receptors and does not affect GABA binding). Buspirone has a high affinity for serotonin receptors in the CNS, but the role it plays is not well understood. Buspirone appears to have mixed agonist/antagonist properties on dopaminergic receptors.

Uses/Indications - Buspirone may be effective in treating certain behavior disorders in dogs and cats; principally those that are fear/phobia related.

Pharmacokinetics - In humans, buspirone is rapidly and completely absorbed, but a high first pass effect limits systemic bioavailability to approximately 5%. Binding to plasma proteins is very high (95%). In rats, highest tissue concentrations are found in the lungs, kidneys, and fat. Lower levels are found in the brain, heart, skeletal muscle, plasma and liver. Both buspirone and its metabolites are distributed into maternal milk. The elimination half-life (in humans) is about 2-4 hours. Buspirone is hepatically metabolized to several metabolites (including one that is active: 1-PP). These metabolites are excreted primarily in the urine.

Contraindications/Precautions/Reproductive Safety - Buspirone should be used with caution with either significant renal or hepatic disease. While buspirone has far less sedating properties than many other like drugs, it should potentially be used in caution in working dogs. While the drug has not been proven to be safe during pregnancy, doses of up to 30 times the labeled dosage in rabbits and rats demonstrated no teratogenic effects.

Adverse Effects/Warnings - Adverse effects are usually minimal with buspirone and it is generally well tolerated. The most likely adverse effect profile seen with buspirone includes dizziness, headache, nausea/anorexia, and restlessness. Other neurologic effects (including sedation) may be noted. Rarely, tachycardias and other cardiovascular symptoms may be present.

Overdosage/Acute Toxicity - Limited information is available. The oral LD_{50} in dogs is: 586 mg/kg. Oral overdoses may produce vomiting, dizziness, drowsiness, miosis and gastric distention. Standard overdose protocols should be followed after ingestion has been determined.

Drug Interactions - **Food** may decrease the rate of absorption, but reduce the first pass metabolism of the drug with a net increase in area under the curve. The clinical significance of this interaction is not thought to be significant and the manufacturer recommends dosing without regard to food. Use of **monoamine oxidase inhibitors** (rarely used in veterinary medicine), including **furazolidone**, with use of buspirone is not recommended because dangerous hypertension may occur.

Doses -
  Dogs:
        For low grade anxieties and fears: 2.5 - 10 mg per dog PO *bid-tid*; must be given every day. In highly fearful situations, may be more effective if combined with either acepromazine or diazepam. (Marder 1991)
  Cats:
      For low grade anxieties and fears:
        a) 2.5 - 15 mg per cat PO *bid-tid*. (Marder 1991)
        b) Initially 2.5 mg per cat *bid* (Kinosian 1994)

Monitoring Parameters - Efficacy & adverse effect profiles.

Dosage Forms/Preparations/FDA Approval Status/Withholding Times -
  Veterinary-Approved Products: None
  Human-Approved Products:
    Buspirone HCl Scored Tablets 5 mg and 10 mg; *BuSpar®* (Mead Johnson); (Rx)

BUSULFAN

Chemistry - An alkylsulfonate antineoplastic agent, busulfan occurs as white, crystalline powder. It is slightly soluble in alcohol and very slightly soluble in water.

Storage/Stability/Compatibility - Busulfan tablets should be stored in well-closed containers at room temperature.

Pharmacology - Busulfan is a bifunctional alkylating agent antineoplastic and is cell cycle-phase nonspecific. The exact mechanism of action has not been determined, but is thought to be due to its alkylating, cross-linking of strands of DNA and myelosuppressive properties. Busulfan's primary activity is against cells of the granulocytic series.

Uses/Indications - Busulfan may be useful in the adjunctive therapy of chronic granulocytic leukemias in small animals.

Pharmacokinetics - Busulfan is well absorbed after oral administration. Distribution characteristics are not well described and it is unknown whether the drug enters the CSF, brain or maternal milk. Busulfan is rapidly hepatically metabolized to at least 12 different metabolites that are slowly excreted into the urine. In humans, serum half life of busulfan averages about 2.5 hours.

Contraindications/Precautions/Reproductive Safety - Busulfan is contraindicated in patients who have shown resistance to the drug in the past. It should only be used by veterinarians with the experience and resources to monitor the toxicity of this agent. The risk versus benefits of therapy must be carefully considered in patients with preexisting bone marrow depression or concurrent infections. Additive bone marrow depression may occur in patients undergoing concomitant radiation therapy.

Busulfan's teratogenic potential has not been well documented, but it is mutagenic in mice and may potentially cause a variety of fetal abnormalities. It is generally recommended to avoid the drug during pregnancy, but because of the seriousness of the diseases treated with busulfan, the potential benefits to the mother must be considered.

Adverse Effects/Warnings - The most commonly associated adverse effect seen with busulfan therapy is myelosuppression. In humans, anemia, leukopenia, and thrombocytopenia may all be noted. Onset of leukopenia is generally 10 to 15 days after initiation of therapy and leukocyte nadirs occurring on average around 11-30 days. Severe bone marrow depression can result in pancytopenia that may take months to years for recovery. In humans, bronchopulmonary dysplasia with pulmonary fibrosis, uric acid nephropathy, and stomatitis have been reported. These effects are more uncommon and generally associated with chronic, higher dose therapy.

Overdosage/Acute Toxicity - There is limited experience with busulfan overdoses. The LD50 in mice is 120 mg/kg. Chronic overdosage is more likely to cause serious bone marrow suppression, than is an acute overdose. However, any overdose, should be treated seriously with standard gut emptying protocols used when appropriate and supportive therapy initiated when required. There is no known specific antidote for busulfan intoxication.

Drug Interactions - Concurrent use with other **bone marrow depressant medications** may result in additive myelosuppression. **Thioguanine** and busulfan used concomitantly may result in hepatotoxicity.

Laboratory Considerations - Busulfan may raise serum **uric acid** levels. Drugs such as allopurinol may be required to control hyperuricemia.

Doses -
 Small Animals:
> For chronic granulocytic leukemias (not during "blastic" phase—of no benefit): 3 -4
> mg/m^2 PO once daily. Discontinue when total white blood cell count reaches approximately 15,000. Repeat as necessary. May require up to two weeks to observe a positive response. If there is too rapid a decline in total WBC's, discontinue drug. (Jacobs, Lumsden et al. 1992)

Monitoring Parameters - 1) CBC; 2) Serum uric acid; 3) Efficacy

Client Information - Clients must understand the importance of both administering busulfan as directed and to report immediately any signs associated with toxicity (*e.g.*, abnormal bleeding, bruising, urination, depression, infection, shortness of breath, etc.).

Dosage Forms/Preparations/FDA Approval Status/Withholding Times -
 Veterinary-Approved Products: None
 Human-Approved Products:
 Busulfan Oral Tablets (scored) 2 mg; *Myleran*® (Glaxo Wellcome); (Rx)

BUTORPHANOL TARTRATE

Chemistry - A synthetic opiate partial agonist, butorphanol tartrate is related structurally to morphine but exhibits pharmacologic actions similar to other partial agonists such as pentazocine or nalbuphine. The compound occurs as a white, crystalline powder that is sparingly soluble in water and insoluble in alcohol. It has a bitter taste and a pK_a of 8.6. The commercial injection has a pH of 3-5.5. One mg of the tartrate is equivalent to 0.68 mg of butorphanol base.

Storage/Stability/Compatibility - The injectable product should be stored out of bright light and at room temperature; avoid freezing.

The injectable product is reported to be **compatible** with the following IV fluids and drugs: acepromazine, atropine sulfate, chlorpromazine, diphenhydramine HCl, droperidol, fentanyl citrate, hydroxyzine HCl, meperidine, morphine sulfate, pentazocine lactate, perphenazine, prochlorperazine, promethazine HCl, scopolamine HBr, and xylazine.

The drug is reportedly **incompatible** with the following agents: dimenhydrinate, and pentobarbital sodium.

Pharmacology - Butorphanol is considered to be, on a weight basis, 4-7 times as potent an analgesic as morphine, 15-30 times as pentazocine, and 30-50 times as meperidine. Its agonist activity is thought to be exerted primarily at the *kappa* and *sigma* receptors and the analgesic actions at sites in the limbic system (sub-cortical level and spinal levels).

The antagonist potency of butorphanol is considered to be approximately 30 times that of pentazocine and 1/40th that of naloxone and will antagonize the effect of true agonists (*e.g.,* morphine, meperidine, oxymorphone).

Besides the analgesic qualities of butorphanol, it possesses significant antitussive activity. In dogs, butorphanol has been shown to elevate CNS respiratory center threshold to CO_2, but unlike opiate agonists, not depress respiratory center sensitivity. Butorphanol, unlike morphine, apparently does not cause histamine release in dogs. CNS depression may occur in dogs, while CNS excitation has been noted (usually at high doses) in horses and dogs.

Although possessing less cardiovascular effects than the classical opiate agonists, butorphanol can cause a decrease in cardiac rate secondary to increased parasympathetic tone and mild decreases in arterial blood pressures.

The risk of causing physical dependence seems to be minimal when butorphanol is used in veterinary patients.

Pharmacokinetics - Butorphanol is absorbed completely in the gut when administered orally, but because of a high first-pass effect only about 1/6th of the administered dose reaches the systemic circulation. The drug has also been shown to be completely absorbed following IM administration.

Butorphanol is well distributed, with highest levels (of the parent compound and metabolites) found in the liver, kidneys, and intestine. Concentrations in the lungs, endocrine tissues, spleen, heart, fat tissue and blood cells are also higher than those found in the plasma. Approximately 80% of the drug is bound to plasma proteins (human data). Butorphanol will cross the placenta and neonatal plasma levels have been roughly equivalent to maternal levels. The drug is also distributed into maternal milk.

Butorphanol is metabolized in the liver, primarily by hydroxylation. Other methods of metabolism include N-dealkylation and conjugation. The metabolites of butorphanol do not exhibit any analgesic activity. These metabolites and the parent compound are mainly excreted into the urine (only 5% is excreted unchanged), but 11-14% of a dose is excreted into the bile and eliminated with the feces.

Following IV doses in horses, the onset of action is approximately 3 minutes with a peak analgesic effect at 15-30 minutes. The duration of action in horses may be up to 4 hours after a single dose.

Uses/Indications - Approved indication for dogs is "for the relief of chronic non-productive cough associated with tracheobronchitis, tracheitis, tonsillitis, laryngitis and pharyngitis originating from inflammatory conditions of the upper respiratory tract" (Package Insert; *Torbutrol*® — Fort Dodge). It is also used in practice in both dogs and cats as a preanesthetic medication, analgesic, and as an antiemetic prior to cisplatin treatment.

The approved indication for horses is "for the relief of pain associated with colic in adult horses and yearlings" (Package Insert; *Torbugesic*® — Fort Dodge). It has also been used clinically as an analgesic in cattle, although published data is apparently lacking.

Contraindications/Precautions - All opiates should be used with caution in patients with hypothyroidism, severe renal insufficiency, adrenocortical insufficiency (Addison's), and in geriatric or severely debilitated patients.

Like other opiates, butorphanol must be used with extreme caution in patients with head trauma, increased CSF pressure or other CNS dysfunction (*e.g.,* coma).

The manufacturer states that butorphanol "should not be used in dogs with a history of liver disease", and because of its effects on suppressing cough, "it should not be used in conditions of the lower respiratory tract associated with copious mucous production." The drug should be used cautiously in dogs with heartworm disease as safety for butorphanol has not been established in these cases.

Although no controlled studies have been performed in domestic animals or humans, the drug has exhibited no evidence of teratogenicity or of causing impaired fertility in laboratory animals. The manufacturer, however, does not recommend its use in pregnant bitches, foals, weanlings (equine), and breeding horses.

The drug is contraindicated in patients having known hypersensitivity to it.

Adverse Effects/Warnings - Adverse effects reported in dogs include, sedation (occasionally), anorexia or diarrhea (rarely).

Adverse effects seen in horses (at usual doses) may include a transient ataxia and sedation. Although reported to have minimal effects, butorphanol has the potential to decrease intestinal motility. Horses may exhibit CNS excitement (tossing and jerking of head, increased ambulation, augmented avoidance response to auditory stimuli) if given high doses (0.2 mg/kg) IV rapidly. Very high doses IV (1 - 2 mg/kg) may lead to the development of nystagmus, salivation, seizures, hyperthermia and decreased GI motility. These effects are considered to be transitory in nature.

Overdosage - Acute life-threatening overdoses with butorphanol should be unlikely. The LD_{50} in dogs is reportedly 50 mg/kg. However, because butorphanol injection is available in two dosage strengths (0.5 mg/ml and 10 mg/ml) for veterinary use, the possibility exists that inadvertent overdoses may occur in small animals. It has been suggested that animals exhibiting symptoms of overdose (CNS effects, cardiovascular changes, and respiratory depression) be treated immediately with intravenous naloxone. Additional supportive measures (*e.g.,* fluids, O_2, vasopressor agents, & mechanical ventilation) may be required. Should seizures occur and persist, diazepam may used for control.

Drug Interactions - Other **CNS depressants** (*e.g.,* anesthetic agents, antihistamines, phenothiazines, barbiturates, tranquilizers, alcohol, etc.) may cause increased CNS or respiratory depression when used with butorphanol, dosage may need to be decreased.

Pancuronium if used with butorphanol may cause increased conjunctical changes.

Doses - Note: All doses are expressed in mg/kg of the <u>base</u> activity. If using the human product (*Stadol*®), 1 mg of tartrate salt = 0.68 mg base.

Dogs:
   As an antitussive:
     a) 0.055 - 0.11 mg/kg SQ q6-12h; treatment should not normally be required for longer than 7 days; or 0.55 mg/kg PO q6-12h; may increase dose to 1.1 mg/kg PO q6-12h (The oral doses correspond to one 5 mg tablet per 20 lbs. and 10 lbs. of body weight, respectively); treatment should not normally be required for longer than 7 days. (Package Insert; *Torbutrol*®; - Fort Dodge)
     b) 0.05 - 0.12 mg/kg PO *bid-tid* (Morgan 1988)
     c) 0.55 mg/kg PO q6h-12h (Ettinger and Barrett 1995)
   As an analgesic:
     a) 0.1 mg/kg IV or 0.4 mg/kg SQ, IM (Morgan 1988)
     b) 0.2 - 0.4 mg/kg q2-5h SQ, IM or IV (Jenkins 1987)
     c) 0.8 - 1.2 mg/kg SQ, IM or IV (Mandsager 1988)
     d) 1 mg per 4.54 kg (10 lbs.) of body weight PO q12h (Kemp 1994)
     e) 0.2 -0.8 mg/kg IV, IM or SubQ (Enos 1993)
   As a preanesthetic:
     a) 0.05 mg/kg IV or 0.4 mg/kg SQ, IM (Morgan 1988)
     b) 0.2 - 0.4 mg/kg IM (with acepromazine 0.02 - 0.04 mg/kg IM) (Reidesel)
   As an anti-emetic prior to cisplatin treatment:
     a) 0.4 mg/kg IM 1/2 hour prior to cisplatin infusion. (Klausner and Bell 1988)

Cats:
   As an analgesic:
     a) 0.1 mg/kg IV or 0.4 mg/kg SQ (Sawyer & Rech, 1987)
     b) 0.4 mg/kg q6h SQ (Jenkins 1987)
     c) 0.4 - 0.8 mg/kg SQ (Mandsager 1988)
     d) 1 mg per cat PO q12h (Kemp 1994)
   As a preanesthetic:
     a) 0.2 - 0.4 mg/kg IM (with glycopyrrolate 0.01 mg/kg IM & ketamine 4 - 10 mg/kg IM) (Reidesel)

Rabbits:
>As an analgesic (post-operative pain): 0.4 mg/kg SubQ q4-6h
>For surgical procedures (in combo with xylazine/ketamine): 0.1 mg/kg once IM or SubQ (Huerkamp 1995)

Cattle:
>As an analgesic for surgery in adult cattle:
>
>a) 20 - 30 mg IV (jugular) (may wish to pretreat with 10mg xylazine) (Powers 1985)

Horses:
>As an analgesic:
>
>a) 0.1 mg/kg IV q3-4h; not to exceed 48 hours (Package Insert; *Torbugesic®*; - Fort Dodge)
>b) 0.02 - 0.05 mg/kg IV (Muir 1987)
>c) 0.01 - 0.1 mg/kg IV (Thurmon and Benson 1987)
>d) 0.02 - 0.1 mg/kg IV; or 0.04 - 0.2 mg/kg IM q3-4h (combined with acepromazine or xylazine) (Orsini 1988)
>
>As a preanesthetic, outpatient surgery, or chemical restraint:
>
>a) 0.01 - 0.04 mg/kg IV (with xylazine 0.1 - 0.5 mg/kg IV) (Orsini 1988)
>
>As an antitussive:
>
>a) 0.02 mg/kg IM *bid-tid* (Orsini 1988)

Birds:
>a) 3 - 4 mg/kg IM. True analgesic effects unknown in avian species, but has no detrimental respiratory or cardiovascular effects. Mild motor deficits may be observed. (Wheler 1993)

Monitoring Parameters -
>1) Analgesic &/or antitussive efficacy
>2) Respiratory rate/depth
>3) Appetite/bowel function
>4) CNS effects

Client Information - Clients should report any significant changes in behavior, appetite, bowel or urinary function in their animals.

Dosage Forms/Preparations/FDA Approval Status/Withholding Times - Note: Butorphanol is a class IV controlled substance. The veterinary products (*Torbutrol®, Torbugesic®*) strengths are listed as base activity. The human product (*Stadol®*) strength is labeled as the tartrate salt.

Veterinary-Approved Products:
>Butorphanol Tartrate Injection; 0.5 mg/ml (activity as base) 10 ml vials; *Torbutrol®* (Fort-Dodge); (Rx) Approved for use in dogs.
>
>Butorphanol Tartrate Injection; 10 mg/ml (activity as base) 50 ml vials; *Torbugesic®* (Fort-Dodge); (Rx) Approved for use in horses not intended for food.
>
>Butorphanol Tartrate Tablets (Veterinary); 1 mg, 5 mg, & 10 mg (activity as base) tablets; bottles of 100; *Torbutrol®* (Fort-Dodge); (Rx) Approved for use in dogs.

Human-Approved Products:
>Butorphanol Tartrate Injection; 1 mg/ml (as tartrate salt; equivalent to 0.68 mg base) in 1 ml vials and 2 mg/ml (as tartrate salt) in 1, 2, & 10 ml vials; *Stadol®* (Mead Johnson); (Rx)
>
>Butorphanol Nasal Spray: 10 mg/ml (2.5 ml metered dose) *Stadol NS®* (Mead Johnson) (Rx)

CALCITONIN SALMON

Chemistry - A polypeptide hormone, calcitonin is a 32-amino acid polypeptide having a molecular weight of about 3600. Calcitonin is available commercially as either calcitonin human, or calcitonin salmon, both of which are synthetically prepared. Potency of calcitonin salmon is expressed in international units (IU). Calcitonin salmon is approximately 50X more potent than calcitonin human on a per weight basis..

Storage/Stability/Compatibility - Calcitonin salmon for injection should be stored in the refrigerator (2-8°C).

Pharmacology - Calcitonin has a multitude of physiologic effects. It principally acts on bone inhibiting osteoclastic bone resorption. By reducing tubular reabsorption of calcium, phosphate, sodium, magnesium, potassium and chloride it promotes their renal excretion. Calcitonin also increases jejunal secretion of water, sodium, potassium and chloride (not calcium).

Uses/Indications - In small animals, calcitonin has been used as adjunctive therapy to control hypercalcemia.

Pharmacokinetics - Calcitonin is destroyed in the gut after oral administration and therefore must be administered parenterally. In humans, the onset of effect after IV administration of calcitonin salmon is immediate. After IM or SubQ administration onset occurs within 15 minutes with maximal effects occurring in about 4 hours. Duration of action is 8-14 hours after IM or SubQ injection. The drug is thought to be rapidly metabolized by the kidneys, in the blood and in peripheral tissues.

Contraindications/Precautions/Reproductive Safety - Calcitonin is contraindicated in animals hypersensitive to it. Patients with a history of hypersensitivity to other proteins may be at risk. Young animals are reportedly up to 100 times more sensitive to calcitonin than are older animals (adults).

There is little information on the reproductive safety of calcitonin. However, it does not cross the placenta. Very high doses have decreased birth weights in laboratory animals, presumably due to the metabolic effects of the drug. Calcitonin has been shown to inhibit lactation.

Adverse Effects/Warnings - There is not a well documented adverse effect profile for calcitonin in domestic animals. Anorexia has been reported in one dog treated with calcitonin. The following effects are documented in humans and potentially could be seen in animals: diarrhea, anorexia, vomiting, swelling and pain at injection site, redness and peripheral paresthesias. Rarely, allergic reactions may occur. Tachyphylaxis (resistance to drug therapy with time) may occur in some dogs treated.

Overdosage/Acute Toxicity - Very limited data available. Nausea and vomiting have been reported after accidental overdose injections.

Drug Interactions - **Vitamin D analogs** and **calcium** products may interfere with the efficacy of calcitonin.

Doses -
Dogs:
For hypervitaminosis D (toxicity):
a) 4 - 6 IU/kg SubQ q12h to q8h (Carothers, Chew et al. 1994b)
b) In animals with severe hypercalcemia (>16 mg/dl) calcitonin may be beneficial when used in combination with furosemide, IV fluids, and prednisone. Initially, give 4 U/kg IV, followed by 4 - 8 U/kg SubQ once or twice daily (dose extrapolated from human information). (Carothers, Chew et al. 1994a)
Reptiles:
a) For hypercalcemia in Green iguanas in combination with fluid therapy: 1.5 IU/kg SubQ q8h for several weeks if necessary. (Gauvin 1993)

Monitoring Parameters - Serum Calcium

Dosage Forms/Preparations/FDA Approval Status/Withholding Times -
Veterinary-Approved Products: None
Human-Approved Products:
Calcitonin Salmon for Injection 200 IU/ml in 2 ml vials; *Calcimar*® (Rhone-Poulenc Rorer); *Micalcin*® (Sandoz); *Salmonine*® (Lennod); *Osteocalcin*® (Arcola); (Rx)
Calcitonin Salmon Nasal Spray: 200 IU/activation (0.09 ml/dose) (in 2 ml metered dose); *Miacalcin*® (Sandoz); (Rx)

Calcium EDTA — see Edetate Calcium Disodium

CALCIUM SALTS
CALCIUM GLUCONATE
CALCIUM GLUCEPTATE
CALCIUM CHLORIDE
CALCIUM LACTATE

Chemistry - Several different salts of calcium are available in various formulations. Calcium gluceptate and calcium chloride are freely soluble in water; calcium lactate is soluble in water; calcium gluconate and calcium glycerophosphate are sparingly soluble in water, and calcium phosphate and carbonate are insoluble in water. Calcium gluconate for injection has a pH of 6-8.2; calcium chloride for injection has a pH of 5.5-7.5; and calcium gluceptate for injection has a pH of 5.6-7.

Storage/Stability/Compatibility - Calcium gluconate tablets should be stored in well-closed containers at room temperature. Calcium lactate tablets should be stored in tight containers at room temperature. Calcium gluconate injection, calcium gluceptate injection, and calcium chloride injection should be stored at room temperature and protected from freezing.

Calcium chloride for injection is reportedly **compatible** with the following intravenous solutions and drugs: amikacin sulfate, ascorbic acid, bretylium tosylate, cephapirin sodium, chloramphenicol sodium succinate, dopamine HCl, hydrocortisone sodium succinate, isoproterenol HCl, lidocaine HCl, methicillin sodium, norepinephrine bitartrate, penicillin G potassium/sodium, pentobarbital sodium, phenobarbital sodium, sodium bicarbonate, verapamil HCl, and vitamin B-complex with C.

Calcium chloride for injection **compatibility information conflicts** or is dependent on diluent or concentration factors with the following drugs or solutions: fat emulsion 10%, dobutamine HCl, oxytetracycline HCl, and tetracycline HCl. Compatibility is dependent upon factors such as pH, concentration, temperature and diluents used. It is suggested to consult specialized references (*e.g., Handbook on Injectable Drugs* by Trissel; see bibliography) for more specific information.

Calcium chloride for injection is reportedly **incompatible** with the following solutions or drugs: amphotericin B, cephalothin sodium, and chlorpheniramine maleate.

Calcium gluceptate for injection is reportedly **compatible** with the following intravenous solutions and drugs: sodium chloride for injection 0.45% and 0.9%, Ringer's injection, lactated Ringer's injection, dextrose 2.5%-10%, dextrose-Ringer's injection, dextrose-lactated Ringer's injection, dextrose-saline combinations, ascorbic acid injection, isoproterenol HCl, lidocaine HCl, norepinephrine bitartrate, phytonadione, and sodium bicarbonate.

Calcium gluceptate for injection is reportedly **incompatible** with the following solutions or drugs: cefamandole naftate, cephalothin sodium, magnesium sulfate, prednisolone sodium succinate, and prochlorperazine edisylate. Compatibility is dependent upon factors such as pH, concentration, temperature and diluents used. It is suggested to consult specialized references (*e.g., Handbook on Injectable Drugs* by Trissel; see bibliography) for more specific information.

Calcium gluconate for injection is reportedly **compatible** with the following intravenous solutions and drugs: sodium chloride for injection 0.9%, lactated Ringer's injection, dextrose 5%-20%, dextrose-lactated Ringer's injection, dextrose-saline combinations, amikacin sulfate, aminophylline, ascorbic acid injection, bretylium tosylate, cephapirin sodium, chloramphenicol sodium succinate, corticotropin, dimenhydrinate, erythromycin gluceptate, heparin sodium, hydrocortisone sodium succinate, lidocaine HCl, methicillin sodium, norepinephrine bitartrate, penicillin G potassium/sodium, phenobarbital sodium, potassium chloride, tobramycin sulfate, vancomycin HCl, verapamil and vitamin B-complex with C.

Calcium gluconate **compatibility information conflicts** or is dependent on diluent or concentration factors with the following drugs or solutions: phosphate salts, oxytetracycline HCl, prochlorperazine edisylate, and tetracycline HCl. Compatibility is dependent upon factors such as pH, concentration, temperature and diluents used. It is suggested to consult specialized references (*e.g., Handbook on Injectable Drugs* by Trissel; see bibliography) for more specific information.

Calcium gluconate is reportedly **incompatible** with the following solutions or drugs: intravenous fat emulsion, amphotericin B, cefamandole naftate, cephalothin sodium, dobutamine HCl, methylprednisolone sodium succinate, and metoclopramide HCl.

Pharmacology - Calcium is an essential element that is required for many functions within the body, including proper nervous and musculoskeletal system function, cell-membrane and capillary permeability, and activation of enzymatic reactions.

Uses/Indications - Calcium salts are used for the prevention or treatment of hypocalcemic conditions.

Pharmacokinetics - Calcium is absorbed in the small intestine in the ionized form only. Presence of vitamin D (in active form) and an acidic pH is necessary for oral absorption. Parathormone (parathyroid hormone) increases with resultant increased calcium absorption in calcium deficiency states and decreases as serum calcium levels rise. Dietary factors (high fiber, phytates, fatty acids), age, drugs (corticosteroids, tetracyclines), disease states (steatorrhea, uremia, renal osteodystrophy, achlorhydria), or decreased serum calcitonin levels may all cause reduced amounts of calcium to be absorbed.

After absorption, ionized calcium enters the extracellular fluid and then is rapidly incorporated into skeletal tissue. Calcium administration does not necessarily stimulate bone formation. Approximately 99% of total body calcium is found in bone. Of circulating calcium, approximately 50% is bound to serum proteins or complexed with anions and 50% is in the ionized form. Total serum calcium is dependent on serum protein concentrations. Total serum calcium changes by approximately 0.8 mg/dl for every 1.09 g/dl change in serum albumin. Calcium crosses the placenta and is distributed into milk.

Calcium is eliminated primarily in the feces, contributed by both unabsorbed calcium and calcium excreted into the bile and pancreatic juice. Only small amounts of the drug are excreted in the urine, as most of the cation filtered by the glomeruli is reabsorbed by the tubules and ascending loop of Henle. Vitamin D, parathormone, and thiazide diuretics decrease the amount of calcium excreted by the kidneys. Loop diuretics (*e.g.,* furosemide), calcitonin, and somatotropin increase calcium renal excretion.

Contraindications/Precautions/Reproductive Safety - Calcium is contraindicated in patients with ventricular fibrillation or with hypercalcemia. Parenteral calcium should not be administered to patients with above normal serum calcium levels. Calcium should be used very cautiously in patients receiving digitalis glycosides, or with cardiac or renal disease. Calcium chloride, because it can be acidifying, should be used with caution in patients with respiratory failure, respiratory acidosis, or renal disease.

Although parenteral calcium products have not been proven to be safe to use during pregnancy, they are often used before, during, and after parturition in cows, ewes, bitches, and queens to treat parturient paresis secondary to hypocalcemia.

Adverse Effects/Warnings - Hypercalcemia can be associated with calcium therapy, particularly in patients with cardiac or renal disease; animals should be adequately monitored. Other effects that may be seen include GI irritation and/or constipation after oral administration, mild to severe tissue reactions after IM or SQ administration of calcium salts and venous irritation after IV administration. Calcium chloride may be more irritating than other parenteral salts and is more likely to cause hypotension. Too rapid intravenous injection of calcium can cause hypotension, cardiac arrhythmias and cardiac arrest.

Should calcium salts be infused perivascularly, first stop the infusion. Ttreatment may then include: infiltrate the affected area with normal saline, corticosteroids administered locally, apply heat and elevate the area, and infiltrate affected area with 1% procaine and hyaluronidase.

Overdosage/Acute Toxicity - Unless other drugs are given concurrently that enhance the absorption of calcium, oral overdoses of calcium containing products are unlikely to cause hypercalcemia. Hypercalcemia can occur with parenteral therapy or oral therapy in combination with vitamin D or increased parathormone levels. Hypercalcemia should be treated by withholding calcium therapy and other calcium elevating drugs (*e.g.,* vitamin D analogs). Mild hypercalcemias generally will resolve without further intervention when renal function is adequate.

More serious hypercalcemias (>12 mg/dl) should generally be treated by hydrating with IV normal saline and administering a loop diuretic (*e.g.,* furosemide) to increase both sodium and calcium excretion. Potassium and magnesium must be monitored and replaced as necessary. ECG should also be monitored during treatment. Corticosteroids, and in humans, calcitonin and hemodialysis have also been employed in treating hypercalcemia.

Drug Interactions - Patients on **digitalis** therapy are more apt to develop arrhythmias if receiving IV calcium—use with caution. Calcium may antagonize the effects of **verapamil (and other calcium-channel blocking agents)**.

Thiazide diuretics used in conjunction with large doses of calcium may cause hypercalcemia.

Oral **magnesium** products with oral calcium may lead to increased serum magnesium and/or calcium, particularly in patients with renal failure. Parenteral calcium can neutralize the effects of hypermagnesemia or magnesium toxicity secondary to parenteral **magnesium sulfate**.

Parenteral calcium may reverse the effects of nondepolarizing **neuromuscular blocking agents** (*e.g.,* metubine, gallamine, pancuronium, atracurium, & vecuronium). Calcium has been reported to prolong or enhance the effects of **tubocurarine**.

Oral calcium can reduce the amount of **phenytoin** or **tetracyclines** absorbed from the GI tract.

Patients receiving both parenteral calcium and **potassium** supplementation may have an increased chance of developing cardiac arrhythmias—use cautiously.

Excessive intake of **vitamin A** may stimulate calcium loss from bone and cause hypercalcemia.

Concurrent use of large doses of **vitamin D** or its analogs may cause enhanced calcium absorption and induce hypercalcemia.

Drug/Laboratory Interactions - Parenteral calcium may cause false-negative results for serum and urinary **magnesium** when using the Titan yellow method of determination.

Doses -
  Dogs:
    For hypocalcemia:
     a) Calcium gluconate injection: 94 - 140 mg/kg IV slowly to effect (intraperitoneal route may also be used). Monitor respirations and cardiac rate and rhythm during administration. (USPC 1990)
     b) For acute hypocalcemia: Calcium gluconate 10% injection: Warm to body temperature and give IV at a rate of 50 - 150 mg/kg (0.5 - 1.5 ml/kg) over 20-30 minutes. If bradycardia develops, halt infusion. Following acute crisis infuse 10 - 15 ml (of a 10% solution) per kg over a 24 hour period. Long term therapy may be accomplished by increasing dietary calcium and using vitamin D. Calcium lactate may be given orally at a rate of 0.5 - 2 g/day. (Seeler and Thurmon 1985)

c) Calcium gluconate 10% 0.5 - 1.5 ml/kg or calcium chloride 10% 1.5 - 3.5 ml (total) IV slowly over 15 minutes; monitor heart rate or ECG during infusion. If ST segment elevation or Q-T interval shortening occur, temporarily discontinue infusion and reinstate at a slower rate when resolved.

Maintenance therapy is dependent on cause of hypocalcemia. Hypoparathyroidism is treated with vitamin D analogs (refer to DHT monograph) with or without oral calcium supplementation. (Russo and Lees 1986)

d) For emergency treatment of tetany and seizures secondary to hypoparathyroidism: Calcium gluconate 10%: 0.5 - 1.5 ml/kg (up to 20 ml) over 15-30 minutes. May repeat at 6-8 hour intervals or give as continuous infusion at 10 - 15 mg/kg/hour. Monitor ECG and stop infusion if S-T segment elevates, Q-T interval shortens, or arrhythmias occur.

For long-term therapy (with DHT—refer to that monograph), calcium supplementation may occasionally be useful. Calcium gluconate at 500 - 750 mg/kg/day divided *tid*, or calcium lactate at 400 - 600 mg/kg/day divided *tid*, or calcium carbonate 100 - 150 mg/kg/day divided *bid*. Monitor serum calcium and adjust as necessary. (Kay and Richter 1988)

For hyperkalemic cardiotoxicity:

a) Secondary to uremic crisis: Correct metabolic acidosis, if present, with sodium bicarbonate (bicarbonate may also be beneficial even if acidosis not present). Calcium gluconate (10%) indicated if serum K+ is > 8 mEq/L. Give at an approximate dose of 0.5 - 1 ml/kg over 10-20 minutes; monitor ECG. Rapidly corrects arrhythmias but effects are very short (10-15 minutes). IV glucose (0.5 - 1 g/kg body weight with or without insulin) also beneficial in increasing intracellular K+ concentrations. (Polzin and Osborne 1985)

Cats:

For hypocalcemia:

a) Calcium gluconate injection: 94 - 140 mg/kg IV slowly to effect (intraperitoneal route may also be used. Monitor respirations and cardiac rate and rhythm during administration. (USPC 1990)

b) For acute hypocalcemia secondary to hypoparathyroidism: Using 10% calcium gluconate injection, give 1 - 1.5 ml/kg IV slowly over 10-20 minutes. Monitor ECG if possible. If bradycardia, or Q-T interval shortening occurs, slow rate or temporarily discontinue. Once life-threatening signs are controlled, add calcium to IV fluids and administer as a slow infusion at 60 - 90 mg/kg/day (of elemental calcium). This converts to 2.5 ml/kg every 6-8 hours of 10% calcium gluconate. Carefully monitor serum calcium (once to twice daily) during this period and adjust dose as required.

Begin oral calcium initially at 50 - 100 mg/kg/day divided 3-4 times daily of elemental calcium and dihydrotachysterol once animal can tolerate oral therapy. Give DHT initially at 0.125 - 0.25 mg PO per day for 2-3 days, then 0.08 - 0.125 mg per day for 2-3 days and finally 0.05 mg PO per day until further dosage adjustments are necessary. As cat's serum calcium is stabilized, intravenous calcium may be reduced and discontinued if tolerated. Stable serum calcium levels (8.5-9.5 mg/dl) are usually achieved in about a week. Continue to monitor and adjust dosages of DHT and calcium to lowest levels to maintain normocalcemia. (Peterson and Randolph 1989) (Note: refer to the DHT monograph for further information.)

c) For hypocalcemia secondary to phosphate enema toxicity or puerperal tetany: follow the guidelines for use of intravenous calcium in "b" above. (Peterson and Randolph 1989)

Cattle:

For hypocalcemia:

a) Calcium gluconate injection: 150 - 250 mg/kg IV slowly to effect (intraperitoneal route may also be used). Monitor respirations and cardiac rate and rhythm during administration. (USPC 1990)

b) Calcium gluconate 23% injection: 250 - 500 ml IV slowly, or IM or SQ (divided and given in several locations, with massage at sites of injection). (Label directions; Calcium Gluc. Injection 23%—TechAmerica)

c) 8 - 12 grams of calcium IV infused over a 5-10 minute period; use a product containing magnesium during the last month of pregnancy if subclinical hypomagnesemia is detected. (Allen and Sansom 1986)

Horses:

For hypocalcemia:

a) Calcium gluconate injection: 150 - 250 mg/kg IV slowly to effect (intraperitoneal route may also be used). Monitor respirations and cardiac rate and rhythm during administration. (USPC 1990)

b) Calcium gluconate 23% injection: 250 - 500 ml IV slowly, or IM or SQ (divided and given in several locations, with massage at sites of injection). (Label directions; Calcium Gluconate Injection 23%—TechAmerica)

c) For lactation tetany: 250 ml per 450 kg body weight of a standard commercially available solution that also contains magnesium and phosphorous IV slowly while ascultating heart. If no improvement after 10 minutes, repeat. Intensity in heart sounds should be noted, with only an infrequent extrasystole. Stop infusion immediately if a pronounced change in rate or rhythm is detected. (Brewer 1987)

Sheep & Goats:

For hypocalcemia:

a) Sheep: Calcium gluconate injection: 150 - 250 mg/kg IV slowly to effect (intraperitoneal route may also be used). Monitor respirations and cardiac rate and rhythm during administration. (USPC 1990)

b) Sheep: Calcium gluconate 23% injection: 25 - 50 ml IV slowly, or IM or SQ (divided and given in several locations, with massage at sites of injection). (Label directions; Calcium Gluconate Injection 23%—TechAmerica)

Swine:

For hypocalcemia:

a) Calcium gluconate injection: 150 - 250 mg/kg IV slowly to effect (intraperitoneal route may also be used). Monitor respirations and cardiac rate and rhythm during administration. (USPC 1990)

b) Calcium gluconate 23% injection: 25 - 50 ml IV slowly, or IM or SQ (divided and given in several locations, with massage at sites of injection). (Label directions; Calcium Gluconate Injection 23%—TechAmerica)

Birds:

For hypocalcemic tetany:

a) Calcium gluconate: 50 - 100 mg/kg IV slowly to effect; may be diluted and given IM if a vein cannot be located. (Clubb 1986)

For egg-bound birds:

a) Initially, calcium gluconate **1%** solution 0.01 - 0.02 ml/g IM. Provide moist heat (80-85°F) and allow 24 hours for bird to pass egg. (Nye 1986)

Reptiles:

a) For egg binding in combination with oxytocin (oxytocin: 1 - 10 IU/kg IM.): Calcium glubionate: 10 -50 mg/kg IM as needed until calcium levels back to normal or egg binding is resolved. Use care when giving multiple injections. Calcium/oxytocin is not as effective in lizards as in other species. (Gauvin 1993)

Monitoring Parameters -

1) Serum calcium
2) Serum magnesium, phosphate, and potassium when indicated
3) Serum PTH (parathormone) if indicated
4) Renal function tests initially and as required
5) ECG during intravenous calcium therapy if possible
6) Urine calcium if hypercalcuria develops

Dosage Forms/Preparations/FDA Approval Status/Withholding Times -

Veterinary-Approved Products (not necessarily a complete list)

Parenteral Products:

Calcium Gluconate (as calcium borogluconate) 23% [230 mg/ml; 20.7 mg (1.06 mEq) calcium per ml]; in 500 ml bottles; Generic; (Rx) Depending on the product, approved for use in cattle, horses, swine, sheep, cats, and dogs. No withdrawal times are required.

Products are also available that include calcium, phosphorus, potassium and/or dextrose; refer to the individual product's labeling for specific dosage information. Trade names for these products include: *Norcalciphos®*—SKB, and *Cal-Dextro® Special, #2, C, & K*—Fort Dodge. They are legend (Rx) drugs.

Oral Products: No products containing only calcium (as a salt) are available commercially with veterinary labeling. There are several products (*e.g., Pet-Cal®* and *Osteoform® Improved*) that contain calcium with phosphorous and vitamin D (plus other ingredients in some preparations).

Human-Approved Products (not a complete list):

Parenteral Products:

Calcium Gluconate Injection 10% [100 mg/ml; 9 mg (0.47 mEq) calcium per ml] in 10 ml amps, 10 & 50 ml, 100 ml, & 200 ml vials; Generic; (Rx)

Calcium Chloride Injection 10% [100 mg/ml; 27.2 mg (1.36 mEq) calcium per ml] in 10 ml amps, vials, and syringes; Generic; (Rx)

Calcium Gluceptate Injection 1.1 g/5 ml in 5 ml amps and 5 ml fill in 10 ml vial; Calcium Gluceptate® (Abbott) (Rx)

Oral Products:

Calcium Gluconate (9% calcium) Tablets: 500 mg (45 mg of calcium), 650 mg (58.5 mg of calcium), 975 mg (87.75 mg calcium), 1 gram (90 mg of calcium); Generic; (OTC)

Calcium Lactate (13% calcium) Tablets: 325 mg (42.25 mg calcium), 650 mg (84.5 mg calcium); Generic; (OTC)

Also available are calcium glubionate syrup, calcium carbonate tablets, suspension & capsules, calcium citrate tablets, dibasic calcium phosphate dihydrate tablets, and tricalcium phosphate tablets.

Camphorated Tincture of Opium — See Paregoric

CAPTOPRIL

Chemistry - Related to a peptide isolated from the venom of a South American pit viper, captopril occurs as a slightly sulfurous smelling, white to off-white, crystalline powder. It is freely soluble in water and in alcohol.

Storage/Stability/Compatibility - Captopril tablets should be stored at a temperature not greater than 30°C, and in tight containers.

Pharmacology - Captopril prevents the formation of angiotensin II (a potent vasoconstrictor) by competing with angiotensin I for the enzyme angiotensin converting enzyme (ACE). ACE has a much higher affinity for captopril than for angiotensin I. Because angiotensin II concentrations are decreased, aldosterone secretion is reduced and plasma renin activity is increased.

The cardiovascular effects of captopril in patients with CHF include decreased total peripheral resistance, pulmonary vascular resistance, mean arterial and right atrial pressures, and pulmonary capillary wedge pressure; no change or decrease in heart rate; and increased cardiac index and output, stroke volume, and exercise tolerance. Renal blood flow can be increased with little changes in hepatic blood flow.

Uses/Indications - The principle uses of captopril in veterinary medicine at present, are as a vasodilator in the treatment of CHF and in the treatment of hypertension. It is being explored as adjunctive treatment in chronic renal failure and in protein losing nephropathies.

Pharmacokinetics - In dogs, approximately 75% of an oral dose is absorbed, but food in the GI tract reduces bioavailability by 30-40%. It is distributed to most tissues (not the CNS) and is 40% bound to plasma proteins in dogs. Captopril crosses the placenta and only about 1% of plasma concentrations are found in milk. The half-life of captopril is about 2.8 hours in dogs and less than 2 hours in humans. The drug is metabolized and renally excreted. More than 95% of a dose is excreted renally, both as unchanged (45-50%) drug and as metabolites. Patients with significant renal dysfunction can have significantly prolonged half-lives.

Contraindications/Precautions - Captopril is contraindicated in patients who have demonstrated hypersensitivity to the ACE inhibitors. It should be used with caution and close supervision, in patients with renal insufficiency and doses may need to be reduced.

Captopril should also be used with caution in patients with hyponatremia or sodium depletion, coronary or cerebrovascular insufficiency, preexisting hematologic abnormalities or a collagen vascular disease (e.g SLE).

Patients with severe CHF should be monitored very closely upon initiation of therapy.

Adverse Effects/Warnings - There have been some reports of hypotension, renal failure, hyperkalemia, vomiting and diarrhea developing in dogs after captopril administration. Although seen in people, skin rashes (4-7% incidence) and neutropenia/agranulocytosis (rare) have not been reported in dogs.

Overdosage - In overdose situations, the primary concern is hypotension; supportive treatment with volume expansion with normal saline is recommended to correct blood pressure. Dogs given 1.5 gm/kg orally developed emesis and decreased blood pressure.

Drug Interactions - Concomitant **diuretics**, or other **vasodilators** may cause hypotension if used with captopril; titrate dosages carefully. Hyperkalemia may develop if given with **potassium** or potassium sparing diuretics (e.g **spironolactone**).

Digoxin levels may increase 15-30% when captopril is added, automatic reduction in dosage is not recommended, but monitoring of serum digoxin levels should be performed.

Non-steroidal anti-inflammatory agents (NSAIDs) may reduce the clinical efficacy of captopril when it is being used as an antihypertensive agent.

Reduced oral absorption of captopril may occur if given concomitantly with **antacids**. It is suggested to separate dosing by at least two hours. **Probenecid** can decrease renal excretion of captopril and possibly enhance the clinical and toxic effects of the drug.

Cimetidine and captopril used concomitantly has caused neurologic dysfunction in two human patients.

Laboratory Interactions - Captopril may cause a false positive **urine acetone test** (sodium nitroprusside reagent). When using **iodohippurate sodium I^{123}/I^{134} or Technetium Tc^{99} pententate renal imaging** in patients with renal artery stenosis, ACE inhibitors may cause a reversible decrease in localization and excretion of these agents in the affected kidney which may lead confusion in test interpretation.

Doses -
   Dogs:
   - a)   1 - 2 mg/kg PO *tid* (start at 1 mg/kg) (Knowlen and Kittleson 1986)
   - b)   0.5 - 2.0 mg/kg PO q8-12h (Bonagura and Muir 1986)
   - c)   For canine dilated cardiomyopathy: 0.5 - 2 mg/kg PO *bid-tid*. Used primarily in dogs refractory to diuretics, other vasodilators, or positive inotropes. (Ogburn 1988)

   Cats:
   - a)   1/4 to 1/2 12.5 mg tablet PO q8-12h (Bonagura 1989)

Monitoring Parameters -
   1) Clinical symptoms of CHF
   2) Serum electrolytes, creatinine, BUN, urine protein
   3) CBC with diff.; periodic
   4) Blood pressure (if treating hypertension or symptoms associated with hypotension arise)

Client Information - Give medication on an empty stomach unless otherwise instructed. Do not abruptly stop or reduce therapy without veterinarian's approval. Contact veterinarian if vomiting or diarrhea persist or are severe, or if animal's condition deteriorates.

Dosage Forms/Preparations/FDA Approval Status/Withholding Times -
   Veterinary-Approved Products: None
   Human-Approved Products:
   Captopril Tablets 12.5, 25, 50, & 100 mg; *Capoten*® (Bristol-Myers Squibb); Generic (Rx)

CARBENICILLIN INDANYL SODIUM

For general information on the penicillins, including adverse effects, contraindications, overdosage, drug interactions and monitoring parameters, refer to the monograph: Penicillins, General Information.

Chemistry - An alpha-carboxypenicillin, carbenicillin is now available only as a an oral dosage form; the sodium salt of the indanyl ester of carbenicillin. It occurs as a bitter-tasting, white to off-white powder that is soluble in water and alcohol. Carbenicillin indanyl sodium may also be known as carindacillin sodium or indanylcarbenicillin sodium.

Storage/Stability/Compatibility - The oral indanyl sodium tablets should be stored in tight containers and protected from temperatures greater than 30°C. The sodium injection powder for reconstitution should be stored at temperatures less than 30°C.

Pharmacology - The alpha-carboxypenicillins, sometimes called anti-pseudomonal penicillins, include both carbenicillin and ticarcillin. These agents have similar spectrums of activity as the aminopenicillins (ampicillin, etc.) including increased activity against many strains of gram negative aerobes not covered by either the natural penicillins or penicillinase-resistant penicillins, including some strains of *E. coli, Klebsiella,* and *Haemophilus*. Additionally, they have activity against several gram negative organisms of the family Enterobacteriaceae, including many strains of *Pseudomonas aeruginosa* and *Acinetobacter*. Like the natural penicillins they are susceptible to inactivation by beta-lactamase-producing bacteria (*e.g., Staph aureus*). Although not as active as the natural penicillins, they do have some activity against many anaerobic bacteria including *Clostridial* organisms.

Uses/Indications - As there are no veterinary-approved carbenicillin products, all uses of this drug are considered extra-label. Generally, carbenicillin is used parenterally in the treatment of systemic *Pseudomonas aeruginosa* infections in small animals, usually in combination with an appropriate aminoglycoside agent. Synergy may occur against some *Pseudomonas* strains when used in combination with aminoglycosides, but *in vitro* inactivation of the aminoglycoside may also occur (see Drug Interactions below) if the drugs are physically mixed together or in patients with severe renal failure.

Because the oral form is poorly absorbed and the drug has a rapid elimination half-life, oral therapy is only indicated for the treatment of susceptible urinary tract (and possibly prostate) infections as levels are too low in serum and other tissues for adequate therapy in other systemic *Pseudomonas* infections.

Pharmacokinetics (specific) - The oral form (indanyl sodium) of the drug is rapidly, but incompletely, absorbed (see above) with only 30-40% of an oral dose absorbed in humans. Peak levels of the indanyl sodium are attained in humans about 30 minutes after administration, but is rapidly hydrolyzed into the base.

Attainable serum levels after oral therapy are generally too low to treat systemic infections, but high levels are achieved in the urine. The volume of distribution is reportedly 0.18-0.2 L/kg in dogs and cats and 0.29-0.4 L/kg in the horse. The drug is 29-60% bound to serum proteins (human). Carbenicillin is thought to cross the placenta and is found in small quantities in milk. In cattle, mastitic milk levels of carbenicillin are approximately twice those found in normal milk, but are too low to treat most causal organisms.

Carbenicillin is eliminated primarily by the kidneys, via both tubular secretion and glomerular filtration. Concurrent probenecid administration can slow elimination and increase blood levels. In humans, about 2-5% of the drug is metabolized by hydrolysis to inactive compounds. The half-life in dogs and cats is reportedly 45-75 minutes and 60-90 minutes in the horse. Clearance is 1.8 ml/kg/min in the dog and 4.6 ml/kg/min in the horse.

Doses -
Dogs:
    For susceptible infections:
      a) For UTI: 15 - 50 mg/kg PO q6-8h (Ford and Aronson 1985)
      b) 15 mg/kg PO, IV *tid* (Morgan 1988)
      c) 55 - 110 mg/kg IV q8h or 55 mg/kg PO q8h (Aronson and Aucoin 1989)

Cats:
    For susceptible infections:
      a) For UTI: 15 - 50 mg/kg PO q6-8h (Ford and Aronson 1985)
      b) 15 mg/kg PO *tid* (Morgan 1988)
      c) 15 mg/kg IV q8h (Upson 1988)
      d) 55 mg/kg PO q8h (Aronson and Aucoin 1989)

Birds:
    For susceptible infections in Psittacines:
      a) 100 - 200 mg/kg PO *bid*; 1/3 tablet added to 4 oz drinking water. Crush tablets and gavage or hide in mash or palatable soft food item. If adding to drinking water, disguise bitter taste by adding *Tang*® or a Pina Colada mix to water. (McDonald 1989)
      b) 200 mg/kg PO for 5-10 days. Crush tablets and apply to favorite food (*e.g.,* cooked sweet potato works well) or mix in mash or hand-feeding formula. (Clubb 1986)

Dosage Forms/Preparations/FDA Approval Status -
Veterinary-Approved Products: None

Human-Approved Products:
    Carbenicillin Indanyl Sodium Coated Oral Tablets 382 mg; *Geocillin*® (Roerig); (Rx)

CARBOPLATIN

Chemistry - Carboplatin, like cisplatin is a platinum-containing antineoplastic agent. It occurs as white to off-white crystalline powder having a solubility of 14 mg/ml in water and is insoluble in alcohol. The commercially available powder for injection contains equal parts of mannitol and carboplatin. After reconstitution with sterile water for injection, a resulting solution of 10 mg/ml of carboplatin has a pH of 5-7 and an osmolality of 94 mOsm/kg.

Storage/Stability/Compatibility - The powder for injection should kept stored at room temperature and protected from light.

After reconstitution, solutions containing 10 mg/ml are stable for at least 8 hours. Some sources say that the solution is stable for up to 24 hours and can be refrigerated, but because there are no preservatives in the solution, the manufacturer recommends discarding unused portions after 8 hours. Previous recommendations to avoid the use of solutions containing sodium chloride to dilute carboplatin, are no longer warranted as only a minimal amount of carboplatin is converted to cisplatin in these solutions.

Because aluminum can displace platinum from carboplatin, the solution should not be prepared, stored or administered where aluminum-containing items can come into contact with the solution. Should carboplatin come into contact with aluminum, a black precipitate will form and the product should not be used.

Pharmacology - Carboplatin's exact mechanism of action is not fully understood. Both carboplatin's and cisplatin's properties are analogous to those of bifunctional alkylating agents producing inter- and intrastrand crosslinks in DNA, thereby inhibiting DNA replication, RNA transcription, and protein synthesis. Carboplatin is cell-cycle nonspecific.

Uses/Indications -Like cisplatin, carboplatin may be useful in a variety of veterinary neoplastic diseases including squamous cell carcinomas, ovarian carcinomas, mediastinal carcinomas, pleural adenocarcinomas, nasal carcinomas and thyroid adenocarcinomas. Carboplatin's primary use currently in small animal medicine is in the adjunctive treatment (post amputation) of osteogenic sarcomas. It's effectiveness in treating transitional cell carcinoma of the bladder has been disappointing thus far. However, carboplatin may have more efficacy against melanomas than does cisplatin.

Carboplatin, unlike cisplatin, appears to be relatively safe to use in cats.

Whether carboplatin is more efficacious than cisplatin for certain cancers does not appear to be decided at this point, but the drug does appear to have fewer adverse effects (less renal toxicity and reduced vomiting) in dogs than does cisplatin. However, it does cost significantly more than cisplatin.

Pharmacokinetics - After IV administration, carboplatin is well distributed throughout the body; highest concentrations are found in the liver, kidney, skin and tumor tissue. The metabolic fate and elimination of carboplatin are complex and the discussion of this aspect of the drugs pharmacokinetics is beyond the scope of this reference. Suffice it to say that the parent drug degrades into platinum and platinum-complexed compounds that are primarily eliminated by kidneys. In dogs, approximately 70% of the platinum administered is secreted in the urine after 72 hours.

Contraindications/Precautions /Reproductive Safety - Carboplatin is contraindicated in patients hypersensitive to it or other platinum-containing compounds. It is also contraindicated in patients with severe bone marrow suppression. Patients with severe carboplatin-induced myelosuppression should be allowed to recover their counts before additional therapy.

Caution is advised in patients with active infections, hearing impairment or preexisting renal or hepatic disease. Dosage may need adjustment in patients with reduced renal function.

Do not give carboplatin IM or SubQ.

Carboplatin is fetotoxic and embryotoxic in rats and the risks of its use during pregnancy should be weighed with its potential benefits. It is unknown whether carboplatin enters maternal milk. In humans, it is recommended to discontinue nursing if the mother is receiving the drug.

Adverse Effects/Warnings - Established adverse effects in dogs include, anorexia, vomiting and bone marrow suppression which is exhibited primarily as thrombocytopenia and/or neutropenia. The nadir of platelet and neutrophil counts generally occur about 14 days post treatment.

Hepatotoxicity (increased serum bilirubin & liver enzymes) is seen in about 15% of human patients treated with carboplatin. Other potential adverse effects include: nephrotoxicity, neuropathies and ototoxicity. These effects occur with carboplatin therapy much less frequently than with cisplatin therapy. Anaphylactoid reactions have been reported rarely in humans that have received platinum-containing compounds (e.g., cisplatin). Hyperuricemia may occur after therapy in a small percentage of patients.

Overdosage - There is limited information available. An overdose of carboplatin would be expected to cause aggravated effects associated with the drug's bone marrow and liver toxicity. Monitor for neurotoxicity, ototoxicity and nephrotoxicity..

Treatment is basically supportive; no specific antidote is available. Plasmapheresis or hemodialysis could potentially be of benefit in removing the drug.

Drug Interactions - The leukopenic or thrombocytopenic effects secondary to carboplatin may be enhanced by **other myelosuppressive medications**. Human patients previously treated with **cisplatin** have an increased risk of developing neurotoxicity or ototoxicity after receiving carboplatin. **Live or killed virus vaccines** administered after carboplatin therapy may not be as effective as the immune-response to these vaccines may be modified by carboplatin therapy. Carboplatin may also potentiate live virus vaccines replication and increase the adverse effects associated with these vaccines.

Doses - Note: Do not confuse cisplatin and carboplatin dosages. Cisplatin dosages are much lower than carboplatin dosages.

Dogs:

a) As adjunctive treatment of osteogenic sarcoma: 300 mg/meter^2 BSA IV every 21 days (Bergman, MacEwen et al. 1996)

  b) As adjunctive treatment of osteogenic sarcoma: 300 mg/meter^2 BSA IV (admixed with D5W and given IV over 15 minutes) usually within 7 days after amputation. Additional treatments given every 21 days for a total of 4 treatments. (Johnston 1997)

  c) As adjunctive treatment of osteogenic sarcoma, melanomas, or various carcinomas: Large Dogs: 350 mg/meter^2 BSA IV (diluted in dextrose) every 3 weeks; Small Dogs: 300 mg/meter^2 BSA IV (diluted in dextrose) every 3 weeks (London and Frimberger 1997)

Cats:

  a) As adjunctive treatment of osteogenic sarcoma, melanomas or various carcinomas: 210 mg/meter^2 BSA IV (diluted in dextrose) every 3 weeks (London and Frimberger 1997)

Monitoring Parameters - 1) CBC; 2) Serum electrolytes, uric acid; 3) Baseline renal and hepatic function tests

Client Information - Clients should fully understand the potential toxicity of this agent and ideally should give informed consent for its use. As carboplatin (and any platinum containing metabolites) are principally excreted in the urine over several days after treatment, clients should be warned to avoid direct contact with patient's urine.

Dosage Forms/Preparations/FDA Approval Status -

  Veterinary-Approved Products: None

  Human-Approved Products:

  Carboplatin Powder for reconstitution and IV Injection 50 mg, 150 mg, & 450 mg vials (contains mannitol); *Paraplatin®* (Bristol-Myers Squibb); (Rx)

    Directions for reconstitution for the 50 mg vial: Add 5 ml of either sterile water for injection, normal saline injection or D5W that will provide a solution containing 10 mg/ml. May infuse directly (usually over 15 minutes) or further dilute. Visually inspect after reconstitution/dilution for discoloration or particulate matter.

CARNITINE
LEVOCARNITINE
L-CARNITINE

Chemistry - Levocarnitine (the L-isomer of carnitine) is an amino acid derivative, synthesized *in vivo* from methionine and lysine. It is required for energy metabolism and has a molecular weight of 161.

Storage/Stability/Compatibility - Levocarnitine capsules, tablets and powder should be stored in well-closed containers at room temperature. The oral solution should be kept in tight containers at room temperature. The injection should be stored at room temperature in the original carton. After opening, discard any unused portion as the injection contains no preservative.

Pharmacology - Levocarnitine is required for normal fat utilization and energy metabolism in mammalian species. It serves to facilitate entry of long-chain fatty acids into cellular mitochondria, where they can be used during oxidation and energy production.

  Severe chronic deficiency is a generally a result of an inborn genetic defect where levocarnitine utilization is impaired and not the result of dietary insufficiency in normal individuals. Effects seen in levocarnitine deficiency may include hypoglycemia, progressive myasthenia, hepatomegaly, CHF, cardiomegaly, hepatic coma, neurologic disturbances, encephalopathy, hypotonia and lethargy.

Uses/Indications - Levocarnitine may be useful as adjunctive therapy of dilated cardiomyopathy in dogs. Up to 90% of dogs with dilated cardiomyopathy may have a carnitine deficiency. Levocarnitine may also protect against doxorubicin-induced cardiomyopathy and reduce risks of myocardial infarction. It may be beneficial in the adjunctive treatment of valproic acid toxicity.

  In cats, levocarnitine has been recommended as being useful as adjunctive therapy in feline hepatic lipidosis by facilitating hepatic lipid metabolism. Its use for this indication is controversial.

Pharmacokinetics - In humans, levocarnitine is absorbed via the GI with a bioavailability of about 15%. Levocarnitine is distributed in milk naturally. Exogenously administered levocarnitine is eliminated by both renal and fecal routes. Plasma levocarnitine levels may be increased in patients with renal failure.

Contraindications/Precautions/Reproductive Safety - Levocarnitine may also be known as Vitamin B$_T$. Products labeled as such may have both D and L racemic forms. Use only Levo-forms as the D- form may competitively inhibit L- uptake with a resulting deficiency. Studies done in rats and rabbits have demonstrated no teratogenic effects and it is generally believed that levocarnitine is safe to use in pregnancy though documented safety during pregnancy has not been established.

Adverse Effects/Warnings - Adverse effect profile is minimal. Gastrointestinal upset is the most likely effect that may be noted. It is usually mild and limited to loose stools or possibly diarrhea; nausea and vomiting are also possible. Human patients have reported increased body odor.

Overdosage/Acute Toxicity - Levocarnitine is a relatively safe drug. Minor overdoses need only to be monitored; with massive overdoses consider gut emptying. Refer to a poison control center for more information.

Drug Interactions - Patients receiving **valproic acid** may require higher dosages of levocarnitine.

Doses -
  Dogs:
      For dogs with myocardial carnitine deficiency associated with dilated cardiomyopathy: 50 - 100 mg/kg PO *tid* (may be mixed in food). (Keene 1992)
  Cats:
      As adjunctive dietary therapy in cats with severe hepatic lipidosis: 250 - 500 mg/day (50 - 100 mg/kg) PO for 2-4 weeks (Use L-carnitine only). (Center 1994)

Monitoring Parameters - 1) Efficacy; 2) Periodic blood chemistries have been recommended for human patients, their value in veterinary medicine is undetermined.

Client Information - Give with meals when possible to reduce likelihood of GI side effects. The majority of dogs responding to carnitine therapy for dilated cardiomyopathy will require other medication to control symptomatology.

Dosage Forms/Preparations/FDA Approval Status/Withholding Times -
  Veterinary-Approved Products: None

  Human-Approved Products:

  Levocarnitine Tablets 330 mg; *Carnitor*® (Sigma-Tau); (Rx)

  Levocarnitine or L-Carnitine Capsules 250 mg; generic; (OTC—as a food supplement)

  Levocarnitine Oral Solution 100 mg/ml in 118 ml bottles; *Carnitor*® (Sigma-Tau); *VitaCarn* (Kendall McGaw); (Rx)

  Levocarnitine Injection 1 g/5 ml in 5 ml amps; *Carnitor*® (Sigma-Tau); (Rx)

  Note: L-carnitine may also be available in bulk powder form from local health food stores

CARPROFEN

Chemistry - A propionic acid derivative non-steroidal antiinflammatory agent, carprofen occurs as a white crystalline compound. It is practically insoluble in water and freely soluble in ethanol at room temperature.

Storage/Stability/Compatibility - The commercially available caplets should be stored at room temperature (15-30°C).

Pharmacology - Like other NSAIDs, carprofen exhibits analgesic, anti-inflammatory, and antipyretic activity probably through its inhibition of cyclooxygenase, phospholipase A_2 and inhibition of prostaglandin synthesis.

Uses/Indications - Carprofen is indicated for the relief of pain and inflammation in dogs. It may also prove to be of benefit in other species as well, but data are scant to support its safe use at this time. In Europe, carprofen is reportedly registered for single dose use in cats, but there have been reported problems (e.g., vomiting) with cats receiving more than a single dose.

Pharmacokinetics - When administered orally to dogs, carprofen is approximately 90% bioavailable. Peak serum levels occur between 1-3 hours post dosing. The drug is highly bound to plasma proteins (99%) and has a low volume of distribution (0.12 - 0.22 l/kg). Carprofen is extensively metabolized in the liver primarily via glucuronidation and oxidative processes. About 70-80% of a dose is eliminated in the feces; 10-20% eliminated in the urine. Some enterohepatic recycling of the drug occurs. Elimination half-life of carprofen in the dog is approximately 8-12 hours.

Contraindications/Precautions/Reproductive Safety - Carprofen is contraindicated in dogs with bleeding disorders (*e.g.,* Von Willebrand's), those that have had prior serious reactions to it or other propionic-class antiinflammatory agents. It should be used with caution in geriatric patients or those with preexisting chronic diseases (*e.g.,* inflammatory bowel disease, renal or hepatic insufficiency).

Adverse Effects/Warnings - Although adverse effects appear to be uncommon with carprofen use in dogs, they can occur. Mild gastrointestinal effects are the most likely to appear, but serious effects (hepatocellular damage and/or renal disease; hematologic and serious gastrointestinal effects) have been reported. Geriatric dogs or dogs with chronic diseases (*e.g.*, inflammatory bowel disease, renal or hepatic insufficiency) may be at greater risk for developing toxicity while taking this drug. Although not proven to be statistically significant, Labrador Retrievers have been associated with 1/3 of the initial cases associated with the reported hepatic syndrome. Before initiating therapy, pre-treatment patient evaluation and discussion with the owner regarding the potential risks versus benefits of therapy are strongly advised.

Overdosage - In dog toxicologic studies, repeated doses of up to 10X resulted in little adversity. Some dogs exhibited hypoalbuminemia, melena or slight increases in ALT. However, post-marketing surveillance suggests that there may be significant interpatient variability in response to acute or chronic overdoses.

Drug Interactions - Note: Although the manufacturer does not list any specific drug interactions in the package insert, it does caution to avoid or closely monitor carprofen's use with other ulcerogenic drugs (*e.g.*, corticosteroids or other NSAIDs).

In humans, there are many interactions possible with NSAIDs. Because clinical experience is limited in dogs, the following may or may not be clinically significant: Because carprofen is highly bound to plasma proteins (99%) it may displace other highly bound drugs. Increased serum levels and duration of actions of **phenytoin, valproic acid, oral anticoagulants**, other **anti-inflammatory agents, salicylates, sulfonamides**, and the **sulfonylurea antidiabetic agents** may occur.

When **aspirin** is used concurrently with carprofen, plasma levels of carprofen could decrease and an increased likelihood of GI adverse effects (blood loss) could occur. Concomitant administration of aspirin with carprofen cannot be recommended.

Probenecid may cause a significant increase in serum levels and half-life of carprofen.

Serious toxicity has occurred when NSAIDs have been used concomitantly with **methotrexate**; use together with extreme caution.

Carprofen may reduce the saluretic and diuretic effects of **furosemide** and increase serum levels of **digoxin**. Use with caution in patients with severe cardiac failure.

Doses -
  Dogs:
      As an antiinflammatory/analgesic:
        a) 2.2 mg/kg PO twice daily; round dose to nearest half caplet increment (Package Insert; *Rimadyl®*—Pfizer)
        b) For surgical pain: 4 mg/kg IV initially once; 2.2 mg/kg PO, IV, subQ or IM, repeat in 12 hours if needed.
           For chronic pain: 2.2 mg/kg PO q12h (Johnson 1996)

  Cats:
      As an antiinflammatory/analgesic: Caution is advised, particularly with long term dosing.
        a) For surgical pain: 4 mg/kg IV initially once; 2.2 mg/kg PO, IV, subQ or IM, repeat in 12 hours if needed.
           For chronic pain: 2.2 mg/kg PO q12h (Johnson 1996)

Monitoring Parameters - 1) Baseline (especially in geriatric dogs or dogs with chronic diseases or those where prolonged treatment is likely): physical exam, CBC, Serum chemistry panel (including liver and renal function tests), UA 2) Clinical efficacy 3) Signs of potential adverse reactions: inappetence, diarrhea, vomiting, melena, polyuria/polydipsia, anemia, jaundice, lethargy, behavior changes, ataxia or seizures 4) Chronic therapy: Consider repeating CBC, UA and serum chemistries on an ongoing basis

Client Information - Although rare, serious adverse effects have been reported with the use of this drug. Clients should be informed of the risks associated with its use and be alerted to monitor for signs of potential adverse effects (see above). Should these signs present, clients should stop the drug immediately and contact their veterinarian.

Dosage Forms/Preparations/FDA Approval Status -
Veterinary-Approved Products:
    Carprofen 25 mg, 75 mg & 100 mg scored caplets in bottles of 100 or 250; *Rimadyl®* (Pfizer); (Rx). Approved for use in dogs.

CEFADROXIL

For general information on the cephalosporins including adverse effects, contraindications, overdosage, drug interactions, and monitoring parameters, refer to the monograph: Cephalosporins, General Information.

Chemistry - A semisynthetic cephalosporin antibiotic, cefadroxil occurs as a white to yellowish-white, crystalline powder that is soluble in water and slightly soluble in alcohol. The commercially available product is available as the monohydrate.

Storage/Stability/Compatibility - Cefadroxil tablets, capsules and powder for oral suspension should be stored at room temperature (15-30°C) in tight containers. After reconstitution, the oral suspension is stable for 14 days when kept refrigerated (2-8°C).

Pharmacology/Spectrum of Activity - A first generation cephalosporin, cefadroxil exhibits activity against the bacteria usually covered by this class. Refer to the monograph: Cephalosporins, General Information for additional information.

Uses/Indications - Cefadroxil is approved for oral therapy in treating susceptible infections of the skin, soft tissue, and genitourinary tract in dogs. It has also been used clinically in cats.

Pharmacokinetics (specific) - Cefadroxil is reportedly well absorbed after oral administration to dogs without regard to feeding state. After an oral dose of 22 mg/kg, peak serum levels of approximately 18.6 micrograms/ml occur within 1-2 hours of dosing. Only about 20% of the drug is bound to canine plasma proteins. The drug is excreted into the urine and has a half-life of about 2 hours. Over 50% of a dose can be recovered unchanged in the urine within 24 hours of dosing.

In cats, the serum half-life has been reported as approximately 3 hours.

Oral absorption of cefadroxil in adult horses after oral suspension was administered was characterized as poor and erratic. In a study done in foals (Duffee, Christensen, and Craig 1989), oral bioavailability ranged from 36-99.8% (mean=58.2%); mean elimination half-life was 3.75 hours after oral dosing.

Doses -
  Dogs:
    For susceptible infections:
      a) 22 mg/kg PO *bid*. Treat skin and soft tissue infections for at least 3 days, and GU infections for at least 7 days. Treat for at least 48 hours after animal is afebrile and asymptomatic. Reevaluate therapy if no response after 3 days of treatment. Maximum therapy is 30 days. (Package Insert; *Cefa-Tabs*®—Fort-Dodge).
      b) 11 - 33 mg/kg PO q8h (Aronson and Aucoin 1989)
      c) 20 mg/kg PO *bid* (q12h) (Morgan 1988), (Jenkins 1987a)
      d) 22 mg/kg PO q8-12h; administer with food if GI upset occurs (Vaden and Papich 1995)

  Cats:
    For susceptible infections:
      a) 11 - 33 mg/kg PO q8h (Aronson and Aucoin 1989)
      b) 22 mg/kg PO q8-12h; administer with food if GI upset occurs (Vaden and Papich 1995)
      c) 10 mg/kg PO q12h (Davis 1985)
      d) 20 mg/kg PO q12-24h (Jenkins 1987a)

Dosage Forms/Preparations/FDA Approval Status/Withholding Times -
  Veterinary-Approved Products:
    Cefadroxil Oral Tablets 50 mg, 100 mg, 200 mg, 1 gram; *Cefa-Tabs*® (Fort-Dodge); (Rx) Approved for use in dogs and cats

    Cefadroxil Powder for Oral Suspension 50 mg/ml in 15 ml and 50 ml btls;*Cefa-Drops* ® (Fort-Dodge) (Rx)

  Human-Approved Products:
    Cefadroxil Oral Tablets 1 gram; *Duri-Cef*® (Mead-Johnson); (Rx) generic (Rx)

    Cefadroxil Oral Capsules 500 mg; *Duri-Cef*® (Mead-Johnson); generic (Rx)

    Cefadroxil Oral Suspension 125 mg/5 ml, 250 mg/5 ml, 500 mg/5 ml;*Duri-Cef*® (Mead-Johnson); generic (Rx)

CEFAZOLIN SODIUM

For general information on the cephalosporins including adverse effects, contraindications, overdosage, drug interactions, and monitoring parameters, refer to the monograph: Cephalosporins, General Information.

Chemistry - An injectable, semi-synthetic cephalosporin antibiotic, cefazolin sodium occurs as a practically odorless or having a faint odor, white to off-white, crystalline powder or lyophilized solid. It is freely soluble in water and very slightly soluble in alcohol. Each gram of the injection contains 2 mEq of sodium. After reconstitution, the solution for injection has a pH of 4.5 - 6 and has a light yellow to yellow color. May also be known as cephazolin sodium in the U.K. and other countries.

Storage/Stability/Compatibility - Cefazolin sodium powder for injection and solutions for injection should be protected from light. The powder for injection should be stored at room temperature (15-30°C); avoid temperatures above 40°C. The frozen solution for injection should be stored at temperatures no higher than -20°C.

After reconstitution, the solution is stable for 24 hours when kept at room temperature and 96 hours if refrigerated. If after reconstitution, the solution is immediately frozen in the original container, the preparation is stable for at least 12 weeks when stored at -20°C.

The following drugs or solutions are reportedly **compatible** with cephapirin: Amino acids 4.25%/dextrose 25%, D_5W in Ringer's, D_5W in Lactated Ringer's, D_5W in sodium chloride 0.2% - 0.9%, D_5W, $D_{10}W$, Ringer's Injection, Lactated Ringer's Injection, normal saline, metronidazole, verapamil HCl and vitamin B-complex.

The following drugs or solutions are reportedly **incompatible** or only compatible in specific situations with cefazolin: amikacin sulfate, amobarbital sodium, ascorbic acid injection, bleomycin sulfate, calcium chloride/gluconate, cimetidine HCl, erythromycin gluceptate, kanamycin sulfate, lidocaine HCl, oxytetracycline HCl, pentobarbital sodium, polymyxin B sulfate, tetracycline HCl and vitamin B-complex with C injection.

Compatibility is dependent upon factors such as pH, concentration, temperature and diluents used. It is suggested to consult specialized references for more specific information (*e.g., Handbook on Injectable Drugs* by Trissel; see bibliography).

Pharmacology/Spectrum of Activity - A first generation cephalosporin, cefazolin exhibits activity against the bacteria usually covered by this class. Because MIC's occasionally differ for cefazolin when compared to either cephalothin/cephapirin, some clinical microbiologists recommend also testing bacterial susceptibilities for this antibiotic. For more specific information, refer to the monograph, Cephalosporins, General Information.

Uses/Indications - In the United States, there are no cefazolin products approved for veterinary species, but it has been used clinically in several species when an short-acting injectable first generation cephalosporin is indicated.

Pharmacokinetics (specific) - Cefazolin is not appreciably absorbed after oral administration and must be given parenterally to achieve therapeutic serum levels. Absorbed drug is excreted unchanged by the kidneys into the urine. Elimination half-lives may be significantly prolonged in patients with severely diminished renal function. Pharmacokinetic parameters for dogs and horses follow:

In dogs, peak levels occur in about 30 minutes after IM administration. The apparent volume of distribution at steady state is 700 ml/kg, total body clearance of 10.4 ml/min/kg with a serum elimination half-life of 48 minutes. Approximately 64% of the clearance can be attributed to renal tubular secretion. The drug is approximately 16-28% bound to plasma proteins in dogs.

In horses, the apparent volume of distribution at steady state is 190 ml/kg, total body clearance of 5.51 ml/min/kg with a serum elimination half-life of 38 minutes when given IV and 84 minutes after IM injection (gluteal muscles). Cefazolin is about 4-8% bound to equine plasma proteins. Because of the significant tubular secretion of the drug, it would be expected that probenecid administration would alter the kinetics of cefazolin. One study performed in horses (Donecker, Sams, and Ashcroft 1986), did not show any effect, but the author's concluded that the dosage of probenecid may have been sub-therapeutic in this species.

In calves, the volume of distribution is 165 ml/kg, and had a terminal elimination half-life of 49-99 minutes after IM administration.

Doses -
   Dogs:
      For susceptible infections:
         a) 20 - 25 mg/kg IM, IV q6-8h (Vaden and Papich 1995)
         b) 10 - 30 mg/kg IM, IV or SQ (Riviere 1989)
         c) 11 - 33 mg/kg IV q8h; 22 - 33 mg/kg IM or SQ q8h (Aronson and Aucoin 1989)
      For surgical prophylaxis (soft-tissue):
         a) 20 mg/kg IV before and then every 2.5 hours during surgery (Rosin et al. 1988)
   Cats:
      For susceptible infections:
         a) 20 - 25 mg/kg IM, IV q6-8h (Vaden and Papich 1995)
         b) 10 - 30 mg/kg IM, IV or SQ (Riviere 1989)
         c) 11 - 33 mg/kg IV q8h; 22 - 33 mg/kg IM or SQ q8h (Aronson and Aucoin 1989)
   Horses:
      For susceptible infections:
         a) Respiratory tract: 11 mg/kg IV or IM q12h (Beech 1987a)

  b) 11 mg/kg IV or IM *qid* (Robinson 1987)
  c) Foals: 20 mg/kg IV q8-12h (Caprile and Short 1987)

Dosage Forms/Preparations/FDA Approval Status -
  Veterinary-Approved Products: None

  Human-Approved Products:
    Cefazolin Sodium Powder for Injection 250 mg (of cefazolin), 500 mg, 1, 5, 10, & 20g; *Ancef®* (SKF); *Kefzol®* (Lilly); *Zolicef®* (Apothecon);*Cefazolin Sodium®* (Apothecon). (Rx)

    Cefazolin Sodium for Injection (IV infusion) 500 mg in 5% Dextrose in Water (of cefazolin), 1 g in 5% Dextrose in Water, 1 g in 10 ml vials; *Ancef®* (SKB), *Kefzol®* (Lilly); (Rx)

CEFOPERAZONE SODIUM

Chemistry - A third generation cephalosporin, cefoperazone sodium contains a piperazine side chain giving it antipseudomonal activity. It occurs as white, crystalline powder and is freely soluble in water and poorly soluble in alcohol. At room temperature, cefoperazone sodium has a maximum solubility in compatible IV solutions of 475 mg/ml (at concentrations >333 mg/ml vigorous and prolonged shaking may be required). Reconstituted solutions of the drug have a pH from 4.5 - 6.5. One gram contains 1.5 mEq of sodium.

Storage/Stability/Compatibility - The sterile powder for injection should be stored at temperatures less than 25°C and protected from light. Once reconstituted, solutions do not need to be protected from light.

  After reconstitution, cefoperazone sodium is generally stable for 24 hours at room temperature and 5 days when refrigerated in a variety of IV solutions (*e.g.*, sterile or bacteriostatic water for injection, dextrose in water/saline/LRS solutions, lactated Ringer's injection, Normasol R, and saline IV solutions). When frozen at -2 to -10°C in dextrose, sodium chloride or sterile water for injection, cefoperazone sodium is stable for 3 weeks (dextrose solutions) to 5 weeks (water or saline solutions).

  Cefoperazone sodium is reportedly **compatible** with cimetidine HCl, clindamycin phosphate, furosemide and heparin sodium, acyclovir sodium, cyclophosphamide, esmolol HCl, famotidine, hydromorphone HCl, magnesium sulfate, and morphine sulfate. It is reportedly **incompatible** with some TPN mixtures, doxapram HCl, gentamicin sulfate, hetastarch, labetolol HCl, meperidine HCl, odansetron HCl, perphenazine, promethazine, and sargostim. Compatibility is dependent upon factors such as pH, concentration, temperature and diluents used. It is suggested to consult specialized references (*e.g., Handbook on Injectable Drugs* by Trissel; see bibliography) for more specific information.

Pharmacology - Cefoperazone is a third generation injectable cephalosporin agent. For more information, refer to the monograph: Cephalosporins, General Information.

Uses/Indications - Cefoperazone is used to treat serious infections, particularly against susceptible *Enterobacteriaceae* not susceptible to other less expensive agents or when aminoglycosides are not indicated (due to their potential toxicity).

Pharmacokinetics - Cefoperazone is not absorbed after oral administration and must be given parenterally. It is widely distributed throughout the body; CSF levels are low if meninges are not inflamed. Cefoperazone crosses the placenta and enters maternal milk in low concentrations; no documented adverse effects to offspring have been noted. Unlike most cephalosporins, cefoperazone is principally excreted in the bile and elimination half-lives are approximately 2 hours in humans. Dosage adjustments generally are not required for patients with renal insufficiency.

Contraindications/Precautions/Reproductive Safety - Only prior allergic reaction to cephalosporins contraindicates cefoperazone's use. In humans documented hypersensitive to penicillin, up to 16% may also be allergic to cephalosporins. The veterinary significance of this is unclear. Because cefoperazone is excreted in the bile, patients with significant hepatic disease or biliary obstruction may have their serum half-lives increase 2 - 4 times above normal. Dosage adjustment may be necessary. Cefoperazone should be used with caution in patients with preexisting bleeding disorders. It contains a thiomethyltetrazole side-chain which has been associated with causing coagulation abnormalities.

  No teratogenic effects were demonstrated in studies in pregnant mice, rats, and monkeys given up to 10 times labeled doses of cefoperazone.

Adverse Effects/Warnings - Cefoperazone is a relatively safe agent. Rarely, hypersensitivity reactions could potentially occur in animals. Because of its thiomethyltetrazole side-chain it may also rarely cause hypoprothrombinemia. Diarrhea secondary to changes in gut flora have been reported. Some human patients demonstrate mild, transient increases in liver enzymes, serum creatinine and BUN. Clinical significance of these effects is in doubt. If administered via the IM route, pain at the injection site has also been noted.

Overdosage/Acute Toxicity - No specific antidotes are available. Overdoses should be monitored and treated symptomatically and supportively if required.

Drug Interactions - A disulfiram-like reaction (anorexia, nausea, vomiting) has been reported in humans who have ingested **alcohol** with 48-72 hours of receiving beta-lactam antibiotics with a thiomethyltetrazole side-chain (*e.g.,* cefamandole, cefoperazone, moxalactam, cefotetan). Because these antibiotics have been associated with bleeding, they should be used cautiously in patients receiving **oral anticoagulants**.

Synergism against some Enterobacteriaceae (*e.g., Pseudomonas aeruginosa*) may be attained if using cefoperazone with a beta-lactamase inhibitor such as **clavulanic acid** or with an **aminoglycoside (*e.g.,* gentamicin, amikacin).** Do not mix cefoperazone in same syringe or IV bag with aminoglycosides as inactivation may occur. Synergy may be unpredictable however and although there have been no reports of additive nephrotoxicity with cefoperazone, some cephalosporins may increase the nephrotoxic potential of aminoglycosides. Probenecid does not have an effect on cefoperazone elimination.

Laboratory Considerations - When using Kirby-Bauer disk diffusion procedures for testing susceptibility, a specific 75 micrograms cefoperazone disk should be used. A cephalosporin-class disk containing cephalothin should not be used to test for cefoperazone susceptibility. An inhibition zone of 21 mm or more indicates susceptibility; 16-20 mm, intermediate; and 15 mm or less, resistant.

When using a dilution susceptibility procedure, an organism with a MIC of 16 micrograms/ml or less is considered susceptible and 64 micrograms/ml or greater is considered resistant. With either method, infections caused by organisms with intermediate susceptibility may be effectively treated if the infection is limited to tissues where the drug is concentrated (*e.g.,* urine, bile) or if a higher than normal dose is used.

In some human patients receiving cefoperazone, a positive direct antiglobulin (**Coombs'**) test has been reported.

Cefoperazone, like most other cephalosporins, may cause a **false-positive urine glucose determination** when using the cupric sulfate solution test (*e.g., Clinitest*®).

Doses -
 Horses:
  For susceptible infections: 30 - 50 mg/kg q8-12h IV or IM (Note: This is a human dose and should be used as a general guideline only) (Walker 1992)
   Monitoring Parameters - 1) Efficacy; 2) PT's, CBC if bleeding occurs

Client Information - Because cefoperazone use is generally associated with inpatient therapy, little client monitoring is required. They should be alert to either bleeding problems or symptoms associated with hypersensitivity.

Dosage Forms/Preparations/FDA Approval Status/Withholding Times -
 Veterinary-Approved Products: None
 Human-Approved Products:
  Cefoperazone Sodium Powder for Injection in 1g, 2g vials. Also available in 1 or 2 gram piggyback containers and in pre-mixed frozen in 50 ml plastic containers *Cefobid*® (Roerig); (Rx)

CEFOTAXIME SODIUM

For general information on the cephalosporins including adverse effects, contraindications, overdosage, drug interactions, and monitoring parameters, refer to the monograph: Cephalosporins, General Information.

Chemistry - A semisynthetic, 3rd generation, aminothiazolyl cephalosporin, cefotaxime sodium occurs as an odorless, white to off-white crystalline powder with a pK_a of 3.4. It is sparingly soluble in water and slightly soluble in alcohol. Potency of cefotaxime sodium is expressed in terms of cefotaxime. One gram of cefotaxime (sodium) contains 2.2 mEq of sodium.

Storage/Stability/Compatibility - Cefotaxime sodium sterile powder for injection should be stored at temperatures of less than 30°C; protect from light. The commercially available frozen injection should be stored at temperatures no greater than -20°C. Depending on storage conditions, the powder or solutions may darken which may indicate a loss in potency.

All commonly used IV fluids and the following drugs are reportedly **compatible** with cefotaxime: metronidazole and verapamil. Compatibility is dependent upon factors such as pH, concentration, temperature and diluents used. It is suggested to consult specialized references for more specific information (*e.g., Handbook on Injectable Drugs* by Trissel; see bibliography).

Pharmacology/Spectrum of Activity - Cefotaxime has a relatively wide spectrum of activity against both gram positive and gram negative bacteria. While less active against *Staphylococcus* *spp.* than the first generation agents, it still has significant activity against those and other gram positive cocci. Cefotaxime, like the other 3rd generation agents, has extended coverage of gram negative aerobes particularly in the family Enterobacteriaceae, including *Klebsiella sp., E. coli, Salmonella, Serratia marcesans, Proteus sp.*, and *Enterobacter sp.*. Cefotaxime's *in vitro* activity against *Pseudomonas aeruginosa* is variable and results are usually disappointing when the drug is used clinically against this organism. Many anaerobes are also susceptible to cefotaxime, including strains of *Bacteroides fragilis, Clostridium sp., Fusobacterium sp., Peptococcus sp.*, and *Peptostreptococcus sp.*.

Because 3rd generation cephalosporins exhibit specific activities against bacteria, a 30 micrograms cefotaxime disk should be used when performing Kirby-Bauer disk susceptibility tests for this antibiotic.

Uses/Indications - In the United States, there are no cefotaxime products approved for veterinary species, but it has been used clinically in several species when an injectable 3rd generation cephalosporin may be indicated.

Pharmacokinetics (specific) - Cefotaxime is not appreciably absorbed after oral administration and must be given parenterally to attain therapeutic serum levels. After administration, the drug is widely distributed in body tissues, including bone, prostatic fluid (human), aqueous humor, bile, ascitic and pleural fluids. Cefotaxime crosses the placenta and activity in amniotic fluid either equals or exceeds that in maternal serum. Cefotaxime also is distributed into milk in low concentrations. In humans, approximately 13-40% of the drug is bound to plasma proteins.

Unlike the first generation cephalosporins (and most 2nd generation agents), cefotaxime will enter the CSF in therapeutic levels (at high dosages) when the patient's meninges are inflamed.

Cefotaxime is partially metabolized by the liver to desacetylcefotaxime which exhibits some antibacterial activity. Desacetylcefotaxime is partially degraded to inactive metabolites by the liver. Cefotaxime and its metabolites are primarily excreted in the urine. Because tubular secretion is involved in the renal excretion of the drug, probenecid has been demonstrated in several species to prolong the serum half-life of cefotaxime.

Pharmacokinetic parameters in certain veterinary species follow: In dogs, the apparent volume of distribution at steady state is 480 ml/kg, and a total body clearance of 10.5 ml/min/kg after intravenous injection. Serum elimination half-lives of 45 minutes when given IV, 50 minutes after IM injection, and 103 minutes after SQ injection have been noted. Bioavailability is about 87% after IM injection and approximately 100% after SQ injection.

In cats, total body clearance is approximately 3 ml/min/kg after intravenous injection and the serum elimination half-life is about 1 hour. Bioavailability is about 93-98% after IM injection.

Doses -
   Dogs:
      For susceptible infections:
         a) For acute pancreatitis: 6 - 40 mg/kg IV or IM *qid* (Morgan 1988)
         b) 27.5 - 55 mg/kg IM, IV or SQ q8h (Aronson and Aucoin 1989)
         c) 25 - 50 mg/kg IV, IM or SQ q8h (Riviere 1989); (Vaden and Papich 1995)

   Cats:
      For susceptible infections:
         a) 27.5 - 55 mg/kg IM, IV or SQ q8h (Aronson and Aucoin 1989)
         b) 25 - 50 mg/kg IV, IM or SQ q8h (Riviere 1989)
         c) 25 - 50 mg/kg IV, IM or SQ q8h (Vaden and Papich 1995)

   Horses:
      For susceptible infections:
         a) Foals: 20 - 30 mg/kg IV q6h (Caprile and Short 1987)

   Birds:
      For susceptible infections:
         a) For most birds: 50 - 100 mg/kg IM *tid*; may be used with aminoglycosides, but nephrotoxicity may occur. Reconstituted vial good for 13 weeks if frozen. (Clubb 1986)
         b) 75 - 100 mg/kg IM or IV q6-8h (Hoeffer 1995)

   Reptiles:
      For susceptible infections:
         a) 20 - 40 mg/kg IM once daily for 7-14 days. (Gauvin 1993)

Dosage Forms/Preparations/FDA Approval Status -
   Veterinary-Approved Products: None

   Human-Approved Products:

   Cefotaxime Sodium Powder for Injection; 500 mg, 1 g (as cefotaxime), 2 g, 10 g; *Claforan®* (Hoechst Marion Roussel); (Rx)

Cefotaxime Sodium for Injection in 5% dextrose bags (50 ml)—frozen; 1 g, 2 g; *Claforan*® (Hoechst Marion Roussel); (Rx)

CEFOXITIN SODIUM

For general information on the cephalosporins including adverse effects, contraindications, over-dosage, drug interactions, and monitoring parameters, refer to the monograph: Cephalosporins, General Information.

Chemistry - Actually a cephamycin, cefoxitin sodium is a semisynthetic antibiotic that is derived from cephamycin C which is produced by *Streptomyces lactamdurans*. It occurs as a white to off-white, somewhat hygroscopic powder or granules with a slight characteristic odor. It is very soluble in water and slightly soluble in alcohol. Each gram of cefoxitin sodium contains 2.3 mEq of sodium.

Storage/Stability/Compatibility - Cefoxitin sodium powder for injection should be stored at temperatures less than 30°C and should not be exposed to temperatures greater than 50°C. The frozen solution for injection should be stored at temperatures no higher than -20°C.

After reconstitution, the solution is stable for 24 hours when kept at room temperature and from 48 hours to 1 week if refrigerated. If after reconstitution the solution is immediately frozen in the original container, the preparation is stable up to 30 weeks when stored at -20°C. Stability is dependent on the diluent used and the reader should refer to the package insert or other specialized references for more information. The powder or reconstituted solution may darken, but this apparently does not affect the potency of the product.

All commonly used IV fluids and the following drugs are reportedly **compatible** with cefoxitin: amikacin sulfate, cimetidine HCl, gentamicin sulfate, kanamycin sulfate, mannitol, metronidazole, mutivitamin infusion concentrate, sodium bicarbonate, tobramycin sulfate and vitamin B-complex with C. Compatibility is dependent upon factors such as pH, concentration, temperature and diluents used. It is suggested to consult specialized references for more specific information (*e.g., Handbook on Injectable Drugs* by Trissel; see bibliography).

Pharmacology/Spectrum of Activity - Although not a true cephalosporin, cefoxitin is usually classified as a 2nd generation agent. Cefoxitin has activity against gram positive cocci, but less so on a per weight basis than the 1st generation agents. Unlike the first generation agents, it has good activity against many strains of *E. coli*, *Klebsiella* and *Proteus* that may be resistant to the first generation agents. In human medicine, cefoxitin's activity against many strains of *Bacteroides fragilis* has placed it in a significant therapeutic role. While *Bacteroides fragilis* has been isolated from anerobic infections in veterinary patients, it may not be as significant a pathogen in veterinary species as in humans.

Because 2nd generation cephalosporins exhibit specific activities against bacteria, a 30-micrograms cefoxitin disk should be used when performing Kirby-Bauer disk susceptibility tests for this antibiotic

Uses/Indications - In the United States, there are no cefoxitin products approved for veterinary species, but it has been used clinically in several species when an injectable second generation cephalosporin may be indicated.

Pharmacokinetics (specific) - Cefoxitin is not appreciably absorbed after oral administration and must be given parenterally to achieve therapeutic serum levels. The absorbed drug is primarily excreted unchanged by the kidneys into the urine via both tubular secretion and glomerular filtration. In humans, approximately 2% of a dose is metabolized to descarbamylcefoxitin, which is inactive. Elimination half-lives may be significantly prolonged in patients with severely diminished renal function.

In horses, the apparent volume of distribution at steady state is 110 ml/kg, total body clearance of 4.32 ml/min/kg with a serum elimination half-life of 49 minutes.

In calves, the volume of distribution is 318 ml/kg, and has a terminal elimination half-life of 67 minutes after IV dosing, and 81 minutes after IM administration. Cefoxitin is approximately 50% bound to calf plasma proteins. Probenecid (40 mg/kg) has been demonstrated to significantly prolong elimination half-lives.

Doses -
  Dogs:
    For susceptible infections:
      a) 6 - 20 mg/kg SQ, IM, IV *tid*; for meningitis: 6 - 40 mg/kg IV *tid-qid* (Morgan 1988)
      b) 11 - 22 mg/kg IV q8h (Aronson and Aucoin 1989)
      c) 10 - 20 mg/kg IV q8h (Riviere 1989)
      d) 30 mg/kg IV q8h (Vaden and Papich 1995)
  Cats:
    For susceptible infections:

    a)   11 - 22 mg/kg IV q8h (Aronson and Aucoin 1989)
    b)   10 - 20 mg/kg IV q8h (Riviere 1989)
    c)   30 mg/kg IV q8h (Vaden and Papich 1995)

Horses:
  For susceptible infections:
    a)   Foals: 20 mg/kg IV q4-6h (Caprile and Short 1987)

Dosage Forms/Preparations/FDA Approval Status -
Veterinary-Approved Products: None

Human-Approved Products:
Cefoxitin Sodium Powder for Injection 1 g (of cefoxitin), 2 g, 10 g
  Mefoxin® (Merck); (Rx)

Cefoxitin Sodium in Dextrose 5% (Frozen) 1 g (20 mg/ml), 2 g (40 mg/ml)
  Mefoxin® (Merck); (Rx)

CEFTIOFUR SODIUM
CEFTIOFUR HCL

For general information on the cephalosporins including adverse effects, contraindications, over-dosage, drug interactions, and monitoring parameters, refer to the monograph: Cephalosporins, General Information.

Chemistry - Ceftiofur sodium and HCl are semisynthetic 3rd generation cephalosporins.

Storage/Stability/Compatibility - Unreconstituted ceftiofur sodium powder for reconstitution should be stored in the refrigerator (2°-8°C). Protect from light. Color of the cake may vary from off-white to tan, but this does not affect potency. After reconstitution with bacteriostatic water for injection or sterile water for injection, the solution is stable for up to 7 days when refrigerated and for 12 hours at room temperature (15-30°C). According to the manufacturer, if a precipitate should form while being stored refrigerated during this time, the product may be used if it goes back into solution after warming. If not, contact the manufacturer. Frozen reconstituted solutions are stable for up to 8 weeks. Thawing may be done at room temperature or by swirling the vial under running warm or hot water.

  The HCl product should be stored at controlled room temperature (20°-25°C; 68°-77°F) and protected from freezing. It should be shaken well before use.

Pharmacology/Spectrum of Activity - Ceftiofur inhibits cell wall synthesis (at stage three) of susceptible multiplying bacteria. Ceftiofur exhibits a spectrum of activity similar to that of cefo-taxime. It has a broad range of in vitro activity against a variety of pathogens, including many species of Pasturella, Streptococcus, Staphylococcus, Salmonella, and E.coli.

Uses/Indications - Ceftiofur sodium/HCl is indicated for treatment of bovine respiratory disease (shipping fever, pneumonia) associated with *Pasturella hemolytica, Pasturella multocida* and *Haemophilus somnus* in lactating or non-lactating cattle and ceftiofur sodium is indicated in horses for respiratory disease associated with *Strep zooepidimicus*:. Ceftiofur HCl is also approved for foot rot in cattle.

  Ceftiofur could potentially be of usefulness in small animal infections as well, but little published data is available to recommend its use.

Pharmacokinetics (specific) - In cattle, ceftiofur sodium and HCl have practically equivalent pharmacokinetic parameters. Peak levels of ceftiofur are slightly higher after IM injection of Naxcel®, but areas under the curve are practically equal as well as elimination half-lives (approx. 9-12 hours).

Doses -
Cattle:
  For labeled indications:
    a)   Naxcel®: 1.1 - 2.2 mg/kg IM once daily for 3 treatments; may give additional doses on 4th and 5th day if response is not satisfactory. Reconstitute 1 g vial with 20 ml and the 4 g vial with 80 ml of either Bacteriostatic Water for Injection or Sterile Water for Injection. (Package Insert; *Naxcel*®—Upjohn)
    b)   Excenel®: 1.1 - 2.2 mg/kg IM or SQ once daily for 3 treatments; may give additional doses on 4th and 5th day if response is not satisfactory. For BRD only: May inject 2.2 mg/kg IM or SQ every other day (days 1 and 3; 48 hour interval). Do not inject more than 15 ml pe IM injection site. (Package Insert; *Excenel*®—Pharmacia/Upjohn)

Horses:
  For respiratory disease associated with *Strep zooepidimicus*::
    a)   Naxcel®: 2.2 - 4.4 mg/kg (2 - 4 ml reconstituted sterile solution per 100 lb. of body weight) with a maximum of 10 ml administered per injection site. Repeat treatment

at 24 hour intervals, continued for 48 hours after symptoms have disappeared. Do not exceed 10 days of treatment. (Package Insert; *Naxcel®*—Upjohn)

Dogs:
For susceptible infections:
  a) The author has received several anecdotal dosages for this product (Naxcel®) in dogs. They range from 2.2 mg/kg subQ once daily for 5-14 days for treatment of UTI to 4.4 - 5.5 mg/kg subQ once daily. Until further data confirms the safety and efficacy of this drug in dogs (and cats); use with caution. (Plumb)

Reptiles:
For susceptible infections:
  a) For chelonians: 4 mg/kg IM once daily for 2 weeks. Commonly used in respiratory infections. (Gauvin 1993)

Dosage Forms/Preparations/FDA Approval Status/Withholding Times -
Veterinary-Approved Products:

Ceftiofur Sodium Powder for Injection 1 g, 4 g vials; *Naxcel®* (Pharmacia&Upjohn); (Rx) Approved for use in cattle and horses. No slaughter withdrawal or milk withholding time are required when administered as labeled.

Ceftiofur HCl Suspension for Injection 50 mg(of ceftiofur)/ml in 100 ml vials; *Excenel®* (Pharmacia&Upjohn); (Rx). Approved for use in cattle. Slaughter withdrawal=48 hours; no milk withholding time required when administered as labeled.

Human-Approved Products: None

CEFTRIAXONE SODIUM

Chemistry - A third generation cephalosporin, ceftriaxone sodium occurs as white to yellowish-orange crystalline powder. It is soluble in water (400 mg/ml at 25°C). Potencies of commercial products are expressed in terms of ceftriaxone. One gram of ceftriaxone sodium contains 3.6 mEq of sodium.

Storage/Stability/Compatibility - The sterile powder for reconstitution should be stored at, or below 25°C and protected from light.

After reconstituting with either 0.9% sodium chloride or D5W, ceftriaxone solutions (at concentrations of approximately 100 mg/ml) are stable for 3 days at room temperature and for 10 days when refrigerated. Solutions of concentrations of 250 mg/ml are stable for 24 hours at room temperature and 3 days when refrigerated. At concentrations of 10-40 mg/ml solutions frozen at -20°C are stable for 26 weeks. The manufacturer does not recommend admixing any other anti-infective drugs with ceftriaxone sodium.

Pharmacology - Ceftriaxone is a third generation injectable cephalosporin agent. For more information, refer to the monograph: Cephalosporins, General Information.

Uses/Indications - Ceftriaxone is used to treat serious infections, particularly against susceptible *Enterobacteriaceae* that are not susceptible to other less expensive agents or when aminoglycosides are not indicated (due to their potential toxicity). Its long half life, good CNS penetration, and activity against *Borrelia burgdorferi* also has made it a potential choice for treating Lyme's disease.

Pharmacokinetics - Ceftriaxone is not absorbed after oral administration and must be given parenterally. It is widely distributed throughout the body; CSF levels are higher when meninges are inflamed. Ceftriaxone crosses the placenta and enters maternal milk in low concentrations; no documented adverse effects to offspring have been noted. Ceftriaxone is excreted by both renal and non-renal mechanisms and in humans, elimination half-lives are approximately 6-11 hours. Dosage adjustments generally are not required for patients with renal insufficiency (unless severely uremic) or with hepatic impairment.

Contraindications/Precautions/Reproductive Safety - Only prior allergic reaction to cephalosporins contraindicates ceftriaxone's use. In humans documented hypersensitive to penicillin, up to 16% may also be allergic to cephalosporins. The veterinary significance of this is unclear.

Although bleeding times have only been reported rarely in humans, ceftriaxone should be used with caution in patients with vitamin K utilization or synthesis abnormalities (*e.g.*, severe hepatic disease).

No teratogenic effects were demonstrated in studies in pregnant mice and rats given up to 20 times labeled doses of ceftriaxone.

Adverse Effects/Warnings - Because veterinary usage of ceftriaxone is very limited, an accurate adverse effect profile has not been determined. The following adverse effects have been reported in humans and may or may not apply to veterinary patients: hematologic effects, including eosinophilia (6%), thrombocytosis (5%), leukopenia (2%) and more rarely, anemia, neutropenia, lymphopenia and thrombocytopenia. Approximately 2-4% of humans get diarrhea. Very high dosages (100 mg/kg/day) in dogs have caused a "sludge" in bile. Hypersensitivity reactions (usually a rash) have been noted. Increased serum concentrations of liver enzymes, BUN, creatinine, and urine casts have been described in about 1-3% of patients. When given IM, pain may be noted at the injection site.

Overdosage/Acute Toxicity - Limited information available; overdoses should be monitored and treated symptomatically and supportively if required.

Drug Interactions - Synergism against some Enterobacteriaceae (*e.g., Pseudomonas aeruginosa*) may be attained if using cefoperazone with an **aminoglycoside (*e.g.,* gentamicin, amikacin).** Organisms with a high degree of resistance to both ceftriaxone and the aminoglycoside are unlikely to be affected when the two drugs are used together.

Probenecid does not have an effect on ceftriaxone elimination.

Laboratory Considerations - When using Kirby-Bauer disk diffusion procedures for testing susceptibility, a specific 30 micrograms ceftriaxone disk should be used. A cephalosporin-class disk containing cephalothin should not be used to test for ceftriaxone susceptibility. An inhibition zone of 18 mm or more indicates susceptibility; 14-17 mm, intermediate; and 13 mm or less, resistant.

When using a dilution susceptibility procedure, an organism with a MIC of 16 micrograms/ml or less is considered susceptible and 64 micrograms/ml or greater is considered resistant. With either method, infections caused by organisms with intermediate susceptibility may be effectively treated if the infection is limited to tissues where the drug is concentrated or if a higher than normal dose is used.

Ceftriaxone, like most other cephalosporins, may cause a **false-positive urine glucose** determination when using the cupric sulfate solution test (*e.g., Clinitest®*).

Ceftriaxone in very high concentrations (50 micrograms/ml or greater) may cause falsely elevated serum creatinine levels when manual methods of testing are used. Automated methods do not appear to be affected.

Doses -
  Dogs/Cats:
    For resistant cases of Lyme Disease when response to other antibiotics is not noted:
      a) 20 mg/kg IV or SubQ q12h for 7-10 days (Greene 1990)

  Horses:
    For susceptible infections: 25 - 50 mg/kg q12h IV or IM (Note: This is a human dose and should be used as a general guideline only) (Walker 1992)

Monitoring Parameters - 1) Efficacy; 2) If long term therapy, occasional CBC, renal function (BUN, Serum Creatinine, urinalysis) and liver enzymes (AST, ALT) may be considered.

Dosage Forms/Preparations/FDA Approval Status/Withholding Times -
  Veterinary-Approved Products: None
  Human-Approved Products:
    Ceftriaxone Powder for Injection 250 mg, 500 mg (as sodium), 1 g, 2g, 10 g; *Cefizox®* (Fujisawa) (Rx)

    Ceftriaxone Injection in 5% dextrose in Water 1 g (as sodium) & 2 g frozen, premixed; *Cefizox®* (Fujisawa) (Rx)

CEPHALEXIN

For general information on the cephalosporins including adverse effects, contraindications, overdosage, drug interactions, and monitoring parameters, refer to the monograph: Cephalosporins, General Information.

Chemistry - A semi-synthetic oral cephalosporin, cephalexin (as the monohydrate) occurs as a white to off-white, crystalline powder. It is slightly soluble in water and practically insoluble in alcohol.

Storage/Stability/Compatibility - Cephalexin tablets, capsules, and powder for oral suspension should be stored at room temperature (15-30°C) in tight containers. After reconstitution, the oral suspension is stable for 2 weeks.

Pharmacology/Spectrum of Activity - A first generation cephalosporin, cephalexin exhibits activity against the bacteria usually covered by this class. Refer to the monograph: Cephalosporins, General Information for more specific information.

Uses/Indications - There are no approved cephalexin products for veterinary use in the United States. It has been used clinically in dogs, cats, horses and birds, however.

Pharmacokinetics (specific) - After oral administration, cephalexin is rapidly and completely absorbed in humans. Cephalexin (base) must be converted to the HCl before absorption can occur and, therefore, absorption can be delayed. There is a form of cephalexin HCl commercially available for oral use which apparently is absorbed more rapidly, but the clinical significance of this is in question.

In a study done in dogs and cats (Silley et al. 1988), peak serum levels reached 18.6 micrograms/ml about 1.8 hours after a mean oral dose of 12.7 mg/kg in dogs, and 18.7 micrograms/ml, 2.6 hours after an oral dose of 22.9 mg/kg in cats. Elimination half-lives ranged from 1-2 hours in both species. Bioavailability was about 75% in both species after oral administration.

In the U.K., an oily suspension of the sodium salt (*Ceporex® Injection*— Glaxovet) is apparently available for IM or SQ injection in animals. In calves, the sodium salt had a 74% bioavailability after IM injection and a serum half-life of about 90 minutes.

Adverse Effects/Warnings - In addition to the adverse effects listed in the general statement on the cephalosporins, cephalexin has reportedly caused salivation, tachypnea and excitability in dogs, and emesis and fever in cats. Nephrotoxicity occurs rarely during therapy with cephalexin, but patients with renal dysfunction, receiving other nephrotoxic drugs or are geriatric may be more susceptible. Interstitial nephritis, a hypersensitivity reaction, has been reported with many of the cephalosporins including cephalexin. The incidence of these effects is not known.

Doses -
Dogs:
For susceptible infections:
    a)   11 - 33 mg/kg PO q8h (Aronson and Aucoin 1989)
    b)   22 mg/kg PO q8h; administer with food if GI upset occurs (Vaden and Papich 1995)
    c)   10 - 30 mg/kg PO q8h (Riviere 1989)
    d)   30 mg/kg PO q12h (Jenkins 1987a)
    e)   For *Staph*. osteomyelitis: 30 mg/kg PO q12h (Ford and Aronson 1985)

Cats:
For susceptible infections:
    a)   11 - 33 mg/kg PO q8h (Aronson and Aucoin 1989)
    b)   22 mg/kg PO q8h; administer with food if GI upset occurs (Vaden and Papich 1995)
    c)   10 - 30 mg/kg PO q8h (Riviere 1989)
    d)   30 mg/kg PO q12h (Jenkins 1987a)

Horses:
For susceptible infections:
    a)   25 mg/kg PO *qid* (Robinson 1987)
    b)   22 - 33 mg/kg PO q6h (Brumbaugh 1987)

Birds:
For susceptible infections:
    a)   35 - 50 mg/kg PO *qid* (using suspension); most preps are well accepted. (Clubb 1986)
    b)   40 - 100 mg/kg q6h PO (Hoeffer 1995)

Dosage Forms/Preparations/FDA Approval Status/Withholding Times -
Veterinary-Approved Products: None

Human-Approved Products:
Cephalexin (monohydrate) Capsules 250 mg, 500 mg and Tablets 250 mg, 500 mg and 1 gram; *Keflex®* (Dista); *Biocef®* (IEL); generic (Rx)

Cephalexin Oral Suspension 125 mg/5ml and 250 mg/5 ml in 100 and 200 ml and UD 5ml; *Keflex®* (Dista); *Biocef®* (IEL); generic (Rx)

CEPHALOSPORINS (GENERAL INFORMATION)

Note: There are presently over 20 different cephalosporin drugs available for either human or veterinary use. Ten separate monographs of cephalosporins that appear to have the most current veterinary use and/or applicability may be found by their generic name. For a more detailed review of cephalosporins in veterinary medicine, the reader is referred to the following article: Caprile, K.A. 1988. The Cephalosporin Antimicrobial Agents: A Comprehensive Review. J Vet Pharmacol Ther 11 (1):1-32.

Pharmacology - The cephalosporin antibiotics are comprised of several different classes of compounds with dissimilar spectrums of activity and pharmacokinetic profiles. All "true" cephalosporins are derived from cephalosporin C which is produced from *Cephalosporium acremonium.*

Cephalosporins are usually bactericidal against susceptible bacteria and act by inhibiting mucopeptide synthesis in the cell wall resulting in a defective barrier and an osmotically unstable spheroplast. The exact mechanism for this effect has not been definitively determined, but beta-lactam antibiotics have been shown to bind to several enzymes (carboxypeptidases, transpeptidases, endopeptidases) within the bacterial cytoplasmic membrane that are involved with cell wall synthesis. The different affinities that various beta-lactam antibiotics have for these enzymes (also known as penicillin-binding proteins; PBPs) help explain the differences in spectrums of activity of these drugs that are not explained by the influence of beta-lactamases. Like other beta-lactam antibiotics, cephalosporins are generally considered to be more effective against actively growing bacteria.

The cephalosporin class of antibiotics is usually divided into three classifications or generations. The so-called first generation of cephalosporins include (routes of administration in parentheses): cephalothin (IM/IV), cefazolin (IM/IV), cephapirin (IM/IV/Intramammary), cephradine (IM/IV/PO), cephalexin (PO) and cefadroxil (PO). While there may be differences in MIC's for individual first generation cephalosporins, their spectrums of activity are quite similar. They possess generally excellent coverage against most gram-positive pathogens and variable to poor coverage against most gram negative pathogens. These drugs are very active *in vitro* against groups A beta-hemolytic and B *Streptococci*, non-enterococcal group D *Streptococci* (*S. bovis*), *Staphylococcus intermedius* and *aureas*, *Proteus mirabilis* and some strains of *E. coli*, *Klebsiella sp.*, *Actinobacillus*, *Pasturella*, *Haemophilus equigenitalis*, *Shigella* and *Salmonella*. With the exception of *Bacteroides fragilis*, most anaerobes are very susceptible to the first generation agents. Most species of *Corynebacteria* are susceptible, but *C. equi* (*Rhodococcus*) is usually resistant. Strains of *Staphylococcus epidermidis* are usually sensitive to the parenterally administered 1st generation drugs, but may have variable susceptibilities to the oral drugs. The following bacteria are regularly resistant to the 1st generation agents: Group D *streptococci/enterococci* (*S. faecalis*, S. *faecium*), Methicillin-resistant *Staphylococci*, indole-positive *Proteus sp.*, *Pseudomonas sp.*, *Enterobacter sp.*, *Serratia sp.* and *Citrobacter sp.*.

The second generation cephalosporins include: cefaclor (PO), cefamandole (IM/IV), cefonicid (IM/IV), ceforanide (IM/IV) and cefuroxime (PO/IM/IV). Although not true cephalosporins (they are actually cephamycins), cefoxitin (IM/IV) and cefotetan (IM/IV) are usually included in this group, although some references categorize cefotetan as a 3rd generation agent. In addition to the gram positive coverage of the 1st generation agents, these agents have expanded gram negative coverage. Cefoxitin and cefotetan also have good activity against *Bacteroides fragilis*. Enough variation exists between these agents in regard to their spectrums of activity against most species of gram negative bacteria, that susceptibility testing is generally required to determine sensitivity. The second generation agents have not found widespread use in most veterinary practices, although cefoxitin has been used somewhat.

The third generation cephalosporins retain the gram positive activity of the first and second generation agents, but in comparison, have much expanded gram negative activity. Included in this group are: cefotaxime (IM/IV), moxalactam (actually a 1-oxa-beta-lacatam; IM/IV), cefoperazone (IM/IV), ceftizoxime (IM/IV), ceftazidime (IM/IV), ceftriaxone (IM/IV), ceftiofur (IM) and cefixime (PO). As with the 2nd generation agents, enough variability exists with individual bacterial sensitivities that susceptibility testing is necessary for most bacteria. Usually only ceftazidime and cefoperazone are active against most strains of *Pseudomonas aeruginosa*. Because of the excellent gram negative coverage of these agents and when compared to the aminoglycosides, their significantly less toxic potential, they have been used on an increasing basis in veterinary medicine. Ceftiofur is approved for use in beef cattle, but its use in other species is hindered by a lack of data on its spectrum of activity or availability of pharmacokinetic profiles.

Uses/Indications - Cephalosporins have been used for a wide range of infections in various species. FDA-approved indications/species, as well as non-approved uses are listed in the Uses/Indications and Dosage sections for each individual drug.

Pharmacokinetics (General)- Until recently, only some first generation cephalosporins were absorbed appreciably after oral administration, but this has changed with the availability of cefuroxime axetil (2nd generation) and cefixime (3rd generation). Depending on the drug, absorption may be delayed, unaltered, or increased if administered with food. There are reported species variations in the oral bioavailability of some cephalosporins which are detailed under each individual drug's monograph.

Cephalosporins are widely distributed to most tissues and fluids, including bone, pleural fluid, pericardial fluid and synovial fluid. Higher levels are found in inflamed than in normal bone. Very high levels are found in the urine, but they penetrate poorly into prostatic tissue and aqueous humor. Bile levels can reach therapeutic concentrations with several of the agents as long as biliary obstruction is not present. With the exception of cefuroxime, no first or second generation cephalosporin enters the CSF (even with inflamed meninges) in therapeutically effective levels. Therapeutic concentrations of cefotaxime, moxalactam, cefuroxime, ceftizoxime, ceftazidime and ceftriaxone can be found in the CSF after parenteral dosing in patients with inflamed meninges. Cephalosporins cross the placenta and fetal serum concentrations can be 10% or more of those found in maternal serum. Cephalosporins enter milk in low concentrations. Protein binding of the drugs is widely variable and species specific. Cephalosporins tend to bind to equine and canine plasma proteins less so then to human plasma proteins.

Cephalosporins and their metabolites (if any) are excreted by the kidneys, via tubular secretion and/or glomerular filtration. Some cephalosporins (*e.g.,* cefotaxime, cefazolin, and cephapirin) are partially metabolized by the liver to desacetyl compounds that may have some antibacterial activity.

Contraindications/Precautions/Reproductive Safety - Cephalosporins are contraindicated in patients who have a history of hypersensitivity to them. Because there may be cross-reactivity, use cephalosporins cautiously in patients who are documented hypersensitive to other beta-lactam antibiotics (*e.g.,* penicillins, cefamycins, carbapenems).

Oral systemic antibiotics should not be administered in patients with septicemia, shock or other grave illnesses as absorption of the medication from the GI tract may be significantly delayed or diminished. Parenteral routes (preferably IV) should be used for these cases.

Cephalosporins have been shown to cross the placenta and safe use of them during pregnancy have not been firmly established, but neither have there been any documented teratogenic problems associated with these drugs. However, use only when the potential benefits outweigh the risks.

Adverse Effects/Warnings - Adverse effects with the cephalosporins are usually not serious and have a relatively low frequency of occurrence.

Hypersensitivity reactions unrelated to dose can occur with these agents and can be manifested as rashes, fever, eosinophilia, lymphadenopathy, or full-blown anaphylaxis. The use of cephalosporins in patients documented to be hypersensitive to penicillin-class antibiotics is controversial. In humans, it is estimated that up to 15% of patients hypersensitive to penicillins will also be hypersensitive to cephalosporins. The incidence of cross-reactivity in veterinary patients is unknown.

Cephalosporins can cause pain at the injection site when administered intramuscularly, although this effect is less so with cefazolin than other agents. Sterile abscesses or other severe local tissue reactions are also possible but are much less common. Thrombophlebitis is also possible after IV administration of these drugs.

When given orally, cephalosporins may cause GI effects (anorexia, vomiting, diarrhea). Administering the drug with a small meal may help alleviate these symptoms. Because the cephalosporins may also alter gut flora, antibiotic-associated diarrhea can occur as well as the selection out of resistant bacteria maintaining residence in the colon of the animal.

While it has been demonstrated that the cephalosporins (particularly cephalothin) have the potential for causing nephrotoxicity, at clinically used doses in patients with normal renal function, risks for this adverse effect occurring appear minimal.

High doses or very prolonged use has been associated with neurotoxicity, neutropenia, agranulocytosis, thrombocytopenia, hepatitis, positive Comb's test, interstitial nephritis, and tubular necrosis. Except for tubular necrosis and neurotoxicity, these effects have an immunologic component.

Some cephalosporins (cefamandole, cefoperazone, moxalactam) that contain a thiomethyltetrazole side chain have been implicated in causing bleeding problems in humans. These drugs are infrequently used in veterinary species at the present time, so any veterinary ramifications of this effect are unclear.

Overdosage/Acute Toxicity - Acute oral cephalosporin overdoses are unlikely to cause significant problems other than GI distress, but other effects are possible (see Adverse effects section).

Drug Interactions - The concurrent use of parenteral **aminoglycosides** or other nephrotoxic drugs (*e.g.,* **amphotericin B**) with cephalosporins is controversial. Potentially, cephalosporins could cause additive nephrotoxicity when used with these drugs, but this interaction has only been well documented with cephaloridine (no longer marketed). Nevertheless, they should be used together cautiously.

In vitro studies have demonstrated that cephalosporins can have synergistic or additive activity against certain bacteria when used with **aminoglycosides, penicillins,** or **chloramphenicol**. However, some clinicians do not recommend using cephalosporins concurrently with **bacteriostatic antibiotics** (*e.g.,* chloramphenicol), particularly in acute infections where the organism is proliferating rapidly.

Probenecid competitively blocks the tubular secretion of most cephalosporins, thereby increasing serum levels and serum half-lives.

A disulfiram-like reaction (anorexia, nausea, vomiting) has been reported in humans who have ingested **alcohol** with 48-72 hours of receiving beta-lactam antibiotics (*e.g.,* cefamandole, cefoperazone, moxalactam, cefotetan) with a thiomethyltetrazole side-chain. Because these antibiotics have been associated with bleeding, they should be used cautiously in patients receiving **oral anticoagulants**.

Drug/Laboratory Interactions - Except for cefotaxime, cephalosporins may cause false-positive **urine glucose determinations** when using cupric sulfate solution (Benedict's Solution, *Clinitest*®). Tests utilizing glucose oxidase (*Tes-Tape*®, *Clinistix*®) are not affected by cephalosporins.

When using the Jaffe reaction to measure **serum or urine creatinine**, cephalosporins (not ceftazidime or cefotaxime) in high dosages may falsely cause elevated values.

In humans, particularly with azotemia, cephalosporins have caused a false-positive direct **Combs' test**. Cephalosporins may also cause falsely elevated **17-ketosteroid** values in urine.

Monitoring Parameters - Because cephalosporins usually have minimal toxicity associated with their use, monitoring for efficacy is usually all that is required. Patients with diminished renal function, may require intensified renal monitoring. Serum levels and therapeutic drug monitoring are not routinely done with these agents.

CEPHALOTHIN SODIUM

For general information on the cephalosporins including adverse effects, contraindications, overdosage, drug interactions, and monitoring parameters, refer to the monograph: Cephalosporins, General Information.

Chemistry - An injectable semi-synthetic cephalosporin antibiotic, cephalothin sodium occurs as a practically odorless, white to off-white, crystalline powder. It is freely soluble in water and very slightly soluble in alcohol. Each gram of the injection contains 2.8 mEq of sodium. After reconstitution the solution for injection has a pH of 6.0-8.5.

Storage/Stability/Compatibility - The sterile powder for injection and reconstitution should be stored at room temperature. After reconstituting with sterile water for injection, cephalothin sodium neutral is stable for 12 hours at room temperature and 96 hours when refrigerated. Precipitates may occur with refrigerated solutions, but can be redissolved with warming and agitation. Solutions may darken, particularly at room temperature, but this does not indicate any loss of potency. In the frozen state, cephalothin sodium solutions are relatively stable.

The following drugs or solutions are reportedly **compatible** with cephalothin: D25W/Amino Acids 4.25%, D5W in Lactated Ringer's, D5W in sodium chloride 0.2% - 0.9%, D5W, D10W, Lactated Ringer's Injection, normal saline, ascorbic acid injection, chloramphenicol sodium succinate, clindamycin phosphate, cytarabine, fluorouracil, heparin sodium, hydrocortisone sodium succinate, magnesium sulfate, metaraminol bitartrate, methotrexate, nitrofurantoin sodium, oxacillin sodium, phytonadione, polymyxin B sulfate, potassium chloride, sodium bicarbonate and vitamin B-complex with C.

The following drugs or solutions are reportedly **incompatible** or only compatible in specific situations with cephalothin: amikacin sulfate, aminophylline, bleomycin sulfate, calcium chloride/gluconate, cimetidine HCl, dopamine HCl, doxorubicin HCl, erythromycin lactobionate, gentamicin sulfate, isoproterenol HCl, kanamycin sulfate, norepinephrine bitartrate, oxytetracycline HCl, penicillin G potassium/sodium, phenobarbital sodium, prochlorperazine edisylate and tetracycline HCl.

Compatibility is dependent upon factors such as pH, concentration, temperature and diluents used. It is suggested to consult specialized references for more specific information (*e.g., Handbook on Injectable Drugs* by Trissel; see bibliography).

Pharmacology/Spectrum of Activity - A first generation cephalosporin, cephalothin exhibits activity against the bacteria usually covered by this class. Refer to the monograph: Cephalosporins, General Information for more specific information.

Uses/Indications - In the United States, there are no cephalothin products approved for veterinary species, but it has been used clinically in several species when a relatively short-acting, injectable, first generation cephalosporin is indicated.

Pharmacokinetics (specific) - Cephalothin is not appreciably absorbed after oral administration and must be given parenterally to achieve therapeutic serum levels. Absorbed drug is partially metabolized by the liver and kidneys to desacetylcephalothin which is about 25% as active an antibacterial as the parent compound. In humans, about 60-95% of the drug is excreted unchanged into the urine and 27-54% of a dose is excreted as the desacetyl metabolite. Elimination half-lives may be significantly prolonged in patients with severely diminished renal function. Pharmacokinetic parameters for dogs and horses follow:

In dogs, the apparent volume of distribution at steady state is 435 ml/kg, total body clearance of 11.6 - 15 ml/min/kg with a serum elimination half-life of 42-51 minutes.

In horses, the apparent volume of distribution at steady state is 145 ml/kg, total body clearance of 13 ml/min/kg with a serum elimination half-life of 15 minutes when given IV and 49 minutes after IM injection. Cephalothin is about 20% bound to equine plasma proteins.

Doses - Note: IM injection may be very painful.

Dogs:
For susceptible infections:
a) 35 mg/kg IM, SQ q8h (Upson 1988)
b) 10 - 30 mg/kg IV or IM q6-8h (Vaden and Papich 1995)
c) 10 - 30 mg/kg IM, IV or SQ (Riviere 1989)
d) 11 - 33 mg/kg IV q8h; 22 - 33 mg/kg IM or SQ q8h (Aronson and Aucoin 1989)
For surgical prophylaxis (soft-tissue):
a) 40 mg/kg IV before and then every 1.5 hours during surgery (Rosin et al. 1988)

Cats:
For susceptible infections:
a) 35 mg/kg IM, SQ q8h (Upson 1988)
b) 10 - 30 mg/kg IV or IM q6-8h (Vaden and Papich 1995)
c) 10 - 30 mg/kg IM, IV or SQ (Riviere 1989)
d) 11 - 33 mg/kg IV q8h; 22 - 33 mg/kg IM or SQ q8h (Aronson and Aucoin 1989)

Cattle:
For susceptible infections:
a) 55 mg/kg SQ q6h (Beech 1987b)

Horses:
For susceptible infections:
a) 11 - 18 mg/kg IM or IV *qid* (Robinson 1987)
b) Foals: 20 - 30 mg/kg IV q6h (Caprile and Short 1987)]
c) 18 mg/kg IM or IV q6h (Beech 1987b)

Birds:
For susceptible infections:
a) 100 mg/kg IM *qid* (Clubb 1986)

Reptiles:
For susceptible infections in most species:
a) 20 - 40 mg/kg IM q12 hours (Gauvin 1993)

Dosage Forms/Preparations/FDA Approval Status -
Veterinary-Approved Products: None

Human-Approved Products:
Cephalothin Sodium Powder for Injection 1 g, 2 g in 10 ml vials and 100 ml piggyback vials and Faspak; *Keflin®, Neutral* (Lilly), generic (Rx)

Cephalothin Sodium Injection 1 g and 2 g in 5% dextrose premixed bags in 50 ml D_5W (frozen); *Cephalothin Sodium®* (Baxter); (Rx)

CEPHAPIRIN SODIUM
CEPHAPIRIN BENZATHINE

For general information on the cephalosporins including adverse effects, contraindications, over-dosage, drug interactions, and monitoring parameters, refer to the monograph: Cephalosporins, General Information.

Chemistry - An injectable semi-synthetic cephalosporin antibiotic, cephapirin sodium occurs as a white to off-white, crystalline powder having a faint odor. It is very soluble in water and slightly soluble in alcohol. Each gram of the injection contains 2.36 mEq of sodium. After reconstitution the solution for injection has a pH of 6.5-8.5. May also be known as cefapirin sodium in the U.K. and other countries.

Storage/Stability/Compatibility - The sterile powder for injection and reconstitution should be stored at room temperature and is stable for 24 months in dry state. After reconstituting with sterile water for injection in concentrations of 50 - 400 mg/ml, cephapirin is stable for 12 hours at room temperature. After reconstituting with bacteriostatic water for injection in concentrations of 250 - 400 mg/ml, cephapirin is stable for 48 hours at room temperature. After reconstituting with sodium chloride 0.9% injection or dextrose 5% in water in concentrations of 20 - 100 mg/ml, cephapirin is stable for 24 hours at room temperature. All of the above solutions are stable for 10 days when stored at 4°C (refrigeration) and may be stable longer when solutions are frozen. Solutions may become yellow, but this does not indicate any loss of potency.

Cephapirin mastitis tubes should be stored at room temperature (15-30°C); avoid excessive heat.

The following drugs or solutions are reportedly **compatible** with cephapirin: D_5W in Ringer's, D_5W in Lactated Ringer's, D_5W in sodium chloride 0.2% - 0.9%, D_5W, $D_{10}W$, $D_{20}W$, Ringer's Injection, Lactated Ringer's Injection, normal saline, bleomycin sulfate, calcium chloride/gluconate, chloramphenicol sodium succinate, diphenhydramine HCl, ergonovine maleate, heparin sodium, hydrocortisone sodium phosphate/succinate, metaraminol bitartrate, oxacillin sodium, penicillin G potassium/sodium, phenobarbital sodium, phytonadione, potassium chloride, sodium bicarbonate, succinylcholine chloride, verapamil HCl, vitamin B-complex with C and warfarin sodium.

The following drugs or solutions are reportedly **incompatible** or only compatible in specific situations with cephapirin: Mannitol 20%, amikacin sulfate, aminophylline, ascorbic acid injection, epinephrine HCl, erythromycin glucuptate, gentamicin sulfate, kanamycin sulfate, nitrofurantoin sodium, norepinephrine bitartrate, oxytetracycline HCl, phenytoin sodium, tetracycline HCl, and thiopental sodium.

Compatibility is dependent upon factors such as pH, concentration, temperature and diluents used. It is suggested to consult specialized references for more specific information (*e.g.,* *Handbook on Injectable Drugs* by Trissel; see bibliography).

Pharmacology/Spectrum of Activity - A first generation cephalosporin, cephapirin exhibits activity against the bacteria usually covered by this class. A cephalothin disk is usually used to determine bacterial susceptibility to this antibiotic when using the Kirby-Bauer method. Refer to the monograph: Cephalosporins, General Information for more specific information.

Uses/Indications - In the United States, there are no parenterally administered cephapirin products approved for veterinary species, but it has been used clinically in several species when a relatively short-acting injectable first generation cephalosporin is indicated.

An intramammary cephapirin sodium product (*Cefa-Lak*®—Fort Dodge) is approved for use in the treatment of mastitis in lactating dairy cows and cephapirin benzathine (*Cefa-Dri*®—Fort Dodge) is approved in dry cows.

Pharmacokinetics (specific) - Cephapirin is not appreciably absorbed after oral administration. In horses, the bioavailability is about 95% after IM injection. The apparent volumes of distribution have been reported as 0.32 L/kg in dogs, 0.335 - 0.399 L/kg in cattle and 0.17 - 0.188 L/kg in horses. The total body clearance of cephapirin is 8.9 ml/min/kg in dogs, 12.66 ml/min/kg in cattle and about 7.8 - 10 ml/min/kg in horses. Serum elimination half-life is about 25 minutes in dogs, 64 - 70 minutes in cattle and 25-55 minutes in horses. Probenecid has been demonstrated to reduce the renal clearance of the drug.

Doses -
Dogs:
   For susceptible infections:
     a)   10 - 30 mg/kg IV or IM q6-8h (Vaden and Papich 1995)
     b)   10 - 30 mg/kg IV, IM, SQ q8h (Riviere 1989)
     c)   11 - 33 mg/kg IV q8h; 22 - 33 mg/kg IM or SQ q8h (Aronson and Aucoin 1989)

Cats:
   For susceptible infections:
     a)   11 - 33 mg/kg IV q8h; 22 - 33 mg/kg IM or SQ q8h (Aronson and Aucoin 1989)
     b)   10 - 30 mg/kg IV, IM, SQ q8h (Riviere 1989)
     c)   10 - 30 mg/kg IV or IM q6-8h (Vaden and Papich 1995)

Cattle:
   For mastitis:
     a)   Lactating cow (*Cefa-Lak*®): After milking out udder, clean and dry teat area. Swab teat tip with alcohol wipe and allow to dry. Insert tip of syringe into teat canal; push plunger to instill entire contents. Massage quarter and do not milk out for 12 hours. May repeat dose q12h. (Label directions; *Cefa-Lak*®—Fort Dodge)
     b)   Dry Cow (*Cefa-Dri*®): Same basic directions as above, but should be done at the time of drying off and not later than 30 days prior to calving. (Label directions; *Cefa-Dri*®—Fort Dodge)

Horses:
   For susceptible infections:
     a)   20 mg/kg IM q8h or q12h if administered with probenecid (50 mg/kg intragastrically). (Juzwiak et al. 1989)
     b)   Foals: 20 - 30 mg/kg IV q6h (Caprile and Short 1987)
     c)   20 mg/kg IM q8h (Brumbaugh 1987)

Dosage Forms/Preparations/FDA Approval Status/Withholding Times -
Veterinary-Approved Products:
   Cephapirin Sodium Mastitis Tube; 200 mg cephapirin per 10 ml tube; *Cefa-Lak*® (Fort Dodge); (OTC) Approved for use in lactating dairy cattle. Milk withdrawal = 96 hours; Slaughter withdrawal = 4 days.

Cephapirin Benzathine Mastitis Tube; 300 mg cephapirin per 10 ml tube; *Cefa-Dri*® (Fort Dodge); (OTC) Approved for use in dry dairy cattle. Milk withdrawal = 72 hours after calving and must not be administered within 30 days of calving; Slaughter withdrawal = 42 days.

Human-Approved Products:
Cephapirin Sodium Powder for Injection 500 mg, 1 g, 2 g, 4 g, 20 g; *Cefadyl*® (Apothecon);*Cephapirin Sodium*® (Lyphomed); , generic; (Rx)

CHARCOAL, ACTIVATED

Chemistry - Activated charcoal occurs as a fine, black, odorless, tasteless powder that is insoluble in water or alcohol. Commercially available activated charcoal products may differ in their adsorptive properties, but one gram must adsorb 100 mg of strychnine sulfate in 50 ml of water to meet USP standards. Activated charcoal has several synonyms including: active carbon, activated carbon, adsorbent charcoal, decolorizing carbon, or medicinal charcoal.

Storage/Stability/Compatibility - Store activated charcoal in well-closed glass or metal containers or in the manufacturer's supplied container.

Pharmacology - Activated charcoal adsorbs many chemicals and drugs in the upper GI tract thereby preventing or reducing their absorption. While activated charcoal also adsorbs various nutrients and enzymes from the gut, when used for acute poisonings, no clinical significance usually results. Activated charcoal reportedly is not effective in adsorbing cyanide, but this has been disputed in a recent study. It also is not very effective in adsorbing alcohols, ferrous sulfate, caustic alkalies, nitrates, sodium chloride/chlorate, petroleum distillates or mineral acids.

Uses/Indications - Activated charcoal is administered orally to adsorb certain drugs or toxins to prevent or reduce their systemic absorption.

Pharmacokinetics - Activated charcoal is not absorbed nor metabolized in the gut.

Contraindications/Precautions/Reproductive Safety - Charcoal should not be used for mineral acids or caustic alkalies as it is ineffective. Although not contraindicated for ethanol, methanol, or iron salts, activated charcoal is not very effective in adsorbing these products and may obscure GI lesions during endoscopy.

Adverse Effects/Warnings - Very rapid GI administration of charcoal can induce emesis. Charcoal can cause either constipation or diarrhea and feces will be black. Products containing sorbitol may cause loose stools and vomiting.
  Charcoal powder is very staining and the dry powder tends to "float" covering wide areas.

Overdosage/Acute Toxicity - None reported when used for acute therapy; see Adverse Effects above for more information.

Drug Interactions - Separate by at least 3 hours administration of any other **orally administered therapeutic agents** from the charcoal dose. Charcoal should not be administered with **dairy products or mineral oil** as the adsorptive properties of the charcoal will be diminished. Do not administer (at the same time) with **syrup of ipecac** as the charcoal can adsorb the ipecac and reduce its efficacy.

Doses -
Dogs & Cats:
  a) 1 gram/5 ml of water; give 10 ml of slurry per kg PO. (Morgan 1988)
  b) For acute poisoning: 2 - 8 g/kg PO once or every 6-8h for 3-5 doses. To enhance excretion of slowly excreted poisons: 0.5 g/kg PO q3h for about 72 hours. (Mount 1989)
  c) 1 - 4 g/kg in 50 - 200 ml of water. Concurrent with or within 30 minutes of giving charcoal, give an osmotic cathartic. Repeated doses of activated charcoal may also bind drugs that are enterohepatically recycled. (Beasley and Dorman 1990)
  d) Administer in a bathtub or other easily cleanable area. Give activated charcoal at 1 - 5 g/kg PO (via stomach tube using either a funnel or large syringe) diluted in water at a concentration of 1 g charcoal/5-10 ml of water. Follow in 30 minutes with sodium sulfate oral cathartic. (Bailey 1989)
Ruminants:
  a) 1 - 3 grams/kg PO (1 gram of charcoal in 3-5 ml of water) via stomach tube; give saline cathartic concurrently. May repeat in 8-12 hours. (Bailey 1986b)
Horses:
  a) Foals: 250 grams (minimum). Adult horses: up to 750 grams. Make a slurry by mixing with up to 4 L (depending on animal's size) of warm water and administer via stomach tube. Leave in stomach for 20-30 minutes and then give a laxative to hasten removal of toxicants. (Oehme 1987b)

Monitoring Parameters - Monitoring for efficacy of charcoal is usually dependent upon the toxin/drug that it is being used for and could include the drug/toxin's serum level, clinical signs, etc.

Client Information - This agent should usually be used with professional supervision, depending on the potential severity of the toxin/overdose. Charcoal can be very staining to fabrics.

Dosage Forms/Preparations/FDA Approval Status/Withholding Times -

Veterinary-Approved Products:

Activated charcoal 47.5%, Kaolin 10% granules (free flowing and wettable) in 1 lb bottles, and 5 kg pails

Toxiban® *Granules* (Vet-A-Mix); (OTC) Indicated for use in both large and small animals.

Activated charcoal 10.4%, Kaolin 6.25% suspension in 240 ml bottles

Toxiban® *Suspension* (Vet-A-Mix); (OTC) Indicated for use in both large and small animals.

Activated Charcoal Aqueous Suspension 50 g in unit dose tube *Liqui-Char-Vet Aqueous Suspension*® (Daniels); (OTC)

Human-Approved Products:

Activated Charcoal Powder in 15, 30, 40 , 120 , 240 g & UD 30 g (Activated charcoal is also available in bulk powder form); Generic, (OTC)

Activated Charcoal Suspension; 25 g in 120 ml bottles, and 50 g in 240 ml bottles; *Actidose-Aqua*® (Paddock) ; (OTC)

Activated Charcoal Suspension with sorbitol; 15 g in 120 ml bottles 25 g in 120 ml bottles, 30 g in 150 ml bottles, and 50 g in 240 ml bottles; *Actidose with Sorbitol*® (Paddock),*CharcoAid*® (Requa); (OTC)

Activated Charcoal Liquid 15 g & 50g with & without sorbitol in 120 ml and 240 ml bottles, 12.5 g in propylene glycol 60 ml bottles, and 25 g in propylene glycol 120 ml bottles; *CharcoAid 2000* ® (Requa) (OTC) Generic; (OTC)

Activated Charcoal Liquid; 12.5 g in 60 ml bottles, 15 g in 75 ml bottles, 25 g in 120 ml bottles, 30 g in 120 ml bottles, & 50 g in 240 ml bottles; *Liqui-Char*® (Jones Medical); (OTC)

Activated Charcoal Granules 15 g in 120 ml bottles; *CharcoAid* 2000® (Requa) (OTC)

CHLORAMBUCIL

Chemistry - A nitrogen mustard derivative antineoplastic agent, chlorambucil occurs as an off-white, slightly granular powder. It is very slightly soluble in water.

Storage/Stability/Compatibility - Chlorambucil tablets should be stored in light-resistant, well-closed containers at room temperature. An expiration date of one year after manufacture is assigned to the commercially available tablets.

Pharmacology - Chlorambucil is a cell-cycle nonspecific alkylating antineoplastic/immunosuppressive agent. Its cytotoxic activity stems from cross-linking with cellular DNA.

Uses/Indications - Chlorambucil may be useful in a variety of neoplastic diseases, including lymphocytic leukemia, multiple myeloma, polycythemia vera, macroglobulinemia, and ovarian adenocarcinoma. It may also be useful as adjunctive therapy for some immune-mediated conditions (*e.g.*, glomerulonephritis, non-erosive arthritis, or immune-mediated skin disease).

Pharmacokinetics - In humans, chlorambucil is rapidly and nearly completely absorbed after oral administration. It is highly bound to plasma proteins. While it is not known whether it crosses the blood-brain barrier, neurological side effects have been reported. Chlorambucil crosses the placenta, but it is not known whether it enters maternal milk. Chlorambucil is extensively metabolized in the liver, primarily to phenylacetic acid mustard, which is active. Phenylacetic acid mustard is further metabolized to other metabolites that are excreted in the urine.

Contraindications/Precautions/Reproductive Safety - Chlorambucil is contraindicated in patients who are hypersensitive to it or have demonstrated resistance to its effects. It should be used with caution in patients with preexisting bone marrow depression or infection, or susceptible to bone marrow depression or infection.

Chlorambucil's teratogenic potential has not been well documented, but it may potentially cause a variety of fetal abnormalities. It is generally recommended to avoid the drug during pregnancy, but because of the seriousness of the diseases treated with chlorambucil, the potential benefits to the mother must be considered. Chlorambucil has been documented to cause irreversible infertility in male humans, particularly when given during pre-puberty and puberty.

Adverse Effects/Warnings - The most commonly associated major adverse effect seen with chlorambucil therapy is myelosuppression manifested by anemia, leukopenia, and thrombocytopenia. It may occur gradually with nadirs occurring usually within 7-14 days of the start of therapy. Recovery generally takes from 7-14 days. Severe bone marrow depression can result in pancytopenia that may take months to years for recovery. In humans, bronchopulmonary dysplasia with pulmonary fibrosis and uric acid nephropathy, have been reported. These effects are more uncommon and generally associated with chronic, higher dose therapy. Hepatotoxicity has been reported rarely in humans. Alopecia and delayed regrowth of shaven fur have been reported in dogs. Poodles or Kerry blues are more likely to be affected than other breeds.

Overdosage/Acute Toxicity - The oral LD$_{50}$ in mice is 123 mg/kg. There has been limited experiences with acute overdoses in humans. Doses of up to 5 mg/kg resulted in neurologic (seizures) toxicity and pancytopenia (nadirs at 1-6 weeks post ingestion). All patients recovered without long term sequelae. Treatment should consist of gut emptying when appropriate (beware of rapidly changing neurologic status if inducing vomiting). Monitoring of CBC's several times a week for several weeks should be performed after overdoses and blood component therapy may be necessary.

Drug Interactions - The principal concern should be the concurrent use with other drugs that are also myelosuppressive, including many of the **other antineoplastics and other bone marrow depressant drugs** (*e.g.*, **chloramphenicol, flucytosine, amphotericin B, or colchicine**). Bone marrow depression may be additive. Use with other **immunosuppressant drugs** (*e.g.*, **azathioprine, cyclophosphamide, corticosteroids**) may increase the risk of infection.

Laboratory Considerations - Chlorambucil may raise serum **uric acid** levels. Drugs such as **allopurinol** may be required to control hyperuricemia in some patients.

Doses -
Dogs:

> For adjunctive therapy (as an immunosuppressant) in the treatment of glomerulonephritis: 0.1 - 0.2 mg/kg PO once daily or every other day. (Vaden and Grauer 1992)
>
> For adjunctive therapy of lymphoreticular neoplasms, macroglobulinemia, and polycythemia vera: 2 - 6 mg/m^2 PO once a day or every other day. (Jacobs, Lumsden et al. 1992)
>
> For lymphoproliferative disease; macroglobulinemia: 2 - 4 mg/m2 PO q24 - 48h. (Gilson and Page 1994)
>
> For chronic lymphocytic leukemia: 20 mg/m^2 PO every 1 -2 weeks or 6 mg/m^2 PO daily. (Vail and Ogilvie 1994)
>
> For treatment of pemphigus complex: Prednisone 2-4 mg/kg PO divided q12h with chlorambucil 0.2 mg/kg q24-48h. (Helton-Rhodes 1994)

Cats:

> For adjunctive immunosuppressive therapy in feline SLE: 0.25 - 0.5 mg/kg PO q48-72 hours. (Thompson 1994)
>
> For treatment of pemphigus complex: Prednisone 2-4 mg/kg PO divided q12h with chlorambucil 0.2 mg/kg q24-48h. (Helton-Rhodes 1994)
>
> For adjunctive treatment of FIP: Predniso(lo)ne 4 mg/kg PO once daily with chlorambucil 20 mg/m^2 every 2-3 weeks. (Weiss 1994)
>
> For chronic lymphocytic leukemia: Chlorambucil at 2 mg/m^2 PO every other day or 20 mg/m^2 every other week; with or without prednisone at 20 mg/m^2 PO every other day. The authors state they have had more success with the high dose-every other week regimen. (Peterson and Couto 1994a)

Horses:

> For adjunctive therapy in treating lymphoma using the LAP protocol: Cytosine arabinoside 200 - 300 mg/m2 SubQ or IM once every 1-2 weeks; Chlorambucil 20 mg/m^2 PO every 2 weeks (alternating with cytosine arabinoside) and Prednisone 1.1 - 2.2 mg/kg PO every other day. If this protocol is not effective (no response seen in 2-4 weeks) add vincristine at 0.5 mg/m^2 IV once a week. Side effects are rare. (Couto 1994)

Monitoring Parameters - 1) Efficacy; 2) CBC, Platelets once weekly (or once stable every other week) during therapy; 3) Uric acid, liver enzymes; if warranted

Client Information - Clients must understand the importance of both administering chlorambucil as directed and to report immediately any signs associated with toxicity (*e.g.*, abnormal bleeding, bruising, urination, depression, infection, shortness of breath, etc.).

**Dosage Forms/Preparations/FDA Approval Status/Withholding Times -
Veterinary-Approved Products**: None
Human-Approved Products:

Chlorambucil Oral Tablets 2 mg; *Leukeran*® (Glaxo Wellcome); (Rx)

CHLORAMPHENICOL
CHLORAMPHENICOL PALMITATE
CHLORAMPHENICOL SODIUM SUCCINATE

Chemistry - Originally isolated from *Streptomyces venezuelae*, chloramphenicol is now produced synthetically. It occurs as fine, white to grayish, yellow white, elongated plates or needle-like crystals with a pK_a of 5.5. It is freely soluble in alcohol and about 2.5 mg are soluble in 1 ml of water at 25°C.

Chloramphenicol palmitate occurs as a bland mild tasting, fine, white, unctuous, crystalline powder having a faint odor. It is insoluble in water and sparingly soluble in alcohol.

Chloramphenicol sodium succinate occurs as a white to light yellow powder. It is freely soluble in both water or alcohol. Commercially available chloramphenicol sodium succinate for injection contains 2.3 mEq of sodium per gram of chloramphenicol.

Storage/Stability/Compatibility - Chloramphenicol capsules and tablets should be stored in tight containers at room temperature (15-30°C). The palmitate oral suspension should be stored in tight containers at room temperature and protected from light or freezing.

The sodium succinate powder for injection should be stored at temperatures less than 40°, and preferably between 15-30°C. After reconstituting the sodium succinate injection with sterile water, the solution is stable for 30 days at room temperature and 6 months if frozen. The solution should be discarded if it becomes cloudy.

The following drugs and solutions are reportedly **compatible** with chloramphenicol sodium succinate injection: all commonly used intravenous fluids, amikacin sulfate, aminophylline, ampicillin sodium (in syringe for 1 hr.) ascorbic acid, calcium chloride/gluconate, cephalothin sodium, cephapirin sodium, colistimethate sodium, corticotropin, cyanocobalamin, dimenhydrinate, dopamine HCl, ephedrine sulfate, heparin sodium, hydrocortisone sodium succinate, hydroxyzine HCl, kanamycin sulfate, lidocaine HCl, magnesium sulfate, metaraminol bitartrate, methicillin sodium, methyldopate HCl, methylprednisolone sodium succinate, metronidazole w/ or w/o sodium bicarbonate, nafcillin sodium, oxacillin sodium, oxytocin, penicillin G potassium/sodium, pentobarbital sodium, phenylephrine HCl w/ or w/o sodium bicarbonate, phytonadione, plasma protein fraction, potassium chloride, promazine HCl, ranitidine HCl, sodium bicarbonate, thiopental sodium, verapamil HCl, and vitamin B-complex with C.

The following drugs and solutions are reportedly **incompatible** (or compatibility data conflicts) with chloramphenicol sodium succinate injection: chlorpromazine HCl, glycopyrrolate, metoclopramide HCl, oxytetracycline HCl, polymyxin B sulfate, prochlorperazine edislyate/mesylate, promethazine HCl, tetracycline HCl, and vancomycin HCl.

Compatibility is dependent upon factors such as pH, concentration, temperature and diluents used. It is suggested to consult specialized references for more specific information (*e.g.*, *Handbook on Injectable Drugs* by Trissel; see bibliography).

Pharmacology - Chloramphenicol usually acts as a bacteriostatic antibiotic, but at higher concentrations or against some very susceptible organisms it can be bactericidal. Chloramphenicol acts by binding to the 50S ribosomal subunit of susceptible bacteria, thereby preventing bacterial protein synthesis. Erythromycin, clindamycin, lincomycin, tylosin, etc., also bind to the same site, but unlike them, chloramphenicol appears to also have an affinity for mitochondrial ribosomes of rapidly proliferating mammalian cells (*e.g.*, bone marrow) which may result in a reversible bone marrow suppression.

Chloramphenicol has a wide spectrum of activity against many gram positive and negative organisms. Gram positive aerobic organisms that are generally susceptible to chloramphenicol include many streptococci and staphylococci. It is also effective against some gram negative aerobes including *Neissiera, Brucella, Salmonella, Shigella,* and *Haemophilus.* Many anaerobic bacteria are sensitive to chloramphenicol, including *Clostridum, Bacteroides* (including *B. fragilis*), *Fusobacterium,* and *Veillonella.* Chloramphenicol also has activity against *Nocardia, Chlamydia, Mycoplasma,* and *Rickettsia.*

Uses/Indications - Chloramphenicol is used for a variety of infections in small animals and horses, particularly those caused by anaerobic bacteria. Because of the human public health implications, the use of chloramphenicol in animals used for food production is banned by the FDA.

Pharmacokinetics - Chloramphenicol is rapidly absorbed after oral administration with peak serum levels occurring approximately 30 minutes after dosing. The palmitate oral suspension produces significantly lower peak serum levels when administered to fasted cats. The sodium succinate salt is rapidly and well absorbed after IM or SQ administration in animals and, contrary to some recommendations, need not be administered only intravenously. The palmitate and sodium succinate is hydrolyzed in the GI tract and liver to the base.

Chloramphenicol is widely distributed throughout the body. Highest levels are found in the liver and kidney, but the drug attains therapeutic levels in most tissues and fluids, including the aqueous and vitreous humor, and synovial fluid. CSF concentrations may be up tp 50% of those in the serum when meninges are uninflamed and higher when meninges are inflamed. A 4-6 hour lag time before CSF peak levels to occur may be seen. Chloramphenicol concentrations in the prostate are approximately 50% of those in the serum. Because only a small amount of the drug is excreted unchanged into the urine in dogs, chloramphenicol may not be the best choice for lower urinary tract infections in that species. The volume of distribution of chloramphenicol has been reported as 1.8 L/kg in the dog, 2.4 L/kg in the cat, and 1.41 L/kg in horses. Chloramphenicol is about 30-60% bound to plasma proteins, enters milk and crosses the placenta.

In most species, chloramphenicol is eliminated primarily by hepatic metabolism via glucuronidative mechanisms. Only about 5-15% of the drug is excreted unchanged in the urine. The cat, having little ability to glucuronidate drugs, excretes 25% or more of a dose as unchanged drug in the urine.

The elimination half-life has been reported as 1.1-5 hours in dogs, <1 hour in foals & ponies, and 4-8 hours in cats. The elimination half-life of chloramphenicol in birds is highly species variable, ranging from 26 minutes in pigeons to nearly 5 hours in bald eagles and peafowl.

The usual serum therapeutic range for chloramphenicol is 5-15 micrograms/ml.

Contraindications/Precautions/Reproductive Safety - Chloramphenicol is contraindicated in patients hypersensitive to it. Because of the potential for hematopoietic toxicity, the drug should be used with extreme caution, if at all, in patients with preexisting hematologic abnormalities, especially a preexisting non-regenerative anemia. The drug should only be used in patients in hepatic failure when no other effective antibiotics are available. Chloramphenicol should be used with caution in patients with impaired hepatic or renal function as drug accumulation may occur. Those patients may need dosing adjustment, and monitoring of blood levels should also be considered in these patients.

Chloramphenicol should be used with caution in neonatal animals, particularly in young kittens. In neonates (humans), circulatory collapse (so-called "Gray-baby syndrome") has occurred with chloramphenicol, probably due to toxic levels accumulating secondary to an inability to conjugate the drug or excrete the conjugate effectively. Because chloramphenicol is found in milk at 50% of serum levels (in humans), the drug should be given with caution to nursing bitches or queens, particularly within the first week after giving birth.

One manufacturer (Osborn) states that chloramphenicol "should not be administered to dogs maintained for breeding purposes". Chloramphenicol has not been determined to be safe for use during pregnancy. The drug may decrease protein synthesis in the fetus, particularly in the bone marrow. It should only be used when the benefits of therapy clearly outweigh the risks..

Adverse Effects/Warnings - While the toxicity of chloramphenicol in humans has been much discussed, the drug is considered by most to have a low order of toxicity in adult companion animals when appropriately dosed.

The development of aplastic anemia reported in humans, does not appear to be a significant problem for veterinary patients. However, a dose-related bone marrow suppression (reversible) is seen in all species, primarily with long-term therapy. Early signs of bone marrow toxicity can include vacuolation of the many of the early cells of the myeloid and erythroid series, lymphocytopenia, and neutropenia.

Other effects that may be noted include, anorexia, vomiting, diarrhea and depression.

It has been said that cats tend to be more sensitive to developing adverse reactions to chloramphenicol than dogs, but this is probably more as a result of the drug's longer half-life in the cat. It is true that cats dosed at 50 mg/kg q12h for 2-3 weeks do develop a high incidence of adverse effects and should be closely monitored when prolonged high-dose therapy is necessary.

Overdosage/Acute Toxicity - Because of the potential for serious bone marrow toxicity, large overdoses of chloramphenicol should be handled by emptying the gut using standard protocols. For more information on the toxicity of chloramphenicol, refer to the Adverse Effects section above.

Drug Interactions - Chloramphenicol can inhibit the hepatic metabolism of several drugs, including **phenytoin, primidone, phenobarbital, pentobarbital,** and **cyclophosphamide**. Chloramphenicol has been demonstrated to prolong the duration of pentobarbital anesthesia by 120% in dogs, and 260% in cats. Phenobarbital may also decrease the plasma concentrations of chloramphenicol. In dogs receiving both chloramphenicol and primidone, anorexia and CNS depression may occur. Serum monitoring of the affected drugs should be considered if any of these drugs are to be used concurrently with chloramphenicol.

The hematologic response to **iron salts** and **Vitamin B$_{12}$** can be decreased when concomitantly administered with chloramphenicol. Chloramphenicol should be used with extreme caution, if at all, with other **drugs that can cause myelosuppression** (*e.g.,* cyclophosphamide).

Penicillin may slightly increase the serum half-life of chloramphenicol. Chloramphenicol may antagonize the bactericidal activity of the **penicillins** or **aminoglycosides**. This antagonism has not been demonstrated *in vivo*, and these drug combinations have been used successfully many times clinically. **Rifampin** may decrease serum chloramphenicol levels. Other antibiotics that bind to the 50S ribosomal subunit of susceptible bacteria (**erythromycin, clindamycin, lincomycin, tylosin**, etc.) may potentially antagonize the activity of chloramphenicol or vice versa, but the clinical significance of this potential interaction has not been determined.

Chloramphenicol may suppress antibody production if given prior to an antigenic stimulus and may affect responses to **vaccinations**. If administered after the antigen challenge, immune response may not be altered. Immunizations should be postponed, if possible, in animals receiving chloramphenicol.

Drug/Laboratory Interactions - False-positive **glucosuria** has been reported, but the incidence is unknown.

Doses -
  Dogs:
    For susceptible infections:
      a) 45 - 60 mg/kg PO q8h; 45 - 60 mg/kg IM, SQ or IV q6-8h (USPC 1990)
      b) 40 - 50 mg/kg IV, IM, SubQ or PO q8h; avoid in young animals or in breeding or pregnant animals; avoid or reduce dosage in animals with severe liver failure. (Vaden and Papich 1995)
      c) 35.75 - 55 mg/kg PO q8h; 16.5 - 22 mg/kg IM, or SQ q8h (Aronson and Aucoin 1989)
      d) For bacterial or Rickettsial infections: 25 - 50 mg/kg PO *tid* (Morgan 1988)
      e) 50 mg/kg PO, IV, IM, SQ q8h (Kirk 1989)
      f) For Rocky Mountain Spotted Fever: 15 - 20 mg/kg q8h PO, IM or IV for 14-21 days (Sellon and Breitschwerdt 1995)

  Cats:
    For susceptible infections:
      a) 25 - 50 mg/kg PO q12h; 12 - 30 mg/kg IM, SQ or IV q12h (USPC 1990)
      b) 50 mg (total dose) IV, IM, SubQ or PO q8h; avoid in young animals or in breeding or pregnant animals; avoid or reduce dosage in animals with severe liver failure. (Vaden and Papich 1995)
      c) For bacterial or Rickettsial infections: 25 mg/kg PO *bid* (Morgan 1988)
      d) 50 mg/kg PO, IV, IM, SQ q12h (Kirk 1989)

  Pocket Pets/Rodents:
    For empiric antibiotic therapy:
      a) Palmitate: 50 mg/kg PO q8h; Succinate: 30 mg/kg IV or IM q8h (Oglesbee 1995)
  Ferrets:
    For proliferative colitis: 10 - 40 mg/kg q8h PO for 2 weeks or 50 mg/kg PO q12h for 10 days. (Fox 1995a)

  Horses:
    For susceptible infections:
      a) 10 - 50 mg/kg PO *qid*. If using palmitate salt, give 20 - 50 mg/kg PO *qid*. For sodium succinate: 20 - 50 mg/kg IM or IV *qid*. (Robinson 1987)
      b) Chloramphenicol sodium succinate: 25 mg/kg IM q8h (Baggot and Prescott 1987)
      c) Foals: Chloramphenicol sodium succinate: 50 mg/kg IV q6-8h (use longer dosage interval in premature foals and those less than 2 days old). (Caprile and Short 1987)
      d) 45 - 60 mg/kg PO q8h; 45 - 60 mg/kg IM, SQ or IV q6-8h (USPC 1990)

  Birds:
    For susceptible infections:
      a) Chloramphenicol sodium succinate: 80 mg/kg IM *bid* - *tid*, 50 mg/kg IV *tid* - *qid*. Chloramphenicol palmitate suspension (30 mg/ml): 0.1 ml/30 grams of body weight *tid* - *qid*. Do not use for initial therapy in life-threatening infections. Must use parenteral form if crop stasis occurs. (Clubb 1986)
      b) Chloramphenicol palmitate suspension (30 mg/ml): 75 mg/kg *tid*; absorption is erratic, but well-tolerated and efficacious in baby birds with enteric infections being hand fed. Will settle out if added to drinking water. (McDonald 1989)
      c) Succinate: 50 mg/kg IM or IV q8h; Palmitate: 75 mg/kg PO q8h (Hoeffer 1995)

Reptiles:

For susceptible infections:

    a) For most species using the sodium succinate salt: 20 - 50 mg/kg IM or SubQ for up to 3 weeks. Chloramphenicol is often a good initial choice until sensitivity results are available. (Gauvin 1993)

Monitoring Parameters -

    1) Clinical efficacy

    2) Adverse effects; chronic therapy should be associated with routine CBC monitoring

Client Information - <u>Must not</u> be used in any animal to be used for food production. There is evidence that humans exposed to chloramphenicol have an increased risk of developing a fatal aplastic anemia. Products should be handled with care. Do not inhale powder and wash hands after handling tablets. Crushed tablets or capsule contents are very bitter tasting and animals may not accept the drug if presented in this manner.

Dosage Forms/Preparations/FDA Approval Status -

  Veterinary-Approved Products:

Note: The oral suspension (palmitate salt) has reportedly been discontinued and the availability of any veterinary-labeled oral dosage form has been sporadic at best.

    Chloramphenicol Oral Tablets 100 mg, 250 mg, 500 mg, 1 gram; Approved for use in dogs only.

    Veterinary-labeled chloramphenicol capsules may also be commercially available.

  Human-Approved Products:

    Chloramphenicol Capsules 250 mg; *Chloromycetin Kapseals*® (Parke-Davis), generic; (Rx)

    Chloramphenicol Sodium Succinate Powder for Injection 100 mg/ml (as sodium succinate) when reconstituted 1 g vials; *Chloromycetin*® *Sodium Succinate* (Parke-Davis), generic; (Rx)

Topical, otic and opthalmic preparations are avalso available.

CHLOROTHIAZIDE
CHLOROTHIAZIDE SODIUM

Chemistry - A thiazide diuretic structurally related to the sulfonamides, chlorothiazide occurs as a white or practically white, odorless, slightly bitter-tasting, crystalline powder. It has a melting point of approximately 355° C. and pK_as of 6.7 and 9.5. It is very slightly soluble in water and slightly soluble in alcohol. The pH of the commercially available oral suspension is from 3.2 to 4.

Chlorothiazide sodium occurs as a white powder that is very soluble in water. The commercial injection is provided as a lyophilized powder mixed with mannitol. Sodium hydroxide is added to adjust the pH to 9.2 - 10 after reconstitution. Approximately 2.4 mEq of sodium is contained in a 500 mg vial.

Storage/Stability/Compatibility - The oral suspension should be protected from freezing. The injectable preparation is stable for 24 hours after reconstitution. If the pH of the reconstituted solution is less than 7.4, precipitation will occur in less than 24 hours.

Chlorothiazide sodium for injection is reportedly **compatible** with the following IV solutions: dextrose and/or saline products for IV infusion (with the exception to many Ionosol and Normosol products), Ringer's injection and Lactated Ringer's, 1/6 M sodium lactate, Dextran 6% with dextrose or sodium chloride, and fructose 10%. It is also reportedly **compatible** with the following drugs: cimetidine HCl, lidocaine HCl, nafcillin sodium, and sodium bicarbonate.

Chlorothiazide sodium is reportedly **incompatible** with the following drugs: amikacin sulfate, chlorpromazine HCl, codeine phosphate, hydralazine HCl, insulin (regular), morphine sulfate, norepinephrine bitartrate, polymyxin B sulfate, procaine HCl, prochlorperazine edisylate and mesylate, promazine HCl, promethazine HCl, streptomycin sulfate, tetracycline HCl, trifluopromazine HCl, and vancomycin HCl.

Pharmacology - Thiazide diuretics act by interfering with the transport of sodium ions across renal tubular epithelium possibly by altering the metabolism of tubular cells. The principle site of action is at the cortical diluting segment of the nephron. Enhanced excretion of sodium, chloride, and water results. Thiazides also increase the excretion of potassium, magnesium, phosphate, iodide, and bromide and decrease the glomerular filtration rate (GFR). Plasma renin and resulting aldosterone levels are increased which contributes to the hypokalemic effects of the thiazides. Bicarbonate excretion is increased, but effects on urine pH are usually minimal. Thiazides initially have a hypercalciuric effect, but with continued therapy, calcium excretion is significantly decreased. Uric acid excretion is also decreased by the thiazides. Thiazides can cause, or exacerbate hyperglycemia in diabetic patients, or induce diabetes mellitus in prediabetic patients.

The antihypertensive effects of thiazides are well known, and these agents are used extensively in human medicine for treating essential hypertension. The exact mechanism of this effect has not been established.

Thiazides paradoxically reduce urine output in patients with diabetes insipidus (DI). They have been used as adjunctive therapy in patients with neurogenic DI and are the only drug therapy for nephrogenic DI.

Uses/Indications - In veterinary medicine, furosemide has largely supplanted the use of thiazides as a general diuretic (edema treatment). Thiazides are still used for the treatment of systemic hypertension, nephrogenic diabetes insipidus, and to help prevent the recurrence of calcium oxalate uroliths in dogs.

Chlorothiazide is approved for use in dairy cattle for the treatment of post parturient udder edema.

Pharmacokinetics - The pharmacokinetics of the thiazides have apparently not been studied in domestic animals. In humans, chlorothiazide is only 10 - 21% absorbed after oral administration. The onset of diuretic activity occurs in 1 to 2 hours and peaks at about 4 hours. The serum half-life is approximately 1-2 hours and the duration of activity is from 6-12 hours. Like all thiazides, the antihypertensive effects of chlorothiazide can take several days to transpire.

Thiazides are found in the milk of lactating humans. Because of the chance of idiosyncratic or hypersensitive reactions, it is recommended that these drugs not be used in lactating females or mothers not nurse if receiving them.

Contraindications/Precautions - Thiazides are contraindicated in patients hypersensitive to any one of these agents or to sulfonamides, and in patients with anuria. They are also contraindicated in pregnant females who are otherwise healthy and have only mild edema. Newborn human infants have developed thrombocytopenia when their mothers received thiazides.

Thiazides should be used with extreme caution, if at all, in patients with severe renal disease or with preexisting electrolyte or water balance abnormalities, impaired hepatic function (may precipitate hepatic coma), hyperuricemia, lupus (SLE) or diabetes mellitus. Patients with conditions that may lead to electrolyte or water balance abnormalities (*e.g.,* vomiting, diarrhea, etc.) should be monitored carefully.

Adverse Effects/Warnings - Hypokalemia is one of the most common adverse effects associated with the thiazides, but rarely causes symptoms or progresses. However, monitoring of potassium is recommended with chronic therapy.

Hypochloremic alkalosis (with hypokalemia) may develop, especially if there are other causes of potassium and chloride loss (*e.g.,* vomiting, diarrhea, potassium-losing nephropathies, etc.) or the patient has cirrhotic liver disease. Dilutional hyponatremia and hypomagnesemia may also occur. Hyperparathyroid-like effects of hypercalcemia and hypophosphatemia have been reported in humans, but have not led to effects such as nephrolithiasis, bone resorption or peptic ulceration.

Hyperuricemia can occur, but is usually asymptomatic.

Other possible adverse effects include GI reactions (vomiting, diarrhea, etc.), hypersensitivity/dermatologic reactions, GU reactions (polyuria), hematologic toxicity, hyperglycemia, hyperlipidemias, and orthostatic hypotension.

Overdosage - Acute overdosage may cause electrolyte and water balance problems, CNS effects (lethargy to coma and seizures), and GI effects (hypermotility, GI distress). Transient increases in BUN have also been reported.

Treatment consists of emptying the gut after recent oral ingestion using standard protocols. Avoid giving concomitant cathartics as they may exacerbate the fluid and electrolyte imbalances that may ensue. Monitor and treat electrolyte and water balance abnormalities supportively. Additionally, monitor respiratory, CNS and cardiovascular status and treat supportively and symptomatically if required.

Drug Interactions - Thiazides used concomitantly with **corticosteroids, corticotropin or amphotericin B** can lead to an increased chance of hypokalemia developing.

Thiazide induced hypokalemia may increase the likelihood of **digitalis** toxicity. **Tubocurarine** or other nondepolarizing neuromuscular blocking agents response or duration may be increased in patients taking thiazide diuretics. **Sulfonamides** may potentiate thiazide activity.

Quinidine half-life may be prolonged by thiazides (thiazides can alkalinize the urine).

Increased hyperglycemia, hyperuricemia and hypotension may occur with concurrent administration with **diazoxide**.

Hypercalcemia may be exacerbated if thiazides are concurrently administered with **Vitamin D or calcium salts**.

Thiazides may alter the requirements of **insulin** or other anti-diabetic agents in diabetic patients.

Laboratory Interactions - Thiazides may decrease **protein-bound iodine** values.

Hydrochlorothiazide may falsely decrease total **urinary estrogen** when using a spectrophoto-metric assay; apparently, chlorothiazide does not interfere with this test.

In asymptomatic patients and those in the developmental stages of acute pancreatitis (humans), thiazides can increase serum **amylase** values.

Thiazides can decrease the renal excretion of **cortisol.**

Doses -
Dogs:
For treatment of nephrogenic diabetes insipidus:
a) 20 - 40 mg/kg PO q12h (Polzin and Osborne 1985), (Nichols 1989)

For treatment of systemic hypertension:
a) 20 - 40 mg/kg PO q12-24h with dietary salt restriction (Cowgill and Kallet 1986)

As a diuretic:
a) 10 - 40 mg/kg PO *bid* (Morgan 1988)

Cattle:
a) 4 - 8 mg/kg once or twice daily PO for adult cattle (Howard 1986)
b) 2 grams PO once or twice daily for 3 - 4 days (Package Insert — *Diuril®* Boluses; MSD)
c) 2 grams PO once to twice daily (Swinyard 1975)

Monitoring Parameters -
1) Serum electrolytes, BUN, creatinine, glucose
2) Hydration status
3) Blood pressure, if indicated
4) Hemograms, if indicated

Client Information - Clients should contact veterinarian if symptoms of water or electrolyte im-balance occur. Symptoms such as excessive thirst, lethargy, lassitude, restlessness, oliguria, GI distress or tachycardia may indicate electrolyte or water balance problem.

Dosage Forms/Preparations/FDA Approval Status/Withholding Times -
Veterinary-Approved Products: None

Human-Approved Products:
Chlorothiazide Tablets 250 mg, 500 mg; *Diuril®* (Merck); *Diurigen®* (Goldline); Generic; (Rx)

Chlorothiazide Oral Suspension 50 mg/ml in 237 ml bottles; *Diuril®* (Merck); (Rx)

Chlorothiazide Sodium Powder for Injection 500 mg vial; *Diuril® Sodium* (Merck); (Rx)

CHLORPHENIRAMINE MALEATE

Chemistry - A propylamine (alkylamine) antihistaminic agent, chlorpheniramine maleate occurs as an odorless, white, crystalline powder with a melting point between 130 - 135° C and a pK_a of 9.2. One gram is soluble in about 4 ml of water, or 10 ml of alcohol. The pH of the commercially available injection is between 4 - 5.2.

Storage/Stability/Compatibility - Chlorpheniramine tablets and sustained-release tablets should be store in tight containers. The sustained-release capsules should be stored in well-closed con-tainers. The oral solution and injectable products should be stored in light-resistant containers; avoid freezing. All chlorpheniramine products should be stored at room temperature (15-30°C).

Chlorpheniramine for injection is reportedly **compatible** with most commonly used IV solu-tions and the following drugs: amikacin sulfate, diatrizoate meglumine 52%/diatrizoate sodium 8% (Renografin-60®), diatrizoate meglumine 34.3%/diatrizoate sodium 35% (*Renovist®*), dia-trizoate sodium 75% (*Hypaque®*), iothalamate meglumine 60% (*Conray®*), and iothalamate sodium 80% (*Angio-Conray®*).

Chlorpheniramine is reportedly **incompatible** with: calcium chloride, kanamycin sulfate, nore-pinephrine bitartrate, pentobarbital sodium, and iodipamide meglumine 52% (*Cholographin®*). Compatibility is dependent upon factors such as pH, concentration, temperature, and diluents used and it is suggested to consult specialized references for more specific information.

Pharmacology - Antihistamines (H$_1$-receptor antagonists) competitively inhibit histamine at H$_1$ receptor sites. They do not inactivate or prevent the release of histamine, but can prevent his-tamine's action on the cell. Besides their antihistaminic activity, these agents all have varying degrees of anticholinergic and CNS activity (sedation). Some antihistamines have antiemetic ac-tivity (*e.g.,* diphenhydramine) or antiseritonin activity (*e.g.,* cyproheptadine, azatadine).

Uses/Indications - Antihistamines are used in veterinary medicine to reduce or help prevent histamine mediated adverse effects.

Pharmacokinetics - Chlorpheniramine pharmacokinetics have not been described in domestic species. In humans, the drug is well absorbed after oral administration, but because of a relatively high degree of metabolism in the GI mucosa and the liver, only about 25-60% of the drug is available to the systemic circulation.

Chlorpheniramine is well distributed after IV injection, the highest distribution of the drug (in rabbits) occurs in the lungs, heart, kidneys, brain, small intestine and spleen. In humans, the apparent steady-state volume of distribution is 2.5 - 3.2 L/kg and it is about 70% bound to plasma proteins. It is unknown if chlorpheniramine is excreted into the milk.

Chlorpheniramine is metabolized in the liver and practically all the drug (as metabolites and unchanged drug) is excreted in the urine. In human patients with normal renal and hepatic function, the terminal serum half-life the drug ranges from 13.2-43 hours.

Contraindications/Precautions - Chlorpheniramine is contraindicated in patients who are hypersensitive to it or other antihistamines in its class. Because of their anticholinergic activity, antihistamines should be used with caution in patients with angle closure glaucoma, prostatic hypertrophy, pyloroduodenal or bladder neck obstruction, and COPD if mucosal secretions are a problem. Additionally, they should be cautiously used in patients with hyperthyroidism, cardiovascular disease or hypertension.

Adverse Effects/Warnings - Most commonly seen adverse effects are CNS depression (lethargy, somnolence) and GI effects (diarrhea, vomiting, anorexia). The sedative effects of antihistamines may diminish with time. Anticholinergic effects (dry mouth, urinary retention) are a possibility.

The sedative effects of antihistamines may adversely affect the performance of working dogs.

Overdosage - Overdosage may cause CNS stimulation (excitement to seizures) or depression (lethargy to coma), anticholinergic effects, respiratory depression, and death. Treatment consists of emptying the gut if the ingestion was oral using standard protocols. Induce emesis if the patient is alert and CNS status is stable. Administration of a saline cathartic and/or activated charcoal may be given after emesis or gastric lavage. Treatment of other symptoms should be performed using symptomatic and supportive therapies. Phenytoin (IV) is recommended in the treatment of seizures caused by antihistamine overdose in humans; barbiturates and diazepam are avoided.

Drug Interactions - Increased sedation can occur if chlorpheniramine is combined with **other CNS depressant drugs**.

Antihistamines may partially counteract the anticoagulation effects of **heparin** or **warfarin**.

Laboratory Interactions - Antihistamines can decrease the wheal and flare response to **antigen skin testing**. In humans, it is suggested that antihistamines be discontinued at least 4 days before testing.

Doses - Note: Contents of sustained-release capsules may be placed on food, but should not be allowed to dissolve before ingestion.

Dogs:
a) 4 - 8 mg PO q12h (Kirk 1986)
b) 2 - 4 mg PO *bid-tid* (Morgan 1988)

Cats:
a) For adjunctive treatment of feline miliary dermatitis: 2 mg PO q12h (Kwochka 1986)
b) 1 - 2 mg PO *bid-tid* (Morgan 1988)

Monitoring Parameters -
1) Clinical efficacy and adverse effects

Client Information/FDA Approval Status - Except in the combination products listed below, no veterinary-approved product is available. Chlorpheniramine is approved for use in humans; the oral dosage forms are either prescription or non-prescription agents, depending on the product's labeling. The injectable products are prescription only.

Dosage Forms/Preparations -

Veterinary-Approved Products:. None None as a single entity. This compound is also found in the veterinary-approved (dogs, cats, horses) products *Diathal*® (Schering) and *Azimycin*® (Schering). *Diathal*® contains: chlorpheniramine maleate 10 mg/ml, procaine penicillin G 200,000 U/ml, dihydrostreptomycin sulfate 250 mg/ml and diphemanil methylsulfate 25 mg/ml. *Azimycin*® contains: chlorpheniramine maleate 10 mg/ml, procaine penicillin G 200,000 U/ml, dihydrostreptomycin sulfate 250 mg/ml, dexamethasone 0.5 mg/ml, and procaine HCl 20 mg/ml.

Human-Approved Products:
Chlorpheniramine Maleate Oral Tablets 2 mg (chewable), 4 mg, 8 mg (timed release), 12 mg (timed release) (OTC)
Chlorpheniramine Maleate Oral Syrup 2 mg/5 ml in 118 ml btls (OTC)

Chlorpheniramine Maleate Injection 10 mg/ml in 30 ml vials & 100 mg/ml in 10 ml vials; (Rx)

There are many registered trade names for chlorpheniramine; a commonly known product is *Chlor-Trimeton*® (Schering). Many combination products are available that combine chlorpheniramine with decongestants, analgesics, and/or antitussives.

CHLORPROMAZINE HCL

Chemistry - A propylamino phenothiazine derivative, chlorpromazine is the prototypic phenothiazine agent. It occurs as a white to slightly creamy white, odorless, bitter tasting, crystalline powder. One gram is soluble in 1 ml of water and 1.5 ml of alcohol. The commercially available injection is a solution of chlorpromazine HCl in sterile water at a pH of 3-5.

Storage/Stability/Compatibility - Protect from light and store at room temperature; avoid freezing the oral solution and injection. Dispense oral solution in amber bottles. Store oral tablets in tight containers. Do not store in plastic syringes or IV bags for prolonged periods of time as the drug may adsorb to plastic.

Chlorpromazine will darken upon prolonged exposure to light; do not use solutions that are darkly colored or if precipitates have formed. A slight yellowish color will not affect potency or efficacy. Alkaline solutions will cause the drug to oxidize.

The following products have been reported to be **compatible** when mixed with chlorpromazine HCl injection: all usual intravenous fluids, ascorbic acid, atropine sulfate, butorphanol tartrate, diphenhydramine, droperidol, fentanyl citrate, glycopyrrolate, heparin sodium, hydromorphone HCl, hydroxyzine HCl, lidocaine HCl, meperidine, metoclopramide, metaraminol bitartrate, morphine sulfate, pentazocine lactate, promazine HCl, promethazine, scopolamine HBr, & tetracycline HCl.

The following products have been reported as being **incompatible** when mixed with chlorpromazine: aminophylline, amphotericin B, chloramphenicol sodium succinate, chlorothiazide sodium, dimenhydrinate, methicillin sodium, methohexital sodium, nafcillin sodium, penicillin g potassium, pentobarbital sodium, phenobarbital sodium, and thiopental sodium. Compatibility is dependent upon factors such as pH, concentration, temperature and diluents used. It is suggested to consult specialized references for more specific information (*e.g., Handbook on Injectable Drugs* by Trissel; see bibliography).

Pharmacology - Once the principle phenothiazine used in veterinary medicine, chlorpromazine has been largely supplanted by acepromazine. It has similar pharmacologic activities as acepromazine, but is less potent and has a longer duration of action. For further information refer to the acepromazine monograph.

Uses/Indications - The clinical use of chlorpromazine as a neuroleptic agent has diminished, but the drug is still used for its antiemetic effects in small animals and occasionally as a preoperative medication and tranquilizer. As an antiemetic, chlorpromazine will inhibit apomorphine-induced emesis in the dog but not the cat. It will also inhibit the emetic effects of morphine in the dog. It does not inhibit emesis caused by copper sulfate, or digitalis glycosides.

Pharmacokinetics - Chlorpromazine is absorbed rapidly after oral administration, but undergoes extensive first pass metabolism in the liver. The drug is also well absorbed after IM injection, but onsets of action are slower than after IV administration.

Chlorpromazine is distributed throughout the body and brain concentrations are higher than those in the plasma. Approximately 95% of chlorpromazine in plasma is bound to plasma proteins (primarily albumin).

The drug is extensively metabolized principally in the liver and kidneys, but little specific information is available regarding its excretion in dogs and cats.

Contraindications/Precautions - Chlorpromazine causes severe muscle discomfort and swelling when injected IM into rabbits; use IV only in this species. See other contraindications/precautions in the acepromazine monograph found earlier in this section.

Adverse Effects/Warnings - In addition to the possible effects listed in the acepromazine monograph, chlorpromazine may cause extrapyrimidal symptoms in the cat when used at high dosages. These symptoms can include tremors, shivering, rigidity & loss of the righting reflexes. Lethargy, diarrhea, and loss of anal sphincter tone may also be seen.

Horses may develop an ataxic reaction with resultant excitation and violent consequences. These ataxic periods may cycle with periods of sedation. Because of this effect, chlorpromazine is rarely used in equine medicine today.

Overdosage - Refer to the information listed in the acepromazine monograph.

Drug Interactions - Phenothiazines should not be given within one month of worming with an **organophosphate agent** as their effects may be potentiated. **Physostigmine** toxicity may be enhanced by chlorpromazine. Toxicity of the herbicide **paraquat** is increased by chlorpromazine.

Other CNS depressant agents (barbiturates, narcotics, anesthetics, etc.) may cause additive CNS depression if used with phenothiazines.

Quinidine given with phenothiazines can cause additive cardiac depression.

Antidiarrheal mixtures (*e.g.,* Kaolin/pectin, bismuth subsalicylate mixtures) and **antacids** may cause reduced GI absorption of oral phenothiazines.

Increased blood levels of both drugs may result if **propranolol** is administered with phenothiazines. Phenothiazines block alpha-adrenergic receptors, if **epinephrine** is then given, unopposed beta-activity causing vasodilation and increased cardiac rate can occur.

Phenytoin metabolism may be decreased if given concurrently with phenothiazines.

Procaine activity may be enhanced by phenothiazines.

Dipyrone used with chlorpromazine has been reported to cause serious hypothermia.

Doses -
Dogs:
    a) 3.3 mg/kg PO once to 4 times daily; 1.1 - 6.6 mg/kg IM once to 4 times daily; 0.55 - 4.4 mg/kg IV once to 4 times daily (Kirk 1986)
    b) As an antiemetic: 0.5 mg/kg IM q8h; 1 mg/kg per rectum q8h (DeNovo 1986)
    c) As a sedative/restraining agent: 3 mg/kg PO q12h; 0.5 mg/kg IM or IV q12h (Davis 1985b)
    d) As a preanesthetic: up to 1.1 mg/kg IM 1 - 1.5 hours prior to surgery (Booth 1988a)
    e) For tranquilization: 0.8 - 2.2 mg/kg PO *bid-tid*
        As an antiemetic: 0.05 mg/kg IV *tid-qid* or 0.5 mg/kg SQ once to 4 times daily.
        For irritable colon syndrome: 0.5 mg/kg IM once to 3 times daily
        As a muscle relaxant during tetanus: 2 mg/kg IM *bid* (Morgan 1988)
    f) As an adjunctive treatment for amphetamine toxicosis: 10 - 18 mg/kg IV (Dumonceaux 1995)
    g) As an antiemetic: 0.2 - 0.4 mg/kg SubQ q8h (Washabau and Elie 1995)

Cats:
    a) 3.3 mg/kg PO once to 4 times daily; 1.1 - 6.6 mg/kg IM once to 4 times daily; 0.55 - 4.4 mg/kg IV once to 4 times daily (Kirk 1986)
    b) As an antiemetic: 0.5 mg/kg IM q8h (DeNovo 1986)
    c) As a sedative/restraining agent: 3 mg/kg PO once daily; 0.5 mg/kg IM or IV once daily (Davis 1985b)
    d) As a preanesthetic: up to 1.1 mg/kg IM one to one and one-half hours prior to surgery (Booth 1988a)
    e) As an antiemetic: 0.2 - 0.4 mg/kg SubQ q8h (Washabau and Elie 1995)

Cattle:
    a) Premedication for cattle undergoing standing procedures: Up to 1 mg/kg IM (may cause regurgitation if animal undergoes general anesthesia) (Hall and Clarke 1983)
    b) 0.22 - 1.0 mg/kg IV; 1.0 - 4.4 mg/kg IM (Howard 1986)

Horses: Note: Because of side effects (ataxia, panic reaction) this drug is not recommended for use in horses; use acepromazine or promazine if phenothiazine therapy is desired.

Swine:
    a) Premedication: 1 mg/kg IM (Hall and Clarke 1983)
    b) 0.55 - 3.3 mg/kg IV; 2 - 4 mg/kg IM (Howard 1986)
    c) Restraint: 1.1 mg/kg IM (effects are at peak in 45-60 minutes);
        Prior to barbiturate anesthesia: 2 - 4 mg/kg IM (Booth 1988a)

Sheep & Goats:
    a) 0.55 - 4.4 mg/kg IV, 2.2 - 6.6 mg/kg IM (Lumb and Jones 1984)
    b) Goats: 2 - 3.5 mg/kg IV q5-6h (Booth 1988a)

Monitoring Parameters -
    1) Cardiac rate/rhythm/blood pressure if indicated and possible to measure
    2) Degree of tranquilization/anti-emetic activity if indicated
    3) Body temperature (especially if ambient temperature is very hot or cold)

Client Information - Avoid getting solutions on hands or clothing as contact dermatitis may develop. May discolor the urine to a pink or red-brown color; this is not abnormal.

Dosage Forms/Preparations -
Veterinary-Approved Products: None
Human-approved Products:

Chlorpromazine Tablets 10 mg, 25 mg, 50 mg, 100 mg, 200 mg; *Thorazine*® (SKF); Generic; (Rx)

Chlorpromazine Extended-release Capsules 30 mg, 75 mg, 150 mg, 200 mg, 300 mg; *Thorazine®* *Spansule®*(SKF); (Rx)

Chlorpromazine Oral Solutions: 2 mg/ml (syrup) in 120 ml bottles; 30 mg/ml (concentrate) in 120 ml bottles, gallons; 100 mg/ml (concentrate) in 60 and 240 ml bottles*Thorazine®* (SKF) ; Generic; (Rx)

Rectal suppositories 25 mg, 100 mg (as base); *Thorazine®* (SKF); (Rx)

Injection 25 mg/ml in 1 & 2 ml amps and cartridges and 10 ml vials; *Thorazine®* (SKF);*Ormazine®* (Hauck); Generic; (Rx)

CHLORPROPAMIDE

Chemistry - An oral sulfonylurea antidiabetic agent, chlorpropamide occurs as a white, crystalline powder having a slight odor. It is practically insoluble in water.

Storage/Stability/Compatibility - Chlorpropamide tablets should be stored in well-closed containers at room temperature.

Pharmacology - Sulfonylureas lower blood glucose concentrations in both diabetic and non-diabetics. The exact mechanism of action is not known, but these agents are thought to exert the effect primarily by stimulating the beta cells in the pancreas to secrete additional endogenous insulin. Ongoing use of the sulfonylureas appear to also enhance peripheral sensitivity to insulin and reduce the production of hepatic basal glucose. The mechanisms causing these effects are yet to be fully explained. Chlorpropamide also has antidiuretic activity, presumably by potentiating vasopressin's effects on the renal tubules. It may also stimulate secretion of vasopressin.

Uses/Indications - While chlorpropamide could potentially be of benefit in the adjunctive treatment of diabetes mellitus in small animals, its use has been primarily for adjunctive therapy in diabetes insipidus in dogs and cats.

Pharmacokinetics - Chlorpropamide is absorbed well from the GI tract. Its distribution characteristics have not been well described, but it is highly bound to plasma proteins and is excreted into milk. Elimination half lives have not been described in domestic animals, but in humans the elimination half life is about 36 hours. The drug is both metabolized in the liver and excreted unchanged. Elimination of chlorpropamide is enhanced in alkaline urine and decreased in acidic urine.

Contraindications/Precautions/Reproductive Safety - Oral antidiabetic agents are considered contraindicated with the following conditions: severe burns, severe trauma, severe infection, diabetic coma or other hypoglycemic conditions, major surgery, ketosis, ketoacidosis or other significant acidotic conditions. Chlorpropamide should only be used when its potential benefits outweigh its risks during untreated adrenal or pituitary insufficiency; thyroid, cardiac, renal or hepatic function impairment; prolonged vomiting; high fever; malnourishment or debilitated condition; or when fluid retention is present.
Safe use during pregnancy has not been established.

Adverse Effects/Warnings - Hypoglycemia is the most common adverse effect noted with this agent. Syndrome of inappropriate antidiuretic hormone (SIADH), anorexia, diarrhea, hepatotoxicity, lassitude or other CNS effects, and hematologic toxicity are all potentially possible, but except for the GI disturbances are less likely to occur than hypoglycemia.

Overdosage/Acute Toxicity - Profound hypoglycemia is the greatest concern after an overdose. Gut emptying protocols should be employed when warranted. Because of its long half life, blood glucose monitoring and treatment with parenteral glucose may be required for several days. Overdoses may also require additional monitoring (blood gases, serum electrolytes) and supportive therapy.

Drug Interactions - A disulfiram-like reaction (anorexia, nausea, vomiting) has been reported in humans who have ingested **alcohol** within 48-72 hours of receiving chlorpropamide.
The following drugs may displace chlorpropamide, or be displaced by chlorpropamide from plasma proteins, thereby causing enhanced pharmacologic effects of the two drugs involved: **chloramphenicol, furazolidone, non-steroidal anti-inflammatory agents, salicylates, sulfonamides, warfarin**.
Beta **adrenergic blocking agents** (*e.g.*, **propranolol**) may affect diabetes (mellitus) control. Chlorpropamide may prolong the duration of action of **barbiturates**. **Probenecid** or **monamine oxidase inhibitors** may increase the hypoglycemic effects of chlorpropamide. **Thiazide diuretics** may exacerbate diabetes mellitus.
Because elimination of chlorpropamide is enhanced in alkaline urine and decreased in acidic urine. **Ammonium chloride** or **vitamin C** may enhance the effects of chlorpropamide and **sodium bicarbonate or other urinary alkalinizers** (citrate solutions) may reduce its effects.

Laboratory Considerations - Chlorpropamide may mildly increase values of liver enzymes, BUN or serum creatinine.

Doses - For adjunctive therapy in diabetes insipidus in dogs and cats. Beneficial effects may be seen in less than 50% of animals treated. A trial period of at least one week of therapy should be given before assessing effect.

Dogs/Cats:
> For adjunctive treatment of diabetes insipidus in animals with partial ADH deficiency: 10-40 mg/kg PO daily. (Randolph and Peterson 1994)

Monitoring Parameters - 1) Serum electrolytes, plasma and urine osmolarity, urine output; if used for DI; 2) Blood Glucose

Dosage Forms/Preparations/FDA Approval Status/Withholding Times -
Veterinary-Approved Products: None
Human-Approved Products:
> Chlorpropamide Tablets 100 mg, 250 mg; *Diabenese*® (Pfizer); Generic; (Rx)

CHLORTETRACYCLINE

Chemistry - A tetracycline antibiotic, chlortetracycline occurs as yellow, odorless crystals. It is slightly soluble in water.

Storage/Stability/Compatibility - Chlortetracycline should be stored in tight containers and protected from light.

For additional information regarding Pharmacology, Indications, Pharmacokinetics, Contraindications, Adverse Effects, etc., see the Tetracycline monograph.

Doses -
Dogs/Cats:
> For susceptible infections:
> a) 25 mg/kg PO q6-8h (Papich 1992)
> b) To prevent recurrence of mycoplasma or chlamydial conjunctivitis in large catteries where topical therapy is impractical: soluble chlortetracycline powder in food at a dose of 50 mg per day per cat for 1 month. (Carro 1994)

Birds:
> For the treatment of chlamydiosis: In small birds add chlortetracycline to food in a concentration of 0.05%; larger psittacines require 1% CTC. (Flammer 1992)

Cattle and Swine:
> For susceptible infections: 6 - 10 mg/kg IV or IM; 10 - 20 mg/kg PO Note: Although not specified in this reference, chlortetracycline is generally administered once daily (Howard 1993)

Dosage Forms/Preparations/FDA Approval Status/Withholding Times -
Veterinary-Approved Products:
> There are several feed additive/water mix preparations available containing chlortetracycline. Trade names may include *Aureomycin*® (Cyanamid), *CTC*® *50* (AL Labs); *Pfichlor*® (Pfizer). See individual labels for more information.

Human-Approved Products:
> A human labeled topical ointment and an ophthalmic ointment are commercially available.

CHORIONIC GONADOTROPIN (HCG)

Chemistry - A gonad-stimulating polypeptide secreted by the placenta, chorionic gonadotropin is obtained from the urine of pregnant women. It occurs as a white or practically white, amorphous, lyophilized powder. It is soluble in water and practically insoluble in alcohol. One International Unit of HCG is equal to one USP unit. There are at least 1500 USP Units per mg.

Chorionic gonadotropin has many synonyms, including human chorionic gonadotropin, HCG, hCG, CG, chorionic gonadotrophin, pregnancy-urine hormone, and PU.

Storage/Stability/Compatibility - Chorionic gonadotropin powder for injection should be stored at room temperature (15-30°C) and protected from light. After reconstitution, the resultant solution is stable for 30-90 days (depending on the product) when stored at 2-15°C.

Pharmacology - HCG mimics quite closely the effects of luteinizing hormone (LH), but also has some FSH-like activity. In males, HCG can stimulate the differentiation of, and androgen production by, testicular interstitial (Leydig) cells. It may also stimulate testicular descent when no anatomical abnormality is present.

In females, HCG will stimulate the corpus luteum to produce progesterone, and can induce ovulation (possibly also in patients with cystic ovaries). In the bitch, HCG will induce estrogen secretion.

Uses/Indications - The veterinary product's labeled indication is for "parenteral use in cows for the treatment of nymphomania (frequent or constant heat) due to cystic ovaries." It has been used for other purposes in several species, refer to the Dosage section for more information.

Pharmacokinetics - HCG is destroyed in the GI tract after oral administration, so it must be given parenterally. After IM injection, peak plasma levels occur in about 6 hours.

HCG is distributed primarily to the ovaries in females and to the testes in males, but some may also be distributed to the proximal tubules in the renal cortex.

HCG is eliminated from the blood in biphasic manner. The initial elimination half-life is about 11 hours and the terminal half-life is approximately 23 hours.

Contraindications/Precautions - In humans, HCG is contraindicated in patients with prostatic carcinoma or other androgen-dependent neoplasias, precocious puberty or having a previous hypersensitivity reaction to HCG. No labeled contraindications for veterinary patients were noted, but the above human contraindications should be used as guidelines.

Antibody production to this hormone has been reported after repetitive use, resulting in diminished effect.

Adverse Effects/Warnings - Potentially, hypersensitivity reactions are possible with this agent. HCG may cause abortion in mares prior to the 35th day of pregnancy, perhaps due to increased estrogen levels. No other reported adverse reactions were noted for veterinary patients.

In humans, HCG has caused pain at the injection site, gynecomastia, headache, depression, irritability and edema.

Overdosage - No overdosage cases have been reported with HCG.

Drug Interactions - No interactions have apparently been reported with HCG.

Doses -

Dogs:

For cryptorchidism:
    a)   500 Units injected twice weekly for 4-6 weeks (McDonald 1988)

For HCG Challenge test (to determine if testicular tissue remains in castrated male dogs; in females to diagnose sexual differentiation disorders or if functional ovarian tissue remains after ovariohysterectomy):
    a)   Male dogs or females with suspected sexual differentiation disorder: Take sample for resting testosterone level. Administer 44 micrograms/kg HCG IM and take a 4 hour post sample.
        Female dogs: 100 - 1000 IU IM during apparent estrous episode. Measure progesterone level in 5-7 days. If above 1.0 ng/ml, this indicates functional ovarian tissue. (Shille and Olson 1989)

To produce luteinization of a persistent follicular cyst:
    a)   500 IU IM; repeat in 48 hours. If effective, will convert from proestrus to estrus in 1-2 days and sexual behavior should stop within 2 weeks. (Barton 1988)

For infertile bitches cycling normally with low progesterone due to lack of corpus luteum formation:
    a)   Next cycle, give 500 IU HCG SQ on days 10-11 of heat cycle or when vaginal smear indicates breeding readiness. Breed 2 days after HCG administration. (Barton and Wolf 1988)

For male infertility secondary to low testosterone, LH and FSH:
    a)   HCG 500 IU SQ twice weekly for 4 weeks. Add PMSG (Pregnant Mare Serum Gonadotropin) 20 IU/kg SQ 3 times weekly. If PMSG is unavailable, use FSH-P at same dose (1 mg FSH = ≈10-14 IU). Continue for 3 months. Once spermatogenesis ensues, may continue with HCG only. (Barton and Wolf 1988)

Cats:

For HCG Challenge test (to determine if testicular tissue remains in castrated male cats; in females to diagnose sexual differentiation disorders or if functional ovarian tissue remains after ovariohysterectomy):
    a)   Male cats or females with suspected sexual differentiation disorder: Take sample for resting testosterone level. Administer 250 micrograms HCG IM and take a 4 hour post sample.
        Queens: 50 - 100 IU IM during apparent estrous episode. Measure progesterone level in 5-7 days. If above 1.0 ng/ml, this indicates functional ovarian tissue. (Shille and Olson 1989)

For infertility in queens due to confirmed ovulation failure:
   a)   100 - 500 IU IM (Barton and Wolf 1988)

To induce ovulation in anestrus queens:
   a)   Give FSH-P 2 mg IM daily (for up to 5 days) until estrus is observed. Give 250 micrograms HCG on first and second day of estrus (Kraemer and Bowen 1986)

After artificial insemination:
   a)   50 - 75 IU IM immediately after insemination; repeat insemination and injection in 24 hours. (Sojka 1986)

Cattle:
   For treatment of ovarian cysts:
   a)   10,000 Units deep IM or 2500 - 5000 Units IV, may repeat in 14 days if animal's behavior or physical exam indicates a need for retreatment. Alternatively, 500 - 2500 Units injected directly into the follicle. (Package Insert; *Follutein®*—Solvay)

Horses:
   For cryptorchidism:
   a)   Foal: 1000 Units injected twice weekly for 4-6 weeks (McDonald 1988) (Note: Many clinicians believe that medical treatment is unwarranted and that surgery should be performed.)

   To induce ovulation in early estrus when one, large dominant follicle that is palpable with a diameter >35 mm is present:
   a)   HCG: 2000 - 3000 IU IV (preferable to treat mare 6 hours before mating) (Hopkins 1987)

   For treatment of persistent follicles during the early transition period:
   a)   1000 - 5000 IU (results are variable). (Van Camp 1986)

   To hasten ovulation and reduce variability of estrus after prostaglandin synchronization:
   a)   HCG: 1500 - 3300 IU 5-6 days after the second prostaglandin treatment or on the first or second day of estrus. (Bristol 1986)

   To induce ovulation after estrus has commenced:
   a)   2500 - 4000 IU IM or SQ; ovulation generally occurs in 24-48 hours (Roberts 1986b)

Sheep & Goats:
   For treatment of cystic follicles in does:
   a)   250 - 1000 Units IV or IM (Smith 1986a)

Dosage Forms/Preparations/FDA Approval Status/Withholding Times - All HCG products are prescription (Rx).
   Chorionic Gonadotropin (HCG) Powder for Injection 5,000 Units per vial with 10 ml of diluent to make 500 Units/ml

   Chorionic Gonadotropin (HCG) Powder for Injection 10,000 Units per vial with 10 ml of diluent to make 1000 Units/ml

   Chorionic Gonadotropin (HCG) Powder for Injection 20,000 Units per vial with 10 ml of diluent to make 2000 Units/ml

   There are several products available with a variety of trade names, as well as many generically labeled products. Two commonly known products are *A.P.L®* (Wyeth-Ayerst) and *Follutein®* (Squibb). Veterinary-Approved Products are known to be available from Solvay (*Follutein®*) and LyphoMed (generically labeled). There are chorionic gonadotropin products approved for use in dairy cattle and beef cattle. There are no withdrawal times for either milk or meat.

CIMETIDINE
CIMETIDINE HCL

Chemistry - An H$_2$- receptor antagonist, cimetidine occurs as a white to off-white, crystalline powder. It has what is described as an "unpleasant" odor and a pK$_a$ of 6.8. Cimetidine is sparingly soluble in water and soluble in alcohol. Cimetidine HCl occurs as white, crystalline powder and is very soluble in water and soluble in alcohol. It has a pK$_a$ of 7.11 and the commercial injection has a pH of 3.8-6.

Storage/Stability/Compatibility - Cimetidine products should be stored protected from light and kept at room temperature. Do not refrigerate the injectable product as precipitation may occur. Oral dosage forms should be stored in tight containers.
   The cimetidine injectable product is **compatible** with the commonly used IV infusions solutions, including amino acid (TPN) solutions, but should be used within 48 hours of dilution. Cimetidine is also reported to be compatible with the following drugs: acetazolamide sodium,

amikacin sulfate, atropine sulfate, carbenicillin disodium, cefoxitin sodium, chlorothiazide sodium, clindamycin phosphate, colistimethate sodium, dexamethasone sodium phosphate, digoxin, epinephrine, erythromycin lactobionate, furosemide, gentamicin sulfate, heparin sodium, insulin (regular), isoproterenol HCl, lidocaine HCl, lincomycin HCl, methylprednisolone sodium succinate, nafcillin sodium, norepinephrine bitartrate, penicillin G potassium/sodium, phytonadione, polymyxin B sulfate, potassium chloride, protamine sulfate, quinidine gluconate, sodium nitroprusside, tetracycline HCl, vancomycin HCl, verapamil HCl, and vitamin B complex (w/ or w/o C).

The following drugs are reported to be either **incompatible** with cimetidine or data are conflicting: amphotericin B, ampicillin sodium, cefamandole naftate, cefazolin sodium, cephalothin sodium, and pentobarbital sodium. Compatibility is dependent upon factors such as pH, concentration, temperature and diluents used. It is suggested to consult specialized references for more specific information (*e.g., Handbook on Injectable Drugs* by Trissel; see bibliography).

Pharmacology - At the H_2 receptors of the parietal cells, cimetidine competitively inhibits histamine, thereby reducing gastric acid output both during basal conditions and when stimulated by food, pentagastrin, histamine or insulin. Gastric emptying time, pancreatic or biliary secretion, and lower esophageal pressures are not altered by cimetidine. By decreasing the amount of gastric juice produced, cimetidine also decreases the amount of pepsin secreted.

Cimetidine has an apparent immunomodulating effect as it has been demonstrated to reverse suppressor T cell-mediated immune suppression. It also possesses weak anti-androgenic activity.

Uses/Indications - In veterinary medicine, cimetidine has been used for the treatment and/or prophylaxis of gastric, abomasal and duodenal ulcers, uremic gastritis, stress-related or drug-induced erosive gastritis, esophagitis, duodenal gastric reflux and esophageal reflux. It has also been employed to treat hypersecretory conditions associated with gastrinomas and systemic mastocytosis. Cimetidine has also been used investigationally as a immunomodulating agent (see doses) in dogs.

Pharmacokinetics - Pharmacokinetic data for veterinary species is limited for this agent. In dogs, the oral bioavailability is reported to be approximately 95%, serum half-life is 1.3 hours and volume of distribution is 1.2 L/kg.

In humans, cimetidine is rapidly and well absorbed after oral administration, but a small amount is metabolized in the liver before entering the systemic circulation (first-pass effect). The oral bioavailability is 70-80%. Food may delay absorption and slightly decrease the amount absorbed, but when given with food, peak levels occur when the stomach is not protected by the buffering capabilities of the ingesta.

Cimetidine is well distributed in body tissues and only 15-20% is bound to plasma proteins. The drug enters milk and crosses the placenta.

Cimetidine is both metabolized in the liver and excreted unchanged by the kidneys. More drug is excreted by the kidneys when administered parenterally (75%) than when given orally (48%). The average serum half-life is 2 hours in humans, but can be prolonged in elderly patients and in those with renal or hepatic disease. Peritoneal dialysis does not appreciably enhance the removal of cimetidine from the body.

Contraindications/Precautions - Cimetidine is contraindicated in patients with known hypersensitivity to the drug.

Cimetidine should be used cautiously in geriatric patients and in patients with significantly impaired hepatic or renal function. In humans meeting these criteria, increased risk of CNS (confusion) effects may occur; dosage reductions may be necessary.

Adverse Effects/Warnings - Adverse effects appear to be very rare in animals at the dosages generally used. Potential adverse effects (documented in humans) that could be seen, include mental confusion, headache (upon discontinuation of the drug), gynecomastia and decreased libido. Rarely, agranulocytosis may develop and if given rapidly IV, transient cardiac arrhythmias may be seen. Pain at the injection site may be noted after IM administration.

Cimetidine does inhibit microsomal enzymes in the liver and may alter the metabolic rates of other drugs (see Drug Interactions below).

Overdosage - Clinical experience with cimetidine overdosage is limited. In laboratory animals, very high dosages have been associated with tachycardia and respiratory failure. Respiratory support and beta-adrenergic blockers have been suggested for use should these symptoms occur.

Drug Interactions - Cimetidine may inhibit the hepatic microsomal enzyme system and thereby reduce the metabolism, prolong serum half-lives, and increase the serum levels of several drugs. It may also reduce the hepatic blood flow and reduce the amount of hepatic extraction of drugs that have a high first-pass effect. The following drugs may be affected: beta-**blockers** (*e.g.,* **propranolol**), **lidocaine, calcium channel blockers** (*e.g.,* **verapamil**), **diazepam (and other benzodiazepines), ethanol, metronidazole, phenytoin, quinidine, theophylline, and warfarin.** Dosage adjustment or increased therapeutic monitoring may be necessary.

Cimetidine may decrease the renal clearance of **procainamide**.

Cimetidine may exacerbate leukopenias when used with other agents that can cause this problem.

Stagger doses (separate by 2 hours if possible) of cimetidine with **antacids, metoclopramide, sucralfate, digoxin,** and **ketoconazole**.

Drug/Laboratory Interactions - Cimetidine may cause small increases in plasma **creatinine** concentrations early in therapy. These increases are generally mild, non-progressive, and have disappeared when therapy is discontinued. Histamine$_2$ blockers may antagonize the effects of histamine and pentagastrin in the **evaluation gastric acid secretion**. After using **allergen extract skin tests**, histamine$_2$ antagonsits may inhibit histamine responses. It is recommended that histamine$_2$ blockers be discontinued at least 24 hours before performing either of these tests.

Doses -
  Dogs:
    For esophagitis:
      a) 5 - 10 mg/kg PO q6h (do not give with antacids) (Jones 1985)
      b) 4 mg/kg PO *qid* (Watrous 1988)

    For prevention of drug-induced gastric erosion/ulceration: 5 mg/kg PO, SQ, *tid* (Schunk 1988)

    For chronic gastritis: 5 - 10 mg/kg PO, IM or IV *tid-qid* (Hall and Twedt 1988)

    For ulcer disease:
      a) 5 - 10 mg/kg PO, IM or IV *tid-qid* (Hall and Twedt 1988)
      b) 4 - 5 mg/kg PO, IV, or SQ *tid-qid* (Chiapella 1988)
      c) 5 mg/kg IV or PO *qid* (Moreland 1988)
      d) 5 - 10 mg/kg PO q6-8h or 10 mg/kg q6h as a slow (over 30 minutes) IV infusion (DeNovo 1986)
      e) 10 mg/kg PO, IM, IV q8h (Matz 1995)

      For gastrinoma: 5 - 15 mg/kg IV, SQ or PO *qid* (Kay, Kruth, and Twedt 1988)

    To prevent histamine-mediated gastric hyperacidity/ulceration secondary to mast cell tumors:
      a) 5 mg/kg q8h (Fox 1995b)
      b) 5 mg/kg PO, IV, *tid-qid* (Stann 1988)

    To decrease gastric acid hypersecretion during the treatment of alkalosis: 5 - 10 mg/kg *tid-qid* (Hardy and Robinson 1986)

    As an immunomodulating agent (reverses suppressor T cell-mediated immune suppression):
      a) 10 - 25 mg/kg PO *bid* (Desiderio and Rankin 1986)
  Cats:
      a) 5 - 10 mg/kg PO q6-8h or 10 mg/kg q6h as a slow (over 30 minutes) IV infusion (DeNovo 1986)

  Cattle:
    To treat abomasal ulcers: 8 - 16 mg/kg *tid* (method of administration not specified); relatively expensive and may be only of minimal value (Whitlock 1986a)

  Horses:
    For foals:
      a) 1000 mg divided *bid* or *tid* PO, IV or IM (Robinson 1987)
      b) 300 - 600 mg PO or IV 4 times a day (Clark and Becht 1987)

  Swine:
    To treat gastric ulcers: 300 mg per animal twice daily (Wass et al. 1986b)

  Reptiles:
    In most species: 4 mg/kg PO q8-12h (Gauvin 1993)

Monitoring Parameters -
  1) Clinical efficacy (dependent on reason for use); monitored by decrease in symptomatology, endoscopic examination, blood in feces, etc.
  2) Adverse effects if noted

Client Information - To maximize the benefit of this medication, it must be administered as prescribed by the veterinarian; symptoms may reoccur if dosages are missed.

Dosage Forms/Preparations/FDA Approval Status/Withholding Times -
  Veterinary-Approved Products: None
  Human-Approved Products:

  Cimetidine Tablets 100 mg, 200 mg, 300 mg, 400 mg, 800 mg; *Tagamet*® HB (SKBeecham) (OTC); *Tagamet*® (SK-Beecham) (Rx); generic (Rx)

Cimetidine HCl Liquid 300 mg (as HCl) per 5 ml; *Tagamet*® (SK-Beecham) (Rx); *Cimetidine Oral Solution*® (Barre-National) (Rx)

Cimetidine HCl for Injection 150 mg/ml in 2 ml vials and 8 ml multiple-dose vials and 8 ml vials; 300 mg (as HCl) in 50 ml 0.9% sodium chloride in premixed single-dose containers; *Tagamet*® (SK-Beecham) (Rx); *Cimetidine*® (Endo) (Rx)

CIPROFLOXACIN

Chemistry - A fluroquinolone antibiotic, ciprofloxacin HCl occurs as a faintly yellowish to yellow, crystalline powder. It is slightly soluble in water. Ciprofloxacin is related structurally to the veterinary-approved drug enrofloxacin (enrofloxacin has an additional ethyl group on the piperazinyl ring).

Storage/Stability/Compatibility - Unless otherwise directed by the manufacturer, ciprofloxacin tablets should be stored in tight containers at temperatures less than 30°C. Protect from strong UV light. The injection should be stored at 5°-25°C and protected from light and freezing.

Pharmacology - Ciprofloxacin is a bactericidal agent. The bactericidal activity of ciprofloxacin is concentration dependent, with susceptible bacteria cell death occurring within 20-30 minutes of exposure. Ciprofloxacin has demonstrated a significant post-antibiotic effect for both gram - and + bacteria and is active in both stationary and growth phases of bacterial replication. Its mechanism of action is not thoroughly understood, but it is believed to act by inhibiting bacterial DNA-gyrase (a type-II topoisomerase), thereby preventing DNA supercoiling and DNA synthesis.

Both enrofloxacin and ciprofloxacin have similar spectrums of activity. These agents have good activity against many gram negative bacilli and cocci, including most species and strains of *Pseudomonas aeruginosa, Klebsiella sp., E. coli, Enterobacter, Campylobacter, Shigella, Salmonella, Aeromonas, Haemophilus, Proteus, Yersinia, Serratia*, and *Vibrio* species. Of the currently commercially available quinolones, ciprofloxacin and enrofloxacin have the lowest MIC values for the majority of these pathogens treated. Other organisms that are generally susceptible include *Brucella sp, Chlamydia trachomatis, Staphylococci* (including penicillinase-producing and methicillin-resistant strains), Mycoplasma, and *Mycobacterium sp.* (not the etiologic agent for Johne's Disease).

The fluroquinolones have variable activity against most *Streptococci* and are not usually recommended to be used for these infections. These drugs have weak activity against most anaerobes and are ineffective in treating anaerobic infections.

Resistance does occur by mutation, particularly with *Pseudomonas aeruginosa, Klebsiella pneumonia, Acinetobacter* and enterococci, but plasmid-mediated resistance is not thought to occur.

Uses/Indications - Because of its similar spectrum of activity, ciprofloxacin could be used as an alternative to enrofloxacin when a larger oral dosage form or intravenous product is desired. But the two compounds cannot be considered equivalent because of pharmacokinetic differences (see below).

Pharmacokinetics - Both enrofloxacin and ciprofloxacin are well absorbed after oral administration in most species. But in dogs, enrofloxacin's bioavailability is about twice that of ciprofloxacin after oral dosing. In humans, the oral bioavailability of ciprofloxacin has been reported to be between 50-85%. Studies of the oral bioavailability in ponies have shown that ciprofloxacin is poorly absorbed (2-12%) while enrofloxacin in foals apparently is well absorbed. In humans, the volume of distribution in adults for ciprofloxacin is about 2-3.5 L/kg and it is approximately 20-40% bound to serum proteins.

Ciprofloxacin is one of the metabolites of enrofloxacin. Approximately 15-50% of the drugs are eliminated unchanged into the urine, by both tubular secretion and glomerular filtration. Enrofloxacin/ciprofloxacin are metabolized to various metabolites that are less active than the parent compounds. Approximately 30-40% of circulating enrofloxacin is metabolized to ciprofloxacin. These metabolites are eliminated both in the urine and feces. Because of the dual (renal and hepatic) means of elimination, patients with severely impaired renal function may have slightly prolonged half-lives and higher serum levels which may not require dosage adjustment.

The pharmacokinetics of ciprofloxacin have been studied in calves and pigs (Nouws et al. 1988). Oral bioavailability is approximately 50% in calves and 40% (only one pig studied) in pigs and it has an elimination half-life of about 2.5 hours in both species. Protein binding was significantly different for each species, with calves having about 70% of the drug bound and pigs only about 23% bound to plasma proteins.

Contraindications/Precautions/Reproductive Safety - Ciprofloxacin, like enrofloxacin should be considered contraindicated in small and medium breed dogs from 2 months to 8 months of age. Bubble-like changes in articular cartilage have been noted when the drug was given at 2-5 times recommend doses for 30 days, although clinical symptoms have only been seen at the 5X dose. Large and giant breed dogs may be in the rapid-growth phase for periods longer than 8 months of age, so longer than 8 months may be necessary to avoid cartilage damage. Quinolones are also contraindicated in patients hypersensitive to them.

Because ciprofloxacin has occasionally been reported to cause crystalluria, animals should not be allowed to become dehydrated during therapy with either ciprofloxacin or enrofloxacin. In humans, ciprofloxacin has been associated with CNS stimulation and should be used with caution in patients with seizure disorders. Patients with severe renal or hepatic impairment may require dosage adjustments to prevent drug accumulation.

Adverse Effects/Warnings - With the exception of potential cartilage abnormalities in young animals (see Contraindications above), the adverse effect profile of fluroquinolones appears to be minimal. GI distress (vomiting, anorexia) is the most common, yet infrequently reported adverse effect. Although not reported thus far in animals, hypersensitivity reactions, crystalluria and CNS effects (dizziness, stimulation) could potentially occur.

Overdosage - Little specific information is available. See the enrofloxacin monograph for more information.

Drug/Drug Interactions - **Antacids** containing cations (Mg^{++}, Al^{+++}, Ca^{++}) may bind to enrofloxacin/ciprofloxacin and prevent its absorption. **Sucralfate** may inhibit absorption of enrofloxacin/ciprofloxacin, separate doses of these drugs by at least 2 hours.

Enrofloxacin/ciprofloxacin administered with **theophylline** may increase theophylline blood levels.

Probenecid blocks tubular secretion of enrofloxacin/ciprofloxacin and may increase its blood level and half-life.

Synergism may occur, but is not predictable, against some bacteria (particularly *Pseudomonas aeruginosa* or other Enterobacteriaceae) with these compounds and **aminoglycosides, 3rd generation cephalosporins agents, and extended-spectrum penicillins**. Although enrofloxacin/ciprofloxacin has minimal activity against anaerobes, *in vitro* synergy has been reported when used with **clindamycin** against strains of *Peptostreptococcus*, *Lactobacillus* and *Bacteroids fragilis*. **Nitrofurantoin** may antagonize the antimicrobial activity of the fluroquinolones and their concomitant use is not recommended. Fluroquinolones may exacerbate the nephrotoxicity of **cyclosporine** (used systemically).

Because the are relatively new additions to the therapeutic armamentarium, more interactions may be forthcoming.

Drug/Laboratory Interactions - In some human patients, the fluroquinolones have caused increases in **liver enzymes, BUN,** and **creatinine** and decreases in **hematocrit**. The clinical relevance of these mild changes is not known at this time.

Doses -
  Dogs:
    For susceptible infections:
      a) Ciprofloxacin: 5 - 15 mg/kg PO q12h
          Avoid or reduce dosage of these drugs in animals with severe renal failure; avoid in young animals or in pregnant or breeding animals (Vaden and Papich 1995)
      b) Ciprofloxacin: 5 - 8 mg/kg PO q12h for UTI; 10 - 15 mg/kg PO q12h for soft tissue and bone infections. (Neer 1988)

  Cats:
    For susceptible infections:
      a) Ciprofloxacin: 5 - 15 mg/kg PO q12h
          Avoid or reduce dosage of these drugs in animals with severe renal failure; avoid in young animals or in pregnant or breeding animals (Vaden and Papich 1995)

  Birds:
    For susceptible gram negative infections:
      a) Using ciprofloxacin 500 mg tablets: 20 - 40 mg/kg PO *bid*. Crushed tablet goes into suspension well, but must be shaken well before administering. (McDonald 1989)
      b) Ciprofloxacin (using crushed tablets): 20 mg/kg PO q12h
          Enrofloxacin: 15 mg/kg PO, or IM or 250 mg/L of drinking water. (Bauck and Hoefer 1993)
      c) Ciprofloxacin (using crushed tablets or suspend) 10 - 15 mg/kg PO q12h (Hoeffer 1995)

Monitoring Parameters - 1) Clinical efficacy; 2) Adverse effects

Dosage Forms/Preparations/FDA Approval Status -
  Veterinary-Approved Products: None

Human-Approved Products:

Ciprofloxacin Oral Tablets 100 mg, 250 mg, 500 mg, 750 mg; *Cipro*® (Bayer); (Rx)

Ciprofloxacin Injection 10 mg/ml (200 mg & 400 mg in 20 ml & 40 ml vials) and 2 mg/ml in 100 ml & 200 ml in 5% dextrose flexible containers; *Cipro I.V.*® (Bayer) (Rx)

CISAPRIDE

Chemistry - An oral GI prokinetic agent, cisapride is a substituted piperidinyl benzamide and is structurally, but not pharmacologically, related to procainamide. It is available commercially as a monohydrate, but potency is expressed in terms of the anhydrate.

Storage/Stability/Compatibility - Unless otherwise instructed by the manufacturer, store cisapride tablets in tight, light-resistant containers at room temperature.

Pharmacology - Cisapride increases lower esophageal peristalsis and sphincter pressure and accelerates gastric emptying. The proposed mechanism of action is that it enhances the release of acetylcholine at the myenteric plexus, but does not induce nicotinic or muscarinic receptor stimulation. Acetylcholinesterase activity is not inhibited. Cisapride blocks dopaminergic receptors to a lesser extent than does metoclopramide and does not increase gastric acid secretion.

Uses/Indications - Cisapride is a new agent. Proposed uses for it in small animals include esophageal reflux and treatment of primary gastric stasis disorders.

Pharmacokinetics - Human data: After oral administration, cisapride is rapidly absorbed with an absolute bioavailability of 35-40%. The drug is highly bound to plasma proteins and apparently extensively distributed throughout the body. Cisapride is extensively metabolized and its elimination half life is about 8-10 hours.

Contraindications/Precautions/Reproductive Safety - Cisapride is contraindicated in patients in whom increased gastrointestinal motility could be harmful (*e.g.*, perforation, obstruction, GI hemorrhage) or those who are hypersensitive to the drug.

Cisapride at high dosages (> 40 mg/kg/day) caused fertility impairment in female rats. At doses 12 to 100 times the maximum recommended, cisapride was embryotoxic and fetotoxic in rabbits and rats. Its use during pregnancy should occur only when the benefits outweigh the risks. Cisapride is excreted in maternal milk in low levels; use with caution in nursing mothers.

Adverse Effects/Warnings - Usage in small animal medicine has been limited to this point and an adverse effect profile has not been determined. As expected in humans, the primary adverse effects are gastrointestinal related with diarrhea and abdominal pain most commonly reported.

Dosage may need to be decreased in patients with severe hepatic impairment.

Overdosage/Acute Toxicity - In one reported human overdose of 540 mg, the patient developed GI distress and urinary frequency. LD$_{50}$ doses in various lab animals range from 160 - 4000 mg/kg. Significant overdoses should be handled using standard gut emptying protocols when appropriate; supportive therapy should be initiated when required.

Drug Interactions - Because cisapride can decrease GI transit times, absorption of other drugs given orally may be affected. **Oral drugs with a narrow therapeutic index** may need serum levels monitored more closely when adding or discontinuing cisapride. Use of **anticholinergic agents** may diminish the effects of cisapride. **Cimetidine** (not ranitidine) may increase cisapride serum levels and cisapride may accelerate **cimetidine** and **ranitidine** absorption thereby enhancing their effects. Cisapride may enhance **anticoagulants'** effects; additional monitoring and anticoagulant dosage adjustments may be required. Cisapride may enhance the sedative effects of **alcohol** or **benzodiazepines**.

Elevated concentrations of cisapride with resultant ventricular arrhythmias may result if coadministered with **ketoconazole**, **itraconazole**, IV **miconazole** or **troleandomycin**. At present, the manufacturer states that cisapride should not be used with these drugs.

Doses -
 Dogs:
 As a promotility agent:
 a) 0.5 mg/kg *tid*; decrease dose if abnormal GI signs or abdominal pain result. (Hall 1994)
 b) To reduce regurgitation associated with megaesophagus: 0.55 mg/kg PO once to three times daily. Practically: 2.5 mg per dose for dogs weighing between 5-10 lbs.; 5 mg per dose for dogs weighing between 11-40 lbs; and 10 mg per dose for dogs greater than 40 lbs. Administer no closer than 30 minutes before feeding. (Tams 1994)
 c) As an antiemetic: 0.1 - 0.5 mg/kg q8h PO (Washabau and Elie 1995)
 Cats:
 For chronic constipation (*e.g.*, megacolon):

    a) In combination with a stool softener (author recommends lactulose at a starting dose of 2 - 3 ml PO *tid*; then adjust prn) and a bulk agent (*e.g.* psyllium or pumpkin pie filling) cisapride is given initially at 2.5 mg (for cats up to 10 pounds) or 5 mg (for cats 11 pounds or heavier) *tid*, 30 minutes before food. Cats weighing greater than 16 pounds may require 7.5 mg. (Tams 1994)

    b) Used adjunctively with conventional dietary therapeutics: 1.25 - 2.5 mg per cat *bid-tid*; cats with hepatic insufficiency should be treated with half the usual dose; probably most effective when given 15 minutes before a meal. (Nixon 1994)

Horses:

As a promotility agent:

    a) Preliminary study: Author states that 0.1 mg/kg was superior to other doses used. No mention of dosage route or frequency was noted. (Roussel 1992)

Monitoring Parameters - Efficacy and adverse effects profile.

Client Information - Because cisapride is a "new" drug, inform client to watch carefully for and report any adverse effects noted.

Dosage Forms/Preparations/FDA Approval Status/Withholding Times -

Veterinary-Approved Products: None

Human-Approved Products:

Cisapride Oral Tablets 10 mg & 20 mg; *Propulsid*® (Janssen); *Prepulsid*® in Canada, New Zealand, etc. (Rx)

Cisapride Suspension: 1 mg/ml in 450 ml bottles; *Propulsid*®(Janssen) (Rx)

CISPLATIN

Chemistry - An inorganic platinum-containing antineoplastic, cisplatin occurs as white powder. One mg is soluble in 1 ml of water or normal saline. The drug is available commercially as powder for injection and as a solution for injection. The powder for injection occurs as a white, lyophilized powder that also contains mannitol, sodium chloride and HCl (to adjust pH). After reconstituting with sterile water for injection a clear solution results having a pH from 3.5-5. Cisplatin injection (premixed solution) has a pH of 3.7-6. Cisplatin may also be known as *cis*-Platinum II, *cis*-DDP, CDDP, *cis*-diamminedichloroplatinum, or DDP.

Storage/Stability/Compatibility - The injection and powder for injection should be stored at room temperature and away from light; do not refrigerate the injection as a precipitate may form. During use, the injection should be protected from direct bright sunlight, but does not need to be protected from normal room incandescent or fluorescent lights.

After reconstituting, the powder for injection is stable for at least 20 hours at room temperature. If using bacteriostatic water for injection to reconstitute the drug to a concentration of 1 mg/ml, solutions are reportedly stable for at least 72 hours at room temperature. Cisplatin is reportedly stable for at least 3 weeks when frozen.

Do not use aluminum hub needles or aluminum containing IV sets as aluminum may displace platinum from the cisplatin molecule with the resulting formation of a black precipitate. Should a precipitate form from either cold temperatures or aluminum contact, discard the solution.

Cisplatin is reportedly **compatible** with the following intravenous solutions and drugs: dextrose/saline combinations, sodium chloride 0.225%-0.9%, magnesium sulfate, and mannitol. It is also compatible in syringes or at Y-sites with: bleomycin sulfate, cyclophosphamide, doxorubicin HCl, droperidol, fluorouracil, furosemide, heparin sodium, leucovorin calcium, methotrexate, mitomycin, vinblastine sulfate, and vincristine sulfate.

Cisplatin **compatibility information conflicts** or is dependent on diluent or concentration factors with the following drugs or solutions: dextrose/saline combinations, dextrose 5% in water, and metoclopramide. Compatibility is dependent upon factors such as pH, concentration, temperature and diluents used. It is suggested to consult specialized references for more specific information (*e.g., Handbook on Injectable Drugs* by Trissel; see bibliography).

Cisplatin is reportedly **incompatible** with the following solutions or drugs: sodium chloride 0.1% and sodium bicarbonate 5%.

Pharmacology - While the exact mechanism of action of cisplatin has not been determined, its properties are analogous to those of bifunctional alkylating agents producing inter- and intrastrand crosslinks in DNA. Cisplatin is cell cycle nonspecific.

Uses/Indications - In veterinary medicine, the use of cisplatin is presently limited to use in dogs. The drug has been or may be useful in a variety of neoplastic diseases including squamous cell carcinomas, transitional cell carcinomas, ovarian carcinomas, mediastinal carcinomas, osteosarcomas, pleural adenocarcinomas, nasal carcinomas and thyroid adenocarcinomas.

Pharmacokinetics - After administration, the drug concentrates in the liver, intestines and kidneys. Platinum will accumulate in the body and may be detected 6 months after a course of therapy has been completed. Cisplatin is highly bound to serum proteins.

In dogs, cisplatin exhibits a biphasic elimination profile. The initial plasma half-life is short (approximately 20 minutes), but the terminal phase is very long (about 120 hours). Approximately 80% of a dose can be recovered as free platinum in the urine within 48 hours of dosing in dogs.

Contraindications/Precautions/Reproductive Safety - Because of severe dose-related primary pulmonary toxicoses (dyspnea, hydrothorax, pulmonary edema, mediastinal edema, and death) associated with cisplatin in cats, the drug is considered contraindicated in this species at the present time. It is presently unknown whether non-toxic doses will have any therapeutic benefits in cats. Cisplatin is also contraindicated in patients with preexisting significant renal impairment, myelosuppression, or a history of hypersensitivity to platinum-containing compounds.

When preparing the product for injection, wear gloves and protective clothing as local reactions may occur with skin or mucous membrane contact. Should accidental exposure occur, wash the area thoroughly with soap and water.

Cisplatin's safe use in pregnancy has not been established. It is teratogenic and embryotoxic in mice. In human men, the drug may cause azoospermia and impaired spermatogenesis.

Adverse Effects/Warnings - In dogs, the most frequent adverse effect seen after cisplatin treatment is vomiting, which usually occurs within 6 hours after dosing and persists for 1-6 hours. Nephrotoxicity may commonly occur unless the animal is adequately diuresed with sodium chloride prior to, and after therapy; diuresis will generally reduce significantly the incidence and severity of nephrotoxicity in the majority of dogs. Other adverse effects that have been reported include hematologic abnormalities (thrombocytopenia and/or granulocytopenia), ototoxicity (high-frequency hearing loss and tinnitus), anorexia, diarrhea (including hemorrhagic diarrhea), seizures, peripheral neuropathies, electrolyte abnormalities, hyperuricemia, increased hepatic enzymes, anaphylactoid reactions and death.

Direct IV infusion over 1-5 minutes should be avoided as it may cause increased nephrotoxicity or ototoxicity.

Overdosage/Acute Toxicity - The minimum lethal dose of cisplatin in dogs is reportedly 2.5 mg/kg ($\approx$80 mg/m^2). Because of the potential for serious toxicity associated with this agent, dosage calculations should be checked thoroughly to avoid overdosing. See Adverse effects above for more information.

Drug Interactions - Cisplatin may reduce serum levels of **phenytoin**.

Because cisplatin can cause significant nephrotoxicity, use of other **nephrotoxic drugs** (*e.g.,* **aminoglycosides, amphotericin B**) within 2 weeks after cisplatin therapy should be avoided.

Doses - For more information, refer to the protocol references found in the appendix or other protocols found in small animal internal medicine references. Additionally, it is strongly recommend to consult the following reference if cisplatin therapy is being considered: Shapiro, W. 1989. Cisplatin Chemotherapy. In Current Veterinary Therapy X: Small Animal Practice. Edited by R. W. Kirk. 497-502. Philadelphia: W.B. Saunders.

Warning: Dogs must undergo saline diuresis before and after cisplatin therapy to reduce the potential for nephrotoxicity development. Some clinicians also recommend using either mannitol and furosemide with saline, but this is somewhat controversial.

Dogs:

For potentially susceptible carcinomas and sarcomas:

    a) 60 mg/m^2 IV over 20 minutes every 3 weeks. Intravenous normal saline is given at 20 ml/kg/hr for 4 hours before and for 2 hours after cisplatin administration. If animal vomits, give chlorpromazine at 0.5 mg/kg IV or SQ; repeat prn to control vomiting. (Knapp et al. 1988)

    c) 30 - 50 mg/m^2 every 3 weeks. Pretreat with fluids at 60 ml/kg for 12 hours before dosing. Give mannitol 0.5 mg/kg 30 minutes before cisplatin. Give cisplatin as a slow drip over 1-6 hours and follow with another 12 hours of fluids at 60 ml/kg. (Macy 1986)

    d) 60 - 70 mg/m^2 IV drip q3-5 weeks. Perform saline diuresis before and after treatment. (MacEwen and Rosenthal 1989)

Monitoring Parameters - Adapted primarily from the reference by Shapiro (Shapiro 1989).

    1) Toxicity. Baseline laboratory data: urinalysis, hemogram, platelet count, serum biochemical and electrolyte determination. Repeat tests before each dose if animal is receiving high-dose therapy ($\approx$monthly) or prn if signs/symptoms of toxicity develop. Animals receiving frequent small doses should be monitored at least weekly. Not recommended to use cisplatin if WBC is <3200/μl, platelets <100,000, creatinine clear-

ance is <1.4 ml/min/kg, or uremia, electrolyte or acid-base imbalance is present. Reduce dose if rapid decreases occur with either WBC or platelets, changes in urine specific gravity or serum electrolytes, elevated serum creatinine or BUN, or if creatinine clearance is >1.4 but <2.9 ml/min/kg.

2) Efficacy. Tumor measurement and radiography at least monthly. In one study (Knapp et al. 1988), the authors state that dogs should be evaluated at 42 days into therapy. Dogs demonstrating complete or partial remission or stable disease should receive additional therapy. Dogs whose disease has progressed should have cisplatin therapy stopped and receive alternate therapies if warranted.

Client Information - Clients must be briefed on the possibilities of severe toxicity developing from this drug, including drug-related mortality.

Dosage Forms/Preparations/FDA Approval Status/Withholding Times -
  Veterinary-Approved Products: None
  Human-Approved Products:
    Cisplatin Injection 1 mg/ml in 50 and 100 ml vials
    Platinol-AQ® (Bristol-Myers Oncology); (Rx)

CITRATE SALTS
POTASSIUM CITRATE
SODIUM CITRATE & CITRIC ACID

Chemistry - Generally used as alkalinizing agents, citric acid and citrate salts are available in several commercially available dosage forms. Citric acid occurs as an odorless or practically odorless, colorless, translucent crystal with a strong acidic taste. It is very soluble in water. Potassium citrate occurs as odorless, transparent crystals or a white, granular powder having a cooling, saline taste. It is freely soluble in water. Sodium citrate occurs as colorless crystals or a white, granular powder. The hydrous form is freely soluble in water. Sodium citrate and citric acid solutions may also be known as Shohl's solution.

Storage/Stability/Compatibility - Store solutions and potassium citrate tablets in tight containers at room temperature unless otherwise recommended by manufacturer.

Pharmacology - Citrate salts are oxidized in the body to bicarbonate, thereby acting as alkalinizing agents. The citric acid component of multi-component products is converted only to carbon dioxide and water and thus, has only a temporary effect on systemic acid-base status.

Uses/Indications - Citrate salts serve as source of bicarbonate; they are more pleasant tasting than bicarbonate preparations making them more palatable. They are used as urinary alkalinizers when an alkaline urine is desirable and in the management of chronic metabolic acidosis accompanied with conditions such as renal tubular acidosis or chronic renal insufficiency. Potassium citrate alone *(Uracit-K®)* has been used for the prevention of calcium oxalate uroliths. The citrate can complex with calcium thereby decreasing urinary concentrations of calcium oxalate. The urinary alkalinizing effects of the citrate also increase the solubility of calcium oxalate.

Pharmacokinetics - Absorption and oxidation are nearly complete after oral administration; less than 5% of a dose is excreted unchanged.

Contraindications/Precautions/Reproductive Safety - Contraindications for products containing sodium citrate and/or potassium citrate: aluminum toxicity, heart failure, severe renal impairment (with azotemia or oliguria), UTI associated with calcium or struvite stones. Additional contraindications for potassium citrate alone include hyperkalemia (or conditions that predispose to hyperkalemia such as adrenal insufficiency, acute dehydration, renal failure, uncontrolled diabetes mellitus), peptic ulcer (particularly with the tablets). The potassium citrate tablets are also contraindicated in patients with delayed gastric emptying conditions, esophageal compression, or intestinal obstruction or stricture. These products should be used with caution (weigh risks vs. benefit) in severe renal tubular acidosis or chronic diarrheal syndromes as they may be ineffective. Sodium citrate products should be used with caution in patients with congestive heart disease.

In dosages not resulting in hypernatremia, hyperkalemia or metabolic alkalosis, these products should not cause fetal harm.

Adverse Effects/Warnings - The primary adverse effects noted with these agents are gastrointestinal in nature, however, most dogs receiving these products tolerate them well. Potassium citrate products have the potential of causing hyperkalemia, especially in susceptible patients. Sodium citrate products may lead to increased fluid retention in patients with cardiac disease. Rarely, metabolic alkalosis could occur.

Overdosage/Acute Toxicity - Overdosage and acute toxicity would generally fall into 4 categories: gastrointestinal distress and ulceration, metabolic alkalosis, hypernatremia (sodium citrate) or hyperkalemia (potassium citrate). Should an overdose occur and there are reasonable expectations of preventing absorption (especially with the tablets), gut emptying protocols should be employed if not contraindicated. Otherwise treat GI effects if necessary with intravenous fluids or other supportive care. Hyperkalemia, hypernatremia and metabolic alkalosis should be treated if warranted. It is suggested to refer to a veterinary poison center, an internal medicine text or other references for additional information for specific treatment modalities for these conditions.

Drug Interactions - Concurrent use with **methenamine** is not recommended as it requires an acidic urine for efficacy. Citrate alkalinizers used with **antacids** (particularly those containing bicarbonate or aluminum salts) may cause systemic alkalosis, and aluminum toxicity (aluminum antacids only) particularly in patients with renal insufficiency. Sodium citrate combined with sodium bicarbonate may cause hypernatremia, and may cause the development of calcium stones in patients with preexisting uric acid stones. When urine is alkalinized by citrate solutions, excretion of certain drugs (*e.g.*, **quinidine, amphetamines, ephedrine, salicylates, tetracycline**) is decreased, and excretion of weakly acidic drugs (*e.g.*, **salicylates**) is increased.

The solubility of **ciprofloxacin & enrofloxacin** is decreased in an alkaline environment. Patients with alkaline urine should be monitored for signs of crystalluria.

With potassium citrate products, the following agents may lead to increases in serum potassium levels (including severe hyperkalemia), particularly in patients with renal insufficiency: **Nonsteroidal antiinflammatory drugs, captopril, enalapril, lisinopril, cyclosporine, digitalis glycosides, potassium-sparing diuretics (*e.g.*, spironolactone), potassium-containing drugs, heparin, and salt substitutes**.

Doses -
  Dogs:
> For adjunctive therapy to inhibit calcium oxalate crystal formation in dogs with hypocitraturia: Using potassium citrate wax-matrix tablets (*Uracit-K®*): 150 mg/kg per day divided into two doses. Crush tablets and mix with food. (Lulich, Osborne et al. 1992)

Monitoring Parameters - Depending on patient's condition, product chosen and reason for use: 1) Serum potassium, sodium, bicarbonate, chloride; 2) Acid/base status; 3) Urine pH, Urinalysis; 4) Serum creatinine, CBC, particularly in chronic renal failure

Dosage Forms/Preparations/FDA Approval Status/Withholding Times -
  Veterinary-Approved Products: None
  Human-Approved Products:

Potassium Citrate Tablets 5 mEq, 10 mEq; *Uracit-K®* (Mission); (Rx)

Potassium Citrate Monohydrate 1110 mg/5 ml & Citric Acid Monohydrate 334 mg/5 ml; *Polycitra®-K Syrup* (Baker Norton); (Rx)

Sodium Citrate Dihydrate 490 mg/5 ml and Citric Acid Monohydrate 640 mg/5 ml; *Oracit®* (Carolina Medical); (Rx)

Sodium Citrate Dihydrate 500 mg/5 ml and Citric Acid Monohydrate 334 mg/5 ml; *Bicitra®* (sugar free) (Baker Norton); (Rx)

Citric Acid monohydrate 334 mg/5 ml, Potassium Citrate monohydrate 550 mg/5 ml and sodium citrate dihydrate 500 mg/5 ml; *Polycitra® Syrup, Polycitra®-LC Syrup* (sugar free) (Baker Norton); (Rx)

Clavulanate/Amoxicillin — See Amoxicillin/Clavulanate

Clavulanate/Ticarcillin — See Ticarcillin /Clavulanate

CLEMASTINE FUMARATE

Chemistry - Also known as meclastine fumarate or mecloprodin fumarate, clemastine fumarate is an ethanolamine antihistamine. It occurs as an odorless, faintly yellow, crystalline powder. It is very slightly soluble in water and sparingly soluble in alcohol.

Tavist-D® contains clemastine fumarate in an immediate release outer shell and phenylpropanolamine HCl in a sustained release inner matrix.

Storage/Stability/Compatibility - Oral tablets and solution should be stored in tight, light resistant containers at room temperature.

Pharmacology - Like other H_1-receptor antihistamines, clemastine acts by competing with histamine for sites on H_1-receptor sites on effector cells. They do not block histamine release, but can antagonize its effects. Clemastine has greater anticholinergic activity, but less sedation than average.

Uses/Indications - Clemastine may be used for symptomatic relief of histamine$_1$-related allergic conditions.

Pharmacokinetics - In humans, clemastine is almost completely absorbed from the GI tract; its distribution is not well characterized, but does distribute into milk. Metabolic fate has not been clearly determined, but it appears to be extensively metabolized and those metabolites are eliminated in the urine. In humans, its duration of action is about 12 hours.

Contraindications/Precautions/Reproductive Safety - Clemastine is contraindicated in patients hypersensitive to it. It should be used with caution in patients with prostatic hypertrophy, bladder neck obstruction, severe cardiac failure, angle-closure glaucoma, or pyeloduodenal obstruction.

Clemastine has been tested in pregnant lab animals in doses up to 312 times labeled without evidence of harm to fetuses. But, because safety has not been established in other species, its use during pregnancy should be weighed carefully. Clemastine enters maternal milk and may potentially cause adverse effects in offspring.

Adverse Effects/Warnings - The most likely adverse effects seen with clemastine are related to its CNS depressant (sedation) and anticholinergic effects (dryness of mucous membranes, etc.).

Overdosage/Acute Toxicity - There are no specific antidotes available. Significant overdoses should be handled using standard gut emptying protocols when appropriate, and supportive therapy initiated when required. The adverse effects seen with overdoses are an extension of the drug's side effects; principally CNS depression (although CNS stimulation may be seen), anticholinergic effects (severe drying of mucous membranes, tachycardia, urinary retention, hyperthermia, etc.) and possibly hypotension. Physostigmine may be considered to treat serious CNS anticholinergic effects and diazepam employed to treat seizures, if necessary.

Drug Interactions - Additive CNS depression may be seen if combining clemastine with other **CNS depressant medications**, such as barbiturates, tranquilizers, etc. **Monoamine oxidase inhibitors** (including **furazolidone**) may intensify the anticholinergic effects of clemastine.

Laboratory Considerations - Because antihistamines can decrease the wheal and flair response to **skin allergen testing**, antihistamines should be discontinued 3 -7 days (depending on the antihistamine used and the reference) before intradermal skin tests.

Doses -
  Dogs:
    As an antihistamine:
      a)   0.5 - 1.5 mg per dog q12h (Paradis and Scott 1992)
      b)   0.05 mg/kg PO q12h (Papich 1992), (White 1994)

Monitoring Parameters - 1) Efficacy; 2) Adverse Effects, if any

Client Information - Clients should understand that antihistamines may be useful for symptomatic relief of allergic symptoms, but are not a cure for the underlying disease.

Dosage Forms/Preparations/FDA Approval Status/Withholding Times -
  Veterinary-Approved Products: None
  Human-Approved Products:
    Clemastine Fumarate Oral Tablets 1.34 mg, 2.68 mg; Oral Solution 0.67 mg/5 ml; *Tavist*® (Sandoz) (Rx), *Antihist-1*® (Various) (OTC);*Tavist-1* ® (Sandoz) (OTC); generic; (Rx)

CLENBUTEROL HCL

Chemistry, Storage/Stability - A beta-2-adrenergic agonist, clenbuterol HCl's chemical name is 1-(4-Amino-3,5-dichlorophenyl)-2-tert-butyl aminoethanol HCl. The commercially available syrup is colorless and should be stored at room temperature (avoid freezing). The manufacturer warns to replace the safety cap on the bottle when not in use.

Pharmacology - Like other beta-2 agonists, clenbuterol is believed to act by stimulating production of cyclic AMP through the activation of adenyl cyclase. By definition, Beta-2 agonists have more smooth muscle relaxation activity (bronchial, vascular and uterine smooth muscle) versus its cardiac effects (Beta 1).

Uses/Indications - Clenbuterol is approved for use in horses as a bronchodilator in the management of airway obstruction, such as chronic obstructive pulmonary disease (COPD).
It has been used as a partitioning agent in food producing animals, but its use for this purpose is banned in the USA as relay toxicity in humans has been documented.

Pharmacokinetics - After oral administration to horses, peak plasma levels of clenbuterol occur 2 hours after administration and the average half life is about 10 hours. The manufacturer states that the duration of effect varies from 6-8 hours.

Contraindications/Precautions/Reproductive Safety - The drug is contraindicated in food producing animals (legal ramifications). It should not be used in pregnant mares near full term as it antagonizes the effects of dinoprost (prostaglandin F$_2$alpha) and oxytocin and can diminish normal uterine contractility. The label states that the drug should not be used in horses suspected of having cardiovascular impairment as tachycardia may occur.

Clenbuterol's safety in breeding stallions and brood mares has not been established.

Adverse Effects/Warnings - Muscle tremors, sweating, restlessness, urticaria and tachycardia may be noted, particularly early in the course of therapy. Creatine kinase elevations have been noted in some horses and rarely ataxia can occur.

Clenbuterol has been touted in some body building circles as an alternative to anabolic steroids for muscle development and body fat reduction, however its safe use for this purpose is in serious question. Be alert for scams to divert legitimately obtained clenbuterol for this purpose.

Overdosage - Some case reports of clenbuterol overdoses have been reported in various species. Depending on dosage and species, emptying gut may be appropriate; otherwise supportive therapy and administration of parenteral beta blockers to control heart rate and rhythm, and elevated blood pressure may be considered.

Drug Interactions - Concomitant administration with **other sympathomimetic amines** (e.g., terbutaline) may enhance the adverse effects of clenbuterol. **Beta blockers** (e.g. propranolol) may antagonize clenbuterol's effects. **Tricyclic antidepressants or monoamine oxidase inhibitors** may potentiate the vascular effects of clenbuterol. Use with inhalation anesthetics (*e.g.*, **halothane, isoflurane, methoxyflurane**), may predispose the patient to ventricular arrhythmias, particularly in patients with preexisting cardiac disease—use cautiously. Use with **digitalis** glycosides may increase the risk of cardiac arrhythmias.

Clenbuterol may antagonize the effects of **dinoprost** (prostaglandin F$_2$alpha) and **oxytocin**.

Doses -

  Horses:

    As a bronchodilator:

      Initially, 0.8 micrograms/kg (practically: 0.5 ml of the commercially available syrup/100 lb. BW) twice daily for 3 days; if no improvement increase to 1.6 micrograms/kg (practically: 1 ml of the commercially available syrup/100 lb. BW) twice daily for 3 days; if no improvement increase to 2.4 micrograms/kg (practically: 1.5 ml of the commercially available syrup/100 lb. BW) twice daily for 3 days; if no improvement increase to 3.2 micrograms/kg (practically: 2 ml of the commercially available syrup/100 lb. BW) twice daily for 3 days; if no improvement discontinue therapy. Recommended duration of therapy is 30 days; then withdraw therapy and reevaluate. If signs return, reinitiate therapy as above. (Package Insert; Ventipulmin®)

Monitoring Parameters - 1) Clinical efficacy; 2) Adverse effects (primarily cardiac rate)

Client Information - Clients should be instructed on the restricted use requirements of this medication and to keep it secure from children or those who may "abuse" it. The drug may prohibited from use by various equine associations (*e.g.*, racing or show).

Dosage Forms/Preparations/FDA Approval Status -

  Veterinary-Approved Products:

    Clenbuterol HCl Oral Syrup 72.5 mcg/ml in 100 ml and 330 ml bottles; *Ventipulmin® Syrup* (Boehringer Ingelheim Vetmedica); (Rx). Approved for use in horses not intended for use as food. Extralabel clenbuterol use is prohibited by federal (USA) law.

  Human-Approved Products: None

Clindamycin HCl
Clindamycin Palmitate HCl
Clindamycin Phosphate

Chemistry - A semisynthetic derivative of lincomycin, clindamycin is available as the hydrochloride hydrate, phosphate ester, and palmitate hydrochloride. Potency of all three salts are expressed as milligrams of clindamycin. The hydrochloride occurs as a white to practically white, crystalline powder. The phosphate occurs as a white to off-white, hygroscopic crystalline powder. The palmitate HCl occurs as a white to off-white amorphous powder. All may have a faint characteristic odor and are freely soluble in water. With the phosphate, about 400 mg are soluble in one ml of water. Clindamycin has a pK$_a$ of 7.45. The commercially available injection has a pH of 5.5-7.

Storage/Stability/Compatibility - Clindamycin capsules and the palmitate powder for oral solution should be stored at room temperature (15-30°C). After reconstitution, the palmitate oral solution (human-product) should not be refrigerated or thickening may occur. It is stable for 2 weeks at room temperature. The veterinary oral solution should be stored at room temperature and has an extended shelf-life.

Clindamycin phosphate injection should be stored at room temperature. If refrigerated or frozen, crystals may form which resolubolize upon warming.

Clindamycin for injection is reportedly **compatible** for at least 24 hours in the following IV infusion solutions: D5W, Dextrose combinations with Ringer's, lactated Ringer's, sodium chloride, D10W, sodium chloride 0.9%, Ringer's injection, and lactated Ringer's injection. Clindamycin for injection is reportedly **compatible** with the following drugs: amikacin sulfate, ampicillin sodium, aztreonam, carbenicillin disodium, cefamandole naftate, cefazolin sodium, cefonicid sodium, cefoperazone sodium, cefotaxime sodium, ceftazidime sodium, ceftizoxime sodium, cefuroxime sodium, cephalothin sodium, cimetidine HCl, gentamicin sulfate, heparin sodium, hydrocortisone sodium succinate, kanamycin sulfate, methylprednisolone sodium succinate, magnesium sulfate, meperidine HCl, metoclopramide HCl, metronidazole, morphine sulfate, penicillin G potassium/sodium, piperacillin sodium, potassium chloride, sodium bicarbonate, tobramycin HCl (not in syringes), verapamil HCl, and vitamin B-complex with C.

Drugs are reportedly **incompatible** with clindamycin include: aminophylline, ranitidine HCl, and ceftriaxone sodium. Compatibility is dependent upon factors such as pH, concentration, temperature and diluents used. It is suggested to consult specialized references for more specific information (*e.g., Handbook on Injectable Drugs* by Trissel; see bibliography).

Pharmacology - The lincosamide antibiotics, lincomycin and clindamycin, share mechanisms of action and have similar spectrums of activity, although lincomycin is usually less active against susceptible organisms. Complete cross-resistance occurs between the two drugs, and at least partial cross-resistance occurs between the lincosamides and erythromycin. They may act as bacteriostatic or bactericidal agents, depending on the concentration of the drug at the infection site, and the susceptibility of the organism. The lincosamides are believed to act by binding to the 50S ribosomal subunit of susceptible bacteria, thereby inhibiting peptide bond formation.

Most aerobic gram positive cocci are susceptible to the lincosamides (*Strep. faecalis* is not) including staphylococci, and streptococci. Other organisms that are generally susceptible include: *Corynebacterium diphtheriae, Nocardia asteroides, Erysepelothrix, Toxoplasma,* and *Mycoplasma sp.* Anaerobic bacteria that are generally susceptible to the lincosamides include: *Clostridium perfringens, C. tetani* (not *C. difficile*), *Bacteroides* (including many strains of *B. fragilis*), *Fusobacterium, Peptostreptococcus, Actinomyces,* and *Peptococcus.*

Uses/Indications - Clindamycin products are approved for use in dogs and humans. The labeled indications for dogs include wounds, abscesses and osteomyelitis caused by *Staphylococcus aureus.* Because clindamycin also has excellent activity against most pathogenic anaerobic organisms, it is also used extensively for those infections. For further information refer to the Dosage or Pharmacology sections.

Pharmacokinetics - The pharmacokinetics of clindamycin have apparently not been extensively studied in veterinary species. Unless otherwise noted, the following information applies to humans. The drug is rapidly absorbed from the gut and about 90% of the total dose is absorbed. Food decreases the rate of absorption, but not the extent. Peak serum levels are attained about 45-60 minutes after oral dosing. IM administration gives peak levels about 1-3 hours post injection.

Clindamycin is distributed into most tissues. Therapeutic levels are achieved in bone, synovial fluid, bile, pleural fluid, peritoneal fluid, skin and heart muscle. Clindamycin also penetrates well into abscesses and white blood cells. CNS levels may reach 40% of those in the serum if meninges are inflamed. Clindamycin is about 93% bound to plasma proteins. The drug crosses the placenta and also can be distributed into milk at concentrations equal to those in the plasma.

Clindamycin is partially metabolized in the liver to both active and inactive metabolites. Unchanged drug and metabolites are excreted in the urine, feces and bile. Half-lives can be prolonged in patients with severe renal or hepatic dysfunction. The elimination half-life of clindamycin in dogs is reportedly 3-5 hours after oral administration and 10-13 hours after subcutaneous administration.

Contraindications/Precautions/Reproductive Safety - Although there have been case reports of parenteral administration of lincosamides to horses, cattle and sheep, the lincosamides are considered to be contraindicated for use in rabbits, hamsters, guinea pigs, horses, and ruminants because of serious gastrointestinal effects that may occur, including death. Clindamycin is contraindicated in patients with known hypersensitivity to it or lincomycin.

The manufacturer recommends using the drug with caution in atopic animals. Patients with very severe renal and/or hepatic disease should receive the drug with caution and the manufacturer suggests monitoring serum clindamycin levels during high-dose therapy in these patients.

Clindamycin crosses the placenta, and cord blood concentrations are approximately 46% of those found in maternal serum. Safe use during pregnancy has not been established, but neither has the drug been implicated in causing teratogenic effects.

Because clindamycin is distributed into milk, nursing puppies or kittens of mothers taking clindamycin may develop diarrheas.

Adverse Effects/Warnings - Adverse effects reported in dogs and cats include gastroenteritis (emesis, loose stools, and infrequently bloody diarrhea in dogs). IM injections reportedly cause pain at the injection site.

Overdosage/Acute Toxicity - There is little information available regarding overdoses of this drug. In dogs, oral doses of up to 300 mg/kg/day for up to one year did not result in toxicity. Dogs receiving 600 mg/kg/day developed anorexia, vomiting and they lost weight.

Drug Interactions - Clindamycin possesses intrinsic neuromuscular blocking activity and should be used cautiously with other **neuromuscular blocking agents**.

Erythromycin and clindamycin have shown antagonism *in vitro*. **Chloramphenicol** and clindamycin may also be antagonistic, but this has not been confirmed.

Unlike lincomycin, clindamycin absorption does not appear to be significantly altered by kaolin.

Drug/Laboratory Interactions - Slight increases in **liver function tests** (AST, ALT, Alk. Phosph.) may occur. There is apparently not any clinical significance associated with these increases.

Doses -
  Dogs:
    For susceptible infections:
      a) 5.5 - 11 mg/kg PO q12h; 11 -16.5 mg/kg SQ q24h (Aronson and Aucoin 1989)
      b) 5 - 11 mg/kg IM, SubQ or PO q12h avoid or reduce dose in patients with severe liver failure (Vaden and Papich 1995)
      c) 10 mg/kg PO or IM q12h (Ford and Aronson 1985)
      d) 5 - 10 mg/kg PO q12h (Jenkins 1987b)
    For treatment of toxoplasmosis:
      a) 10 - 40 mg/kg/day PO divided *tid-qid*. (Murtaugh 1988)
  Cats:
    For susceptible infections:
      a) 5.5 - 11 mg/kg PO q12h; 11 -16.5 mg/kg SQ q24h (Aronson and Aucoin 1989)
      b) 5 - 11 mg/kg SubQ or PO q12h (Vaden and Papich 1995)
      c) 10 mg/kg PO or IM q12h (Ford and Aronson 1985)
      d) 5 - 10 mg/kg PO q12h (Jenkins 1987b)
    For treatment of toxoplasmosis:
      a) 25 mg/kg PO divided into 2-3 doses per day for 4 weeks (Lappin 1995)

Monitoring Parameters -
  1) Clinical efficacy
  2) Adverse effects; particularly severe diarrheas
  3) Manufacturer recommends doing periodic liver and kidney function tests and blood counts if therapy persists for more than 30 days.

Client Information - Clients should be instructed to report the incidence of severe, protracted or bloody diarrhea to the veterinarian.

Dosage Forms/Preparations/FDA Approval Status/Withholding Times -
Veterinary-Approved Products:
  Clindamycin (as the HCl) Oral Capsules 25 mg, 75 mg, 150 mg
    Antirobe® (Upjohn); (Rx) Approved for use in dogs.
  Clindamycin (as the HCl) Oral Solution 25 mg/ml in 20 ml bottles
    Antirobe® Aquadrops (Upjohn); Generic; (Rx) Approved for use in dogs.
Human-Approved Products:
  Clindamycin (as the HCl) Oral Capsules 75 mg, 150 mg, 300 mg
    Cleocin® (Upjohn); generic (Rx)
  Clindamycin (as the palmitate HCl) Granules for oral solution 75 mg/5 ml (15 mg/ml) (as palmitate) in 100 ml bottles; *Cleocin® Pediatric* (Upjohn); (Rx)
  Clindamycin (as the Phosphate) Injection 150 mg/ml in 2, 4, 6, and 60 ml vials 4, 6 ml ADD-Vantage vials, 50 ml Galaxy plastic containers and 60 ml pharmacy bulk packages; *Cleocin® Phosphate* (Upjohn); (Rx); generic (Rx)
  Also available in topical and vaginal preparations.

CLIOQUINOL

Chemistry - Also known as iodochlorhydroxyquin, clioquinol possesses antibacterial, antifungal and amoebicidal activity. It occurs as a tasteless, voluminous, yellowish white to brownish yellow powder that has a slight characteristic odor. The drug is practically insoluble in water and alcohol.

Storage/Stability/Compatibility - Unless otherwise directed, store clioquinol boluses at room temperature and protect from light.

Pharmacology - Information on the mechanism of action of clioquinol was not located, but its action is probably due to its iodine content. It is reportedly active against some cocci, *E. coli*, yeasts, and some protozoal parasites, particularly *Trichomonas sp.*.

Uses/Indications - Clioquinol boluses are approved for oral use in horses to treat diarrheas that have failed to respond to regular forms of treatment, particularly if caused by some protozoal organisms. Clioquinol was once used orally in humans to treat diarrhea, but severe neurotoxic reactions have eliminated its use in humans, except as a topical antifungal.

Pharmacokinetics - The drug is only minimally absorbed after oral administration in horses. No other information was noted.

Contraindications/Precautions/Reproductive Safety - Not to be used in horses intended for food. No other information located.

Adverse Effects/Warnings - The manufacturer does not list any adverse effects for this product when used orally in horses. In humans, subacute myelo-opticoneuropathy was seen in many patients taking the drug orally for prolonged periods of time. It is unknown if the drug causes neurotoxic effects in horses. Topical administration for 28 days of the 3% topical preparation has caused toxicity in dogs.

Overdosage/Acute Toxicity - No specific information located regarding overdosage in horses. Iodism or potentially neurotoxic reactions (see Adverse effects above) could result.

Drug Interactions; **Drug/Laboratory Interactions** - None located, but the iodine component of the drug may affect some thyroid function tests.

Doses -
  Horses:
    For chronic diarrhea in horses:
      a) 1 bolus (10 g) for a 1000 lb horse PO daily until feces become formed. Then reduce dose and give daily or reduce dose and give on alternate days or even less frequently.
         (Package insert; *Rheaform*® *Boluses*—Solvay)

Monitoring Parameters -
  1) Clinical efficacy
  2) Occasional neurological evaluations recommended with prolonged therapy

Dosage Forms/Preparations/FDA Approval Status/Withholding Times -
Veterinary-Approved Products: Note: Current marketing status is unknown.
  Clioquinol Oral Boluses 10 g; *Rheaform*® *Boluses* (Fort Dodge); (Rx) Approved for use in horses.

  Human-Approved Products: No systemic products approved in the United States. Topical formulations are available.

CLOMIPRAMINE HCL

Chemistry - A dibenzazepine-derivative tricyclic antidepressant, clomipramine HCl occurs as a white to off-white crystalline powder and is freely soluble in water.

Storage/Stability/Compatibility - The commercially available capsules should be stored at temperatures less than 30°C in tight containers and protected from moisture. An expiration date of 3 years from the date of manufacture is assigned to the commercially available capsules.

Pharmacology - While the exact mechanism of action of tricyclic antidepressants is not fully understood, it is believed that their most significant effects result from their action in preventing the reuptake of norepinephrine and serotonin at the neuronal membrane. Clomipramine is apparently a selective inhibitor of serotonin (5-HT) reuptake.

Uses/Indications - In veterinary medicine, clomipramine is used primarily in dogs as a treatment for obsessive compulsive disorders (ritualistic stereotypical behaviors) and may also be useful for dominance aggression and anxiety (separation).

Clomipramine may also be useful in cats, but cats tend to be more sensitive to tricyclics antidepressant drugs and the commercially available dosage forms preclude convenient dosing in this species.

Pharmacokinetics - While no dog or cat pharmacokinetic data was located, in humans the drug is well absorbed from the GI tract, but a substantial first pass effect reduces its systemic bioavailability to approximately 50%. The presence of food in the gut apparently does not significantly alter its absorption.

Clomipramine is highly lipophilic and widely distributed throughout the body with an apparent volume of distribution of 17 L/kg. The drug crosses the placenta and into maternal milk. Plasma levels have been detected in nursing babies of mothers taking the drug. Both clomipramine and its active metabolite (desmethylclomipramine) cross the blood-brain barrier and significant levels are found in the brain. It should be noted that although therapeutic effects may take several weeks to be seen, adverse effects may occur early on in treatment.

Clomipramine is metabolized principally in the liver to several metabolites including desmethylclomipramine, which is active. About two-thirds of these metabolites are eliminated in the urine and the rest in the feces. After a single dose, the elimination half life of clomipramine averages 32 hours and desmethylclomipramine averages 69 hours, but there is wide interpatient variation.

Contraindications/Precautions/Reproductive Safety - These agents are contraindicated if prior sensitivity has been noted with any other tricyclic. Concomitant use with monoamine oxidase inhibitors is generally contraindicated.

In humans, these drugs (tricyclic antidepressants) may lower seizure threshold. Use with caution in animals with preexisting seizure disorders. Because of their anticholinergic effects use with caution in patients with decreased GI motility, urinary retention, cardiac rhythm disturbances or increased intraocular pressure. In humans tricyclic antidepressants have caused hepatic abnormalities. Baseline and annual monitoring of liver enzymes is suggested for animals receiving clomipramine long term. Tricyclics should be used cautiously in patients with hyperthyroidism or those that are receiving thyroid supplementation as there may be an increased risk of cardiac rhythm abnormalities developing.

No teratogenic effects were noted in mice and rats given clomipramine at dosages of up 20X usual maximum human dosage. Data in other domestic species appear to be lacking.

Adverse Effects/Warnings - The primary adverse effects reported thus far with the use of clomipramine in dogs is sedation and some anticholinergic (dry mouth etc.) effects. Cardiac effects such as tachycardia secondary to the drugs anticholinergic activity may also result.

Cats have been reported to be more susceptible to the adverse effects of clomipramine than are dogs.

Overdosage - Overdosage with tricyclics can be life-threatening (arrhythmias, cardiorespiratory collapse). Because the toxicities and therapies for treatment are complicated and controversial, it is recommended to contact a poison control center for further information in any potential overdose situation.

Drug Interactions - Because of additive effects, use clomipramine cautiously with other agents with **anticholinergic** or **CNS depressant** effects. Tricyclic antidepressants used with **antithyroid** agents may increase the potential risk of agranulocytosis. **Cimetidine** may inhibit tricyclic antidepressant metabolism and increase the risk of toxicity. Use in combination with **sympathomimetic agents** may increase the risk of cardiac effects (arrhythmias, hypertension, hyperpyrexia). Concomitant use with **monoamine oxidase inhibitors** (including selegiline/deprenyl) is generally contraindicated.

Laboratory Considerations - Tricyclics can widen QRS complexes, prolong PR intervals and invert or flatten T-waves on **ECG**. The response to **metapyrone** may be decreased by clomipramine. Tricyclics may alter (increase or decrease) **blood glucose** levels.

Doses -

Dogs:
a) For treatment of male dimorphic behaviors (urine marking, mounting, roaming, intermale aggression); fearful/fear aggression behaviors; noise phobias; obsessive/compulsive behaviors (self-mutilation, excessive grooming, stereotypies): 1 mg/kg PO every 12 hours for 2 weeks; then 2 mg/kg PO q12h for 2 weeks, then 3 mg/kg PO q12h for 4 weeks and maintain. May take 4-6 weeks to see apparent improvement. (Overall 1997)
b) 1 - 3 mg/kg once daily; may take 2-3 weeks to see effect (Line 1998)

Cats:
a) For urine marking/spraying; inter-cat aggression related to social hierarchy± redirected aggression; compulsive grooming/wool sucking: 0.5 mg/kg once daily PO (Overall 1997)

Monitoring Parameters - 1) Clinical efficacy; 2) Adverse Effects: Baseline liver function tests; EKG

Dosage Forms/Preparations/FDA Approval Status -
  Veterinary-Approved Products: None
  Human-Approved Products:
    Clomipramine Oral Capsules 25 mg, 50 mg, 75 mg; *Anafranil*®(Ciba); Generic (Rx)

CLONAZEPAM

Chemistry - A benzodiazepine anticonvulsant, clonazepam occurs as an off-white to light yellow, crystalline powder having a faint odor. It is insoluble in water and slightly soluble in alcohol.

Storage/Stability/Compatibility - Tablets should be stored in air-tight, light resistant containers at room temperature. After manufacture, a 5 year expiration date is assigned.

Pharmacology - The subcortical levels (primarily limbic, thalamic, and hypothalamic) of the CNS are depressed by diazepam and other benzodiazepines thus producing the anxiolytic, sedative, skeletal muscle relaxant, and anticonvulsant effects seen. The exact mechanism of action is unknown, but postulated mechanisms include: antagonism of serotonin, increased release of and/or facilitation of gamma-aminobutyric acid (GABA) activity and diminished release or turnover of acetylcholine in the CNS. Benzodiazepine specific receptors have been located in the mammalian brain, kidney, liver, lung and heart. In all species studied, receptors are lacking in the white matter.

Uses/Indications - Clonazepam is used primarily as an adjunctive anticonvulsant in dogs not controlled with other more standard therapies. Like diazepam, it may also be useful in the treatment of status epilepticus.

Pharmacokinetics - In humans, the drug is well absorbed from the GI tract; crosses the blood-brain barrier and placenta; is metabolized in the liver to several metabolites that are excreted in the urine. Peak serum levels occur about 3 hours after oral dosing. Half-lives range from 19-40 hours.

Contraindications/Precautions/Reproductive Safety - Clonazepam is contraindicated in patients who are hypersensitive to it or other benzodiazepines, have significant liver dysfunction or have acute narrow angle glaucoma. Benzodiazepines have been reported to exacerbate myasthenia gravis.

  Safe use during pregnancy has not been established; adverse effects have been seen in rabbits and rats. It is not known if the drug enters maternal milk, however several other benzodiazepines have been documented to enter maternal milk.

Adverse Effects/Warnings - There is very limited information on the adverse effect profile of this drug in domestic animals. Sedation (or excitement) and ataxia may occur. Clonazepam has been reported to cause a multitude of various adverse effects in humans. Some of the more significant ones include increased salivation, hypersecretion in upper respiratory passages, GI effects (vomiting, constipation, diarrhea, etc.), transient elevations of liver enzymes, hematologic effects (anemia, leukopenia, thrombocytopenia, etc.). Tolerance (usually noted after 3 months of therapy) to the anticonvulsant effects has been reported in dogs.

  Patients discontinuing clonazepam, particularly those who have been on the drug chronically at high dosages, should be tapered off or status epilepticus may be precipitated. Vomiting and diarrhea may occur during this process.

Overdosage/Acute Toxicity - When used alone, clonazepam overdoses are generally limited to significant CNS depression (confusion, coma, decreased reflexes, etc). Treatment of significant oral overdoses consists of standard protocols for removing and/or binding the drug in the gut and supportive systemic measures. The use of analeptic agents (CNS stimulants such as caffeine, amphetamines, etc.) are generally not recommended.

Drug Interactions - If administered with other **CNS depressant agents (barbiturates, narcotics, anesthetics**, etc.) additive effects may occur. If used with phenytoin, increased serum phenytoin levels and decreased clonazepam levels may occur.

  Rifampin may induce hepatic microsomal enzymes and decrease the pharmacologic effects of benzodiazepines. **Cimetidine or Erythromycin** has been reported to decrease the metabolism of benzodiazepines.

Laboratory Considerations - Benzodiazepines may decrease the thyroidal uptake of I^{123} or I^{131}.

Doses -
 Dogs:
   As an adjunctive medication in the treatment of seizures:
     a) 0.5 mg/kg PO q8-12h (Papich 1992)
     b) 0.5 mg/kg q12h (Fenner 1994)
     c) 0.5 mg/kg PO *bid-tid*; may need to lower phenobarbital dose by 10-20%. (Neer 1994)

Monitoring Parameters - 1) Efficacy; 2) Adverse Effects. The therapeutic blood level has been reported as 0.015 - 0.07 micrograms/ml.

Client Information - A major factor in anticonvulsant therapy failure is lack of compliance with the prescribed therapy. Owners must be counseled on the importance of giving doses regularly.

Dosage Forms/Preparations/FDA Approval Status/Withholding Times -
 Veterinary-Approved Products: None
 Human-Approved Products:
   Clonazepam Oral Tablets 0.5 mg, 1 mg, 2 mg; *Klonopin*® (Roche) (Rx);*Clonazepam*® (Lemmon) (Rx)
   All clonazepam products are controlled drugs (C-IV).

Cloprostenol Sodium

Chemistry - A synthetic prostaglandin of the F class, cloprostenol sodium occurs as a white or almost white, amorphous, hygroscopic powder. It is freely soluble in water and alcohol. Potency of the commercially available product is expressed in terms of cloprostenol.

Storage/Stability/Compatibility - Cloprostenol sodium should be stored at room temperature (15-30°C); protect from light.

Pharmacology - Prostaglandin F_{2alpha} and its analogues cloprostenol and fluprostenol are powerful luteolytic agents. They cause rapid regression of the corpus luteum and arrest its secretory activity. These prostaglandins also have direct stimulating effect on uterine smooth muscle causing contraction and a relaxant effect on the cervix.
 In normally cycling animals, estrus will generally occur 2-5 days after treatment. In pregnant cattle treated between 10-150 days of gestation, abortion will usually occur 2-3 days after injection.

Uses/Indications - Cloprostenol (*Estrumate*®—Miles) is approved for use in beef or dairy cattle to induce luteolysis. It is recommended by the manufacturer for unobserved or undetected estrus in cows cycling normally, pyometra or chronic endometritis, expulsion of mummified fetus, luteal cysts, induced abortions after mismating and to schedule estrus and ovulation for controlled breeding.

Pharmacokinetics - No information was located on the pharmacokinetics of cloprostenol.

Contraindications/Precautions - Cloprostenol is contraindicated in pregnant animals when abortion or induced parturition is not desired.

Adverse Effects/Warnings - The manufacturer does not list any adverse effects for this product when used as labeled. If used after the 5th month of gestation, increased risk of dystocia and decreased efficacy occur.
 Do not administer IV.
 Women of child-bearing age, persons with asthma or other respiratory diseases should use extreme caution when handling cloprostenol as the drug may induce abortion or acute bronchoconstriction. Cloprostenol is readily absorbed through the skin and must be washed off immediately with soap and water.

Overdosage - The manufacturer states that at doses of 50 and 100 times those recommended, cattle may show symptoms of uneasiness, slight frothing and milk let-down.
 Overdoses of cloprostenol or other synthetic prostaglandin F_{2alpha} analogs in small animals reportedly can result in shock and death.

Drug Interactions - Other **oxytocic agents**' activity may be enhanced by cloprostenol.

Doses -
 Cattle:
   For treatment of pyometra:
     a) 500 micrograms IM (up to 97% efficacy) (McCormack 1986)
   For pyometra or chronic endometritis, mummified fetus (manual assistance may be required to remove from vagina), luteal cysts:
     a) 500 micrograms IM (Package Insert; *Estrumate*®—Miles/Mobay)

For unobserved or undetected estrus in cows with continued ovarian cyclicity an a mature corpus luteum:

    a) 500 micrograms IM; estrus should commence in 2-5 days at which time the animal may be inseminated. If estrus detection is not possible or practical animal may be inseminated twice at 72 and 96 hours post injection. (Package Insert; *Estrumate*®—Miles/Mobay)

For abortion, from one week after mating to approximately the 150th day of gestation:

    a) 500 micrograms IM; abortion generally takes place in 4-5 days after injection. (Package Insert; *Estrumate*®—Miles/Mobay)

For controlled breeding:

    a) Single injection method: Use only animals with mature corpus luteum. Examine rectally to determine corpus luteum maturity, anatomic normality, and lack of pregnancy. Give 500 micrograms cloprostenol IM. Estrus should occur in 2-5 days. Inseminate at usual time after detecting estrus, or inseminate once at 72 hours post injection, or twice at 72 and 96 hours post injection.

        Double injection method: Examine rectally to determine if animal is anatomically normal, not pregnant, and cycling normally. Give 500 micrograms IM. Repeat dose 11 days later. Estrus should occur in 2-5 days after second injection. Inseminate at usual time after detecting estrus, or inseminate once at 72 hours post second injection, or twice at 72 and 96 hours post second injection.

        Animals that come into estrus after first injection may be inseminated at the usual time after detecting estrus.

        Any controlled breeding program should be completed by either observing animals and re-inseminating or hand mating after returning to estrus, or turning in clean-up bull(s) five to seven days after the last injection of cloprostenol to cover any animals returning to estrus. (Package Insert; *Estrumate*®—Miles/Mobay)

Horses:

To cause abortion prior to the twelfth day of gestation:

    a) 100 micrograms IM, most effective day 7 or 8 post estrus. Mare will usually return to estrus within 5 days. (Lofstedt 1986)

Swine:

To induce parturition in sows:

    a) 175 micrograms IM; give 2 days or less before anticipated date of farrowing. Farrowing generally occurs in approximately 36 hours after injection. (Pugh 1982)

Sheep & Goats:

To induce parturition in does:

    a) 62.5 - 125 micrograms IM at 144 days of gestation in early morning. Deliveries will peak at 30-35 hours after injection. Maintain goat in usual surrounding and minimize outside disturbances. (Williams 1986)

Client Information - Cloprostenol should be used by individuals familiar with its use and precautions. Pregnant women, asthmatics or other persons with bronchial diseases should handle this product with extreme caution. Any accidental exposure to skin should be washed off immediately.

Dosage Forms/Preparations/FDA Approval Status/Withholding Times -

  Veterinary-Approved Products:

  Cloprostenol Sodium Injection Equiv. to 250 micrograms/ml cloprostenol in 10 ml or 20 ml vials; *Estrumate*® (Bayer); (Rx) Approved for use in beef and dairy cattle. No preslaughter withdrawal nor milk withdrawal is required; no specific tolerance for cloprostenol residues have been published.

  Human-Approved Products: None

CLORAZEPATE DIPOTASSIUM

Chemistry - A benzodiazepine anxiolytic, sedative-hypnotic and anticonvulsant, clorazepate dipotassium occurs as a light yellow, fine powder that is very soluble in water and slightly soluble in alcohol.

Storage/Stability/Compatibility - Capsules and tablets should be stored in tight, light resistant containers at room temperature. Clorazepate dipotassium is unstable in the presence of water. It has been recommended to keep the dessicant packets in with the original container of the capsules and tablets and to consider adding a dessicant packet to the prescription vial when dispensing large quantities of tablets or capsules to the client.

Pharmacology - The subcortical levels (primarily limbic, thalamic, and hypothalamic) of the CNS are depressed by clorazepate and other benzodiazepines thus producing the anxiolytic, sedative, skeletal muscle relaxant and anticonvulsant effects seen. The exact mechanism of action is unknown, but postulated mechanisms include: antagonism of serotonin, increased release of and/or facilitation of gamma-aminobutyric acid (GABA) activity and diminished release or turnover of acetylcholine in the CNS. Benzodiazepine specific receptors have been located in the mammalian brain, kidney, liver, lung and heart. In all species studied, receptors are lacking in the white matter.

Uses/Indications - Clorazepate has been used in dogs both as an adjunctive anticonvulsant (usually in conjunction with phenobarbital) and in the treatment of behavior disorders, primarily those that are anxiety or phobia-related. In dogs, clorazepate has been reported to be less prone to developing tolerance to its anticonvulsant effects than is clonazepam.

Pharmacokinetics - Clorazepate is one of the most rapidly absorbed oral benzodiazepines and, therefore, has a rapid onset of action. Peak serum levels generally occur within 1-2 hours. Clorazepate's distribution characteristics are not well described. Clorazepate is metabolized to desmethyldiazepam and other metabolites. Desmethyldiazepam is active and has a very long half life (in humans up to 100 hours). In dogs, the sustained release preparation apparently offers no pharmacokinetic advantage over the non-sustained preparations (Brown and Forrester 1989).

Contraindications/Precautions/Reproductive Safety - Clorazepate is contraindicated in patients who are hypersensitive to it or other benzodiazepines, have significant liver dysfunction or have acute narrow angle glaucoma. Benzodiazepines have been reported to exacerbate myasthenia gravis.

Safe use during pregnancy has not been established; teratogenic effects of similar benzodiazepines have been noted in rabbits and rats. It is not known if the drug enters maternal milk, however desmethyldiazepam (an active metabolite of clorazepate) and several other benzodiazepines have been documented to enter maternal milk.

Adverse Effects/Warnings - In dogs, the most likely adverse effects seen include sedation and ataxia. These effects apparently occur infrequently, are mild and usually transient. Many other adverse effects are potentially possible; see the clonazepam monograph for more information.

Use with caution in dogs displaying fear-induced aggression, as they actually provoke dogs to attack.

Overdosage/Acute Toxicity - When used alone, clorazepate overdoses are generally limited to significant CNS depression (confusion, coma, decreased reflexes, etc). Treatment of significant oral overdoses consists of standard protocols for removing and/or binding the drug in the gut and supportive systemic measures. The use of analeptic agents (CNS stimulants such as caffeine, amphetamines, etc) are generally not recommended.

Drug Interactions - If administered with other **CNS depressant agents (barbiturates, narcotics, anesthetics,** etc.) additive effects may occur. If used with phenytoin, increased serum phenytoin levels and decreased clorazepate levels may occur.

Rifampin may induce hepatic microsomal enzymes and decrease the pharmacologic effects of benzodiazepines. **Cimetidine or Erythromycin** has been reported to decrease the metabolism of benzodiazepines.

Antacids do not affect the degree of absorption of clorazepate, but may decrease the rate of conversion of clorazepate to desmethyldiazepam (active metabolite). It is unlikely this interaction is of clinical significance.

Laboratory Considerations - Benzodiazepines may decrease the thyroidal uptake of I^{123} or I^{131}. Clorazepate may increase serum alkaline phosphatase and serum cholesterol levels; clinical significance is unclear.

Doses -
  Dogs:
    As an adjunctive medication in the treatment of seizures:
      a) 2 mg/kg PO q12h (Papich 1992)
      b) 1 -2 mg/kg PO q12h (Fenner 1994)
      c) 0.5 mg/kg PO *bid-tid*; may need to lower phenobarbital dose by 10-20%. (Neer 1994)
    As adjunctive therapy for the treatment of fears and phobias:
      a) 11.25 - 22.5 mg per dog PO once to twice daily (recommends the sustained delivery - *"Tranxene®-SD"*) product. (Marder 1991)
      b) Using the sustained delivery product (*"Tranxene®-SD"*), initially give 22.5 mg for large dogs, 11.25 mg for medium dogs and 5.6 mg for small dogs PO; adjust dosage according dog's response. (Shull-Selcer and Stagg 1991)

Monitoring Parameters -1) Efficacy; 2) Adverse Effects

Client Information - A major factor in anticonvulsant therapy failure is lack of compliance with the prescribed therapy. Owners must be counseled on the importance of giving doses regularly.

Dosage Forms/Preparations/FDA Approval Status/Withholding Times -
   Veterinary-Approved Products: None
   Human-Approved Products:
      Note: All clorazepate products are controlled drugs (C-IV).
      Clorazepate dipotassium capsules 3.75 mg, 7.5 mg, 15 mg; generic; (Rx)

      Clorazepate dipotassium tablets sustained-release (single dose) 11.25 mg, 22.5 mg; *Tranxene-SD*® (Abbott); (Rx);*Tranxene-SD Half Strength*® (Abbott) (Rx)

      Clorazepate dipotassium tablets 3.75 mg, 7.5 mg, 11.25 mg, 15 mg, 22.5 mg; *Tranxene*® (Abbott),*Gen-Xene*®(Alra), generic; (Rx)

CLORSULON

Chemistry - A benzenesulfonamide, clorsulon has a chemical name of 4-amino-6-trichloroethenyl-1,3-benzenedisulfonamide.

Storage/Stability/Compatibility - Unless otherwise instructed by the manufacturer, clorsulon should be stored at room temperature (15-30°C).

Pharmacology - In susceptible flukes, clorsulon inhibits the glycolytic enzymes 3-phosphoglycerate kinase and phosphoglyceromutase, thereby blocking the Emden-Myerhof glycolytic pathway. The fluke is deprived of its main metabolic energy source and dies.

Uses/Indications - Clorsulon is approved for use in the treatment of immature and adult forms of *Fasciola hepatica* (Liver fluke) in cattle. It is not effective against immature flukes less than 8 weeks old. It also has activity against *Fasciola gigantica*. Although not approved, the drug has been used in practice in various other species (*e.g.,* sheep, llamas). It has activity against *F. magna* in sheep, but is not completely effective in eradicating the organism after a single dose, thereby severely limiting its clinical usefulness against this parasite. Clorsulon is also not effective against the rumen fluke (*Paramphistomum*).

Pharmacokinetics - After oral administration to cattle, the drug is absorbed rapidly with peak levels occurring in about 4 hours. Approximately 75% of the circulating drug is found in the plasma and 25% in erythrocytes. At 8-12 hours after administration, clorsulon levels peak in the fluke.

Contraindications/Precautions/Reproductive Safety - No milk withdrawal time has been determined, and the drug is labeled not to be used in female dairy cattle of breeding age.
   Clorsulon is considered to be safe to use in pregnant or breeding animals.

Adverse Effects/Warnings - When used as directed adverse effects are unlikely to occur with this agent.

Overdosage/Acute Toxicity - Clorsulon is very safe when administered orally to cattle or sheep. Doses of up to 400 mg/kg have not produced toxicity in sheep. A dose that is toxic in cattle has also not been determined.

Drug Interactions & Drug/Laboratory Interactions - None identified.

Doses -
   Cattle:
      For *Fasciola hepatica* infections:
         a) 7 mg/kg PO; deposit suspension over the back of the tongue. (Label directions; *Curatrem*®—MSD-AgVet)

   Sheep:
      For *Fasciola hepatica* infections:
         a) 7 mg/kg PO. (Roberson 1988a)

   Llamas:
      For *Fasciola hepatica* infections:
         a) 7 mg/kg PO. (Fowler 1989)

Monitoring Parameters -
   1) Clinical efficacy

Client Information - Shake well before using.

Dosage Forms/Preparations/FDA Approval Status/Withholding Times -
   Clorsulon 8.5% (85 mg/ml) Oral Drench in quarts or gallons; *Curatrem*® (Rhone Merieux); (OTC) Approved for use in beef and non-lactating dairy cattle. Slaughter withdrawal= 8 days.

CLOXACILLIN SODIUM
CLOXACILLIN BENZATHINE

For general information on the penicillins, including adverse effects, contraindications, overdosage, drug interactions and monitoring parameters, refer to the monograph: Penicillins, General Information.

Chemistry - An isoxazolyl-penicillin, cloxacillin sodium is a semisynthetic penicillinase-resistant penicillin. It is available commercially as the monohydrate sodium salt which occurs as an odorless, bitter-tasting, white, crystalline powder. It is freely soluble in water and soluble in alcohol and has a pK_a of 2.7. One mg of cloxacillin sodium contains not less than 825 micrograms of cloxacillin.

Cloxacillin sodium may also be known as sodium cloxacillin, chlorphenylmethyl isoxazolyl penicillin sodium or methylchlorophenyl isoxazolyl penicillin sodium.

Cloxacillin benzathine occurs as white or almost white powder that is slightly soluble in water and alcohol. A 1% (10 mg/ml) suspension has a pH from 3-6.5.

Storage/Stability/Compatibility - Cloxacillin sodium capsules and powder for oral solution should be stored at temperatures less than 40°C and preferably at room temperature (15-30°C). After reconstituting, refrigerate any remaining oral solution and discard after 14 days. If stored at room temperature, the oral solution is stable for 3 days.

Unless otherwise instructed by the manufacturer, cloxacillin benzathine mastitis syringes should be stored at temperatures less than 25°C in tight containers.

Pharmacology/Uses/Indications - Cloxacillin, dicloxacillin and oxacillin have nearly identical spectrums of activity and can be considered therapeutically equivalent when comparing *in vitro* activity. These penicillinase-resistant penicillins have a more narrow spectrum of activity than the natural penicillins. Their antimicrobial efficacy is aimed directly against penicillinase-producing strains of gram positive cocci, particularly *Staphylococcal* species. They are sometimes called anti-staphylococcal penicillins. There are documented strains of Staphylococcus that are resistant to these drugs (so-called methicillin-resistant *Staph*), but these strains have not as yet been a major problem in veterinary species. While this class of penicillins do have activity against some other gram positive and gram negative aerobes and anaerobes, other antibiotics (penicillins and otherwise) are usually better choices. The penicillinase-resistant penicillins are inactive against *Rickettsia*, mycobacteria, fungi, *Mycoplasma* and viruses.

The veterinary use of these agents has been primarily in the treatment of bone, skin, and other soft tissue infections in small animals when penicillinase-producing *Staphylococcus* species have been isolated, or in the treatment of mastitis with cloxacillin in dairy cattle.

Pharmacokinetics (specific) - Cloxacillin is only available in oral and intramammary dosage forms. Cloxacillin sodium is resistant to acid inactivation in the gut, but is only partially absorbed. The bioavailability after oral administration in humans has been reported to range from 37-60%, and if given with food, both the rate and extent of absorption is decreased.

The drug is distributed to the liver, kidneys, bone, bile, pleural fluid, synovial fluid and ascitic fluid. Only minimal amounts are distributed into the CSF, as with the other penicillins. In humans, approximately 90-95% of the drug is bound to plasma proteins.

Cloxacillin is partially metabolized to both active and inactive metabolites. These metabolites and the parent compound are rapidly excreted in the urine via both glomerular filtration and tubular secretion mechanisms. A small amount of the drug is also excreted in the feces via biliary elimination. The serum half-life in humans with normal renal function ranges from about 24-48 minutes. In dogs, 30 minutes has been reported as the elimination half-life.

Doses - Author's (Plumb) note: Injectable form is not available in the U.S.A.

  Dogs:
    For susceptible infections:
      a) 20 - 40 mg/kg PO q8h (Vaden and Papich 1995)
      b) 10 - 15 mg/kg q6h PO, IV, or IM (Greene 1984)
      c) For *Staph.* diskospondylitis or skin infections: 10 mg/kg PO *qid* (Morgan 1988)
      d) For *Staph.* osteomyelitis: 10 mg/kg PO q6h (Ford and Aronson 1985)
      e) For *Staph.* diskospondylitis: 10 mg/kg *qid* PO for 4-6 weeks (Kornegay 1986)

  Cats:
    For susceptible infections:
      a) 20 - 40 mg/kg PO or IM q6-8h (Papich 1988)
      b) 10 - 15 mg/kg q6h PO, IV, or IM (Greene 1984)
      c) For *Staph.* diskospondylitis or skin infections: 10 mg/kg PO *qid* (Morgan 1988)
      d) For *Staph.* osteomyelitis: 10 mg/kg PO q6h (Ford and Aronson 1985)
      e) 10 mg/kg PO, IM, or IV q6h (Kirk 1989)

Cattle:
>   For mastitis (treatment or prophylaxis) caused by susceptible organisms:
>   a)   Lactating cow (using lactating cow formula; *Dari-Clox®*): After milking out and dis-
>   infecting teat, instill contents of syringe; massage. Repeat q12h for 3 total doses.
>   Dry (non-lactating) cows (using dry cow formula; benzathine): After last milking (or
>   early in the dry period), instill contents of syringe and massage into each quarter.
>   (Package inserts; *Dari-Clox®*, *Orbenin-DC®*—Beecham; *Dri-Clox®*—Fort Dodge)

Client Information - Unless otherwise instructed by the veterinarian, this drug should be given
orally on an empty stomach, at least 1 hour before feeding or 2 hours after. Keep oral solution in
the refrigerator and discard any unused suspension after 14 days.

Dosage Forms/Preparations/FDA Approval Status/Withholding Times -
Veterinary-Approved Products:
>   Cloxacillin Benzathine 500 mg (of cloxacillin) in a peanut-oil gel; 10 ml syringe for intra-
>   mammary infusion
>   *Orbenin-DC®* (Pfizer), *Dry-Clox®* (Fort Dodge); (Rx) Approved for use in dairy cows
>   during the dry period (immediately after last milking or early in the dry period). Do not
>   use within 30 days prior to calving (28 days for *Orbenin-DC®*). Slaughter withdrawal =
>   30 days (28 days for *Orbenin-DC®*). A tolerance of 0.01 ppm has been established for
>   negligible residues in uncooked edible meat and milk from cattle.
>   Cloxacillin Sodium 200 mg (of cloxacillin) in vegetable oils; 10 ml syringe for intramammary
>   infusion
>   *Dari-Clox®* (Pfizer); (Rx) Approved for use in lactating dairy cows. Milk withdrawal = 48
>   hours; Slaughter withdrawal = 10 days.

Human-Approved Products:
>   Cloxacillin Sodium Capsules 250 mg, 500 mg; *Tegopen®* (Apothecon) (Rx),*Cloxapen®* (SK-
>   Beecham) (Rx), generic; (Rx)
>   Cloxacillin Sodium Powder for Oral Solution 125 mg/5 ml in 100 & 200 ml bottles;
>   *Tegopen®* (Apothecon) (Rx), generic; (Rx)

CODEINE PHOSPHATE

Chemistry - A phenanthrene-derivative opiate agonist, codeine is available as the base and three
separate salts. Codeine base is slightly soluble in water and freely soluble in alcohol. Codeine
phosphate occurs as fine, white, needle-like crystals or white, crystalline powder. It is freely soluble in water. Codeine sulfate's appearance is similar to codeine phosphate, but it is soluble in
water.

Storage/Stability/Compatibility - Codeine phosphate and sulfate tablets should be stored in
light-resistant, well-closed containers at room temperature. Codeine phosphate injection should
be stored at room temperature (avoid freezing) and protected from light. Do not use the injection
if it is discolored or contains a precipitate.

   Codeine phosphate injection is reportedly compatible with glycopyrrolate or hydroxyzine HCl.
It is reportedly incompatible with aminophylline, ammonium chloride, amobarbital sodium,
chlorothiazide sodium, heparin sodium, methicillin sodium, pentobarbital sodium, phenobarbital
sodium, phenytoin sodium, secobarbital sodium, sodium bicarbonate, sodium iodide, and
thiopental sodium.

Pharmacology - Codeine possesses activity similar to other opiate agonists. It is a good antitussive and a mild analgesic. It produces similar respiratory depression as does morphine at
equianalgesic dosages. For further information on opiate pharmacology, refer to: Opiate
Agonists, Pharmacology.

Uses/Indications - In small animal medicine, codeine is used principally as an oral analgesic
when salicylates are not effective and parenteral opiates are not warranted. It may also be useful
as an antitussive or as an antidiarrheal.

Pharmacokinetics - No information was located specifically for domestic animals. The following information is human data unless otherwise noted. After oral administration, codeine salts are
rapidly absorbed. It is about 2/3's as effective after oral administration when compared with parenteral administration. After oral dosing, onset of action is usually within 30 minutes and analgesic effects persist for 4-6 hours. Codeine is metabolized in the liver and then excreted into the
urine.

Contraindications/Precautions/Reproductive Safety - All opiates should be used with caution
in patients with hypothyroidism, severe renal insufficiency, adrenocortical insufficiency
(Addison's disease) and in geriatric or severely debilitated patients. Codeine is contraindicated in
cases where the patient is hypersensitive to narcotic analgesics, or in patients taking monamine

oxidase inhibitors (MAOIs). It is also contraindicated in patients with diarrhea caused by a toxic ingestion until the toxin is eliminated from the GI tract or when used repeatedly in patients with severe inflammatory bowel disease.

Codeine should be used with caution in patients with head injuries or increased intracranial pressure and acute abdominal conditions (*e.g.,* colic) as it may obscure the diagnosis or clinical course of these conditions. It should be used with extreme caution in patients suffering from respiratory disease or from acute respiratory dysfunction (*e.g.,* pulmonary edema secondary to smoke inhalation).

Opiate analgesics are also contraindicated in patients who have been stung by the scorpion species *Centruroides sculpturatus* Ewing and *C. gertschi* Stahnke as they may potentiate these venoms.

Do not use the combination product containing acetaminophen in cats.

Opiates cross the placenta. Very high doses in mice have caused delayed ossification. Use during pregnancy only when the benefits outweigh the risks, particularly with chronic use. Although codeine enters maternal milk, no documented problems have been associated with its use in nursing mothers.

Adverse Effects/Warnings - Codeine generally is well tolerated, but adverse effects are possible, particularly at higher dosages or with repeated use. Sedation is the most likely effect seen. Potential gastrointestinal effects include anorexia, vomiting, constipation, ileus, and biliary and pancreatic duct spasms. Respiratory depression is generally not noted unless the patient receives high doses or is at risk (see contraindications above).

In cats, opiates may also cause CNS stimulation with hyperexcitability, tremors and seizures possible.

Overdosage/Acute Toxicity - Opiate overdosage may produce profound respiratory and/or CNS depression in most species. Other effects can include cardiovascular collapse, hypothermia, and skeletal muscle hypotonia. Oral ingestions of codeine should be removed when possible using standard gut removal protocols. Because rapid changes in CNS status may occur, inducing vomiting should be attempted with caution. Naloxone is the agent of choice in treating respiratory depression. In massive overdoses, naloxone doses may need to be repeated and animals should be closely observed as naloxone's effects may diminish before subtoxic levels of codeine are attained. Mechanical respiratory support should also be considered in cases of severe respiratory depression. Serious overdoses involving any of the opiates should be closely monitored; it is suggested to contact an animal poison center for further information.

Drug Interactions - Other **CNS depressants** (*e.g.,* anesthetic agents, antihistamines, phenothiazines, barbiturates, tranquilizers, alcohol, etc.) may cause increased CNS or respiratory depression when used with meperidine. **Anticholinergic drugs** used with codeine may increase the chances of constipation developing.

In humans, meperidine (a compound related to codeine) is contraindicated in patients for at least 14 days after receiving **monamine oxidase (MOA) inhibitors** (rarely used in veterinary medicine). Some human patients have exhibited signs of opiate overdose after receiving therapeutic doses of meperidine while on these agents.

Laboratory Considerations - Plasma **amylase** and **lipase** values may be increased for up to 24 hours following administration of opiate analgesics as they may increase biliary tract pressure.

Doses -
  Dogs:
    As an antitussive:
      a) 0.1 - 0.3 mg/kg PO q6-8h (Papich 1992)
      b) 1 - 2 mg/kg PO q6-12h (Fenner 1994)
    As an analgesic:
      a) 0.5 - 1 mg/kg PO q6-8h (Papich 1992)
      b) In combination with acetaminophen: Using a 60 mg codeine and 300 mg acetaminophen fixed-dose tablet (*e.g., Tylenol*® *#4*), give 1 - 2 mg/kg (of the codeine) PO q6-8h. Using codeine alone: 1 - 4 mg/kg PO q1-6 hours (Hansen 1994)
    As an antidiarrheal:
      a) 0.25 - 0.5 mg/kg PO q6-8h (Sherding and Johnson 1994a)

Monitoring Parameters - 1) Efficacy; 2) Adverse Effects (see above)

Client Information - Keep out of reach of children. Have client monitor for efficacy and changes in mentition or GI effects.

Dosage Forms/Preparations/FDA Approval Status/Withholding Times -
  Veterinary-Approved Products: None

Human-Approved Products:
There are many products available containing codeine. The following is a partial listing:
Codeine Phosphate Oral Tablets 30 mg, 60 mg; generic (Rx) C-II
Codeine Sulfate Oral Tablets 15 mg, 30 mg, 60 mg; (Generic); (Rx) C-II
Codeine Phosphate Parenteral Injection 30 mg/ml, 60 mg/ml; generic. (Rx) C-II
Codeine Phosphate 7.5 mg (#1), 15 mg (#2), 30 mg (#3), 60 mg (#4) with Acetaminophen 300 mg tablets; *Tylenol® with Codeine #'s 1, 2, 3, 4* (McNeil), Generic; (Rx); C-III
Codeine Phosphate 15 mg (#2), 30 mg (#3), 60 mg (#4) with Aspirin 320 mg tablets; *Empirin with Codeine #'s 2, 3, 4* (Glaxo Wellcome), Generic; (Rx); C-III

Note: Codeine-only products are Class-II controlled substances. Combination products with aspirin or acetaminophen are Class-III. Codeine containing cough syrups are either Class-V or Class-III, depending on the state.

COLCHICINE

Chemistry - An antigout drug possessing many other pharmacologic effects, colchicine occurs as a pale yellow, amorphous powder or scales. It is soluble in water and freely soluble in alcohol.

Storage/Stability/Compatibility - Colchicine tablets should be stored in tight, light resistant containers. The injection should be diluted only in 0.9% sodium chloride for injection or sterile water for injection. Do not use D5W or bacteriostatic sodium chloride for injection as precipitation may occur. Do not use solutions that have become turbid.

Pharmacology; Uses/Indications - Colchicine is best known for its antigout activity in humans. The mechanism for this effect is not totally understood, but it probably is related to the drug's ability to reduce the inflammatory response to the disposition of monosodium urate crystals. Colchicine inhibits cell division during metaphase by interfering with sol-gel formation and the mitotic spindle.

In veterinary medicine, colchicine has been proposed as a treatment in small animals for amyloidosis. Colchicine apparently blocks the synthesis and secretion of serum amyloid A (SAA; an acute-phase reactant protein) by hepatocytes thereby preventing the formation of amyloid-enhancing factor and preventing amyloid disposition. For colchicine to be effective however, it must be given early in the course of the disease and it will be ineffective once renal failure has occurred.

Colchicine has also been proposed for treating chronic hepatic fibrosis presumably by decreasing the formation and increasing the breakdown of collagen.

Pharmacokinetics - No information was located specifically for domestic animals, the following information is human/lab animal data unless otherwise noted. After oral administration, colchicine is absorbed from the GI tract. Some of the absorbed drug is metabolized in the liver (first-pass effect). These metabolites and unchanged drug are re-secreted into the GI tract via biliary secretions where it is reabsorbed. This "recycling" phenomena may explain the intestinal manifestations noted with colchicine toxicity. Colchicine is distributed into several tissues, but is concentrated in leukocytes. Plasma half-life is about 20 minutes, but leukocyte half-life is approximately 60 hours. Colchicine is deacetylated in the liver and also metabolized in other tissues. While most of a dose (as colchicine and metabolites) is excreted in the feces, some is excreted in the urine. More may be excreted in the urine in patients with hepatic disease. Patients with severe renal disease may have prolonged half-lives.

Contraindications/Precautions/Reproductive Safety - Colchicine is contraindicated in patients with serious renal, GI, or cardiac dysfunction and should be used with caution in patients in early stages of these disorders. It should also be used with caution in geriatric or debilitated patients.

Because colchicine has been demonstrated to be teratogenic in laboratory animals (mice and hamsters) it should be used during pregnancy only when its potential benefits outweigh its risks. It is unknown if colchicine enters maternal milk; use cautiously in nursing mothers. Colchicine may decrease spermatogenesis.

Adverse Effects/Warnings - There has been very little experience with colchicine in domestic animals. There are reports that colchicine can cause nausea, vomiting and diarrhea in dogs. The following adverse effects have been noted in humans and may not accurately reflect its use in dogs or cats. GI effects have been noted (abdominal pain, anorexia, vomiting, diarrhea). Because these symptoms are an early sign of toxicity it is recommended to discontinue therapy should they occur. Prolonged administration has caused bone marrow depression. Severe local irritation has been noted if extravasation occurs after intravenous administration; thrombophlebitis has also been reported.

Overdosage/Acute Toxicity - Colchicine can be a very toxic drug after relatively small overdoses. Deaths in humans have been reported with a single oral ingestion of as little as 7 mg, but 65 mg is considered the lethal dose in an adult human. GI manifestations are usually the presenting symptoms seen. These can range from anorexia and vomiting to bloody diarrhea or paralytic ileus. Renal failure, hepatotoxicity, pancytopenia, paralysis, shock and vascular collapse may also occur.

There is no specific antidote to colchicine. Gut removal techniques should be employed when applicable. Because of the extensive GI "recycling" of the drug, repeated doses of activated charcoal and a saline cathartic may reduce systemic absorption. Other treatment is symptomatic and supportive. Dialysis (peritoneal) may be of benefit.

Drug Interactions - **Non-steroidal anti-inflammatory agents, especially phenylbutazone** may increase the risks of thrombocytopenia, leukopenia or bone marrow depression development when used concurrently with colchicine. Many **antineoplastics and other bone marrow depressant drugs (*e.g.*, chloramphenicol, flucytosine, amphotericin B)** may cause additive myelosuppression when used with colchicine. Colchicine may enhance the activity of **sympathomimetic agents and CNS depressants**; clinical significance is unknown.

Laboratory Considerations - Colchicine may cause false-positive results when testing for **erythrocytes or hemoglobin in urine**. Colchicine may interfere with **17-hydroxycorticosteroid** determinations in urine if using the Reddy, Jenkins, and Thorn procedure. Colchicine may cause increased serum values of **alkaline phosphatase**.

Doses -
Colchicine may have some efficacy in the treatment of amyloidosis, but veterinary dosages are apparently unavailable at this time.

Dogs:
For the adjunctive treatment of hepatic cirrhosis/fibrosis:
a) 0.025 - 0.03 mg/kg/day PO. Benefit is unproven. (Johnson and Sherding 1994)
b) 0.025 mg/kg PO per day; more evaluation on efficacy needed. (Rutgers 1994)
c) 0.03 mg/kg PO once daily (Leveille-Webster and Center 1995)

Monitoring Parameters - 1) Efficacy; 2) Adverse Effects (see above); 3) CBC

Client Information - Clients should be informed of the "investigational" nature of colchicine use in dogs and should be informed of the potential adverse effects that may be seen. They should report changes in appetite or other GI effects immediately.

Dosage Forms/Preparations/FDA Approval Status/Withholding Times -
Veterinary-Approved Products: None
Human-Approved Products:
Colchicine Tablets 0.5 mg, 0.6 mg; *Colchicine®* (Abbott) (Rx); Generic; (Rx)
Colchicine Injection 0.5 mg/ml in 2 ml amps; (Lilly); (Rx)

Co-Trimoxazole; Co-trimazine — See Sulfa/Trimethoprim

CORTICOTROPIN (ACTH)

Chemistry - A 39 amino acid polypeptide, corticotropin is secreted from the anterior pituitary. The first 24 amino acids (from the N-terminal end of the chain) define its biologic activity. While human, sheep, cattle and swine corticotropin have different structures, the first 24 amino acids are the same and, therefore, biologic activity is thought to be identical. Commercial sources of ACTH generally are obtained from porcine pituitaries. One USP unit of corticotropin is equivalent to 1 mg of the international standard.

Corticotropin is available commercially as corticotropin for injection, repository corticotropin for injection, and corticotropin zinc hydroxide suspension. Corticotropin is commonly called ACTH (abbreviated from adrenocorticotropic hormone). Repository corticotropin is often called ACTH gel and is the most commonly used ACTH product in veterinary medicine.

Storage/Stability/Compatibility - Corticotropin for injection (aqueous) can be stored at room temperature (15-30°C) before reconstitution. After reconstitution, it should be refrigerated and used within 24 hours. Repository corticotropin injection should be stored in the refrigerator (2-8°C). To allow ease in withdrawing the gel into a syringe, the vial may be warmed with warm water prior to use.

Pharmacology - ACTH stimulates the adrenal cortex (principally the zona fasiculata) to stimulate the production and release of glucocorticoids (primarily cortisol in mammals and corticosterone in birds). ACTH release is controlled by corticotropin-releasing factor (CRF) activated in the central nervous system and via a negative feedback pathway, whereby either endogenous or exogenous glucocorticoids suppresses ACTH release.

Uses/Indications - In veterinary medicine, an ACTH product (*Adrenomone®*—Summit Hill) is approved for use in dogs, cats, and beef or dairy cattle for stimulation of the adrenal cortex when there is a deficiency of ACTH, and as a therapeutic agent in primary bovine ketosis. In practice however, it tends to be used most often in the diagnosis of hyper- or hypoadrenocorticism (ACTH-stimulation test) and to monitor the response to mitotane therapy in Cushing's syndrome.

ACTH has been used for several purposes in human medicine for its corticosteroid stimulating properties, but as it must be injected, it is not commonly employed.

Pharmacokinetics - Because it is rapidly degraded by proteolytic enzymes in the gut, ACTH cannot be administered PO. It is not effective if administered topically to the skin or eye.

After IM injection in humans, repository corticotropin injection is absorbed over 8-16 hours. The elimination half-life of circulating ACTH is about 15 minutes, but because of the slow absorption after IM injection of the gel, effects may persist up to 24 hours.

Contraindications/Precautions - When used for diagnostic purposes, it is unlikely that increases in serum cortisol levels induced by ACTH will have significant deleterious effects on conditions where increased cortisol levels are contraindicated (*e.g.,* systemic fungal infections, osteoporosis, peptic ulcer disease, etc.). ACTH gel should not be used in patients hypersensitive to porcine proteins.

ACTH should only be used during pregnancy when the potential benefits outweigh the risks. It may be embryocidal. Neonates born from mothers receiving ACTH should be observed for signs of adrenocortical insufficiency.

Adverse Effects/Warnings - Prolonged use may result in fluid and electrolyte disturbances and other adverse effects. If using on a chronic basis, refer to the human literature for an extensive listing of potential adverse reactions. The veterinary manufacturer suggests giving potassium supplementation with chronic therapy.

Do not administer the repository form (gel) IV.

Overdosage - When used for diagnostic purposes, acute inadvertent overdoses are unlikely to cause any significant adverse effects. Monitor as required and treat symptomatically if necessary.

Drug Interactions - Glucocorticoids may alter the insulin requirements of diabetics. When used chronically, there are several potential interactions with ACTH including **barbiturates, phenytoin, rifampin, cyclophosphamide, estrogens, ulcerogenic drugs** (*e.g.,* **ASA, NSAIDs), potassium-depleting diuretics/drugs** (*e.g.,* **amphotericin B) and oral anticoagulants**. If the drug is to be used for purposes other than diagnostic purposes and the animal is receiving or will receive one of drugs listed above, refer to an appropriate reference (see bibliography) for further information.

Drug/Laboratory Interactions - ACTH may decrease ^{131}I uptake by the thyroid gland. ACTH may suppress **skin test reactions** and interfere with **urinary estrogen** determinations.

Doses - Obtain specific information from the laboratory on sample handling and laboratory normals for cortisol when doing ACTH stimulation tests. ACTH is quite unstable in unfrozen plasma.

Dogs:
ACTH Stimulation Test:
   a) Draw baseline blood sample for cortisol determination and administer 2.2 Units/kg of ACTH gel IM. Draw sample 120 minutes after injection. (Feldman and Peterson 1984), (Kemppainen and Zerbe 1989b)
   b) Draw baseline blood sample for cortisol determination and administer 0.5 Units/kg of ACTH gel IM. Draw sample 120 minutes after injection.
      Normals: Pre-ACTH 1.1-8.0 micrograms/dl; Post-ACTH 6.2-16.8 micrograms/dl.
      Hyperadrenocorticism: Pre-ACTH 4.0-10.8 micrograms/dl; Post-ACTH 11.7-50 micrograms/dl.
      Hypoadrenocorticism: Pre-ACTH and Post-ACTH: ≤ 1.0 micrograms/dl. (Morgan 1988)

Cats:
ACTH Stimulation Test:
   a) Draw baseline blood sample for cortisol determination and administer 2.2 Units/kg of ACTH gel IM. Draw samples at 60 minutes and 120 minutes after injection. (Peterson and Randolph 1989), (Kemppainen and Zerbe 1989b)
   b) Draw baseline blood sample for cortisol determination and administer 0.5 Units/kg of ACTH gel IM. Draw sample 120 minutes after injection.
      Normals: Pre-ACTH 0.33-2.6 micrograms/dl; Post-ACTH 4.8-7.6 micrograms/dl.
      Hyperadrenocorticism: Pre-ACTH 4.0-10.8 micrograms/dl; Post-ACTH 11.7-50 micrograms/dl.
      Hypoadrenocorticism: Pre-ACTH and Post-ACTH: ≤ 1.0 micrograms/dl. (Morgan 1988)

Cattle:
For ACTH deficiency or for primary bovine ketosis:
  a) 200 - 600 Units initially followed by daily or semi-daily dose of 200 - 300 Units (Package Insert; *Adrenomone*®—Summit Hill)
  b) 200 Units IM daily (Howard 1986)

Horses:
ACTH Stimulation Test:
  a) Draw baseline blood sample for cortisol determination and administer 1 Unit/kg IM of ACTH gel. Draw second sample 8 hours later. Normal stimulation will result in serum cortisol levels will increase 2-3 times. Horses with pituitary tumors will increase cortisol fourfold after ACTH. (Beech 1987b)

Birds:
ACTH Stimulation Test:
  a) Draw baseline blood sample for corticosterone (not cortisol) determination and administer 16 - 25 Units IM. Draw second sample 1-2 hours later. Normal baseline corticosterone levels vary with regard to species, but generally range from 1.5 - 7 ng/ml. After ACTH, corticosterone levels generally increase by 5 - 10 times those of baseline. Specific values are listed in the reference. (Lothrop and Harrison 1986)

Dosage Forms/Preparations/FDA Approval Status/Withholding Times -
Veterinary-Approved Products:
Corticotropin, Repository for Injection; 40 Units/ml and 80 Units/ml in 5 ml an d10 ml vials;
ACTH Gel (Anthony); *Adrenomone*® (Summit Hill) (Rx) Approved for use in dogs, cats, and beef or dairy cattle.

Human-Approved Products:
Corticotropin Powder for Injection; 25 Units per vial, and 40 Units per vial
  Acthar® (Rorer) (Rx) *ACTH* ®(Parke-Davis); (Rx); generic (Rx)

Corticotropin, Repository for Injection; 40 Units/ml and 80 Units/ml in 1 ml and 5 ml vials
  H.P. Acthar® *Gel* (Rorer) (Rx), *ACTH-80*®(Various); (Rx)

CYCLOPHOSPHAMIDE

Chemistry - A nitrogen-mustard derivative, cyclophosphamide occurs as a white, crystalline powder that is soluble in water and alcohol. The commercially available injection has pH of 3 to 7.5. Cyclophosphamide may also be known as CPM, CTX or CYT.

Storage/Stability/Compatibility - Cyclophosphamide tablets and powder for injection should be stored at temperatures less than 25°C. They may be exposed to temperatures up to 30°C for brief periods, but should not be exposed to temperatures above 30°C. Tablets should be stored in tight containers. The commercially available tablets (*Cytoxan*®) are manufactured in bi-level manner with a white tablet containing the cyclophosphamide found within a surrounding flecked outer tablet. Therefore, the person administering the drug need not protect their hands from cyclophosphamide exposure unless the tablets are split or crushed.

Cyclophosphamide injection may be dissolved in aromatic elixir to be used as an oral solution. When refrigerated, it is stable for 14 days.

After reconstituting the powder for injection with either sterile water for injection or bacteriostatic water for injection the product should be used within 24 hours if stored at room temperature and within 6 days if refrigerated.

Cyclophosphamide is reportedly **compatible** with the following intravenous solutions and drugs: Amino acids 4.25%/dextrose 25%, D5 in normal saline, D5W, sodium chloride 0.9%. It is also compatible in syringes or at Y-sites for brief periods with the following: bleomycin sulfate, cisplatin, doxorubicin HCl, droperidol, flurouracil, furosemide, heparin sodium, leucovorin calcium, methotrexate sodium, metoclopramide HCl, mitomycin, vinblastine sulfate, and vincristine sulfate. Compatibility is dependent upon factors such as pH, concentration, temperature and diluents used. It is suggested to consult specialized references for more specific information (*e.g.*, *Handbook on Injectable Drugs* by Trissel; see bibliography).

Pharmacology - While commonly categorized as an alkylating agent, the parent compound (cyclophosphamide) is not, but cyclophosphamide's metabolites such as phosphoramide mustard do act as alkylating agents interfering with DNA replication, RNA transcription and replication, and ultimately disrupting nucleic acid function. The cytotoxic properties of cyclophosphamide are also enhanced by phosphorylating activity the drug possesses.

Cyclophosphamide has marked immunosuppressive activity and both white cells and antibody production are decreased, but the exact mechanisms for this activity have not been fully elucidated.

Uses/Indications - In veterinary medicine, cyclophosphamide is used primarily in small animals, both as an antineoplastic agent and an immunosuppressant. Refer to the Dosages section below or the Protocols (at the end of this section), for more information. Cyclophosphamide has also been used as a chemical shearing agent in sheep.

Pharmacokinetics - While the pharmacokinetics of cyclophosphamide have not been detailed in dogs or cats, it is presumed that the drug is handled in a manner similar to humans. The drug is well absorbed after oral administration with peak levels occurring about 1 hour after dosing. Cyclophosphamide and its metabolites are distributed throughout the body, including the CSF (albeit in subtherapeutic levels). The drug is only minimally protein bound and is distributed into milk and presumed to cross the placenta.

Cyclophosphamide is metabolized in the liver to several metabolites. Which metabolites account for which portion of the cytotoxic properties of the drug are a source of controversy. After IV injection, the serum half-life of cyclophosphamide is approximately 4-65 hours, but drug/metabolites can be detected up to 72 hours after administration. The majority of the drug is excreted as metabolites and unchanged drug in the urine.

Contraindications/Precautions/Reproductive Safety - There are no absolute contraindications to the use of cyclophosphamide, but it must be used with caution in patients with leukopenia, thrombocytopenia, previous radiotherapy, impaired hepatic or renal function, or in those for whom immunosuppression may be dangerous (*e.g.,* infected patients).

Because of the potential for development of serious Adverse effects, cyclophosphamide should only be used in patients who can be adequately and regularly monitored.

Cyclophosphamide's safe use in pregnancy has not been established and it is potentially teratogenic and embryotoxic. Cyclophosphamide may induce sterility (may be temporary) in male animals.

Adverse Effects/Warnings - Primary adverse effects in animals associated with cyclophosphamide are myelosuppression, gastroenterocolitis (nausea, vomiting, diarrhea), alopecia (especially in breeds where haircoat continually grows, *e.g.,* Poodles, Old English Sheepdogs), and hemorrhagic cystitis.

Cyclophosphamide's myelosuppressant effects primarily impact the white cells lines, but may also effect red cell and platelet production. The nadir for leukocytes occurs generally between 7-14 days after dosing and may require up to 4 weeks for recovery.

Sterile hemorrhagic cystitis induced by cyclophosphamide is thought to be caused by the metabolite acrolein. Up to 30% of dogs receiving long-term (>2 months) cyclophosphamide can develop this problem. In cats, cyclophosphamide-induced-cystitis (CIC) is rare. Initial symptoms may present as hematuria and dysuria. Because bacterial cystitis is not uncommon in immuno-suppressed patients, it must be ruled out by taking urine cultures. Diagnosis of CIC is made by a negative urine culture and inflammatory urine sediment found during urinalysis. Because bladder fibrosis and/or transitional cell carcinoma of the bladder is also associated with cyclophosphamide use, these may need to be ruled out by contrast radiography. It is believed that the incidence of CIC may be minimized by increasing urine production and frequent voiding. The drug should be given in the morning and animals should be encouraged to drink/urinate whenever possible. Recommendations for treatment of CIC include discontinuation of the cyclophosphamide, furosemide, and corticosteroids. Refractory cases have been treated by surgical debridement, 1% formalin or 25% DMSO instillation in the bladder.

Other adverse effects that may be noted with CTX therapy include pulmonary infiltrates and fibrosis, depression, immune-suppression with hyponatremia, and leukemia.

In recovering dogs with immune-mediated hemolytic anemia, taper the withdrawal of the drug slowly over several months and monitor for early signs of relapse. Rapid withdrawal can lead to a rebound hyperimmune response.

Overdosage/Acute Toxicity - There is only limited information on acute overdoses of this drug. The lethal dose in the dogs has been reported as 40 mg/kg IV. If an oral overdose occurs, the animal should be hospitalized for supportive care.

Drug Interactions - **Phenobarbital** (or other barbiturates) given chronically may increase the rate of metabolism of cyclophosphamide via microsomal enzyme induction and increase the likelihood of toxicity development.

Allopurinol and thiazide diuretics may increase the myelosuppression caused by cyclophosphamide.

The absorption of orally administered **digoxin** tablets and elixir may be decreased when cyclophosphamide is also being given. This effect may even occur several days after the cyclophosphamide was administered.

Succinylcholine metabolism may be slowed with resulting prolongation of effects, as cyclophosphamide may decrease the levels of circulating pseudocholinesterases.

Use caution when using cyclophosphamide with other **cardiotoxic agents** (*e.g.,* **doxorubicin**) as potentiation of cardiotoxicity may occur.

Drug/Laboratory Interactions - **Uric acid** levels (blood and urine) may be increased after cyclophosphamide use. The immunosuppressant properties of cyclophosphamide may cause false negative **skin test** results to a variety of antigens, including tuberculin, Candida, and Trichophyton.

Doses - For more information, refer to the protocol references found in the appendix or other protocols found in numerous references, including: *Handbook of Small Animal Practice* (Ogilvie 1988), (Cotter 1988), (Stann 1988a); *Handbook of Small Animal Therapeutics* (Rosenthal 1985); *Current Veterinary Therapy X: Small Animal Practice* (Helfand 1989), (Matus 1989); and *Textbook of Veterinary Internal Medicine, 3rd Edition* (Couto 1989a).

Dogs:

For susceptible neoplastic diseases:
a) 50 mg/m^2 PO or IV 4 days/week. (MacEwen and Rosenthal 1989)
b) 50 mg/m^2 PO or IV 4 days/week or 200 mg/m^2 IV weekly. (Rosenthal 1985)
c) For multiple myeloma in patients refractory to melphalan: 1 mg/kg PO once daily. For macroglobulinemia in patients refractory to chlorambucil: 1 mg/kg PO once daily. (Hurvitz and Johnessee 1985)

As an immunosuppressant:
a) For adjunctive therapy for immune-mediated hemolytic anemia (probably should be reserved for dogs w/fulminant intravascular hemolysis, autoagglutination or those that require repeated transfusion or have persistant reticulocytopenia): Initially at 2 mg/kg/day IV or PO for 4 days; no treatment for 3 days and then repeat cycle. (Bucheler and Cotter 1995)
b) For immune-mediated hemolytic anemia: 50 mg/m^2 for 4 consecutive days per week. May be overtreatment; efficacy not proven. (Weiser 1989a)
c) For immune-mediated hemolytic anemia if glucocorticoids unsuccessful: Add cyclophosphamide at 2.2 mg/kg (50 mg/m^2) PO or IV once daily for 4 consecutive days of each week. Discontinue CTX when PCV increases significantly and attempt to slowly reduce steroids dose and D/C eventually, if possible. (Thompson 1989b)
c) For immune-mediated hemolytic anemia: Usually steroids used initially, but cyclophosphamide (&/or azathioprine) may be indicated early in therapy for cases with severe hemolysis and agglutination. Cyclophosphamide 2 mg/kg PO once daily for 4 days, stop for 3 days, then repeat. Animals should receive steroids, CTX, and azathioprine if they exhibit massive agglutination and intravascular hemolysis (poor prognosis). (Maggio-Price 1988)
d) For immune-mediated thrombocytopenia: If corticosteroids ineffective, may use either vincristine, azathioprine or cyclophosphamide. CTX dose: 50 mg/m^2 PO once daily for 3-4 days/week. May give initial doses IV. Decrease dose if renal or hepatic impairment exists. After 1-4 weeks, taper dose and discontinue after platelet count is >100,000/µl. Serious bleeding secondary to thrombocytopenia and hemorrhagic cystitis can occur; use cautiously. (Young 1988)
e) For rheumatoid arthritis: In conjunction with a glucocorticoid (predniso(lo)ne); give CTX PO once daily in the AM for 4 consecutive days each week at 2.5 mg/kg if weighs <10 kg, 2 mg/kg if 10-35 kg, and 1.5 mg/kg if >35 kg. Discontinue: 1 month after remission of synovial inflammation (determined from joint tap), after 4 months of treatment, or if hemorrhagic cystitis develops. If cystitis develops, switch to azathioprine. (Tangner and Hulse 1988)
f) For polymyositis: In conjunction with steroids, if steroids alone are ineffective: 1 mg/kg PO once daily for 4 days, then off 3 days. Decrease concurrent prednisone dose to 1 mg/kg/day. (Knaack 1988)

Cats:

For susceptible neoplastic diseases:
a) For advanced mammary carcinoma: Doxorubicin: 30 mg/m^2 IV every 3 weeks up to 4-8 treatments. Cyclophosphamide: 100 mg/m^2 PO once daily on days 3, 4, 5, and 6 after doxorubicin. (Loar 1988)

As an immunosuppressant:
a) Give 2.5 mg/kg once daily PO for 4 consecutive days out of 7 for up to 3 weeks. Alternatively, 7 mg/kg IV may be given once a week. (Hurvitz and Johnessee 1985)
b) For immune-mediated hemolytic anemia: 50 mg/m^2 for 4 consecutive days per week. May be overtreatment; efficacy not proven. (Weiser 1989a)
c) For rheumatoid arthritis: In conjunction with a glucocorticoid (predniso(lo)ne); give CTX PO once daily in the AM for 4 consecutive days each week at 2.5 mg/kg. Discontinue 1 month after remission of synovial inflammation (determined from joint

tap), after 4 months of treatment, or if hemorrhagic cystitis develops. If cystitis develops, switch to azathioprine. (Tangner and Hulse 1988)

Sheep:
As a chemical defleecing agent:
a) 25 mg/kg PO once (McConnell and Hughey 1989)

Monitoring Parameters -
1) Efficacy. See the Protocol section or refer to the references from the Dosage section above for more information.
2) Toxicity, see Adverse Effects above. Regular hemograms and urinalyses are mandatory.

Client Information - Clients must be briefed on the possibilities of severe toxicity developing from this drug, including drug-related mortality. Clients should contact veterinarian should the animal exhibit any symptoms of abnormal bleeding and/or bruising.

Although no special precautions are necessary with handling intact tablets, direct exposure should be avoided to split or crushed tablets, oral elixir, or the animal's urine or feces. Should exposure occur, wash the area thoroughly with soap and water.

Dosage Forms/Preparations/FDA Approval Status/Withholding Times -
Veterinary-Approved Products: None

Human-Approved Products:
Cyclophosphamide Tablets 25 mg, 50 mg; *Cytoxan*® (Mead Johnson Oncology); (Rx)

Cyclophosphamide Powder for Injection 100 mg, 200 mg, 500 mg, 1 g and 2 g vials;*Cytoxan*® (with sodium chloride) and*Cytoxan*® *Lyophilized* (with mannitol) (Mead Johnson Oncology) (Rx), *Neosar*® (Pharmacia & Upjohn) (Rx)

CYPROHEPTADINE HCL

Chemistry - An antihistamine that also possesses serotonin antagonist properties, cyproheptadine HCl occurs as a white to slightly yellow crystalline powder. Approximately 3.64 mg are soluble in one ml of water and 28.6 mg in one ml of alcohol.

Storage/Stability/Compatibility - Cyproheptadine HCl tablets and oral solution should be stored at room temperature and freezing should be avoided.

Pharmacology - Like other H_1-receptor antihistamines, cyproheptadine acts by competing with histamine for sites on H_1-receptor sites on effector cells. Antihistamines do not block histamine release, but can antagonize its effects. Cyproheptadine also possesses potent antiserotonin activity and reportedly has calcium channel blocking action as well.

Uses/Indications - Cyproheptadine may be useful as an antihistamine, and may also be employed in cats as an appetite stimulant. The drug may be useful as adjunctive therapy for Cushing's syndrome, probably as a result of its antiserotonin activity. But one study demonstrated efficacy in less than 10% of dogs treated for pituitary dependent adrenocorticism.

Pharmacokinetics - Limited data available. Cyproheptadine is well absorbed after oral administration. Its distribution characteristics are not well described. Cyproheptadine is apparently nearly completely metabolized in the liver and these metabolites are then excreted in the urine. Elimination is reduced in renal failure.

Contraindications/Precautions/Reproductive Safety - Cyproheptadine is contraindicated in patients hypersensitive to it. It should be used with caution in patients with prostatic hypertrophy, bladder neck obstruction, severe cardiac failure, angle-closure glaucoma, or pyeloduodenal obstruction.

Cyproheptadine has been tested in pregnant lab animals in doses up to 32 times labeled dose without evidence of harm to fetuses. But, because safety has not been established in other species, its use during pregnancy should be weighed carefully. It is unknown whether cyproheptadine enters maternal milk or may potentially cause adverse effects in offspring; use with caution.

Adverse Effects/Warnings - The most likely adverse effects seen with cyproheptadine are related to its CNS depressant (sedation) and anticholinergic (dryness of mucous membranes, etc.) effects. At higher dosages, cyproheptadine has caused significant polyphagia in dogs.

Overdosage/Acute Toxicity - There are no specific antidotes available. Significant overdoses should be handled using standard gut emptying protocols when appropriate and supportive therapy when required. The adverse effects seen with overdoses are an extension of the drug's side effects, principally CNS depression (although CNS stimulation may be seen), anticholinergic effects (severe drying of mucous membranes, tachycardia, urinary retention, hyperthermia, etc.)

and possibly hypotension. Physostigmine may be considered to treat serious CNS anticholinergic effects, and diazepam employed to treat seizures, if necessary.

Drug Interactions - Additive CNS depression may be seen if combining cyproheptadine with other **CNS depressant medications**, such as barbiturates, tranquilizers, etc. **Monoamine oxidase inhibitors** (including **furazolidone**) may intensify the anticholinergic effects of antihistamines. Cyproheptadine may increase amylase and prolactin serum levels when administered with **thyrotropin-releasing hormone**.

Laboratory Considerations - Because antihistamines can decrease the wheal and flair response to **skin allergen testing**, antihistamines should be discontinued from 3 -7 days (depending on the antihistamine used and the reference) before intradermal skin tests.

Doses -
  Dogs:
    As an antihistamine:
      a) 1.1 mg/kg PO q8-12h (Papich 1992)
      b) 0.3 - 2 mg/kg PO *bid* (Bevier 1990)

  Cats:
    As an appetite stimulant:
      a) 2 - 4 mg per cat PO once or twice daily (Davenport 1994)
      b) 2 mg per cat every 12 hours; may take up to 24 hours for a response. Give at this dosage for one week and then taper. (Forney and Allen 1992)

Monitoring Parameters - 1) Efficacy; 2) Adverse Effects, if any

Client Information - Clients should understand that antihistamines may be useful for symptomatic relief of allergic symptoms, but are not a cure for the underlying disease.

Dosage Forms/Preparations/FDA Approval Status/Withholding Times -
  Veterinary-Approved Products: None
  Human-Approved Products:
    Cyproheptadine Oral Tablets 4 mg, Cyproheptadine Syrup 2 mg/5 ml; *Periactin*® (Merck) (Rx), generic; (Rx)

CYTARABINE

Chemistry - A synthetic pyrimidine nucleoside antimetabolite, cytarabine occurs as an odorless, white to off-white, crystalline powder with a pK_a of 4.35. It is freely soluble in water and slightly soluble in alcohol. Cytarabine is also commonly known as ARA-C or Cytosine Arabinoside. It may also be known as 1-beta-D-Arabinofuranosylcytosine or Arabinosylcytosine.

Storage/Stability/Compatibility - Cytarabine sterile powder for injection should be stored at room temperature (15-30°C). After reconstituting with bacteriostatic water for injection, solutions are stable for at least 48 hours when stored at room temperature. One study however, demonstrated that the reconstituted solution retains 90% of its potency for up to 17 days when stored at room temperature. If the solution develops a slight haze, the drug should be discarded.

Cytarabine is reportedly **compatible** with the following intravenous solutions and drugs: amino acids 4.25%/dextrose 25%, dextrose containing solutions, dextrose-saline combinations, dextrose-lactated Ringer's injection combinations, Ringer's injection, lactated Ringer's injection, sodium chloride 0.9%, sodium lactate 1/6 M, corticotropin, lincomycin HCl, methotrexate sodium, metoclopramide HCl, potassium chloride, prednisolone sodium phosphate, sodium bicarbonate, and vincristine sulfate.

Cytarabine **compatibility information conflicts** or is dependent on diluent or concentration factors with the following drugs or solutions: cephalothin sodium, gentamicin sulfate, hydrocortisone sodium succinate, and methylprednisolone sodium succinate. Compatibility is dependent upon factors such as pH, concentration, temperature and diluents used. It is suggested to consult specialized references for more specific information (*e.g., Handbook on Injectable Drugs* by Trissel; see bibliography).

Cytarabine is reportedly **incompatible** with the following solutions or drugs: carbenicillin disodium, fluorouracil, regular insulin, nafcillin sodium, oxacillin sodium, and penicillin G sodium.

Pharmacology - Cytarabine is converted intracellularly into cytarabine triphosphate which apparently competes with deoxycytidine triphosphate, thereby inhibiting DNA polymerase with resulting inhibition of DNA synthesis. Cytarabine is cell phase specific, and acts principally during the S-phase (DNA synthesis). It may also, under certain conditions, block cells from the G_1 phase to the S phase.

Uses/Indications - In veterinary medicine, cytarabine is used primarily in small animals as an antineoplastic agent for lymphoreticular neoplasms, myeloproliferative disease and CNS lymphoma. Refer to the Dosages below or the Protocols (at the end of this section), for more information.

Pharmacokinetics - Cytarabine has very poor systemic availability after oral administration and is only used parenterally. Following IM or SQ injections, the drug peaks in the plasma within 20-60 minutes, but levels attained are much lower than with an equivalent IV dose.

Cytarabine is distributed widely throughout the body, but crosses into the CNS in only a limited manner. If given via continuous IV infusion, CSF levels are higher than with IV bolus injection and can reach 40-60% of those levels found in the plasma. In humans, cytarabine is only about 13% bound to plasma proteins. The drug apparently crosses the placenta, but it is not known if it enters milk.

Circulating cytarabine is rapidly metabolized by the enzyme cytidine deaminase, principally in the liver, but also in the kidneys, intestinal mucosa, and granulocytes, to the inactive metabolite ara-U (uracil arabinoside). About 80% of a dose is excreted in the urine within 24 hours as both ara-U ($\approx$90%) and unchanged cytarabine ($\approx$10%).

Contraindications/Precautions/Reproductive Safety - Cytarabine is contraindicated in patients hypersensitive to it. Because of the potential for development of serious adverse reactions, cytarabine should only be used in patients who can be adequately and regularly monitored.

The person preparing or administering cytarabine for injection, need not observe any special handling precautions other than wearing gloves. However, should any contamination occur, thoroughly wash off the drug from skin or mucous membranes.

Cytarabine's safe use in pregnancy has not been established and it is potentially teratogenic and embryotoxic.

Adverse Effects/Warnings - The principal adverse effects of cytarabine is myelosuppression (with leukopenia being most prevalent), but anemia and thrombocytopenia can also be seen. Myelosuppressive effects are more pronounced with IV administration and reach a nadir at 5-7 days, and generally recover at 7-14 days.

GI disturbances (anorexia, nausea, vomiting, diarrhea), conjunctivitis, oral ulceration, hepatotoxicity and fever may also be noted with cytarabine therapy. Anaphylaxis has been reported, but is believed to occur very rarely.

Cytarabine is a mutagenic and potentially carcinogenic agent.

Overdosage/Acute Toxicity - Cytarabine efficacy and toxicity (see Adverse Effects) are dependent not only on the dose, but also the rate the drug is given. In dogs, the IV LD_{50} is 384 mg/kg when given over 12 hours and 48 mg/kg when infused IV over 120 hours. Should an inadvertent overdose occur, supportive therapy should be instituted.

Drug Interactions - Presumably due to causing alterations in the intestinal mucosa, cytarabine may decrease the amount of **digoxin** (tablets only) that is absorbed after oral dosing. This effect may persist for several days after cytarabine has been discontinued.

Limited studies have indicated that cytarabine may antagonize the anti-infective activity of **gentamicin** or **flucytosine**. Animals receiving either of these drugs with cytarabine should be closely monitored for decreased anti-infective efficacy.

Drug/Laboratory Interactions - None reported.

Doses - For more information, refer to the protocol references found in the appendix or other protocols found in numerous references, including: *Handbook of Small Animal Practice* (Stann 1988a); *Handbook of Small Animal Therapeutics* (Rosenthal 1985); and *Textbook of Veterinary Internal Medicine, 3rd Edition* (Couto 1989a).

Dogs:
   For susceptible neoplastic diseases:
   a) 100 mg/m^2 IV or SQ once daily for 2-4 days; repeat *prn* 20 mg/m^2 intrathecally for 1-5 days. (Thompson 1989a)
   b) 100 mg/m^2 IV (slowly), IM, or SQ once daily for 4 days, if no toxicity develops may increase dose by 50%. (Coppoc 1988)

Cats:
   For susceptible neoplastic diseases:
   a) 100 mg/m^2 IV or SQ once daily for 2-4 days; repeat *prn* 20 mg/m^2 intrathecally for 1-5 days. (Thompson 1989a)
   b) 100 mg/m^2 once daily for 2 days; 10 mg/m^2 once daily for 2 weeks. (Couto 1989b)

Monitoring Parameters -
   1) Efficacy; see the Protocol section or refer to the references from the Dosage section above for more information.
   2) Toxicity; see Adverse Effects above. Regular hemograms are mandatory. Periodic liver and kidney function tests are suggested.

Client Information - Clients must be briefed on the possibilities of severe toxicity developing from this drug, including drug-related mortality. Clients should contact the veterinarian should the patient exhibit any symptoms of profound depression, abnormal bleeding and/or bruising.

Dosage Forms/Preparations/FDA Approval Status/Withholding Times -
   Veterinary-Approved Products: None
   Human-Approved Products:
      Cytarabine Powder for Injection 100 mg, 500 mg, 1 g & 2 g in vials; *Cytosar-U®* (Upjohn) (Rx); generic (Rx)
      Cytarabine Injection 20 mg/ml in 5 ml vials and 50 ml bulk vials; *Tarabine PRS®* (Adria) (Rx)

CYTHIOATE

Chemistry - Cythioate is an oral organophosphate agent.

Storage/Stability/Compatibility - Unless otherwise noted by the manufacturer store products in tight, light resistant containers at room temperature.

Pharmacology - After being distributed into body fluids, cythioate is ingested by fleas, ticks and demodectic mites. It then inhibits acetylcholinesterase thereby interfering with neuromuscular transmission.

Uses/Indications - Cythioate is approved for use for flea control in dogs of all ages. It may also be useful in treating tick infestations and the control od demodectic mites.

Pharmacokinetics - No information located.

Contraindications/Precautions/Reproductive Safety - Cythioate is contraindicated in greyhounds (no information located on safety in other sight hound breeds). It is also contraindicated in sick, debilitated, stressed (recovering from surgery, etc.), anemic or pregnant animals.

Adverse Effects/Warnings - Cythioate is relatively safe and at recommended doses should be devoid of adverse effects in otherwise healthy dogs. At higher doses and in susceptible dogs, muscle tremors and hyperexcitability may be noted.
   Repeated or prolonged dosing may lead to adverse effects. The manufacturer warns against using cythioate simultaneously with other drugs, insecticides, pesticides or chemicals having cholinesterase inhibiting activity and using within a few days before or after using any other cholinesterase inhibitor.

Overdosage/Acute Toxicity - If overdoses occur, vomiting, tremors, hyperexcitability, salivation and diarrhea may occur. The manufacturer recommends treating with atropine at 0.22 mg/kg IM at 15-30 minute intervals depending upon the severity of the symptoms. Use of succinylcholine, theophylline/aminophylline, reserpine, and respiratory depressant drugs (*e.g.,* narcotics, phenothiazines) should be avoided in patients with organophosphate toxicity. If an ingestion occurs by a human, contact a poison control center, physician or hospital emergency room.

Drug Interactions - **Acepromazine or other phenothiazines** should not be given within one month of worming with an organophosphate agent as their effects may be potentiated. Because of its anticholinesterase activity, avoid the use of organophosphates with **DMSO**. Cythioate could theoretically enhance the toxic effects of **levamisole**. **Pyrantel Pamoate (or tartrate)** adverse effects could be intensified if used concomitantly with an organophosphate. Patients receiving organophosphate anthelmintics should not receive **succinylcholine** or other depolarizing muscle relaxants for at least 48 hours. Drugs such as **morphine, neostigmine, physostigmine** and **pyridostigmine** should be avoided when using organophosphates as they can inhibit cholinesterase.

Doses -
   Dogs:
      For flea control:
         a) Tablets: one 30 mg tablet for each 20 lbs of body weight once every third day or twice a week.
            Liquid: 1 ml (16 mg) PO for each 10 lbs of body weight once every third day or twice a week. Apply to food and mix thoroughly. The first week of therapy will kill 95% of fleas. Additional treatments for several weeks are necessary to remove fleas that reinfest dogs from the environment. (Package insert; *Proban®*—Miles)

Monitoring Parameters - 1) Efficacy; 2) Adverse effects

Client Information - Keep out of reach of children. Be sure client understands dosing recommendations and the importance of not exceeding them.

Dosage Forms/Preparations/FDA Approval Status/Withholding Times -
Veterinary-Approved Products:
  Cythioate Tablets 30 mg, 90 mg Cythioate Oral Liquid 1.6% (w/w) (16 mg/ml) in 25 ml
      and 120 ml containers; *Proban*® (Bayer); (Rx)
  Human-Approved Products: None

d-Panthenol —see Dexpanthenol

DACARBAZINE

Chemistry - An antineoplastic agent, dacarbazine occurs as a colorless to ivory colored crystalline solid. It is slightly soluble in water or alcohol. After reconstituting with sterile water, the injection has a pH of 3-4. Dacarbazine may also be known as DTIC, DIC, or imidazole carboxamide.

Storage/Stability/Compatibility - The powder for injection should be protected from light and kept refrigerated. If exposed to heat the powder may change color from ivory to pink, indicating some decomposition.

  After reconstituting with sterile water for injection the resultant solution is stable for up to 72 hours if kept refrigerated or up to 8 hours at room temperature. If further diluted (up to 500 ml) with either D5W or normal saline the solution is stable for at least 24 hours when refrigerated (8 hours at room temperature under normal room lighting).

Pharmacology - The mechanism for dacarbazine's antineoplastic activity has not been precisely determined, but it is believed the drug acts as an alkylating agent. It possesses minimal immunosuppressant activity and is probably not a cell cycle-phase specific drug.

Uses/Indications - Dacarbazine has been used to treat lymphoreticular neoplasms in dogs. It has minimal activity against osteosarcomas and malignant melanomas.

Pharmacokinetics - Dacarbazine (DTIC) is poorly absorbed from the GI tract and is administered intravenously. The drug's distribution characteristics are not well known, but it is only slightly bound to plasma proteins and probably concentrates in the liver. Only limited amounts cross the blood-brain barrier and it is unknown if it crosses the placenta or enters maternal milk. Dacarbazine is extensively metabolized in the liver and is excreted in the urine via tubular secretion.

Contraindications/Precautions/Reproductive Safety - Dacarbazine (DTIC) is contraindicated in patients who are hypersensitive to it. DTIC can cause life-threatening toxicity. It should only be used where adequate monitoring and support can be administered. It should be used with caution in patients with preexisting bone marrow depression, hepatic or renal dysfunction, or infection.

  DTIC is teratogenic in rats at higher than clinically used dosages. It should be used during pregnancy only when the potential benefits outweigh its risks. While it is unknown if DTIC enters maternal milk, the potential carcinogenicity of the drug warrants using extreme caution in allowing the mother to continue nursing while receiving DTIC.

Adverse Effects/Warnings - Gastrointestinal toxicity (including vomiting, anorexia, diarrhea) can be commonly seen after administration. Bone marrow toxicity is usually asymptomatic with leukocyte and platelet nadirs seen several weeks after therapy. Occasionally severe hematopoietic toxicity can occur with fatal consequences. Other delayed toxic effects can include, alopecia, severe hepatotoxicity, renal impairment, and photosensitivity reactions. These delayed reactions are more rarely seen.

  Because DTIC can cause extensive pain and tissue damage, avoid extravasation injuries. Severe pain at the injection site can occur if giving the concentrated drug; dilution and administration by IV infusion is recommended.

  There is increasing evidence that chronic exposure by health care-givers to antineoplastic drugs increases the mutagenic, teratogenic and carcinogenic risks associated with these agents. Proper precautions in the handing, preparation, administration and disposal of these drugs and supplies associated with their use is strongly recommended.

Overdosage/Acute Toxicity - Because of the toxic potential of this agent, iatrogenic overdoses must be avoided. Recheck dosage calculations. See Adverse Effects above for additional information on toxicity.

Drug Interactions - Drugs that induce liver microsomal enzymes (*e.g.*, **phenobarbital**) may increase the metabolism of DTIC. **Other bone marrow depressant drugs** (*e.g.*, **other neoplastics, chloramphenicol, flucytosine, amphotericin B or colchicine**) may cause additive myelosuppression when used with DTIC.

Doses -
  Dogs:
    For lymphoreticular neoplasms:
      a) 200 - 250 mg/m2 IV once daily for 5 days; repeat cycle every 21 days. (Jacobs, Lumsden et al. 1992)
    For soft tissue sarcomas:
      a) As part of the ADIC protocol: Dacarbazine 1000 mg/m^2 IV drip over 6-8 hours, repeat every 3 weeks; Doxorubicin 30 mg/m^2 IV every 3 weeks; trimethoprim/sulfadiazine 15 mg/kg PO q12h. (Peterson and Couto 1994b)

Monitoring Parameters - 1) Efficacy; 2) Toxicity, including CBC with differential and platelets; renal and hepatic function tests

Client Information - Inform clients of the potential toxicities and risks associated with this therapy and to report immediately any signs associated with serious toxicity (*e.g.*, bloody vomiting or diarrhea, abnormal bleeding, bruising, urination, depression, infection, shortness of breath, etc.).

Dosage Forms/Preparations/FDA Approval Status/Withholding Times -
  Veterinary-Approved Products: None
  Human-Approved Products:
    Dacarbazine Parenteral (IV use) Injection 10 mg/ml in 10 & 20 ml vials ; *DTIC-Dome*® (Bayer); (Rx)

DACTINOMYCIN

Chemistry - An antibiotic antineoplastic agent, dactinomycin (also known as actinomycin D) occurs as a bright red, crystalline powder. It is somewhat hygroscopic and soluble in water at 10°C and slightly soluble at 37°C. The commercially available preparation is a yellow lyophilized mixture of dactinomycin and mannitol.

Storage/Stability/Compatibility - The commercially available powder should be stored at room temperature and protected from light. When reconstituting, sterile water for injection without preservatives must be used as preservatives may cause precipitation. After reconstituting, the manufacturer recommends using the solution immediately and discarding any unused portion as the solution does not contain any preservatives. The reconstituted solution may be added to D5W or normal saline IV infusions. IV fluid sterilizing filters (cellulose ester membrane) may partially remove dactinomycin.

Pharmacology - Dactinomycin is an antibiotic antineoplastic. While it has activity against gram positive bacteria, the drug's toxicity precludes its use for this purpose. Dactinomycin's exact mechanism of action for its antineoplastic activity has not been determined, but it apparently inhibits DNA-dependent RNA synthesis. Dactinomycin forms a complex with DNA and interferes with DNA's template activity. Dactinomycin also possesses immunosuppressing and some hypocalcemic activity.

Uses/Indications - Dactinomycin has been used as adjunctive treatment of lymphoreticular neoplasms, bone and soft tissue sarcomas, and malignant melanomas in small animals.

Pharmacokinetics - Because dactinomycin is poorly absorbed it must be given IV. It is rapidly distributed and high concentrations may be found in bone marrow and nucleated cells. Dactinomycin crosses the placenta, but it is unknown whether it enters maternal milk. The majority of the drug is excreted unchanged in the bile and urine.

Contraindications/Precautions/Reproductive Safety - Dactinomycin can cause life-threatening toxicity. It should only be used where adequate monitoring and support can be administered. Dactinomycin is contraindicated in patients who are hypersensitive to it. It should be used with caution in patients with preexisting bone marrow depression, hepatic dysfunction, or infection.

  Dactinomycin has been demonstrated to be embryotoxic and teratogenic in rats, rabbits and hamsters at higher than clinically used dosages. It should be used during pregnancy only when the potential benefits outweigh its risks. While it is unknown if dactinomycin enters maternal milk, the potential mutagenicity and carcinogenicity of the drug warrants using extreme caution in allowing the mother to continue nursing while receiving dactinomycin.

Adverse Effects/Warnings - Adverse effects that may be seen more frequently include anemia, leukopenia, thrombocytopenia (or other signs of bone marrow depression), ulcerative stomatitis or other GI ulceration. Because dactinomycin may cause increased serum uric acid levels, allopurinol may be required to prevent urate stone formation in susceptible patients. Hepatotoxicity is potentially possible with this agent.

Because dactinomycin can cause extensive pain and tissue damage, avoid extravasation injuries. Dilution and administration by IV infusion is recommended or to administer slowly into a running IV line; use the "two-needle" technique.

There is increasing evidence that chronic exposure by health care-givers to antineoplastic drugs increases the mutagenic, teratogenic and carcinogenic risks associated with these agents. Proper precautions in the handing, preparation, administration and disposal of these drugs and supplies associated with their use is strongly recommended.

Overdosage/Acute Toxicity - Because of the toxic potential of this agent, iatrogenic overdoses must be avoided. Recheck dosage calculations. See Adverse Effects above for additional information on toxicity.

Drug Interactions - **Other bone marrow depressant drugs** (*e.g.*, **other neoplastics, chloramphenicol, flucytosine, amphotericin B or colchicine**) may cause additive myelosuppression when used with dactinomycin. Additive cardiotoxicity may occur if used concurrently or sequentially with **doxorubicin**. Patients requiring **vitamin K**, may require higher dosages when receiving dactinomycin.

Laboratory Considerations - Dactinomycin may interfere with determination of **antibacterial drug levels** if using bioassay techniques.

Doses - Also see the section on antineoplastic protocols found in the appendix.

a) 0.7 mg/m^2 IV every 7 days (Jacobs, Lumsden et al. 1992)

Monitoring Parameters - 1) Efficacy; 2) Toxicity: including CBC with differential and platelets; hepatic function tests; check inside patient's mouth for ulceration

Client Information - Inform clients of the potential toxicities and risks associated with this therapy and to report immediately any signs associated with serious toxicity (*e.g.*, bloody vomiting or diarrhea, abnormal bleeding, bruising, urination, depression, infection, shortness of breath, etc.).

Dosage Forms/Preparations/FDA Approval Status/Withholding Times -
   Veterinary-Approved Products: None
   Human-Approved Products:
   Dactinomycin for Injection 500 micrograms (with 20 mg mannitol); *Cosmogen*® (MSD); (Rx)

DANAZOL

Chemistry - A synthetic derivative of ethisterone (ethinyl testosterone), danazol occurs as a white to pale yellow, crystalline powder. It is practically insoluble in water and sparingly soluble in alcohol.

Storage/Stability/Compatibility - Danazol capsules should be stored in well-closed containers at room temperature.

Pharmacology - Danazol is a synthetic androgen with weak androgenic effects. It suppresses the pituitary-ovarian axis. Danazol probably directly inhibits the synthesis of sex steroids and binds to sex steroid receptors in tissues, where it may express anabolic, weak androgenic, and antiestrogenic effects.

Uses/Indications - In veterinary medicine, danazol is primarily used as adjunctive therapy (with corticosteroids) in the treatment of canine immune-mediated thrombocytopenia and hemolytic anemia. There is apparently synergism when danazol is combined with corticosteroids for these indications. Once remission is attained, some dogs may have their dosage reduced or other medications may be eliminated and be controlled with danazol alone. In humans, danazol has been used for the treatment of endometriosis, fibrocystic breast disease, idiopathic thrombocytopenic purpura and a variety of other conditions.

Pharmacokinetics - There is very limited data available. Danazol is absorbed from the GI tract, but appears to be a rate limited process as increasing the dosage does not yield a corresponding increase in serum level. Distribution information is practically nonexistent; the drug apparently crosses the placenta. Danazol is believed to be principally metabolized in the liver. In humans, half-lives average about 4-5 hours.

Contraindications/Precautions/Reproductive Safety - Danazol should be used in patients with severe cardiac, renal or hepatic function impairment, or undiagnosed abnormal vaginal bleeding only when its benefits outweigh its risks.

Because of documented teratogenic effects, danazol is considered contraindicated during pregnancy. While it is unknown if danazol enters maternal milk, the potential adverse effects associated with androgens in young animals warrants that caution be used.

Adverse Effects/Warnings - Hepatotoxicity (incidence rare) is the most significant of the adverse effects that have been reported thus far in dogs. Otherwise virilization in females is the most likely other effect that may be seen. Rarely, danazol may cause weight gain, or lethargy.

Human patients have developed vaginitis. Other potential adverse effects include edema, testicular atrophy, hirsutism or alopecia.

Overdosage/Acute Toxicity - No information was located. Significant overdoses should initially be handled by contacting an animal poison control center and initiate gut emptying protocols when applicable.

Drug Interactions - Concomitant use of danazol with **anticoagulants** may enhance the anticoagulant effect because danazol may decrease the synthesis of procoagulant factors in the liver. In diabetics, danazol may affect **insulin** requirements (doses may need to be increased) by affecting carbohydrate metabolism.

Laboratory Considerations - Danazol may decrease total **serum thyroxine (T4) and increase T3 uptake**; because thyroid-binding globulin is decreased free T4 and TSH remain normal. **ALT (SGPT) and AST (SGOT)** may increase early in therapy but decrease towards baseline later in therapy. After discontinuation of danazol, levels usually return to baseline.

Doses -
  Dogs:
    For adjunctive treatment of immune-mediated hemolytic anemia or thrombocytopenia:
      a) 5 mg/kg PO q12h; usually used for the first two weeks of therapy in combination with corticosteroids. (Thompson 1994)
      b) 10 - 20 mg/kg/day (divided *bid - tid*) (Dougherty 1994)
      c) Initially, (in addition to prednis(ol)one) danazol may be given at 10 mg/kg/day PO. Once anemia improves, corticosteroids may be slowly tapered and eventually DC'd. When remission maintained by danazol alone, may lower to 5 mg/kg/day. Slowly taper after 2-3 months of normal hemograms with frequent monitoring of hemograms. (Bucheler and Cotter 1995)

  Cats:
    For adjunctive treatment of immune-mediated hemolytic anemia:
      a) 5 mg/kg PO twice daily (Loar 1994)

Monitoring Parameters - For autoimmune hematologic disorders: 1) Efficacy (CBC, platelets, etc.); 2) Hepatic function, baseline and at regular intervals while on therapy.

Client Information - Clients should be informed that it may take several (2-3) months to see a positive response with this drug. They should monitor for hepatotoxicity (jaundice) or changes in hematologic status (bleeding, tarry stools, etc.).

Dosage Forms/Preparations/FDA Approval Status/Withholding Times -
  Veterinary-Approved Products: None
  Human-Approved Products:
    Danazol Oral Capsules 50 mg, 100 mg, 200 mg; *Danocrine*® (Sanofi-Winthrop), generic; (Rx)

DANTROLENE SODIUM

Chemistry - A hydantoin derivative which is dissimilar structurally and pharmacologically from other skeletal muscle relaxant drugs, dantrolene sodium is a weak acid with a pK_a of 7.5. It occurs as an odorless, tasteless, orange, fine powder that is slightly soluble in water. It rapidly hydrolyzes in aqueous solutions to the free acid form which precipitates out of solution.

Storage/Stability/Compatibility - Dantrolene capsules should be stored in well-closed containers at room temperature. Dantrolene powder for injection should be stored at temperatures less than 30°C and protected from prolonged exposure to light. After reconstitution, the powder for injection should be used within 6 hours when stored at room temperature and should be protected from direct light. It is not compatible with either normal saline or D5W injection.

Pharmacology - Dantrolene exhibits muscle relaxation activity by direct action on muscle. While the exact mechanism is not well understood, it probably acts on skeletal muscle by interfering with the release of calcium from the sarcoplasmic reticulum. It has no discernible effects on the respiratory or cardiovascular systems, but can drowsiness and dizziness. The reasons for these CNS effects are not known.

Uses/Indications - In humans, oral dantrolene is indicated primarily for the treatment associated with upper motor neuron disorders (*e.g.,* multiple sclerosis, cerebral palsy, spinal cord injuries, etc.). In veterinary medicine, its proposed indications include the prevention and treatment of malignant hyperthermia syndrome in various species, the treatment of functional urethral obstruction due to increased external urethral tone in dogs and cats, the prevention and treatment of equine post-anesthetic myositis (PAM) and equine exertional rhabdomyolysis. It has also been recommended to be used in the treatment of bites from Black Widow Spiders in small animals and in the treatment of porcine stress syndrome.

Pharmacokinetics - The bioavailability of dantrolene after oral administration in humans is only about 35% and after intragastric administration to horses, approximately 39%. The drug is fairly slowly absorbed, with peak levels occurring about 5 hours after oral administration (humans) and 1.5 hours in horses. The drug is substantially bound to plasma proteins (principally albumin), but many drugs may displace it from such (see Drug Interactions).

Dantrolene is rapidly eliminated from the horse (t1/2≈130 minutes). The elimination half-life in humans is approximately 8 hours. Dantrolene is metabolized in the liver and the metabolites are excreted in the urine. Only about 1% of the parent drug is excreted unchanged in the urine and bile.

Contraindications/Precautions - Because dantrolene can cause hepatotoxicity, it should be used with extreme caution in patients with preexisting liver disease. It should be used with caution in patients with severe cardiac dysfunction or pulmonary disease. The safe use of dantrolene during pregnancy has not been determined.

Adverse Effects/Warnings - The most significant adverse reaction with dantrolene therapy is hepatotoxicity. In humans, it is most commonly associated with high dose chronic therapy, but may also be seen after short high dose therapy. The incidence of this reaction is unknown in veterinary medicine, but must be monitored for.

More common, but less significant are the CNS associated signs of sedation, dizziness, headache, etc. and GI effects (nausea, vomiting, constipation). Also seen are increased urinary frequency, and possibly hypotension.

Overdosage - There is no specific antidotal therapy to dantrolene overdoses, therefore remove the drug from the gut if possible and treat supportively.

Drug Interactions - Dantrolene may be displaced from plasma proteins by **warfarin** with increased effects or adverse reactions resulting. Diazepam, phenytoin or phenylbutazone have not been demonstrated to alter the plasma protein binding of dantrolene.

Increased risks of hepatotoxicity from dantrolene have been seen in women >35 years of age who are also receiving **estrogen** therapy. The veterinary significance is unknown for this potential interaction.

Increased sedation may be seen if **tranquilizing agents** are used concomitantly with dantrolene.

Doses -
  Dogs:
    For treatment of functional urethral obstruction due to increased external urethral tone:
      a) 1 - 5 mg/kg PO q8h (Polzin and Osborne 1985), (Chew, DiBartola, and Fenner 1986)
      b) 3 - 15 mg/kg PO divided *bid-tid* (Morgan 1988)
    For adjunctive treatment of Black Widow Spider bite:
      a) 1 mg/kg IV; followed by 1 mg/kg PO q4h (Bailey 1986a)
  Cats:
    For treatment of functional urethral obstruction due to increased external urethral tone:
      a) 0.5 - 2 mg/kg PO q8h (Polzin and Osborne 1985)
  Horses:
    For treatment of acute rhabdomyolosis:
      a) 15 - 25 mg/kg slow IV *qid* (Robinson 1987)
    For prevention of rhabdomyolysis:
      a) 2 mg/kg PO once daily (Robinson 1987)
    For prevention of post-anesthetic myositis (PAM):
      a) 10 mg/kg PO (intragastric) 1.5 hours before surgery. This should give peak levels at the time surgery begins and maintain postulated therapeutic levels for an additional 2 hours. The intragastric preparation was made by dissolving/suspending the contents of oral capsules into 500 ml of normal saline. Should further doses be warranted, additional doses of 2.5 mg/kg PO (intragastric) q60 minutes can be given.
        Alternatively, IV doses of 1.9 mg/kg loading will give therapeutic levels but will only persist for about 20 minutes. An IV dose of 4 mg/kg will maintain therapeutic levels for about 2 hours but peak levels will be quite high. (Court et al. 1987)
  Swine:
    Prevention or treatment of malignant hyperthermia:
      a) 3.5 mg/kg IV (Booth 1988a)
Monitoring Parameters -
Depending on the reason for use:
  1) Baseline and periodic liver function tests (ALT, AST, Alk Phos, etc) if projecting to be used chronically or using high dosages
  2) Body temperature (malignant hyperthermia)
  3) Urine volume, frequency, continence

Client Information - This drug should only be used by professionals familiar with its use.

Dosage Forms/Preparations/FDA Approval Status/Withholding Times -
  Veterinary-Approved Products: None
  Human-Approved Products:
  Human-Approved Products:

    Dantrolene Sodium 25 mg, 50 mg, 100 mg capsules; *Dantrium*® (Procter & Gamble Pharm.) (Rx)

    Dantrolene Sodium for Injection 20 mg per vial (with mannitol 3 g.); *Dantrium*® *Intravenous* (Procter & Gamble Pharm.) (Rx)

Note: Because of the expense, minimum order quantity, and non-returnable nature of the commercially available intravenous product, it is not well suited for veterinary use.

DECOQUINATE

Chemistry - A coccidiostat, decoquinate occurs as a cream to buff-colored fine amorphous powder having a slight odor. It is insoluble in water.

Storage/Stability/Compatibility - Decoquinate is reportedly incompatible with strong bases or oxidizing material. Follow label storage directions; store in a cool, dry place. *Deccox*® is labeled as being compatible (and cleared for use) with bacitracin zinc (with or without roxarsone), chlortetracycline, and lincomycin.

Pharmacology - Decoquinate is 4-hydroxy quinolone agent that has anticoccidial activity. Decoquinate act on the sporozoite stage of the life cycle. The sporozoite apparently can still penetrate the host intestinal cell, but further development is prevented. The mechanism of action for decoquinate is to disrupt electron transport in the mitochondrial cytochrome system of coccidia.

Uses/Indications - Decoquinate is labelled for use in cattle for the prevention of coccidiosis in either ruminating or non-ruminating calves, cattle or young goats caused by the species *E. christenseni* or *E. ninakohlyakimoviae* . It is used for prevention of coccidiosis in broilers caused by *E. tenella, E. necatrix, E. acervulina, E. mivati, E. maxima* or *E. burnetti.*

Pharmacokinetics - No information located.

Contraindications/Precautions/Reproductive Safety - Decoquinate is not effective for treating clinical coccidiosis and has no efficacy against adult coccidia. Decoquinate is not approved for use in animals producing milk for food or in laying chickens.

Adverse Effects/Warnings - No adverse effects listed when given as directed.

Overdosage/Acute Toxicity - No specific information located. Decoquinate is considered to have a wide safety margin.

Drug Interactions/Laboratory Considerations - None located.

Doses -
  Dogs:
    For coccidiosis:
      a) Prophylaxis: 50 mg/kg PO once daily (Matz 1995)
  Cattle:
    For prophylaxis of coccidiosis:
      a) Using the 6% premix: 0.5 mg/kg per day in feed for at least 28 days. (Penzhorn and Swan 1993) (McDougald and Roberson 1988)
  Goats:
    For prophylaxis of coccidiosis:
      a) 0.5 mg/kg per day in feed during periods of exposure. (Bretzlaff 1993)
  Llamas:
    For prophylaxis of coccidiosis:
      a) Using the 6% premix: 0.5 mg/kg per day in feed for at least 28 days. (Johnson 1993)

Client Information - Decoquinate should be used for at least 4 weeks when used for preventing coccidiosis outbreaks.

Dosage Forms/Preparations/FDA Approval Status/Withholding Times -
  Veterinary-Approved Products:
    Decoquinate 6% (27.2 grams per lb.) Feed Additive (with corn meal, soybean oil, lecithin and silicon dioxide) in 50 LB bags; *Deccox*® (Rhone-Poulenc); (OTC) Approved for use in cattle (not lactating dairy cattle), goats (not lactating dairy goats) and poultry (not laying chickens).

Decoquinate 10X (2.271 grams per lb.) Feed Additive (with vitamins A, D3, E) in 20 LB. buckets; *Deccox 10X®* (Vedco); (OTC) Approved for use in cattle (not lactating dairy cattle), goats (not lactating dairy goats).

Decoquinate 568 mg per pound Top Dress (with vitamins A, D3, E) in 20 LB buckets; *Deccox Top Dress®* (Vedco); (OTC) Approved for use in cattle (not lactating dairy cattle), goats (not lactating dairy goats).

Human-Approved Products: None

DEFEROXAMINE MESYLATE

Chemistry - An iron chelating agent, deferoxamine mesylate occurs as a white to off-white powder that is freely soluble in alcohol or water. Deferoxamine may also be known as desferoxamine mesylate or by the abbreviation DFO.

Storage/Stability/Compatibility - Store at room temperature. After reconstitution with sterile water for injection, the solution may be stored at room temperature, protected from light for up to one week. It is recommended not to mix this agent with other drugs; do not use if solution is turbid. Dilution in either normal saline, lactated Ringer's or dextrose 5% has been recommended when administering as an intravenous infusion.

Pharmacology - Deferoxamine (DFO) binds ferric (Fe^{+++}) ions to its three hydroxamic groups forming ferrioxamine. This forms a stable, water soluble compound that is readily excreted by the kidneys. DFO does not appear to chelate other trace metals (except aluminum) or electrolytes in clinically significant quantities.

Uses/Indications - Deferoxamine is used for the treatment of either acute or chronic iron toxicity. It is being evaluated as an iron chelator for adjunctive treatment of acute cardiac ischemia and as a chelator for aluminum toxicity.

Pharmacokinetics - DFO is poorly absorbed from the GI and is usually given parenterally. The drug is widely distributed in the body. DFO and ferrioxamine are excreted primarily in the urine. Ferrioxamine will give the urine a reddish color (*"vin rosé"*) which indicates iron removal.

Contraindications/Precautions/Reproductive Safety - DFO is contraindicated in patients with severe renal failure, unless dialysis is used to remove ferrioxamine.

Because deferoxamine has caused skeletal abnormalities in animals at dosages just above those recommended for iron toxicity, it should be used during pregnancy only when its benefits outweigh it risks.

Adverse Effects/Warnings - There is little veterinary experience with this drug. Potential adverse effects include, allergic reactions, auditory neurotoxicity (particularly with chronic, high-dose therapy), pain or swelling at injection sites, and GI distress. Too rapid IV injection may cause rapid heart rates, convulsions, hypotension, hives, and wheezing.

Oral administration of DFO is controversial. Some have recommended oral administration after oral iron ingestions, but DFO may actually increase the amount of iron absorbed from the gut. At present, oral sodium bicarbonate solution 5% given as a gastric lavage is probably a better treatment in reducing oral absorption of iron.

Overdosage/Acute Toxicity - See above adverse effects. Chronic high dose use may also lead to hypocalcemia and thrombocytopenia.

Drug Interactions - **Vitamin C** may be synergistic with deferoxamine in removing iron, but may in fact, lead to increased tissue iron toxicity especially in cardiac muscle. It should be used with caution, particularly in patients with preexisting cardiac disease.

Laboratory Considerations - DFO may interfere (falsely low values) with **colorimetric iron assays**. It may also cause falsely high **total iron binding capacity (TIBC)** measurements.

Doses -
Dogs/Cats:
In dogs at risk for, or exhibiting signs of severe iron toxicosis:
    a) Initiate ASAP or at least within 12 hours of ingestion; give as a constant rate infusion at 15 mg/kg/hour. More rapid infusion may precipitate arrhythmias or aggravate hypotension. If constant rate infusion is not possible or are unable to monitor pt. during infusion, give 40 mg/kg IM q4-8h, depending on clinical status. Continue therapy until serum iron levels are below 300 microliters/dl or decrease below the TIBC, whichever is lower. Chelation theRApy may require 2-3 days of therapy. Following recovery, monitor for signs of GI obstruction, which may develop 4-6 weeks post-ingestion. (Greentree and Hall 1995)

Experimentally, as a ferric ion chelator during treatment of cardiac arrest:
    a) 5 - 15 mg/kg IV, IM or SubQ. (Muir 1994)

    b)   10 mg/kg IV, IM q2h twice, then *tid* for 24 hours. (Hackett and Van pelt 1995)

Experimentally, as a ferric ion chelator to prevent re-perfusion injuries secondary to gastric dilatation volvulus (GDV):

    a)   50 mg/kg IV over 5 minutes (Lantz, Badylak et al. 1992)

Monitoring Parameters - For iron overload: 1) Efficacy (serum ferritin, serum iron, TIBC, are recommended to monitor iron overload); 2) Adverse effects (see above); additionally, if chronic iron overload: eye examinations (iron toxicity and its subsequent removal may adversely affect vision)

Dosage Forms/Preparations/FDA Approval Status/Withholding Times -
  Veterinary-Approved Products: None

  Human-Approved Products:

  Deferoxamine Mesylate Powder for Injection 500 mg vials; *Desferal® Mesylate* (Ciba); (Rx)

Dermcaps® - see Fatty Acids

DES — see Diethylstilbesterol

DESMOPRESSIN ACETATE

Chemistry - A synthetic polypeptide related to arginine vasopressin (antidiuretic hormone), desmopressin acetate occurs as a fluffy white powder having a bitter taste. The commercially available nasal solution has HCl added and the pH is approximately 4. This preparation also contains chlorobutonal 0.5% as a preservative.

Storage/Stability/Compatibility - The nasal solution should be stored in the refrigerator (2-8°C). It has an expiration date of one year after manufacture. While the nasal solution should be stored in the refrigerator, it is stable at room temperature for 3 weeks in the unopened bottle. The product for injection should be stored refrigerated (4°C); do not freeze.

Pharmacology - Desmopressin is related structurally to arginine vasopressin, but it has more antidiuretic activity and less vasopressor properties on a per weight basis. Desmopressin increases water reabsorption by the collecting ducts in the kidneys, thereby increasing urine osmolality and decreasing net urine production. Therapeutic doses do not directly affect either urinary sodium or potassium excretion.

  Desmopressin also causes a dose-dependent increase in plasma factor VIII and plasminogen factor. It also causes smaller increases in factor VIII-related antigen and ristocetin cofactor activities.

Uses/Indications - Desmopressin has been found to be useful in the treatment of central diabetes insipidus in small animals. It may be useful in treating Von Willebrand's disease, but its short duration of activity (2-4 hours) in this condition, resistance development, and expense limit its usefulness for this disorder.

Pharmacokinetics - Because desmopressin is destroyed in the GI tract, it must be given parenterally or topically. In humans, intranasal administration is commonly used, while in veterinary medicine topical administration to the conjunctiva is preferred. The onset of antidiuretic action in dogs usually occurs within one hour of administration, peaks in 2-8 hours and may persist for up to 24 hours. Distribution characteristics of desmopressin are not well described, but it does enter maternal milk. The metabolic fate is also not well understood. Terminal half lives in humans after IV administration are from 0.4 - 4 hours.

Contraindications/Precautions/Reproductive Safety - Desmopressin is contraindicated in patients hypersensitive to it. It should not be used for treatment of type IIB or platelet-type (pseudo) Von Willebrand's disease as platelet-aggregation and thrombocytopenia may occur. German shorthair pointers apparently can have this type of vWD. Desmopressin should be used with caution in patient's susceptible to thrombotic events.

  Safe use during pregnancy has not been established; however safe doses of up to 125 times the average human antidiuretic dose have been given to rats and rabbits without demonstration of fetal harm.

Adverse Effects/Warnings - Side effects in small animals apparently are uncommon. Occasionally eye irritation may occur after conjunctival administration. Hypersensitivity reactions are possible. Humans using the drug have complained about increased headache frequency.

Overdosage/Acute Toxicity - Dosages that are too high may lead to fluid retention and hyponatremia. Dosage reduction and fluid restriction may be employed to treat. Adequate monitoring should be performed.

Drug Interactions - **Chlorpropamide, carbamazepine, clofibrate, fludrocortisone,** or **urea** may enhance the antidiuretic effects of desmopressin. **Lithium,** large doses of **epinephrine, demeclocycline, heparin or alcohol** may decrease the antidiuretic effects of desmopressin.

Laboratory Considerations - See Monitoring Parameters

Doses -
  Dogs:
      For treatment of diabetes insipidus:
          a) Initially, 1 - 2 micrograms SubQ or 1 - 2 drops of the nasal spray intraconjunctivally once or twice daily respectively. Adjust dose as necessary. Watch for signs of water intoxication and hyponatremia. (Nichols 1992)
          b) 1 - 4 drops topically of the nasal solution in the conjunctival sac every 12-24 hours. Adjust dose to control polyuria/polydipsia. (Randolph and Peterson 1994)

      For treatment of Von Willebrand's disease:
          a) 1 micrograms/kg SubQ gives a duration of action of 3-4 hours; repeated dosages within 24 hours does not prolong response time. (Brooks 1994)

  Cats:
      To help differentiate central diabetes insipidus from the nephrogenic form: 1 drop into the conjunctival sac twice daily for 2-3 days; a dramatic reduction in water intake or a 50% or greater increase in urine concentration gives strong evidence for a deficit in ADH production. For treatment of central DI: 1 - 2 drops into the conjunctival sac once or twice a day; duration of activity 8-24 hours. (Bruyette 1991)

Monitoring Parameters - For Central DI: Serum electrolytes, urine osmolality and/or urine volume; For Von Willebrand's disease: Bleeding times

Client Information - Keep solutions refrigerated whenever possible. Instruct clients on the importance of compliance with this drug; it is a treatment, not a cure for the condition. Clients should be counseled on the expense associated with using this drug long-term.

Dosage Forms/Preparations/FDA Approval Status/Withholding Times -
  Veterinary-Approved Products: None
  Human-Approved Products:
  Desmopressin Acetate Nasal Solution 10 micrograms/0.1 ml metered dose (0.01%) in 2.5 or 5 ml bottles and 1.5 mg/ml in 2.5 ml bottles *DDAVP® Nasal Spray* (Rhone-Poulenc Rorer); (Rx);*Stimate®* (Armour) (Rx)

  Desmopressin Acetate Parenteral Injection 4 micrograms/ml in 1 ml amps and 10 ml multiple dose vials; *DDAVP®* (Rhone-Poulenc Rorer); (Rx)

  Desmopressin Acetate Tablets 0.1 mg & 0.2 mg *DDAVP®* (Rhone-Poulenc Rorer) (Rx)

DESOXYCORTICOSTERONE PIVALATE
DOCP

Chemistry - A mineralocorticoid, desoxycorticosterone pivalate (DOCP) occurs as a white or creamy white powder that is odorless and stable in air. It is practically insoluble in water, slightly soluble in alcohol and vegetable oils. The injectable product is a white aqueous suspension and has a pH between 5 - 8.5.

Storage/Stability/Compatibility - Store the injectable suspension at room temperature and protect from light or freezing. Do not mix with any other agent.

Pharmacology - Desoxycorticosterone pivalate (DOCP) is a long-acting mineralocorticoid agent. The site of action of mineralocorticoids is at the renal distal tubule where it increases the absorption of sodium. Mineralocorticoids also enhance potassium and hydrogen ion excretion. To be effective, mineralocorticoids require a functioning kidney.

Uses/Indications - DOCP is indicated for the treatment of adrenocortical insufficiency in dogs.

Pharmacokinetics - Little information is available. It is injected IM as a microcrystalline depot for slow dissolution into the circulation. DOCP usually has a duration of action in dogs for 21-30 days after injection.

Contraindications/Precautions/Reproductive Safety - The drug is labeled as being contraindicated in dogs suffereing from congestive hear failure, severe renal disease or edema.

  The manufacturer states that the drug should not be used in pregnanat dogs as safe use during pregnancy has not been established; use in pregnant animals when the potential benefits outweigh the risks.

Adverse Effects/Warnings - Occasionally, irritation at the site of injection may occur. Adverse effects of DOCP are generally a result of excessive dosage (see Overdosage below). Because some animals may be more (or less) sensitive to the effects of the drug, "cookbook" dosing without ongoing monitoring is inappropriate. Some animals may require additional supplementation with a glucocorticoid agent on an ongoing basis. All animals with hypoadrenocorticism should receive additional glucocorticoids (2-10 times basal) during periods of stress or acute illness.

Do not administer DOCP IV as acute collapse and shock may result. If given IV, treat immediately for shock with IV fluids and glucocorticoids.

Overdosage/Acute Toxicity - Overdosage may cause polyuria, polydipsia, hypernatremia, hypertension, edema and hypokalemia. Cardiac enlargement is possible with prolonged overdoses. Electrolytes should be aggressively monitored and potassium may need to be supplemented. Patients should have the drug discontinued until symptoms and signs associated with overdosage have resolved and then restart the drug at a lower dosage.

Drug Interactions - Patients may develop hypokalemia if mineralocorticoids are administered concomitantly with **amphotericin B** or **potassium-depleting diuretics** (*e.g.,* thiazides, furosemide). As **diuretics** can cause a loss of sodium, they may counteract the effects DOCP.

Potentially, DOCP could increase the **insulin** requirements of diabetic patients or reduce **salicylate** blood levels. The clinical significance of these potential interactions with DOCP have not been determined.

Because DOCP may cause hypokalemia, it should be used with caution and with increased monitoring when used in patients receiving **digitalis glycosides**.

Doses -
  Dogs:
    Note: Dosage requirements are variable and should be individualized to the patient.
    For hypoadrenocorticism:
      a) Initially, inject 2.2 mg/kg IM every 25 days. Monitor (serum potassium and sodium) and adjust as necessary. Most patients are well controlled at doses of 1.1 - 2.2 mg/kg given every 21-30 days. (Proposed Package Insert for DOCP. **Note:** Not final and not FDA-approved; refer to actual package insert for approved dose)
      b) Initially, inject 2.2 mg/kg IM every 25 days. Because it has little or no glucocorticoid activity, add prednisone or prednisolone at 0.2 mg/kg PO daily. Adjust dosages until dog is stable and otherwise healthy. Then slowly reduce glucocorticoid to a minimal or zero dosage. Perhaps one-half of all dogs will require no routine glucocorticoid, but should have it available for emergencies. Monitor (serum potassium and sodium, BUN) and adjust as necessary. (Feldman, Nelson et al. 1992)
      c) 1 - 2 mg/kg IM every 3-4 weeks (some dogs require up to 3 mg/kg) (Nichols, Peterson et al. 1994)

Monitoring Parameters - 1) Serum electrolytes, BUN, creatinine; initially every 1-2 weeks, then once stabilized every 3-4 months; 2) Weight, PE for edema

Client Information - Clients should be familiar with the symptoms associated with both hypoadrenocorticism (*e.g.,* weakness, depression, anorexia, vomiting, diarrhea, etc.) and DOCP overdosage (*e.g.,* edema) and report these to the veterinarian immediately. If client is injecting the drug at home, instruct in proper technique for IM administration. Vial should be shaken vigorously to suspend the microcrystals.

Dosage Forms/Preparations/FDA Approval Status -
  Veterinary-Approved Products:
    Desoxycorticosterone Pivalate Injectable Suspension 25 mg/ml in 4 ml vials; *Percorten-V®* (Novartis); (Rx) Approved for use in dogs.

  Human-Approved Products: None

DETOMIDINE HCL

Chemistry - An imidazoline derivative alpha$_2$-adrenergic agonist, detomidine HCl occurs as a white crystalline substance that is soluble in water.

Storage/Stability/Compatibility - Detomidine HCl for injection should be stored at room temperature (15-30°C) and be protected from light.

Pharmacology - Detomidine, like xylazine is an alpha$_2$-adrenergic agonist that produces a dose-dependent sedative and analgesic effect, but also has cardiac and respiratory effects. For more information refer to the xylazine monograph or the adverse effects section below.

Uses/Indications - At the present time detomidine is only approved for use as a sedative analgesic in horses, but it also has been used clinically in other species.

Pharmacokinetics - Detomidine is well absorbed after oral administration, but is used only parenterally at the present time. The drug is apparently rapidly distributed into tissues, including the brain after parenteral administration and is extensively metabolized and then excreted primarily into the urine.

Contraindications/Precautions/Reproductive Safety - Detomidine is contraindicated in horses with preexisting AV or SA heart block, severe coronary insufficiency, cerebrovascular disease, respiratory disease or chronic renal failure. It should be used with caution in animals with endotoxic or traumatic shock or approaching shock, and advanced hepatic or renal disease. Horses who are stressed due to temperature extremes, fatigue, or high altitude should also receive the drug with caution.

Although animals may appear to be deeply sedated, some may respond to external stimuli; use appropriate caution. The manufacturer recommends allowing the horse to stand quietly for 5 minutes prior to injection and for 10-15 minutes after injection to improve the effect of the drug. After administering detomidine, protect the animal from temperature extremes.

Adverse Effects/Warnings - Detomidine can cause an initial rise in blood pressure which is then followed by bradycardia and heart block. Atropine at 0.02 mg/kg IV has been successfully used to prevent or correct the bradycardia that may be seen when the detomidine is used at labeled dosages. Also, piloerection, sweating, salivation, slight muscle tremors, and penile prolapse may all be noted after injection.

Overdosage/Acute Toxicity - The manufacturer states that detomidine is tolerated by horses at doses 5 times (0.2 mg/kg) the high dose level (0.04 mg/kg). Doses of 0.4 mg/kg given daily for 3 consecutive days produced microscopic foci of myocardial necrosis in 1 of 8 horses tested. Doses of 10-40 times those recommended can cause severe respiratory and cardiovascular changes which can become irreversible and cause death. Yohimbine theoretically could be used to reverse some or all of the effects of the drug, but not enough clinical experience has been reported to make any recommendations for its use at this time.

Drug Interactions - The manufacturer warns against using this agent with intravenous **potentiated sulfonamides (e.g., trimethoprim/sulfa)** as fatal dysrhythmias may occur, and to use with extreme caution in combination with **other sedative or analgesic drugs**. Because this is a relatively new drug, more interactions may be forthcoming; refer to the xylazine monograph for more information on interactions with alpha$_2$-adrenergic agonists.

Doses -
  Horses:
    For sedation/analgesia:
      a) 20 - 40 micrograms/kg (0.02 - 0.04 mg/kg) IV or IM (IV only for analgesia). Effects generally occur within 2-5 minutes. Lower dose will generally provide 30-90 minutes of sedation and 30-45 minutes of analgesia. The higher dose will generally provide 90-120 minutes of sedation and 45-75 minutes of analgesia. Allow animal to rest quietly prior to and after injection. (Package insert; *Dormosedan®*—SKB)

  Cattle:
    For sedation/analgesia:
      a) 30 - 60 micrograms/kg (0.03 - 0.06 mg/kg) IV or IM (Not approved). (Alitalo 1986)

Monitoring Parameters -
  1) Level of sedation, analgesia
  2) Cardiac rate/rhythm; blood pressure if indicated

Client Information - This drug should be used in a professionally supervised setting by individuals familiar with its properties.

Dosage Forms/Preparations/FDA Approval Status/Withholding Times -
  Veterinary-Approved Products:
  Detomidine HCl for Injection 10 mg/ml in 5 and 20 ml vials
    Dormosedan® (Pfizer); (Rx) Approved for use in horses.
    The trade name, *Domosedan®* may be used in countries outside of the United States.

  Human-Approved Products: None

DEXAMETHASONE
DEXAMETHASONE SODIUM PHOSPHATE
DEXAMETHASONE 21-ISONICOTINATE

Note: For more information refer to the monograph: Glucocorticoids, General Information.

Chemistry - A synthetic glucocorticoid, dexamethasone occurs as an odorless, white to practically white, crystalline powder that melts with some decomposition at about 250°C. It is practically insoluble in water and sparingly soluble in alcohol. Dexamethasone sodium phosphate occurs as an odorless or having a slight odor, white to slightly yellow, hygroscopic powder. One gram of is soluble in about 2 ml of water; it is slightly soluble in alcohol. Dexamethasone 21-isonicotinate occurs as a nearly odorless and tasteless, white to slight yellow, crystalline powder.

1.3 mg of dexamethasone sodium phosphate is equivalent to 1 mg of dexamethasone; 4 mg/ml of dexamethasone sodium phosphate injection is approximately equivalent to 3 mg/ml of dexamethasone.

Storage/Stability/Compatibility - Dexamethasone is heat labile and should be stored at room temperature (15-30°C) unless otherwise directed by the manufacturer. Dexamethasone sodium phosphate injection should be protected from light. Dexamethasone tablets should be stored in well-closed containers.

Dexamethasone sodium phosphate for injection is reportedly **compatible** with the following drugs: amikacin sulfate, aminophylline, bleomycin sulfate, cimetidine HCl, glycopyrrolate, lidocaine HCl, nafcillin sodium, netilmicin sulfate, prochlorperazine edisylate and verapamil.

It is reportedly **incompatible** with: daunorubicin HCl, doxorubicin HCl, metaraminol bitartrate, and vancomycin. Compatibility is dependent upon factors such as pH, concentration, temperature and diluents used. It is suggested to consult specialized references for more specific information (*e.g., Handbook on Injectable Drugs* by Trissel; see bibliography).

Contraindications/Precautions - Because dexamethasone has negligible mineralocorticoid effect, it should generally not be used alone in the treatment of adrenal insufficiency. For more information refer to the Glucocorticoid monograph.

Doses -
  Dogs:
    Low-Dose Dexamethasone Suppression Test:
      a) Draw pre-sample. Inject 0.01 - 0.015 mg/kg dexamethasone IV (may dilute dexamethasone 1:10 with sterile saline to insure accurate dosing). Collect samples at 4 hrs. and 8 hrs. post dexamethasone. Usual pre-dose cortisol normals: 0.5 - 4.0 micrograms/dl; post-dexamethasone normals: less than 1.5 micrograms/dl. (Kemppainen and Zerbe 1989a)
      b) Draw pre-sample in AM. Inject 0.01 mg/kg dexamethasone sodium phosphate IV. Draw sample 8 hours post injection. (Feldman 1989), (Morgan 1988), (Feldman, Schrader, and Twedt 1988)

    High-Dose Dexamethasone Suppression Test:
      a) Draw pre-dose sample. Inject 0.1 or 1.0 mg/kg IV dexamethasone. Draw post-dose samples at 4 hours and 8 hours. Use 1.0 mg/kg dose if not suppressed at lower dose (0.1 mg/kg). Use 1.0 mg/kg dose with caution in patients with diabetes mellitus and if cortisol values are greater than 12 micrograms/dl. (Kemppainen and Zerbe 1989a)
      b) Draw pre-dose sample. Administer 0.1 mg/kg IV dexamethasone sodium phosphate. Draw second sample 8 hours post injection. (Feldman 1989)
      c) Draw pre-dose sample. Administer 0.1 mg/kg IV dexamethasone sodium phosphate. Draw second sample 4 hours post injection. (Morgan 1988)
      d) Draw pre-dose sample. Administer 0.1 mg/kg IV dexamethasone sodium phosphate. Draw second sample 4 or 8 hours post injection. (Feldman, Schrader, and Twedt 1988)

    Combined Dexamethasone Suppression-ACTH Stimulation test:
    (Note: Many clinicians do not recommend using this test)
      a) Draw pre-dose sample. Administer 0.1 mg/kg IV dexamethasone; collect post-dexamethasone sample 4 hours later. Immediately give ACTH (gel) 2.2 IU/kg IM. Collect post-ACTH sample 2 hours later. (Kemppainen and Zerbe 1989a)

    For toy breed dogs with hydrocephalus:
      a) 0.25 mg/kg *tid - qid*; reduce dose slowly over 2-4 weeks. (Simpson 1989)

    For adjunctive therapy of craniocerebral/spinal trauma:
      a) If patient's condition is not improved 30 minutes after receiving water soluble glucocorticoids: 2 mg/kg by slow IV infusion. If patient continues to deteriorate, additional therapy is warranted. (Shores 1989)
      b) Initially, 0.2 mg/kg bolus, then 0.2 mg/kg daily in 2-3 divided doses. If animal is in shock, give 2.0 mg/kg initially. (Fenner 1986a)
      c) For spinal cord trauma: 2 - 3 mg/kg IV followed in 6-8 hours by 1 mg/kg SQ or IV *bid-tid* for 24 hours. Then 0.2 mg/kg SQ or IV *bid-tid* for 2-3 days. Then 0.1 mg/kg IV or SQ *bid-tid* for 3-5 days. (Schunk 1988a)

    To reduce intracerebral pressure and edema:
      a) In the palliative therapy of intracranial neoplasms: 0.25 - 2.0 mg/kg q6h IV in acute episodes .(LeCouteur and Turrel 1986)
      b) In the adjunctive therapy of status epilepticus: 2 mg/kg IV initially; repeat in 6-8 hours with 1 mg/kg. Follow with tapering doses. (Schunk 1988b)

For adjunctive therapy of fibrocartilaginous embolic myopathy:
    a) 2.2 mg/kg IV, then 6-8 hours later give 1 mg/kg SQ. Repeat 1 mg/kg SQ in 12 hours, then give 0.1 mg/kg SQ *bid* for 3-5 days. (Schunk 1988a)

For patients with thoracolumbar intervertebral disk disease and acute onset of paraparesis:
    a) 2 mg/kg IV followed in 6-8 hours with 0.5 - 1.0 mg/kg SQ, *bid-tid* for 24 hours, then 0.1 mg/kg SQ or PO *bid* for 3-5 days. (Schunk 1988a)

For medical therapy of cervical spondylopathy:
    a) With an acute onset or sudden worsening with moderate to marked tetraparesis: 2.2 mg/kg IV once followed in 6-8 hours by 1 mg/kg SQ *bid* for two doses. Then 0.1 - 0.2 mg/kg PO or SQ twice a day for 3-5 days. (Schunk 1988a)

For adjunctive therapy of shock:
    a) Dexamethasone sodium phosphate: 4 - 6 mg/kg IV (Kemppainen 1986)

For initial adjunctive treatment of acute adrenocortical collapse:
    a) Dexamethasone: 0.5 - 1.0 mg/kg IV or Dexamethasone Sodium phosphate 2 - 4 mg/kg IV. (Schrader 1986), (Feldman, Schrader, and Twedt 1988)

For treatment of acquired thrombocytopenia:
    a) 0.25 - 0.3 mg/kg IV or SQ once, then 0.1 - 0.15 mg/kg SQ or PO twice a day for 7 days. Decrease oral dose by 1/2 every 5-7 days for 3 weeks, then go to alternate day therapy for 6 weeks. (Dodds 1988)

For adjunctive therapy of endotoxemia secondary to acute gastric dilatation-volvulus:
    a) 5 mg/kg slowly IV (Bellah 1988)

For adjunctive therapy of cholecalciferol (*Quintox®*, *Rampage®*) toxicity:
    a) 1 mg/kg SQ divided *qid* (Grauer and Hjelle 1988b)

For labeled indications (anti-inflammatory/glucocorticoid agent) for dexamethasone injection (*Azium®*):
    a) 0.5 - 1 mg IV or IM; may be repeated for 3-5 days. (Package Insert; *Azium®*— Schering)

For labeled indications (anti-inflammatory/glucocorticoid agent) for dexamethasone tablets (*Azium®*):
    a) 0.25 - 1.25 mg daily in single or two divided doses (Package Insert; *Azium® Tablets*— Schering)

For labeled indications (various inflammatory conditions associated with the musculoskeletal system) for dexamethasone 21-isonicotinate (*Voren®*):
    a) 0.25 - 1 mg IM; may repeat for 3-5 days. (Package Insert; *Voren®*— Bio-ceutic)

Cats:
High-Dose Dexamethasone Suppression Test:
    a) As a screening test for feline hyperadrenocorticism: 0.1 mg/kg IV. A dose of 1 mg/kg IV may differentiate pituitary-dependent hyperadrenocorticism (PDH) from an adrenal tumor. (Zerbe 1989)

Combined Dexamethasone Suppression-ACTH Stimulation test:
    a) Collect blood sample, then give dexamethasone 0.1 mg IV, collect sample 2 hours after dexamethasone. Immediately give ACTH (2.2 IU/kg) and collect samples 1 and 2 hours post ACTH. (Zerbe 1989)

For endotoxic or septicemic shock:
    a) Dexamethasone sodium succinate: 5 mg/kg IV (Jenkins 1985)

As adjunctive therapy for feline neoplasias (lymphosarcoma, acute lymphoid leukemia, mast cell neoplasms):
    a) 2 - 6 mg/m^2 q24-48h PO, SQ or IV (Couto 1989)

For adjunctive emergency treatment of feline asthma:
    a) 1 mg/kg IV (sodium phosphate salt) (Noone 1986)

For chronic therapy of feline allergic bronchitis:
    a) 0.25 mg PO once to 3 times daily. Once patient stabilizes, attempt to reduce dose; keep on alternate-day therapy for at least 1-2 months after symptoms have initially resolved. (Bauer 1988)

For alternative therapy for idiopathic feline miliary dermatitis:
    a) 1 mg PO once daily for 7 days, then 1 mg PO twice a week. May need to add progestational agent. (Kwochka 1986)

For labeled indications (anti-inflammatory agent) for dexamethasone injection (*Azium®*):

a) 0.125 - 0.5 mg IV or IM; may be repeated for 3-5 days. (Package Insert; *Azium*®—Schering)

For labeled indications (anti-inflammatory/glucocorticoid agent) for dexamethasone tablets (*Azium*®):

a) 0.125 - 0.5 mg daily in single or divided doses (Package Insert; *Azium*® *Tablets*—Schering)

For labeled indications (various inflammatory conditions associated with the musculoskeletal system) for dexamethasone 21-isonicotinate (*Voren*®):

a) 0.125 - 0.5 mg IM; may repeat for 3-5 days. (Package Insert; *Voren*®— Bio-ceutic)

Cattle:

For adjunctive therapy of insect bites or stings:

a) 2 mg/kg IM or IV q4h (use epinephrine if anaphylaxis develops) (Fowler 1993)

For adjunctive therapy of cerebral edema secondary to polioencephalomalacia:

a) 1 - 2 mg/kg intravenously (Dill 1986)

For adjunctive therapy of radial nerve injury, or femoral nerve paralysis:

a) Adult cattle (400-800 kg and not pregnant): 20 - 40 mg IM or IV; Calves: 10 mg IM or IV. Taper or discontinue therapy in 2-3 days. Many cases require only a single dose. (Rebhun 1986)

For adjunctive therapy of obturator nerve paralysis:

a) 10 - 40 mg parenterally once daily for 2-3 days then discontinue. (Rebhun 1986)

For adjunctive therapy of peroneal nerve injuries:

a) 10 - 30 mg parenterally for acute cases when not contraindicated due to pregnancy or infection. (Rebhun 1986)

For elective inducement of parturition or termination of pregnancy:

a) For abortion: 25 mg parenterally with 25 mg prostaglandin $F_{2\alpha}$ after 150 days of gestation. For inducement or parturition from 8th month of gestation on: 20 mg IM. (Drost 1986)

b) For inducement of parturition when given within 2 weeks of normal term: 20 - 30 mg IM (Barth 1986)

For adjunctive therapy of aseptic laminitis:

a) 5 - 20 mg IM or IV; continue therapy for 2-3 days (Berg 1986)

For primary bovine ketosis:

a) 5 - 20 mg IV or IM (Package Insert; *Azium*®— Schering)

Horses:

For glucocorticoid therapy:

a) 0.05 - 0.2 mg/kg once daily IV, IM or PO (Robinson 1987)

Dexamethasone suppression test:

a) 20 mg IM. Normal values: Cortisol levels decrease 50% in 2 hours, 70% in 4 hours, and 80% at 6 hours. At 24 hours levels are still depressed about 30% of original value. (Beech 1987b)

For labeled indications (various inflammatory conditions associated with the musculoskeletal system) for dexamethasone 21-isonicotinate (*Voren*®):

a) 5 - 20 mg IM; may repeat. (Package Insert; *Voren*®— Bio-ceutic)

For labeled indications (anti-inflammatory/glucocorticoid agent) for dexamethasone injection (*Azium*®):

a) 2.5 - 5 mg IV or IM. (Package Insert; *Azium*®— Schering)

For labeled indications (anti-inflammatory/glucocorticoid agent) for dexamethasone sodium phosphate injection (*Azium*®-*SP*):

a) 2.5 - 5 mg IV. (Package Insert; *Azium*®— Schering)

Swine:

For glucocorticoid therapy:

a) 1 - 10 mg IV or IM (Howard 1986)

Llamas:

For adjunctive therapy of anaphylaxis:

a) 2 mg/kg IV (Smith 1989)

Birds:
> For shock, trauma, gram negative endotoxemia:
>> a) Dexamethasone 2 mg/ml injection: 2 - 4 mg/kg IM or IV once, twice or three times daily. Taper off drug when using long-term. (Clubb 1986)

Reptiles:
> a) For septic shock in most species: Using Dexamethasone Sodium Phosphate:0.1 - 0.25 mg/kg IV or IM (Gauvin 1993)

Dosage Forms/Preparations/Approval Status/Withdrawal Times-
Veterinary-Approved Products:

Dexamethasone Oral Tablets 0.25 mg; *Azium*® *Tablets* (Schering), generic; (Rx) Approved for use in dogs and cats

Dexamethasone Chewable Tablets; *Pet-Derm III* ® (Pfizer) (Rx). 0.25 mg scored tablets. Approved for dogs only.

Dexamethasone Injection 2 mg/ml; *Azium*® *Solution* (Schering),*Dexameth-a-Vet*® (Anthony) (Rx) generic; (Rx) Approved for use in dogs, cats, horses and cattle. There are no withdrawal times required when used in cattle.

Dexamethasone Sodium Phosphate Injection 4 mg/ml (equivalent to 3 mg/ml dexamethasone); *Azium*® *SP Injection* (Schering), *Dex-A-Vet Injection* (Anthony), generic; (Rx) Approved for use in horses.

Human-Approved Products: All require a presecription (Rx); many different trade named products are available.
Tablets: 0.25 mg, 0.5 mg, 0.75 mg, 1 mg, 1.5 mg, 2 mg, 4 mg, & 6 mg
Oral Elixir/Solution: 0.5 mg/5 ml, 0.5 mg/0.5 ml
Dexamethasone Acetate Injection: 8 mg/ml, 16 mg/ml
Dexamethasone Sodium Phosphate Injection: 4 mg/ml, 10 mg/ml, 20 mg/ml, 24 mg/ml

DEXPANTHENOL
D-PANTHENOL

Chemistry - The alcohol of D-pantothenic acid, dexpanthenol occurs as a slightly bitter-tasting, clear, viscous, somewhat hygroscopic liquid. It is freely soluble in water or alcohol.

Storage/Stability/Compatibility - Dexpanthenol should be protected from both freezing and excessive heat. It is incompatible with strong acids and alkalis.

Pharmacology - A precursor to pantothenic acid, dexpanthenol acts as a precursor to coenzyyme A which is necessary for acetylation reactions to occur during gluconeogenesis and in the production acetylcholine. It has been postulated that post-surgical ileus can be prevented by giving high doses of dexpanthenol by assuring adequate levels of acetylcholine. However, one study in normal horses (Adams, Lamar, and Masty 1984) failed to demonstrate any effect of dexpanthenol on peristalsis.

Uses/Indications - Dexpanthenol has been suggested for use in intestinal atony or distension, postoperative retention of flatus and feces, prophylaxis and treatment of paralytic ileus after abdominal surgery or traumatic injuries, equine colic (not due to mechanical obstruction) and any other condition when there is an impairment of smooth muscle function. Controlled studies are lacking with regard to proving the efficacy of the drug for any of these indications.

Pharmacokinetics - Dexpanthenol is rapidly converted to pantothenic acid *in vivo*, which is widely distributed throughout the body, primarily as coenzyme A.

Contraindications/Precautions - Dexpanthenol is contraindicated in ileus secondary to mechanical obstruction or in cases of colic caused by the treatment of cholinergic anthelmintics. It is also contraindicated in humans with hemophilia as it may exacerbate bleeding.
Safety in use during pregnancy has not been established.

Adverse Effects/Warnings - Adverse reactions are reportedly rare. Hypersensitivity reactions have been reported in humans, but may have been due to the preservative agents found in the injectable product. Potentially, GI cramping and diarrhea are possible.

Overdosage - The drug is considered non-toxic even when administered in high doses.

Drug Interactions - The manufacturer's have recommended that dexpanthenol not be administered within 12 hours of **neostigmine** or other parasympathomimetic agents and within 1 hour of receiving **succinylcholine**. The clinical significance of these potential interactions have not been documented, however.

Doses -
Dogs, Cats:
> a) 11 mg/kg IM; repeat if indicated at 4-6 hour intervals (Rossoff 1974)

b) 11 mg/kg IM; may be repeated in 2 hours after initial injection and followed every 6-8 hours until condition is alleviated. The time interval and duration of therapy will depend upon the degree of severity that the animal is exhibiting from the clinical standpoint. (Label Instructions; d-Panthenol Injectable - Vedco)

Horses:
a) 2.5 grams IV or IM; repeat if indicated at 4-6 hour intervals (Rossoff 1974), (Label Instructions; d-Panthenol Injectable - Vedco)

Monitoring Parameters -
1) Clinical Efficacy

Client Information - Should be used in a professionally-monitored situation where gastrointestinal motility can be monitored.

Dosage Forms/Preparations/FDA Approval Status/Withholding Times -
Veterinary-Approved Products:
Dexpanthenol Injection 250 mg/ml in 100 ml vials (Veterinary labeled)
Generic; (Rx) Approved for use in dogs, cats, and horses.

Human-Approved Products:
Dexpanthenol Injection 250 mg/ml in 2 ml amps, 2 ml & 10 ml vials, UD Stat-Pak 2 ml disp syringes; *Ilopan*® (Adria), Generic; (Rx)

Dextrose — see the appendix (Tables of Parenteral Fluids)

DEXTRAN 70

Note: Dextran is also available as Dextran 40 and Dextran 75. Because Dextran 70 is the most commonly version used in veterinary medicine, the following monograph is limited to it alone.

Chemistry - A branched polysaccharide used intravenously as a plasma volume expander, dextran 70 occurs as a white to light yellow amorphous powder. It is freely soluble in water and insoluble in alcohol. Dextran 70 contains (on average) molecules of 70,000 daltons. Each 500 ml of the commercially available 6% dextran 70 in normal saline provides 77 mEq of sodium.

Storage/Stability/Compatibility - Dextran 70 injection should be stored at room temperature; preferably in an area with little temperature variability. While only clear solutions should be used, dextran flakes can form but can be resolubolized by heating the solution in a boiling water bath until clear, or autoclaving at 110°C for 15 minutes. Dextran 70 is compatible with many other solutions and drugs; refer to specialized references (e.g. Trissel) for more information.

Pharmacology - Dextran 70 has osmotic effects similarly to albumin. Dextran's colloidal osmotic effect draws fluid into the vascular system from the interstitial spaces, resulting in increased circulating blood volume.

Uses/Indications - Dextran 70 is a relatively low cost colloid for the adjunctive treatment of hypovolemic shock.

Pharmacokinetics - After IV infusion, circulating blood volume is increased maximally within one hour and effects can persist for 24 hours or more. Approximately 20-30% of a given dose remains in the intravascular compartment at 24 hours and it may be detected in the blood 4-6 weeks after dosing. Dextran 70 is slowly degraded to glucose by dextranase in the spleen and then metabolized to carbon dioxide and water. A small amount may be excreted directly into the gut and eliminated in the feces.

Contraindications/Precautions/Reproductive Safety - Patients overly susceptible to circulatory overload (severe heart or renal failure) should receive dextran 70 with great caution. Dextran 70 is contraindicated in patients with severe coagulopathies and should be used with caution in patients with thrombocytopenia as it can interfere with platelet function. Do not give dextran IM. Patients on strict sodium restriction should receive dextran cautiously as a 500 ml bag contains 77 mEq of sodium

Adverse Effects/Warnings - Moderate to life threatening reactions appear to rare in the dog. Dextran 70 may increase bleeding time and decrease von Willebrand's factor antigen and factor VIII activity. This apparently does not usually cause clinical bleeding in dogs.

Anaphylactoid reactions are not that rare in humans, but apparently are very rare in dogs. Dextran 70 has only been rarely associated with acute renal failure, unlike dextran 40. In humans, GI effects (abdominal pain, nausea/vomiting) have been reported with use of dextran 70.

Overdosage - The drug should be dosed and monitored carefully as volume overload may result.

Drug Interactions - Dextran reportedly has no drug interactions that are clinically significant.

Lab Interactions - Dextran 70 may interfere with **blood cross-matching** as it can cross-link with red blood cells and appear as rouleaux formation. Isotonic saline may be used to negate this effect. Blood **glucose** levels may be increased as dextran is degraded. Falsely elevated **bilirubin** levels may be noted; reason unknown.

Doses -

Dogs:

a) Up to 40 ml/kg/day; not to be infused faster than 5 ml/kg/hr (Haskins 1992)

b) 20 ml/kg; bolus to effect (Eastlake and Snyder 1998)

Monitoring Parameters - Other than the regular monitoring performed in patients that would require volume expansion therapy, there is no inordinate monitoring required specific to dextran therapy.

Dosage Forms/Preparations/FDA Approval Status -

Veterinary-Approved Products: None

Human-Approved Products:

6% Dextran-70 in normal saline (0.9% NaCl) in 500 ml; *Dextran 70* (McGaw); *Gentran® 70* (Baxter) *Macrodex®* (Medisan); (Rx)

6% Dextran-70 in D5W in 500 ml; *Macrodex®* (Medisan); (Rx)

DIAZEPAM

Chemistry - A benzodiazepine, diazepam is a white to yellow, practically odorless crystalline powder with a melting point between 131°-135°C and pK_a of 3.4. Diazepam is tasteless initially, but a bitter after-taste develops. One gram is soluble in 333 ml of water, 25 ml of alcohol, and it is sparingly soluble in propylene glycol. The pH of the commercially prepared injectable solution is adjusted with benzoic acid/sodium benzoate to 6.2-6.9. It consists of a 5 mg/ml solution with 40% propylene glycol, 10% ethanol, 5% sodium benzoate/benzoic acid buffer, and 1.5% benzyl alcohol as a preservative.

Storage/Stability/Compatibility - All diazepam products should be stored at room temperature (15°-30°C). The injection should be kept from freezing and protected from light. The oral dosage forms (tablets/capsules) should be stored in tight containers and protected from light.

Because diazepam may adsorb to plastic, it should not be stored drawn up into plastic syringes. The drug may also significantly adsorb to IV solution plastic (PVC) bags and to the infusion tubing. This adsorption appears to be dependent on several factors (temperature, concentration, flow rates, line length, etc.).

The manufacturers of injectable diazepam do not recommend the drug be mixed with any other medication or IV diluent. The drug has been successfully diluted to concentrations of 5 mg/50 ml or 5 mg/100 ml in normal saline, lactated Ringer's and D5W. Differing results have occurred with different manufacturer's products. Do not administer if a precipitate forms and does not clear.

Pharmacology - The subcortical levels (primarily limbic, thalamic, and hypothalamic) of the CNS are depressed by diazepam and other benzodiazepines thus producing the anxiolytic, sedative, skeletal muscle relaxant, and anticonvulsant effects seen. The exact mechanism of action is unknown, but postulated mechanisms include: antagonism of serotonin, increased release of and/or facilitation of gamma-aminobutyric acid (GABA) activity, and diminished release or turnover of acetylcholine in the CNS. Benzodiazepine specific receptors have been located in the mammalian brain, kidney, liver, lung, and heart. In all species studied, receptors are lacking in the white matter.

Uses/Indications - Diazepam is used clinically for its anxiolytic, muscle relaxant, hypnotic, appetite stimulant, and anticonvulsant activities. Refer to the dosage section for those and other suggested indications and doses for each species.

Pharmacokinetics - Diazepam is rapidly absorbed following oral administration. Peak plasma levels occur within 30 minutes to 2 hours after oral dosing. The drug is slowly (slower than oral) and incompletely absorbed following IM administration.

Diazepam is highly lipid soluble and is widely distributed throughout the body. It readily crosses the blood-brain barrier and is fairly highly bound to plasma proteins. In the horse at a serum of concentration of 75 ng/ml, 87% of the drug is bound to plasma proteins. In humans, this value has been reported to be 98-99%.

Diazepam is metabolized in the liver to several metabolites, including desmethyldiazepam (nordiazepam), temazepam, and oxazepam, all of which are pharmacologically active. These are eventually conjugated with glucuronide and eliminated primarily in the urine. Because of the active metabolites, serum values of diazepam are not useful in predicting efficacy. Serum half-lives (approximated) have been reported for diazepam and metabolites in dogs, cats, and horses:

	Dogs	Cats	Horses	Humans
Diazepam	2.5 - 3.2 hrs	5.5 hrs	7 - 22 hrs	20 - 50 hrs
Nordiazepam	3 hrs	21.3 hrs		30 - 200 hrs

Contraindications/Precautions - Slowly inject intravenously. This is particularly true when using a small vein for access or in small animals. Diazepam may cause significant thrombophlebitis. Too rapid of an injection of intravenous diazepam in small animals or neonates, may cause cardiotoxicity secondary to the propylene glycol in the formulation. Intra-carotid artery injections must be avoided.

Use cautiously in patients with hepatic or renal disease and in debilitated or geriatric patients. the drug should be administered to patients in coma, shock or with significant respiratory depression very cautiously. It is contraindicated in patients with known hypersensitivity to the drug. Benzodiazepines may impair the abilities of working animals. If administering the drug IV, be prepared to administer cardiovascular or respiratory support.

Diazepam has been implicated in causing congenital abnormalities in humans if administered during the first trimester of pregnancy. Infants born of mothers receiving large doses of benzodiazepines shortly before delivery have been reported to suffer from apnea, impaired metabolic response to cold stress, difficulty in feeding, hyperbilirubinemia, hypotonia, etc. Withdrawal symptoms have occurred in infants whose mothers chronically took benzodiazepines during pregnancy. The veterinary significance of these effects is unclear, but the use of these agents during the first trimester of pregnancy should only occur when the benefits clearly outweigh the risks associated with their use. Benzodiazepines and their metabolites are distributed into milk and may cause CNS effects in nursing neonates.

Adverse Effects/Warnings - In horses, diazepam may cause muscle fasiculations, weakness and ataxia at doses sufficient to cause sedation. Doses greater than 0.2 mg/kg may induce recumbency as a result of its muscle relaxant properties and general CNS depressant effects.

Cats may exhibit changes in behavior (irritability, depression, aberrant demeanor) after receiving diazepam. There have been recent reports of cats developing hepatic failure after receiving oral diazepam for several days; until this potential adverse effect is confirmed or refuted, use with caution in cats.

Dogs may exhibit a contradictory response (CNS excitement) following administration of diazepam. The effects with regard to sedation and tranquilization are extremely variable with each dog. Because of this individual variation, diazepam is not an ideal sedating agent for this species.

Overdosage - When administered alone, diazepam overdoses are generally limited to significant CNS depression (confusion, coma, decreased reflexes, etc). Hypotension, respiratory depression, and cardiac arrest have been reported in human patients, but apparently are quite rare.

Treatment of acute toxicity consists of standard protocols for removing and/or binding the drug in the gut if taken orally, and supportive systemic measures. The use of analeptic agents (CNS stimulants such as caffeine) are generally not recommended.

Drug Interactions - Metabolism of diazepam may be decreased and excessive sedation may occur if given with the following drugs: **cimetidine, erythromycin, isoniazid, ketoconazole, propranolol, & valproic acid**.

If administered with other **CNS depressant agents (barbiturates, narcotics, anesthetics**, etc.) additive effects may occur.

Antacids may slow the rate, but not the extent of oral absorption; administer 2 hours apart to avoid this potential interaction.

The pharmacologic effects of **digoxin** may be increased; monitor serum digoxin levels or symptoms of toxicity.

Rifampin may induce hepatic microsomal enzymes and decrease the pharmacologic effects of benzodiazepines.

Laboratory Interactions: Patients receiving diazepam, may show false negative **urine glucose** results if using *Diastix®* or *Clinistix®* tests.

Doses -
  Dogs:
     As a restraining agent/sedative:
        a) 0.2 - 0.6 mg/kg IV (Morgan 1988)
        b) 0.25 mg/kg PO q8h (Davis 1985a)
     For treatment of seizures:
        a) 1 - 4 mg/kg divided into 3-4 doses daily (Morgan 1988)
        b) For adjunctive treatment of seizure disorders: 2.5 - 15 mg *tid* (Bunch 1986)
     For status epilepticus:
        a) 0.5 - 1.0 mg/kg IV in increments of 5 - 10 mg, to effect (Morgan 1988)

   b) Up to 10 mg IV; not more than 3 doses (Kay and Aucoin 1985)

   c) For post-myelographic seizures: 0.4 mg/kg IV (slowly); if no effect use phenobarbital or pentobarbital (Walter, Feeney, and Johnston 1986)

   d) For metaldehyde, strychnine or brucine induced seizures/tremors: 2 - 5 mg/kg IV (Bailey 1986a)

   e) For methylxanthine (*e.g.,* theophylline) induced seizures: 0.5 - 2.0 mg/kg IV (if unsuccessful use phenobarbital at 6 mg/kg IV q6-12h) (Hooser and Beasley 1986)

   f) For salicylate toxicity induced seizures: 2.5 - 20 mg IV or PO (Handagama 1986)

   g) Seizures secondary to CNS trauma: 0.25 - 0.5 mg/kg IV (Fenner 1986)

For white shaker dog syndrome:

   a) 0.25 mg/kg PO *tid-qid* (Morgan 1988)

For Scotty cramp:

   a) 0.5 - 2.0 mg/kg IV to effect or PO *tid* (Morgan 1988)

As a preanesthetic:

   a) 0.1 mg/kg IV slowly (Morgan 1988)

For irritable colon syndrome:

   a) 0.15 mg/kg PO *tid* (Morgan 1988)

For functional urethral obstruction/urethral sphincter hypertonus:

   a) 2 - 10 mg q8h (Polzin and Osborne 1985)

   b) 2 - 10 mg PO *tid*; 0.5 mg/kg IV (Chew, DiBartola, and Fenner 1986)

For separation anxiety:

   a) 0.5 - 2.2 mg/kg PO *prn* (Morgan 1988)

Cats:

As an appetite stimulant:

   a) 0.05 - 0.15 mg/kg IV once daily to every other day or 1 mg PO once daily (Morgan 1988)

   b) 0.05 - 0.4 mg/kg IV, IM or PO. After IV administration eating may begin a few seconds; have food readily available. (Booth 1988a)

Status epilepticus:

   a) 0.5 - 1.0 mg/kg IV in increments of 5 - 10 mg, to effect (Morgan 1988)

Urine marking and anxiety:

   a) 1 - 2 mg PO *bid* (Morgan 1988)

For salicylate toxicity induced seizures:

   a) 2.5 - 5 mg IV or PO (Handagama 1986)

For adjunctive treatment of feline psychogenic alopecia and dermatitis:

   a) 1 - 2 mg PO *bid* (Walton 1986)

For treatment of seizure disorders:

   a) 2.5 - 5 mg *tid* (Bunch 1986)

   b) 1 - 4 mg/kg divided into 3-4 doses daily (Morgan 1988)

   c) 0.5 - 1.0 mg/kg PO daily (Schwartz-Porsche 1986)

Functional urethral obstruction/urethral sphincter hypertonus:

   a) 2 - 5 mg PO *tid*; 0.5 mg/kg IV (Chew, DiBartola, and Fenner 1986)

Cattle:

Sedative in calves:

   a) 0.4 mg/kg IV (Booth 1988a)

As a tranquilizer:

   a) 0.55 - 1.1 mg/kg IM (Lumb and Jones 1984)

Treatment of CNS hyperactivity and seizures:

   a) 0.5 - 1.5 mg/kg IM or IV (Bailey 1986b)

Rabbits:

As a tranquilizer (to increase relaxation of lightly anesthetized animals and permit ET intubation): 1 mg/kg IV prn (Huerkamp 1995)

Horses:

For seizures:

   a) Foals: 0.05 - 0.4 mg/kg IV; repeat in 30 minutes if necessary;
       Adults: 25 - 50 mg IV; repeat in 30 minutes if necessary. (Sweeney and Hansen 1987)

Treatment of seizures secondary to intraarterial injection of xylazine or other similar agents:

   a) 0.10 - 0.15 mg/kg IV (Thurmon and Benson 1987)

As an appetite stimulant:

a) 0.02 mg/kg IV; immediately after dosing offer animal food. Keep loud noises and distractions to a minimum. If effective, usually only 2-3 treatments in a 24-48 hour period is required. (Ralston 1987)

Swine:
For tranquilization:
a) 5.5 mg/kg IM (will develop posterior ataxia in 5 minutes and then recumbency within 10 minutes) (Booth 1988a)
b) 0.55 - 1.1 mg/kg IM (Lumb and Jones 1984)

For sedation prior to pentobarbital anesthesia:
a) 8.5 mg/kg IM (maximized at 30 minutes; reduces pentobarbital dose by 50%) (Booth 1988a)

For treatment of CNS hyperactivity and seizures:
a) 0.5 - 1.5 mg/kg IM or IV (Howard 1986)

Sheep:
As a tranquilizer:
a) 0.55 - 1.1 mg/kg IM (Lumb and Jones 1984)

Goats:
For Bermuda grass induced toxicosis and tremors:
a) 0.8 mg/kg IV (Booth 1988a)

To stimulate appetite:
a) 0.04 mg/kg IV; offer food immediately, duration of effect may last up to 45 minutes. (Booth 1988a)

Monitoring Parameters - Horses should be observed carefully after receiving this drug.

Client Information - Keep out of reach of children and in tightly closed containers.

Dosage Forms/Preparations/FDA Approval Status/Withholding Times -
Veterinary-Approved Products: None
Human-Approved Products:

Diazepam oral tablets 2 mg, 5 mg, 10 mg; *Valium*® (Roche); Generic; (Rx)

Diazepam timed-release oral capsules 15 mg; *Valrelease*® (Roche); (Rx)

Diazepam oral solution 1 mg/ml in 500 ml containers and unit-dose (5 & 10 mg) 5 mg/ml in 30 ml dropper bottle; *Diazepam Intensol*® (Roxane); *Generic* (Rx)

Diazepam Injection 5 mg/ml in 2 ml amps & syringes & 1, 2, 10 ml vials, 2 ml Tel-E-Ject; Emulsified Injection: 5 mg/ml in 3 ml vials; *Valium*® (Roche); *Zetran*® (Hauck);*Dizac*® (Ohmeda); Generic; (Rx)

Diazepam is a **Class-IV controlled substance**.

DIAZOXIDE, ORAL

Chemistry - Related structurally to the thiazide diuretics, diazoxide occurs as an odorless, white to creamy-white, crystalline powder with a melting point of about 330°. It is practically insoluble to sparingly soluble in water and slightly soluble in alcohol.

Storage/Stability/Compatibility - Diazoxide capsules and oral suspensions should be stored at 2-30°C and protected from light. Protect solutions/suspensions from freezing. Do not use darkened solutions/suspensions as they may be subpotent.

Pharmacology - Although related structurally to the thiazide diuretics, diazoxide does not possess any appreciable diuretic activity. By directly causing a vasodilatory effect on the smooth muscle in peripheral arterioles, diazoxide reduces peripheral resistance and blood pressure. To treat malignant hypertension, intravenous diazoxide is generally required for maximal response.

Diazoxide also exhibits hyperglycemic activity by directly inhibiting pancreatic insulin secretion. This action may be a result of the drug's capability to decrease the intracellular release of ionized calcium, thereby preventing the release of insulin from the insulin granules. Diazoxide does not apparently affect the synthesis of insulin, nor does it possess any antineoplastic activity. Diazoxide also enhances hyperglycemia by stimulating the beta-adrenergic system, thereby stimulating epinephrine release and inhibiting the uptake of glucose by cells.

Uses/Indications - Oral diazoxide is used in canine medicine for the treatment of hypoglycemia secondary to hyperinsulin secretion (*e.g.,* insulinoma). Insulinomas are apparently very rare in the cat, and there is little experience with this drug in that species.

Pharmacokinetics - The serum half-life of diazoxide has been reported to be about 5 hours in the dog; other pharmacokinetic parameters in the dog appear to be unavailable. In humans, serum diazoxide (at 10 mg/kg PO) levels peaked at about 12 hours after dosing with capsules. It is unknown what blood levels are required to obtain hyperglycemic effects. Highest concentrations of diazoxide are found in the kidneys with high levels also found in the liver and adrenal glands. Approximately 90% of the drug is bound to plasma proteins and it crosses the placenta and into the CNS. It is not known if diazoxideis distributed into milk. Diazoxide is partially metabolized in the liver and is excreted as both metabolites and unchanged drug by the kidneys. Serum half-life of the drug is prolonged in patients with renal impairment.

Contraindications/Precautions - Diazoxide should not be used in patients with functional hypoglycemia or for treating hypoglycemia secondary to insulin overdosage in diabetic patients. Unless the potential advantages outweigh the risks, do not use in patients hypersensitive to thiazide diuretics.

Because diazoxide can cause sodium and water retention, use cautiously in patients with congestive heart failure or with renal disease.

Adverse Effects/Warnings - When used to treat insulinomas in dogs, most commonly seen adverse reactions include anorexia, vomiting and/or diarrhea. Other effects that may be seen include tachycardia, hematologic abnormalities (agranulocytosis, aplastic anemia, thrombocytopenia), diabetes mellitus, cataracts (secondary to hyperglycemia?), and sodium and water retention.

Administering the drug with meals or temporarily reducing the dose may alleviate the gastrointestinal side effects. Adverse effects may be more readily noted in dogs with concurrent hepatic disease.

Overdosage - Acute overdosage may result in severe hyperglycemia and ketoacidosis. Treatment should include insulin (see previous monograph) and fluid and electrolytes. Intensive and prolonged monitoring is recommended.

Drug Interactions - Thiazide diuretics may potentiate the hyperglycemic effects of oral diazoxide. Some clinicians have recommended using hydrochlorothiazide (2 - 4 mg/kg/day PO) in combination with diazoxide, if diazoxide is ineffective alone to increase blood glucose levels. Caution: hypotension may occur.

Diazoxide may displace **warfarin** or **bilirubin** from plasma proteins. **Phenothiazines** (*e.g.,* chlorpromazine) may enhance the hyperglycemic effects of diazoxide. Diazoxide may increase the metabolism, or decrease the protein binding of **phenytoin**.

alpha-adrenergic agents (*e.g.,* **phenoxybenzamine**) may decrease the effectiveness of diazoxide in increasing glucose levels.

Diazoxide may enhance the hypotensive actions of **other hypotensive agents** (*e.g.,* hydralazine, prazosin, etc.)

Drug/Laboratory Interactions - Diazoxide will cause a false-negative insulin response to **glucagon**.

Doses -
  Dogs:
    For hypoglycemia secondary to insulin secreting islet cell tumors:
      a) 10 mg/kg divided twice daily PO with meals; may increase dose up to 60 mg/kg to alleviate signs of hypoglycemia, if tolerated. (Lothrop 1989)
      b) 10 mg/kg/day initially, may increase gradually up to 40 mg/kg/day if needed. (Leifer 1986)
      c) If after frequent feedings (4-6 small meals per day) and glucocorticoids (prednisone 1.1 - 4.4 mg/kg/day) alone fail to control hypoglycemia or dog develops "Cushinoid" appearance, add diazoxide (reduce prednisone dose if "Cushinoid") initially at 10 mg/kg divided twice a day. May gradually increase dosage to 60 mg/kg/day as tolerated and add hydrochlorothiazide (2 - 4 mg/kg/day). (Feldman and Nelson 1987c)

    For adjunctive therapy of hypoglycemia secondary to insulin secreting non-islet cell (extrapancreatic) tumors:
      a) Diazoxide 5-13 mg/kg PO *tid* (may add hydrochlorothiazide 2 - 4 mg/kg/day) (Weller 1988)

Monitoring Parameters -
    1) Blood (serum) glucose
    2) CBC (at least q3-4 months)
    3) Physical exam (monitor for symptoms of other adverse effects—see above)

Client Information - Clients should be instructed to monitor for symptoms of hyper- or hypoglycemia, abnormal bleeding, GI disturbances, etc.

Dosage Forms/Preparations/FDA Approval Status/Withholding Times -
  Veterinary-Approved Products: None
  Human-Approved Products:
Finding a supply of this medication may be a problem.

Diazoxide Oral Capsules 50 mg; Diazoxide Oral Suspension 50 mg/ml in 30 ml dropper bottles; *Proglycem*® (Baker Norton); (Rx)

Also available as 50 mg tablets in the U.K. as *Eudemine*® (Allan & Hanburys).

DICHLORPHENAMIDE

Chemistry - A carbonic anhydrase inhibitor, dichlorphenamide occurs as a white or nearly white, crystalline powder with a melting range of 235-240°C, and pK_as of 7.4 and 8.6. It is very slightly soluble in water and soluble in alcohol.

Storage/Stability/Compatibility - Store tablets in well-closed containers and at room temperature. An expiration date of 5 years after the date of manufacture is assigned to the commercially available tablets.

Pharmacology - See the discussion listed in the acetazolamide monograph immediately prior to this one.

Uses/Indications - Dichlorphenamide is used for the medical treatment of glaucoma.

Pharmacokinetics - The pharmacokinetics of this agent have apparently not been studied in domestic animals. One report (Roberts 1985) states that after a dose of 2.2 mg/kg, the onset of action is 30 minutes, maximal effect in 2-4 hours, and duration of action is 6-12 hours in small animals.

Contraindications/Precautions, Adverse Effects/Warnings, Overdosage, & Drug Interactions - See the discussion in the acetazolamide monograph found immediately prior to this one.

Doses -
  Dogs:
> a) 2 - 5 mg/kg PO q8h (Davis 1985)
> b) 10 - 15 mg/kg per day divided 2-3 times daily (Brooks 1986)
> c) 2 - 5 mg/kg PO divided *tid* (Wyman 1986)
> d) 2 - 4 mg/kg PO *bid-tid* (Morgan 1988)

  Cats:
> a) 10 - 25 mg (total) q8h PO (Davis 1985)
> b) 1 mg/kg PO *bid-tid* (Morgan 1988)

Monitoring Parameters -
  1) Intraocular pressure/tonometry
  2) Serum electrolytes
  3) Baseline CBC with differential and periodic retests if using chronically.
  4) Other adverse effects

Client Information - If GI upset occurs, give with food. Notify veterinarian if abnormal bleeding or bruising occurs or if animal develops tremors or a rash.

Dosage Forms/Preparations/FDA Approval Status/Withholding Times -
  Veterinary-Approved Products: None
  Human-Approved Products: At the time this edition went to press, there were rumors that the manufacturer was discontinuing this product and it may not be available.
    Dichlorphenamide 50 mg Tablets (scored); *Daranide*® (Merck); (Rx)

DICHLORVOS

Chemistry - An organophosphate insecticide, dichlorvos is also known as 2,2,-dichlorovinyl dimethyl phosphate or DDVP.

Storage/Stability/Compatibility - Dichlorvos tablets and capsules should be kept refrigerated (2-8°C). Dichlorvos feed additives should not be stored at temperatures below freezing. Dichlorvos is sensitive to hydrolysis if exposed to moisture and to oxidizing agents.

Pharmacology - Like other organophosphate agents, dichlorvos inhibits acetylcholinesterase interfering with neuromuscular transmission in susceptible parasites.

Uses/Indications - Dichlorvos is indicated for use internally in dogs and cats for the treatment of roundworms (*Toxocara canis, Toxocara cati, Toxacaris leonina*) and hookworms (*Ancylostoma caninum, Ancylostoma tubaeforme, Uncinaria stenocephala*). It is effective in swine against *Ascaris, Trichuris, Ascarops strongylina* and *Oesophagostomum spp.*. In horses, dichlorvos is labeled as being effective for the treatment and control of bots, pinworms, large and small bloodworms and large roundworms. It is also used as a premise spray to keep fly populations controlled and as a flea and tick collar for dogs and cats.

Pharmacokinetics - Specific information was not located for this agent.

Contraindications/Precautions/Reproductive Safety - Do not administer to horses suffering from heaves, colic, diarrhea, constipation, or infectious diseases until these conditions have been corrected. In dogs and cats, dichlorvos is contraindicated in animals exhibiting symptoms of severe constipation, intestinal impaction, liver dysfunction, circulatory failure, or to animals exposed to, or showing signs of infection. Dogs infected with D. immitis should not receive dichlorvos. Dichlorvos should not be used in conjunction with any other anthelmintics, taeniacides, filaricides (DEC exempted) or within a few days of other medications that inhibit cholinesterase (see drug interactions below).

Studies performed in target species have demonstrated no teratogenic effects at usual doses.

Adverse Effects/Warnings - Adverse effects are generally dose-related and may include those listed below in the Overdosage/Acute Toxicity section. Cats, young animals, or debilitated animals may be more susceptible to toxic effects. Use in young kittens, cats with any other concurrent diseases or debilitated or animals otherwise stressed, should probably be avoided.

Overdosage/Acute Toxicity - If overdoses occur, vomiting, tremors, bradycardia, respiratory distress, hyperexcitability, salivation and diarrhea may occur. Atropine (see atropine and pralidoxime monographs for more information) may be antidotal. Use of succinylcholine, theophylline, aminophylline, reserpine, or respiratory depressant drugs (*e.g.,* narcotics, phenothiazines) should be avoided in patients with organophosphate toxicity. If an ingestion occurs by a human, contact a poison control center, physician or hospital emergency room.

Drug Interactions - **Acepromazine or other phenothiazines** should not be given within one month of worming with an organophosphate agent as their effects may be potentiated. Because of its anticholinesterase activity, avoid the use of organophosphates with **DMSO**. Cythioate could theoretically enhance the toxic effects of **levamisole**. **Pyrantel Pamoate (or tartrate)** adverse effects could be intensified if used concomitantly with an organophosphate. Patients receiving organophosphate anthelmintics should not receive **succinylcholine** or other depolarizing muscle relaxants for at least 48 hours. Drugs such as **morphine, neostigmine, physostigmine** and **pyridostigmine** should be avoided when using organophosphates as they can inhibit cholinesterase.

Doses -
Dogs:
> a) 26.4 - 33 mg/kg PO (Papich 1992)
> b) Adults: 27 - 33 mg/kg; Puppies: 11 mg/kg (Sherding and Johnson 1994a)

Cats:
> a) 11 mg/kg PO (Papich 1992), (Sherding and Johnson 1994a)

Pocket Pets:
> Including rats, gerbils, mice, Guinea pig, hamsters, chinchillas for fleas/lice: Hang 5 cm of a dichlorvos strip 6 inches above cage for 24 hours, twice weekly for 3 weeks. (Anderson 1994)

Large Animals:
> Read and follow label directions, including any withdrawal times stated.

Monitoring Parameters - 1) Efficacy; 2) Adverse Effects

Client Information - Keep out of reach of children. Handling of dichlorvos liquid preparations (*e.g.,* premise spray) must be done with extreme care; follow all label directions! Oral pellets are non-digestible and may be seen in the animals feces.

Dosage Forms/Preparations/FDA Approval Status/Withholding Times -
Veterinary-Approved Products:
> Dichlorvos Oral: Tablets 10 mg, 20 mg; Capsules 68 mg, 136 mg, 204 mg; Pellets (in packets) 136 mg, 204 mg, 544 mg; *Task*® & *Task*® *Tabs* (Fermenta); (Rx). Approved for use in dogs (Capsules, Pellets and Tabs) and cats (Tabs Only).

> Dichlorvos Oral Equine Wormer 78 g/pkt; *Cutter Dichlorvos Horse Wormer*® (Miles); (OTC)

> Dichlorvos Feed Additives: *Atgard*® *C* (Fermenta); (OTC); *Atgard*® *Swine Wormer* (Fermenta); (OTC)

> Also available in a 9.6% flea and tick collar for dogs and cats: *Pet Insecticide Collar* (Fermenta); (OTC) and a 40.2% concentrate for premise spraying in 5 gallon containers: *Vapona*® *Concentrate* (Fermenta); (OTC).

Human-Approved Products: None

DICLOXACILLIN SODIUM

For general information on the penicillins, including adverse effects, contraindications, overdosage, drug interactions and monitoring parameters, refer to the monograph: Penicillins, General Information..

Chemistry - An isoxazolyl-penicillin, dicloxacillin sodium is a semisynthetic penicillinase-resistant penicillin. It is available commercially as the monohydrate sodium salt which occurs as a white to off-white, crystalline powder that is freely soluble in water and has a pK_a of 2.7-2.8. One mg of dicloxacillin sodium contains not less than 850 micrograms of dicloxacillin.

Dicloxacillin sodium may also be known as sodium dicloxacillin, dichlorphenylmethyl isoxazolyl penicillin sodium or methyldichlorophenyl isoxazolyl penicillin sodium.

Storage/Stability/Compatibility - Dicloxacillin sodium capsules and powder for oral suspension should be stored at temperatures less than 40°C and preferably at room temperature (15-30°C). After reconstituting, any remaining oral suspension should be refrigerated and discard after 14 days. If kept at room temperature, the oral suspension is stable for 7 days.

Pharmacology/Uses/Indications - Refer to the Cloxacillin monograph for information regarding this drug.

Pharmacokinetics (specific) - Dicloxacillin is only available in oral dosage forms. Dicloxacillin sodium is resistant to acid inactivation in the gut, but is only partially absorbed. The bioavailability after oral administration in humans has been reported to range from 35-76% and, if given with food, both the rate and extent of absorption is decreased.

The drug is distributed to the liver, kidneys, bone, bile, pleural fluid, synovial fluid and ascitic fluid. However, one manufacturer states that levels of the drug that are achieved in ascitic fluid are not clinically therapeutic. As with the other penicillins, only minimal amounts are distributed into the CSF. In humans, approximately 95-99% of the drug is bound to plasma proteins.

Dicloxacillin is partially metabolized to both active and inactive metabolites. These metabolites and the parent compound are rapidly excreted in the urine via both glomerular filtration and tubular secretion mechanisms. A small amount of the drug is also excreted in the feces via biliary elimination. The serum half-life in humans with normal renal function ranges from about 24-48 minutes. In dogs, 20-40 minutes has been reported as the elimination half-life.

Doses -
Dogs:
For susceptible infections:
    a) 11 - 25 mg/kg PO q8h (Papich 1988)
    b) 10 - 50 mg/kg q8h PO (Greene 1984)
    c) For resistant *Staph.* infections: 10 - 20 mg/kg PO *tid-qid* (Morgan 1988)
    d) 10 - 25 mg/kg PO q8h (Ford and Aronson 1985)
    e) 27.5 - 33 mg/kg PO q8h (Aronson and Aucoin 1989)
    f) 11 - 55 mg/kg PO q8h (Kirk 1989)

Cats:
For susceptible infections:
    a) 11 - 25 mg/kg PO q8h (Papich 1988)
    b) 10 - 50 mg/kg q8h PO (Greene 1984)
    c) For resistant *Staph.* infections: 10 - 20 mg/kg PO *tid-qid* (Morgan 1988)
    d) 10 - 25 mg/kg PO q8h (Ford and Aronson 1985)
    e) 11 - 55 mg/kg PO q8h (Kirk 1989)
    f) 27.5 - 33 mg/kg PO q8h (Aronson and Aucoin 1989)

Client Information - Unless otherwise instructed by the veterinarian, this drug should be given on an empty stomach, at least 1 hour before feeding or 2 hours after. Keep oral suspension in the refrigerator and discard any unused suspension after 14 days. If the suspension is stored at room temperature it should be discarded after 7 days.

Dosage Forms/Preparations/FDA Approval Status -
  Veterinary-Approved Products: None
  Human-Approved Products:
    Dicloxacillin Sodium Capsules 125 mg, 250 mg, 500 mg; *Dynapen®* (Apothecon) (Rx), *Dycill®* (SK-Beecham) (Rx), *Pathocil®* (Wyeth-Ayerst); generic; (Rx)
    Dicloxacillin Sodium Powder for Oral Suspension 62.5 mg/5 ml reconstituted in 80, 100, and 200 mls; *Pathocil®* (Wyeth-Ayerst); (Rx)

DIETHYLCARBAMAZINE CITRATE

Chemistry - A piperazine derivative, diethylcarbamazine citrate (DEC) occurs as a white, slightly hygroscopic, crystalline powder that is either odorless or has a slight odor and a melting point of approximately 138°C. It is very soluble in water and slightly soluble (1 gram in 35 ml) in alcohol.

Storage/Stability/Compatibility - Unless otherwise specified by the manufacturer, diethylcarbamazine products should be stored in tight containers at room temperature and protected from light.

Pharmacology - The exact mechanism of how DEC exerts in its anti-filaricidal (early larval stages of D. immitis) and anti-nematodal effects is not clearly understood. It is believed that DEC acts on the parasite's nervous system in a nicotinic-like fashion, thereby paralyzing it.

Uses/Indications - DEC is approved (depending on product) for use for the prophylaxis of heartworm disease (*D. immitis*), and/or the treatment of ascariasis in dogs. The drug is also used in ferrets and zoo animals susceptible to heartworm. DEC is used in dogs at higher dosages as alternative therapy for several other parasites (see Dosage section below). Some products may be labeled for use in cats to treat ascarid infections.

In the U.K., DEC is used as an injectable product to control parasitic bronchitis (*Dictyocaulus viviparous*) in sheep and cattle.

In humans, DEC is indicated as a filaricidal for the treatment of *Wucheria bancrofti, Brugia malayi, Loa loa* and *Onchocerca volvulus*.

Pharmacokinetics - DEC is rapidly absorbed after oral administration, with peak serum levels occurring in about 3 hours. The drug is distributed to all tissues and organs except fat. DEC is rapidly metabolized and is primarily excreted in the urine (70% of a dose within 24 hours) as metabolites or unchanged drug (10-25% of a dose).

Contraindications/Precautions/Reproductive Safety - Diethylcarbamazine is contraindicated in dogs with microfilaria, as a shock-like reaction can occur in dogs with microfilaria who are treated with DEC. This effect may only be seen in 0.3 - 5% of dogs, but the potential seriousness of the reaction precludes its use in all dogs with microfilaria. Dogs cleared of adult worms and microfilaria may be started on DEC therapy for prophylaxis. Microfilaria detected in dogs who have undergone aldulticide and microfilaricide therapy and are receiving DEC prophylaxis, should have the DEC stopped until existing microfilaria are eliminated.

DEC has been reported to cause infertility problems in male dogs, but these reports are rare. Controlled studies have not found any adverse effects on semen volume, pH, sperm counts or motility.

DEC alone is reportedly safe to use in pregnant dogs throughout the gestational period.

Adverse Effects/Warnings - When used at recommended doses for heartworm prophylaxis, adverse effects are very uncommon for DEC. Some dogs develop diarrhea or vomiting while on the drug, which may necessitate discontinuation. GI effects are more predominant when used at higher dosages for the treatment of ascarids or other susceptible parasites. Giving with food or soon after eating may alleviate GI disturbances. Case reports of fixed drug eruptions after DEC have also been reported in dogs.

In microfilaria positive dogs who receive DEC, an anaphylactoid reaction can be seen within 20 minutes of dosing. Systems affected or symptoms seen may include GI (salivation, diarrhea, emesis), CNS (depression, ataxia, prostration, lethargy), shock (pale mucous membranes, weak pulses, tachycardia, dyspnea), hepatic (increased liver enzymes) or DIC. The reaction generally peaks within 1-2 hours after the dose and death can occur. Treatment is basically supportive, using fluid therapy and intravenous corticosteroids.

In addition to the adverse effects above, the following have been reported with combination products that contain DEC: DEC/Styrylpyridium (*Styrid® Caricide®*): gastroenteritis, teratogenesis, sterilization and thrombocytopenia. DEC/Oxibendazole (*Filaribits® Plus*) has been implicated in causing periportal hepatitis in dogs.

Overdosage/Acute Toxicity - DEC is considered to be a relatively non-toxic compound, but quantitative data regarding its toxicity was not found. In dogs, large overdoses generally result in vomiting or depression. Inducement of vomiting or absorption reduction measures (activated charcoal, cathartics) could be considered for very large ingestions. Symptoms, should they occur, should be handled in a supportive manner.

Drug Interactions - If used with diethylcarbamazine, other **nicotine-like compounds** (*e.g., **pyrantel, morantel, levamisole*) could theoretically enhance the toxic effects of each other; use with DEC only with intensified monitoring.

Doses -
  Dogs:
    For heartworm prophylaxis:
      a) 6.6 mg/kg PO once a day preceding infection and for 60 days following last exposure to mosquitos. In dogs who become microfilaremic while on DEC, may continue, but do not interrupt daily DEC therapy. (Knight 1988)

    b) 6.6 mg/kg PO daily from beginning of mosquito season and for two months thereafter. Should be given year-round in areas where mosquitos are active throughout the year. Re-examine 3 months after starting therapy and at 6 month intervals for microfilaria. (Todd, Paul, and DiPietro 1985)

    c) 2.5 - 3 mg/kg PO daily; begin prior to mosquito season. (Rawlings and Calvert 1989)

    d) 5 - 7 mg/kg PO daily. Begin before infection is likely and continue 60 days after mosquito season. Some areas will require year-round treatment. (Calvert and Rawlings 1986)

For treatment of susceptible parasites (other than heartworm—must not be used in microfilaria positive patients):

    a) For ascarids: 55- 110 mg/kg PO; may be used as a preventative for ascaridiasis when dosed at 6.6 mg/kg PO per day. (Todd, Paul, and DiPietro 1985)

    b) For lungworms (*Crenosoma vulpis*): 80 mg/kg PO q12h for 3 days. (Todd, Paul, and DiPietro 1985)

Cats:
For Ascarids:
    a) 55 - 110 mg/kg PO (Todd, Paul, and DiPietro 1985)

Ferrets:
For heartworm prophylaxis:
    a) 5.5 mg/kg PO once a day. (Randolph 1986)

Cattle:
For the treatment of early stages of *Dictyocaulus viviparous* infestations:
    a) 22 mg/kg IM for 3 successive days; or 44 mg/kg IM once. (Note: DEC is available in an injectable dosage form containing 400 mg/ml in the U.K., no approved injectable form is available in the U.S.A.) (Brander, Pugh, and Bywater 1982)

Monitoring Parameters -
    1) Microfilaria, when used for heartworm prophylaxis
    2) Clinical efficacy, when used as an anthelmintic

Client Information - Give all doses as directed. Dogs must be checked for microfilaria before restarting DEC in the spring. Dogs receiving DEC year around should be checked every six months.

Dosage Forms/Preparations/FDA Approval Status/Withholding Times - All DEC products are available via prescription only (Rx).

Veterinary-Approved Products:

Diethylcarbamazine Citrate Tablets (plain or film-coated) 50 mg, 100 mg, 200 mg, 300 mg, 400 mg (Rx)

Diethylcarbamazine Citrate Chewable Tablets 60 mg, 120 mg, 180 mg; *Filaribits*® (SKB)

Diethylcarbamazine Citrate Oral Liquid (Syrup) 60 mg/ml

Diethylcarbamazine Citrate Combination Products (refer to product literature for more information): *Filaribits*® *Plus* (Pfizer) Tablets containing Diethylcarbamazine Citrate/Oxibendazole in 60 mg/45 mg, 180 mg/136 mg strengths.

Human-Approved Products:

Diethylcarbamazine Citrate Tablets 50 mg; *Hetrazan*® (Lederle); (Rx)

DIETHYLSTILBESTROL
DES

Chemistry - A synthetic nonsteroidal estrogen agent, diethylstilbestrol occurs as an odorless, white, crystalline powder with a melting range of 169°-175°C. It is practically insoluble in water; soluble in alcohol or fatty oils. Diethylstilbestrol is also known as DES or Stilbestrol.

Storage/Stability/Compatibility - All commercially available DES tablets (plain tablets, enteric-coated tablets) should be stored at room temperature (15-30°C) in well-closed containers.

Pharmacology - Estrogens are necessary for the normal growth and development of the female sex organs and in some species contribute to the development and maintenance of secondary female sex characteristics. Estrogens cause increased cell height and secretions of the cervical mucosa, thickening of the vaginal mucosa, endometrial proliferation and increased uterine tone.

Estrogens have effects on the skeletal system. They increase calcium deposition, accelerate epiphyseal closure and increase bone formation. Estrogens have a slight anabolic effect and can increase sodium and water retention.

Estrogens affect the release of gonadotropins from the pituitary gland, which can cause inhibition of lactation, inhibition of ovulation and inhibition of androgen secretion.

Excessive estrogen will delay the transport of the ovum and prevent it from reaching the uterus at the appropriate time for implantation. DES also possess antineoplastic activity against some types of neoplasias (perianal gland adenoma and prostatic hyperplasia). It affects mRNA and protein synthesis in the cell nucleus and is cell cycle nonspecific.

Uses/Indications - DES has been used in estrogen responsive incontinence in spayed female dogs and in the prevention of pregnancy after mismating in female dogs and cats. Its use alone for prevention of mismating is controversial as its efficacy is in doubt.

DES is used in canine medicine for the treatment of certain estrogen-responsive neoplasias (see Pharmacology and Doses below). The use of DES for these conditions is controversial because of the risks associated with therapy.

One author (Teske 1986) states that in small animals, "because of the alternatives and its possible side effects, estrogen is only indicated for treating mismating". Another (Olson et al. 1986), states that in dogs, "owners should be routinely discouraged from having their bitches undergo abortion with estrogens."

Pharmacokinetics - DES is well absorbed from the GI tract of monogastric animals. It is slowly metabolized by the liver, primarily to a glucuronide form and then excreted in the urine and feces.

Contraindications/Precautions - DES is contraindicated during pregnancy, as it has been demonstrated to cause fetal malformations of the genitourinary system.

Estrogens have been documented to be carcinogenic at low levels in some laboratory animals. Because of the potential for danger to the public health, DES must not be used in animals to be used for human consumption.

Adverse Effects/Warnings - In cats and dogs estrogens are considered to be toxic to the bone marrow and can cause blood dyscrasias. Blood dyscrasias are more prevalent in older animals and if higher dosages are used. Initially, a thrombocytosis and/or leukocytosis may be noted, but thrombocytopenia/leukopenias will gradually develop. Changes in a peripheral blood smear may be apparent within two weeks after estrogen administration. Chronic estrogen toxicity may be characterized by a normochromic, normocytic anemia, thrombocytopenia and neutropenia. Bone marrow depression may be transient and begin to resolve within 30 - 40 days or may persist or progress to a fatal aplastic anemia. Doses of 2.2 mg/kg per day have caused death in cats secondary to bone marrow toxicity.

In cats, daily administration of DES has resulted in pancreatic, hepatic and cardiac lesions.

Estrogens may cause cystic endometrial hyperplasia and pyometra. After therapy is initiated, an open-cervix pyometra may be noted 1-6 weeks after therapy.

When used chronically in male animals, feminization may occur. In females, signs of estrus may occur and persist for 7-10 days.

Experimental administration of DES to female dogs as young as 8 months. of age have induced malignant ovarian adenocarcinomas. Doses ranging from 60 to 495 mg given over 1 month to 4 years were implicated in causing these tumors.

Overdosage - Acute overdosage in humans with estrogens has resulted in nausea, vomiting and withdrawal bleeding in females. No information was located regarding acute overdose in veterinary patients, however, the reader is referred to the warnings and adverse effects listed above.

Drug Interactions - **Rifampin** may decrease estrogen activity if administered concomitantly. This is presumably due to microsmal enzyme induction with resultant increase in estrogen metabolism. Other known enzyme inducers (*e.g.,* **phenobarbital, phenylbutazone**, etc.), may have a similar effect, but clinical significance is unclear.

Enhanced glucocorticoid effects may result if estrogens are used concomitantly with **corticosteroid agents**. It has been postulated that estrogens may either alter the protein binding of corticosteroids and/or decrease their metabolism. Corticosteroid dosage adjustment may be necessary when estrogen therapy is either started or discontinued.

Oral anticoagulant activity may be decreased if estrogens are administered concurrently. Increases in anticoagulant dosage may be necessary if adding estrogens.

Drug/Laboratory Interactions - Estrogens in combination with progestins (*e.g.,* oral contraceptives) have been demonstrated in humans to increase **thyroxine-binding globulin (TBG)** with resultant increases in total circulating thyroid hormone. Decreased **T_3 resin uptake** also occurs, but free T_4 levels are unaltered.

Doses -
  Dogs:
    For pregnancy avoidance after mismating:
      a) 0.1 - 1 mg PO for 5 days if animal is presented 24-48 hours after coitus. If animal is presented later than 5 days post-coitus: 1 - 2 mg PO for 5 days after ECP therapy (0.044 mg/kg (ECP) IM once during 3-5 days of standing heat or within 72 hours of mismating) (Woody 1988)

For treatment of perianal gland adenomas and prostatic hyperplasias:
   a) 0.1 - 1 mg PO q24-48h (Thompson 1989)
   b) 1 mg PO q72h; or 1.1 mg/kg once. Do not administer more than 25 mg. (Rosenthal 1985)

For treatment of estrogen-responsive incontinence:
   a) Initially 0.1 - 1 mg PO daily for 3-5 days, followed by maintenance therapy of approximately 1 mg PO per week. Some animals may require much higher initial dosages to obtain a response. Maximum initial doses of 0.1 - 0.3 mg/kg once daily for 7 days, then reduce to once weekly. All maintenance doses should be gradually reduced to the lowest effective dose. (Polzin and Osborne 1985)
   b) 0.1 - 1 mg PO per day for 3-5 days, then 1 mg once weekly (LaBato 1988)
   c) 0.1 - 1 mg PO for 3-5 days followed by 1 mg every week or less often. Some animals may require more than 1 mg weekly to maintain. (Chew, DiBartola, and Fenner 1986)

Monitoring Parameters - When therapy is either at high dosages or chronic; see Adverse effects for more information.
   Done at least monthly:
     1) Packed Cell Volumes (PCV)
     2) White blood cell counts (CBC)
     3) Platelet counts
   Baseline, one month after therapy, and repeated 2 months after cessation of therapy if abnormal:
     1) Liver function tests

Client Information - Contact veterinarian if signs and symptoms of lethargy, diarrhea, vomiting, abnormal discharge from vulva, excessive water consumption and urination or abnormal bleeding occur.

Dosage Forms/Preparations/FDA Approval Status/Withholding Times -
 Veterinary-Approved Products: None
 Human-Approved Products: At the time of writing, no commercially available regular oral DES products are available in the USA, however compounded preparations may be available from a variety of compounding pharmacies.

   Diethylstilbestrol Diphosphate Injection 50 mg/ml in 5 ml amps: .i.*Stilphostrol*;® (Miles) (Rx)

   Diethylstilbestrol Diphosphate 50 mg Tablets; *Stilphostrol*® (Miles) (Rx)

DIFLOXACIN HCL

Chemistry/Storage/Stability/Compatibility - A 4-fluroquinolone antibiotic, difloxacin HCl commercially available tablets should be stored between 15-30°C (59-86°F) and protected from excessive heat.

Pharmacology - Like other drugs in its class, difloxacin is a concentration-dependent bactericidal agent. It acts by inhibiting bacterial DNA-gyrase (a type-II topoisomerase), thereby preventing DNA supercoiling and DNA synthesis. The net result is disruption of bacterial cell replication.
  Difloxacin has good activity against many gram negative and gram positive bacilli and cocci, including most species and strains of *Klebsiella spp., Staphylococcus spp., E. coli, Enterobacter, Campylobacter, Shigella, Proteus, Pasturella* species. Some strains of *Pseudomonas aeruginosa* and *Pseudomonas species* are resistant and most *Enterococcus spp.* are resistant. Like other fluroquinolones, difloxacin has weak activity against most anaerobes and is not a good choice when treating known or suspected anaerobic infections.
  Development of bacterial resistance to 4-fluroquinolones can occur.

Uses/Indications - Difloxacin is indicated for treatment in dogs for bacterial infections susceptible to it.

Pharmacokinetics - After oral administration in dogs, difloxacin serum levels peak about 3 hours post dosing. The drug is well distributed (V_d=2.8 L/kg) in dogs and marginally bound to plasma proteins (16-52% in dogs). Difloxacin is eliminated by the kidneys and high levels are attained in the urine. Serum half life is about 9 hours in dogs. Urine levels remain well above MIC's for susceptible organisms for at least 24 hours after dosing.

Contraindications/Precautions/Reproductive Safety - Difloxacin, like other fluroquinolones can cause arthropathies in immature, growing animals. Because dogs appear to be more sensitive to this effect, the manufacturer states that the drug is contraindicated in immature dogs during the rapid growth phase (between 2-8 months in small and medium-sized breeds and up to 18 months in large and giant breeds). The drug should also be considered to be contraindicated in dogs known to be hypersensitive to difloxacin or other drugs in its class (quinolones).

The manufacturer states that difloxacin should be used with caution in animals with known or suspected CNS disorders (e.g., seizure disorders) as rarely drugs in this class have been associated with CNS stimulation and seizures.

While difloxacin may find use in other species, early anectdotal reports are that it can cause nausea and vomiting in cats.

Safety in breeding or pregnant dogs has not been established. It is not known whether orbifloxacin enters maternal milk.

Adverse Effects/Warnings - While the manufacturer reports that only self-limited gastrointestinal effects (anorexia, vomiting, diarrhea) were reported during clinical studies (at 5 mg/kg dosing) in adult animals, higher doses or additional experience with use of the drug may demonstrate additional adverse effects.

Overdosage - Dogs receiving up to 2.5X (25 mg/kg) for 30 days did not demonstrate overly significant adverse effects. Facial erythema/edema, diarrhea, decreased appetite and weight loss were noted.

Drug Interactions - **Antacids** or other agents containing divalent or trivalent cations (Mg^{++}, Al^{+++}, Ca^{++}) may bind to difloxacin and prevent its absorption. **Sucralfate** may inhibit absorption of difloxacin; separate doses of these drugs by at least 2 hours, if both are required.

Difloxacin administered with **theophylline** may increase theophylline blood levels.

Probenecid may block the tubular secretion of difloxacin and may increase its blood level and half-life.

Synergism may occur, but is not predictable, against some bacteria (particularly *Pseudomonas aeruginosa* or other Enterobacteriaceae) with these compounds and **aminoglycosides, 3rd generation cephalosporins agents, and extended-spectrum penicillins**. Although difloxacin apparently has minimal activity against anaerobes, *in vitro* synergy has been reported when other fluroquinolones have been used with **clindamycin** against strains of *Peptostreptococcus*, *Lactobacillus* and *Bacteroids fragilis*. **Nitrofurantoin** may antagonize the antimicrobial activity of the fluroquinolones and their concomitant use is not recommended. Fluroquinolones may exacerbate the nephrotoxicity of **cyclosporine** (used systemically).

The manufacturer reports that difloxacin was used concurrently in field trials with a variety of drugs including heartworm preventative, thyroid hormones, ectoparasiticides, antiseizure drugs, anesthetics, antihistamines, and topical antibiotic/antiinflammatory preps without untoward effects.

Doses -

Dogs:
> For susceptible infections:
>> a) 5 mg/kg - 10 mg/kg once daily PO for 2 - 3 days beyond the cessation of clinical signs to a maximum of 30 days therapy. (Package Insert—Dicural®)

Monitoring Parameters/Client Information - Efficacy is the most important monitoring parameter. Clients should be instructed on the importance of giving the medication as instructed and not to discontinue it on their own.

Dosage Forms/Preparations/FDA Approval Status -
Veterinary-Approved Products:
Difloxacin Oral Scored Tablets: 11.4 mg & 45.4 mg in btls of 100 & 500; 136 mg (dbl. scored) in btls of 50 & 250; *Dicural*® (Fort Dodge); (Rx). Approved for use in dogs. Federal law prohibits the use of the drug in food-producing animals.

Human-Approved Products: None

DIGITOXIN

Chemistry - A cardiac glycoside, digitoxin occurs as a bitter tasting, odorless, white to pale buff colored, microcrystalline powder. It is practically insoluble in water and one gram is soluble in approximately 150 ml of alcohol.

Storage/Stability/Compatibility - Digitoxin tablets should be stored at room temperature (15-30°C) and kept in well-closed containers. Digitoxin injection is hydrolyzed at pH's less than 3. It is said to be compatible with most available IV solutions and it is not compatible with acids or alkalies.

Uses/Indications - Like digoxin, digitoxin is indicated for heart failure or atrial arrhythmias, but because it is metabolized by the liver to a greater extent, some clinicians feel that it should be used instead of digoxin in patients with diminished renal function. Others believe that digoxin may be used in these patients if adequate serum level monitoring is performed and dosage adjustments are made as necessary. Digitoxin is not routinely used in cats and some clinicians state it is contraindicated in this species.

Pharmacokinetics - Digitoxin has only one steroidal hydroxyl group (versus two for digoxin) and therefore is much less polar. It is rapidly and nearly completely absorbed in the small intestine after oral administration. It is unknown if the presence of food alters either the rate or extent of absorption.

Digitoxin is highly protein bound (97% in humans, 70-90% in dogs) and values generally are the same in uremic patients. It is unknown if digitoxin enters the milk.

Digitoxin is extensively metabolized and the elimination half-life usually remains unchanged in renal failure patients. The elimination half-life in dogs has been reported range from 8-49 hours. Like digoxin, this apparent interpatient variability suggests that digitoxin serum levels msut be monitored to optimize therapy and reduce the chance for toxicity. Digitoxin is usually not recommended for use in cats because of its "very long" half-life, but one study reported a $t_{1/2}$ of only 32 hours, although other values have been reported to be longer than 100 hours.

Pharmacology, Contraindications/Precautions,
Adverse Effects/Warnings, Overdosage, Drug Interactions -
See the information listed for digoxin.

Doses -
  Dogs:
     a) 0.033 - 0.11 mg/kg/day PO divided *bid* (Kirk 1986)
     b) 0.03 - 0.04 mg/kg *bid* to *tid* (Kittleson 1985a)
     c) Oral maintenance: 0.04 - 0.1 mg/kg/day divided q8h; Rapid intravenous digitalization for atrial arrhythmias: 0.01 - 0.03 mg/kg divided; give 1/2 of above dose IV and wait for 30-60 minutes and give 1/4th the dose IV; wait another 30-60 minutes and give the remainder if necessary. (Miller 1985)
     d) 0.022 mg/kg q8-12h PO; puppies can tolerate higher dosages than mature dogs (McConnell and Hughey 1987)

  Cats: Note: Many cardiologists feel that digitoxin should not be used in cats. If used in cats, diligent monitoring is required.
     a) 0.0055 mg/kg q12h (use tablets only) (Kirk 1986)
     b) 0.005 - 0.015 mg/kg PO once daily (Morgan 1988)

  Horses:
     a) 0.03 - 0.06 mg/kg PO for digitalization; 0.01 mg/kg PO for maintenance (Robinson 1987)

Monitoring Parameters -
  1) Serum levels
     Because of this drug's narrow therapeutic index, and interpatient variability, it is strongly recommended to monitor serum levels to help guide therapy. Unless the patient (dog) received an initial loading dose, at least 36 hours should pass after starting therapy to monitor serum levels to allow levels to approach steady-state. Suggested therapeutic serum levels in the dog are 15-35 ng/ml (Neff-Davis 1985). Toxicity is usually associated with levels greater than 40 ng/ml. Levels at the higher end of the suggested range may be necessary to treat some atrial arrhythmias, but may also result in higher incidences of adverse effects. Usually a trough level (just before next dose or at least 4-10 hours after the last dose) is recommended.
  2) Appetite/weight
  3) Cardiac rate, ECG changes
  4) Serum electrolytes
  5) Clinical efficacy for CHF (improved perfusion, decreased edema, increased venous (or arterial) O_2 levels).

Client Information - Contact veterinarian if animal displays changes in behavior, vomits, has diarrhea, lack of appetite, symptoms of colic (horses), becomes lethargic or depressed.

Dosage Forms/Preparations/FDA Approval Status/Withholding Times -
  Veterinary-Approved Products: None
  Human-Approved Products:
    Digitoxin Tablets 0.05 mg, 0.1 mg; *Crystodigin*® (Lilly); (Rx)

DIGOXIN

Chemistry - A cardiac glycoside, digoxin occurs as bitter tasting, clear to white crystals or as white, crystalline powder. It is practically insoluble in water, slightly soluble in diluted alcohol, and very slightly soluble in 40% propylene glycol solution. Above 235°C it melts with decomposition.

The commercial injection consists of a 40% propylene glycol, 10% alcohol solution having a pH of 6.6-7.4.

Storage/Stability/Compatibility - Digoxin tablets, capsules, elixir and injection should be stored at room temperature (15-30°C) and protected from light.

At pH's from 5-8, digoxin is stable, but in solutions with a pH of less than 3, it is hydrolyzed.

The injectable product is compatible with most commercially available IV solutions, including lactated Ringer's, D5W, and normal saline. To prevent the possibility of precipitation occurring, one manufacturer (Glaxo Wellcome) recommends that the injection be diluted by a volume at least 4 times with either sterile water, D5W, or normal saline. Digoxin injection has been demonstrated to be **compatible** with bretylium tosylate, cimetidine HCl, lidocaine HCl, and verapamil HCl.

Digoxin is **incompatible** with dobutamine HCl, acids and alkalies. The manufacturer does not recommend mixing digoxin injection with other medications. Compatibility is dependent upon factors such as pH, concentration, temperature, diluents used and it is suggested to consult specialized references for more specific information.

Pharmacology - The pharmacology of the digitalis glycosides have been extensively studied, but a thorough discussion is beyond the scope of this reference. Suffice it to say that digitalis glycosides cause the following effects in patients with a failing heart: increased myocardial contractility (inotropism) with increased cardiac output; increased diuresis with reduction of edema secondary to a decrease in sympathetic tone; reduction in heart size, heart rate, blood volume, and pulmonary and venous pressures; and (usually) no net change in myocardial oxygen demand.

The digitalis glycosides also have several electrocardiac effects, including: decreased conduction velocity through the AV node, and prolonged effective refractory period (ERP). They may also increase the PR interval, decrease the QT interval and cause ST segment depression.

The exact mechanism of action of these agents have not been fully described, but their ability to increase the availability of Ca^{++} to myocardial fibers and to inhibit Na^{+}-K^{+}-ATPase with resultant increased intracellular Na^{+} and reduced K^{+} probably largely explain their actions.

For additional information, it is suggested to refer to a pharmacology text.

Uses/Indications - The veterinary indications for digitalis glycosides include treatment of congestive heart failure, atrial fibrillation or flutter, and supraventricular tachycardias.

Pharmacokinetics - Absorption following oral administration occurs in the small intestine and is variable dependent upon the oral dosage form used (see Dosage Forms below). Food may delay, but does not alter the extent of absorption. Peak serum levels generally occur within 45-60 minutes after oral elixir, and at about 90 minutes after oral tablet administration. In patients receiving an initial oral dose of digoxin, peak effects may occur in 6-8 hours after the dose.

The drug is distributed widely throughout the body with highest levels found in kidneys, heart, intestine, stomach, liver and skeletal muscle. Lowest concentrations are found in the brain and the plasma. At therapeutic levels, approximately 20-30% of the drug is bound to plasma proteins. Because only small amounts are found in fat, obese patients may receive too high dosages if dosing is based on total body weight versus lean body weight.

Digoxin is metabolized slightly, but the primary method of elimination is renal excretion both by glomerular filtration and tubular secretion. As a result, dosage adjustments must be made in patients with significant renal disease. Values reported for the elimination half-life of digoxin in dogs have been highly variable, with values reported from 14.4-56 hours. Elimination half-lives reported in other species include: Cats≈33.3±9.5 hrs; Sheep≈7.15 hrs.; Horses≈16.9 - 23.2 hrs.; and Cattle≈7.8 hrs.

Contraindications/Precautions - Digitalis cardioglycosides are contraindicated in patients with ventricular fibrillation or in digitalis intoxication. They should be used with extreme caution in patients with glomerulonephritis and heart failure or with idiopathic hypertrophic subaortic stenosis (IHSS). They should be used with caution in patients with severe pulmonary disease, hypoxia, acute myocarditis, myxedema, or acute myocardial infarction, frequent ventricular premature contractions, ventricular tachycardias, chronic constrictive pericarditis or incomplete AV block. They may be used in patients with stable, complete AV block or severe bradycardia with heart failure if the block was not caused by the cardiac glycoside.

When used to treat atrial fibrillation or flutter prior to administration with an antiarrhythmic agent that has anticholinergic activity (*e.g.,* quinidine, procainamide, disopyramide), digitalis glycosides will reduce, but not eliminate the increased ventricular rates that may be produced by those agents. Since digitalis glycosides may cause increased vagal tone, they should be used with caution in patients with increased carotid sinus sensitivity.

Elective cardioversion of patients with atrial fibrillation should be postponed until digitalis glycosides have been withheld for 1-2 days, and should not be attempted in patients with signs of digitalis toxicity.

Because digoxin is principally eliminated by the kidneys, it should be used with caution and serum levels monitored in patients with renal disease. Animals that are hypernatremic, hypokalemic, hypercalcemic, hyper- or hypothyroid may require smaller dosages; monitor carefully.

The veterinary elixir is available in two separate concentrations, do not confuse the two.

Adverse Effects/Warnings - Adverse effects of digoxin are usually associated with high or toxic serum levels and are categorized into cardiac and extracardiac signs and symptoms. There are species differences with regard to the sensitivity to digoxin's toxic effects also. Cats are relatively sensitive to digoxin while dogs tend to be more tolerant of high serum levels.

Cardiac effects may be seen before other extra-cardiac symptoms and may include almost every type of cardiac arrhythmia described with a resultant worsening of heart failure symptoms. More common arrhythmias or ECG changes seen, include complete or incomplete heart block, bigeminy, ST segment changes, paroxysmal ventricular or atrial tachycardias with block, and multifocal premature ventricular contractions. Because these effects can also be caused by worsening heart disease, it may be difficult to determine if they are a result of the disease process or of digitalis intoxication. If in doubt, monitor serum levels or stop digoxin therapy temporarily.

Extracardiac symptoms most commonly seen in veterinary medicine include mild GI upset, anorexia, weight loss and diarrhea. Vomiting has been associated with IV injections and should not cause anxiety nor alarm. Ocular and neurologic effects are routinely seen in humans, but are not prevalent in animals or are not detected.

Overdosage - Symptoms of chronic toxicity are discussed above. In dogs the acute toxic dose after IV administration has been reported to be 0.177 mg/kg.

Treatment of chronic digoxin toxicity is dictated by the severity of the signs and symptoms associated with it. Many patients will do well after temporarily stopping the drug and reevaluating the dosage regimen.

If an acute ingestion has recently occurred and no present cardiotoxic or neurologic signs (coma, seizures, etc.) have been manifested, emptying the stomach may be indicated followed with activated charcoal administration. Because digoxin can be slowly absorbed and there is some enterohepatic recirculation of the drug, repeated charcoal administration may be beneficial even if the ingestion occurred well before treatment. Anion-exchange resins such as colestipol or cholestyramine have also been suggested to reduce the absorption and enterohepatic circulation of digoxin and digitoxin, but are not readily available in most veterinary practices. These agents may be of more benefit to adsorb less polar compounds such as digitoxin.

Dependent on the type of cardiotoxicity, supportive and symptomatic therapy should be implemented. Serum electrolyte concentrations, drug level if available on a "stat" basis, arterial blood gases if available, and continuous ECG monitoring should be instituted. Acid-base, hypoxia, and fluid and electrolyte imbalances should be corrected. The use of potassium in normokalemic patients is very controversial and should only be attempted with constant monitoring and clinical expertise.

The use of specific antiarrhythmic agents in treating life-threatening digitalis-induced arrhythmias may be necessary. Phenytoin, lidocaine, and propranolol are most commonly employed for these arrhythmias. Atropine may be used to treat sinus bradycardia, SA arrest, or 2nd or 3rd degree AV block.

Digoxin immune Fab is a promising treatment for digoxin or digitoxin life-threatening toxicity. It is produced from specific digoxin antibodies from sheep and will bind directly to the drug, inactivating it. It is extremely expensive however and veterinary experience with it is extremely limited.

Drug Interactions - Many digoxin interactions are listed in human medicine, the following may be of importance in veterinary medicine: **Antacids, cimetidine, metoclopramide, neomycin (oral), chemotherapy agents** (*e.g.,* **cyclophosphamide, doxorubicin, vinca alkaloids, cytarabine**) may decrease the amount of digoxin absorbed from the GI tract.

The following agents may either increase the serum level, decrease the elimination rate, or enhance the toxic effects of digoxin: **diazepam, quinidine, anticholinergics, succinylcholine, verapamil, tetracycline and erythromycin.**

Patients on digoxin that receive **thyroid replacement therapy** may need their digoxin dosage adjusted.

Penicillamine may decrease serum levels of digoxin independent of route of digoxin dosing.

Drugs that can affect electrolyte balance can alter the efficacy or enhance the toxic effects of digoxin. **Diuretics (furosemide, thiazides)** may predispose the patient to digitalis toxicity. Other drugs which can deplete body potassium (**amphotericin B, glucocorticoids, ACTH, laxatives, sodium polystyrene sulfonate**) or decrease extracellular potassium (**glucagon, high dose IV dextrose, dextrose/insulin infusions**) may also predispose patients to toxic effects of digitalis drugs. **Spironolactone** may enhance or decrease the toxic effects of digoxin.

Refer to specialized references for more information.

Doses -
Dogs:
- a) 0.22 mg/m^2 of body surface area *bid* (Note: body surface area from weight conversion chart may be found in the appnedix) (Kittleson and Knowlen 1986)
- b) Oral maintenance dose: 0.01 - 0.02 mg/kg divided *bid*, monitor and adjust dosage *prn*. Rapid oral digitalization: 0.02 - 0.06 mg/kg divided *bid* the first day and then a maintenance dose. (Kittleson 1985b)
- c) Rapid intravenous digitalization for atrial arrhythmias: 0.01 - 0.02 mg/kg divided; give 1/2 of above dose IV and wait for 30-60 minutes and give 1/4th the dose IV; wait another 30-60 minutes and give the remainder if necessary. (Miller 1985)
- d) Elixir: 0.005 - 0.008 mg/kg PO *bid*; Tablets: 0.005 - 0.01 mg/kg PO *bid* (Moses 1988)
- e) Elixir: 0.18 mg/m^2 PO *bid*; Tablet dose same as "a" above (Kittleson 1985a)
- f) For canine dilated cardiomyopathy: 0.01 - 0.02 mg/kg PO divided *bid*; maintain serum levels between 1-2 ng/ml. (Ogburn 1988)

Cats: (Note: cats dislike the taste of the elixir)
- a) Elixir: 0.003 - 0.004 mg/kg PO *bid* (Moses 1988)
- b) Tablets: 0.005 - 0.008 mg/kg/day PO divided *bid*;
  alternatively: For cats weighing:
  2-3 kg = 1/4 of a 0.125 mg tablet every other day.
  4-5 kg = 1/4 of a 0.125 mg tablet every day.
  6 kg or > = 1/4 of a 0.125 mg tablet *bid* (Kittleson 1985a)
- c) Oral maintenance 0.007 - 0.015 mg/kg once daily to every other day. Rapid IV: 0.005 mg/kg lean body weight divided between three doses (1/2 the dose initially, then 60 minutes later another 1/4 of the dose, 60 minutes later the remainder (if necessary) or to effect. Stop if marked bradycardia, diminished AV conduction, other digoxin related arrhythmias or clinical signs of toxicity are present. Begin oral therapy as soon as the last IV dose is completed. (Miller 1985)

Cattle:
- a) 0.25 mg/100 lbs body weight (not destroyed in rumen), titrate dose to normalize atrial rate; not excreted in milk (McConnell and Hughey 1987)

Horses:
- a) 0.022 mg/kg daily orally (maintenance) (McConnell and Hughey 1987)
- b) 0.06 - 0.08 mg/kg PO q8h for 5-6 doses to digitalize, then 0.01 - 0.02 mg/kg PO maintenance. (Hilwig 1987)

Note: a case report of serious digoxin toxicity in a horse has been reported following 0.035 - 0.07 mg/kg/day for 5 days; digitalize with caution.

Birds:
- a) Using 0.5 mg/ml elixir, 4 drops in 2oz of water as the sole water source, change daily) (McConnell and Hughey 1987)

Monitoring Parameters -
1) Serum levels
   Because of the significant interpatient pharmacokinetic variation seen with this drug and its narrow therapeutic index, it is strongly recommended to monitor serum levels to help guide therapy. Unless the patient received an initial loading dose, at least 6 days should pass after beginning therapy to monitor serum levels as to allow levels to approach steady-state. Suggested therapeutic serum levels in the dog are 0.9 - 3.0 ng/ml and 0.9 - 2.0 ng/ml in cat (Neff-Davis 1985). For other species, values from 0.5 - 2.0 ng/ml can be used as guidelines. Levels at the higher end of the suggested range may be necessary to treat some atrial arrhythmias, but may also result in higher incidences of adverse effects. Usually a trough level (just before next dose or at least 8 hours after last dose) is recommended.
2) Appetite/weight
3) Cardiac rate, ECG changes
4) Serum electrolytes
5) Clinical efficacy for CHF (improved perfusion, decreased edema, increased venous (or arterial) O$_2$ levels).

Client Information - Contact veterinarian if animal displays changes in behavior, vomits, has diarrhea, lack of appetite, symptoms of colic (horses), becomes lethargic or depressed.

Dosage Forms/Preparations/FDA Approval Status/Withholding Times -
There are bioavailability differences between dosage forms and in tablets produced by different manufacturers. It is recommended that tablets be used from a manufacturer that the clinician has confidence in and that brands not be routinely interchanged. Should a change in dosage forms be

desired, the following bioavailability differences can be used as guidelines in altering the dose: Intravenous = 100%, IM ≈ 80%, Oral tablets ≈ 60%, Oral elixir ≈ 75%, Oral capsules ≈ 90-100%. The bioavailability of digoxin in veterinary species has only been studied in a limited manner. One study in dogs yielded similar values as those above for oral tablets and elixir, but in horses only about 20% of an intragastric dose was bioavailable.

Veterinary-Approved Products:

Digoxin Elixir 0.05 mg/ml 60 ml dropper bottle; *Cardoxin*® *LS* (Evsco); (Rx)

Digoxin Elixir 0.15 mg/ml in 60 ml dropper bottle; *Cardoxin*® (Evsco); (Rx)

Digoxin tablets and elixir have been approved for veterinary use, but no species are listed in the indications. There are no drug residue data for meat or milk published and no meat or milk withdrawal times are available.

Human-Approved Products:

Digoxin for Injection 0.1 mg/ ml in 1 ml amps & 0.25 mg/ml in 2 ml amps, & 1 & 2 ml Tubex; *Lanoxin*® (Glaxo Wellcome), *Digoxin*® (Elkins-Sinn) and (Wyeth-Ayerst) (Rx)

Digoxin tablets 0.125 mg, 0.25 mg and 0.5 mg; *Lanoxin*® (Glaxo Wellcome), generic; (Rx)

Digoxin capsules 0.05 mg, 0.1 mg, 0.2 mg; *Lanoxicaps*® (Glaxo Wellcome); (Rx)

Digoxin Elixir Pediatric 0.05 mg/ml in 60 ml dropper bottle, 50 ml and UD 2.5 & 5 ml; *Lanoxin*® (Glaxo Wellcome); (Rx); generic (Rx)

DIHYDROTACHYSTEROL
DHT

Chemistry - A vitamin D analog, dihydrotachysterol (DHT) occurs as odorless, colorless or white crystals, or crystalline white powder. It is practically insoluble in water, sparingly soluble in vegetable oils, and soluble in alcohol. Dihydrotachysterol may also be known as DHT, dichysterol, or dihydrotachysterol$_2$.

Storage/Stability/Compatibility - All DHT products should be stored at room temperature (15-30°C). Capsules or tablets should be stored in well-closed, light-resistant containers and the oral concentrate should be stored in tight, light-resistant containers.

Pharmacology - DHT is hydroxylated in the liver to 25-hydroxy-dihydrotachysterol which is the active form of the drug and is an analog of 1,25-dihydroxyvitamin D. Vitamin D is considered a hormone and, in conjunction with parathormone (PTH) and calcitonin, regulates calcium homeostasis in the body. Active analogues (or metabolites) of vitamin D enhance calcium absorption from the GI tract, promote reabsorption of calcium by the renal tubules, and increase the rate of accretion and resorption of minerals in bone.

Uses/Indications - DHT is used in small animals to treat hypocalcemia secondary to hypoparathyroidism or severe renal disease.

Pharmacokinetics - If fat absorption is normal, vitamin D analogs are readily absorbed from the GI tract (small intestine). Bile is required for adequate absorption and patients with steatorrhea, liver or biliary disease will have diminished absorption. DHT is hydroxylated in the liver to 25-hydroxy-dihydrotachysterol which is the active form of the drug. Unlike some other forms of vitamin D, DHT does not require parathormone activation in the kidneys.

Contraindications/Precautions/Reproductive Safety - DHT is contraindicated in patients with hypercalcemia, vitamin D toxicity, malabsorption syndrome, or abnormal sensitivity to the effects of vitamin D. It should be used with extreme caution in patients with hyperphosphatemia (many clinicians believe hyperphosphatemia or a combined calcium/phosphorous product of > 70 mg/dl is a contraindication to its use), or in patients with renal dysfunction (when receiving the drug for non-renal indications).

Adverse Effects/Warnings - Hypercalcemia, nephrocalcinosis and hyperphosphatemia are potential complications of DHT therapy. Symptoms of hypercalcemia include polydipsia, polyuria and anorexia. Monitoring of serum calcium levels is mandatory while using this drug

Overdosage/Acute Toxicity - Acute ingestions should be managed using established protocols for removal or prevention of the drug being absorbed from the GI. Orally administered mineral oil may reduce absorption and enhance fecal elimination.

Hypercalcemia secondary to chronic dosing of the drug should be treated by first temporarily discontinuing DHT and exogenous calcium therapy. If the hypercalcemia is severe, furosemide, calcium-free IV fluids (*e.g.,* normal saline), urine acidification, and corticosteroids may be employed. Because of the long duration of action of DHT (up to one week), hypercalcemia may persist. Restart DHT/calcium therapy at a reduced dosage with diligent monitoring when calcium serum levels return to the normal range.

Drug Interactions - Magnesium containing antacids may cause hypermagnesemia when used with vitamin D analogs.

Thiazide diuretics may cause hypercalcemia when given in conjunction with Vitamin D analogs.

Corticosteroids can nullify the effects of vitamin D analogs.

Phenytoin, barbiturates or primidone may induce hepatic enzyme systems and increase the metabolism of Vitamin D analogs thus decreasing their activity.

Patients on **verapamil or digoxin** are sensitive to the effects of hypercalcemia; intensified monitoring is required.

Mineral oil, sucralfate, cholestyramine, or colestipol may reduce the amount of drug absorbed.

Drug/Laboratory Interactions - Serum cholesterol levels may be falsely elevated by vitamin D analogs when using the Zlatkis-Zak reaction for determination.

Doses -
Vitamin D therapy for hypocalcemic conditions is often used with exogenously administered calcium products. Refer to the calcium monograph or the references cited below for further information.

Dogs:
For hypocalcemia secondary to hypoparathyroidism:
    a) Once life-threatening signs of hypocalcemia have been controlled with intravenous calcium, give DHT initially at 0.03 - 0.06 mg/kg/day PO for 2-3 days, then 0.02 - 0.03 mg/kg/day for 2-3 days, and finally 0.01 mg/kg/day until further dosage adjustments are required. Stable serum calcium levels (8.5-9.5 mg/dl) are usually achieved in a week. Determine serum calcium levels twice daily during initial treatment period until levels have stabilized in the low-normal range. (Peterson 1986)
    b) 0.007 - 0.010 mg/kg PO once daily (maintenance dose); may require 1-2 weeks to restore normocalcemia. (Mulnix 1985)
    c) For **secondary hypoparathyroidism**: During initial loading period with calcium and DHT, monitor serum calcium 1-2 times daily for 5-10 days. Give loading dose of DHT at 0.02 - 0.05 mg/kg PO once daily for 2-3 days, then 0.01 - 0.03 mg/kg PO once daily for 1 week. After a low normal serum calcium is achieved, give 0.01 mg/kg PO once every other day and then every third day etc., until it can be finally stopped. Dose should be individualized for each animal. During loading period, calcium should be given at 25 - 50 mg (elemental calcium)/kg/day divided 2-4 times a day. After 1 week, decrease dose to 15 - 25 mg (elemental calcium)/kg/day divided and gradually reduce. The goal is to keep serum calcium levels in the low-normal range (7.5 - 9.5 mg/dl) so that the remaining parathyroid tissue will respond via feedback mechanisms.

        For **primary hypoparathyroidism** (animals will require therapy for life): Loading regimen is the same as for secondary hypoparathyroidism. Then DHT may be given at 0.01 mg/kg PO once daily and eventually every other day if serum calcium levels permit. Reduce oral calcium supplementation to as low a dose as possible; may consider replacing pharmaceuticals with a high calcium diet. Monitoring of calcium levels may be reduced to 1-2 times per month after loading regimen is completed and animal is relatively stable. Dosage adjustments of either DHT or calcium should be made in increments of about 25%. Eventually, animal may only need to be monitored (serum calcium) only several times a year. (Meuten and Armstrong 1989)

For hypocalcemia secondary to severe renal failure:
    a) After hyperphosphatemia is controlled (do not use calcium and vitamin D if calcium/phosphate product is in excess of 70 mg/dl), use oral calcium carbonate therapy. If calcium alone does not resolve hypocalcemia add DHT at 0.125 mg per dog PO 3 times per week. Adjust dose based on serial calcium determinations. Maximum effect may require 2-4 weeks and duration may persist up to 1 week after treatment is discontinued. (Allen 1989)
    b) In combination with calcium therapy, give DHT initially at 0.03 mg/kg/day for 2 days, then 0.02 mg/kg/day for 2 days, then 0.01 mg/kg/day maintenance dose. (Kay and Richter 1988)

Cats:
For hypocalcemia secondary to hypoparathyroidism:
    a) For secondary hypoparathyroidism: As per dogs in "c" above. Dosage is empirical. Cats with hypoparathyroidism secondary to thyroidectomy may require treatment for several months. (Meuten and Armstrong 1989)
    b) In combination with calcium therapy (initially at 50 - 100 mg/kg/day divided 3-4 times daily of elemental calcium), give DHT initially at 0.125 - 0.25 mg PO per day

for 2-3 days, then 0.08 - 0.125 mg per day for 2-3 days and finally 0.05 mg PO per day until further dosage adjustments are necessary. Stable serum calcium levels (8.5-9.5 mg/dl) are usually achieved in about a week. Continue to monitor and adjust dosages of DHT and calcium to lowest levels to maintain normocalcemia. (Peterson and Randolph 1989) (Note: refer to the calcium monograph for further information.)

Monitoring Parameters -
1) Serum calcium levels should be monitored closely (some clinicians recommend twice daily) during the initial treatment period. When the animal is stabilized frequency may be reduced, but never discontinued. All animals receiving DHT therapy should have calcium levels determined at least 2-4 times yearly.
2) Serum phosphorous (particularly in renal failure patients)

Client Information - Clients should be briefed on the symptoms of hypercalcemia (polydipsia, polyuria, anorexia) and hypocalcemia (muscle tremors, twitching, tetany, weakness, stiff gait, ataxia, behavioral changes, and seizures) and instructed to report these symptoms to the veterinarian.

Dosage Forms/Preparations/FDA Approval Status/Withholding Times -
Veterinary-Approved Products: None
Human-Approved Products:

Dihydrotachysterol Oral Tablets 0.125 mg, 0.2 mg, 0.4 mg; *DHT® Tablets* (Roxane); (Rx)

Dihydrotachysterol Oral Capsules 0.125 mg; *Hytakerol®* (Winthrop)

Dihydrotachysterol Oral Concentrate Solution 0.2 mg/ml in 30 ml bottles, and 0.25 mg/ml (in oil) in 15 ml bottles; *DHT® Intensol* (Roxane), *Hytakerol®* (Winthrop); (Rx)

DILTIAZEM HCL

Chemistry - A calcium channel blocker, diltiazem HCl occurs as a white to off-white crystalline powder having a bitter taste. It is soluble in water and alcohol. Potencies may be expressed in terms of base (active moiety) and the salt. Dosages are generally expressed in terms of the salt. Diltiazem is also known as latiazem HCl.

Storage/Stability/Compatibility - Diltiazem oral products should be stored at room temperature in tight, light resistant containers.

Pharmacology - Diltiazem is a calcium-channel blocker similar in action to drugs such as verapamil or nifedipine. While the exact mechanism is unknown, diltiazem inhibits the transmembrane influx of extracellular calcium ions in myocardial cells and vascular smooth muscle, but does not alter serum calcium concentrations. The net effects of this action is to inhibit the cardiac and vascular smooth muscle contractility, thereby dilating main systemic and coronary arteries. Total peripheral resistance, blood pressure and cardiac afterload are all reduced.

Diltiazem also has effects on cardiac conduction. It slows AV node conduction and prolongs refractory times. Diltiazem rarely affects SA node conduction, but in patients with Sick Sinus Syndrome, resting heart rates may be reduced.

Although diltiazem can cause negative inotropic effects, it is rarely of clinical importance (unlike verapamil or nifedipine). Diltiazem apparently does not affect plasma renin or aldosterone concentrations nor affect blood glucose or insulin concentrations.

Uses/Indications - Diltiazem may be useful in the treatment of atrial fibrillation, supraventricular tachycardias, and hypertrophic cardiomyopathy. For specific information, refer to the Dosages section.

Pharmacokinetics - After an oral dose, about 80% of the dose is absorbed rapidly from the gut, but because of a high first pass effect only about half of that absorbed reaches the systemic circulation. Approximately 75% of the drug is bound to serum proteins in humans. Diltiazem enters maternal milk in concentrations approximating those found in the plasma. Diltiazem is rapidly and almost completely metabolized in the liver. Serum half lives in humans range from 3.5 to 10 hours. Renal impairment may only slightly increase half lives.

Contraindications/Precautions/Reproductive Safety - Diltiazem is contraindicated in patients with severe hypotension (<90 mm Hg systolic), sick sinus syndrome or 2nd or 3rd degree AV block (unless a functioning pacemaker is in place), acute MI, radiographically documented pulmonary congestion, or if the patient is hypersensitive to it.

Diltiazem should be used with caution in geriatric patients or those with heart failure (particularly if also receiving beta blockers), or hepatic or renal impairment.

High doses in rodents have resulted in increased fetal deaths and skeletal abnormalities. Use during pregnancy only when the benefits outweigh the potential risks.

Adverse Effects/Warnings - Experience in both dogs and cats is limited. At usual doses, bradycardia is the most prominent side effect reported in dogs thus far. Specific adverse effects in cats are not well described. Potentially, GI distress, hypotension, heart block or other rhythm distur-bances, CNS effects, rashes, or elevations in liver function tests could occur in either species.

Overdosage/Acute Toxicity - The oral LD$_{50}$ in dogs has been reported as >50 mg/kg. Symptoms noted after overdosage may include heart block, bradycardia, hypotension, and heart failure. Treatment should consist of gut emptying protocols when warranted, and supportive and symptomatic treatment. Atropine may be used to treat bradycardias or 2nd or 3rd degree AV block. If these do not respond to vagal blockade, isoproterenol may be tried (with caution). Fixed block may require cardiac pacing. Inotropics (*e.g.,* dobutamine, dopamine, isoproterenol) and pressors (*e.g.,* dopamine, norepinephrine) may be required to treat heart failure and hypotension. A slow intravenous calcium infusion (1 ml/10 kg body weight of 10% calcium gluconate) may also be useful for severe acute toxicity.

Drug Interactions - While data conflicts regarding whether diltiazem affects **digoxin** pharma-cokinetics, diligent monitoring of digoxin serum concentrations should be performed. Diltiazem may increase the likelihood of bradycardia, AV block or CHF developing in patients also receiv-ing beta **blockers (including ophthalmic** beta **blockers)**. Additionally, diltiazem may substan-tially increase the bioavailability of **propranolol. Cimetidine** may increase plasma diltiazem concentrations; increased monitoring of diltiazem's effects are warranted. **Ranitidine** may also affect diltiazem concentrations, but to a lesser extent. Diltiazem may affect **cyclosporin** or **quinidine** serum concentrations; increased monitoring and dosage adjustments may be required.

Doses -
  Dogs:
    For treatment of supraventricular tachyarrhthymias:
    a) 0.5 - 1 (up to 1.5) mg/kg PO q8h (Pion 1992)
    b) For atrial fibrillation with rapid ventricular response in dogs with dilated cardiomy-opathy: 0.4 - 0.5 mg/kg PO *tid*; increase dosage gradually every 2-3 days while pa-tient is observed for deterioration of cardiovascular function. Dosages above 1 mg/kg are not recommended. (Calvert 1992)
    c) Initially give a 0.25 mg/kg IV bolus over 2 minutes. Repeat 0.25 mg/kg IV bolus ev-ery 15 minutes until conversion occurs or total dosage of 0.75 mg/kg has been given. (Russell and Rush 1995)
    For supraventricular arrhythmias, hypertrophic cardiomyopathy, hypertension:
    a) 0.5 - 1.5 mg/kg PO q8h; titrate upwards to effect (Miller, Tilley et al. 1994)

  Cats:
    For treatment of supraventricular tachyarrhythmias:
    a) 0.5 - 1 (up to 1.5) mg/kg PO q8h (Pion 1992)

    For treatment of hypertrophic cardiomyopathy:
    a) 7.5 mg PO *tid* (Pion 1992)
    b) 1.75 - 2.5 mg/kg PO *tid* (Bright 1992)
    c) Initially 7.5 mg (1/4th of a 30 mg tablet) PO q8h; may be given as initial therapy in asymptomatic cats or added to therapy in cats responding poorly to furosemide or enalapril. (Bonagura and Lehmkuhl 1994)

    For supraventricular arrhythmias, hypertrophic cardiomyopathy, hypertension:
    a) 0.5 - 2.5 mg/kg PO q8h (Miller, Tilley et al. 1994)

Monitoring Parameters - 1) ECG/Heart Rate; 2) Blood Pressure; 3) Adverse Effects

Client Information - Inform clients of potential adverse effects. Stress compliance.

Dosage Forms/Preparations/FDA Approval Status/Withholding Times -
  Veterinary-Approved Products: None
  Human-Approved Products:

  Diltiazem Tablets 30 mg, 60 mg, 90 mg, and 120 mg; *Cardizem*® (Hoechst Marion Roussel) (Marion Merrell Dow, generic; (Rx)

  Diltiazem Extended-Release Tablets: 120 mg, 180 mg, & 240 mg; *Tiamate*® (Hoechst Marion Roussel) (Rx)

  Diltiazem Oral Capsules Extended Release 60 mg, 90 mg, 120 mg, 180 mg, 240 mg, 300 mg, 360 mg; *Cardizem*® SR (Hoechst Marion Roussel); (Rx);*Cardizem CD*® (Hoechst Marion Roussel) (Rx);*Dilacor XR*® (Rhone-Poulenc Rorer) (Rx);*Tiazac*® (Forest) (Rx); generic (Rx)

  Diltiazem Injection 5 mg/ml in 5 ml & 10 ml vials; *Cardizem*® (Hoechst Marion Roussel);*Diltiazem*® (Bedford Labs) (Rx)

DIMENHYDRINATE

Chemistry - An ethanolamine derivative antihistamine, dimenhydrinate contains approximately 54% diphenhydramine and 46% 8-chlorotheophylline. It occurs as an odorless, bitter and numbing-tasting, white crystalline powder with a melting range of 102°-107°C. Dimenhydrinate is slightly soluble in water and is freely soluble in propylene glycol or alcohol. The pH of the commercially available injection ranges from 6.4 to 7.2.

Storage/Stability/Compatibility - Dimenhydrinate products should be stored at room temperature; avoid freezing the oral solution and injectable products. The oral solution should be stored in tight containers and tablets stored in well-closed containers.

Dimenhydrinate injection is reportedly **compatible** with all commonly used intravenous replenishment solutions and the following drugs: amikacin sulfate, atropine sulfate, calcium gluconate, chloramphenicol sodium succinate, corticotropin, ditrizoate meglumine and sodium, diphenhydramine HCl, droperidol, fentanyl citrate, heparin sodium, iothalamate meglumine and sodium, meperidine HCl, methicillin sodium, metoclopramide, morphine sulfate, norepinephrine bitartrate, oxytetracycline HCl, penicillin G potassium, pentazocine lactate, perphenazine, phenobarbital sodium, potassium chloride, scopolamine HBr, vancomycin HCl and vitamin B-complex w/ vitamin C.

The following drugs are either **incompatible** or compatible only in certain concentrations with dimenhydrinate: aminophylline, ammonium chloride, amobarbital sodium, butorphanol tartrate, glycopyrrolate, hydrocortisone sodium succinate, hydroxyzine, iodipamide meglumine, pentobarbital sodium, prochlorperazine edisylate, promazine HCl, promethazine HCl, tetracycline HCl, and thiopental sodium. Compatibility is dependent upon factors such as pH, concentration, temperature, and diluents used and it is suggested to consult specialized references for more specific information.

Pharmacology - Dimenhydrinate has antihistaminic, antiemetic, anticholinergic, CNS depressant and local anesthetic effects. These principle pharmacologic actions are thought to be a result of only the diphenhydramine moiety. Used most commonly for its antiemetic/-motion sickness effects, dimenhydrinate's exact mechanism of action for this indication is unknown, but the drug does inhibit vestibular stimulation. The anticholinergic actions of dimenhydrinate may play a role in blocking acetylcholine stimulation of the vestibular and reticular systems. Tolerance to the CNS depressant effects can ensue after a few days of therapy and antiemetic effectiveness also may diminish with prolonged use.

Uses/Indications - In veterinary medicine, dimenhydrinate is used primarily for its antiemetic effects in the prophylactic treatment of motion sickness in dogs and cats.

Pharmacokinetics - The pharmacokinetics of this agent have apparently not been studied in veterinary species. In humans, the drug is well absorbed after oral administration with antiemetic effects occurring within 30 minutes of administration. Antiemetic effects occur almost immediately after IV injection. The duration of effect is usually 3-6 hours.

Diphenhydramine is metabolized in the liver, and the majority of the drug is excreted as metabolites into the urine. The terminal elimination half-life in adult humans ranges from 2.4 - 9.3 hours.

Contraindications/Precautions - Dimenhydrinate is contraindicated in patients who are hypersensitive to it or to other antihistamines in its class. Because of their anticholinergic activity, antihistamines should be used with caution in patients with angle closure glaucoma, prostatic hypertrophy, pyloroduodenal or bladder neck obstruction, and COPD if mucosal secretions are a problem. Additionally, they should be used with caution in patients with hyperthyroidism, seizure disorders, cardiovascular disease or hypertension. It may mask the symptoms of ototoxicity and should therefore be used with this knowledge when concomitantly administering with ototoxic drugs.

Adverse Effects/Warnings - Most common adverse reactions seen are CNS depression (lethargy, somnolence) and anticholinergic effects (dry mouth, urinary retention). GI effects (diarrhea, vomiting, anorexia) are less common, but have been noted.

The sedative effects of antihistamines, may adversely affect the performance of working dogs. The sedative effects of antihistamines may diminish with time.

Overdosage - Overdosage may cause CNS stimulation (excitement to seizures) or depression (lethargy to coma), anticholinergic effects, respiratory depression and death. Treatment consists of emptying the gut if the ingestion was oral. Induce emesis if the patient is alert and CNS status is stable. Administration of a saline cathartic and/or activated charcoal may be given after emesis or gastric lavage. Treatment of other symptoms should be performed using symptomatic and supportive therapies. Phenytoin (IV) is recommended in the treatment of seizures caused by antihistamine overdose in humans; use of barbiturates and diazepam are avoided.

Drug Interactions - Increased sedation can occur if dimenhydrinate (diphenhydramine) is combined with **other CNS depressant drugs**. Antihistamines may partially counteract the anticoagulation effects of **heparin** or **warfarin**. Diphenhydramine may enhance the effects of **epinephrine**.

Dimenhydrinate may potentiate the anticholinergic effects of other **anticholinergic drugs**. Dimenhydrinate has been demonstrated to induce hepatic microsomal enzymes in animals (species not specified); the clinical implications of this effect are unclear.

Laboratory Interactions - Antihistamines can decrease the wheal and flare response to **antigen skin testing**. In humans, it is suggested that antihistamines be discontinued at least 4 days before testing.

Doses -

  Dogs:
    For prevention and treatment of motion sickness:
      a) 8 mg/kg PO q8h (Jones 1985), (DeNovo 1986)
      b) 25 - 50 mg PO once to 3 times a day (Morgan 1988)
      c) 4 - 8 mg/kg PO q8h (Washabau and Elie 1995)

  Cats:
    For prevention and treatment of motion sickness:
      a) 12.5 mg (total dose) PO q8h (Davis 1985b)
      b) 12.5 mg PO once to 3 times a day (Morgan 1988)
      c) 8 mg/kg PO q8h (DeNovo 1986)
      d) 4 - 8 mg/kg PO q8h (Washabau and Elie 1995)

Monitoring Parameters -
  1) Clinical efficacy and adverse effects (sedation, anticholinergic signs, etc.)

Dosage Forms/Preparations/FDA Approval Status/Withholding Times -
  Veterinary-Approved Products: None
  Human-Approved Products:

  Dimenhydrinate Tablets or capsules 50 mg; Commonly known as *Dramamine®* (Upjohn) (OTC); Many other OTC products also available

  Dimenhydrinate Oral Liquid 12.5 mg/4 ml, 12.5 mg/5 ml and 15.62 mg/5 ml; in pints and gallons and in 90 ml, 120 ml and 480 ml bottles *Children's Dramamine®* (Upjohn) (OTC); generic (OTC)

  Dimenhydrinate Injection 50 mg/ml; in 1 ml amps and vials, 5 & 10 ml vials; *Dramamine®* (Upjohn); Generic; (Rx)

DIMERCAPROL
BAL

Chemistry - A dithiol chelating agent, dimercaprol occurs as a colorless or nearly colorless, viscous liquid that is soluble in alcohol, vegetable oils, and water, but is unstable in aqueous solutions. It has a very disagreeable mercaptan-like odor. The commercially available injection is a peanut oil and benzyl benzoate solution. Although the solution may be turbid or contain small amounts of flocculent material or sediment, this does not mean the solution is deteriorating.

  Dimercaprol may also be known as BAL, British Anti-Lewisite, dimercaptopropanol, or dithioglycerol.

Storage/Stability/Compatibility - Dimercaprol injection should be stored below 40°C; preferably at room temperature (15-30°C).

Pharmacology - The sulfhydryl groups found on dimercaprol form heterocyclic ring complexes with heavy metals, principally arsenic, lead, mercury and gold. This binding helps prevent or reduce heavy metal binding to sulfhydryl-dependent enzymes. Different metals have differing affinities for both dimercaprol and sulfhydryl-dependent enzymes and the drug is relatively ineffective in chelating some metals (*e.g.,* selenium). Chelation to dimercaprol is not irreversible and metals can dissociate from the complex as dimercaprol concentrations decrease, in an acidic environment, or if oxidized. The dimercaprol-metal complex is excreted via renal and fecal routes.

Uses/Indications - The principal use of dimercaprol in veterinary medicine is in treating intoxications caused by arsenical compounds. It is occasionally used for lead, mercury and gold intoxication.

Pharmacokinetics - After IM injection, peak blood levels occur in 30-60 minutes. The drug is slowly absorbed through the skin after topical administration.

  Dimercaprol is distributed throughout the body, including the brain. Highest tissue levels are found in the liver and kidneys.

Non-metal bound drug is rapidly metabolized to inactive compounds and excreted in the urine, bile and feces. In humans, the duration of action is thought to be about 4 hours, with the drug completely eliminated within 6-24 hours.

Contraindications/Precautions/Reproductive Safety - Dimercaprol is contraindicated in patients with impaired hepatic function, unless secondary to acute arsenic toxicity. The drug is also contraindicated in iron, cadmium, and selenium poisoning as the chelated complex can be more toxic than the metal alone.

Because dimercaprol is potentially nephrotoxic, it should be used cautiously in patients with impaired renal function. In order to protect the kidneys, the urine should be alkalinized to prevent the chelated drug from dissociating in the urine. Animals with diminished renal function or who develop renal dysfunction while on therapy should either have the dosage adjusted or discontinue therapy dependent on the clinical situation.

Adverse Effects/Warnings - IM injections are necessary with this compound but can be very painful, particularly if the drug is not administered deeply. Vomiting and seizures can occur with higher dosages. Transient increases in blood pressure with concomitant tachycardia has been reported. Most adverse effects are transient in nature as the drug is eliminated rapidly.

Dimercaprol is potentially nephrotoxic.

Overdosage/Acute Toxicity - Symptoms of dimercaprol overdosage in animals include vomiting, seizures, tremors, coma and death. No specific doses were located to correspond with these symptoms, however.

Drug Interactions - Because dimercaprol can form a toxic complex with certain metals (cadmium, selenium, uranium and iron). Do not administer with **iron or selenium salts**. At least 24 hours should pass after the last dimercaprol dose, before iron or selenium therapy is begun.

Drug/Laboratory Interactions - Iodine I[131] thyroidal uptake values may be decreased during or immediately following dimercaprol therapy as it interferes with normal iodine accumulation by the thyroid.

Doses -
Dogs & Cats:
For arsenic toxicity:
 a) Intensive supportive care is required. Give dimercaprol as early as possible after exposure at 2.5 - 5 mg/kg IM. The 5 mg/kg dose should only be used for acute cases and only for the first day of therapy. Repeat doses at 4 hour intervals for the first 2 days; every 8 hours on the third day, and twice daily for the next 10 days until recovery. Give with sodium thiosulfate: 40 - 50 mg/kg IV as a 20% solution *bid-tid* until recovery. (Neiger 1989)
 b) Cats: If ingestion was recent, use emetics or gastric lavage to help prevent arsenic absorption. If clinical signs are present and ingestion was within 36 hours, begin dimercaprol therapy at 2.5 - 5 mg/kg IM q4h for the first 2 days, the q12h until recovery. Fluid therapy should be instituted to prevent dehydration and maintain renal function. (Reid and Oehme 1989)
 c) 4 mg/kg IM q4-6h; do not give for more than 4 continuous days. (Grauer and Hjelle 1988c)
 d) Loading dose of 5 mg/kg IM (acute cases only) followed by 2.5 mg/kg IM q3-4h for two days, then progressively lengthen the dosing interval to q12h until recovery is evident. (Mount 1989)

Food Animals:
For arsenic toxicity:
 a) 3 mg/kg IM q4h for first 2 days, then q6h on the third day, then *bid* for 10 days until recovery. (Hatch 1988a)
 b) 4 - 5 mg/kg initially, then 2 - 3 mg/kg IM q4-6h for the first day and 1 mg/kg for at least 2 more days. May be beneficial in animals poisoned with inorganic arsenic compounds, but not organic arsenicals. (Furr and Buck 1986)
For mercury toxicity:
 a) For bovine or swine: 3 mg/kg IM four times daily for 3 days, then twice daily for 10 days. Treatment is often unsuccessful. (Osweiler and Hook 1986)
Horses:
For arsenic toxicity:
 a) Dimercaprol therapy in horses is difficult because it must be used acutely and any substantial delays in treatment significantly decrease its effectiveness, as well as the amounts of dimercaprol that are required and the necessity to inject the drug IM. If available, the dose is: 5 mg/kg IM initially, followed by 3 mg/kg IM q6h for the remainder of the first day, then 1 mg/kg IM q6h for two or more additional days, as

needed. (Oehme 1987a) (Note: Refer to this reference for additional information on the use of sodium thiosulfate and protective laxative therapy.)

Monitoring Parameters -
1) Liver function
2) Renal function
3) Hemogram
4) Hydration and perfusion status
5) Electrolytes and acid/base status
6) Urinary pH

Client Information - Because of the potential toxicity of this agent and the seriousness of most heavy metal intoxications, this drug should be used with close professional supervision only. Dimercaprol can impart a strong, unpleasant mercaptan-like odor to the animal's breath.

Dosage Forms/Preparations/FDA Approval Status/Withholding Times -
Veterinary-Approved Products: None
Human-Approved Products:
Dimercaprol Injection 100 mg/ml (for IM use only) in 3 ml amps; *BAL in Oil®* (Becton Dickinson); (Rx)

DIMETHYL SULFOXIDE
DMSO

Chemistry - DMSO is a clear, colorless to straw-yellow liquid. It is dipolar, aprotic (acts as a Lewis base) and extremely hygroscopic. It has a melting/freezing point of 18.5°C, boiling point of 189°C, and a molecular weight of 78.1. It is miscible with water (heat is produced), alcohol, acetone, chloroform, ether and many organic solvents. A 2.15% solution in water is isotonic with serum.

Storage/Stability/Compatibility - Must be stored in airtight containers and away from light. As DMSO may react with some plastics, it should be stored in glass or in the container provided by the manufacturer. If DMSO is allowed to contact room air it will self-dilute to a concentration of 66-67%. DMSO is apparently compatible with many compounds, but because of the chances for accidental percutaneous absorption of potentially toxic compounds, the admixing of DMSO with other compounds is not to be done casually.

Pharmacology - The pharmacologic effects of DMSO are diverse. DMSO traps free radical hydroxide and its metabolite, dimethyl sulfide (DMS) traps free radical oxygen. It appears that these actions help to explain some of the anti-inflammatory, cryopreservative, antiischemic, and radioprotective qualities of DMSO.

DMSO will easily penetrate the skin. It also serves as a carrier agent in promoting the percutaneous absorption of other compounds (including drugs and toxins) that normally would not penetrate. Drugs such as insulin, heparin, phenylbutazone, and sulfonamides may all be absorbed systemically when mixed with DMSO and applied to the skin.

DMSO has weak antibacterial activity when used clinically and possible clinical efficacy when used topically as an antifungal. The mechanism for these antimicrobial effects have not been elucidated.

The anti-inflammatory/analgesic properties of DMSO have been thoroughly investigated. DMSO appears to be more effective an anti-inflammatory agent when used for acute inflammation versus chronic inflammatory conditions. The analgesic effects of DMSO has been compared to that produced by narcotic analgesics and is efficacious for both acute and chronic musculoskeletal pain.

DMSO decreases platelet aggregation, but reports on its effects on coagulability have been conflicting, as has its effect on the myocardium. DMSO has diuretic activity independent of the method of administration. It also provokes histamine release from mast cells, which probably contributes to the local vasodilatory effects seen after topical administration.

DMSO also apparently has some anticholinesterase activity and enhances prostaglandin E, but blocks the synthesis of prostaglandins E_2, $F_{2-alpha}$, H_2, and G_2. It inhibits the enzyme alcohol dehydrogenase, which not only is responsible for the metabolism of alcohol, but also the metabolism of ethylene glycol into toxic metabolites.

Uses/Indications - Purported uses for DMSO are rampant, but the only FDA-approved veterinary indication for DMSO is: "...as a topical application to reduce acute swelling due to trauma" (Package Insert - *Domoso®* — Syntex). Other possible indications for DMSO include: adjunctive treatment in transient ischemic conditions, CNS trauma and cerebral edema, skin ulcers/wounds/burns, adjunctive therapy in intestinal surgeries, and analgesia for post-operative or intractable pain, amyloidosis in dogs, reduction of mammary engorgement in the nursing bitch, enhancement of antibiotic penetration in mastitis in cattle, and limitation of tissue damage following extravasation injuries secondary to chemotherapeutic agents.

DMSO's effect on alcohol dehydrogenase, may make it useful in the treatment of ethylene glycol poisoning, but this has not been sufficiently studied as of yet. DMSO's attributes as a potential carrier of therapeutic agents across the skin and into the systemic circulation and its synergistic effects with other agents are potentially exciting, but require much more study before they can be routinely recommended.

While the potential indications for DMSO are many, unfortunately, the lack of well-controlled studies leave many more questions than answers regarding this drug.

Pharmacokinetics - DMSO is well absorbed after topical administration, especially at concentrations between 80-100%. It is extensively and rapidly distributed to virtually every area of the body. After IV administration to horses, the serum half-life was approximately 9 hours. DMSO is metabolized to dimethyl sulfide (DMS) and is primarily excreted by the kidneys, although biliary and respiratory excretion also takes place.

In cattle, the drug is eliminated quite rapidly and after 20 days no detectable drug or metabolites are found in milk, urine, blood, or tissues.

Contraindications/Precautions - Wear rubber gloves when applying topically, and apply with clean or sterile cotton to minimize the chances for contaminating with potentially harmful substances. Apply only to clean, dry areas to avoid carrying other chemicals into the systemic circulation.

DMSO may mask existing pathology with its anti-inflammatory and analgesic activity.

At high doses DMSO has been shown to be teratogenic in hamsters and chicks, but not in mice, rats or rabbits; weigh the risks versus benefits when using in pregnant animals.

Because DMSO may degranulate mast cells, animals with mastocytomas should only receive DMSO with extreme caution. DMSO should be used cautiously in animals suffering from dehydration or shock as its diuretic and peripheral vasodilatory effects may exacerbate these conditions.

Adverse Effects/Warnings - When used as labeled, DMSO appears to be an extremely safe drug. Local effects ("burning", erythema, vesiculation, dry skin, local allergic reactions) and garlic or oyster-like breath odor are the most likely adverse effects. They are transient and quickly resolve when therapy is discontinued. Lenticular changes, which may result in myopia, have been noted primarily in dogs and rabbits when DMSO is used chronically and at high doses. These effects are slowly reversible after the drug is discontinued.

When DMSO is administered intravenously to horses it may cause hemolysis and hemoglobinuria. These effects can be minimized by using concentrations of 20% or less (not less than 2% in water) and slowly administering.

Reports of hepatotoxicity and renal toxicity have also been reported for various species and dosages. These occur fairly rarely and some clinicians actually believe DMSO has a protective effect on ischemically insulted renal tissue.

Overdosage - The reported LD_{50}'s following IV dosage in dogs and cats are: Cats $\approx$ 4 g/kg, and Dogs $\approx$ 2.5 g/kg. Signs of toxicity include: sedation and hematuria at non-lethal doses; coma, seizures, opisthotonus, dyspnea and pulmonary edema at higher dosages. Should an acute overdosage be encountered, treat supportively.

Drug Interactions - Because of its anticholinesterase activity, avoid the use of **organophosphates** or **other cholinesterase inhibitors** with DMSO. A fatality secondary to mercury intoxication was reported when DMSO was mixed with a **mercury salt** "red blister" and applied topically to the leg of a horse. Because it inhibits alcohol dehydrogenase, DMSO may prolong the effects of **alcohol. Insulin, corticosteroids** (including endogenous steroids), and **atropine** may be potentiated by DMSO.

Doses -

 Dogs:
  a) Liberal application should be administered topically to the skin over the affected area 3-4 times daily. Total daily dosage should not exceed 20 grams (or mls of liquid) and therapy should not exceed 14 days. (Package Insert - *Domoso*®; Syntex Animal Health)
  b) An investigational protocol for the treatment of increased CSF pressure secondary to CNS trauma: 1 gram of DMSO/kg body weight IV over 45 minutes. A 10% solution may be prepared by diluting 32 ml of the 90% solution into 250 ml of sterile water for injection; approximately 290 ml of 10% DMSO solution results. Caution: the LD_{50} for DMSO in dogs is 2.5 grams/kg. (Plumb 1988)

 Horses:
  a) Liberal application should be administered topically to the skin over the affected area 2-3 times daily. Total daily dosage should not exceed 100 grams (or mls of liquid)

and therapy should not exceed 30 days. (Package Insert - *Domoso*®; Syntex Animal Health)

b) For treatment of cerebral edema secondary to eastern equine encephalitis (EEE): 1 g/kg as a 20% solution in D5W IV over 30 minutes once daily for up to 3 days. (Wilson 1987)

c) Adjunctive treatment of equine protozoal myeloencephalitis (EPM): 1 g/kg as a 20% solution in D5W IV over 30 minutes once to twice daily. (Brewer 1987)

d) For spinal cord injury: 1 gm/kg IV as a 20% solution in saline once daily for 3 days, then every other day for 6 days (Robinson 1987)

e) For cantharidin poisoning: 0.9 gm/kg IV as a 10% solution in polyionic fluids (Schmitz and Reagor 1987)

f) 0.25 - 1.0 grams/kg diluted in normal saline or D5W at a concentration of not more than 20%. Concentrations greater than 10% should be given <u>slowly</u> IV. Generally felt that the higher dosages are necessary to treat increased intracranial pressure and cerebral edema with twice daily dosing. At U of Minn. usual dose is 110 ml in 1 liter of saline (10%) given daily to an average sized horse. (Plumb 1988)

Monitoring Parameters -
1) Efficacy
2) Hemoglobinuria/hematocrit if indicated
3) Ophthalmic exams with high doses or chronic use in the dog

Client Information/FDA Approval Status - Do not use non-medical grades of DMSO as they may contain harmful impurities. Wear rubber gloves when applying topically. DMSO should be applied with clean or sterile cotton to minimize the chances for contaminating with potentially harmful substances. Apply only to clean, dry skin. Use in well ventilated area; avoid inhalation and contact with eyes. May damage some fabrics. Keep lid tightly on container when not in use. Keep out of reach of children. Do not mix with any other substance without veterinarian's approval.

Selected DMSO products are approved for use in dogs and in horses not intended for food purposes. It is a veterinary prescription (Rx) drug.

Dosage Forms/Preparations -
Veterinary Approved Products:

Dimethyl Sulfoxide Veterinary Gel 90%; Domoso® (Fort Dodge) Gel 90% (medical grade) in 60 g., and 120 g. tubes, and 425 g. jars.

Dimethyl Sulfoxide Veterinary Solution 90%; Domoso® (Fort Dodge) 90% (medical grade) in 4 oz spray bottle, 16 oz., and 1 gallon bottles

Human Approved Products:

Dimethylsulfoxide Solution 50 % aqueous solution in 50 mls and 70% solution in 250 mls; *Rimso-50*® (Research Industries) (Rx);*Rimso-50*® (Roberts);*Kemsol*® (Horner); (Rx)

Note: A topical otic product, *Synotic*® (Fort Dodge) which contains: DMSO 60% and fluocinolone acetonide 0.01% is also available for veterinary use. Supplied in 8 ml and 60 ml dropper bottles.

For more information, refer to the excellent article reviewing DMSO by Brayton. (Brayton, CF. Dimethyl Sulfoxide (DMSO): A Review, Cornell Vet., 1986, 76; 61-90)

DINOPROST TROMETHAMINE
PROSTAGLANDIN F$_{2\alpha}$TROMETHAMINE

Chemistry - The tromethamine (THAM) salt of the naturally occurring prostaglandin F$_{2alpha}$, dinoprost tromethamine occurs as a white to off-white, very hygroscopic, crystalline powder with a melting point of about 100°C. One gram is soluble in about 5 ml of water. 1.3 micrograms of dinoprost tromethamine is equivalent to 1 micrograms of dinoprost. Dinoprost tromethamine may also be known as dinoprost trometamol, PGF$_{2alpha}$ THAM, or prostaglandin F$_{2alpha}$ tromethamine.

Storage/Stability/Compatibility - Dinoprost for injection should be stored at room temperature (15-30°C) in airtight containers. The human-approved product is recommended to be stored under refrigeration. Dinoprost is considered to be relatively insensitive to heat, light, and alkalis.

Pharmacology - Prostaglandin F$_{2alpha}$ has several pharmacologic effects on the female reproductive system, including stimulation of myometrial activity, relaxation of the cervix, inhibition of steroidogenesis by corpora lutea, and can potentially lyse corpora lutea.

Uses/Indications - *Lutalyse*® (Upjohn) is labeled for use in cattle as a luteolytic agent for estrous synchronization, unobserved (silent) estrous in lactating dairy cattle, pyometra, and as an abortifacient in feedlot and non-lactating dairy cattle. It is labeled in swine to act as a parturitient inducing agent. The product is labeled for use in mares as a luteolytic agent to control the time of estrus in cycling mares and to assist in inducing estrus in "difficult to breed mares."

Unlabeled uses of dinoprost include its use in small animals as an abortifacient agent and as adjunctive medical therapy in pyometra. Although not approved, dinoprost is used also in sheep and goat reproductive medicine.

Pharmacokinetics - In studies done in rodents, dinoprost was demonstrated to distribute very rapidly to tissues after injection. In cattle, the serum half-life of dinoprost has been stated to be only "minutes" long.

Contraindications/Precautions - Unless being used as an abortifacient or parturition inducer, dinoprost should not be used during pregnancy in all species. Dinoprost is contraindicated in animals with bronchoconstrictive respiratory disease (*e.g.,* asthma, "heavey" horses). It should not be administered intravenously.

In swine, dinoprost should not be administered prior to 3 days of normal predicted farrowing as increased neonatal mortality may result.

According to the manufacturer, dinoprost is contraindicated in mares with acute or subacute disorders of the vascular system, GI tract, respiratory system or reproductive tract.

Dinoprost should be used with extreme caution, if at all, in dogs or cats greater than 8 years old, or with preexisting cardiopulmonary or other serious disease (liver, kidney, etc.). Some clinicians regard closed-cervix pyometra as a relative contraindication to the use of dinoprost.

Adverse Effects/Warnings - In cattle, increased temperature has been reported when administered in overdose (5-10X recommended doses) quantities. Limited salivation and bacterial infections at the injection site have been reported. If administered intravenously, increased heart rates have been noted.

In mares, transient decreased body (rectal) temperature and sweating have been reported most often. Less frequently, increased respiratory and heart rates, ataxia, abdominal pain and lying down have also been noted. These effects are generally seen within 15 minutes of administration and resolve within an hour.

In swine, dinoprost has caused erythema and pruritis, urination, defecation, slight ataxia, hyperpnea, dyspnea, nesting behavior, abdominal muscle spasms, tail movements, increased vocalization and salivation. These effects may last up to 3 hours. At doses of 10 times recommended, vomiting may be seen in swine.

In dogs and cats, dinoprost can cause abdominal pain, emesis, defecation, urination, pupillary dilation followed by constriction, tachycardias, restlessness and anxiety, fever, hypersalivation, dyspnea and panting. Cats may also exhibit increased vocalization and intense grooming behavior. Severity of effects is generally dose dependent. Defecation can be seen even with very low dosages. Reactions generally appear in 5-120 minutes after administration and may persist for 20-30 minutes. Fatalities have occurred (especially in dogs) after use. Dogs and cats should be monitored for cardiorespiratory effects, especially after receiving higher dosages.

When used as an abortifacient in humans, dinoprost causes nausea, vomiting or diarrhea in about 50% of patients.

Overdosage - Dogs are apparently more sensitive to the toxic effects of dinoprost than other species. The LD$_{50}$ in the bitch has been reported to be 5.13 mg/kg after SQ injection which may be only 5X greater than the recommended dose by some clinicians.

In cattle, swine, and horses, dinoprost's effects when administered in overdose quantities are outlined above in the Adverse effects section. If symptoms are severe in any species and require treatment; supportive therapy is recommended.

Drug Interactions - Other **oxytocic agents**' activity may be enhanced by dinoprost. Reduced effect of dinoprost would be expected with concomitant administration of a **progestin**.

Doses -

  Dogs:

    For treatment of pyometra:

      a) 0.25 mg/kg SQ once a day for 5 days. Give bactericidal antibiotics concurrently. Not recommended in animal > 8 yrs. old or if severely ill. Closed-cervix pyometra is a relative contraindication. (Nelson 1988)

      b) 0.025 - 0.25 mg/kg every 12 hours to effect. Initially use lower dosage to determine adverse effects on patient. Dosage depends on adverse effects and clinical condition of animal. For small dogs and cats: Dilute 1 ml (5 mg) of dinoprost injection to 25 ml with sterile water for injection, which will yield a concentration of 0.2 mg/ml (200 micrograms/ml). Adjunctive therapy includes systemic antibiotics (*e.g.,* chloramphenicol, trimethoprim/sulfa, ampicillin) and anterior vaginal douches with 200-500

ml warm 1% tamed iodine (povidone iodine) solution daily during prostaglandin treatment. (Lein 1986)
c) 0.05 mg/kg (50 micrograms/kg) every 12 hours (Wheaton 1989)

For treatment of cystic endometrial hyperplasia-pyometra:
a) 0.1 - 0.25 mg/kg once daily until discharge stops, but not for more than 5 days; reexamine in 2 weeks. If discharge has recurred, treat at 0.25 - 0.5 mg/kg as above. Do not give a third course of therapy. Concurrent antibiotic treatment is necessary. (Shille 1986)

As an abortifacient:
a) All doses are quoted using the THAM salt (Lutalyse®):
During the first half of gestation: 250 micrograms/kg every 12 hours SubQ for 4 days, starting at least 5 days after cytologic diestrus. After the eighth injection, draw blood sample for serum progesterone concentration. Examine several weeks post treatment to verify pregnancy termination (failures have been reported).
During second half of gestation: Verify preganancy (palpation/ultrasound). Inject 250 micrograms/kg SubQ every 12 hours until abortion is complete. Treatment efficacy is determined by monitoring the completeness of pregnancy termination. (Root and Johnston 1995)
b) In healthy bitches from midgestation to term: 25 - 250 micrograms/kg IM twice a day. Hospitalization and close monitoring essential. Vaginoscopy done daily to detect dilation of cervix. Radiography or ultrosonagraphy done every 3-5 days during treatment to determine if abortion is complete. (Lein 1986)

Cats:
For treatment of pyometra:
a) Initially 0.1 mg/kg SQ, then 0.25 mg/kg SQ once a day for 5 days. Give bactericidal antibiotics concurrently. Not recommended in animals > 8 yrs. old or if severely ill. Closed-cervix pyometra is a relative contraindication. Reevaluate in 2 weeks; retreat for 5 more days if necessary. (Nelson 1988), (Feldman and Nelson 1989)
b) Same as for dogs above (Lein 1986)

As an abortifacient:
a) After day 40 of gestation: 0.5 - 1.0 mg/kg SQ initially and then 24 hours later. Abortion generally ensues in 8-24 hours. (Woody 1988)

Cattle:
For estrus synchronization in beef cattle and non-lactating dairy heifers:
a) 25 mg IM either once or twice at a 10-12 day interval. If using single injection method, breed at usual time relative to estrus. If using dual dose method, breed at either the usual time relative to estrus, or about 80 hours after the second injection. (Package Insert; *Lutalyse*®—Upjohn)

For unobserved (silent) estrus in lactating dairy cattle with a corpus luteum:
a) 25 mg IM. Breed cows as they are detected in estrus. If estrus not detected, breed at 80 hours post injection. If cow returns to estrus, breed at usual time relative to estrus. (Package Insert; *Lutalyse*®—Upjohn)

For pyometra:
a) 25 mg IM. Uterus begins evacuating within 24 hours of injection. (McCormack 1986), (Package Insert; *Lutalyse*®—Upjohn)

As an abortifacient:
a) Between 5-150 days of gestation: 25 - 30 mg IM
After 150 days of gestation: 25 mg dexamethasone with 25 mg dinoprost (efficacy up to 95%) (Drost 1986)
b) 25 mg IM during the first 100 days of gestation (Package Insert; *Lutalyse*®—Upjohn)

To induce parturition:
a) 25 - 30 mg IM; delivery will occur in about 72 hours (Drost 1986)

Horses:
To induce cyclic activity in animals who are acyclic due to persistent corpus lutea:
a) 5 mg IM; most effective in mares with corpora lutea older than 5 days and who have progesterone levels >1 ng/ml (4 ng/ml even better). (Rossdale 1987)

For difficult to breed mares secondary to progesterone levels consistent with the presence of a functional corpus luteum:
a) 1 mg per 45 kg body weight IM (Package Insert; *Lutalyse*®—Upjohn)

For controlling time of estrus of estrous cycling mares:

    a) 1 mg per 45 kg body weight IM. When treated during diestrus, most mares return to estrus in 2-4 days and ovulate 8-12 days after treatment. (Package Insert; *Lutalyse*®—Upjohn)

As an abortifacient:
    a) Prior to the 12th day of pregnancy: 5 mg IM
    After the 4th month of pregnancy: 1 mg per 45 kg body weight (1 mg per 100 pounds) daily until abortion takes place. (Lofstedt 1986)
    b) From day 80-300: 2.5 mg q12h; approximately 4 injections required on average to induce abortion (Roberts 1986a)

For estrus synchronization in normally cycling mares:
    a) Three methods:
    1) Two injection method— On day 1 give 5 mg dinoprost and again on day 16. Most (60%) mares will begin estrus 4 days after the second injection and about 90% will show estrous behavior by the 6th day after the second injection. Breed using AI every second day during estrus or inseminate at predetermined times without estrus detection. Alternatively, an IM injection of HCG (2500-3300 Units) can be added on the first or second day (usually day 21) of estrus to hasten ovulation. Breed using AI on days 20, 22, 24, and 26. This may be of more benefit when used early in the breeding season.

    2) Progestagen/Prostaglandin method— Give altrenogest (0.44 mg/kg) for 8-12 days PO. On last day of altrenogest therapy (usually day 10) give dinoprost *(dose not noted, but suggest using same dose as "1" above)*. Majority of mares will show estrus 2-5 days after last treatment. Inseminante every 2 days after detection of estrus. Synchronization may be improved by giving 2500 IU of HCG IM on first or second day of estrus or 5-7 days after altrenogest is withdrawn.

    3) On day 1, inject 150 mg progesterone and 10 mg estradiol-17beta daily for 10 days. On last day, also give dinoprost *(dose not noted, but suggest using same dose as "1" above)*. Perform AI on alternate days after estrus detection or on days 19, 21, and 23. (Bristol 1987)

Swine:

For estrus synchronization (grouping):
    a) At 15-55 days of gestation 15 mg dinoprost IM, followed in 12 hours by 10 mg IM. Animals will abort and return to estrus in 4-5 days. Close observation of estrus over several days is needed. (Carson 1986)

As an abortifacient:
    a) 5 - 10 mg IM; abortion occurs in 24-48 hours and estrus occurs 4-5 days later. (Drost 1986)

To induce parturition:
    a) 10 - 25 mg IM from 2-6 days before expected parturition; farrowing usually occurs 24-36 hours later. (Drost 1986)

Sheep & Goats:

For estrus synchronization in cycling ewes and does:
    a) Ewes: Give 8 mg IM on day 5 of estrous cycle and repeat in 11 days. Estrus will begin approximately 2 days after last injection.
    Does: Give 8 mg IM on day 4 of estrous cycle and repeat in 11 days. Estrus will begin approximately 2 days after last injection. (Carson 1986)

To induce estrous in does (weighing up to 65 kg):
    a) 2.5 mg on days 4-17 of estrous cycle.

As an abortifacient:
    a) Doe: 5 - 10 mg IM throughout entire pregnancy. Abortion takes place in 4-5 days.
    Ewe (during first two months of pregnancy): 10 - 15 mg IM; abortion takes place within 72 hours. (Drost 1986)

To induce parturition:
    a) Does: 2.5 - 5.0 mg IM on day 144; parturition occurs in 28-57 hours. (Ott 1986a)
    b) Does: 2.5 - 20 mg on days 144-149. Higher dosage (20 mg) yields more predictable interval from injection to delivery ($\approx$32 hours). (Ott 1986b)

For chronic metritis/pyometra:
    a) Doe: 2.5 - 5.0 mg SQ with systemic antibiotics (Franklin 1986b)

Monitoring Parameters - Depending on use, see above. Monitoring for adverse effects is especially important in small animals.

Client Information - Dinoprost should be used by individuals familiar with its use and precautions. Pregnant women, asthmatics or other persons with bronchial diseases should handle this product with extreme caution. Any accidental exposure to skin should be washed off immediately.

Dosage Forms/Preparations/FDA Approval Status/Withholding Times -
Veterinary-Approved Products:

Dinoprost Tromethamine for injection, equivalent to 5 mg/ml of dinoprost in 10 ml and 30 ml vials; *Lutalyse®* (Upjohn); (Rx) Approved for use in beef and non-lactating dairy cattle, swine and mares. No preslaughter withdrawal or milk withdrawal is required when used as labeled; no specific tolerance for dinoprost residues have been published. It is not for use in horses intended for food

Human-Approved Products: None

DIPHENHYDRAMINE HCL

Chemistry - An ethanolamine-derivative antihistamine, diphenhydramine HCl occurs as an odorless, white, crystalline powder which will slowly darken upon exposure to light. It has a melting range of 167 - 172° C. One gram is soluble in about 1 ml of water or 2 ml of alcohol. Diphenhydramine HCl has a pK_a of about 9, and the commercially available injection has its pH adjusted to 5-6.

Storage/Stability/Compatibility - Preparations containing diphenhydramine should be stored at room temperature (15-30°C) and solutions should be protected from freezing. Tablets and oral solutions should be kept in well-closed containers. Capsules and the elixir should be stored in tight containers.

Diphenhydramine for injection is reportedly **compatible** with all commonly used IV solutions and the following drugs: amikacin sulfate, aminophylline, ascorbic acid injection, atropine sulfate, bleomycin sulfate, butorphanol tartrate, cephapirin sodium, chlorpromazine HCl, colistimethate sodium, diatrizoate meglumine/sodium, dimenhydrinate, droperidol, erythromycin lactobionate, fentanyl citrate, glycopyrrolate, hydromorphone HCl, hydroxyzine HCl, iothalamate meglumine/sodium, lidocaine HCl, meperidine HCl, methicillin sodium, metoclopramide, methyldopate HCl, morphine sulfate, nafcillin sodium, netilmicin sulfate, penicillin G potassium/sodium, pentazocine lactate, perphenazine, polymyxin B sulfate, prochlorperazine edisylate, promazine HCl, promethazine HCl, scopolamine HBr, tetracycline HCl and vitamin B complex w/C. Compatibility is dependent upon factors such as pH, concentration, temperature, and diluents used and it is suggested to consult specialized references for more specific information.

Diphenhydramine is reportedly **incompatible** with the following drugs: amobarbital sodium, amphotericin B, cephalothin sodium, hydrocortisone sodium succinate, iodipamide meglumine, pentobarbital sodium, secobarbital sodium, and thiopental sodium.

Pharmacology - Like other antihistamines, diphenhydramine competitively inhibits histamine at H_1 receptors. In addition; it also has substantial sedative, anticholinergic, antitussive, and antiemetic effects.

Uses/Indications - In veterinary medicine, diphenhydramine is used principally for its antihistaminic effects, but also for its other pharmacologic actions as well. Its sedative effects can be of benefit in treating the agitation (pruritis, etc.) associated with allergic responses. It has also been used for treatment and prevention of motion sickness and as an antiemetic in small animals. It has also been suggested for use as adjunctive treatment of aseptic laminitis in cattle. For other suggested uses, refer to the Dosage section below.

Pharmacokinetics - The pharmacokinetics of this agent have apparently not been studied in domestic animals. In humans, diphenhydramine is well absorbed after oral administration, but because of a relatively high first-pass effect, only about 40-60% reaches the systemic circulation.

Following IV administration in rats, diphenhydramine reaches its highest levels in the spleen, lungs and brain. The drug is distributed into milk, but has not been measured quantitatively. In humans, diphenhydramine crosses the placenta and is approximately 80% bound to plasma proteins.

Diphenhydramine is metabolized in the liver and the majority of the drug is excreted as metabolites into the urine. The terminal elimination half-life in adult humans ranges from 2.4-9.3 hours.

Contraindications/Precautions - Diphenhydramine is contraindicated in patients who are hypersensitive to it or other antihistamines in its class. Because of their anticholinergic activity, antihistamines should be used with caution in patients with angle closure glaucoma, prostatic hypertrophy, pyloroduodenal or bladder neck obstruction, and COPD if mucosal secretions are a problem. Additionally, they should be used with caution in patients with hyperthyroidism, cardiovascular disease or hypertension.

Adverse Effects/Warnings - The most commonly seen adverse effects are CNS depression (lethargy, somnolence), and anticholinergic effects (dry mouth, urinary retention). The sedative effects of antihistamines may diminish with time. GI effects (diarrhea, vomiting, anorexia), are a possibility.

The sedative effects of antihistamines may adversely affect the performance of working dogs.

Overdosage - Overdosage can cause CNS stimulation (excitement to seizures) or depression (lethargy to coma), anticholinergic effects, respiratory depression and death. Treatment consists of emptying the gut if the ingestion was oral using standard protocols. Induce emesis if the patient is alert and CNS status is stable. Administration of a saline cathartic and/or activated charcoal may be given after emesis or gastric lavage. Treatment of other symptoms should be performed using symptomatic and supportive therapies. Phenytoin (IV) is recommended in the treatment of seizures caused by antihistamine overdose in humans; barbiturates and diazepam should be avoided.

Drug Interactions - Increased sedation can occur if diphenhydramine is combined with **other CNS depressant drugs**.

Antihistamines may partially counteract the anticoagulation effects of **heparin** or **warfarin**.

Diphenhydramine may enhance the effects of **epinephrine**.

Laboratory Interactions - Antihistamines can decrease the wheal and flare response to **antigen skin testing**. In humans, it is suggested that antihistamines be discontinued at least 4 days before testing.

Doses -

Dogs:

Prevention of motion sickness/antiemetic:
a) 2 - 4 mg/kg PO, IM q8h (Washabau and Elie 1995)
b) 2 - 4 mg/kg PO q8h (DeNovo 1986)

For treatment of extrapyrimidal effects secondary to phenothiazines:
a) 2 - 5 mg/kg IV (Bailey 1986)

For adjunctive treatment (of tremors) secondary to organophosphate or carbamate poisoning:
a) 4 mg/kg PO (Carson 1986)
b) 1 - 4 mg/kg PO *tid* (reduces nicotinic receptor overload) (Grauer and Hjelle 1988)

For prevention of allergic reactions secondary to doxorubicin therapy:
a) For dogs up to 20 lbs = 10 mg IV;
for dogs 20 - 60 lbs = 20 mg IV;
for dogs over 60 lbs. = 30 mg IV. Give prior to doxorubicin administration. (Klausner and Bell 1988)
b) 1 mg/kg IV with 5 mg/kg cimetidine before therapy. (Coppoc 1988)

For severe urticaria and angioedema:
a) 2 mg/kg IM *bid prn* (with steroids: prednisone 2 mg/kg IM *bid* and epinephrine 1:10,000: 0.5 - 2.0 ml SQ) (Giger and Werner 1988)

For canine atopy/allergic inhalant dermatitis:
a) 2 mg/kg PO *tid* (effectiveness is questionable, but may be tried) (Giger and Werner 1988)

For preoperative therapy for splenic mast cell tumors:
a) 2.2 mg/kg IM *bid* (with cimetidine 5 mg/kg PO, IV *tid-qid*) (Stann 1988)

For treatment of the reverse sneeze syndrome:
a) 25 mg PO *tid -qid*, dosage is usually decreased to once or twice a week for maintenance. (Prueter 1988a)

As an antipruritic:
a) 25 - 50 mg PO *bid-tid* (Morgan 1988)

Cats:

For severe urticaria and angioedema:
a) 2 mg/kg IM *bid prn* (with steroids: prednisone 2 mg/kg IM *bid* and epinephrine 1:10,000: 0.5 - 2.0 ml SQ) (Giger and Werner 1988)

Prevention of motion sickness/antiemetic:
a) 2 - 4 mg/kg PO, IM q8h (Washabau and Elie 1995)
b) 2 - 4 mg/kg PO q8h (DeNovo 1986)

Horses:
> For adjunctive therapy of anaphylaxis:
>> a) 0.25 - 1 mg/kg IV or IM (Evans 1996)

Cattle:
> For adjunctive therapy of anaphylaxis:
>> a) 0.5 - 1 mg/kg IM or IV (used with epinephrine and steroids) (Clark 1986)
>
> For adjunctive therapy of aseptic laminitis:
>> a) During the acute phase (with corticosteroids): 55 - 110 mg/100 kg body weight IV or IM (Berg 1986)

Monitoring Parameters -
> 1) Clinical efficacy and adverse effects

Client Information/FDA Approval Status - Diphenhydramine is approved for use in humans. The oral dosage forms are either prescription or non-prescription agents, depending on the product's labeling. The injectable products are prescription only.

Dosage Forms/Preparations -
Veterinary-Approved Products: None
Human-Approved Products:
> Diphenhydramine HCl Capsules 25 mg, 50 mg; 12.5 mg chewable) & 50 mg Tablets
>
> Diphenhydramine HCl Oral Elixir or Syrup 12.5 mg/5 ml (2.5 mg/ml) in 4 oz, pint and gallon bottles
>
> Diphenhydramine Injection 10 mg/ml in 10 ml or 30 ml vials; 50 mg/ml in 1 ml amps and 10 ml vials

Diphenhydramine is available under several trade names; a commonly known product is *Benadryl*® (Parke-Davis).

Diphenoxalate HCl/Atropine - see Opiate Antidiarrheals

Diphenylhydantoin - see Phenytoin

DISOPYRAMIDE PHOSPHATE

Chemistry - Structurally dissimilar from other available antiarrhythmic agents, disopyramide phosphate occurs as a white or practically white crystalline powder with a pK_a of 10.4. It is freely soluble in water and slightly soluble in alcohol.

Storage/Stability/Compatibility - Disopyramide capsules should be stored at room temperature (15-30°C) and in well-closed containers. An extemporaneously prepared suspension of 1-10 mg/ml of disopyramide (from capsules) in cherry syrup has been shown to be stable for one month if stored in amber bottles and refrigerated (2-8°C).

Pharmacology - Considered to be a class Ia (membrane-stabilizing) antiarrhythmic, with actions similar to either quinidine or procainamide, disopyramide reduces myocardial excitability and conduction velocity and also possesses anticholinergic activity (150 mg of disopyramide ≈ 0.09 mg of atropine) which may contribute to the effects of the drug.

The exact mechanism of action of the drug has not been established. Disopyramide's cardiac electrophysiologic effects include: 1) shortened sinus node recovery time 2) increased atrial and ventricular refractory times 3) decreased conduction velocity through the atria and ventricles 4) decreased automaticity of ectopic atrial or ventricular pacemakers.

Disopyramide has direct negative inotropic effects. It generally has minimal effects on resting heart rates or blood pressure. Systemic peripheral resistance may increase by 20%.

Uses/Indications - Indicated for the oral treatment or prevention of ventricular tachyarrhythmias in the dog. Because of its negative inotropic effects and short half-life in the dog, disopyramide is generally considered to be a 2nd or 3rd line agent for veterinary (canine) use. A controlled release product is available which may useful, but has not been extensively evaluated in the dog.

Pharmacokinetics - In humans, disopyramide is rapidly absorbed following oral administration with peak levels occurring within 2-3 hours after the conventional capsules are administered. Peak levels occur at about 6 hours post dose with the controlled-release capsules.

Disopyramide is distributed throughout the body in the extracellular water and is not extensively bound to tissues. Binding to plasma proteins is variable and dependent on the drug's concentration. At therapeutic levels it is approximately 50-65% plasma protein bound (human data). Disopyramide crosses the placenta and milk concentrations may exceed those found in the plasma.

Disopyramide is metabolized in the liver, but 40-65% of it is excreted unchanged in the urine. Patients with renal disease may need dosage adjustments made to prevent drug accumulation.

The half-life of the drug is approximately 7 hours in humans with normal renal function, but only 2-3 hours in the dog.

Contraindications/Precautions - Disopyramide should usually not be used in patients with glaucoma (closed-angle), urinary retention, or myasthenia gravis because of its anticholinergic effects.

Disopyramide is contraindicated in 2nd or 3rd degree AV block (unless pacemaker inserted), cardiogenic shock, or if the patient is hypersensitive to the drug.

Disopyramide should not be used in patients with severe uncompensated or poorly compensated cardiac failure or hypotension because of its negative inotropic effects. Patients with atrial fibrillation or flutter must be digitalized before therapy so as to negate beyond acceptable increased ventricular response after disopyramide therapy. Disopyramide should be used with caution in patients with sick sinus syndrome, bundle branch block, or Wolff-Parkinson-White (WPW) syndrome.

Use of disopyramide with other class 1A antiarrhythmics or propranolol may cause additive negative inotropic effects (see Drug Interactions).

Disopyramide should be used with caution (and possibly at a reduced dosage) in patients with hepatic or renal disease.

Adverse Effects/Warnings - Most common adverse reactions are secondary to disopyramide's anticholinergic effects (dry mouth, eyes, nose; constipation; urinary hesitancy or retention) and cardiovascular effects (edema, hypotension, dyspnea, syncope, conduction disturbances (AV block). Other adverse effects that have been reported in humans include: GI effects (vomiting, diarrhea, etc.), intrahepatic cholestasis, hypoglycemia, fatigue, headache, muscle weakness and pain. In contrast to the urinary hesitancy effects, disopyramide can also cause urinary frequency and urgency.

Overdosage - Symptoms of overdosage/toxicity include: anticholinergic effects, apnea, loss of consciousness, hypotension, cardiac conduction disturbances and arrhythmias, widening of the QRS complex and QT interval, bradycardia, congestive heart failure, seizures, asystole, and death.

Treatment consists initially of prompt gastric emptying, charcoal, and cathartics. Followed by vigorous symptomatic therapy using, if necessary, cardiac glycosides, vasopressors and sympathomimetics, diuretics, mechanically assisted respiration, and endocardial pacing. Disopyramide can be removed with hemodialysis.

Drug Interactions - Do not use disopyramide within 48 hours of using **verapamil**.

Additive or antagonistic cardiac effects may occur as well as additive toxic effects (e.g negative inotropism) when disopyramide is used with **other Class I antiarrhythmic agents** (*e.g.,* **procainamide, quinidine, lidocaine, phenytoin) or propranolol**; use with caution.

Oral anticoagulant (warfarin) doses may need to be adjusted when adding disopyramide.

Disopyramide's metabolism may be increased by drugs that induce microsomal enzymes (*e.g.,* **phenobarbital, phenytoin**). Serum levels may need to be monitored and dosages adjusted.

Additive anticholinergic effects may be encountered if used concomitantly with other **anticholinergics (atropine, glycopyrrolate)**.

Doses -
  Dogs:
>   a) 7 - 30 mg/kg q2h PO (Wilcke 1985)
>   b) For dogs >18kg: 100 mg PO *tid-qid* (Morgan 1988)
>   c) 6 - 15 mg/kg PO q8h (Kirk 1986)
>   d) For ventricular arrhythmias: 11 - 22 mg/kg q8h PO (q12h if using long-acting product). May use in conjunction with quinidine or procainamide. (Ettinger 1989)

Monitoring Parameters -
>   1) ECG
>   2) Blood pressure if possible
>   3) Symptoms of adverse effects (see above); liver function tests if chronic therapy
>   4) Serum levels if indicated (lack of efficacy, toxicity)
>   Therapeutic levels in humans have been reported to be between 2 - 7 micrograms/ml and toxic levels are considered to above 9 micrograms/ml. Levels of up to 7 micrograms/ml may be necessary to treat and prevent the recurrence of refractory ventricular tachycardias.

Client Information - Contact veterinarian if animal has persistent problems with difficult urination, dry mouth, vomiting, constipation, becomes lethargic or depressed, or has difficulty breathing.

Dosage Forms/Preparations/FDA Approval Status/Withholding Times -

Veterinary-Approved Products: None

Human-Approved Products:

Disopyramide Phosphate Capsules 100 mg, 150 mg; *Norpace*® (Searle), Generic; (Rx)

Disopyramide Phosphate Capsules Extended-Release 100 mg, 150 mg; *Norpace CR*® (Searle); (Rx); Generic (Rx)

dl-Methionine - see Methionine

DMSO - see Dimethyl Sulfoxide

DOBUTAMINE HCL

Chemistry - Dobutamine HCl is a synthetic inotropic agent related structurally to dopamine. It occurs as a white, to off-white, crystalline powder with a pK_a of 9.4. Dobutamine is sparingly soluble in water and alcohol.

Storage/Stability/Compatibility - Dobutamine injection should be stored at room temperature (15-30°C). It must be further diluted before administration (see Preparation of Solution below); diluted solutions should be used within 24 hours.

Dobutamine is compatible with the usually used IV solutions (D5W, sodium chloride 0.45% & 0.9%, dextrose-saline combinations, lactated Ringer's) and is reported to be **compatible** with the following drugs: amiodarone HCl, atropine sulfate, dopamine HCl, epinephrine HCl, hydralazine HCl, isoproterenol HCl, lidocaine HCl, meperidine HCl, metaraminol bitartrate, morphine sulfate, nitroglycerin, norepinephrine (levarterenol) bitartrate, phentolamine mesylate, phenylephrine HCl, procainamide HCl, propranolol HCl, and verapamil HCl.

Dobutamine may be **incompatible** with the following agents: aminophylline, bretylium tosylate, bumetamide, calcium chloride or gluconate, diazepam, digoxin, furosemide, heparin (inconsistent results), regular insulin, magnesium sulfate, phenytoin sodium, potassium chloride (at high concentrations only - 160 mEq/l), potassium phosphate, and sodium bicarbonate.

Pharmacology - Dobutamine is considered a direct beta₁-adrenergic agonist. It also has mild beta₂- and alpha₁-adrenergic effects at therapeutic doses. These effects tend to balance one another and cause little direct effect on the systemic vasculature. In contrast to dopamine, dobutamine does not cause the release of norepinephrine. It has relatively mild chronotropic, arrhythmogenic, and vasodilative effects.

Increased myocardial contractility and stroke volumes result in increased cardiac output. Decreases in left ventricular filling pressures (wedge pressures) and total peripheral resistance occur in patients with a failing heart. Blood pressure and cardiac rate generally are unaltered or slightly increased because of increased cardiac output. Increased myocardial contractility may increase myocardial oxygen demand and coronary blood flow.

Uses/Indications - Dobutamine is used as a rapid-acting injectable positive inotropic agent for short term treatment of heart failure.

Pharmacokinetics - Because it is rapidly metabolized in the GI tract and is not available after oral administration, dobutamine is only administered intravenously (as a constant infusion). After intravenous administration, the onset of action generally occurs within 2 minutes and peaks after 10 minutes.

Dobutamine is metabolized rapidly in the liver and other tissues and has a plasma half-life of approximately 2 minutes in humans. The drug's effects diminish rapidly after cessation of therapy.

Pharmacokinetic data for domestic animals is apparently unavailable. It is unknown if dobutamine crosses the placenta or into milk.

Contraindications/Precautions - Dobutamine is contraindicated in patients with known hypersensitivity to the drug or with idiopathic hypertropic subaortic stenosis (IHSS). The injectable formulation contains sodium bisulfite as a preservative which has been documented to cause allergic-type reactions in some human patients. Hypovolemic states must be corrected before administering dobutamine. Because it may increase myocardial oxygen demand and increase infarct size, dobutamine should be used very cautiously after myocardial infarction. Dobutamine can enhance atrioventricular conduction, animals with atrial fibrillation should be digitalized prior to receiving dobutamine.

Adverse Effects/Warnings - The most commonly reported adverse effects in humans are: ectopic beats, increased heart rate, increased blood pressure, chest pain, and palpitations. Similar adverse effects could be expected for veterinary patients. At usual doses these effects are generally mild and will not necessitate halting therapy, but dosage reductions should be performed. Other, more rare adverse effects reported include: nausea, headache, vomiting, leg cramps, paresthesias, and dyspnea.

Overdosage - Symptoms reported with excessive dosage include tachycardias, increased blood pressure, nervousness, and fatigue. Because of the drug's short duration of action, temporarily halting therapy is usually all that is required to reverse these effects.

Drug Interactions - beta-**Blockers** (*e.g.,* **propranolol**) may antagonize the cardiac effects of dobutamine, and result in a preponderance of alpha adrenergic effects and increased total peripheral resistance.

Use of **halothane or cyclopropane** with dobutamine may result in increased incidences of ventricular arrhythmias.

Synergistic effects (increased cardiac output and reduced wedge pressure) may result if dobutamine is used with **nitroprusside**.

Insulin requirements may increase in diabetic patients receiving dobutamine.

Oxytocic drugs may induce severe hypertension when used with dobutamine in obstetric patients.

Doses - Dobutamine is administered as a constant rate intravenous infusion only.

Dogs:
- a) 5 - 20 micrograms/kg/min IV infusion; rates above 20 micrograms/kg/min may be associated with tachycardia (Kittleson 1985b)
- b) 2 - 20 micrograms/kg/min IV infusion (Morgan 1988)

Cats:
No specific doses for cats were located, but the lower dosage range for dogs could be used as a guideline to initiate therapy. One route of metabolism for dobutamine is by glucuronidation, so half-lives in cats may be longer than in other species. Monitor and use with caution.

Horses:
- a) 1 - 5 micrograms/kg/minute (Muir and McGuirk 1987b)
- b) 2 - 10 micrograms/kg/minute IV infusion (Robinson 1987)

Monitoring Parameters -
1) Heart rate and rhythm, blood pressure if possible
2) Urine flow
3) Ideally, measurement of central venous or pulmonary wedge pressures and cardiac output

Client Information - This drug should only be used by professionals familiar with its use and in a setting where adequate patient monitoring can be performed.

Dosage Forms/Preparations/FDA Approval Status/Withholding Times -
Veterinary-Approved Products: None
Human-Approved Products:
Dobutamine HCl Injection 12.5 mg/ml in 20 ml vial; *Dobutrex*® (Lilly); Generic (Rx)

Preparation of Solution - The solution for injection must be further diluted to a concentration no greater than 5 mg/ml (total of at least 50 ml of diluent) before administering.

Generally, it is added to D5W, normal saline (if not severely sodium restricted) or other compatible IV solution. The following approximate concentrations will result if 1 vial (250 mg) is added either 250, 500, or 1000 ml IV solutions:

1 vial (250 mg) in: 250 ml ≈ 1000micrograms/ml
"   500 ml ≈ 500micrograms/ml
"   1000 ml ≈ 250micrograms/ml

A mechanical fluid administration control device should be used, if available, to administer dobutamine. When using a mini-drip IV administration set (60 drops ≈ 1 ml), 1 drop contains approximately 8.3 micrograms at the 500 micrograms/ml concentration.

DOCUSATE SODIUM
DOCUSATE CALCIUM
DOCUSATE POTASSIUM

Chemistry - Docusate is available in sodium, potassium, and calcium salts. They are anionic, surface-active agents and possess wetting and emulsifying properties.

Docusate sodium (also known as dioctyl sodium succinate, DSS, or DOSS) occurs as a white, wax-like plastic solid with a characteristic odor. One gram is soluble in approximately 70 ml of water and it is freely soluble in alcohol and glycerin. Solutions are clear and have a bitter taste.

Docusate calcium (also known as dioctyl calcium succinate) occurs as a white, amorphous solid with a characteristic odor (octyl alcohol). It is very slightly soluble in water, but freely soluble in alcohol.

Docusate potassium (also known as dioctyl potassium succinate) occurs as a white, amorphous solid with a characteristic odor (octyl alcohol). It is sparingly soluble in water and soluble in alcohol.

Storage/Stability/Compatibility - Capsules of salts of docusate should be stored in tight containers at room temperature. Temperatures above 86°F can soften or melt soft gelatin capsules. Docusate sodium solutions should be stored in tight containers and the syrup should be stored in tight, light-resistant containers.

Pharmacology - Docusate salts reduce surface tension and allow water and fat to penetrate the ingesta and formed feces, thereby softening the stool. Recent *in vivo* studies have also demonstrated that docusate also increases cAMP concentrations in colonic mucosal cells which may increase both ion secretion and fluid permeability from these cells into the colon lumen.

Uses/Indications - Docusate is used in small animals when feces are hard or dry, or in anorectal conditions when passing firm feces would be painful or detrimental. Docusate is used alone and in combination with mineral oil in treating fecal impactions in horses.

Pharmacokinetics - It is unknown how much docusate is absorbed after oral administration, but it is believed that some is absorbed from the small intestine and is then excreted into the bile.

Contraindications/Precautions - Use with caution in patients with pre-existing fluid or electrolyte abnormalities; monitor.

Adverse Effects/Warnings - At usual doses, clinically significant adverse effects should be very rare. Cramping, diarrhea and intestinal mucosal damage are possible. The liquid preparations may cause throat irritation if administered by mouth.

Overdosage - In horses, single doses of 0.65 - 1 gm/kg have caused dehydration, intestinal mucosal damage, and death. Because of the secretory effects that high dose docusate can produce, hydration and electrolyte status should be monitored and treated if necessary.

Drug Interactions - Theoretically, **mineral oil** should not be given with docusate (DSS) as enhanced absorption of the mineral oil could occur. However, this interaction does not appear to be of significant clinical concern with large animals. It is less clear whether there is a significant problem in using this combination in small animals and the concurrent use of these agents together in dogs or cats cannot be recommended. If it is deemed necessary to use both docusate and mineral oil in small animals, separate doses by at least two hours.

Doses -
  Dogs:
    Docusate Sodium:
      a) 2 mg/kg PO (Davis 1985a)
      b) One to four 50 mg capsules PO once daily (Burrows 1986)
      c) 50 - 300 mg PO q12h (Kirk 1989)
      d) Small Dog: 25 mg PO once to twice daily
         Medium/large Dog: 50 mg PO once to twice daily (Morgan 1988)
      e) 250 mg/12 ml glycerin disposable enema syringe (Disposaject®; P-M): Insert rectally and express contents; may repeat in one hour (Package Insert)

    Docusate Calcium:
      a) Two to three 50 mg capsules or one 240 mg capsule PO once daily (Burrows 1986)
      b) One or two 50 mg capsules q12-24h PO (Kirk 1989)

  Cats:
    Docusate Sodium:
      a) 50 mg PO per day; 5 - 10 ml of *Colace®* (strength not specified) as an enema (Sherding 1989)
      b) 2 mg/kg PO (Davis 1985a)
      c) 50 mg capsule once daily PO (Burrows 1986)
      d) 50 - 100 mg q 12-24h PO (Kirk 1989)
      e) 25 mg PO once to twice daily (Morgan 1988)
      f) 250 mg/12 ml glycerin disposable enema syringe (Disposaject®; P-M): Insert rectally and express contents; may repeat in one hour (Package Insert)

    Docusate Calcium:
      a) 50 - 100 mg PO per day (Sherding 1989)
      b) One to two 50 mg capsules PO once daily (Burrows 1986)
      c) 50 mg q12-24h PO (Kirk 1989)

Horses:
- a) 10 - 20 mg/kg diluted in 2 L of warm water PO; may repeat in 48 hours. (Clark and Becht 1987)
- b) 7.5 - 30 grams (150 - 600 mls of a 5% solution) PO; or 3 - 5 grams (60 - 100 mls of 5% solution) if used with mineral oil. (Sellers and Lowe 1987)

Monitoring Parameters -1) Clinical efficacy; hydration and electrolyte status if indicated

Client Information - Unless otherwise directed, give this medication on an empty stomach. Do not give with other laxative agents without the approval of the veterinarian.

Dosage Forms/Preparations/FDA Approval Status/Withholding Times - There are several docusate products marketed for veterinary use; their approval status is unknown. Docusate products are available without prescription (OTC).

Docusate Sodium 100 mg Tablets & Docusate Sodium Capsules 50 mg, 100 mg, 240 mg, 250 mg, 300 mg; Softgel 100 mg

Docusate Sodium Syrup 20 mg/4 ml in 473 ml; 50 mg/15 ml in UD 15 & 30 ml, 60 mg/15 ml in 240 ml, pt and gal.; 150 mg/15 ml in pt and gal.

Docusate Sodium Liquid/Solution 50 mg/ml and 100 mg/ml in 60 ml and gal.; Veterinary products for use in large animals are generally available in gallons in concentrations of either 5% (50 mg/ml) or 10% (100 mg/ml). There are many trade names for docusate sodium, perhaps the best known is *Colace*® (Bristol-Meyers Squibb). It is also available generically.

Docusate Calcium 50 mg and 240 mg capsules (human-labeled); There are many trade names for docusate calcium, perhaps the best known is *Surfak*® (Hoechst). It is also available generically.

Docusate Potassium Tablets 100 mg & Docusate Potassium Capsules 240 mg; *Kasof*® (Stuart), *Dialose*® (Stuart), Generic

DOPAMINE HCL

Chemistry - An endogenous catecholamine which is the immediate precursor to norepinephrine, dopamine (as the HCl salt) occurs as a white to off-white crystalline powder. It is freely soluble in water and soluble in alcohol. The injectable concentrated solution has a pH of 2.5 - 5.5 and may contain an antioxidant (sodium bisulfate). The pH of the ready-to-use injectable products in dextrose have a pH from 3 - 5.

Storage/Stability/Compatibility - Dopamine injectable products should be protected from light. Solutions that are pink, yellow, brown or purple indicate decomposition of the drug. Solutions that are darker than a light yellow should be discarded. Dopamine solutions should be stored at room temperature (15-30°C).

After dilution in a common IV solution (not 5% bicarbonate), dopamine is stable for at least 24 hours at room temperature, but it is recommended to dilute the drug just prior to use. Dopamine is stable in solutions with a pH of less than 6.4, and most stable at pH's less than 5. It is oxidized at alkaline pH.

Dopamine is reported to be **compatible** with the following IV fluids: D5 in LRS, D5 in half-normal saline, D5 in normal saline, D5W, mannitol 20% in water, lactated Ringer's, normal saline, and 1/6M sodium lactate. Dopamine is reported to be compatible with the following drugs: aminophylline, bretylium tosylate, calcium chloride, carbenicillin disodium, cephalothin sodium neutral, chloramphenicol sodium succinate, dobutamine HCl, gentamicin sulfate (gentamicin potency retained for only 6 hours), heparin sodium, hydrocortisone sodium succinate, kanamycin sulfate, lidocaine HCl, methylprednisolone sodium succinate, oxacillin sodium, potassium chloride, tetracycline HCl, and verapamil HCl.

Dopamine is reported to be **incompatible** with: Amphotericin B, ampicillin sodium, iron salts, metronidazole w/sodium bicarbonate, penicillin G potassium, and sodium bicarbonate. Compatibility is dependent upon factors such as pH, concentration, temperature, and diluents used and it is suggested to consult specialized references for more specific information.

Pharmacology - Dopamine is a precursor to norepinephrine and acts directly and indirectly (by releasing norepinephrine) on both alpha and beta1 receptors. Dopamine also has dopaminergic effects.

At very low IV doses, 0.5 - 2 micrograms/kg/min, dopamine acts predominantly on dopaminergic receptors and dilates the renal, mesenteric, coronary, and intracerebral vascular beds. At doses from 2 - 10 micrograms/kg/min, dopamine also stimulates beta1 adrenergic receptors. The net effect at this dosage range is to exert positive cardiac inotropic activity, increase organ perfusion, renal blood flow and urine production. At these lower doses, systemic vascular resistance remains largely unchanged. At higher doses, >10-12 micrograms/kg/min, the dopaminergic effects are overridden by alpha effects. Systemic peripheral resistance is increased and hypotension may be corrected in cases where systemic vascular resistance is diminished. Renal and peripheral blood flow are thus decreased.

Uses/Indications - Dopamine should be used only in critical care settings where adequate monitoring can be provided. It is used to correct the hemodynamic imbalances present in shock after adequate fluid volume replacement, to treat oliguric renal failure, and, occasionally, as adjunctive therapy for the treatment of acute heart failure.

Pharmacokinetics - Dopamine is not administered orally as it is rapidly metabolized in the GI tract. After IV administration, the onset of action is usually within 5 minutes and persists for less than 10 minutes after the infusion has stopped.

Dopamine is widely distributed in the body, but does not cross the blood-brain barrier in appreciable quantities. It is unknown if dopamine crosses the placenta.

The plasma half-life of dopamine is approximately 2 minutes. It is metabolized in the kidney, liver, and plasma by monoamine oxidase (MAO) and catechol-*O*-methyltransferase (COMT) to inactive compounds. Up to 25% of a dose of dopamine is metabolized to norepinephrine in the adrenergic nerve terminals. In human patients receiving monoamine oxidase inhibitors, dopamine's duration of activity can be as long as one hour.

Contraindications/Precautions - Dopamine is contraindicated in patients with pheochromocytoma, ventricular fibrillation, and uncorrected tachyarrhythmias. It is not a substitute for adequate fluid, electrolyte or blood product replacement therapy and should be used with caution in patients with ischemic heart disease or an occlusive vascular disease. Decrease dose or discontinue the drug should symptoms occur implicating dopamine as the cause of reduced circulation to the extremities or the heart. The drug should be discontinued or dosage reduced should arrhythmias (PVC's) occur.

Adverse Effects/Warnings - Most frequent adverse effects seen include nausea and vomiting, ectopic beats, tachycardia, palpitation, hypotension, hypertension, dyspnea, headache and vasoconstriction.

Extravasation injuries with dopamine can be very serious with necrosis and sloughing of surrounding tissue. Patient's IV sites should be routinely monitored. Should extravasation occur, infiltrate the site (ischemic areas) with a solution of 5-10 mg phentolamine (Regitine®) in 10-15 ml of normal saline. A syringe with a fine needle should be used to infiltrate the site with many injections.

Overdosage - Accidental overdosage is manifested by excessive blood pressure elevation (see adverse effects above). Treatment consists only of temporarily discontinuing therapy since dopamine's duration of activity is so brief. Should the patients condition fail to stabilize, the use of phentolamine has been suggested for use.

Drug Interactions - **Oxytocic drugs** may cause severe hypertension when used with dopamine.
Dopamine may reverse the effects of beta-**blocking agents**.

Monoamine oxidase inhibitors (rarely used in veterinary medicine), can significantly prolong and enhance the effects on dopamine.

Use of **halothane or cyclopropane** may result in increased myocardial sensitization to the catecholamines; dopamine-induced ventricular arrhythmias may be treated with propranolol.

Seizures, hypotension, and bradycardia have been reported if dopamine is used concurrently with **phenytoin**.

In animals (species not specified), the renal and mesenteric vasodilitation effects of dopamine have been antagonized by **butyrephenones** (*e.g.,* **haloperidol), opiates, and phenothiazines**.

Doses -

To prepare solution: Add contents of vial to either 250 ml, 500 ml, or 1000 ml of normal saline, D5W, lactated Ringers injection, or other compatible IV fluid. If adding a 200 mg vial (5 ml @40 mg/ml) to a one liter bag, the resultant solution will contain an approximate concentration of 200 micrograms/ml. If using a mini-drip IV set (60 drops/ml), each drop will contain approximately 3.3 micrograms. In small dogs and cats it may be necessary to use less dopamine so the final concentration will be less; in large animals, a higher concentration may be necessary.

Usual Doses:

The dosage of dopamine is determined by its indication (for more information refer to the pharmacology section above). Use an IV pump or other flow controlling device to increase precision in dosing.

For adjunctive therapy for oliguric renal failure:
   a) Low doses (2 - 5 micrograms/kg/min) with diuretics (furosemide) are used to attempt to convert a patient from an oliguric state to a non-oliguric one.

For adjunctive therapy for acute heart failure:
   a) IV infusion of 1 - 10 (some say up to 15 micrograms/kg/min) micrograms/kg/min.

For treatment of severe hypotension/shock: (Note: Dopamine is not a substitute for adequate volume replacement therapy when indicated.)

    a) 1- 20 micrograms/kg/min IV infusion. Although 20 micrograms/kg/min is listed here as the upper limit of dosing, some human patients with severe circulatory decompensation have required doses greater than 50 micrograms/kg/min. While discontinuing an infusion, it may be necessary to gradually withdraw the drug to a dose not less than 5 micrograms/kg/min and expand blood volume with IV fluids.

Monitoring Parameters -
1) Urine flow
2) Cardiac rate/rhythm
3) Blood pressure
4) IV site

Client Information - Dopamine should be used only in an intensive care setting or where adequate monitoring is possible.

Dosage Forms/Preparations/FDA Approval Status/Withholding Times -

Veterinary-Approved Products: None

Human-Approved Products:

Dopamine HCl for Injection 40 mg/ml, 80 mg/ml and 160 mg/ml in 5 ml, 10ml & 20 ml vials or 5 and 10 ml-syringes; *Intropin®* (Faulding); *Dopamine HCL®* (Abbott); Generic; (Rx)

Dopamine HCl in 5% dextrose for infusion 0.8 mg/ml, 1.6 mg/ml, 3.2 mg/ml in 250 and 500 ml bags; (Abbott) (Rx)

DORAMECTIN

Chemistry/Storage/Stability/Compatibility - An avermectin antiparasitic compound, doramectin is isolated from fermentations from the soil organism *Streptomyces avermitilis*. The commercially available injectable solution is a colorless to pale yellow, sterile solution. The injectable solution should be stored below 86°F (30°C).

Pharmacology - The primary mode of action of avermectins like doramectin is to affect chloride ion channel activity in the nervous system of nematodes and arthropods. Doramectin binds to receptors that increase membrane permeability to chloride ions. This inhibits the electrical activity of nerve cells in nematodes and muscle cells in arthropods and causes paralysis and death of the parasites. Avermectins also enhance the release of gamma amino butyric acid (GABA) at presynaptic neurons. GABA acts as an inhibitory neurotransmitter and blocks the post-synaptic stimulation of the adjacent neuron in nematodes or the muscle fiber in arthropods. Avermectins are generally not toxic to mammals as they do not have glutamate-gated chloride channels and these compounds do not readily cross the blood-brain barrier where mammalian GABA receptors occur.

Uses/Indications - Doramectin injection is indicated for the treatment and control of the following endo- and ectoparasites in cattle: roundworms (adults and some fourth stage larvae)— *Ostertagia ostertagi* (including inhibited larvae), *O. lyrata, Haemonchus placei, Trichostrongylus axei, T. colubriformis, T. longispicularis, Cooperia oncophora, C. pectinata, C. punctata, C. surnabada (syn. mcmasteri), Bunostomum phlebotomum, Strongyloides papillosus, Oesophagostomum radiatum, Trichuris spp.,*; lungworms (adults and fourth stage larvae)— *Dictyocaulus viviparus*; eyeworms (adults)—*Thelazia spp.*; grubs (parasitic stages)—*Hypoderma bovis, H. lineatum* ; lice—*Haematopinus eurysternus, Linognathus vituli, Solenopotes capillatus*; and mange mites—*Psoroptes bovis, Sarcoptes scabiei*.

The manufacturer states the doramectin protects cattle against infection or reinfection with *Ostertagia ostertagi* for up to 21 days.

Pharmacokinetics - After subcutaneous injection, the time to peak plasma concentration in cattle is about 5 days. Bioavailability is for practical purposes, equal with subQ and IM injections.

Contraindications/Precautions/Reproductive Safety - The manufacturer warns to not use in other animal species as severe adverse reactions, including fatalities in dogs, may result.

  Studies performed in breeding animals (bulls, and cows in early and late pregnancy), at a dose of 3X recommended had no effect on breeding performance.

Adverse Effects/Warnings - No listed adverse effects. Intramuscular injections may have a higher incidence of injection site blemishes at slaughter than do subcutaneous injections.

Overdosage - In field trials, no toxic signs were seen in cattle given up to 25X the recommended dose. In breeding animals (bulls, and cows in early and late pregnancy), a dose 3 times the recommended dose had no effect on breeding performance.

Drug Interactions - None noted.

Doses -
 Cattle:
     For labeled indications: 200 mcg/kg (1 ml per 110 lb. body weight)) SubQ or IM.
     Injections should be made using 16 to 18 gauge needles. Subcutaneous injections
     should be administered under the loose skin in front of or behind the shoulder.
     Intramuscular injections should be administered into the muscular region of the neck.
     Beef Quality Assurance guidelines recommend subcutaneous administration as the
     preferred route. (Label Directions; *Dectomax®*—Pfizer)

Monitoring Parameters - Efficacy

Client Information/Withdrawal Times - Cattle must not be slaughtered for human consumption within 35 days of treatment. Not for use in female dairy cattle 20 months of age or older. A withdrawal period has not been established for this product in pre-ruminating calves. Should not be used in calves to be processed for veal.

Dosage Forms/Preparations/FDA Approval Status -
 Human-Approved Products: None
 Veterinary-Approved Products:
    Doramectin 10 mg/ml Injectable Solution in 100 ml, 250 ml, and 500 ml multi-dose vials;
    Dectomax® (Pfizer); (OTC). Approved for use in cattle (see limitations in Client
    Information above).

DOXAPRAM HCL

Chemistry - Doxapram HCl is a white to off-white, odorless, crystalline powder that is stable in light and air. It is soluble in water, sparingly soluble in alcohol and practically insoluble in ether. Injectable products have a pH from 3.5-5. Benzyl alcohol or chlorobutanol is added as a preservative agent in the commercially available injections.

Storage/Stability/Compatibility - Store at room temperature and avoid freezing solution. Do not mix with alkaline solutions (*e.g.,* thiopental, aminophylline, sodium bicarbonate). Doxapram is **compatible** with D5W or normal saline.

Pharmacology - Doxapram is a general CNS stimulant, with all levels of the CNS affected. The effects of respiratory stimulation are a result of direct stimulation of the medullary respiratory centers and possibly through the reflex activation of carotid and aortic chemoreceptors. Transient increases in respiratory rate and volume occur, but increases in arterial oxygenation usually do not ensue. This is because doxapram usually increases the work associated with respirations with resultant increased oxygen consumption and carbon dioxide production.

Pharmacokinetics - Little pharmacokinetic data appears to be published for domestic animals. Onset of effect in humans and animals after IV injection usually occurs within 2 minutes. The drug is well distributed into tissues. In dogs, doxapram is rapidly metabolized and most is excreted as metabolites in the urine within 24-48 hours after administration. Small quantities of metabolites may be excreted up to 120 hours after dosing.

Uses/Indications - The manufacturer of *Dopram®-V* lists the following indications:
  For Dogs, Cats, and Horses: To stimulate respiration during and after general anesthesia and/or to speed awakening and reflexes after anesthesia.
  For Neonatal Dogs and Cats: Initiate or stimulate respirations following dystocia or cesarean section.
  Doxopram also has been used for treatment of CNS depression in food animals (not approved) and has been suggested as a treatment of respiratory depression in small animals caused by reactions to radiopaque contrast media or for barbiturate overdosage (see precautions below).

Contraindications/Precautions - Doxapram should not be used as a substitute for aggressive artificial (mechanical) respiratory support in instances of severe respiratory depression.
  Contraindications from the human literature include: seizure disorders, head trauma, uncompensated heart failure, severe hypertension, cardiovascular accidents, respiratory failure secondary to neuromuscular disorders, airway obstruction, pulmonary embolism, pneumothorax, acute asthma, dyspnea, or whenever hypoxia is not associated with hypercapnea. Doxapram should be used with caution in patients with history of asthma, arrhythmias, or tachycardias. It should be used with extreme caution in patients with cerebral edema or increased CSF pressure, pheochromocytoma or hyperthyroidism. Patients who have a history of hypersensitivity to the drug or are receiving mechanical ventilation should not receive doxapram. The above contraindications/precautions are not listed in the veterinary product literature provided by the manufacturer.
  Avoid the use of a single injection site for a prolonged period of time or extravasation when administering intravenously. However, subcutaneous injection has been recommended for use in neonatal feline and canine patients.

Adverse Effects/Warnings - Hypertension, arrhythmias, seizures, and hyperventilation leading to respiratory alkalosis has been reported. These effects are most probable with repeated or high doses. The drug reportedly has a narrow margin of safety when used in humans.

Safety of doxopram has not been established in pregnant animals. The potential risks versus benefits should be weighed before using.

Overdosage - Symptoms of overdosage include: hypertension, skeletal muscle hyperactivity, tachycardia, and generalized CNS excitation including seizures. Treatment is supportive. Drugs such as short acting IV barbiturates may be used to help decrease CNS hyperactivity. Oxygen therapy may be necessary.

Drug Interactions - Additive pressor effects may occur with **sympathomimetic** agents

Doxapram may mask the effects of **muscle relaxant** drugs.

Doxapram may increase epinephrine release; therefore use should be delayed for approximately 10 minutes after discontinuation of anesthetic agents (*e.g.,* **halothane, enflurane**) that have been demonstrated to sensitize the myocardium to catecholamines.

Doses -
Dogs, Cats:
    a) 1 - 5 mg/kg IV; may repeat prn. To stimulate respirations in newborns: 1- 2 drops under tongue or 0.1 ml IV in umbilical vein (should be used with caution if product contains benzyl alcohol as a preservative). (Package Insert; *Dopram®-V* - Robins)
    b) Cats: 5 - 10 mg/kg IV (Boothe 1990)

Rabbits/Rodents:
For respiratory depression:
    a) Rabbits: 2 - 5 mg/kg SubQ or IV q15 minutes
        Rodents: 2 - 5 mg/kg SubQ q15 minutes (Huerkamp 1995)

Cattle, Swine:
    a) 5 - 10 mg/kg IV (Howard 1986)

Horses:
    a) 0.5 - 1 mg/kg IV at 5 minute intervals (do not exceed 2 mg/kg in foals); For foal resuscitation: 0.02 - 0.05 mg/kg/min IV (Robinson 1987)

Monitoring Parameters -
    1) Respiratory rate
    2) Cardiac rate and rhythm
    3) Blood gases if available and indicated
    4) CNS level of excitation
    5) Blood pressure if possible and indicated

Client Information- This agent should be used in an inpatient setting or with direct professional supervision.

Dosage Forms/Preparations/FDA Approval Status/Withholding Times -
Veterinary-Approved Products:
Doxapram HCl for Injection: 20 mg/ml; 20 ml multi-dose vial; *Dopram-V®* (Fort Dodge); (Rx) Approved for use in dogs, cats & horses

Human-Approved Products:-
Doxapram HCl for Injection: 20 mg/ml in 20 ml vial; *Dopram®* (Robins); (Rx) ; generic, (Rx)

DOXEPIN HCL

Chemistry - A dibenzoxazepine derivative tricyclic antidepressant, doxepin HCl occurs as a white powder that is freely soluble in alcohol.

Storage/Stability/Compatibility - Store products in protected from direct sunlight in tight, light-resistant containers at room temperature.

Pharmacology - Doxepin is a tricyclic agent that has a antihistaminic, anticholinergic, and alpha1-adrenergic blocking activity. In the CNS, doxepin inhibits the reuptake of norepinephrine and serotonin (5-HT) by the presynaptic neuronal membrane, thereby increasing their synaptic concentrations. Doxepin is considered to be a moderate inhibitor of norepinephrine and weak inhibitor of serotonin.

Uses/Indications - The primary use for doxepin in veterinary medicine is the adjunctive therapy of psychogenic dermatoses, particularly those that have an anxiety component.

Pharmacokinetics - Doxepin appears to be well absorbed after oral administration. Doxepin and its *N*-demethylated active metabolite are distributed into milk. The drug is extensively metabolized in the liver.

Contraindications/Precautions/Reproductive Safety - These agents are contraindicated if prior sensitivity has been noted with any other tricyclic. Concomitant use with monoamine oxidase inhibitors is generally contraindicated. Doxepin is probably contraindicated in dogs with urinary retention or glaucoma.

Rodent studies have demonstrated no teratogenic effects, but safety during pregnancy has not been established. Doxepin is excreted into milk, and one case report of sedation and respiratory depression in the infant has been reported.

Adverse Effects/Warnings - While doxepin has less potential for cardiac adverse effects than many other tricyclics, it can cause ventricular arrhythmias, particularly after overdoses. In dogs, it may also cause hyperexcitability, GI distress, or lethargy. However, potential adverse effects can run the entire gamut of systems. Refer to other human drug references for additional information.

Overdosage/Acute Toxicity - Overdosage with tricyclics can be life-threatening (arrhythmias, cardiorespiratory collapse). Because the toxicities and therapies for treatment are complicated and controversial, it is recommended to contact an animal poison control center for further information in any potential overdose situation.

Drug Interactions - Because of additive effects, use doxepin cautiously with other agents with **anticholinergic** or **CNS depressant** effects. Tricyclic antidepressants used with antithyroid agents may increase the potential risk of agranulocytosis. **Cimetidine** may inhibit tricyclic antidepressant metabolism and increase the risk of toxicity. Use in combination with **sympathomimetic agents** may increase the risk of cardiac effects (arrhythmias, hypertension, hyperpyrexia). Concomitant use with **monoamine oxidase inhibitors** is generally contraindicated.

Laboratory Considerations - Tricyclics can widen QRS complexes, prolong PR intervals and invert or flatten T-waves on **ECG**. Tricyclics may alter (increase or decrease) **blood glucose** levels.

Doses -
Dogs:
For treatment of psychogenic dermatoses: 3 - 5 mg/kg PO q12h; maximum dose is 150 mg (per dog) q12h. (Shanley and Overall 1992)

For antihistaminic effects in treatment of atopy: 0.5 - 1 mg/kg q12h PO (White 1994)

Monitoring Parameters - 1) Efficacy; 2) Adverse effects

Client Information - Inform clients that several weeks may be required before efficacy is noted and to continue dosing as prescribed. All tricyclics should be dispensed in child-resistant packaging and kept well away from children or pets.

Dosage Forms/Preparations/FDA Approval Status/Withholding Times -
Veterinary-Approved Products: None
Human-Approved Products:

Doxepin Oral Capsules, 10 mg, 25 mg, 50 mg, 75 mg, 100 mg, 150 mg; *Sinequan®* (Roerig); generic; (Rx)

Doxepin Oral Concentrate, 10 mg/ml, 25 mg, 50 mg, 75 mg, 100 mg, 150 mg; *Sinequan®* *Concentrate* (Roerig), generic; (Rx)

DOXORUBICIN HCL

Chemistry - An anthracycline glycoside antibiotic antineoplastic, doxorubicin HCl occurs as a lyophilized, red-orange powder that is freely soluble in water, slightly soluble in normal saline, and very slightly soluble in alcohol. The commercially available powder for injection also contains lactose and methylparaben to aid dissolution. After reconstituting, the solution has a pH from 3.8 - 6.5. The commercially available solution for injection has a pH of approximately 3. Doxorubicin HCl may also be known as Hydroxydaunomycin HCl, Hydroxydaunorubicin HCl, ADR, or as the commonly known proprietary product, *Adriamycin®* (Adria).

Storage/Stability/Compatibility - The commercially available solution for injection is stable for 18 months when stored in the refrigerator (2-8°C) and protected from light.

Lyophilized powder for injection should be stored away from direct sunlight and in a dry place. After reconstituting with sodium chloride 0.9%, the single-use lyophilized powder product is reportedly stable for 24 hours at room temperature and 48 hours when refrigerated. The manufacturer recommends protecting from sunlight. They also recommend not freezing the product and discarding any unused portion. However, one study found that powder reconstituted with sterile water to a concentration of 2 mg/ml lost only about 1.5% of its potency per month over 6 months when stored in the refrigerator. When frozen at -20°C, no potency loss after 30 days was detected and sterility was maintained by filtering the drug through a 0.22µm filter before injection.

The manufacturer states that after reconstitution, the multi-dose vials may be stored for up to 7 days at room temperature in normal room light, and for up to 15 days in the refrigerator.

Doxorubicin HCl is reportedly **compatible** with the following intravenous solutions and drugs: dextrose 3.3% in sodium chloride 3%, D5W, Normosol R (pH 7.4), lactated Ringer's injection, and sodium chloride 0.9%. In syringes with: bleomycin sulfate, cisplatin, cyclophosphamide, droperidol, fluorouracil, leucovorin calcium, methotrexate sodium, metoclopramide HCl, mito-mycin, and vincristine sulfate. The drug is compatible during Y-site injection with bleomycin sulfate, cisplatin, cyclophosphamide, droperidol, fluorouracil, leucovorin calcium, methotrexate sodium, metoclopramide HCl, mitomycin, vinblastine sulfate and vincristine sulfate.

Doxorubicin HCl **compatibility information conflicts** or is dependent on diluent or concentra-tion factors with the following drugs or solutions: vinblastine sulfate (in syringes and as an IV additive). Compatibility is dependent upon factors such as pH, concentration, temperature and diluents used. It is suggested to consult specialized references for more specific information (*e.g., Handbook on Injectable Drugs* by Trissel; see bibliography).

Doxorubicin HCl is reportedly **incompatible** with the following solutions or drugs: amino-phylline, cephalothin sodium, dexamethasone sodium phosphate, diazepam, fluorouracil (as an IV additive only), furosemide, heparin sodium and hydrocortisone sodium succinate.

Pharmacology - Although possessing antimicrobial properties, doxorubicin's cytotoxic effects precludes its use as an anti-infective agent. The drug causes inhibition of DNA synthesis, DNA-dependent RNA synthesis and protein synthesis, but the precise mechanism(s) for these effects is (are) not well understood. The drug acts throughout the cell cycle and also possesses some im-munosuppressant activity.

Doxorubicin is most cytotoxic to cardiac cells, followed by melanoma, sarcoma cells, and nor-mal muscle and skin fibroblasts. Other rapidly proliferating "normal" cells, such as bone marrow, hair follicles, GI mucosa, may also be affected by the drug.

Uses/Indications - Doxorubicin is perhaps the most widely used antineoplastic agent at present in small animal medicine. It may be useful in the treatment of a variety of carcinomas and sar-comas in both the dog and cat. Refer to the Dosage references or the Protocols found in the ap-pendix for more information.

Pharmacokinetics - Doxorubicin must be administered IV as it is not absorbed from the GI tract and is extremely irritating to tissues if administered SQ or IM. After IV injection, the drug is rapidly and widely distributed, but does not appreciably enter the CSF. It is highly bound to tis-sue and plasma proteins, probably crosses the placenta and is distributed into milk.

Doxorubicin is metabolized extensively by the liver and other tissues via aldo-keto reductase primarily to doxorubicinol, which is active. Other inactive metabolites are also formed. Doxorubicin and its metabolites are primarily excreted in the bile and feces. Only about 5% of the drug is excreted in the urine within 5 days of dosing. Doxorubicin is eliminated in a triphasic manner. During the first phase ($t_{1/2} \approx 0.6$ hours) doxorubicin is rapidly metabolized, via the "first pass" effect followed by a second phase ($t_{1/2} \approx 3.3$ hours). The third phase has a much slower elimination half-life (17 hours for doxorubicin and 32 hours for metabolites), presumably due to the slow release of the drug from tissue proteins.

Contraindications/Precautions/Reproductive Safety - Doxorubicin is contraindicated or rela-tively contraindicated (measure risk vs. benefit) in patients with myelosuppression, impaired car-diac function, or who have reached the total cumulative dose level of doxorubicin and/or daunorubicin. It should be used with caution in patients with hyperuricemia/hyperuricuria, or impaired hepatic function. Dosage adjustments are necessary in patients with hepatic impair-ment.

Because doxorubicin can be very irritating to skin, gloves should be worn when administering or preparing the drug. Ideally, doxorubicin injection should be prepared in a vertical laminar flow hood. Should accidental skin or mucous membrane contact occur, wash the area immediately using soap and copious amounts of water.

Doxorubicin is teratogenic and embryotoxic in laboratory animals. It is unknown if it affects male fertility.

Adverse Effects/Warnings - Doxorubicin may cause several adverse effects including bone marrow suppression, cardiac toxicity, alopecia, gastroenteritis (vomiting, diarrhea) and stomati-tis.

An immediate hypersensitivity reaction may be seen, characterized by urticaria, facial swelling, vomiting, arrhythmias (see below) and/or hypotension. Pretreatment with a histamine$_1$ blocker such as diphenhydramine (IV prior to treatment at 10 mg for dogs up to 9 kg; 20 mg for dogs 9-27 kg; and 30 mg for dogs over 27 kg) or alternatively, dexamethasone (0.55 mg/kg IV), is often recommended to reduce or eliminate these effects.

Cardiac toxicity of doxorubicin falls into two categories, acute and cumulative. Acute cardiac toxicity may occur during IV administration or several hours subsequent, and is manifested by cardiac arrest preceded by ECG changes (T-wave flattening, S-T depression, voltage reduction, arrhythmias). Rarely, an acute hypertensive crisis has been noted after infusion. Acute cardiac toxicity does not preclude further use of the drug, but additional treatment should be delayed. The administration of diphenhydramine and/or glucocorticoids before doxorubicin administration may prevent these effects.

Cumulative cardiac toxicity requires halting any further therapy and can be extremely serious. Diffuse cardiomyopathy with severe congestive heart failure refractory to traditional therapies is generally noted. It is believed that the risk of cardiac toxicity is greatly increased in dogs when the cumulative dose exceeds 250 mg/m^2, but may be seen at doses as low as 100 mg/m^2. Therefore, it is not recommended to exceed 240 mg/m^2 total dose in dogs. It is unknown what the incidence of cardiotoxicity or the dosage ceiling for doxorubicin is in cats, but most clinicians believe that 240 mg/m^2 should also be used as the upper limit cumulative dose in cats.

In cats, doxorubicin is a potential nephrotoxin and they should have renal function monitored before and during therapy.

Doxorubicin should be administered IV slowly, over at least 10 minutes, in a free flowing line.

Extravasation injuries secondary to perivascular administration of doxorubicin can be quite serious, with severe tissue ulceration and necrosis possible. Prevention of extravasation should be a priority and animals should be frequently checked during the infusion. Should extravasation occur, one author (Coppoc 1988) makes the following recommendations for veterinary patients: Immediately flood the area with 5 ml of sodium bicarbonate injection 8.4%, 15-30 ml of 0.9% sodium chloride, and 4 mg dexamethasone. Then apply a steroid/DMSO (*concentrations not noted*) solution topically to the site and cover with an occlusive dressing (*e.g.,* plastic wrap). Continue to treat using the occlusive dressing for 3-5 days. In humans with severe extravasation injuries due to doxorubicin, site excision and plastic surgery has been necessary.

Overdosage/Acute Toxicity - Inadvertent acute overdosage may be manifested by exacerbations of the adverse effects outlined above. A lethal dose for dogs has been reported as 72 mg/m^2 (O'Keefe and Harris 1990). Supportive and symptomatic therapy is suggested should an overdose occur.

Drug Interactions - Although doxorubicin is used in conjunction with other antineoplastic agents, toxicity may be also be potentiated. This is particularly true (in humans) with **cyclophosphamide**. Doxorubicin may exacerbate cyclophosphamide-induced hemorrhagic cystitis and **mercaptopurine**-associated hepatotoxicity. Cyclophosphamide may also potentiate the cardiotoxic effects of doxorubicin.

Drug/Laboratory Interactions - Doxorubicin may significantly increase both blood and urine concentrations of **uric acid**.

Doses - For maximum effect, doxorubicin is most commonly employed as part of a multi-drug protocol. For more information, refer to the protocols found in the appendix or other protocols found in numerous references, including: *Handbook of Small Animal Practice* (Stann 1988b); *Handbook of Small Animal Therapeutics* (Rosenthal 1985); *Current Veterinary Therapy X: Small Animal Practice* (Helfand 1989), (Matus 1989); and *Textbook of Veterinary Internal Medicine, 3rd Edition* (Couto 1989a).

  Dogs:
    For susceptible neoplasms:
      a) 30 mg/m^2 IV or intracavitary every 21 days or 10 mg/m^2 IV every 7 days. Maximum cumulative dose: 240 mg/m^2. Pretreat with antihistamine. (Thompson 1989a)
      b) 30 mg/m^2 IV every 21 days. Maximum cumulative dose: 200 mg/m^2. (Macy 1986)
      b) 30 mg/m^2 IV every 21 days. Maximum cumulative dose: 240 mg/m^2. (MacEwen and Rosenthal 1989)

  Cats:
    For susceptible neoplasms:
      a) For lymphosarcoma, carcinomas, sarcomas, myeloma, and leukemias: 20 - 30 mg/m^2 every 3-4 weeks. (Couto 1989b)

Monitoring Parameters -
  1) Efficacy
  2) Toxicity
      a) CBC with platelets
      b) Dogs with pre-existing heart disease should be monitored with regular ECG's (insensitive to early toxic changes caused doxorubicin) and/or echocardiogram
      c) Evaluate hepatic function prior to therapy
      d) Urinalyses and serum creatinine/BUN in cats

Client Information - Clients must be briefed on the possibilities of severe toxicity developing from this drug, including drug-related mortality. Clients should contact the veterinarian should the patient exhibit any symptoms of profound depression, abnormal bleeding (including bloody diarrhea) and/or bruising.

Doxorubicin may cause urine to be colored orange to red for 1-2 days after dosing. Mild anorexia and occasional vomiting are commonly seen 2-5 days post-therapy. Avoid handling urine of treated dogs.

Dosage Forms/Preparations/FDA Approval Status/Withholding Times -
Veterinary-Approved Products: None.
Human-Approved Products:

Doxorubicin HCl Lyophilized Powder for Injection 10 mg, 20 mg, 50 mg, 100 mg, & 150 mg vials; *Adriamycin RDF®* (Pharmacia); *Doxorubicin HCL®* (Cetus), *Adriamycin PFS®* (Pharmacia); *Rubex®* (Bristol-Myers Oncology); generic; (Rx). Reconstitute with appropriate amount of 0.9% sodium chloride for final concentration of 2 mg/ml.

Doxorubicin HCl Injection 2 mg/ml in 5, 10, 20, 25 ml & 100 ml (preservative free) vials; *Adriamycin PFS®* ((Pharmacia); *Doxorubicin HCl®* (Cetus); *Doxil®* (Sequus); (Rx)

DOXYCYCLINE CALCIUM
DOXYCYCLINE HYCLATE
DOXYCYCLINE MONOHYDRATE

Chemistry - A semi-synthetic tetracycline that is derived from oxytetracycline, doxycycline is available as hyclate, calcium and monohydrate salts. The hyclate salt is used in the injectable dosage form and in oral tablets and capsules. It occurs as a yellow, crystalline powder that is soluble in water and slightly soluble in alcohol. After reconstitution with sterile water, the hyclate injection has a pH of 1.8-3.3. Doxycycline hyclate may also be known as doxycycline hydrochloride.

The monohydrate salt is found in the oral powder for reconstitution. It occurs as a yellow, crystalline powder that is very slightly soluble in water and sparingly soluble in alcohol. The calcium salt is formed *in situ* during manufacturing. It is found in the commercially available oral syrup.

Storage/Stability/Compatibility - Doxycycline hyclate tablets and capsules should be stored in tight, light resistant containers at temperatures less than 30°C, and preferably at room temperature (15-30°C). After reconstituting with water, the monohydrate oral suspension is stable for 14 days when stored at room temperature.

The hyclate injection when reconstituted with a suitable diluent (*e.g.,* D5W, Ringer's injection, Sodium Chloride 0.9%, or Plasma-Lyte 56 in D5W) to a concentration of 0.1 to 1 mg/ml may be stored for 72 hours if refrigerated. Frozen reconstituted solutions (10 mg/ml in sterile water) are stable for at least 8 weeks if kept at -20°C, but should not be refrozen once thawed. If solutions are stored at room temperature, different manufacturers give different recommendations regarding stability, ranging from 12-48 hours. Infusions should generally be completed within 12 hours of administration.

Doxycycline hyclate for injection is reportedly **compatible** with the following IV infusion solutions and drugs: D5W, Ringer's injection, sodium chloride 0.9%, or Plasma-Lyte 56 in D5W, Plasma-Lyte 148 in D5W, Normosol M in D5W, Normosol R in D5W, invert sugar 10%, acyclovir sodium, hydromorphone HCl, magnesium sulfate, meperidine HCl, morphine sulfate, perphenazine and ranitidine HCl. Compatibility is dependent upon factors such as pH, concentration, temperature and diluents used. It is suggested to consult specialized references for more specific information (*e.g., Handbook on Injectable Drugs* by Trissel; see bibliography).

Pharmacology - Tetracyclines generally act as bacteriostatic antibiotics and inhibit protein synthesis by reversibly binding to 30S ribosomal subunits of susceptible organisms, thereby preventing binding to those ribosomes of aminoacyl transfer-RNA. Tetracyclines also are believed to reversibly bind to 50S ribosomes and additionally alter cytoplasmic membrane permeability in susceptible organisms. In high concentrations, tetracyclines can also inhibit protein synthesis by mammalian cells.

As a class, the tetracyclines have activity against most *mycoplasma*, spirochetes (including the Lyme disease organism), *Chlamydia* and *Rickettsia*. Against gram positive bacteria, the tetracyclines have activity against some strains of *staphylococcus* and *streptococci*, but resistance of these organisms is increasing. Gram positive bacteria that are usually covered by tetracyclines, include *Actinomyces sp., Bacillus anthracis, Clostridium perfringens* and *tetani, Listeria monocytogenes* and *Nocardia*. Among gram negative bacteria that tetracyclines usually have *in vitro* and *in vivo* activity against, include *Bordetella sp., Brucella, Bartonella, Haemophilus sp., Pasturella multocida, Shigella,* and *Yersinia pestis*. Many or most strains of *E. coli, Klebsiella,*

Bacteroides, Enterobacter, Proteus and *Pseudomonas aeruginosa* are resistant to the tetracyclines.

Doxycycline generally has very similar activity as other tetracyclines against susceptible organisms, but some strains of bacteria may be more susceptible to doxycycline or minocycline and additional *in vitro* testing may be required.

Uses/Indications - Although there are no veterinary-approved doxycycline products available, its favorable pharmacokinetic parameters (longer half-life, higher CNS penetration) when compared to either tetracycline HCl or oxytetracycline HCl make it a reasonable choice to use in small animals when a tetracycline is indicated, particularly when a tetracycline is indicated in an azotemic patient. Because there is apparently less clinical experience with this agent in small animals than with either tetracycline or oxytetracycline, some caution should be employed before routinely using.

In avian species, some clinicians feel that doxycycline is the drug of choice in the oral treatment of psittacosis, particularly when treating only a few birds.

Pharmacokinetics - Doxycycline is well absorbed after oral administration. Bioavailability is 90-100% in humans. No bioavailability data was located for veterinary species, but it is thought that the drug is also readily absorbed in monogastric animals. Unlike tetracycline HCl or oxytetracycline, doxycycline absorption may only be reduced by 20% by either food or dairy products in the gut. This is not considered to be clinically important.

Tetracyclines as a class, are widely distributed to the heart, kidney, lungs, muscle, pleural fluid, bronchial secretions, sputum, bile, saliva, synovial fluid, ascitic fluid, and aqueous and vitreous humor. Doxycycline is more lipid soluble and penetrates body tissues and fluids better than tetracycline HCl or oxytetracycline, including to the CSF, prostate and eye. While CSF levels are generally insufficient to treat most bacterial infections, doxycycline has been shown to be efficacious in the treatment of the CNS effects associated with Lyme disease in humans. The volume of distribution at steady-state in dogs is approximately 1.5 L/kg. Doxycycline is bound to plasma proteins in varying amounts dependent upon species. The drug is approximately 25-93% bound to plasma proteins in humans, 75-86% in dogs, and about 93% in cattle and pigs.

Doxycycline's elimination from the body is relatively unique. The drug is primarily excreted into the feces via non-biliary routes in an inactive form. It is thought that the drug is partially inactivated in the intestine by chelate formation and then excreted into the intestinal lumen. In dogs, about 75% of a given dose is handled in this manner. Renal excretion of doxycycline can only account for about 25% of a dose in dogs, and biliary excretion less than 5%. The serum half-life of doxycycline in dogs is approximately 10-12 hours and a clearance of about 1.7 ml/kg/min. In calves, the drug has similar pharmacokinetic values. Doxycycline does not accumulate in patients with renal dysfunction.

Contraindications/Precautions/Reproductive Safety - Doxycycline is contraindicated in patients hypersensitive to it. Because tetracyclines can retard fetal skeletal development and discolor deciduous teeth, they should only be used in the last half of pregnancy when the benefits outweigh the fetal risks. Doxycycline is considered to be less likely to cause these abnormalities than other more water soluble tetracyclines (*e.g.*, tetracycline, oxytetracycline). Unlike either oxytetracycline or tetracycline, doxycycline can be used in patients with renal insufficiency.

Until further studies documenting the safety of intravenous doxycycline in horses are done, the parenteral route of administering this drug in horses should be considered contraindicated.

Adverse Effects/Warnings - The most commonly reported sided effects of oral doxycycline therapy in dogs and cats are nausea and vomiting. To alleviate these effects, the drug could be given with food without clinically significant reductions in drug absorption.

Tetracycline therapy (especially long-term) may result in overgrowth (superinfections) of non-susceptible bacteria or fungi.

In humans, doxycycline (or other tetracyclines) has also been associated with photosensitivity reactions and, rarely, hepatotoxicity or blood dyscrasias.

Intravenous injection of even relatively low doses of doxycycline has been associated with cardiac arrhythmias, collapse and death in horses.

Overdosage/Acute Toxicity - With the exception of intravenous dosing in horses (see above), doxycycline is apparently quite safe in most mild overdose situations. Oral overdoses would most likely be associated with GI disturbances (vomiting, anorexia, and/or diarrhea). Although doxycycline is less vulnerable to chelation with cations than other tetracyclines, oral administration of divalent or trivalent cation antacids may bind some of the drug and reduce GI distress. Should the patient develop severe emesis or diarrhea, fluids and electrolytes should be monitored and replaced if necessary.

Rapid intravenous injection of doxycycline has induced transient collapse and cardiac arrhythmias in several species, presumably due to chelation with intravascular calcium ions. If overdose quantities are inadvertently administered, these effects may be more pronounced.

Drug Interactions - When orally administered, tetracyclines can chelate **divalent or trivalent cations** which can decrease the absorption of the tetracycline or the other drug if it contains these cations. Oral antacids, saline cathartics or other GI products containing aluminum, calcium, magnesium, zinc or bismuth cations are most commonly associated with this interaction. Doxycycline has a relatively low affinity for calcium ions, but it is recommended that all oral tetracyclines be given at least 1-2 hours before or after the cation-containing product.

Oral iron products are also associated with decreased tetracycline absorption, and administration of iron salts should preferably be given 3 hours before or 2 hours after the tetracycline dose. **Oral sodium bicarbonate, kaolin, pectin, or bismuth subsalicylate** may impair tetracycline absorption when given together orally.

Bacteriostatic drugs like the tetracyclines, may interfere with bactericidal activity of the **penicillins, cephalosporins,** and **aminoglycosides**. There is some amount of controversy regarding the actual clinical significance of this interaction, however.

Tetracyclines may increase the bioavailability of **digoxin** in a small percentage of patients (human) and lead to digoxin toxicity. These effects may persist for months after discontinuation of the tetracycline.

Tetracyclines may depress plasma prothrombin activity and patients on **anticoagulant** (*e.g.,* **warfarin**) therapy may need dosage adjustment. Tetracyclines have been reported to increase the nephrotoxic effects of **methoxyflurane** and tetracycline HCl or Oxytetracycline are not recommended to used with methoxyflurane.

GI side effects may be increased if tetracyclines are administered concurrently with **theophylline** products.

Tetracyclines have reportedly reduced **insulin** requirements in diabetic patients, but this interaction is yet to be confirmed with controlled studies.

Drug/Laboratory Interactions - Tetracyclines (not minocycline) may cause falsely elevated values of **urine catecholamines** when using fluorometric methods of determination.

Tetracyclines reportedly can cause false-positive **urine glucose** results if using the cupric sulfate method of determination (Benedict's reagent, *Clinitest*®), but this may be the result of ascorbic acid which is found in some parenteral formulations of tetracyclines. Tetracyclines have also reportedly caused false-negative results in determining urine glucose when using the glucose oxidase method (*Clinistix*®, *Tes-Tape*®).

Doses -
Dogs:
For susceptible infections:
a) 5 mg/kg PO or IV q12h; administer with food if GI upset occurs; avoid in young animals; avoid or reduce dose in animals with severe liver disease (Vaden and Papich 1995)
b) For canine ehrlichiosis: 5 - 10 mg/kg every 12-24 hours for 2-3 months (duration of treatment based upon preliminary data). (Greene 1995)
c) For canine ehrlichiosis: 5 mg/kg PO, IV once daily for 7 days in acute cases, and 10 mg/kg PO once daily for 7-21 days in chronic cases. (Morgan 1988)
d) For Lyme Disease: 10 mg/kg PO q24h for 21-28 days (Appel and Jacobson 1995)
e) For salmon poisoning disease: 10 mg/kg IV twice a day for at least 7 days. (Rikihisa and Zimmerman 1995)

Cats:
For susceptible infections:
a) 5 mg/kg PO or IV q12h; administer with food if GI upset occurs; avoid in young animals; avoid or reduce dose in animals with severe liver disease (Vaden and Papich 1995)
b) 5 mg/kg PO q12h (Davis 1985)
c) For feline ehrlichiosis: 5 mg/kg twice daily (Kordick, Lappin et al. 1995)

Horses:
Warning: Doxycycline intravenously in horses has been associated with fatalities. Until further work is done demonstrating the safety of this drug, it cannot be recommended for parenteral use in this species.

Birds:
For Psittacosis (Chlamydiosis):
a) In psittacines: 25 mg/kg PO *bid* or 50 mg/kg PO once daily using the oral syrup or suspension. Emesis may occur. Increase dosage if giving with gavage formula. In critically ill birds (either confirmed or suspected of psittacosis) 20 mg/kg IV once only may be administered; followed with oral therapy. (McDonald 1989)
b) In psittacines: 17.6 - 26.4 mg/kg PO *bid* using the oral syrup or suspension. For initial therapy in severe cases: 22 - 44 mg/kg IV once or twice; do not give IM. Long term

therapy (45 days) can be given as 200 mg (from capsules) per pound of food. (Clubb 1986)

    c) Using the oral liquid/suspension: 50 mg/kg PO every 24 hours, or divided every 12 hours (use less for macaws).

       Using the hyclate salt on on corn, beans, rice and oatmeal: 1 gram per kg of feed.

       Using the injectable product (*Vibaravenos®*-may not be available commercially in the USA): 100 mg/kg IM once weekly (75 mg/kg IM once weekly in macaws and lovebirds) (Bauck and Hoefer 1993)

Reptiles:
    For susceptible infections:
    a) For chelonians: 10 mg/kg PO once daily for 4 weeks. Useful for bacterial respiratory infections in tortoises having suspected Mycoplasma infections.

       In most species: 10 mg/kg PO once daily for 10-45 days (Gauvin 1993)

Monitoring Parameters -
    1) Clinical efficacy
    2) Adverse effects

Client Information - Oral doxycycline products may be administered without regard to feeding. Milk or other dairy products do not significantly alter the amount of doxycycline absorbed.

Dosage Forms/Preparations/FDA Approval Status/Withholding Times -
   Veterinary-Approved Products: None

Human-Approved Products:

Doxycycline (as the hyclate) Tablets and Capsules 50 mg, 100 mg; *Vibramycin®*(Pfizer); *Doxychel® Hyclate* (Rachelle), *Doxy Caps®* (Edwards); *Bio-Tab®* (Inter. Ethical Labs); *Vibra-Tabs®* (Pfizer); generic; (Rx)

Doxycycline (as monohydrate) Tablets and Capsules 50 mg, 100 mg; *Monodox®* (Oclassen) (Rx)

Doxycycline coated pellets (as hyclate) 100 mg; *Doryx®* (Parke-Davis) (Rx)

Doxycycline (as the monohydrate) Powder for Oral Suspension 5 mg/ml 25 mg/5 ml after re-constitution in 60 ml bottles
   Vibramycin® (Pfizer); (Rx)

Doxycycline (as the calcium salt) Oral Syrup 10 mg/ml in 50 ml bottles. *Vibramycin®* (Pfizer); (Rx)

Doxycycline (as the hyclate) Powder for Injection 100 mg and 200 mg vials
   Vibramycin® IV (Roerig); *Doxychel® Hyclate* (Rachelle); *Doxy 100 & 200* (Lyphomed); generic; (Rx)

DOXYLAMINE SUCCINATE

Chemistry - An ethanolamine-derivative antihistamine, doxylamine succinate occurs as a white to creamy-white powder with a characteristic odor. It has a melting range of 103-108°C and pK_a values of 5.8 and 9.3. Doxylamine succinate has solubilities of 0.5 g/ml in alcohol and 1 g/ml in water. The commercially available injection has an approximate pH of 4.8 - 5.2.

Storage/Stability/Compatibility - Tablets should be stored in well-closed, light-resistant packaging at room temperature. No information on the storage, stability, or compatibility was found regarding the injectable product.

Pharmacology - Like other antihistamines, doxylamine competitively inhibits histamine at H_1 receptors. It also has substantial sedative and anticholinergic effects.

Uses/Indications - This drug is recommended (by the manufacturer) "for use in conditions in which antihistaminic therapy may be expected to alleviate some signs of disease in dogs, cats, and horses."

Pharmacokinetics - Pharmacokinetic parameters are apparently unavailable for domestic animals. Doxylamine has a serum half-life of approximately 10 hours in human adults.

Contraindications/Precautions - The manufacturer recommends that the injectable product should not be administered by the IV route in dogs or cats, and that IM and SQ injection sites be divided. Inject slowly IV in horses. Do not use in horses intended for food purposes.

  Doxylamine is also contraindicated in patients who are hypersensitive to it or other antihistamines in its class. Because of their anticholinergic activity, antihistamines should be used with caution in patients with angle closure glaucoma, prostatic hypertrophy, pyloroduodenal or bladder neck obstruction, and COPD if mucosal secretions are a problem. Additionally, they should be used with caution in patients with hyperthyroidism, cardiovascular disease or hypertension.

Adverse Effects/Warnings - The manufacturer lists CNS depression, incoordination and GI disturbances as adverse effects at therapeutic dosages.

Overdosage - The manufacturer includes CNS stimulation (excitement, seizures) and ataxia as symptoms associated with overdosage. Treatment should be supportive, as outlined in the previous antihistamine monographs.

Drug Interactions - Potential drug interactions for doxylamine include, increased sedation if doxylamine is combined with **other CNS depressant drugs**.
   Antihistamines may partially counteract the anticoagulation effects of **heparin** or **warfarin**.
   Doxylamine may enhance the effects of **epinephrine**.

Laboratory Interactions - Antihistamines can decrease the wheal and flare response to **antigen skin testing**. In humans, it is suggested that antihistamines be discontinued at least 4 days before testing.

Doses -
   Dogs:
   a) 1.1 - 2.2 mg/kg IM or SQ q8-12h *prn* (Package Insert; *A-H*® *Injection* - Coopers Animal Health)
   b) 1.1 - 2.2 mg/kg IM, SQ, or PO q8h (Schultz 1986)

   Cats:
   a) 1.1 - 2.2 mg/kg IM or SQ q8-12h *prn* (Package Insert; *A-H*® *Injection* - Coopers Animal Health)
   b) 1.1 - 2.2 mg/kg IM, SQ, or PO q8h (Schultz 1986)

   Horses:
   a) 0.55 mg/kg IV(slowly), IM or SQ q8-12h *prn*. For maintenance therapy: 2.2 - 4.4 mg/kg/day PO divided into 3 or 4 daily doses. (Package Insert; *A-H*® *Injection* - Coopers Animal Health)
   b) 0.55 mg/kg q8-12h IM or SQ (Schultz 1986)

   Bovine:
   a) 200 - 300 mg q8-12h PO, IM or SQ (Schultz 1986)

   Sheep, Swine:
   a) 100 mg q8-12h PO, IM or SQ (Schultz 1986)

Monitoring Parameters -
   1) Efficacy/Adverse effects

Dosage Forms/Preparations/FDA Approval Status -
   Veterinary-Approved Products:
   Doxylamine Succinate for Injection 11.36 mg/ml; 250 ml vials; *A-H*® *Injection* (Schering); (Rx) Approved for use in dogs, cats, and horses (not intended for food purposes).

   Doxylamine Succinate Tablets 25 mg, 100 mg; bottles of 50; *A-H*® *Tablets* (Schering); (Rx) Approved for use in dogs, cats, and horses (not intended for food purposes).

   Human-Approved Products: None

Droperidol - see Fentanyl/Droperidol

EDETATE CALCIUM DISODIUM
CALCIUM EDTA

Chemistry - A heavy metal chelating agent, edetate calcium disodium (CaEDTA) occurs as an odorless, white, crystalline powder or granules and is a mixture of dihydrate and trihydrate forms. It has a slight saline taste and is slightly hygroscopic. CaEDTA is freely soluble in water and very slightly soluble in alcohol. The commercially available injection (human) has a pH of 6.5-8 and has approximately 5.3 mEq of sodium per gram of CaEDTA.
   Edetate calcium disodium has several synonyms including: calcium disodium edathamil, Calcium EDTA (CaEDTA), calcium disodium edetate, calcium edetate, calcium disodium ethylenediaminetetra-acetate and sodium calcium edetate.

Storage/Stability/Compatibility - CaEDTA should be stored at temperatures less than 40°, and preferably at room temperature (15-30°C). The injection can be diluted with either normal saline or 5% dextrose.

Pharmacology - The calcium in CaEDTA can be displaced by divalent or trivalent metals to form a stable water soluble complex that can be excreted in the urine. One gram of CaEDTA can theoretically bind 620 mg of lead, but in reality only about 5 mg per gram is actually excreted into the urine in lead poisoned patients. In addition to chelating lead, CaEDTA also chelates and eliminates zinc from the body. CaEDTA also binds cadmium, copper, iron and manganese, but to a much lesser extent than either lead or zinc. CaEDTA is relatively ineffective for use in treating mercury, gold or arsenic poisoning.

Uses/Indications - CaEDTA is used as a chelating agent in the treatment of lead poisoning.

Pharmacokinetics - CaEDTA is well absorbed after either IM or SQ administration. It is distributed primarily in the extracellular fluid. Unlike dimercaprol, CaEDTA does not penetrate erythrocytes or enter the CNS in appreciable amounts. The drug is rapidly excreted renally, either as unchanged drug or chelated with metals. Changes in urine pH or urine flow do not significantly alter the rate of excretion. Decreased renal function can cause accumulation of the drug and can increase its nephrotoxic potential. In humans with normal renal function, the average elimination half-life of CaEDTA is 20-60 minutes after IV administration, and 1.5 hours after IM administration.

Contraindications/Precautions/Reproductive Safety - CaEDTA is contraindicated in patients with anuria. It should be used with extreme caution and with dosage adjustment in patients with diminished renal function.

Most small animal clinicians recommend using the SQ route when treating small animals as IV administration of CaEDTA has been associated with abrupt increases in CSF pressure and death in children with lead-induced cerebral edema.

Adverse Effects/Warnings - The most serious of adverse effect associated with this compound is renal toxicity (renal tubular necrosis), but in dogs CaEDTA also can cause depression and GI symptoms. GI symptoms (vomiting, diarrhea) in dogs may be alleviated by zinc supplementation.

Do not administer CaEDTA orally as it may increase the amount of lead absorbed from the GI tract.

Animals with symptoms of cerebral edema should not be overhydrated.

Chronic therapy may lead to zinc deficiency; zinc supplementation should be considered in these animals.

Overdosage/Acute Toxicity - Doses greater than 12 g/kg are lethal in dogs; refer to Adverse Effects for more information.

Drug Interactions - Concurrent administration of CaEDTA with **zinc insulin preparations (NPH, PZI)** will decrease the sustained action of the insulin preparation.

The renal toxicity of CaEDTA may be enhanced by the concomitant administration of **glucocorticoids**.

Use with caution with **other nephrotoxic compounds** (*e.g.,* aminoglycosides, amphotericin B).

Drug/Laboratory Interactions - CaEDTA may cause increased **urine glucose** values and/or cause inverted T-waves on **ECG**.

Doses -

The manufacturer of the injectable (human) product recommends diluting the injection to a concentration of 2 - 4 mg/ml with either normal saline or 5% dextrose when used for intravenous use. Because the injection is painful when given IM, 1 ml of procaine HCl 1% is recommended to be added to each ml of injection before administering IM.

Dogs & Cats:
    For lead poisoning:
        a) Be sure there is no lead in GI tract before using. Give 100 mg/kg SQ divided into 4 daily doses in 5% dextrose for 5 days. May require second course of treatment, particularly if blood lead levels >0.10 ppm. Do not exceed 2 g/day and do not treat for more than 5 consecutive days. (Grauer and Hjelle 1988b)
        b) Dilute to a one percent solution (10 mg/ml) with either normal saline or D$_5$W and give 27.5 mg/kg SQ q6h for five days and then give 5 days rest; repeat if necessary. Alternately, may give 50 mg/kg SQ q12h for 5 days if q6h is too inconvenient. (Mount 1989)
        c) Cats: 27.5 mg/kg in 15 ml D$_5$W SQ *qid* for 5 days. Recheck blood lead 2-3 weeks later and repeat therapy (with either CaEDTA or penicillamine) if greater than 0.2 ppm. (Reid and Oehme 1989)
    For zinc toxicity:
        a) 100mg/kg divided into four SubQ doses per day. Dilute in D5W to reduce local irritation at site of injection.. Exact dosage is not known nor how long therapy should continue. If possible, monitor serum zinc concentrations and maintain animal's hydration status. (Meurs and Breitschwerdt 1995)

Horses:

For lead poisoning:

a) Remove animal from source of lead. If severely affected give CaEDTA at 75 mg/kg IV slowly in D_5W or saline daily for 4-5 days (may divide daily dose into 2-3 administrations per day). Stop therapy for 2 days and repeat for another 4-5 days. Give adequate supportive and nutritional therapy. (Oehme 1987d)

Food Animals:

For lead poisoning:

a) Cattle: 67 mg/kg slow IV twice daily for 2 days; withhold dose for 2 days and then give again for 2 days. Cattle may require 10-14 days to recover and may require several series of treatments. (Bailey 1986b)

b) Cattle: 73.3 mg/kg/day slow IV divided 2-3 times a day for 3-5 days. If additional therapy is required, a 2 day rest period followed by another 5 day treatment regimen is recommended. (Sexton and Buck 1986)

Birds:

a) For lead poisoning in psittacines: 35 mg/kg IM *bid* for 5-7 days. After initial therapy, may give orally until all lead fragments are dissolved and/or passed from GI tract. (McDonald 1989)

Monitoring Parameters -

1) Blood lead or zinc (serial), and/or urine *d*-ALA
2) Renal function tests, urinalyses, hydration status
3) Serum phosphorus and calcium values
4) Periodic cardiac rate/rhythm monitoring may be warranted during administration

Client Information - Because of the potential toxicity of this agent and the seriousness of most heavy metal intoxications, this drug should be used with close professional supervision only.

Dosage Forms/Preparations/FDA Approval Status/Withholding Times -

Note: Do not confuse with Edetate Disodium which should <u>not</u> be used for lead poisoning as it may cause severe hypocalcemia.

Veterinary-Approved Products:

Edetate Calcium Disodium Injection 50 mg/ml in 500 ml single dose vials. *Meta-Dote®* (Anthony) (Rx). Approved for use in cattle, horses, goats, sheep and swine. Not intended for use on animals to be used as food.

Human-Approved Products:

Edetate Calcium Disodium Injection 200 mg/ml in 5 ml amps (1 gram/amp); *Calcium Disodium Versenate®* (3M Pharm.) (Rx)

EDROPHONIUM CHLORIDE

Chemistry - A synthetic quanternary ammonium cholinergic (parasympathomimetic) agent, edrophonium chloride occurs as a white crystalline powder having a bitter taste. Approximately 2 grams are soluble in one ml of water. The injection has a pH of approximately 5.4.

Storage/Stability/Compatibility - Edrophonium chloride injection should be stored at room temperature. It is reportedly compatible at Y-site injections with Heparin Sodium, Hydrocortisone sodium succinate, potassium chloride and vitamin B complex with C. Compatibility is dependent upon factors such as pH, concentration, temperature and diluents used. It is suggested to consult specialized references (*e.g., Handbook on Injectable Drugs* by Trissel; see bibliography) for more specific information.

Pharmacology - Edrophonium is an anticholinesterase agent that is very short acting. It briefly attaches to acetylcholinesterase, thereby inhibiting its hydrolytic activity on acetylcholine. As acetylcholine accumulates, the following signs and symptoms may be noted: miosis, increased skeletal and intestinal muscle tone, bronchoconstriction, ureter constriction, salivation, sweating (in animals with sweat glands), and bradycardia.

Uses/Indications - The primary use for edrophonium is in the diagnosis of myasthenia gravis. It is also used for the reversal of nondepolarizing agents (*e.g.,* vecuronium, pancuronium, metocurine, atracurium, gallamine or tubocurarine). Because of its short duration of action, its clinical usefulness for this indication is questionable as longer acting drugs such as neostigmine or pyridostigmine may be more useful. Edrophonium may also be useful in the diagnosis and treatment of some supraventricular arrhythmias, particularly when other more traditional treatments are ineffective and in a controlled intensive care-type setting.

Pharmacokinetics - Edrophonium is only effective when given parenterally. After IV administration, it begins to have effects on skeletal muscle within one minute and effects may persist for up to 10 minutes. Myasthenic patients may have effects persisting longer after the first dose. Edrophonium's exact metabolic fate and excretion characteristics have not been well described.

Contraindications/Precautions/Reproductive Safety - Edrophonium is considered relatively contraindicated in patients with bronchial asthma, or mechanical urinary or intestinal tract obstruction. It should be used with caution (with adequate monitoring and treatment available) in patients with bradycardias or atrioventricular block. Some human patients are documented to be hypersensitive to the drug and exhibit severe cholinergic reactions.

Edrophonium's safety profile during pregnancy is not established; use only when necessary. It is unknown whether edrophonium enters maternal milk. While no problems have been documented in nursing humans or animals, its safety has not been established.

Adverse Effects/Warnings - Adverse effects associated with edrophonium are generally dose related and cholinergic in nature. Although usually mild and easily treated with a "tincture of time", severe adverse effects are possible with large overdoses (see below).

Overdosage/Acute Toxicity - Overdosage of edrophonium may induce a cholinergic crisis. Symptoms of cholinergic toxicity can include GI effects (nausea, vomiting, diarrhea), salivation, sweating (in animals able to do so), respiratory effects (increased bronchial secretions, bronchospasm, pulmonary edema, respiratory paralysis), ophthalmic effects (miosis, blurred vision, lacrimation), cardiovascular effects (bradycardia or tachycardia, cardiospasm, hypotension, cardiac arrest), muscle cramps and weakness.

Treatment of edrophonium overdosage, consists of both respiratory and cardiac supportive therapy and atropine if necessary. Refer to the atropine monograph for more information on its use for cholinergic toxicity.

Drug Interactions - Edrophonium's cardiac effects may be increased in patients receiving **digoxin**; excessive slowing of heart rate may occur. **Drugs that possess some neuromuscular blocking activity** (*e.g.,* aminoglycoside antibiotics, some antiarrhythmic and anesthetic drugs) may necessitate increased dosages of edrophonium in treating or diagnosing myasthenic patients. Edrophonium may prolong the Phase I block of **depolarizing muscle relaxants** (*e.g.,* succinylcholine, decamethonium). Pyridostigmine antagonizes the actions of **non-depolarizing neuromuscular blocking agents (pancuronium, tubocurarine, gallamine, vecuronium, atracurium,** etc.). **Atropine** will antagonize the muscarinic effects of edrophonium, but concurrent use should be used cautiously as atropine can mask the early symptoms of cholinergic crisis. Theoretically, **dexpanthenol** may have additive effects when used with edrophonium.

Doses -
Dogs:
    For presumptive diagnosis of myasthenia gravis (MG):
        a) Inject 0.1 - 0.2 mg/kg IV; short term increased muscle strength is seen in a positive (not necessarily specific for MG, both false positives and negatives) test. (Shelton 1992)
        b) 0.11 - 0.22 mg/kg IV (Papich 1992)

Cats:
    For presumptive diagnosis of myasthenia gravis (MG):
        a) 2.5 mg IV (Papich 1992)
        b) 0.25 - 0.5 mg per cat IV (Joseph, Carrillo et al. 1988)

Monitoring Parameters - Dependent on its indication. See doses above.

Client Information - Edrophonium is a drug that should be used in a controlled clinical setting. Clients should be briefed on the side effects that can occur with its use.

Dosage Forms/Preparations/FDA Approval Status/Withholding Times -
Veterinary-Approved Products: None
Human-Approved Products:

Edrophonium Chloride for Injection 10 mg/ml in one ml amps and 10 ml & 15 ml vials; *Tensilon*® (ICN), *Enlon*® (Ohmeda); *Reversol*® (Organon); (Rx)

Edrophonium Chloride for Injection 10 mg/ml with 0.14 mg/ml Atropine Sulfate; in 5 ml amps and 15 ml vials *Enlon-Plus*® (Ohmeda); (Rx)

EFA-Caps® **- see Fatty Acids**

ENALAPRIL MALEATE
ENALAPRILAT

Chemistry - Angiotensin-converting enzyme (ACE) inhibitors, enalapril maleate and enalaprilat are structurally related to captopril. Enalapril is a prodrug and is converted *in vivo* by the liver to enalaprilat. Enalapril maleate occurs as a white to off white crystalline powder. 25 mg are soluble in one ml of water. Enalaprilat occurs as a white to off white crystalline powder that is slightly soluble in water.

Storage/Stability/Compatibility - The commercially available tablets should be stored at temperatures less than 30°C and in tight containers. When stored properly, the tablets have an expiration date of 30 months after manufacture.

Enalaprilat injection should be stored at temperatures less than 30°C. After dilution with D5W, normal saline, or D5 in lactated Ringer's it is stable for up to 24 hours at room temperature. Enalaprilat has been documented to be incompatible with amphotericin B or phenytoin sodium. Many other mediations have been noted to be compatible with enalaprilat at various concentrations. Compatibility is dependent upon factors such as pH, concentration, temperature and diluents used. It is suggested to consult specialized references (*e.g., Handbook on Injectable Drugs* by Trissel; see bibliography) for more specific information.

Pharmacology - Enalapril is converted in the liver to the active compound enalaprilat. Enalaprilat prevents the formation of angiotensin II (a potent vasoconstrictor) by competing with angiotensin I for the enzyme angiotensin converting enzyme (ACE). ACE has a much higher affinity for enalaprilat than for angiotensin I. Because angiotensin II concentrations are decreased, aldosterone secretion is reduced and plasma renin activity is increased.

The cardiovascular effects of enalaprilat in patients with CHF include decreased total peripheral resistance, pulmonary vascular resistance, mean arterial and right atrial pressures, and pulmonary capillary wedge pressure, no change or decrease in heart rate, and increased cardiac index and output, stroke volume, and exercise tolerance. Renal blood flow can be increased with little change in hepatic blood flow.

Uses/Indications - The principle uses of enalapril/enalaprilat in veterinary medicine at present are as a vasodilator in the treatment of heart failure and in the treatment of hypertension. It may also be of benefit in treating the effects associated with valvular heart disease, and left to right shunts. It is being explored as adjunctive treatment in chronic renal failure and in protein losing nephropathies.

Pharmacokinetics - Enalapril/enalaprilat has different pharmacokinetic properties than captopril in dogs. It has a slower onset of action (4-6 hours), but a longer duration of action (12-14 hours). In humans, enalapril is well absorbed after oral administration, but enalaprilat is not. Both enalapril and enalaprilat are distributed poorly into the CNS and are distributed into milk in trace amounts. Enalaprilat crosses the placenta. In humans, the half life of enalapril is about 2 hours; enalaprilat about 11 hours. Half lives are increased in patients with renal failure or severe CHF.

Contraindications/Precautions/Reproductive Safety - Enalaprilat is contraindicated in patients who have demonstrated hypersensitivity to the ACE inhibitors. It should be used with caution and close supervision, in patients with renal insufficiency and doses may need to be reduced.

Enalaprilat should also be used with caution in patients with hyponatremia or sodium depletion, coronary or cerebrovascular insufficiency, preexisting hematologic abnormalities or a collagen vascular disease (*e.g.,* SLE). Patients with severe CHF should be monitored very closely upon initiation of therapy.

Enalapril crosses the placenta. High doses in rodents have caused decreased fetal weights and increases in fetal and maternal death rates; teratogenic effects have not been reported.

Adverse Effects/Warnings - Enalapril/enalaprilat's adverse effect profile in dogs is principally GI distress (anorexia, vomiting, diarrhea). Potentially, hypotension, renal dysfunction and hyperkalemia could occur. Because it lacks a sulfhydryl group (unlike captopril), there is less likelihood that immune-mediated reactions will occur, but rashes, neutropenia and agranulocytosis have been reported in humans.

Overdosage/Acute Toxicity - In dogs, a dose of 200 mg/kg was lethal, but 100 mg/kg was not. In overdose situations, the primary concern is hypotension; supportive treatment with volume expansion with normal saline is recommended to correct blood pressure. Because of the drug's long duration of action, prolonged monitoring and treatment may be required. Recent overdoses, should be managed using gut emptying protocols when warranted.

Drug Interactions - Concomitant **diuretics** or other **vasodilators** may cause hypotension if used with enalapril/enalaprilat; titrate dosages carefully. Some clinicians recommend reducing **furosemide** doses (by 25 - 50%) when adding enalapril to therapy in CHF.

Hyperkalemia may develop if given with **potassium** or **potassium sparing diuretics** (*e.g.,* **spironolactone**).

Non-steroidal anti-inflammatory agents (NSAIDs) may reduce the clinical efficacy of enalapril/enalaprilat when it is being used as an antihypertensive agent. Indomethacin appears to be most likely to evoke this problem.

Laboratory Considerations - When using **iodohippurate sodium I^{123}/I^{134} or Technetium Tc^{99} pententate renal imaging** in patients with renal artery stenosis, ACE inhibitors may cause a reversible decrease in localization and excretion of these agents in the affected kidney which may lead to confusion in test interpretation.

Doses -
  Dogs:
    a) As a vasodilator in heart failure: 0.5 - 1 mg/kg q12-24h (DeLellis and Kittleson 1992)
    b) 0.25 - 0.5 mg/kg PO once to twice a day (Muir and Bonagura 1994)
    c) For adjunctive treatment of heart failure: 0.5 mg/kg once daily initially with or without food. If response is inadequate increase to 0.5 mg/kg *bid* (Package Insert—*Enacard®*-Merck)

  Cats:
    a) As a vasodilator in heart failure: Initially, 0.25 mg/kg q12-24h (DeLellis and Kittleson 1992)
    b) 0.25 - 0.5 mg/kg PO once to twice a day (Muir and Bonagura 1994)

Monitoring Parameters - 1) Clinical symptoms of CHF; 2) Serum electrolytes, creatinine, BUN, urine protein 3) CBC with differential.; periodic 4) Blood pressure (if treating hypertension or symptoms associated with hypotension arise)

Client Information - Give medication on an empty stomach unless otherwise instructed. Do not abruptly stop or reduce therapy without veterinarian's approval. Contact veterinarian if vomiting or diarrhea persist or are severe or if animal's condition deteriorates.

Dosage Forms/Preparations/FDA Approval Status/Withholding Times -
  Veterinary-Approved Products:
    Enalapril Maleate Tablets 1 mg, 2.5 mg, 5 mg, 10 mg, 20 mg; *Enacard®* (Merck); (Rx) Approved for use in dogs.

  Human-Approved Products:
    Enalapril Maleate Tablets 2.5 mg, 5 mg, 10 mg, 20 mg; *Vasotec®* (Merck; Frosst-Canada); (Rx);

    Enalaprilat Injection (for IV use) equivalent to 1.25 mg/ml in 1 and 2 ml vials; *Vasotec® I.V.* (Merck); (Rx)

ENROFLOXACIN

Chemistry - A fluoroquinolone antibiotic, enrofloxacin occurs as a pale yellow, crystalline powder. It is slightly soluble in water. Enrofloxacin is related structurally to the human-approved drug ciprofloxacin (enrofloxacin has an additional ethyl group on the piperazinyl ring).

Storage/Stability/Compatibility - Unless otherwise directed by the manufacturer, enrofloxacin tablets should be stored in tight containers at temperatures less than 30°C. Protect from strong UV light.

Pharmacology - Enrofloxacin is a bactericidal agent. The bactericidal activity of enrofloxacin is concentration dependent, with susceptible bacteria cell death occuring within 20-30 minutes of exposure. Enrofloxacin has demonstrated a significant post-antibiotic effect for both gram - and + bacteria and is active in both stationary and growth phases of bacterial replication.

Its mechanism of action is not thoroughly understood, but it is believed to act by inhibiting bacterial DNA-gyrase (a type-II topoisomerase), thereby preventing DNA supercoiling and DNA synthesis.

Both enrofloxacin and ciprofloxacin have similar spectrums of activity. These agents have good activity against many gram negative bacilli and cocci, including most species and strains of *Pseudomonas aeruginosa, Klebsiella sp., E. coli, Enterobacter, Campylobacter, Shigella, Salmonella, Aeromonas, Haemophilus, Proteus, Yersinia, Serratia*, and *Vibrio* species. Of the currently commercially available quinolones, ciprofloxacin and enrofloxacin have the lowest MIC values for the majority of these pathogens treated. Other organisms that are generally susceptible include *Brucella sp, Chlamydia trachomatis, Staphylococci* (including penicillinase-producing and methicillin-resistant strains), Mycoplasma, and *Mycobacterium sp.* (not the etiologic agent for Johne's Disease).

The fluoroquinolones have variable activity against most *Streptococci* and are not usually recommended to be used for these infections. These drugs have weak activity against most anaerobes and are ineffective in treating anaerobic infections.

Resistance does occur by mutation, particularly with *Pseudomonas aeruginosa, Klebsiella pneumonia, Acinetobacter* and enterococci, but plasmid-mediated resistance is not thought to occur.

Uses/Indications - Enrofloxacin is approved for use in dogs and cats (oral only) for the management of of diseases assicaited with bacteria susceptible to enrofloxacin. It is also been approved for use in cattle (not dairy cattle or veal calves) and for chickens and turkeys.

Pharmacokinetics - Both enrofloxacin and ciprofloxacin are well absorbed after oral administration in most species. But in dogs, enrofloxacin's bioavailability (approximately 80%) is about twice that of ciprofloxacin after oral dosing. 50% of Cmax is reportedly attained within 15 minutes of dosing and peak levels (Cmax) occur within one hour of dosing. The presence of food in the stomach may delay the rate, but not the extent of absorption.

Enrofloxacin/ciprofloxacin are distributed throughout the body. Volume of distribution in dogs is at least 2.8 L/kg. Only about 27% is bound to canine plasma proteins. Highest concentrations are found in the bile, kidney, liver, lungs, and reproductive system (including prostatic fluid and tissue). Therapeutic levels are also attained in bone, synovial fluid, skin, muscle, aqueous humor and pleural fluid. Low concentrations are found in the CSF, and levels may only reach 6-10% of those found in the serum.

Enrofloxacin/ciprofloxacin is eliminated via both renal and non-renal mechanisms. Approximately 15-50% of the drugs are eliminated unchanged into the urine, by both tubular secretion and glomerular filtration. Enrofloxacin/ciprofloxacin are metabolized to various metabolites that are less active than the parent compounds. Approximately 30-40% of circulating enrofloxacin is metabolized to ciprofloxacin. These metabolites are eliminated both in the urine and feces. Because of the dual (renal and hepatic) means of elimination, patients with severely impaired renal function may have slightly prolonged half-lives and higher serum levels which may not require dosage adjustment. The elimination half-lives in dogs are approximately 4-5 hours and in cats, 6 hours.

Contraindications/Precautions/Reproductive Safety - Enrofloxacin is contraindicated in small and medium breed dogs from 2 months to 8 months of age. Bubble-like changes in articular cartilage have been noted when the drug was given at 2-5 times recommend doses for 30 days, although clinical symptoms have only been seen at the 5X dose. Large and giant breed dogs may be in the rapid-growth phase for periods longer than 8 months of age, so longer than 8 months may be necessary to avoid cartilage damage. Quinolones are also contraindicated in patients hypersensitive to them.

Because ciprofloxacin has occasionally been reported to cause crystalluria, animals should not be allowed to become dehydrated during therapy with either ciprofloxacin or enrofloxacin. In humans, ciprofloxacin has been associated with CNS stimulation and should be used with caution in patients with seizure disorders. Patients with severe renal or hepatic impairment may require dosage adjustments to prevent drug accumulation.

The safety of enrofloxacin in pregnant dogs has been investigated. Breeding, pregnant and lactating dogs receiving up to 15 mg/kg day demonstrated no treatement related effects. However, because of the risks of cartilage abnormalities in young animals, the fluoroquinolones are not generally recommended to be used during pregnancy unless the benefits of therapy clearly outweigh the risks. Limited studies in male dogs at various dosages have indicated no effects on male breeding performance. Safety in breeding, pregnant, or lactating cats has not been established.

Adverse Effects/Warnings - With the exception of potential cartilage abnormalities in young animals (see Contraindications above), the adverse effect profile of these drugs appears to be minimal. GI distress (vomiting, anorexia) is the most common, yet infrequently reported adverse effect. Although not reported thus far in animals, hypersensitivity reactions, crystalluria and CNS effects (dizziness, stimulation) could potentially occur.

Overdosage/Acute Toxicity - It is unlikely an acute overdose of either compound would result in symptoms more serious than either anorexia and vomiting. Dogs receiving 10 times the labeled dosage rate of enrofloxacin for at least 14 days developed only vomiting and anorexia. Death did occur in some dogs when fed 25 times the labeled rate for 11 days, however.

Drug Interactions - **Antacids** containing cations (Mg^{++}, Al^{+++}, Ca^{++}) may bind to enrofloxacin/ciprofloxacin and prevent its absorption. **Sucralfate** may inhibit absorption of enrofloxacin/ciprofloxacin, separate doses of these drugs by at least 2 hours.

Enrofloxacin/ciprofloxacin administered with **theophylline** may increase theophylline blood levels.

Probenecid blocks tubular secretion of enrofloxacin/ciprofloxacin and may increase its blood level and half-life.

Synergism may occur, but is not predictable, against some bacteria (particularly *Pseudomonas aeruginosa* or other Enterobacteriaceae) with these compounds and **aminoglycosides, 3rd generation cephalosporins agents, and extended-spectrum penicillins**. Although enrofloxacin/ciprofloxacin has minimal activity against anaerobes, *in vitro* synergy has been reported when used with **clindamycin** against strains of *Peptostreptococcus, Lactobacillus* and *Bacteroids fragilis*. **Nitrofurantoin** may antagonize the antimicrobial activity of the fluoroquinolones and their concomitant use is not recommended. Fluoroquinolones may exacerbate the nephrotoxicity of **cyclosporine** (used systemically).

Because the fluoroquinolones are relatively new additions to the therapeutic armamentarium, more interactions may be forthcoming.

Drug/Laboratory Interactions - In some human patients, the fluoroquinolones have caused increases in **liver enzymes, BUN,** and **creatinine** and decreases in **hematocrit**. The clinical relevance of these mild changes is not known at this time.

Doses -
Dogs:
   For susceptible infections:
   a) 5- 20 mg/kg per day PO, may be given once daily or divided and given twice daily (q12h). Treatment should continue for at least 2-3 days beyond cessation of clinical signs, to a maximum duration of therapy is 30 days. (Package insert; Baytril®—Bayer)
   b) Enrofloxacin: 2.5 mg/kg PO q12h up to 10 days. Injectable product is to be given IM for the first dose and then followed by oral therapy. (Package insert; *Baytril®*—Miles)
   d) Enrofloxacin: 2.5 - 5 mg/kg PO or IM q12 h
   Avoid or reduce dosage of these drugs in animals with severe renal failure; avoid in young animals or in pregnant or breeding animals (Vaden and Papich 1995)

Cats:
   For susceptible infections:
   a) 5- 20 mg/kg per day PO, may be given once daily or divided and given twice daily (q12h). Treatment should continue for at least 2-3 days beyond cessation of clinical signs, to a maximum duration of therapy is 30 days. (Package insert; Baytril®—Bayer)
   b) Enrofloxacin: 2.5 - 5 mg/kg PO or IM q12 h
   Avoid or reduce dosage of these drugs in animals with severe renal failure; avoid in young animals or in pregnant or breeding animals (Vaden and Papich 1995)

Pocket Pets/Rodents:
   For empiric antibiotic therapy:
   a) 5 - 15 mg/kg q12h PO; tablets may be crushed and mixed with simple syrup (Oglesbee 1995)

Horses:
   Note: Usage of enrofloxacin in horses is controversial. While there has been much discussion regarding the potential for cartilage abnormalities or other arthropathies in horses, objective data are lacking. At the present time however, it probably should only be used in adult horses when other antibiotics are inappropriate with the client informed of, and agrees to accept the risks for any potential adverse effects.
   a) 2.5 mg/kg q12h (Whittem 1993)

Cattle:
   Enrofloxacin (Baytril® 100) has very recently been approved for the treatment of bovine respiratory disease associated with *Pasteurella haemolytica, Pasteurella multocida*, and *Haemophilus sommus*. It is administered by injection and is intended to be used for the treatment of individual animals. The reprted dosage is: 2.5 - 5 mg/kg subQ once daily for 3-5 days or 7.5 - 12.5 mg/kg once. The product is prescription only and is not for use in cattle intended for dairy production or in veal calves. Animals intended for human consumption must not be slaughtered within 28 days from the last treatment. Extralabel use of fluoroquinolones in food animals has been prohibited by the FDA.

Birds:
   For susceptible gram negative infections:
   a) Using ciprofloxacin 500 mg tablets: 20 - 40 mg/kg PO *bid*. Crushed tablet goes into suspension well, but must be shaken well before administering. (McDonald 1989)
   b) Ciprofloxacin (using crushed tablets): 20 mg/kg PO q12h
   Enrofloxacin: 15 mg/kg PO, or IM or 250 mg/L of drinking water. (Bauck and Hoefer 1993)
   c) Ciprofloxacin (using crushed tablets or suspend) 10 - 15 mg/kg PO q12h (Hoeffer 1995)

A method to make a 10.2 mg/ml **oral suspension** of enrofloxacin has been described: Make a stock solution of "HMC 0.15%" by mixing 7.5 ml of *Lubrivet®* with 92.5 ml of water. Crush three (3) whole 68 mg tablets with a "pinch" of citric acid. Add crushed mixture to a dispensing vial and and 15 ml of "HMC0.15%". Shake well to dissolve tablet coating. *qs ad* to 20 ml with "HMC 0.15%" and allow to stand at room temperature for 30 minutes to allow tablet coating to completely diossolve. Shake well before use and keep refrigerated. A

14 day expiration date has been assigned. By crushing six (6) tablets a 20.4 mg/ml suspension may be compounded using the same technique.

Note: 3.23% concentrate is also available and is approved for use (in drinking water at either 25 or 50 ppm for 3-7 days) in chickens and turkeys.

Reptiles:
For susceptible infections:
   a) For most species: For respiratory infections:5 mg/kg IM every 5 days for 25 days; For chronic respiratory infections in tortoises: 15 mg/kg IM every 72 hours for 5-7 treatments. (Gauvin 1993)

Monitoring Parameters -1) Clinical efficacy; 2) Adverse effects

Client Information - Do not crush tablets as drug is very bitter tasting.

Dosage Forms/Preparations/FDA Approval Status/Withholding Times -
Veterinary-Approved Products: (Note: See additional dosage forms in the dosage section for cattle and birds)

Enrofloxacin Oral Tablets 22.7 mg, 68 mg; *Baytril®* (Miles); (Rx) Approved for use in dogs and cats.

Enrofloxacin Injection 22.7 mg/ml in 20 ml vials; *Baytril®* (Miles); (Rx) Approved for use in dogs. A non-approved method for diluting the IM injectable product for IV administration has been described: Dilute 1 part of *Baytril®* injection with 2 parts of sterile water for injection and administer IV over 20 minutes or so.

Human-Approved Products: None. Note: Use of enrofloxacin by humans cannot be recommmended due to a high degree of CNS effects.

EPHEDRINE SULFATE

Chemistry - A sympathomimetic alkaloid, ephedrine sulfate occurs as fine, odorless, white crystals or powder. Approximately 770 mg are soluble in one ml of water. The commercially available injection has a pH of 4.5-7.

Storage/Stability/Compatibility - Store ephedrine sulfate products in tight, light resistant containers at room temperature unless otherwise directed.

Pharmacology - While the exact mechanism of ephedrine's actions are undetermined, it is believed that it indirectly stimulates both alpha-, beta$_1$, beta$_2$-adrenergic receptors by causing the release of norepinephrine. Prolonged use or excessive dosing frequency can deplete norepinephrine from its storage sites and tachyphylaxis (decreased response) may ensue. Tachyphylaxis has not been documented in dogs or cats, however, when used for urethral sphincter hypotonus.
  Pharmacologic effects of ephedrine include increased vasoconstriction, heart rate, coronary blood flow, blood pressure, mild CNS stimulation, and decreased bronchoconstriction, nasal congestion and appetite. Ephedrine can also increase urethral sphincter tone and produce closure of the bladder neck; its principle veterinary indications are as a result of these effects.

Uses/Indications - Ephedrine is used chiefly for the treatment of urethral sphincter hypotonus and resulting incontinence in dogs and cats. It has also been used in an attempt to treat nasal congestion and/or bronchoconstriction in small animals. It potentially could be used parenterally as a pressor agent in the treatment of shock, but veterinary use is very limited for this indication.

Pharmacokinetics - Ephedrine is rapidly absorbed after oral or parenteral administration. Although not confirmed, ephedrine is thought to cross both the blood-brain barrier and the placenta. Ephedrine is metabolized in the liver and excreted unchanged in the urine. Urine pH may significantly alter excretion characteristics. In humans: at urine pH of 5, half life is about 3 hours; at urine pH of 6.3, half life is about 6 hours.

Contraindications/Precautions/Reproductive Safety - Ephedrine is contraindicated in patients with severe cardiovascular disease, particularly with arrhythmias. Ephedrine should be used with caution in patients with glaucoma, prostatic hypertrophy, hyperthyroidism, diabetes mellitus, cardiovascular disorders or hypertension. Ephedrine's effects on fertility, pregnancy or fetal safety are not known. Use with caution during pregnancy. The drug is excreted in milk and may have deleterious effects on nursing animals.

Adverse Effects/Warnings - Most likely side effects include restlessness, irritability, tachycardia, hypertension. Anorexia may be a problem in some animals.

Overdosage - Symptoms of overdosage may consist of an exacerbation of the adverse effects listed above or, if a very large overdose, severe cardiovascular (hypertension to rebound hypotension, bradycardias to tachycardias, and cardiovascular collapse) or CNS effects (stimulation to coma) can be seen.

If the overdose was recent, empty the stomach using the usual precautions and administer charcoal and a cathartic. Treat symptoms supportively as they occur.

Drug Interactions - Ephedrine should not be administered with other **sympathomimetic agents** (*e.g.,* **phenylpropanolamine**) as increased toxicity may result.

Ephedrine should not be given within two weeks of a patient receiving **monoamine oxidase inhibitors**.

An increased chance of hypertension developing can result if ephedrine is given concomitantly with **indomethacin (or other NSAIDs, including aspirin), reserpine, tricyclic antidepressants, or ganglionic blocking agents**.

An increased risk of arrhythmias developing can occur if ephedrine is administered to patients who have received **cyclopropane** or a **halogenated hydrocarbon anesthetic agent**. Propranolol may be administered should these occur.

Urinary alkalinizers (*e.g.,* sodium bicarbonate, citrates, carbonic anhydrase inhibitors) may reduce the urinary excretion of ephedrine and prolong its duration of activity. Dosage adjustments may be required to avoid toxic symptoms.

Concomitant use of ephedrine with beta **blockers** may diminish the effects of both drugs.

An increased risk of arrhythmias may occur if ephedrine is used concurrently with **digitalis glycosides**.

Laboratory Considerations - beta adrenergic agonists may decrease **serum potassium** concentrations. Clinical relevance is uncommon.

Doses -
Dogs:
  For treatment of bronchospasm:
    a) For maintenance therapy: 1 - 2 mg/kg PO q8-12h (McKiernan 1992)
    b) 2 mg/kg PO q8-12h (Bonagura 1994)
  For treatment of urinary incontinence responsive to adrenergic drugs:
    a) 4 mg/kg or 12.5 - 50 mg PO per dog q8-12h. (Papich 1992)
    b) 5 - 15 mg PO q8h (Labato 1994)
Cats:
  For treatment of bronchospasm:
    a) For emergency treatment 2- 5 mg PO (McKiernan 1992)
  For treatment of urinary incontinence responsive to adrenergic drugs:
    a) 2 - 4 mg/kg PO q8-12h. (Papich 1992)
    b) 2 - 4 mg PO q8h (Labato 1994)

Monitoring Parameters - 1) Clinical effectiveness; 2) Adverse effects (see above)

Client Information - For this drug to be effective, it must be administered as directed by the veterinarian; missed doses will negate its effect. It may take several days for the full benefit of the drug to take place. Contact veterinarian if the animal demonstrates ongoing changes in behavior (restlessness, irritability) or if incontinence persists or increases.

Dosage Forms/Preparations/FDA Approval Status/Withholding Times -
  Veterinary-Approved Products: None
  Human-Approved Products:
  Ephedrine Sulfate Oral Capsules 25 mg (OTC), 50 mg (Rx); generic
  Ephedrine Sulfate Injection 25 mg/ml in 1 ml amps
  Ephedrine Sulfate Injection 50 mg/ml in 1 ml amps, 10 ml vials and 10 ml disposable syringes; *Ephedrine Sulfate*® (Lilly); generic (Rx)

EPINEPHRINE

Chemistry - An endogenous catecholamine, epinephrine occurs as white to nearly white, microcrystalline powder or granules. It is only very slightly soluble in water, but it readily forms water soluble salts (*e.g.,* HCl) when combined with acids. Both the commercial products and endogenous epinephrine are in the levo form, which is about 15 times more active than the dextro-isomer. The pH of commercial injections are from 2.5 - 5. Epinephrine is sometimes known as Adrenalin.

Storage/Stability/Compatibility - Epinephrine HCl for injection should be stored in tight containers and protected from light. Epinephrine will darken (oxidation) upon exposure to light and air. Do not use the injection if it is pink, brown or contains a precipitate. The stability of the injection is dependent on the form and the preservatives present, and may vary from one manufacturer to another. Epinephrine is rapidly destroyed by alkalies, or oxidizing agents.

Epinephrine HCl is reported to be **compatible** with the following intravenous solutions: Dextran 6% in dextrose 5%, Dextran 6% in normal saline, dextrose-Ringer's combinations, dextrose-lactated Ringer's combinations, dextrose-saline combinations, dextrose 2.5%, dextrose 5% (becomes unstable at a pH > 5.5), dextrose 10%, Ringer's injection, lactated Ringer's injection, normal saline, and sodium lactate 1/6 M.   Epinephrine HCl is reportedly **compatible** with the following drugs: amikacin sulfate, cimetidine HCl, dobutamine HCl, metaraminol bitartrate, and verapamil HCl.

Epinephrine HCl is reported to be **incompatible** with the following intravenous solutions: Ionosol-D-CM, Ionosol-PSL (Darrow's), Ionosol-T w/ dextrose 5% (Note: other Ionosol product are compatible), sodium chloride 5%, and sodium bicarbonate 5%. Epinephrine HCl is reportedly **incompatible** with the following drugs: aminophylline, cephapirin sodium, hyaluronidase, mephentermine sulfate, sodium bicarbonate, and warfarin sodium. Compatibility is dependent upon factors such as pH, concentration, temperature, and diluents used and it is suggested to consult specialized references for more specific information.

Pharmacology - Epinephrine is an endogenous adrenergic agent that has both alpha and beta activity. It relaxes smooth muscle in the bronchi and the iris, antagonizes the effects of histamine, increases glycogenolysis, and raises blood sugar. If given by rapid IV injection it causes direct stimulation of the heart (increased heart rate and contractility), and increases systolic blood pressure. If given slowly IV, it usually produces a modest rise in systolic pressure and a decrease in diastolic blood pressure. Total peripheral resistance is decreased because of beta effects.

Uses/Indications - Epinephrine is employed primarily in veterinary medicine as a treatment for anaphylaxis and in cardiac resuscitation. Because of its vasocontrictive properties, epinephrine is also added to local anesthetics to retard systemic absorption and prolong effect.

Pharmacokinetics - Epinephrine is well absorbed following IM or SQ administration. IM injections are slightly faster absorbed than SQ administration; absorption can be expedited by massaging the injection site. Epinephrine is rapidly metabolized in the GI tract and liver after oral administration and is not effective via this route. Following SQ injection, the onset of action is generally within 5-10 minutes. The onset of action following IV administration is immediate and intensified.

Epinephrine does not cross the blood-brain barrier, but does cross the placenta and is distributed into milk.

Epinephrine's actions are ended primarily by the uptake and metabolism of the drug into sympathetic nerve endings. Metabolism takes place in both the liver and other tissues by monoamine oxidase (MAO) and catechol-*O*-methyltransferase (COMT) to inactive metabolites.

Contraindications/Precautions - Epinephrine is contraindicated in patients with narrow-angle glaucoma, hypersensitivity to epinephrine, shock due to non-anaphylactoid causes, during general anesthesia with halogenated hydrocarbons or cyclopropane, during labor (may delay the second stage) and in cardiac dilatation or coronary insufficiency. Epinephrine should also not be used in cases where vasopressor drugs are contraindicated (*e.g.,* thyrotoxicosis, diabetes, hypertension, toxemia of pregnancy). It should not be injected with local anesthetics into small appendages of the body (*e.g.,* toes, ears, etc.) because of the chance of necrosis and sloughing.

Use epinephrine with caution in cases of hypovolemia; it is not a substitute for adequate fluid replacement therapy. It should be used with extreme caution in patients with a prefibrillatory cardiac rhythm, because of its excitatory effects on the heart. While epinephrine's usefulness in asystole is well documented, it also can cause ventricular fibrillation; use cautiously in cases of ventricular fibrillation.

Adverse Effects/Warnings - Epinephrine can induce a feeling of fear or anxiety, tremor, excitability, vomiting, hypertension (overdosage), arrhythmias (especially if patient has organic heart disease or has received another drug that sensitizes the heart to arrhythmias), hyperuricemia, and lactic acidosis (prolonged use or overdosage). Repeated injections can cause necrosis at the injection site.

Overdosage - Symptoms seen with overdosage or inadvertent IV administration of SQ or IM dosages can include: sharp rises in systolic, diastolic, and venous blood pressures, cardiac arrhythmias, pulmonary edema and dyspnea, vomiting, headache, and chest pain. Cerebral hemorrhages may result because of the increased blood pressures. Renal failure, metabolic acidosis and cold skin may also result.

Because epinephrine has a relatively short duration of effect, treatment is mainly supportive. If necessary, the use an alpha-adrenergic blocker (*e.g.,* phentolamine) or a beta-adrenergic blocker (*e.g.,* propranolol) can be considered to treat severe hypertension and cardiac arrhythmias. Prolonged periods of hypotension may follow, which may require treatment with norepinephrine.

Drug Interactions - Do not use with other **sympathomimetic amines** (*e.g.,* **isoproterenol**) because of additive effects and toxicity.

Certain **antihistamines (diphenhydramine, chlorpheniramine, etc.) and l-thyroxine** may potentiate the effects of epinephrine.

Propranolol (or other beta-blockers) may potentiate hypertension, and antagonize epinephrine's cardiac and bronchodilating effects by blocking the beta effects of epinephrine.

Nitrates, alpha-blocking agents, or diuretics may negate or diminish the pressor effects of epinephrine.

When epinephrine is used with drugs that sensitize the myocardium (**halothane, high doses of digoxin**) monitor for signs of arrhythmias. Hypertension may result if epinephrine is used with **oxytocic agents**.

Doses -
Note: Be certain when preparing injection that you do not confuse 1:1000 (1 mg/ml) with 1:10,000 (0.1 mg/ml) concentrations. To convert a 1:1000 solution to a 1:10,000 solution for IV or intratracheal use, dilute each ml with 9 ml of normal saline for injection. Epinephrine is only one aspect of treating cardiac arrest, refer to specialized references or protocols for more information.

Dogs:
Cardiac resuscitation (asystole):
a) 0.05 - 0.5 mg (0.5 - 5 ml) of 1:10,000 solution intratracheally or intravenously. May need to repeat every 5 minutes. If intratracheal of IV sites are inaccessible, the intracardiac (IC) route may be used. IC dose is 0.5 to 5 micrograms/kg (0.0005 to 0.005 mg/kg). (Wingfield 1985)
b) 0.2 ml/kg intratracheally of a 1:10,000 solution (Moses 1988)

For anaphylaxis:
a) 0.01 - 0.02 mg/kg IV; or the dosage may be doubled and given via the endotracheal tube if IV line is not yet established. In less severe cases, may be given IM or SubQ (Cohen 1995)
b) Dilute 1 ml of 1:1,000 in 10 mls of saline and give 1 ml/10 kg body weight IV or IM. May repeat q5-15 minutes. (Kittleson 1985a)

Cats:
For cardiac resuscitation:
a) 0.05 - 0.5 mg (0.5 - 5 ml) of 1:10,000 solution intratracheally or intravenously. May need to repeat every 5 minutes. If intratracheal or IV sites are inaccessible, the intracardiac (IC) route may be used. IC dose is 0.5 to 5 micrograms/kg (0.0005 to 0.005 mg/kg). (Wingfield 1985)

For bronchoconstriction/anaphylaxis:
a) 0.01 - 0.02 mg/kg IV; or the dosage may be doubled and given via the endotracheal tube if IV line is not yet established. In less severe cases, may be given IM or SubQ (Cohen 1995)

For feline asthma/anaphylaxis:
a) 0.1 ml of a 1:1,000 dilution SQ or IV (Noone 1986)
b) 0.1 mg SQ q4-6h or 0.2 mg in 100 ml of D5W IV *tid-tid prn* (Morgan 1988)
c) Dilute 1 ml of 1:1,000 in 10 mls of saline and give 1 ml/10 kg body weight IV or IM. May repeat q5-15 minutes. (Kittleson 1985a)

Horses:
For anaphylaxis:
a) 3 - 5 ml of 1:1,000 per 450 kg of body weight either IM or SQ. For foal resuscitation: 0.1 ml/kg of 1:1,000 IV (preferably diluted with saline) (Robinson 1987)

Ruminants, Swine:
For treatment of anaphylaxis:
a) 0.5 - 1.0 ml/100 lbs. body weight of 1:1,000 SQ or IM; dilute to 1:10,000 if using IV; may be repeated at 15 minute intervals Often used in conjunction with corticosteroids and diphenhydramine (Clark 1986)

Monitoring Parameters -
1) Cardiac rate/rhythm
2) Respiratory rate/auscultation during anaphylaxis
3) Urine flow if possible
4) Blood pressure, and blood gases if indicated and if possible

Client Information - Pre-loaded syringes containing an appropriate amount of epinephrine may be dispensed to clients for treatment of anaphylaxis in animals with known hypersensitivity. Anaphylactic symptoms (depending on species) should be discussed. Clients should be instructed in proper injection technique (IM or SQ) and storage conditions for epinephrine. Do not use epinephrine if it is outdated , discolored or contains a precipitate.

Federal (U.S.A.) law restricts this drug to use by or on the order of a licensed veterinarian.

Dosage Forms/Preparations/FDA Approval Status/Withholding Times -
  Veterinary-Approved and Human-Approved Products: Epinephrine is approved for use in dogs, cats, horses, cattle, sheep, and swine.

    Epinephrine HCl for Injection 0.1 mg/ml (1:10,000) in 10 ml syringes (human-label); (Rx)

    Epinephrine HCl for Injection 1 mg/ml (1:1,000) in 1 ml amps & syringes and 10 ml, 30 ml and 100 ml vials; *Adrenalin Chloride*® (P-D); Veterinary-labeled generic; (Rx)

    It is also available in products labeled for human use as a powder form (aerosol) for inhalation, and a sterile suspension for injection. Epinephrine bitartrate is available as a powder form (aerosol) for inhalation. Epinephrine HCl is also available as a solution for nebulization and in automatically injecting syringes for treatment of hypersensitivity reactions.

EPOETIN ALFA
EPOETIN BETA
ERYTHROPOIETIN
EPO
r-HuEPO

Chemistry - A biosynthetic form of the glycoprotein human hormone erythropoietin, epoetin alfa (EPO) has a molecular weight of approximately 30,000. It is commercially available as a sterile, preservative-free, colorless solution. Sodium chloride solution is added to adjust tonicity and is buffered with sodium citrate:citric acid. Human albumin (2.5 mg per vial) is also added to the solution.

Storage/Stability/Compatibility - The injectable solution should be stored in the refrigerator (2-8°C); do not freeze. Do not shake the solution as denaturation of the protein with resultant loss of activity may occur. If light exposure is limited to 24 hours or less, no effects on potency should occur. When stored as directed, the solution has an expiration of date of 2 years after manufacture. Do not mix with other drugs or use the same IV tubing where other drugs are running. Because the solution contains no preservatives, the manufacturer recommends using each vial only as a single use.
  A method of diluting the Amgen product to facilitate giving very small dosages has been described (Grodsky 1994). Using a 1:20 dilution (1 part Epogen® to 19 parts bacteriostatic normal saline does not require any additional albumin to prevent binding of the drug to container. No data is available commenting on this dilution's stability.

Pharmacology - Erythropoietin is a naturally occurring substance produced in the kidney and is considered a hormone as it regulates erythropoiesis. It stimulates erythrocyte production by stimulating the differentiation and proliferation of committed red cell precursors. EPO also stimulates the release of reticulocytes.
  Recombinant Human EPO alfa (r-HuEPO-alpha) serves as a substitute for endogenous EPO, primarily in patients with renal disease. It is believed that various uremic toxins may be responsible for the decreased production of EPO by the kidney.

Uses/Indications - EPO has been used to treat dogs and cats for anemia associated with chronic renal failure. Some clinicians state that because of the expense and potential risks associated with its use, PCV's should be in the "teens" before considering beginning EPO therapy.

Pharmacokinetics - EPO is only absorbed after parenteral administration. It s unclear whether the drug crosses the placenta or enters milk. The drug's metabolic fate is unknown. In patients with chronic renal failure, half lives are prolonged approximately 20% over those with normal renal function.

Contraindications/Precautions/Reproductive Safety - EPO is contraindicated in patients with uncontrolled hypertension or in those who are hypersensitive to it (see Adverse Effects below). EPO cannot be recommended for use in equines.
  Some teratogenic effects (decrease in body weight gain, delayed ossification, etc) have been noted in pregnant rats given high dosages. Rabbits receiving 500 mg/kg during days 6-18 of gestation showed no untoward effects on offspring. However, use during pregnancy only when benefits outweigh the potential risks.

Adverse Effects/Warnings - In dogs and cats, the most troublesome aspect of EPO therapy is the development of autoantibodies with resultant resistance to further treatment. Perhaps up to 30% of all patients will develop antibodies significant enough to cause profound anemia, arrestment of erythropoiesis and transfusion dependency. Should a patient develop refractory anemia while receiving adequate EPO doses and have normal iron metabolism, a bone marrow aspirate should be considered. A myeloid:erythroid ratio of greater than 6 predicts significant autoantibody formation and contraindicates further EPO therapy. Some clinicians believe that the drug (EPO) should be withdrawn if PCV starts to drop while on therapy.

Other effects reported include systemic hypertension, seizures and iron depletion. Local reactions at injection sites (which may be a predictor of antibody formation), fever, arthralgia, and mucocutaneous ulcers are also possible. Other effects that have been noted that may be a result of the animal's disease (or compounded by such), include cardiac disease (may be related to hypertension associated with chronic renal failure). In humans, hyperkalemia, seizures, and iron deficiency have been reported.

Overdosage/Acute Toxicity - Acute overdoses appear to be relatively free of adverse effects. Single doses of up to 1600 Units/kg in humans demonstrated no untoward signs of toxicity. Chronic overdoses may lead to polycythemia or other adverse effects. Cautious phlebotomy may be employed should polycythemia occur.

Drug Interactions - **Androgens (*e.g.,* nandrolone)** may potentially increase the response to EPO (Note: this effect has not been confirmed in well-controlled studies nor has the safety of this combination been determined). One case report has noted that EPO and **desmopressin** used together reduced the bleeding time in one human patient with end-stage renal disease. **Probenecid** has been demonstrated to reduce the renal tubular excretion of EPO; clinical significance is unclear at this time.

Laboratory Considerations - No laboratory interactions of major clinical importance have yet been described. EPO can affect several lab test values via its pharmacologic effect. See Pharmacology, Adverse Effects and Monitoring Parameters sections for more details.

Doses -
Dogs:
    As adjunctive therapy for the treatment of anemia associated with end-stage renal disease:
    a) Initially, 100 Units/kg SubQ 3 times weekly, this dose is maintained for the first 12 weeks of therapy or until the target hematocrit of 37-45% is attained. Once the lower range of the target hematocrit is attained, the dosing interval is changed to twice weekly (or once weekly if polycythemia needs to be prevented.) If anemia recurs with twice weekly injections, three times weekly injections are reinstituted. If adequate control is not achieved with these dosing intervals, then dose may be increased by an additional 25 - 50 Units/kg. Maintenance doses usually fall in the 75 - 100 mg/kg twice to three times weekly range. Do not adjust dosage more often than once every three weeks (due to the long lag time for a response). If an adequate response is not achieved, reevaluate for iron deficiency, other blood loss, hemolysis, or infectious, neoplastic or inflammatory disease processes that could retard erythropoiesis. (Cowgill 1992)

Cats:
    As adjunctive therapy for the treatment of anemia associated with end-stage renal disease:
    a) As above, but the target hematocrit is: 30 - 40%. (Cowgill 1992)

Monitoring Parameters - 1) Hematocrit; PCV; (Initially weekly, then when dose and HCt is stable, at 1-2 month intervals); 2) Blood Pressure (initially, at least monthly then every 1-2 months thereafter); 3) Renal Function Status; 4) Iron status (serum iron, TIBC), RBC indices (initially and regularly during therapy to insure adequate iron availability)

Client Information - Clients should be made aware of the "investigational nature" of this agent and should understand the potential risks as well as the benefits of therapy. For outpatient administration, training in proper injection techniques, drug handling and storage considerations should be performed.

Dosage Forms/Preparations/FDA Approval Status/Withholding Times -
Veterinary-Approved Products: None
Human-Approved Products:
    Epoetin Alfa for Injection 2000 Units/ml, 3000 Units/ml, 4000 Units/ml, 10,000 Units/ml and 20,000 units/ml in 1 ml & 2 ml (10,000U only) vials; *Epogen*® (Amgen), *Procrit*® (Ortho Biotech); (Rx)

EPRINOMECTIN

Chemistry/Storage/Stability- A member of the avermectin-class of antiparasitic agents, eprinomectin is also known as MK-397 or 4-epi-acetylamino-4-deoxy-avermectin B1. The commercially available product should be stored protected from light and kept at 86°F (30°C) or less. Storage at up to 104°F (40°C) is permitted for a short period of time.

Pharmacology - Eprinomectin binds selectively to glutamate-gated chloride ion channels which occur in invertebrate nerve and muscle cells. This leads to an increase in cell membrane permeability to chloride ions leading to paralysis and death of the parasite. Like ivermectin, eprinomectin also enhances the release of gamma amino butyric acid (GABA) at presynaptic neurons. GABA acts as an inhibitory neurotransmitter and blocks the post-synaptic stimulation of the adjacent neuron in nematodes or the muscle fiber in arthropods. These compounds are generally not toxic to mammals as they do not have glutamate-gated chloride channels and these compounds do not readily cross the blood-brain barrier.

Uses/Indications - In cattle, eprinomectin is indicated for a variety gastrointestinal roundworms including adult and L4 stages of *Haemonchus placei, Ostertagia ostertagi, Trichostrongylus axei* and *colubriformis, Cooperia oncophora/punctata/surnabada, Nematodirus helvetianus, Oesophagostomum radiatum, Bunostomun phlebotomum* and *Trichuris spp.* (adults only); cattle grubs; lice; mange mites; horn flies (for 7 days after treatment) and lungworms (*Dictyocaulus vivaparus*—for 21 days after treatment).

Pharmacokinetics - No information located.

Contraindications/Precautions/Reproductive Safety - Do not give orally or intravenously. Up to 3X dosage demonstrated no adverse effect on breeding performance of cows or bulls.

Adverse Effects/Warnings - At the time of writing, no adverse reactions have been reported.

Overdosage - Calves given up to 5X dosage showed no signs of adverse effects. One subject (of 6) showed signs of mydriasis when give a 10X dose.

Drug Interactions - No interactions noted.

Doses -
> **Cattle**: For labeled indications: 1 ml per 10 kg (22 lb) body weight applied topically along backline in a narrow strip from the withers to the tailhead. (*Eprinex*® Package Insert—Merck)

Client Information/Residue Warnings - When used as labeled, there are no milk or meat withdrawal times required. Weather conditions (including rainfall) during administration do not affect efficacy. Do not apply to backline if covered with mud or manure. Dispose of containers in an approved landfill or by incineration; do not contaminate water as eprinomectin may adversely affect fish and aquatic organisms.

Dosage Forms/Preparations/FDA Approval Status -
Veterinary-Approved Products:
> Eprinomectin Topical (Pour-On) Solution 5 mg/ml in 250 ml and 1 liter bottle with a squeeze-measure-pour-system, or a 2.5 L or 5 L collapsible pack for use with appropriate automatic dosing equipment; *Eprinex*® (Merck); (OTC). Approved for use in beef or dairy cattle.

Epsom Salts - see Magnesium Sulfate

EPSIPRANTEL

Chemistry - A pyrazino-benzazepine oral cesticide, epsiprantel occurs as a white powder that is sparingly soluble in water.

Storage/Stability/Compatibility - Tablets should be stored at room temperature.

Pharmacology - Epsiprantel's exact mechanism of action against cestodes has not been determined. The tapeworm's ability to regulate calcium is apparently affected, causing tetany and disruption of attachment to the host. Also, alteration to the integument make the worm vulnerable to digestion by the host animal.

Uses/Indications - Epsiprantel is indicated for the treatment (removal) of *Dipylidium caninum* and Taenia *pisiformis* in dogs, and *Dipylidium caninum* and *Taenia taeniaeformis* in cats.

Pharmacokinetics - Unlike praziquantel, epsiprantel is absorbed only very poorly after oral administration and the bulk of the drug is eliminated in the feces. Less than 0.1% of the drug is recovered in the urine after dosing. No metabolites have thus far been detected.

Contraindications/Precautions/Reproductive Safety - There are no labeled contraindications to this drug, but the manufacturer states not to use it in puppies or kittens less than 7 weeks of age. Safety for use in pregnant or breeding animals has also not been determined, but teratogenic effects would be highly unlikely since the drug is so poorly absorbed.

Adverse Effects/Warnings - Adverse effects would be unexpected with this agent, although vomiting and/or diarrhea could potentially occur. Because the drug has been just released at the time of writing this monograph, further adverse effects may be reported as more experience is obtained.

Overdosage/Acute Toxicity - Acute toxicity resulting from an inadvertant overdose is highly unlikely. Doses as high as 36X the recommended dose resulted only in vomiting in some of the kittens tested. Single doses of 36X those recommended in dogs caused no adverse effects.

Drug Interactions; Drug/Laboratory Interactions - None reported thus far.

Doses -
  Dogs:
      a) 5.5 mg/kg PO once (Package insert; *Cestex*®—Beecham)
  Cats:
      a) 2.75 mg/kg PO once (Package insert; *Cestex*®—Beecham)

Monitoring Parameters -
      1) Clinical efficacy

Client Information - Fasting is not required nor is it recommended before dosing. Because the worm may be partially or completely digested, worm fragments may not be seen in the feces after treating. A single dose is usually effective, but measures should be taken to prevent reinfection, particularly against *D. caninum*.

Dosage Forms/Preparations/FDA Approval Status/Withholding Times -
  Veterinary-Approved Products:
      Epsiprantel Oral Tablets (Film-coated) 12.5, 25, 50 and 100 mg; *Cestex*® (Pfizer), (Rx) Approved for use in dogs and cats.
  Human-Approved Products - None

ERYTHROMYCIN
ERYTHROMYCIN ESTOLATE
ERYTHROMYCIN ETHYLSUCCINATE
ERYTHROMYCIN LACTOBIONATE
ERYTHROMYCIN GLUCEPTATE

Chemistry - A macrolide antibiotic produced from *Streptomyces erythreus*, erythromycin is a weak base that is available commercially in several salts and esters. It has a pK_a of 8.9.

Erythromycin base occurs as a bitter-tasting, odorless or practically odorless, white to slight yellow, crystalline powder. Approximately 1 mg is soluble in 1 ml of water; it is soluble in alcohol.

Erythromycin estolate occurs as a practically tasteless and odorless, white, crystalline powder. It is practically insoluble in water and approximately 50 mg are soluble in 1 ml of alcohol. Erythromycin estolate may also be known as erythromycin propionate lauryl sulfate.

Erythromycin ethylsuccinate occurs as a practically tasteless and odorless, white to slight yellow, crystalline powder. It is very slightly soluble in water and freely soluble in alcohol.

Erythromycin lactobionate occurs as white to slightly yellow crystals or powder. It may have a faint odor and is freely soluble in water and alcohol.

Erythromycin gluceptate occurs as a practically odorless, white, slightly hygroscopic powder that is freely soluble in water and alcohol. It may also be known as erythromycin glucoheptonate.

Storage/Stability/Compatibility - Erythromycin (base) capsules and tablets should be stored in tight containers at room temperature (15-30°C). Erythromycin estolate preparations should be protected from light. To retain palatability, the oral suspensions should be refrigerated.

Erythromycin ethylsuccinate tablets and powder for oral suspension should be stored in tight containers at room temperature. The commercially available oral suspension should be stored in the refrigerator to preserve palatability. After dispensing, the oral suspensions are stable for at least 14 days at room temperature, but individual products may have longer labeled stabilities.

Erythromycin lactobionate powder for injection should be stored at room temperature. For initial reconstitution (vials), only sterile water for injection should be used. After reconstitution, the drug is stable for 24 hours at room temperature and 2 weeks if refrigerated. To prepare for administration via continuous or intermittent infusion, the drug is further diluted in 0.9% sodium chloride, Lactated Ringer's, or *Normosol-R*. Other infusion solutions may be used, but first must be buffered with 4% sodium bicarbonate injection (1 ml per 100 ml of solution). At pH's of <5.5, the drug is unstable and loses potency rapidly. Many drugs are physically incompatible with erythromycin lactobionate; refer to an appropriate reference (*e.g.,* Trissell—see bibliography) for more information.

Erythromycin gluceptate powder for injection should be stored at room temperature. For initial reconstitution (vials), only sterile water for injection (without preservatives) should be used. After reconstitution, the drug is stable for 7 days if refrigerated. Many drugs are physically incompatible with erythromycin gluceptate; refer to an appropriate reference (*e.g.,* Trissell—see bibliography) for more information.

Pharmacology - Erythromycin is usually a bacteriostatic agent, but in high concentrations or against highly susceptible organisms it may be bactericidal. The macrolides (erythromycin and tylosin) are believed to act by binding to the 50S ribosomal subunit of susceptible bacteria, thereby inhibiting peptide bond formation.

Erythromycin has *in vitro* activity against gram positive cocci (staphylococci, streptococci), gram positive bacilli (*Bacillus anthracis, Corynebacterium, Clostridium sp.*, (not *C. difficile*), *Listeria, Erysipelothrix*), some strains of gram negative bacilli, including *Haemophilus, Pasturella,* and *Brucella.* Some strains of *Actinomyces, Mycoplasma, Chlamydia, Ureaplasma,* and Rickettsia are also inhibited by erythromycin. Most strains of the family Enterobacteriaceae (*Pseudomonas, E. coli, Klebsiella,* etc.) are resistant to erythromycin.

Erythromycin is less active at low pH's and many clinicians suggest alkalinizing the urine if using the drug to treat UTI's.

Uses/Indications - Erythromycin is approved for use to treat infections caused by susceptible organisms in dogs, cats, swine, sheep, and cattle. It is often employed when an animal is hypersensitive to penicillins or if other antibiotics are ineffective against a certain organism.

Erythromycin is at the present time considered to be the treatment of choice (with rifampin) for the treatment of *C. (Rhodococcus) equi* infections in foals.

Pharmacokinetics - Erythromycin is absorbed after oral administration in the upper small intestine. Several factors can influence the bioavailability of erythromycin, including salt form, dosage form, GI acidity, food in the stomach, and stomach emptying time. Both erythromycin base and stearate are susceptible to acid degradation, and enteric coatings are often used to alleviate this. Both the ethylsuccinate and estolate forms are dissociated in the upper small intestine and then absorbed. After IM or SQ injection of the polyethylene-based veterinary product (*Erythro®-200; Gallimycin®-200*) in cattle, absorption is very slow. Bioavailabilities are only about 40% after SQ injection, and 65% after IM injection.

Erythromycin is distributed throughout the body into most fluids and tissues including the prostate, macrophages, and leukocytes. CSF levels are poor. Erythromycin may be 73-81% bound to serum proteins and the estolate salt, 96% bound. Erythromycin will cross the placenta and levels of 5-20% of those in the mother's serum can be found in the fetal circulation. Erythromycin levels of about 50% of those found in the serum can be detected in milk. The volume of distribution for erythromycin in dogs is reportedly 2 L/kg, 3.7 - 7.2 L/kg in foals, 2.3 L/kg in mares, and 0.8 L/kg in cattle.

Erythromycin is primarily excreted unchanged in the bile, but is also partly metabolized by the liver via *N*-demethylation to inactive metabolites. Some of the drug is reabsorbed after biliary excretion. Only about 2-5% of a dose is excreted unchanged in the urine.

The reported elimination half-life of erythromycin in various species are: 60-90 minutes in dogs and cats, 60-70 minutes in foals and mares, and 190 minutes in cattle.

Contraindications/Precautions/Reproductive Safety - Erythromycin is contraindicated in patients hypersensitive to it. In humans, the estolate form has been associated rarely with the development of cholestatic hepatitis. This effect has not apparently been reported in veterinary species, but the estolate should probably be avoided in patients with preexisting liver dysfunction.

Many clinicians believe that erythromycin is contraindicated in adult horses (see Adverse Effects below), and oral erythromycin should not be used in ruminants as severe diarrheas may result.

While erythromycin has not demonstrated teratogenic effects in rats and the drug is not thought to posses serious teratogenic potential, it should only be used during pregnancy when the benefits outweigh the risks.

Adverse Effects/Warnings - Adverse effects are relatively infrequent with erythromycin when used in small animals, swine, sheep, or cattle. When injected IM, local reactions and pain at the injection site may occur. Oral erythromycin may cause GI disturbances with diarrhea, anorexia, and vomiting occasionally seen. Rectal edema and partial anal prolapse have been associated with erythromycin in swine. Intravenous injections must be given very slowly, as the intravenous forms can readily cause thrombophlebitis. Allergic reactions can occur, but are thought to be very rare.

Oral erythromycin should not be used in ruminants as severe diarrheas may result.

In foals treated with erythromycin, a mild, self-limiting diarrhea may occasionally occur. Adult horses may develop severe, sometimes fatal diarrheas from erythromycin and the use of the drug in adults is very controversial.

Erythromycin may alter temperature homeostasis in foals. Foals between the ages of 2 and 4 months old have been reported to develop hyperthermia with associated respiratory distress and tachypnea. Physically cooling off these animals is reported to be successful in controlling this effect.

Overdosage/Acute Toxicity - With the exception of the adverse effects outlined above, erythromycin is apparently quite non-toxic. However, shock reactions have been reported in baby pigs receiving erythromycin overdosages.

Drug Interactions - Because erythromycin, the **lincosamides** (**clindamycin, lincomycin**), and **chloramphenicol** all bind to the 50S ribosomal subunit, competition for binding can occur and some clinicians state these drugs should not be used concurrently. *In vitro* synergy with other antimicrobials (*e.g.,* sulfonamides, rifampin) has been reported with erythromycin. The concomitant use of erythromycin with bactericidal antibiotics (*e.g.,* penicillin) is controversial, but documentation of either clinical synergy, additive activity, or antagonism is apparently lacking.

Decreased clearance of **theophylline** may occur with resultant toxicity in patients receiving erythromycin (particularly high dosages). Patients should be monitored for symptoms of theophylline toxicity and serum theophylline levels monitored if necessary.

Patients stabilized on **warfarin** anticoagulant therapy may develop prolonged prothrombin times and bleeding when erythromycin is added. Enhanced monitoring is recommended.

The metabolism of **methylprednisolone** may be inhibited by concurrent administration of erythromycin. The clinical significance of this interaction is unknown.

Erythromycin may increase the bioavailability of **digoxin** in a small percentage of human patients and can lead to digoxin toxicity. Veterinary significance of this interaction is questionable.

Interactions have also been reported with erythromycin and the following human drugs (rarely used in veterinary species—refer to other references if necessary): **carbamazepine, cyclosporine** (systemic), and **triazolam**.

Drug/Laboratory Interactions - Erythromycin may cause falsely elevated values of **AST** (SGOT), and **ALT** (SGPT) when using colorimetric assays.

Fluorometric determinations of **urinary catecholamines** can be altered by concomitant erythromycin administration.

Doses -

Dogs:
> For susceptible infections:
> > a) 5 - 20 mg/kg PO q8h (Ford and Aronson 1985)
> > b) 10 mg/kg PO *tid* (Morgan 1988)
> > c) 10 mg/kg PO q8h (Kirk 1989)
> > d) 12 - 22 mg/kg PO q8h (Aronson and Aucoin 1989)

Cats:
> For susceptible infections:
> > a) 5 - 20 mg/kg PO q8h (Ford and Aronson 1985)
> > b) 15 mg/kg PO q8h (Jenkins 1987b)
> > c) 10 mg/kg PO *tid* (Morgan 1988)
> > d) 10 mg/kg PO q8h (Kirk 1989)
> > e) 12 - 22 mg/kg PO q8h (Aronson and Aucoin 1989)

Birds:
> For susceptible infections:
> > a) Oral suspension: 60 mg/kg PO q12h (Hoeffer 1995)

Cattle:
> For susceptible infections:
> > a) 4 - 8 mg/kg IM q12-24h (Jenkins 1987b)
> > b) For bronchopneumonia and fibrinous pneumonia in cattle associated with bacteria sensitive to erythromycin and resistant to sulfas, penicillin G and tetracyclines: Using *Erythro-200®*: 44 mg/kg IM q24h usually for a maximum of 4 days. Inject no more than 10 ml at any one site. Do not inject at any site previously used. Severe local tissue reactions may occur. Recommend a 30 day slaughter withdrawal at this dosage. (Hjerpe 1986)
>
> For mastitis:
> > a) Dry cow (using dry cow formula): Milk out affected quarter, clean and disinfect. Infuse contents of one syringe into each affected quarter at time of drying off. Close teat orifice with gentle pressure and massage udder.
> > Lactating cow (using lactating cow formula): As above, but repeat after each milking for 3 milkings. (Label directions; *Erythro®-Dry & Erythro®-36*—Ceva)

Horses:
> For treatment of *C. (Rhodococcus) equi* infections in foals:
> > a) Erythromycin estolate or ethylsuccinate: 25 mg/kg PO *tid* with rifampin: 5 mg/kg PO *tid*. (Hillidge and Zertuche 1987)

    b) Erythromycin estolate: 25 mg/kg PO q6h
        Erythromycin gluceptate: 5 mg/kg IV q4-6h (Caprile and Short 1987)
    c) Erythromycin estolate: 25 mg/kg PO *qid*
        Erythromycin gluceptate: 5 mg/kg IV 4-6 times daily
        Erythromycin base (veterinary) injectable: 10 mg/kg IM *bid* (Prescott, Hoover, and Dohoo 1983)

For susceptible infections:
    a) Erythromycin estolate: 25 mg/kg PO q6h
        Erythromycin ethylsuccinate: 25 mg/kg PO q8h
        Erythromycin gluceptate: 5 mg/kg IV q4-6h
        Erythromycin lactobionate: 3 - 5 mg/kg IV q6-8h (Brumbaugh 1987)

Swine:
    For susceptible infections:
    a) For respiratory infections: 2.2 - 6.6 mg/kg IM once daily
        For scours in young pigs: 22 mg/kg IM in one or more daily doses. (Label directions; *Erythro®-100* & *Erythro®-200*—Ceva)

Sheep:
    For susceptible infections:
    For respiratory infections in older animals: 2.2 mg/kg IM once daily as indicated.
    For prevention of "dysentery" in newborn lambs when the likely causative agent is susceptible to erythromycin: 123 mg/kg IM once soon after birth. (Label directions; *Erythro®-100* & *Erythro®-200*—Ceva)

Monitoring Parameters -
    1) Clinical efficacy
    2) Adverse effects (periodic liver function tests if patient receiving erythromycin estolate long-term; may not be necessary for foals receiving erythromycin and rifampin for *Rhodococcus* infections)

Client Information - The intramuscular 100 mg/ml (*Erythro-100®*) & 200 mg/ml products (*Erythro-200®*) have quite specific instructions on where and how to inject the drug. Refer to the label directions or package insert for more information before using.

Dosage Forms/Preparations/FDA Approval Status/Withholding Times -
Veterinary-Approved Products:
Erythromycin 100 mg/ml for IM Injection (with 2% butyl aminobenzoate as a local anesthetic) in 100 ml vials
    Erythro-100® (Rhone Merieux); (OTC) Approved for use in dogs, cats, cattle, sheep, and swine. Milk withdrawal = 72 hours. Slaughter withdrawal for cattle, sheep, swine = 48 hours.

Erythromycin 200 mg/ml for IM Injection in 100 ml, 250 ml, and 500 ml vials
    Erythro-200® (Rhone Merieux); (OTC) Approved for use in cattle, sheep, and swine. Milk withdrawal = 72 hours. Slaughter withdrawal for cattle =14 days (21 days to avoid excessive trimming). Slaughter withdrawal for sheep = 3 days (10 days to avoid excessive trimming). Slaughter withdrawal for swine = 7 days (10 days to avoid excessive trimming).

Erythromycin Mastitis Infusion Tube for Dry Cows; 600 mg erythromycin per 12 ml tube
    Erythro®-Dry (Rhone Merieux); (OTC) Approved for use in dry dairy cattle. Milk withdrawal = 36 hours. Slaughter withdrawal = 14 days nor within 96 hours of calving. Calves born to treated cows may not be slaughtered for food at less than 10 days of age.

Erythromycin Mastitis Infusion Tube for Lactating Cows; 50 mg/ml of erythromycin per 6 ml tube
    Erythro®-36 (Rhone Merieux); (OTC) Approved for use in dry dairy cattle. Milk withdrawal = 36 hours. Slaughter withdrawal = 14 days.

There are also several erythromycin premixes alone and in combination with other drugs for use in swine and/or poultry.

Human-Approved Products:
Erythromycin Base Oral Tablets enteric-coated 250 mg, 500 mg; *Ery-Tab®* (Abbott); *E-Mycin®* (Boots), *Robimycin® Robitabs®* (Robins);*E-Base®* (Barr); (Rx)

Erythromycin Base Oral Tablets film-coated 250 mg, 500 mg
    Erythromycin Film-Tabs® (Abbott); (Rx)

Erythromycin Base Oral Capsules delayed release enteric-coated pellets 250 mg; *Eryc®* (Parke-Davis); (Rx)

Erythromycin Base Delayed Relased Tablets 333 mg, generic, (Rx)

Erythromycin Base Tablets with polymer coated particles 500 mg; *PCE Dispertab* ® (Abbott) (Rx)

Erythromycin Base Oral Capsules delayed release 250 mg; generic (Rx)

Erythromycin Estolate Tablets 500 mg (as estolate) *Ilosone*® (Dista) (Rx)

Erythromycin Estolate Capsules 250 mg (as estolate); *Ilosone Pulvules*® (Dista) (Rx); generic, (Rx)

Erythromycin Estolate Suspension: 125 mg (as estolate) per 5 ml in 480 mls and 250 mg (as estolate) per 5 ml in 100 & 480 mls; *Ilosone*® (Dista); generic, (Rx)

Erythromycin Stearate Film-coated tablets 250 mg, 500 mg; generic; (Rx)

Erythromycin Ethylsuccinate Chewable Tablets: 200 mg (as ethylsuccinate; equiv. to 125 mg of base); *EryPed*® (Abbott) (Rx)

Erythromycin Ethylsuccinate Tablets: 400 mg (as ethylsuccinate); *E.E.S. 400;* generic, (Rx)

Oral Suspension: 40 mg/ml (equiv. to 25 mg/ml base), 80 mg/ml (equiv. to 50 mg/ml base) in 100, 200, 480, and 500 ml bottles; 100 mg per 2.5 ml in 50 mls, 200 & 400 mg (as ethyl-succinate) per 5 ml in 60, 100, 200 and 480 ml and UD 5 ml (100's); *EryPed Drops*® (Abbott); *EryPed 400*® (Abbott); *E.E.S. 400*; generic (Rx)

Powder for Oral Suspension: 200 mg (as ethylsuccinate) per 5 ml when reconstituted in 100 & 200 mls ; *E.E.S. Granules*® (Abbott) (Rx)

Granules for Oral Suspension: 400 mg (as ethylsuccinate) per 5 ml when reconstituted; *EryPed Drops* ® (Abbott)

Erythromycin Lactobionate Powder for Injection: 500 mg & 1 g (as lactobionate); generic (Rx)

Erythromycin Lactobionate Injection: 1 g erythromycin (as gluceptate) per vial in 30 mls; *Ilotycin Gluceptate*® (Dista) (Rx)

ESMOLOL HCL

Chemistry - A short acting beta1 adrenergic blocker, esmolol occurs as white or off white crystalline powder. It is not as lipophilic as either labetolol or propranolol, but is comparable to acebutolol. 650 mg is soluble in one ml of water and 350 mg is soluble in one ml of alcohol.

Storage/Stability/Compatibility - The concentrate for injection should be stored at room temperature; freezing does not adversely affect the potency of the drug. It is a clear, colorless to light yellow solution. Expiration dates of 3 years are assigned after manufacture.

After diluted to a concentration of 10 mg/ml esmolol HCl is stable (at refrigeration temperatures or room temperature) for at least 24 hours in commonly used IV solutions. At this concentration it is reportedly compatible with digoxin, dopamine, fentanyl, lidocaine, morphine sulfate,, nitroglycerin and nitroprusside. Compatibility is dependent upon factors such as pH, concentration, temperature and diluents used. It is suggested to consult specialized references (*e.g., Handbook on Injectable Drugs* by Trissel; see bibliography) for more specific information.

Pharmacology - Esmolol primarily blocks both beta1 adrenergic receptors in the myocardium. At clinically used doses, esmolol does not have any intrinsic sympathomimetic activity (ISA) and unlike propranolol, it does not possess membrane-stabilizing effects (quinidine-like) nor bronchoconstrictive effects. Cardiovascular effects secondary to esmolol include: negative inotropic and chronotropic activity which can lead to reduced myocardial oxygen demand. Systolic and diastolic blood pressures are reduced at rest and during exercise. Esmolol's antiarrhythmic effect is thought to be due to its blockade of adrenergic stimulation of cardiac pacemaker potentials. Esmolol increases sinus cycle length, slows AV node conduction and prolongs sinus node recovery time.

Uses/Indications - Esmolol may be used as test drug to indicate whether beta blocker therapy is warranted as an antiarrhythmic agent or as an infusion in the short term treatment of supraventricular tachyarrhythmias (*e.g.,* atrial fibrillation/flutter, sinus tachycardia).

Pharmacokinetics - Esmolol is administered via the IV route. After injection it is rapidly and widely distributed, but not appreciably to the CNS, spleen or testes. The distribution half life is about 2 minutes. Steady-state blood levels occur in about 5 minutes if a loading dose was given or about 30 minutes if no load was given. It is unknown whether the drug crosses the placenta or enters milk. Esmolol is rapidly metabolized in the blood by esterases. Renal or hepatic dysfunction do not appreciably alter elimination characteristics. Terminal half life is about 10 minutes and duration of action after discontinuing IV infusion is about 10-20 minutes.

Contraindications/Precautions/Reproductive Safety - Esmolol is contraindicated in patients with overt cardiac failure, 2nd or 3rd degree AV block, sinus bradycardia, or in cardiogenic shock. It should be used with caution (weigh benefit vs. risk) in patients with CHF, bronchoconstrictive lung disease or with diabetes mellitus.

Studies done in rats and rabbits demonstrated no teratogenic effects at doses up to 3 times the maximum human maintenance dose (MHMD). Higher doses (8 times or more MHMD) demonstrated some maternal death and fetal resorption.

Adverse Effects/Warnings - At usual doses adverse effects are uncommon and generally an extension of the drug's pharmacologic effects. Hypotension (with resultant symptoms) and bradycardia are the most likely adverse effects seen. These are generally mild and transient in nature. Esmolol may mask certain symptoms of developing hypoglycemia (such as increased heart rate or blood pressure).

Overdosage/Acute Toxicity - The IV LD_{50} in dogs is approximately 32 mg/kg. Dogs receiving 2 mg/kg per minute for one hour showed no adverse effects; doses of 3 mg/kg/minute for one hour produced ataxia and salivation and 4 mg/kg/minute for one hour caused muscular rigidity, tremors, seizures, ptosis, vomiting, hyperpnea, vocalizations and prostration. These effects all resolved within 90 minutes of the end of infusion. Because of the short duration of action of the drug, discontinuation or dosage reduction may be all that is required. Otherwise symptomatic and supportive treatment may be initiated.

Drug Interactions - As esmolol may increase serum **digoxin** levels up to 20%, it should be used with caution in digitalized patients with increased monitoring when necessary. Titrate esmolol dosage carefully in patients also receiving **morphine**. Morphine may increase steady-state esmolol serum concentrations up to 50%. **Succinylcholine**'s neuromuscular blockade effects may be prolonged when esmolol is used, but this effect is probably not relevant clinically. If esmolol is used with **sympathomimetic amines or xanthines** (*e.g.*, theophylline, aminophylline) mutual inhibition of effects may occur. Concurrent use of monoamine oxidase inhibitors (including **furazolidone**) with esmolol is not recommended due to potentially hypertension occurring.

Doses -
 Dogs:
　　For ultra-short acting beta blockade (for treating or assisting in treatment of ventricular arrhythmias):
　　a) 0.5 mg/kg IV slow load, then 50 - 200 micrograms/kg/min infusion. (Hamlin 1992)
　　b) Give incremental doses of 0.05 - 0.1 mg/kg boluses every 5 minutes to a maximum dose of 0.5 mg/kg; or as an infusion of 50 - 200 micrograms/kg/min. If arrhythmia conversion does not occur, then other drugs with negative inotropic effects (e.g. diltiazem or verapamil) may be given 30 minutes after esmolol administration. (Russell and Rush 1995)

Monitoring Parameters - 1) Blood Pressure; 2) ECG; 3) Heart Rate

Client Information - Esmolol should only be used in an in-patient setting where appropriate monitoring is available.

Dosage Forms/Preparations/FDA Approval Status/Withholding Times -
 Veterinary-Approved Products: None
 Human-Approved Products:
　Esmolol HCl Injection 10 mg/ml in 10 ml vials & 250 mg/ml in 10 ml amps;*Brevibloc*® (Ohmeda); (Rx)

ESTRADIOL CYPIONATE

Chemistry - Estradiol is a naturally occurring steroidal estrogen. Estradiol cypionate is produced by esterifying estradiol with cyclopentanepropionic acid, and occurs as a white to practically white, crystalline powder. It is either odorless or may have a slight odor and has a melting range of 149-153°C. Less than 0.1 mg/ml is soluble in water and 25 mg/ml is soluble in alcohol. Estradiol cypionate is sparingly soluble in vegetable oils.

Storage/Stability/Compatibility - Estradiol cypionate should be stored in light-resistant containers at temperatures of less than 40°C, preferably at room temperature (15-30°C); avoid freezing.

Commercially available injectable solutions of estradiol cypionate are sterile solutions in a vegetable oil (usually cottonseed oil); they may contain chlorobutanol as a preservative.

It is not recommended to mix estradiol cypionate with other medications.

Pharmacology - The most active endogenous estrogen, estradiol possesses the pharmacologic profile expected of the estrogen class. Estrogens are necessary for the normal growth and development of the female sex organs and in some species contribute to the development and maintenance of secondary female sex characteristics. Estrogens cause increased cell height and secretions of the cervical mucosa, thickening of the vaginal mucosa, endometrial proliferation and increased uterine tone.

Estrogens have effects on the skeletal system. They increase calcium deposition, accelerate epiphyseal closure and increase bone formation. Estrogens have a slight anabolic effect and can increase sodium and water retention.

Estrogens affect the release of gonadotropins from the pituitary gland. This can cause inhibition of lactation, inhibition of ovulation and inhibition of androgen secretion.

Uses/Indications - For mares, indications for the use of estradiol include, induction of estrus during the non-breeding or breeding seasons and to enhance the mare's uterine defense mechanism. Estradiol cypionate has also been used as an abortifacient agent (see warnings below) in cattle, cats and dogs.

One product (*ECP®* — Upjohn) approved for use in breeding cattle, indications listed in its package insert for use in bovine medicine include:

To correct anestrus (absence of heat period) in the absence of follicular cysts in some cases.

To treat cattle having persistent corpus luteum due to certain causes.

To expel purulent material from the uterus in pyometra of cows.

To stimulate uterine expulsion of retained placentas and mummified fetuses.

Pharmacokinetics - No specific information was located regarding the pharmacokinetics of estradiol in veterinary species. In humans, estrogen in oil solutions after IM administration are absorbed promptly and absorption continues over several days. Esterified estrogens (*e.g.,* estradiol cypionate) have delayed absorption after IM administration. Estrogens are distributed throughout the body and accumulate in adipose tissue. Elimination of the steroidal estrogens occurs principally by hepatic metabolism. Estrogens and their metabolites are primarily excreted in the urine, but are also excreted into the bile, where most is reabsorbed from the GI.

Contraindications/Precautions - Estradiol is contraindicated during pregnancy. It has been demonstrated to cause fetal malformations of the genitourinary system and to induce bone marrow depression in the fetus.

In cases of prolonged corpus luteum in cows, thorough uterine exam should be completed to determine if endometritis or a fetus is present

Adverse Effects/Warnings - Estrogens have been associated with severe adverse reactions in small animals; see the Adverse Effects section in the DES monograph (prior to this one) for more information.

In cattle, prolonged estrus, genital irritation, decreased milk flow, precocious development and follicular cysts may develop after estrogen therapy. These effects may be secondary to overdosage and dosage adjustment may reduce or eliminate them.

Overdosage - No reports of inadvertent acute overdosage in veterinary patients was located; see Adverse Effects above.

Drug Interactions - **Rifampin** may decrease estrogen activity if administered concomitantly. This is presumably due to microsmal enzyme induction with resultant increase in estrogen metabolism. Other known enzyme inducers (*e.g.,* **phenobarbital, phenylbutazone**, etc.), may have a similar effect, but clinical significance is unclear.

Enhanced glucocorticoid effects may result if estrogens are used concomitantly with **corticosteroid agents**. It has been postulated that estrogens may either alter the protein binding of corticosteroids and/or decrease their metabolism. Corticosteroid dosage adjustment may be necessary when estrogen therapy is either started or discontinued.

Oral anticoagulant activity may be decreased if estrogens are administered concurrently. Increases in anticoagulant dosage may be necessary if adding estrogens.

Drug/Laboratory Interactions - Estrogens in combination with progestins (*e.g.,* oral contraceptives) have been demonstrated in humans to increase **thyroxine-binding globulin** (TBG) with resultant increases in total circulating thyroid hormone. Decrease **T3 resin uptake** also occurs, but free T4 levels are unaltered. It is unclear if estradiol affects these laboratory tests.

Doses -
  Dogs:
      For pregnancy avoidance after mismating:
        a) 0.02 mg/kg (ECP) IM within 72 hours of mating (Burke 1986)
        b) 0.044 mg/kg (ECP) IM once during 3-5 days of standing heat or within 72 hours of mismating (Woody 1988)
        c) 0.044 mg/kg (ECP), not to exceed 1 mg total dose, IM once administered during estrus or early diestrus. (Olson et al. 1986)

Cats:
For pregnancy avoidance after mismating:
a) 0.125 - 0.25 mg (ECP) IM within 40 hours of mating (Wildt 1986)
b) 0.125 - 0.25 mg (ECP) IM within 3-5 days of coitus (Woody 1988)

Cattle:
a) To terminate pregnancy by causing the regression of the corpus luteum: 4 - 8 mg IM if given with 4 days of unwanted breeding. During the 4th to 7th months of pregnancy: 20 mg IM; may require repeated doses for 2-3 days. If used after the 7 months of pregnancy, dystocia, metritis, and retained placenta are common adverse effects. (Drost 1986)
b) Cows: Anestrus: 3 - 5 mg IM; Pyometra: 10 mg IM; Retained placenta: 10 mg IM; Persistent corpus luteum: 4 mg IM; Mummified fetus: 10 mg IM.
Heifers: Anestrus: 3 mg IM. (Package Insert; *ECP*® — Upjohn)

Horses:
For induction of estrus during the non-breeding season:
a) 10 mg estradiol cypionate will result in estrus 2-3 days after treatment (Squires and McKinnon 1987)

For induction of estrus in mares with "silent heat" during breeding season:
a) 1 mg estradiol (Squires and McKinnon 1987)

To enhance the mare's uterine defense mechanism:
a) 1 - 2 mg estradiol daily for 3-5 days (Squires and McKinnon 1987)

Monitoring Parameters - When therapy is either at high dosages or chronic; see adverse effects for more information.
Done at least monthly:
1) Packed Cell Volumes (PCV)
2) White blood cell counts (CBC)
3) Platelet counts
Baseline, one month after therapy, and repeated 2 months after cessation of therapy if abnormal:
1) Liver function tests

Dosage Forms/Preparations/FDA Approval Status/Withholding Times -
Veterinary-Approved Products:
Estradiol Cypionate in Oil for Injection 2 mg/ml in 50 ml vials
ECP® (Upjohn), Generic; (Rx) Approved for use in cattle. No slaughter withdrawal times were located for these products.

Human-Approved Products:
Estradiol Cypionate in Oil for Injection 5 mg/ml in 5 & 10 ml vials)
Generic; Many trade names; (Rx)

ETHACRYNIC ACID

Chemistry - A loop diuretic, ethacrynic acid occurs as a white or nearly white, odorless or practically odorless crystalline powder. It is very slightly soluble in water and freely soluble in alcohol.

Storage/Stability/Compatibility - Ethacrynic acid tablets should be stored at room temperature in well-closed containers. An expiration date of 5 years is assigned at the time of manufacture.

Pharmacology - Ethacrynic acid reduces the absorption of electrolytes in the ascending section of the loop of Henle, decreases the reabsorption of both sodium (to a much greater extent than the thiazides) and chloride, increases the excretion of potassium in the distal renal tubule, and directly effects electrolyte transport in the proximal tubule. The exact mechanisms of ethacrynic acid's effects have not been established. It has no effect on carbonic anhydrase nor does it antagonize aldosterone. Ethacrynic acid increases renal excretion of water, sodium, potassium, chloride, calcium, magnesium, hydrogen, ammonium and bicarbonate.

Uses/Indications - Ethacrynic acid is a loop diuretic that shares the same indications as furosemide (congestive cardiomyopathy, pulmonary edema, hypercalcuric nephropathy, uremia, as adjunctive therapy in hyperkalemia and, occasionally, as an antihypertensive agent). Its use has been largely supplanted in the armamentarium by furosemide for these indications.
Ethacrynic acid may be useful in the treatment of nephrogenic diabetes insipidus as it may cause a paradoxical decrease in urine volume. Other uses include the adjunctive treatment of hypercalcemia and to increase the excretion of bromide in the treatment of bromide toxicity.

Pharmacokinetics - Ethacrynic acid is absorbed rapidly and nearly completely from the GI tract. It does not enter the CNS and accumulates in the liver. It is unknown if etha-crynic acid crosses the placenta or enters milk. Ethacrynic acid is metabolized in the liver and also secreted via the proximal tubules into the urine. Serum half lives in humans average around one hour. Duration of effect is about 6-8 hours after oral dosing and about 2 hours after IV administration.

Contraindications/Precautions/Reproductive Safety - Ethacrynic acid is contraindicated in patients with anuria, who are hypersensitive to the drug or have seriously depleted electrolytes. Ethacrynic acid is also contraindicated in human infants (safety not established).

Ethacrynic acid should be used with caution in patients with preexisting electrolyte or water balance abnormalities, impaired hepatic function (may precipitate hepatic coma) and diabetes mellitus. Patients with conditions that may lead to electrolyte or water balance abnormalities (*e.g.,* vomiting, diarrhea, etc.) should be monitored carefully.

A study where pregnant dogs received 5 mg/kg daily demonstrated no teratogenic effects or effects on the pregnancy. It is unknown whether the drug enters milk.

Adverse Effects/Warnings - Ethacrynic acid may induce fluid and electrolyte abnormalities. Patients should be monitored for hydration status and electrolyte imbalances (especially potassium, calcium and sodium). Other potential adverse effects include ototoxicity (especially in cats with high dose IV therapy), gastrointestinal disturbances, hematologic effects (anemia, leukopenia), weakness and restlessness. Ethacrynic acid is thought to have a greater incidence of ototoxicity and GI effects than furosemide.

Overdosage/Acute Toxicity - The LD_{50} in dogs after oral administration is > 1000 mg/kg and after IV injection > 300 mg/kg. Chronic overdosing at 10 mg/kg for six months in dogs led to development of calcification and scarring of the renal parenchyma.

Acute overdosage may cause electrolyte and water balance problems, CNS effects (lethargy to coma and seizures) and cardiovascular collapse.

Treatment consists of emptying the gut after recent oral ingestion, using standard protocols. Avoid giving concomitant cathartics as they may exacerbate the fluid and electrolyte imbalances that can occur. Aggressively monitor and treat electrolyte and water balance abnormalities supportively. Additionally, monitor respiratory, CNS, and cardiovascular status. Treat supportively and symptomatically if necessary.

Drug Interactions - Pharmacologic effects of **theophylline** may be enhanced when given with ethacrynic acid. Ototoxicity and nephrotoxicity associated with the **aminoglycoside antibiotics** may be increased when ethacrynic acid is also used. If used concomitantly with **corticosteroids, corticotropin or amphotericin B,** ethacrynic acid may increase the chance of hypokalemia development. Ethacrynic acid-induced hypokalemia may increase chances of **digitalis** toxicity. There may be an increased risk of GI hemorrhage when ethacrynic acid is used with **corticosteroids**. Patients on **aspirin** therapy may need dosage adjustment as ethacrynic acid competes for renal excretory sites. Ethacrynic acid may inhibit the muscle relaxation qualities of **tubocurarine**, but increase the effects of **succinylcholine**. Enhanced effects may occur if ethacrynic acid is used concomitantly with **other diuretics**. The uricosuric effects of **probenecid** or **sulfinpyrazone** may be inhibited by ethacrynic acid. Ethacrynic acid may alter the requirements of **insulin** or other anti-diabetic agents in diabetic patients.

Doses -
  Dogs/Cats:
      a) 0.2 - 0.4 mg/kg IM or IV q4-12h (Allen, Pringle et al. 1993)

Monitoring Parameters - 1) Serum electrolytes, BUN, creatinine, glucose; 2) Hydration status; 3) Blood pressure, if indicated; 4) Symptoms of edema, patient weight, if indicated; 5) Evaluation of ototoxicity, particularly with prolonged therapy or in cats

Client Information - Recommend to administer dosage with meals when possible. Clients should contact veterinarian if symptoms of water or electrolyte imbalance occur. Symptoms such as excessive thirst, lethargy, lassitude, restlessness, oliguria, GI distress or tachycardia may indicate electrolyte or water balance problems.

Dosage Forms/Preparations/FDA Approval Status/Withholding Times -
  Veterinary-Approved Products: None
  Human-Approved Products:
    Ethacrynic acid Oral Tablets 25 mg, 50 mg; *Edecrin*® (Merck) (Rx)

    Ethacrynate Sodium Powder for Injection (for IV use only) equiv. to 50 mg ethacrynic acid/50 ml vial; *Edecrin Sodium*® (Merck); (Rx)

ETHANOL
ALCOHOL, ETHYL
ETHYL ALCOHOL

Chemistry - A transparent, colorless, volatile liquid having a characteristic odor and a burning taste, ethyl alcohol is miscible with water and many other solvents.

Storage/Stability/Compatibility - Alcohol should be protected from extreme heat or from freezing. Do not use unless the solution is clear. Alcohol may precipitate many drugs, do not administer other medications in the alcohol infusion solution unless compatibility is documented (see *Trissell* or other references for additional information).

Pharmacology - By competitively inhibiting alcohol dehydrogenase, alcohol can prevent the formation of ethylene glycol to its toxic metabolites (glycoaldehyde, glycolate, glyoxalate, and oxalic acid). This allows the ethylene glycol to be principally excreted in the urine unchanged. A similar scenario exists for the treatment of methanol poisoning. For alcohol to be effective however, it must be given very early after ingestion. It is seldom useful if started 8 hours after a significant ingestion.

Uses/Indications - The principal use of ethanol in veterinary medicine is in the treatment of ethylene glycol or methanol toxicity. While there is much interest in the use of 4-methyl pyrazole for ethylene glycol poisoning, alcohol is a readily available and economical alternative when patients present within a few hours after ingestion.

Ethyl alcohol is also used in aerosol form as a mucokinetic agent in horses.

Pharmacokinetics - Alcohol is well absorbed orally, but is administered intravenously for toxicity treatment. It rapidly distributes throughout the body and crosses the blood-brain barrier. Alcohol crosses the placenta.

Contraindications/Precautions/Reproductive Safety - Because ethylene glycol and methanol intoxications are life threatening, there are no absolute contraindications to ethanol's use for these indications.

Alcohol's safety during pregnancy has not been established for short term use. Use only when necessary.

Adverse Effects/Warnings - The systemic adverse effects of alcohol are quite well known. The CNS depression associated with the high levels used to treat ethylene glycol and methanol toxicity can confuse the clinical monitoring of these toxicities. Ethanol's affects on antidiuretic hormone may enhance diuresis. As both ethylene glycol and methanol may also cause diuresis, fluid and electrolyte therapy requirements need to be monitored and dealt with. Pulmonary edema may result. Other adverse affects include pain and infection at the injection site and phlebitis. Extravasation should be watched for and avoided.

When aerosolized in horses, irritation and bronchoconstriction may result.

Overdosage/Acute Toxicity - If symptoms of overdosage occur, either slow the infusion or discontinue temporarily. Alcohol blood levels may be used to monitor both efficacy and toxicity of alcohol.

Drug Interactions - A disulfiram reaction (tachycardia, vomiting, weakness) may occur if alcohol is used concomitantly with the following drugs: **chlorpropamide, metronidazole, furazolidone,** cephalosporins having methyltetrazolethiol side chain (**cefamandole, cefoperazone, cefotetan, moxalactam**). Alcohol may cause additive CNS depression when used with other **CNS depressant drugs** (*e.g.,* **barbiturates, benzodiazepines, phenothiazines, etc.**). Alcohol may affect glucose metabolism and affect i**nsulin or oral antidiabetic agents** effect. Alcohol may increase the severity of side effects seen with **bromocriptine.**

Doses -
Dogs:
> For ethylene glycol poisoning:
>> a) As a 20% solution, give 5.5 ml/kg IV q4h for 5 treatments, then q6h for four additional treatments. (Forrester and Lees 1994)

Cats:
> For ethylene glycol poisoning:
>> a) As a 20% solution, give 5 ml/kg IV q6h for 5 treatments, then q8h for four additional treatments. (Forrester and Lees 1994)

Monitoring Parameters - 1) Alcohol blood levels (and ethylene glycol or methanol levels); 2) Degree of CNS effect

Client Information - Systemically administered alcohol should be given in a controlled clinical environment.

Dosage Forms/Preparations/FDA Approval Status/Withholding Times -
Veterinary-Approved Products: None
Human-Approved Products:
   Alcohol (Ethanol) in Dextrose Infusions
      5% Alcohol & 5% Dextrose in Water (450 Cal/L 1114 mOsm/L) in 1000 mls (Abbott, Clintec) (Rx)
      5% Alcohol & 5% Dextrose in Water (450 Cal/L, 1125 mOsm/L) in 1000 mls (McGaw) (Rx)
      10% Alcohol & 5% Dextrose in Water (720 Cal/L, 1995 mOsm/L) in 1000 mls (McGaw) (Rx)

Note: Since alcohol infusions are generally only used in veterinary medicine for the treatment of ethylene glycol/methanol toxicity and obtaining medical or laboratory grade alcohol or the above mentioned products can be very difficult in an emergency situation, veterinarians have had to often improvise. One improvisation that has been successful, albeit not pharmaceutically elegant, is to use commercially available vodka diluted in an appropriate IV solution. Should this be necessary, it is recommended that an in-line filter be used for the IV. For information on obtaining tax-free alcohol for medicinal purposes contact a regional office of the Bureau of Alcohol, Tobacco, and Firearms.

ETHYLISOBUTRAZINE HCL

Chemistry - Ethylisobutrazine is a phenothiazine derivative with similar actions as acepromazine. Its chemical name is 2-ethyl-10-(3-dimethylamino-2-methypropyl) phenothiazine.

Storage/Stability/Compatibility - Should be protected from light and excessive heat. Injectable solution should be a colorless to light yellow or amber color. Discard if color deviates from above.

Pharmacology - The pharmacologic actions of ethylisobutrazine reportedly are very similar to other phenothiazines (*e.g.,* acepromazine), but clinical experience with this agent is much less than with acepromazine. For further information on the pharmacologic activity of phenothiazines, please refer to the acepromazine monograph.

Uses/Indications - Ethylisobutrazine is only approved for use in dogs. Approved indications include "..as an aid in controlling intractable patients during many common clinical procedures such as examinations, grooming and administration of medications; to control excessive barking in kennels; to control vomiting associated with motion sickness and with administration of anthelmintics; as an aid in the management of pruritis associated with severe dermatoses, especially those with a tendency toward self-mutilation" (Package Insert; *Diquel*®—Coopers).

Pharmacokinetics - No pharmocokinetic information was located for this agent.

Contraindications/Precautions - Not recommended for use in species other than dogs. Please refer to acepromazine monograph immediately preceding this one for more information regarding phenothiazines. The manufacturer also cautions to carefully observe patients receiving chronic therapy for blood dyscrasias and allergic reactions.

Adverse Effects/Warnings - Refer to the acepromazine monograph for more information regarding phenothiazines.

Overdosage - No information on overdoses was located regarding this agent; refer to the information for acepromazine for general guidelines regarding phenothiazine overdoses.

Drug Interactions - Ethylisobutrazine should not be given within one month of worming with an **organophosphate agent** as their effects may be potentiated. **Other CNS depressant agents (barbiturates, narcotics, anesthetics**, etc.) may cause additive CNS depression if used with ethylisobutrazine.
   Quinidine when given with phenothiazines may cause additive cardiac depression.
   Antidiarrheal mixtures (*e.g.,* Kaolin/pectin, bismuth subsalicylate mixtures) and **antacids** may cause reduced GI absorption of oral phenothiazines. Increased blood levels of both drugs may result if **propranolol** is administered with phenothiazines. Phenothiazines block alpha-adrenergic receptors which, if **epinephrine** is given, can lead to unopposed beta-activity causing vasodilation and increased cardiac rate.
   Phenytoin metabolism may be decreased if given concurrently with phenothiazines.
   Procaine activity may be enhanced by phenothiazines.

Doses -
  Dogs:
      a) 4.4 - 11 mg/kg IM or PO, or 2.2 - 4.4 mg/kg IV. Duration and degree of tranquilization may be varied between 6-72 hours by adjusting dosage. Young animals may require lower dosages. When used as a preoperative medication, the general anesthetic

dosage should be reduced and administered carefully to effect. (Package Insert; *Diquel®*— Coopers)

Monitoring Parameters -
1) Cardiac rate/rhythm/blood pressure if indicated and possible to measure
2) Degree of tranquilization
3) Body temperature (especially if ambient temperature is very hot or cold)

Client Information - Keep tablets stored in tight, child-resistant containers. Do not freeze injectable preparation. See monitoring parameters above. May discolor the urine to a pink or red-brown color; this is not abnormal.

Dosage Forms/Preparations/FDA Approval Status/Withholding Times -
Veterinary-Approved Products:

Ethylisobutrazine HCl Injection 50 mg/ml in 100 ml vials; *Diquel®* (Schering-Plough); (Rx) Approved for use in dogs.

Ethylisobutrazine HCl tablets (scored) 50 mg in bottles of 50; *Diquel®* (Schering-Plough); (Rx) Approved for use in dogs.

Human-Approved Products: None

ETIDRONATE DISODIUM

Chemistry - An analog of pyrophosphate, etidronate disodium (also known as EHDP, Na_2EHDP, or sodium etidronate) is a biphosphonate agent that occurs as a white powder and is freely soluble in water. Unlike pyrophosphate, etidronate is resistant to enzymatic degradation in the gut.

Storage/Stability/Compatibility - Store tablets in tight containers at room temperature. After dilution, the injectable product is stable for 48 hours at room temperature.

Pharmacology - Etidronate's primary site of action is bone. It reduces normal and abnormal bone resorption. This effect can reduce hypercalcemia associated with malignant neoplasms. Etidronate can also increase serum phosphate concentrations, presumably by increasing the renal tubular reabsorption of phosphate. Some early studies in lab animals suggest that etidronate may inhibit the formation of bone metastases with some tumor types.

Uses/Indications - The primary use in small animals at this time for etidronate is in the treatment of severe hypercalcemia associated with neoplastic disease. Etidronate is also indicated in humans for the treatment of Paget's disease and heterotopic ossification (*e.g.*, after total hip replacement). It is being evaluated for the treatment of osteoporosis in humans as well.

Pharmacokinetics - Oral absorption is poor and dose dependent. As little as 1% of a dose (smaller doses) may be absorbed; with higher doses, 6-10% may be absorbed. After oral dosing, the drug is rapidly cleared from blood and 50% of the drug absorbed goes into bone. At usual doses, it appears that etidronate does not cross the placenta. Duration of effect may be very prolonged. In humans, effects have persisted for up to one year after discontinuation in patient's with Paget's disease. Effects for hypercalcemia may last for 11 days. Absorbed etidronate is excreted unchanged by the kidneys. Approximately 50% of the absorbed dose is excreted within 24 hours, the remainder is chemisorbed to bone and then slowly eliminated.

Contraindications/Precautions/Reproductive Safety - Etidronate is considered contraindicated for the treatment of hypercalcemia in patients with renal function impairment (serum creatinines > 5 mg/dl). Risk vs. benefit should be carefully considered in patients with bone fractures (delays healing), enterocolitis (higher risk of diarrhea), cardiac failure (especially with parenteral etidronate as patients may not tolerate the extra fluid load) or in patients with renal function impairment (serum creatinines 2.5 - 5 mg/dl).

Etidronate's safety during pregnancy has not been established. Rabbits given oral doses 5 times those recommended in humans, demonstrated no overt problems with offspring. Rats given very large doses IV, showed skeletal malformations. It is unknown if the drug enters milk.

Adverse Effects/Warnings - Adverse effects are not well described in small animals. In humans, diarrhea and nausea (with higher oral doses), and bone pain/tenderness are most the likely adverse effects reported.

Do not confuse etidronate with **etretinate or etomidate**.

Overdosage/Acute Toxicity - Very little information is available at this time. Overdoses may result in hypocalcemia (ECG changes may occur), bleeding problems (secondary to rapid chelation of calcium) and proximal renal tubule damage.

Use standard gut emptying protocols after oral ingestion when warranted. IV calcium administration (*e.g.*, calcium gluconate) may be used to reverse hypocalcemia. Intensive monitoring is suggested.

Drug Interactions - Absorption of oral etidronate may be inhibited by **antacids (containing calcium, magnesium or aluminum), milk or other foods high in calcium content, or mineral supplements or medications containing iron, magnesium, calcium or aluminum**. Separate etidronate doses from these substances by at least two hours.

Laboratory Considerations - Etidronate may interfere with bone uptake of **technetium Tc 99m medronate or technetium Tc 99m oxidronate**

Doses -
   Dogs:
      For severe hypercalcemia associated with neoplastic disease:
         a) 5 mg/kg/day PO (Papich 1992)

   Cats:
      For severe hypercalcemia associated with neoplastic disease:
         a) 10 mg/kg/day PO (Papich 1992)

Monitoring Parameters - Serum calcium; serum protein

Client Information - Recommend to give dose on an empty stomach. If anorexia or vomiting occur; notify veterinarian.

Dosage Forms/Preparations/FDA Approval Status/Withholding Times -
   Veterinary-Approved Products: None
   Human-Approved Products:
      Etidronate Disodium Tablets 200 mg, 400 mg; *Didronel*® (Procter & Gamble); (Rx)

      Etidronate Disodium for Injection (for IV infusion only) 50 mg/ml (300 mg/amp) in 6 ml amps; *Didronel*® *I.V. Infusion* ((MGI Pharma) (Rx)

ETODOLAC

Chemistry/Storage/Stability/Compatibility - An indole acetic acid derivative non-steroidal antiinflammatory agent (NSAID), etodolac occurs as a white, crystalline compound that is insoluble in water, but soluble in alcohol or DMSO.

The commercially available veterinary tablets should be stored at controlled room temperature (15-30°C).

Pharmacology - Like other NSAIDs, etodolac has analgesic, antiinflammatory and antipyrexic activity. Etodolac appears to be more selective for inhibition of cyclooxygenase-2 than cyclooxygenase-1. This means that the drug should possess greater inhibition of the prostaglandins involved with pain and inflammation than those involved with cytoprotection of the GI tract and renal tissue. Etodolac is also thought to inhibit macrophage chemotaxis, which may explain some of its antiinflammatory activity.

Uses/Indications - Etodolac is labeled for the management of pain and inflammation associated with osteoarthritis in dogs. It may find uses however for a variety of conditions where pain and/or inflammation should be treated.

Pharmacokinetics - After oral administration to healthy dogs, etodolac is rapidly and nearly completely absorbed. The presence of food may alter the rate, but not the extent of absorption. Peak serum levels occur about 2 hours post dosing. Etodolac is highly bound to serum proteins. The drug is primarily excreted via the bile into the feces. Glucuronide conjugates have been detected in the bile but not the urine. Elimination half life in dogs varies depending whether food is present in the gut, which may affect the rate of enterohepatic circulation of the drug. These values range from about 8 hours (fasted) to 12 hours (non-fasted).

Contraindications/Precautions/Reproductive Safety - Etodolac is contraindicated in dogs previously found to be hypersensitive to it. It should be used with caution in dogs with preexisting or occult GI, hepatic, cardiovascular or hematologic abnormalities as NSAIDs may exacerbate these conditions. Patients may be more susceptible to renal injury from etodolac if they are dehydrated, on diuretics, or have preexisting renal, hepatic or cardiovascular dysfunction.

Safety of etodolac hs not been established in dogs less than 12 months of age. Safe use has also not been established in breeding, pregnant, or lactating dogs. Use only when the benefits clearly outweigh the potential risks of use in these animals.

Adverse Effects/Warnings - In clinical field studies, etodolac's primary adverse effect was vomiting/regurgitation, reported in about 5% of dogs tested. Diarrhea, lethargy, and hypoproteinemia were also reported in a small number of dogs. Urticaria, behavioral changes and inappetence were reported in less than 1% of dogs treated. It must be remembered however, that as the drug is used in many more dogs for significant periods of time, additional adverse effects may surface.

The manufacturer warns to terminate therapy if inappetence, vomiting, fecal abnormalities or anemia are observed.

Overdosage - Limited information is available, but in a safety study where dogs were given 40 mg/kg/day (2.7X) GI ulcers, weight loss, emesis and local occult blood were noted. Doses of 80 mg/kg/day (5.3X), caused 6 of 8 dogs to either die or become moribund secondary to GI ulceration. It should be noted that these were not single dose overdoses. However, they do demonstrate that there is relatively narrow therapeutic window for the drug in dogs and that doses should be carefully determined (*i.e.*, do not confuse mg/kg dosages with mg/lb).

Drug Interactions - Note: Although the manufacturer does not list any specific drug interactions in the package insert, it does caution to avoid or closely monitor etodolac's use with other drugs, especially those that are also highly protein bound. It also recommends closely monitoring, or avoiding using etodolac with any other ulcerogenic drugs (*e.g.*, corticosteroids, other NSAIDs).

In humans, there are many interactions possible with NSAIDs. Because clinical experience is limited in dogs, the following may or may not be clinically significant. Because etodolac is highly bound to plasma proteins, it may displace other highly bound drugs. Increased serum levels and duration of actions of **phenytoin, valproic acid, oral anticoagulants**, other **anti-inflammatory agents, salicylates, sulfonamides**, and the **sulfonylurea antidiabetic agents** may occur.

When **aspirin** is used concurrently with etodolac, plasma levels of etodolac could decrease and an increased likelihood of GI adverse effects (blood loss) could occur. Concomitant administration of aspirin with etodolac cannot be recommended.

Probenecid may cause a significant increase in serum levels and half-life of etodolac.

Serious toxicity has occurred when NSAIDs have been used concomitantly with **methotrexate**; use together with extreme caution.

Etodolac may reduce the saluretic and diuretic effects of **furosemide** and increase serum levels of **digoxin**. Use with caution in patients with severe cardiac failure.

Doses -

Dogs:

    a) For treatment of pain and inflammation associated with osteoarthritis: 10 - 15 mg/kg PO once daily. Dogs less than 5 kg cannot be accurately dosed with EtoGesic®. Adjust dose to obtain satisfactory response, but do not exceed 15 mg/kg. For long term therapy, reduce dose level to minimum effective dosage. (Package Insert; *EtoGesic*®—Fort Dodge)

Monitoring Parameters - Efficacy and adverse effects

Client Information - Because etodolac is a new drug for use in dogs, clients should be cautioned to monitor and report any significant change in the animal's health to the veterinarian.

Dosage Forms/Preparations/FDA Approval Status -

Veterinary-Approved Products:

Etodolac 150 mg and 300 mg scored tablets in bottles of 100 & 250; *EtoGesic*® (Fort Dodge); (Rx) Approved for use in dogs.

Human-Approved Products:

Etodolac 200 mg, 300 mg oral capsules and 400 mg, 500mg tablets; *Lodine*® (Wyeth-Ayerst); Rx

ETRETINATE
ACITRETIN

Note: Etretinate has recently been withdrawn from the market by its manufacturer and replaced with acitretin. Acitretin is an active metabolite of etritinate and has the same indications, but acitretin is reportedly dosed at a rate of 2/3's that of etrinate. For example, if the dose for etrinate is 2 mg/kg, then acitretin would be dosed at 1.32 mg/kg. Until a full monograph for acitretin can be written, use with extreme caution and refer to other current sources for information.

Pharmacology - Etretinate is a synthetic retinoid agent that may be useful in the treatment of several disorders related to abnormal keratinization and/or sebaceous gland abnormalities in small animals. The drug apparently has some anti-inflammatory activity, but its exact mechanism of action is not known.

Uses/Indications - Etretinate may be useful in the treatment of canine lamellar ichthyosis, solar-induced precancerous lesions in Dalmatians or in bull Terriers, actinic keratoses, squamous cell carcinomas, and intracutaneous cornifying epitheliomas (multiple keratoacanthomas).

While the drugs has been effective in treating idiopathic seborrhea (particularly in cocker spaniels), it is not effective in treating the ceruminous otitis that may also be present. Results have been disappointing in treating idiopathic seborrheas seen in basset hounds and West Highland terriers.

Etretinate's usage in cats is very limited, but it has shown some usefulness in treating paraneoplastic actinic keratosis, solar-induced squamous cell carcinoma and Bowen's Disease in this species.

Pharmacokinetics - Etretinate absorption is enhanced by high lipid content in the gut. After absorption, a high first pass effect in the liver limits etretinate amounts available to the systemic circulation. However, the acid form metabolite formed from this first pass effect is pharmacologically active. Etretinate and the active metabolite are highly bound to plasma proteins. The drug is subsequently metabolized to conjugate forms that are excreted in the bile and urine. Terminal half life can be very long probably due to storage in adipose tissue. In humans, terminal half life after six months of therapy is approximately 120 days.

Contraindications/Precautions/Reproductive Safety - Etretinate should only be used when the potential benefits outweigh the risks when the following conditions exist: cardiovascular disease, hypertriglyceridemia or sensitivity to etretinate.

Etretinate is a known teratogen. Major anomalies have been reported in children of women taking the medication. It should also be considered to be absolutely contraindicated in pregnant veterinary patients. Etretinate is excreted in rat milk. At this time, it is not recommended to be used in nursing mothers.

Adverse Effects/Warnings - At the present time, veterinary experience with this medication is limited, but incidence of adverse effects appear to less in companion animals than in people. Most animals treated (thus far) do not exhibit adverse effects. Potential adverse effects include: anorexia/vomiting/diarrhea, cracking of foot pads, pruritus, ventral abdominal erythema, polydipsia, lassitude, joint pain/stiffness, eyelid abnormalities and conjunctivitis (KCS), swollen tongue, and behavioral changes.

The most common adverse effect seen in cats is anorexia with resultant weight loss. If cats develop adverse effects, the time between doses may be prolonged (e.g., Every other week give every other day) to reduce the total dose given.

Do not confuse etretinate with **etidronate disodium** or **etomidate**.

Overdosage/Acute Toxicity - There appears to be very limited information on overdoses with this agent. Because of the drug's potential adverse effects, gut emptying should be considered with acute overdoses when warranted.

Drug Interactions - Etretinate used with **other retinoids** (isotretinoin, tretinoin, or vitamin A) may cause additive toxic effects. There may be increased potential for hepatotoxicity when etretinate is used with methotrexate or other **hepatotoxic drugs** (*e.g.*, anabolic steroids, androgens, asparaginase, erythromycins, estrogens, fluconazole, halothane, ketoconazole, sulfonamides or valproic acid); use with caution and increase monitoring. Use with **tetracyclines** may increase the potential for the occurrence of pseudotumor cerebri (cerebral edema and increased CSF pressure).

Laboratory Considerations - In humans, etretinate has caused significant increases in **plasma triglyceride, serum cholesterol, serum ALT (SGPT), serum AST (SGOT) and serum LDH concentrations. Serum HDL** (high density lipoprotein) concentrations may be decreased. Veterinary significance of these effects are unclear.

Doses -
Dogs:
  For treating seborrhea:
    a) In American cocker spaniels: 0.75 - 1 mg/kg PO once daily; may require long term therapy. (Kwochka 1992)
    b) 1 mg/kg PO once daily (q24h); response is seen within 2 months (Kwochka 1994)

  For treatment of primary seborrhea in cocker spaniels; primary keratinization disorders/ichthyosis; Schnauzer comedo syndrome; hair follicle dysplasias: 1 mg/kg once daily or divided q12h PO.

  For Sebaceous adenitis in Akitas or Samoyeds; Multiple infundibular keratanizing acanthomas: 1 - 2 mg/kg once daily or divided q12h PO.

  For actinic keratosis/solar-induced squamous cell carcinoma; epitheliotrophic lymphoma: 2 mg/kg once daily or divided q12h PO. (Power and Ihrke 1995)

  For sebaceous adenitis:
    a) 1 - 2 mg/kg PO once daily; may be useful particularly in long-coated breeds (Kwochka 1994)

Cats:
  For actinic keratosis/solar-induced squamous cell carcinoma; or Bowen's Disease: 10 mg/cat once daily PO. (Power and Ihrke 1995)

Monitoring Parameters - 1) Efficacy; 2) Liver function tests (baseline and if symptoms appear) 3) Schirmer tear tests (monthly—especially in older dogs)

Client Information - Acitretin should be handled by pregnant women in the household with extreme care, if at all. Veterinarians must take the personal responsibility to educate clients of the potential risk of ingestion by pregnant females.

Milk or high fat foods will increase the absorption of etretinate. To reduce variability of absorption, either have clients consistently give with meals or not. Long term therapy can be quite expensive.

Dosage Forms/Preparations/FDA Approval Status/Withholding Times -
  Veterinary-Approved Products: None
  Human-Approved Products:
    Acitretin 10 mg, 25 mg Capsules; Soriatane® (Roche); (Rx)

EUTHANASIA AGENTS CONTAINING PENTOBARBITAL

For therapeutic uses (other than euthanasia) of pentobarbital, see the main pentobarbital monograph for this agent. The sections on chemistry, storage, pharmacokinetics, overdosage, drug interactions, and monitoring parameters can be found in the main pentobarbital monograph also.

Pharmacology - Pentobarbital causes death by severely depressing the medullary respiratory and vasomotor centers when administered at high doses. Cardiac activity may persist for several minutes following administration.

Phenytoin is added to *Beuthanasia®-D Special* (Schering) and lidocaine to *FP-3®* (Vortech) for their added cardiac depressant effects and to denature the compounds from a Class-II controlled substance to Class-III drugs. Pentobarbital is also known as pentobarbitone.

Uses/Indications - For rapid, humane euthanasia in animals not intended for food purposes. Individual products may be approved for use in specific species. Barbituric acid derivatives are considered to be the "preferred method of euthanasia of individual dogs, cats, and other small animals." (AVMA Panel on Euthanasia, 1986).

Contraindications/Precautions - Must not be used in animals to be used for food purposes (human or animal consumption). Should be stored in such a manner that these products will not be confused with therapeutic agents. Extreme care in handling filled syringes and proper disposal of used injection equipment must be undertaken. Avoid any contact with open wounds or accidental injection. Keep out of reach of children.

Prior use of a tranquilizing agent may be necessary when the animal is in pain or agitated.

Adverse Effects/Warnings - Minor muscle twitching may occur after injection. Death may be delayed or not accomplished if injection given perivascularly.

Doses - Because different products have different concentrations, please refer to the information provided with the product in use.
  Dogs:
        Pentobarbital sodium (as a single agent): Approximately 120 mg/kg for the first 4.5 kg of body weight, and 60 mg/kg for every 4.5 kg of body weight thereafter. Preferably administer IV.

        Pentobarbital sodium with phenytoin (*Beuthanasia®-D Special*): 1 ml for each 4.5 kg of body weight
  Cats:
        Pentobarbital sodium (as a single agent): Approximately 120 mg/kg for the first 4.5 kg of body weight, and 60 mg/kg for every 4.5 kg of body weight thereafter. Administer IV.

        Pentobarbital sodium with phenytoin (*Beuthanasia®-D Special*): 1 ml for each 4.5 kg of body weight (not approved for use in this species)
Large Animals: (Note: **must not** be used in animals to be consumed by either humans or other animals). Depending on product concentration, most animals require 10 - 15 ml per 100 pounds of body weight.
Monitoring Parameters -
    1) Respiratory, cardiac rate, corneal reflex

Client Information - Must be administered by an individual familiar with its use. Inform client observing euthanasia, that animal may give a terminal gasp after becoming unconscious.

Dosage Forms/Preparations - See other pentobarbital dosage forms under the main monograph for lower concentration products.

  Pentobarbital Sodium for Injection (Euthanasia)
    Sleepaway® (Fort Dodge) 260 mg/ml; 100 ml vials; C-II
    Euthanasia-6® (Anthony) 390 mg/kg; 100 ml, 250 ml vials; C-II

Euthanasia Solution (Vet-Labs) 324 mg/ml; 100 ml vials; C-II

Pentobarbital Sodium 390 mg/ml/Phenytoin Sodium 50 mg/ml for Injection (Euthanasia)
  Beuthanasia® *-D Special* (Schering) 100 ml vials; C-III

Pentobarbital Sodium 390 mg/ml/Lidocaine 20 mg/ml for Injection (Euthanasia)
  FP-3® (Vortech) 100ml vials; C-III

All products are controlled substances and require a prescription. Pentobarbital alone is a Class-II controlled substance, combination products are generally Class-III.

Another barbiturate combination product similar to *Beuthanasia*®-D or *FP-3*® is: *Repose*® (Syntex) which contains 400 mg/ml secobarbital and 25 mg/ml dibucaine. The suggested dose for euthanasia in dogs and cats is: 0.22 ml/kg body weight IV.

FAMOTIDINE

Chemistry - An H_2-receptor antagonist, famotidine occurs as a white to pale yellow, crystalline powder. It is odorless, but has a bitter taste. 740 micrograms are soluble in one ml of water.

Storage/Stability/Compatibility - Tablets should be stored in well-closed, light-resistant containers at room temperature. Tablets are assigned an expiration date of 30 months after date of manufacture.

The powder for oral suspension should be stored in tight containers at temperatures less than 40°C. After reconstitution, the resultant suspension is stable for 30 days when stored at temperatures less than 30°C.; do not freeze.

Famotidine injection should be stored in the refrigerator (2-8°C). It is compatible with most commonly used IV infusion solutions and is stable for 48 hours at room temperature when diluted in these solutions.

Pharmacology - At the H_2 receptors of the parietal cells, famotidine competitively inhibits histamine, thereby reducing gastric acid output both during basal conditions and when stimulated by food, pentagastrin, histamine or insulin. Gastric emptying time, pancreatic or biliary secretion, and lower esophageal pressures are not altered by famotidine . By decreasing the amount of gastric juice produced, H_2-blockers also decrease the amount of pepsin secreted.

Uses/Indications - In veterinary medicine, famotidine may be useful for the treatment and/or prophylaxis of gastric, abomasal and duodenal ulcers, uremic gastritis, stress-related or drug-induced erosive gastritis, esophagitis, duodenal gastric reflux and esophageal reflux.

Although there is less veterinary experience with this agent than with either ranitidine or cimetidine, it has some potential advantages in that it suffers from fewer documented drug interaction problems and may suppress acid production longer than with either cimetidine or ranitidine. The clinical advantage of using famotidine over either drug has not been confirmed.

Pharmacokinetics - Famotidine is not completely absorbed after oral administration, but undergoes only minimal first-pass metabolism. In humans, systemic bioavailability is about 40-50%. Distribution characteristics are not well described. In rats, the drug concentrates in the liver, pancreas, kidney and submandibular gland. Only about 15-20% is bound to plasma proteins. In rats, the drug does not cross the blood brain barrier nor the placenta. It is distributed into milk. When the drug is administered orally, about 1/3 is excreted unchanged in the urine and the remainder primarily metabolized in the liver and then excreted in the urine. After intravenous dosing, about 2/3's of a dose is excreted unchanged.

The pharmacokinetics of famotidine, ranitidine, and cimetidine have been investigated (Duran and Ravis 1993) in horses After a single IV dosage, elimination half lives of cimetidine, ranitidine and famotidine all were in the 2-3 hour range and were not significantly different. Of the three drugs tested, famotidine had a larger volume of distribution (4.28 L/kg) than either cimetidine (1.14 L/kg) or ranitidine (2.04 L/kg). Bioavailability of each of the drugs was low; famotidine (13%), ranitidine (13.5%) and cimetidine (30%).

Contraindications/Precautions/Reproductive Safety - Famotidine is contraindicated in patients with known hypersensitivity to the drug.

Famotidine should be used cautiously in geriatric patients and in patients with significantly impaired hepatic or renal function. Famotidine may have negative inotropic effects and have some cardioarrhythmogenic properties. Use with caution in patients with cardiac disease.

In lab animal studies, famotidine demonstrated no detectable harm to offspring. Large doses may affect the mother's food intake and weight gain during pregnancy which may indirectly be harmful. Use in pregnancy when potential benefits outweigh the risks. In rats nursing from mothers receiving very high doses of famotidine, transient decreases in weight gain occurred.

Adverse Effects/Warnings - Because there is limited experience with this drug, its adverse effect profile has not been determined for veterinary species. Other H_2 blockers have been demonstrated to be relatively safe and exhibit minimal adverse effects. Potential adverse effects (documented in humans) that could be seen include GI effects (anorexia, vomiting, diarrhea), headache, or dry mouth or skin. Rarely, agranulocytosis may develop particularly when used concomitantly with other drugs that can cause bone marrow depression.

There have been reports of famotidine causing intravascular hemolysis when given intravenously to cats.

Overdosage/Acute Toxicity - The minimum acute lethal dose in dogs is reported to be >2 grams/kg for oral doses and approximately 300 mg/kg for intravenous doses. IV doses in dogs ranging from 5-200 mg/kg IV caused vomiting, restlessness, mucous membrane pallor and redness of the mouth and ears. Higher doses caused hypotension, tachycardia and collapse.

Because of this wide margin of safety associated with the drug, most overdoses should require only monitoring. In massive oral overdoses, gut emptying protocols should be considered and supportive therapy initiated when warranted.

Drug Interactions - Stagger doses (separate by 2 hours if possible) of famotidine with **antacids, metoclopramide, sucralfate, digoxin,** and **ketoconazole**. Famotidine may exacerbate leukopenias when used with other **bone marrow suppressing drugs**.

Unlike cimetidine or ranitidine, famotidine does not appear to inhibit hepatic cytochrome P-450 enzyme systems and dosage adjustments of other drugs (*e.g.,* warfarin, theophylline, diazepam, procainamide, phenytoin) that are metabolized by this metabolic pathway should usually not be required.

Laboratory Considerations - Histamine$_2$ blockers may antagonize the effects of histamine and pentagastrin in the **evaluation gastric acid secretion**. After using **allergen extract skin tests**, histamine$_2$ antagonists may inhibit histamine responses. It is recommended that histamine$_2$ blockers be discontinued at least 24 hours before performing either of these tests.

Doses -
  Dogs:
    As an adjunct in ulcer treatment:
      a) 0.5 mg/kg PO, SubQ, IM, IV q12-24 hours (Matz 1995)
      b) 0.5 - 1 mg/kg PO or IV once or twice daily (Johnson, Sherding et al. 1994)
  Cats:
    As an adjunct in ulcer treatment:
      a) 0.5 mg/kg PO, SubQ, IM, IV q12-24 hours (Matz 1995)
        Note: See the warning above about use IV in cats.
  Horses:
    As an adjunct in ulcer treatment:
      a) IV doses: 0.23 mg/kg IV q8h or 0.35 mg/kg IV q12h. Oral doses: 1.88 mg/kg PO q8h or 2.8 mg/kg PO q12h. (Duran and Ravis 1993)

Monitoring Parameters - 1) Clinical efficacy (dependent on reason for use); monitored by decrease in symptomatology, endoscopic examination, blood in feces, etc.; 2) Adverse effects, if noted

Client Information - To maximize the benefit of this medication, it must be administered as prescribed by the veterinarian; symptoms may reoccur if dosages are missed.

Dosage Forms/Preparations/FDA Approval Status/Withholding Times -
  Veterinary-Approved Products: None
  Human-Approved Products:
    Famotidine Film-coated Tablets 10 mg, 20 mg, 40 mg; *Pepcid*®. (Merck) (Rx);*Pepcid AC Acid Controller*® (J & J Merck); (Rx)

    Famotidine Oral Powder for Suspension 40 mg/5 ml (400 mg total); *Pepcid*®. (Merck); (Rx)

    Famotidine Injection 10 mg/ml in 2 ml single dose vials and 4 ml multidose vials; premixed - 20 mg per 50 ml in 0.9% NaCl *Pepcid*® *I.V.*.(Merck) (Rx)

FATTY ACIDS, ESSENTIAL/OMEGA
FISH OIL/VEGETABLE OIL DIETARY SUPPLEMENTS

Chemistry - The commercially available veterinary products generally contain a combination of fish oil (eicosapentaenoic and docosahexanoic acids), vegetable oil (gamma linolenic acid) which serve as essential fatty acids. They may also contain vitamin E (d-alpha tocopherol) and vitamin A.

Storage/Stability/Compatibility - The oral capsules should be stored in tight containers and protected from heat (cool, dry place).

Pharmacology - The exact pharmacologic actions of these products are not well described; particularly in light of the combination nature of the commercial products being marketed it is difficult to ascertain which compounds may be responsible for their proposed efficacy.

Fish oils affect arachidonic acid levels in plasma lipids and platelet membranes. They may affect production of inflammatory prostaglandins in the body, thereby reducing inflammation and pruritus. Linolenic or linoleic acids may be used as an essential fatty acid source which are necessary for normal skin and haircoats.

Uses/Indications - These products are generally indicated for the treatment of pruritus associated with atopy, and idiopathic seborrhea; and pruritus in cats for the adjunctive treatment of miliary dermatitis and eosinophilic granuloma complex.

Contraindications/Precautions/Reproductive Safety - Safe use in pregnancy has not been established; these products are not recommended for use in pregnant human patients.

Adverse Effects/Warnings - At high dosages, GI disturbances (*e.g.,* vomiting, diarrhea) may be seen. Rarely, some dogs become lethargic or more pruritic. In human patients, increased bleeding times and decreased platelet aggregation have been noted with use of fish oils; use with caution in patients with coagulopathies.

Overdosage/Acute Toxicity - With products containing vitamin A, acute toxicosis may result after accidental overdoses. Contact a poison control center for additional information.

Drug Interactions - Because of potential affects on bleeding times, use with caution in patients receiving anticoagulant medications such as **aspirin**, **warfarin** or **heparin**.

Doses -
  Dogs & Cats:
> Because of the unique nature of each commercially available product, see the actual label directions of that product for specific dosage recommendations.

Monitoring Parameters - Efficacy/Adverse Effects

Dosage Forms/Preparations/FDA Approval Status/Withholding Times -
  Veterinary-Approved Products:
  EFA-Caps® (Allerderm/Virbac); (OTC); Contains: Eicosapentaenoic acid 50 mg, Docosahexanoic acid 25 mg, Gamma linolenic acid 10 mg, Vitamin E 11 I.U. and vitamin A 850 I.U.

  EFA-Caps® *HP* (Allerderm/Virbac); (OTC); Contains: Eicosapentaenoic acid 100 mg, Docosahexanoic acid 60 mg, Gamma linolenic acid 30 mg, Vitamin E 11 I.U. and vitamin A 850 I.U.

  EFA Liquid (Allerderm/Virbac); (OTC); Contains: Vitamin E 1.8 U/ml, vitamin A 230 U/ml, Vitamin D2 54 U/ml in a base containing linoleic, linolenic, arachidonic, oleic, palmitoleic, and clupanodonic acids. Does not contain fish oil.

  Dermcaps®, *Dermcaps*® *ES*, and *Dermcaps*® *ES Liquid* (DVM); (OTC): all contain fish oil and vitamin E, but the exact concentrations are not listed on the label.

  Human-Approved Products:
  There are many fish oil capsules available without prescription having various trade names.

FEBANTEL

Chemistry - A phenylguanidine anthelmintic, febantel occurs as a colorless powder. It is insoluble in water and alcohol. Structurally, febantel is related to the benzimidazoles. As febantel is at least partially metabolized to fenbendazole and oxibendazole *in vivo*, it is sometimes categorized as a probenzimidazole agent.

Storage/Stability/Compatibility - Febantel (alone) should be stored at room temperature.

Partially used febantel (*Rintal*®) syringes may be stored for up to one year if capped tightly and expiration date is not exceeded. When mixed extemporaneously with trichlorfon (*Combot*®), it should be stored tightly sealed and used within 6 days if kept at room temperature and within 2 months if refrigerated. Mix well before administering.

Pharmacology - The mode of action of this agent is thought to be via inhibition of fumarate reductase in the worm, thereby blocking glucose uptake. The majority of the activity is believed to be derived from the active metabolites, fenbendazole and oxfendazole.

Uses/Indications - Febantel paste and oral (tube) suspension is indicated (labeled) for the treatment of large and small strongyles (*Strongulus vulgaris*, *S. edentatus*, *S. equinus*), ascarids (*P. equorum*—adult and sexually immature forms), and pinworms (*Oxyuris equi*—adult and 4th stage larva) in horses. In combination with trichlorfon (*Combotel*®), it is indicated (labeled) for the removal of the mouth and stomach stages of bots (*Gastrophilus intestinalis*, *G. nasalis*).

Febantel (in combination with praziquantel—*Vercom®*) is indicated (labeled) for the following intestinal parasites in dogs and puppies: hookworms (*Ancylostoma caninum*), roundworms (*Toxocara canis*), whipworms (*Trichuris vulpus*) and tapeworms (*Dipylidium caninum & Taenia pisiformis*).

Febantel (in combination with praziquantel—*Vercom®*) is indicated (labeled) for the following intestinal parasites in cats and kittens: hookworms (*Ancylostoma tubaeforme*), roundworms (*Toxocara canti*) and tapeworms (*Dipylidium caninum & Taenia taeniaeformis*).

Although not approved for use in cattle or sheep, febantel has greater than 85% efficacy against the following helminths in those species: Abomasal nematodes, small intestinal nematodes, large intestinal nematodes (*Oesophogostomum spp.*), lungworms and trematodes (*F. hepatica*— 4 week to 15 week stages; not in sheep).

Pharmacokinetics - In the horse, febantel is apparently readily absorbed from the GI tract and is rapidly metabolized to fenbendazole-sulphone, fenbendazole and oxibendazole. Febantel is also absorbed from the intestine in cattle and sheep. Sheep apparently absorb and metabolize the drug faster than do cattle. Maximum plasma concentrations occur 6-12 hours after dosing in sheep and 12-24 hours in cattle.

Contraindications/Precautions - When used alone in horses, the manufacturer lists no contraindications to the use of the drug. It is considered to be safe in breeding stallions and pregnant mares. The combination product (*Combotel®*) is labeled as being contraindicated in horses "...suffering from colic, diarrhea, constipation, or infectious disease until such conditions have been corrected."

The combination product (*Vercom®*) is contraindicated in pregnant small animals.

Adverse Effects/Warnings - When used at recommended dosages in horses, adverse reactions are unlikely to occur. Anaphylaxis is listed as a possible reaction, but case reports documenting this were not found in the literature. At very high doses (8 times labeled), a self-limiting diarrhea has been described.

Adverse effects in horses with the combination product *Combotel®*, include mouth irritation with resultant salivation, occasional diarrhea and colic. Adverse effects are more likely to occur if given on an empty stomach or if feed is withheld prior to dosing.

In dogs and cats, *Vercom®* (febantel & praziquantel) is unlikely to cause serious adverse effects at usual doses. Dogs may exhibit salivation, anorexia, emesis or gagging, and diarrhea or soft stools. Incidence of these effects was less than 3% of dogs treated in clinical trials. Cats may show signs (less than 10% incidence) of salivation, vomiting, depression and rejection of the paste. These effects are described as mild and self-limiting.

Overdosage/Toxicity - In horses, febantel has a reported 40X margin of safety after a single oral dose. Slightly decreased red blood cell counts, hemoglobin and hematocrit may be noted for 3 weeks after this dosage. Repeated doses of 8X recommended resulted only in a self-limiting diarrhea.

While, in horses there is a considerable safety factor for febantel, there is much less so for trichlorfon (in *Combotel®*). For more information on the toxicity for this compound (trichlorfon) refer to its monograph found later in this section.

The LD_{50} in dogs is greater than 10 g/kg of febantel. When administered at 15X recommended dose to mature dogs and cats, or 10X recommended dose to puppies or kittens for 6 days, transient salivation, diarrhea, vomiting and anorexia were noted. In dogs receiving 5 or 10 mg/kg PO for 90 days, testicular and prostatic hypoplasia were noted.

Drug Interactions, **Drug/Laboratory Interactions** - None reported.

Doses -
  Dogs:
    In combination with praziquantel (*Vercom®*) for labeled parasites (see Indications):
    a) Older than 6 months of age: 10 mg/kg (febantel)/1 mg/kg (praziquantel) PO for 3 days
       Puppies: 15 mg/kg (febantel)/1.5 mg/kg (praziquantel) PO for 3 days. (Package insert; *Vercom® Paste*—Miles)
  Cats:
    In combination with praziquantel (*Vercom®*) for labeled parasites (see Indications):
    a) Older than 6 months of age: 10 mg/kg (febantel)/1 mg/kg (praziquantel) PO for 3 days
       Kittens: 15 mg/kg (febantel)/1.5 mg/kg (praziquantel) PO for 3 days. (Package insert; *Vercom® Paste*—Miles)

Ruminants:
   For removal of GI nematodes:
      a) 5 - 10 mg/kg PO (Blagburn et al. 1989)
      b) 10 mg/kg PO (Roberson 1988b)

Horses:
   For labeled indications:
      a) 6 mg/kg PO or tube; retreat in 6-8 weeks if reinfection is likely to occur. (Robinson 1987), (Package Inserts; *Rintal*® Paste & Suspension—Miles)

Monitoring Parameters -1) Efficacy; 2) Adverse effects, if severe

Client Information - Clients should be informed on general measures to reduce exposure to helminth eggs and larva. Dogs with concomitant flea and *Dipylidium caninum* infestations should have measures taken to remove the fleas from the animal and the environment.

Dosage Forms/Preparations/FDA Approval Status -
  Veterinary-Approved Products:
    Febantel Oral Paste 45.5%; 6 gram, and 36 gram (multi-dose) syringe
      Rintal® Paste (Bayer), (OTC) Approved for use in horses.
    Febantel Suspension 93 mg/ml (9.3%) in 26 fl. oz. bottles
      Rintal® Suspension (Bayer); (Rx) Approved for use in horses.
    Febantel 3.4% (34 mg/gram) and Praziquantel 0.34% (3.4 mg/gram) Oral paste syringe; 4.8 g, 12 g, and 36 g syringes
      Vercom® Paste (Bayer); (Rx) Approved for use in dogs, cats, puppies, and kittens.

    Praziquantel/pyrantel pamoate plus febantel; *Drontal Plus Tablets*® (Bayer) (Rx) small, medium and large dog sizes

    May also be known as *Amatron*® or *Bayverm*® in the U.K..

  Human-Approved Products: None

FENBENDAZOLE

Chemistry - A benzimidazole anthelmintic, fenbendazole occurs as a white, crystalline powder. It is only slightly soluble in water.

Storage/Stability/Compatibility - Fenbendazole products should be stored at room temperature.

Uses/Indications - Fenbendazole is indicated (labeled) for the removal of the following parasites in **dogs**: ascarids (*Toxocara canis, T. leonina*), Hookworms (*Ancylostoma caninum, Uncinaria stenocephala*), whipworms (*Trichuris vulpis*), and tapeworms (*Taenia pisiformis*). It is not effective against *Dipylidium caninum*. Fenbendazole has also been used clinically to treat *Capillaria aerophilia*:, *Filaroides hirthi* and *Paragonimus kellicoti* infections in dogs.

Fenbendazole is indicated (labeled) for the removal of the following parasites in **cattle**: Adult forms of: *Haemonchus contortus, Ostertagia ostertagi, Trichostrongylus axei, Bunostomum phlebotomum, Nematodirus helvetianus, Cooperia spp., Trichostrongylus colubriformis, Oesophagostomum radiatum* and *Dictyocaulus vivaparus*. It is also effective against most immature stages of the above listed parasites. Although not approved, it also has good activity against *Moniezia spp.*, and arrested 4th stage forms of *Ostertagia ostertagi*.

Fenbendazole is indicated (labeled) for the removal of the following parasites in **horses**: large strongyles (*S. edentatus, S. equinus, S. vulgaris*), small strongyles (*Cyathostomum spp., Cylicocylus spp., Cylicostephanus spp.,Triodontaphorus spp.*) and pinworms (*Oxyuris equi*).

Fenbendazole is indicated (labeled) for the removal of the following parasites in **swine**: large roundworms (*Ascaris suum*), lungworms (*Metastrongylus apri*), nodular worms (*Oesphagostomum dentatum, O. quadrispinulatum*), small stomach worms (*Hyostrongylus rubidus*), whipworms (*Trichuris suis*) and kidney worms (*Stephanuris dentatus*; both mature and immature).

Although not approved, fenbendazole has been used in **cats, sheep, goats, pet birds and llamas**. See Dosage section for more information.

Fenbendazole is considered to be safe to use in pregnant bitches and is generally considered to be safe to use in pregnancy for all species.

Pharmacokinetics - Fenbendazole is only marginally absorbed after oral administration. After oral dosing in calves and horses, peak blood levels of 0.11 micrograms/ml and 0.07 micrograms/ml respectively, were measured. Absorbed fenbendazole is metabolized (and vice-versa) to the active compound, oxfendazole (sulfoxide) and the sulfone. In sheep, cattle, and pigs, 44-50% of a dose of fenbendazole is excreted unchanged in the feces, and <1% in the urine.

Contraindications/Precautions - Fenbendazole is not approved for use in lactating dairy cattle or for horses intended for food purposes.

Adverse Effects/Warnings - At usual doses, fenbendazole generally does not cause any adverse effects. Hypersensitivity reactions secondary to antigen release by dying parasites may occur; particularly at high dosages. Vomiting may infrequently occur in dogs or cats receiving fenbendazole.

  Single doses (even at exaggerated doses) are not effective in dogs and cats; must treat for 3 days.

Overdosage/Toxicity - Fenbendazole is apparently well tolerated at doses up to 100X recommended. The LD_{50} in laboratory animals exceeds 10 grams/kg when administered PO. It is unlikely an acute overdosage would lead to clinical symptoms.

Drug Interactions - Oxfendazole or fenbendazole should not be given concurrently with the **bromsalan flukicides (Dibromsalan, Tribromsalan)**. Abortions in cattle and death in sheep have been reported after using these compounds together.

Doses -
  Dogs:
  For susceptible Ascarids, hookworms, whipworms, and tapeworms (*Taenia spp.* only):
  a) 50 mg/kg PO for 3 consecutive days. (Package insert; Panacur®—Hoechst), (Cornelius and Roberson 1986)
  b) 55 mg/kg PO for 3 days (5 days for *Taenia*). (Chiapella 1988), (Reinemeyer 1985)
  For *Ascarids*:
  a) 50 mg/kg PO once daily for 3 days. (Todd, Paul, and DiPietro 1985)
  For *Capillaria plica*:
  a) 50 mg/kg once daily for 3 days; repeat a single 50 mg/kg dose 3 weeks later. (Todd, Paul, and DiPietro 1985)
  b) 50 mg/kg PO daily for 3-10 days. (Brown and Prestwood 1986)
  For *Capillaria aerophilia*:
  a) 25 - 50 mg/kg q12h for 10-14 days. (Hawkins, Ettinger, and Suter 1989)
  b) 50 mg/kg PO once daily for 10-14 days (Reinemeyer 1995)
  For *Filaroides hirthi*:
  a) 50 mg/kg PO once daily for 14 days. Symptoms may worsen during therapy, presumably due to a reaction when the worm dies. (Hawkins, Ettinger, and Suter 1989)
  b) 50 mg/kg PO once daily for 10-14 days(Reinemeyer 1995)
  For *Taenia spp.* tapeworms (not effective against *Dipylidium caninum*):
  a) 50 mg/kg PO for 3 days. (Todd, Paul, and DiPietro 1985)
  For *Paragonimus kellicoti*:
  a) 50 - 100 mg/kg PO divided twice daily for 10-14 days. (Todd, Paul, and DiPietro 1985)
  b) 50 mg/kg PO once daily for 10-14 days(Reinemeyer 1995)
  For *Trichuris* Colitis: Typhlitis:
  a) 50 mg/kg PO once daily for 3 consecutive days; repeat in 2-3 weeks and again in 2 months. (DeNovo 1988)
  For *Crenosoma vulpis:*
  a) 50 mg/kg PO once daily for 3 days(Reinemeyer 1995)
  For *Giardia:*
  a) 50 mg/kg PO once daily for 3 days (Barr and Bowman 1994)
  For *Eucoleus boehmi*:
  a) 50 mg/kg PO once daily for 10-14 days; improvement may only be temporary (Reinemeyer 1995)
  Cats:
  For susceptible Ascarids, hookworms, *Strongyloides*, and tapeworms (*Taenia spp.* only):
  a) 50 mg/kg PO for 5 days. (Dimski 1989)
  For lungworms (*Aelurostrongylus abstrusus*):
  a) 20 mg/kg PO once daily for 5 days; repeat after 5 days. (Todd, Paul, and DiPietro 1985)
  b) 25 - 50 mg/kg q12h for 10-14 days. (Hawkins, Ettinger, and Suter 1989)
  c) 50 mg/kg PO for 10 days. (Pechman 1989)
  d) 20 mg/kg PO once daily for 5 days; repeat in 5 days(Reinemeyer 1995)
  For lungworms (*Capillaria aerophilia*):
  a) 50 mg/kg PO for 10 days. (Pechman 1989)
  b) 50 mg/kg PO once daily for 10-14 days(Reinemeyer 1995)

For *Capillaria feliscati*:
  a) 25 mg/kg *bid* PO for 3-10 days. (Brown and Prestwood 1986)
  b) 25 mg/kg PO q12h for 10 days. (Brown and Barsanti 1989)

For *Paragonimus kellicoti*:
  a) 50 mg/kg PO daily for 10 days. (Pechman 1989)
  b) 50 mg/kg PO once daily for 10-14 days(Reinemeyer 1995)

Cattle:
  For removal/control of *Haemonchus contortus, Ostertagia ostertagi, Trichostrongylus axei, Bunostomum phlebotomum, Nematodirus helvetianus, Cooperia spp., Trichostrongylus colubriformis, Oesophagostomum radiatum, and Dictyocaulus vivaparus:*
  a) 5 mg/kg PO (Paul 1986)
  b) 7.5 mg/kg PO (Roberson 1988b)

  For *Moniezia spp.*, and arrested 4th stage forms of *Ostertagia ostertagi*:
  a) 10 mg/kg PO (Paul 1986), (Roberson 1988b)

Horses:
  For susceptible parasites:
  a) 5 mg/kg PO; 10 mg/kg once daily for 5 days to treat *S. vulgaris* in foals. (Robinson 1987)
  b) 5 mg/kg PO; 10 mg/kg for ascarids. (Roberson 1988b)
  c) For treatment of migrating large strongyles: 50 mg/kg PO for 3 consecutive days, or 10 mg/kg for 5 consecutive days. (Herd 1987)

Swine:
  For susceptible parasites:
  a) 5 mg/kg PO; 3 mg/kg in feed for 3 days; 10 mg/kg for ascarids (Roberson 1988b)
  b) For whipworms in potbellied pigs: 9 mg/kg PO for days (Braun 1995)

Sheep & Goats:
  For susceptible parasites:
  a) 5 mg/kg in feed for 3 days. (Roberson 1988b)

Llamas:
  For susceptible parasites:
  a) 10 - 15 mg/kg PO (as paste or suspension). (Fowler 1989)
  b) 5 - 10 mg/kg PO for 1-3 days. Fenbendazole and ivermectin are the most effective and safest anthelmintics for use in llamas. (Cheney and Allen 1989)

Birds:
  a) For *Ascaris*: 10 - 50 mg/kg PO once; repeat in 10 days. Do not use during molt (may cause stunted feathers) or while nesting.
      For flukes or microfilaria: 10 - 50 mg/kg PO once daily for 3 days.
      For *Capillaria*: 10 - 50 mg/kg PO once daily for 5 days. Is not effective against gizzard worms in finches. (Clubb 1986)
  b) For nematodes, some trematodes: 10 -50 mg/kg PO once daily for 3-5 days; 20 - 100 mg/kg oral single dose range; 125 mg/L of drinking water for 5 days (50 mg/L for 5 days in finches); or 100 mg/kg of feed for 5 days. Not recommended to be used in breeding season during molting. (Marshall 1993)

Reptiles:
  For susceptible infections:
  a) For most species: 50 - 100 mg/kg PO once; repeat in 2-3 weeks; very effective against *strongyloides*. (Gauvin 1993)

Dosage Forms/Preparations/FDA Approval Status -
Veterinary-Approved Products:
  Fenbendazole Granules 222 mg/gram (22.2%) in 0.18 oz & 1 g, 2 g, 4 g packets and 1 lb jars; *Panacur*® *Granules* 22.2% (Hoechst). (Rx) Approved for use in dogs.

  Fenbendazole Granules 222 mg/gram (22.2%); *Panacur*® *Granules* 22.2% (Hoechst). (OTC) Approved for use in horses not intended for food.

  Fenbendazole Suspension 100 mg/ml (10%); available in both equine and bovine labeled products; *Panacur*® *Suspension* (Hoechst). (Rx) Approved for use in horses (not intended for food) and cattle   Slaughter withdrawal=8 days (cattle). *Safe-Guard*® Suspension (Hoechst) (OTC) Approved for use in beef and dairy cattle. Slaughter withdrawal = 8 days

  Fenbendazole Paste 100 mg/gram (10%); available in both equine and bovine labeled products and sizes. *Panacur*® *Paste* (Hoechst). (OTC) Approved for use in horses (not intended for food) and cattle. Slaughter withdrawal=8 days (cattle). *Safe Guard Paste*® (Hoechst) (OTC)

Approved for use in horses not intended for food and cattle. Slaughter withdrawal = 8 days; no milk withdrawal time.

Fenbendazole Medicated Block 750 mg/lb.; 25 lb. block; *Safe-Guard Sweetlix*® (Hoechst); (OTC) Approved for use in beef cattle. Slaughter withdrawal= 16 days.

Fenbendazole Type B Medicated Feed

Safe-Guard EZ Scoop Swine Dewormer® (Hoechst) (OTC). 1.8% Fenbendazole No slaughter withdrawal time required

Safe-Guard 0.96% Scoop Dewormer® (Hoechst) (OTC) Approved for use in cattle. No milk withdrawal time; slaughter withdrawal time=13 days

Fenbendazole Type C Medicated Feed

Safe-Guard Free-choice Cattle Dewormer® (Hoechst) (OTC). 0.50% Fenbendazole (2.27 g/lb) Approved for use in beef and dairy cattle. No milk withdrawal time.

Safe-Guard 35% Salt Free-choice Cattle Dewormer® (Hoechst) (OTC) 1.9 g/lb Fenbendazole. Approved for use in dairy and beef cattle. Slaughter withdrawal time=13 days; no milk withdrawal time.

Fenbendazole Pellets

Safe-Guard 0.5% Cattle Top Dress® (Hoechst) (OTC) Slaughter withdrawal time=13 days; no milk withdrawal period

Safe-Guard 1.96% Scoop Dewormer Mini Pellets® (Hoechst) (OTC) Approved for use in beef and dairy cattle. No milk withdrawal time; slaughter withdrawal time=13 days

Fenbendazole Premix 20% Type A (200 mg/gram)

Safe-Guard Premix® (Hoechst). (OTC) Approved for use in swine. dairy and beef cattle, zoo & wildlife animals. Slaughter withdrawal for cattle = 13 days; no milk withdrawal time. Slaughter withdrawal for swine=none. Wildlife animal slaughter (hunting) withdrawal = 14 days.

Human-Approved Products: None

FENPROSTALENE

Chemistry - Fenprostalene is a methyl ester synthetic analogue of prostaglandin F_{2alpha}. No other information was located on the chemistry of the compound.

Storage/Stability/Compatibility - Fenprostalene injection should be stored at room temperature. At temperatures below 5°C, the commercial product may congeal, but stability and potency are unaffected. Viscosity should normalize after rewarming the vial.

Pharmacology - Fenprostalene exhibits pharmacologic actions similar to those of other prostaglandins of the F series. Effects on the female reproductive system include stimulation of myometrial activity, relaxation of the cervix, inhibition of steroidogenesis by corpora lutea, and potentially lysing corpora lutea.

Uses/Indications - Fenprostalene is labeled for use as an abortifacient in feedlot heifers during the first 150 days of gestation and for estrus synchronization in beef and non-lactating dairy cattle.

Pharmacokinetics - The pharmacokinetics of fenprostalene have been studied in lactating dairy cattle (Tomlinson, Spires, and Bowen 1985). The drug is apparently more slowly absorbed and eliminated than other prostaglandins. The percentage of drug excreted in the milk was not appreciably greater than other prostaglandins and is practically gone 48 hours after injection.

Contraindications/Precautions - Unless being used as an abortifacient or parturition inducer, fenprostalene should not be used during pregnancy in all species. Fenprostalene is contraindicated in animals with bronchoconstrictive respiratory disease (*e.g.,* asthma, "heavey" horses).

Give fenprostalene via the subcutaneous route only; do not administer intravenously nor intramuscularly. When injecting use a 16 gauge 1/2 - 3/4 inch needle. Suggested areas of injection are the neck, area behind shoulder or escutcheon (areas with freer movement between skin and underlying tissues).

Adverse Effects/Warnings - The adverse reaction reported with fenprostalene is a local reaction with possible bacterial infection at the injection site. Rarely, the infection may disseminate systemically and result in mortality.

Overdosage - No information was located. Should an inadvertent overdose occur, it is suggested to monitor the animal carefully and treat supportively if necessary.

Drug Interactions - Other **oxytocic agents**' activity may be enhanced by fenprostalene. Reduced effect of fenprostalene would be expected with concomitant administration of a **progestin**.

Doses-
  Cattle:
    To induce abortion in feedlot heifers at 150 days or less of gestation:
      a)   1 mg SQ. Approximately 92% success rate. Abortion occurs on average 5 days after administration. (Package Insert; *Bovilene*®—Syntex)
    For estrus synchronization in beef cattle and non-lactating dairy cattle:
      a)   Single injection method: Use only animals with mature corpus luteum. Examine rectally to determine corpus luteum maturity, anatomic normality, and lack of pregnancy. Give 1 mg SQ. Estrus should occur in 1-5 days. Breed at usual time after detecting estrus.

        Double injection method: Examine rectally to determine if animal is anatomically normal, not pregnant, and cycling normally. Give 1 mg SQ. Animals detected in estrus after the first injection may be bred at the usual time relative to estrus. Those not entering estrus should be given a repeat dose 11-13 days after the first injection. Estrus should occur in 2-5 days after second injection. Breed at usual time after detecting estrus or inseminate once at 80 hours post second injection, or twice at 72 and 96 hours post second injection.

        Any controlled breeding program should be completed by either observing animals (particularly during the 3rd week after treatment) and re-inseminating or hand mating after returning to estrus, or turning in clean-up bull(s) to cover any animals returning to estrus. (Package Insert; *Bovilene*®—Syntex)

Client Information - Fenprostalene should only be used by individuals familiar with its use and precautions. Pregnant women, asthmatics or other persons with bronchial diseases should handle this product with extreme caution. Any accidental exposure to skin should be washed off immediately using soap and water.

Dosage Forms/Preparations/FDA Approval Status/Withholding Times -
  Veterinary-Approved Products:
    Fenprostalene for Injection 0.5 mg/ml (500 micrograms/ml) in 20 ml and 50 ml vials; *Bovilene*® (Fort Dodge); (Rx) Approved for use in beef cattle and non-lactating dairy cattle. No preslaughter withdrawal is required when used as labeled. In uncooked edible tissues of cattle, safe concentrations for total residues have been reported to be 10 parts per billion (ppb) in muscle, 20 ppb in liver, 30 ppb in kidney, 40 ppb in fat and 100 ppb at the injection site.
  Human-Approved Products: None

FENTANYL, TRANSDERMAL

Note: A separate monograph for fentanyl/droperidol (Innovar®) follows this one.

Chemistry - Fentanyl citrate, a very potent opiate agonist, occurs as a white, crystalline powder. It is sparingly soluble in water and soluble in alcohol. It is odorless and tasteless (not recommended for taste test because of extreme potency) with a pK_a of 8.3 and a melting point between 147°-152°C.

Storage/Stability/Compatibility - Fentanyl transdermal patches should be stored at temperatures less than 25°C and applied immediately after removing from the individually sealed package.

Pharmacology - Fentanyl is a *mu* opiate agonist. The pharmacology of the opiate agonists are discussed in more detail in the monograph, Narcotic (opiate) Agonist Analgesics.

Uses/Indications - In veterinary medicine, fentanyl transdermal patches are used primarily in dogs and cats and have been shown to be useful for the adjunctive control of postoperative pain and in the control of severe pain associated with chronic pain, dull pain and non-specific, widespread pain (*e.g.,* associated with cancer, pancreatitis, aortic thromboemboli, peritonitis, etc.). Although clinical use in dogs and cats has been limited, thus far transdermal fentanyl has overall been clinically effective and has not had substantial adverse effect problems.

In humans, significant respiratory depression with use of the patches after surgery has precluded from using them post-operatively, but this has not been a significant problem in veterinary medicine.

Pharmacokinetics - There have been limited pharmacokinetic studies performed with transdermal fentanyl patches in dogs and cats. While therapeutic levels of fentanyl are attained, there is a significant interpatient variability with both the time to achieve therapeutic levels and the levels themselves. Cats tend to achieve therapeutic levels faster than do dogs and in dogs, the patch should be applied 24 hours in advance of need if possible, minimum of 12 hours pre-need. Most cats attain therapeutic benefit in about 6 hours after application. While applied, duration of action persists for at least 72 hours (usually for at least 104 hours). Duration of action is generally longer in cats than in dogs.

Contraindications/Precautions - Use cautiously with other CNS depressants, dosages of other opiates may need to be reduced when given with fentanyl transdermal, particularly several hours after application of the patch. Transdermal fentanyl should be used cautiously in geriatric, very ill or debilitated patients and those with a preexisting respiratory problem. Febrile patients may have increased absorption of fentanyl and will require increased monitoring should application be made.

Safe use in pregnancy has not been established.

Adverse Effects/Warnings - Respiratory depression and bradycardia associated with fentanyl patches are the most concerning adverse effects, but incidence of these effects have not been widespread thus far when used alone (without other opiates or other respiratory and cardiodepressant medications). Rashes at the patch site have been reported and should they occur, the patch should be removed. If an additional patch is warranted, a different site should be chosen. Urine retention and constipation may occur. Consider removing patch in patients developing a fever after application, as fentanyl absorption may increase. Some patients exhibit dysphoria after application; acepromazine or other mild tranquilizer may alleviate dysphoria.

Overdosage - Overdosage may produce profound respiratory and/or CNS depression in most species. Newborns may be more susceptible to these effects than adult animals. Other toxic effects may include cardiovascular collapse, tremors, neck rigidity, and seizures. Naloxone is the agent of choice in treating respiratory depression. In massive overdoses, naloxone doses may need to be repeated, animals should be closely observed as naloxone's effects may diminish before sub-toxic levels of fentanyl are attained. Mechanical respiratory support should also be considered in cases of severe respiratory depression.

Drug Interactions - For opiates (fentanyl): Other **CNS depressants** (*e.g.,* anesthetic agents, antihistamines, phenothiazines, barbiturates, tranquilizers, alcohol, etc.) may cause increased CNS or respiratory depression when used with opiates. Opiate analgesics are contraindicated in patients receiving **monamine oxidase (MOA) inhibitors** (rarely used in veterinary medicine) for at least 14 days after receiving MOA inhibitors (in humans).

Laboratory Interactions - Plasma **amylase** and **lipase** values may be increased for up to 24 hours following administration of opiate analgesics as they may increase biliary tract pressure.

Doses -

    Dogs/Cats: The following dosage regimen is used at the University of Minnesota Veterinary Teaching Hospital and is adapted from a presentation by Dr. Lynelle Graham:

In acutely painful patients provide alternative analgesia (injectable opioids, epidural opioids or constant rate infusion of opioids) until "lag" phase is completed (usually 6 hours in cats and a minimum of 12 hours in dogs).

Patch Size:

Patient	Dose	Fentanyl Content
Small Dogs ** (<5kg) & Cats	25 mcg/hr	2.5 mg
Dogs: 5-10 kg	25 mcg/hr	2.5 mg
Dogs: 10-20 kg	50 mcg/hr	5 mg
Dogs: 20-30 kg	75 mcg/hr	7.5 mg
Dogs: >30 kg	100 mcg/hr	10 mg

** Small dogs and cats may be dosed with 1/2 patch, but the patch **should not be cut in half!** Cover 1/2 the gel membrane with tape. "Half-patch dosing" is suggested for pediatric, geriatric and systemically ill cats and small dogs.

Patch may be placed either at dorsal or lateral cervical area, the lateral thorax or the inguinal area. If the neck is used, collars/leashes cannot be placed over the patch. Thorax is easily used and contact maximized (especially in cats), but can be difficult to bandage and the bald spot and change in hair growth/color may bother some clients. Inguinal area may be difficult to see and assess and some patients can lick/chew at the area. Regardless of site chosen, it must be clean and dry at the time of application and while the patch is attached. Do not place where a heating pad may come into contact. Site should be closely clipped with at least a 1 cm margin around the patch. Do not shave as cuts, abrasions or wounds can alter the absorption of fentanyl. After clipping, wipe with damp cloth to remove small hairs and skin debris; do not scrub or surgically prepare the site. Allow to completely dry.

Remove occlusive membrane from patch by folding back the edge and gently tear away the membrane to expose the sticky surface. Be careful not to expose your skin to the gel surface. Place patch over clipped area and hold it in place for 2-3 minutes to maximize adherence.

Use a slightly padded bandage or transparent dressing used with medical adhesive spray to assure adherence and to keep it dry. Check every few hours to ensure proper placement and adherence.

Dispose of used patches in a safe and effective manner.

Monitoring Parameters - 1) analgesic efficacy 2) heart rate and respiratory rate

Client Information - Explain carefully to clients how to apply (if applicable), remove and dispose of patches. Should accidental human skin contact occur, wash with water (only; no soap, etc.). Consider making application, removal and disposal an outpatient procedure, thereby bypassing concerns with clients.

Dosage Forms/Preparations/FDA Approval Status/Withholding Times -

Veterinary-Approved Products: None:

Human-Approved Products:

Transdermal: 2.5 mg (10 cm^2; 25 mcg/hr); 5 mg (20 cm^2; 50 mcg/hr); 7.5 mg (30 cm^2; 75 mcg/hr); 10 mg (40 cm^2; 100 mcg/hr); *Duragesic®-25* (etc.), (Janssen); (Rx) C-II

All fentanyl products are Class-II controlled substances.

FENTANYL CITRATE/DROPERIDOL

Chemistry - Fentanyl citrate, a very potent opiate agonist, occurs as a white, crystalline powder. It is sparingly soluble in water and soluble in alcohol. It is odorless and tasteless (not recommended for taste test because of extreme potency) with a pK$_a$ of 8.3 and a melting point between 147°-152°C.

Droperidol, a butyrophenone neuroleptic agent, occurs as a white to light tan, amorphous or macrocrystalline powder. One gram is soluble in 10 L of water and 600 ml of alcohol. It is odorless and tasteless (not recommended for taste test because of extreme potency) with a pK$_a$ of 7.6 and a melting point between 144°-148°C.

The combination commercially available products (*Innovar®* and *Innovar®-Vet*) have pH's of approximately 3-3.5.

Storage/Stability/Compatibility - Intact ampules and vials should be stored at room temperature and out of light. *Innovar®* has been reported to be **compatible** when mixed with the following agents: D5W, lactated Ringer's, D5 in lactated Ringer's, normal saline, benzquinamide, glycopyrrolate, heparin sodium, hydrocortisone sodium succinate, potassium chloride, and sodium bicarbonate. Compatibility is dependent upon factors such as pH, concentration, temperature and diluents used, and it is suggested to consult specialized references (*e.g., Handbook on Injectable Dugs* by Trissel; see bibliography) for more specific information.

Pharmacology - The butyrephenones (*e.g.,* droperidol) as a class cause tranquilization and sedation (sedation may be less so than with the phenothiazines), anti-emetic activity, reduced motor activity, and inhibition of CNS catecholamines (dopamine, norepinephrine). The pharmacology of the opiate agonists are discussed in more detail in the monograph, Narcotic (opiate) Agonist Analgesics. When used together droperidol/fentanyl will induce considerable neuroleptanalgesia. The actions of droperidol are said to potentiate the analgesic effects of fentanyl.

In dogs, *Innovar®* can cause decreased heart rates secondary to increased vagal tone and a decrease in arterial blood pressures. In cats, increased heart rates can be noted as well as a decrease in blood pressure.

Uses/Indications - Droperidol/fentanyl is approved in veterinary medicine only for use in the dog. It is indicated alone as a combination analgesic/tranquilizer for minor surgical, dental and orthopedic procedures and manipulations of short duration or (in combination with other general anesthetics) for major surgical procedures. It is condsidered by some clinicians to be the drug of choice as a chemical restraining agent in aggresive dogs. Fentanyl/droperidol has also been used as a tranquilizer/analgesic in cats.

Pharmacokinetics - No veterinary references regarding the pharmacokinetics of these agents were located. The onset of action after IV administration in dogs occurs within minutes and slightly longer after IM administration. In cats, after SQ injection, the onset of effect occurs within 20-30 minutes. Both drugs are metabolized in the liver and are eliminated in the urine (both as metabolites and unchanged drug). Duration of effect (at usual doses) after IM administration in dogs is generally 30-40 minutes, most animals will be sedated for several hours after anesthetic actions have ceased. Approximately 1.5 hours are necessary for dogs to recover after IV administration.

Contraindications/Precautions - This combination is not approved for use in food producing animals. Use cautiously with other CNS depressants, dosages of other anesthetics may need to be reduced when given after *Innovar®*. Pentobarbital dosages (for anesthesia) must be reduced for 4

hours after *Innovar®*. Perivascular injections may be irritating to surrounding tissue; avoid extravasation. Australian terriers may be resistant to the neuroleptanalgesic effects of *Innovar®* at usual doses, but exhibit side effects of tremors, excessive salivation, bradycardia, and diarrhea.

Adverse Effects/Warnings - In dogs, adverse effects with *Innovar®* are usually dose related and most commonly observed at the higher end of the dosing range. They include defecation, flatulence, respiratory depression, panting, nystagmus, head tremors, pain after IM injection, and personality changes (rare). Bradycardia and salivation can be seen if the animal is not pretreated with atropine or other anticholinergic agents. Animals may show a startle reaction following stimuli (*e.g.,* loud noises) and rarely seizures may develop.

A syndrome described as "woody chest" can occur after rapid IV administration. The thoracic musculature becomes very rigid and interferes with normal breathing, but can be treated with naloxone, or mechanical ventilation and muscle relaxant agents.

CNS stimulation, ataxia, and abnormal behavior (squealing, "goose-stepping", stumbling into objects) can be seen in pigs following IM administration.

IM or SQ injection may cause irritation and pain at the injection site.

Overdosage - Overdosage may produce profound respiratory and/or CNS depression in most species. Newborns may be more susceptible to these effects than adult animals. Other toxic effects may include cardiovascular collapse, tremors, neck rigidity, and seizures. Naloxone is the agent of choice in treating respiratory depression. In massive overdoses, naloxone doses may need to be repeated, animals should be closely observed as naloxone's effects may diminish before sub-toxic levels of fentanyl are attained. Mechanical respiratory support should also be considered in cases of severe respiratory depression. 4-aminopyridine has been demonstrated to act as an antagonist to droperidol in the dog at a dose 0.5 mg/kg IV, but it is not available in an approved commercially available dosage form.

Pentobarbital (6.6 mg/kg) has been suggested as a treatment for CNS effects (seizures) and extension and rigidity of the neck. Extreme caution must be used as barbiturates and narcotics can have additive respiratory depression effects.

Drug Interactions - For opiates (fentanyl): Other **CNS depressants** (*e.g.,* anesthetic agents, antihistamines, phenothiazines, barbiturates, tranquilizers, alcohol, etc.) may cause increased CNS or respiratory depression when used with opiates. Opiate analgesics are contraindicated in patients receiving **monamine oxidase (MOA) inhibitors** (rarely used in veterinary medicine) for at least 14 days after receiving MOA inhibitors (in humans).

For butyrephenones (droperidol): **CNS depressant agents (barbiturates, narcotics, anesthetics**, etc.) may cause additive CNS depression if used with butyrephenones.

Laboratory Interactions - Plasma **amylase** and **lipase** values may be increased for up to 24 hours following administration of opiate analgesics as they may increase biliary tract pressure.

Doses -

Caution: Doses are for the veterinary product (*Innovar-Vet®*) which is **8X** more concentrated than the human labeled product (*Innovar®*).

Dogs: To prevent bradycardia and excessive salivation, atropine (0.045 mg/kg SQ) or glycopyrrolate should generally be given 15 minutes prior to IV administration or concurrently with IM dose.

    a) For analgesia and tranquilization: 1 ml per 6.8 - 9.1 kg (0.11 - 0.15 ml/kg) IM or 1 ml per 11.35 - 27 kg (0.037 - 0.088 ml/kg) IV (Package Insert: *Innovar®-Vet*—P/M; Mallinckrodt)

    b) For general anesthesia: 1 ml per 18.2 kg (40 lbs.) IM; or 1 ml per 11.35 - 27.3 kg (25 - 60 lbs) IV. Followed by a general anesthetic (barbiturate, halothane, etc.) in 10 minutes after IM injection and 1 minute after IV injection. (Package Insert; *Innovar®-Vet*—P/M; Mallinckrodt)

    c) For tranquilization: 0.3 - 0.5 ml per 55 kg IV
       As a preanesthetic: 1 ml per 20 kg IM
       As an anesthetic for gastric dilatation: 1 ml per 10 - 30 kg.; dilute in 20 ml of saline, give IV slowly (Morgan 1988)

Cats:

    a) 1 ml/9 kg body weight (*Innovar®-Vet*) SQ; maximal effects occur between 30-60 minutes (Grandy and Heath 1987)

Monitoring Parameters -
    1) Level of neuroleptanalgesia
    2) Respiratory/cardiovascular status

Client Information - This drug should only be used by professionals familiar with its effects in a setting where adequate respiratory support can be performed.

Dosage Forms/Preparations/FDA Approval Status/Withholding Times -
Note: The veterinary approved product (*Innovar®-Vet*) is 8 times more concentrated than the human approved product. Do not confuse the two.

Veterinary-Approved Products: Note; this product may no longer be marketed.
Fentanyl citrate 0.4 mg/ml and Droperidol 20 mg/ml for Injection in 20 ml vials
Innovar®-Vet (Schering Plough); (Rx) Approved for use in dogs.

Human-Approved Products:
0.05 mg fentanyl (as citrate) and 2.5 mg droperidol per ml in 2 & 5 ml amps; *Innovar®* (Janssen); (Rx);*Fentanyl Citrate and Droperidol®* (Astra) (Rx)

Innovar® and *Innovar®-Vet* are Class-II controlled substances.

FENTHION

Chemistry - A topical organophosphate antiparasiticide, fenthion occurs as a yellowish-brown almost odorless, oily liquid. It is miscible with alcohol, but practically immiscible with water.

Storage/Stability/Compatibility - Follow storage and disposal directions as per each product's label. Do not mix with other agents.

Pharmacology - Fenthion is topically administered organophosphate. Organophosphates act by inhibiting acetylcholinesterase, thereby interfering with neuromuscular transmission of susceptible parasites.

Uses/Indications - In dogs, fenthion (*Pro-Spot®*) is indicated for the topical treatment of fleas. In cattle (non-lactating), fenthion is used in treating and controlling lice and cattle grub infestations. In swine, it is used for the control of lice.

Pharmacokinetics - No information was located.

Contraindications/Precautions/Reproductive Safety - Do not use on dogs less than 10 weeks of age or on stressed, sick or convalescing animals. Fenthion's safety on breeding males or on pregnant females has not been established.
  Do not treat calves less than 3 months old, or on stressed, sick or convalescing animals. Do not use in lactating animals. Do not treat cattle within 10 days of dehorning, shipping, weaning, or exposure to contagious or infectious disease.

Adverse Effects/Warnings - In dogs, adverse effects reported after using Pro-Spot® include anorexia, vomiting, loose stools/diarrhea, and intermittent coughing.
  In cattle, fenthion may cause bloat, excessive salivation and posterior paralysis. The manufacturer states that should such effects occur, it is highly probable that a host-parasite reaction exists. If a host-parasite reaction occurs, the manufacturer recommends not using atropine (unless a gross overdose) or stomach tubes to relieve bloat (trocarization may be useful). Anti-inflammatory agents may be useful.

Overdosage/Acute Toxicity - If overdoses occur, vomiting, tremors, hyperexcitability, salivation and diarrhea may occur. Cattle may present symptoms of frequent defecation, urination, salivation, muscular weakness or twitching. Use of succinylcholine, theophylline/aminophylline, reserpine, and respiratory depressant drugs (*e.g.*, narcotics, phenothiazines) should be avoided in patients with organophosphate toxicity. Treatment of organophosphate toxicity may range from careful observation if symptoms are mild and not progressing, to treatment with atropine and pralidoxime. Refer to those two monographs for more information on their use. If an ingestion or exposure occurs in a human, contact a poison control center, physician or hospital emergency room.

Drug Interactions - Acepromazine or other phenothiazines should not be given within one month of using an organophosphate agent as their effects may be potentiated. Because of its anticholinesterase activity, avoid the use of organophosphates with **DMSO**. Fenthion could theoretically enhance the toxic effects of **levamisole. Pyrantel Pamoate (or tartrate)** adverse effects could be intensified if used concomitantly with an organophosphate. Patients using organophosphates should not receive **succinylcholine** or other depolarizing muscle relaxants for at least 48 hours. Drugs such as **morphine, neostigmine, physostigmine** and **pyridostigmine** should be avoided when using organophosphates as they can inhibit cholinesterase.

Doses -
  Dogs:
      a) Read and follow directions for *Pro-Spot®*; Weigh animals prior to dosing. Be certain of the dose and the product you are using (there are two *Pro-Spot®* concentrations and five separate products available—see below). The labeled dose is: 4 - 8 mg/kg topically, not more often than once every two weeks.

Food Animals:
 Thoroughly read and follow label directions for use, including withdrawal times.

Monitoring Parameters - 1) Efficacy; 2) Adverse effects

Client Information - Thoroughly read label directions. Keep out of reach of children. Be sure client understands dosing recommendations and the importance of not exceeding them. Clients should report adverse effects immediately to veterinarian.

Dosage Forms/Preparations/FDA Approval Status/Withholding Times -
 Veterinary-Approved Products:

 Fenthion 20% Topical; *Spotton*® (Miles); (OTC) Approved for use in beef cattle and dairy cattle not of breeding age. Slaughter withdrawal = 45 days.

 Fenthion 3% Topical; *Tiguvon*® *(Cattle)* (Miles); (OTC) Approved for use in beef cattle and non-lactating dairy cattle. Slaughter withdrawal = 35 days after first treatment; if second treatment required = 45 days.

 Fenthion 3% Topical; *Tiguvon*® *(Swine)* (Miles); (OTC) Approved for use in swine. Slaughter withdrawal = 14 days.

 5.6% Topical: *Pro-Spot*® *10 & 20*; Fenthion 13.8%: *Pro-Spot*® *40, 80 & 160*; (Miles); (Rx) Approved for use in dogs.

Human-Approved Products: None

FERROUS SULFATE

Chemistry - An orally available iron supplement, ferrous sulfate occurs as odorless, pale-bluish-green, crystals or granules having a saline, styptic taste. In dry air the drug is efflorescent. If exposed to moisture or moist air, the drug is rapidly oxidized to a brownish-yellow ferric compound which should not be used medicinally. Exposure to light or an alkaline medium will enhance the conversion from the ferrous to ferric state.

 Ferrous sulfate is available commercially in two forms, a "regular" and a "dried" form. Regular ferrous sulfate contains 7 molecules of water of hydration and is freely soluble in water and insoluble in alcohol. Ferrous sulfate contains approximately 200 mg of elemental iron per gram. Dried ferrous sulfate consists primarily of the monohydrate with some tetrahydrate. It is slowly soluble in water and insoluble in water. Dried ferrous sulfate contains 300 mg of elemental iron per gram. Ferrous sulfate, dried may also be know as ferrous sulfate, exsiccated.

Storage/Stability/Compatibility - Unless otherwise instructed, store ferrous sulfate preparations in tight, light-resistant containers.

Pharmacology - Iron is necessary for myoglobin and hemoglobin in the transport and utilization of oxygen. While neither stimulating erythropoiesis nor correcting hemoglobin abnormalities not caused by iron deficiency, iron administration does correct both physical symptoms and decreased hemoglobin levels secondary to iron deficiency.

 Ionized iron is also a component in the enzymes cytochrome oxidase, succinic dehydrogenase, and xanthine oxidase.

Uses/Indications - While iron is a necessary trace element in all hemoglobin-utilizing animals, the use of therapeutic dosages of ferrous sulfate (or other oral iron) preparations in veterinary medicine is limited primarily to the treatment of iron-deficiency anemias in dogs (usually due to chronic blood loss), although it may occasionally be used in other species. Injectable iron products are usually used in the treatment of iron deficiency anemias associated with newborn animals.

Pharmacokinetics - Oral absorption of iron salts is complex and is determined by a variety of factors, including diet, iron stores present, degree of erythropoiesis, and dose. Iron is thought to be absorbed throughout the GI tract, but is most absorbed in the duodenum and proximal jejunum. Food in the GI tract may reduce the amount absorbed.

 After absorption, the ferrous iron is immediately bound to transferrin, and is transported to the bone marrow and eventually incorporated into hemoglobin. Iron metabolism occurs in a nearly closed system. Because iron liberated by the destruction of hemoglobin is reused by the body and only small amounts are lost by the body via hair and nail growth, normal skin desquamation and GI tract sloughing, normal dietary intake usually is sufficient to maintain iron homeostasis.

Contraindications/Precautions/Reproductive Safety - Ferrous sulfate (or other oral iron products) are considered contraindicated in patients with hemosiderosis, hemochromotosis, hemolytic anemias, or known hypersensitivity to any component of the product. Because of the GI irritating properties of the drugs, oral iron products are also considered contraindicated by some clinicians in patients with GI ulcerative diseases.

Adverse Effects/Warnings - Adverse effects associated with non-toxic doses are usually limited to mild gastrointestinal upset. Division of the daily dosage may reduce this effect, but dosage reduction may also be necessary in some animals.

Overdosage/Acute Toxicity - Ingestion of iron containing products may result in serious toxicity. While lethal doses are not readily available in domestic species, as little as 400 mg (of elemental iron) is potentially fatal in a child. Initial symptoms of acute iron poisoning usually present as an acute onset of gastrointestinal irritation and distress (vomiting—possibly hemorrhagic, abdominal pain, diarrhea). The onset of these effects may be seen within 30 minutes of ingestion, but also can be delayed for several hours. Peripheral vascular collapse may rapidly follow with symptoms of depression, weak and/or rapid pulse, hypotension, cyanosis, ataxia, and coma possible. Some patients do not exhibit this phase of toxicity and may be asymptomatic for 12-48 hours after ingestion, when another critical phase may occur. This phase may be exhibited by pulmonary edema, vasomotor collapse, cyanosis, pulmonary edema, fulminant hepatic failure, coma and death. Animals who survive this phase may exhibit long-term sequelae, including gastric scarring and contraction and have persistent digestive disturbances.

Because an acute onset of gastroenteritis may be associated with a multitude of causes, diagnosis of iron intoxication may be difficult unless the animal has been observed ingesting the product or physical evidence suggests ingestion. Ferrous sulfate (and gluconate) tablets are radiopaque, and often can be observed on abdominal radiographs. Serum iron levels and total iron binding capacity (TIBC) may also be helpful in determining the diagnosis, but must be done on an emergency basis to have any clinical benefit.

Treatment of iron intoxication must be handled as an emergency. In humans who have ingested 10 mg/kg or more of elemental iron within 4 hours of presentation, the stomach is emptied, preferably using gastric lavage with a large bore tube to remove tablet fragments. It is generally recommended to avoid using emetics in patients who already have had episodes of hemorrhagic vomiting. These patients are lavaged using tepid water or 1-5% sodium bicarbonate solution.

In dogs, one author (Mount 1989), has recommended using oral milk of magnesia to help bind the drug, administering apomorphine if appropriate to help dislodge tablets, and to instill a gastric lavage slurry of 50% sodium bicarbonate with a portion left in the stomach.

Deferoxamine is useful in chelating iron that has been absorbed. After chelation, a water soluble complex forms that is rapidly eliminated by the kidneys. Dosage recommendations for iron intoxicated dogs are:

    a) In severely affected animals: 40 mg/kg IV at a rate not exceeding 15 mg/kg/hr (avoiding hypotension); repeat every 4-12 hours at 20 mg/kg as determined by animal's response.

    In less acutely afflicted animals: 20 mg/kg q4-12h IM or SQ q3-12h.

    Three days of therapy may be required in severely poisoned animals. (Mount 1989)

    b) Initially, 10 mg/kg IM or IV for 2 doses, 2 hours apart. After the second dose has been given, the urine should be examined. If no color change is seen after the second dose and the animal is not exhibiting clinical signs or symptoms or intoxication, no further treatment is required. If the urine is a reddish-orange color, a significant amount of iron has been ingested and treatment should continue at 10 mg/kg q8h for 24 hours. Do not exceed 80 mg/kg total dose of deferoxamine in 24 hours. Continue to monitor carefully, particularly for shock. (Papich 1990)

In addition to chelation therapy, other supportive measures may be necessary, including treatment of acidosis, prophylactic antibiotics, oxygen, treatment for shock, coagulation abnormalities, seizures and/or hyperthermia. After the acute phases have resolved, dietary evaluation and management may be required.

Drug Interactions - Oral iron preparations can bind to orally administered **tetracyclines**, thereby decreasing the absorption of both compounds. If both drugs are necessary, give the tetracycline dose 2 hours before or 3 hours after the iron dose.

Because **chloramphenicol** may delay the response to iron administration, avoid using chloramphenicol in patients with iron deficiency anemia.

Iron can decrease the efficacy of **penicillamine**, probably by decreasing its absorption. Doses of the two drugs should be spaced as far apart as possible, should both be required.

Antacids, **eggs**, or **milk** administered concurrently with oral iron preparations can reduce the bioavailability of the iron. Separate iron doses from these items as far apart as possible.

Iron salts may precipitate **phosphate** in the GI tract.

Drug/Laboratory Interactions - Large doses of oral iron can color the feces black and cause false-positives with the **guiaic test for occult blood** in the feces. Iron does not usually affect the benzidine test for occult blood.

Doses - Caution: Unless otherwise noted, doses are for ferrous sulfate (regular—not dried). Dosing of oral iron products can be confusing; some authors state doses in terms of the iron salt and some state doses in terms of elemental iron. For the doses below, assume that the doses are for ferrous sulfate and not elemental iron, unless specified.

Dogs:

For iron deficiency anemia:

a) 100 - 300 mg PO once daily (Kirk 1986), (Morgan 1988)

Warning: in CVT X: Small Animal Practice (Kirk 1989): The dosage listed in the back of the book is for 100 - 300 **mg/kg** PO q24h, but it is believed that this dose is erroneous, as these doses would most probably be toxic and possibly fatal.

b) 60 - 300 mg PO per day for 2 weeks or more. (Adams 1988a)

c) First correct underlying cause of blood loss, then give ferrous sulfate at 100 - 300 mg per day PO. Absorption is enhanced if administered 1 hour before or several hours after feeding. Reduce dosage if GI side effects occur. (Harvey, French, and Meyer 1982)

Cats:

For iron deficiency anemia:

a) 50 - 100 mg PO once daily (Kirk 1986), (Morgan 1988)

b) 30 - 200 mg PO per day for 2 weeks or more. (Adams 1988a)

Cattle:

As a hematinic:

a) 8 - 15 g PO per day for 2 weeks or more. (Adams 1988a)

Horses:

As a hematinic:

a) 2 - 8 g PO per day for 2 weeks or more. (Adams 1988a)

Swine:

As a hematinic:

a) 0.5 - 2 g PO per day for 2 weeks or more. (Adams 1988a)

Sheep:

As a hematinic:

a) 0.5 - 2 g PO per day for 2 weeks or more. (Adams 1988a)

Monitoring Parameters -

1) Efficacy; adverse effects

a) hemograms

b) serum iron and total iron binding capacity, if necessary. Normal serum iron values for dogs and cats are reported as 80-180 micrograms/dl and 70-140 micrograms/dl, respectively. Total iron binding for dogs and cats are reported as 280-340 micrograms/dl and 270-400 micrograms/dl, respectively. (Morgan 1988)

Client Information - Because of the potential for serious toxicity when overdoses of oral iron-containing products are ingested by either children or animals, these products should be kept well out of reach of children and pets.

Dosage Forms/Preparations/FDA Approval Status/Withholding Times -

Veterinary-Approved Products: No veterinary-approved products containing only ferrous sulfate could be located, but there are many multivitamin with iron containing products available.

Human-Approved Products:

Ferrous Sulfate Tablets (20% elemental iron) 195 mg (39 mg iron), 300 mg (60 mg iron), 324 mg (65 mg iron); *Mol-Iron*®(Schering-Plough); *Feratab*® (Upsher-Smith); generic (OTC)

Ferrous Sulfate Caplets: 160 mg (50 mg iron); *Fe50* ® (Northampton) (OTC)

Ferrous Sulfate Capsules: 250 mg (50 mg iron);*Ferospace*® (Hudson); generic, (OTC)

Ferrous Sulfate Tablets Timed-Release 525 mg (105 mg iron); *Fero-Gradumet*® *Filmtabs*® (Abbott) (OTC)

Ferrous Sulfate Syrup 18 mg/ml (3.6 mg iron/ml) in pints; *Fer-In-Sol*® (Mead Johnson Nutritionals); (OTC)

Ferrous Sulfate Elixir 44 mg/ml (8.8 mg iron/ml) in pints and gallons 220 mg (44 mg iron) per 5 ml in pints and gallons

Feosol® (SKBeecham); (OTC); generic (OTC)

Ferrous Sulfate Drops 125 mg/ml (25 mg iron/ml) in 50 ml *Fer-In-Sol*® (Mead Johnson Nutritionals), *Fer-Iron*® (various generics), (OTC)

Ferrous Sulfate, Dried (exissicated) Capsules 190 mg (60 mg iron); *Fer-In-Sol*® (Mead Johnson Nutritionals); (OTC)

Ferrous Sulfate, Dried (exissicated) Capsules Timed-Release 159 mg (50 mg iron); 250 mg dried ferrous sulfate equivalent (50 mg iron); *Feosol*®(SK-Beecham); *Ferralyn Lanacaps*® (Lannett); *Ferra-TD*® (Goldline); generic (OTC)

Ferrous Sulfate, Dried (exissicated) Tablets 200 mg (65 mg iron); *Feosol*® (SK-Beecham); (OTC)

Ferrous Sulfate, Dried (exissicated) Tablets, Slow-Release 160 mg (50 mg iron); *Slow FE*® (Ciba Consumer); (OTC)

FINASTERIDE

Chemistry - Finasteride is a 4-azasteroid synthetic drug that inhibits 5 alpha-dihydroreductase (DH) and has a molecular weight of 372.55.

Storage/Stability/Compatibility - Store tablets below 30°C in tight containers and protected from light.

Pharmacology - Finasteride specifically and totally inhibits 5-alpha-reductase. This enzyme is responsible for metabolizing testosterone to dihydrotestosterone (DHT) in the prostate, liver and skin. DHT is a potent androgen and is the primary hormone responsible for the development of the prostate.

Uses/Indications - Finasteride is a new compound for use in humans to treat benign prostatic hypertrophy. It potentially may be useful in treating the same condition in canine patients. Because of the drug's relative expense and the long duration of therapy required to see a response, its usefulness may be limited in veterinary medicine.

Pharmacokinetics - Finasteride is absorbed after oral administration and in humans about 65% is bioavailable. The presence of food does not affect absorption. It is distributed across the blood-brain barrier and is found in seminal fluid. In humans, about 90% is bound to plasma proteins. Finasteride is metabolized in the liver and the half life is about 6 hours. Metabolites are excreted in the urine and feces. In humans, a single daily dose suppresses DHT concentrations for 24 hours.

Contraindications/Precautions/Reproductive Safety - Finasteride is contraindicated in patients hypersensitive to it. It should be used with caution in patients with significant hepatic impairment as metabolism of the drug may be reduced. Finasteride should be used in males only; do not use in sexually developing animals.

Adverse Effects/Warnings - The adverse effects reported in humans thus far has been very limited, mild and transient. Decreased libido, decreased ejaculate volume, and impotence have been reported.

Overdosage/Acute Toxicity - No information was located.

Drug Interactions - Anticholinergic drugs, adrenergic or xanthine-derivative bronchodilators may precipitate or aggravate urinary retention thereby negating the effects of the drug.

Doses -
  Dogs:
    For benign prostatic hyperplasia:
      a) 5 mg PO once daily; preliminary results. Lower doses may be effective, but dose response studies have not been reported. (Klausner, Bell et al. 1994)

Monitoring Parameters - Efficacy: Prostate exam

Client Information - Clients should understand that therapy may be prolonged before efficacy can be determined and that regular dosing compliance is mandatory.

Dosage Forms/Preparations/FDA Approval Status/Withholding Times -
  Veterinary-Approved Products: None
  Human-Approved Products:
    Finasteride Oral Tablets 5 mg; *Proscar*® (Merck); (Rx)

FIPRONIL

Chemistry/Storage/Stability/Compatibility - Fipronil is a phenylpyrazole antiparasitic agent. The commercially available topical products should be stored at room temperature, unless otherwise directed by the manufacturer. Commercially available solutions are flammable; keep away from heat and open flame.

Pharmacology - Fipronil's mechanism of action in invertebrates is to interfere with the passage of chloride ions in GABA regulated chloride channels, thereby disrupting CNS activity.

Uses/Indications - In the USA, Fipronil is indicated for the treatment of fleas and ticks in dogs and cats. It may be of use in other species as well, but available safety and efficacy data is not readily accessible.

Pharmacokinetics - The manufacturer states that fipronil collects in the oils of the skin and hair follicles and continues to be released over a period a time resulting in long residual activity. Topically applied, the drug apparently spreads over the body in approximately 24 hours via translocation.

Contraindications/Precautions/Reproductive Safety - Do not use on kittens less than 12 weeks of age and on puppies less than 10 weeks old. While temporary irritation may occur at the site of administration, animals who have demonstrated sensitivity reactions to fipronil or any of the ingredients in the products, should probably not be retreated.

The manufacturer warns that the product may be harmful to debilitated, aged, pregnant, or nursing animals.

Adverse Effects/Warnings - Rarely, hypersensitivity has been reported. Temporary irritation may occur at the site of administration.

Overdosage - No adverse effects have been reported in studies where 5X the maximum dose was administered to dogs and cats. Dogs fed 640 mg/kg and cats fed 320 mg/kg of fipronil showed no significant adverse effects.

Drug Interactions - Although the manufacturer does not list any known drug interactions, it warns that certain medications can interact with insecticides.

Doses - Note: Refer to the package information for specific instructions on application of fipronil products.

Dogs:
> For areas where high risk of infestation, if dog allergic to fleas or where tick control is needed: Apply *Frontline® Top Spot* once a month.
> For areas with less severe flea infestations, animals without flea dermatitis and where ticks are not a threat: Apply *Frontline® Top Spot* once every 2-3 months. (Label Information—*Frontline® Top Spot*; Merial)
> Spray: Intervals as above. 1.5 -3 ml per lb of body weight (1-2 pumps/lb. using the 250 ml btl. and 3-6 pumps/lb. using the 100 ml btl.). Pets with long or dense hair coats receive the higher dose rate.

Cats:
> For flea and tick control: Apply *Frontline® Top Spot* once a month. (Label Information—*Frontline® Top Spot*; Merial)
> Spray: Intervals as above. 1.5 -3 ml per lb of body weight (1-2 pumps/lb. using the 250 ml btl. and 3-6 pumps/lb. using the 100 ml btl.). Pets with long or dense hair coats receive the higher dose rate.

Monitoring Parameters - Efficacy

Client Information - Keep product away from children. Do not contaminate food, water or feed and dispose of container properly. Avoid human contact and wear latex gloves when applying/spraying. Avoid contact with animal until dry.

Remains effective after bathing (but do not shampoo within 48 hours of application), water immersion or exposure to sunlight. Spotted areas may appear wet or oily for up to 24 hours after application. Do not reapply for 30 days.

Dosage Forms/Preparations/EPA Approval Status -
Veterinary-Approved Products:
Fipronil Topical Solution 9.7% available in cards of 3 pipettes in 0.5 ml (cats/kittens; green), 0.67 ml (dogs up to 22 lb.; gold), 1.34 ml (dogs 23 - 44lbs; blue), 2.68 ml (dogs 45-88 lb.; purple); *Frontline® Top Spot* (Merial); (OTC) Approved for use in dogs and cats.

Fipronil Topical Spray 0.29% available in 100 ml (cat/small dog—each spray delivers 0.5 ml) and 250 ml (large dog—each trigger spray delivers 1.5 ml) spray btls; *Frontline® Spray Treatment* (Merial); (OTC) Approved for use in dogs and cats.

FLORFENICOL

Chemistry/Storage/Stability/Compatibility - A fluorinated analog of thiamphenicol, florfenicol is commercially available as light yellow to straw-colored injectable solution also containing n-ethyl-2-pyrolidone, propylene glycol and polyethylene glycol. It should be stored between 2°-30°C (36°-86°F).

Pharmacology - Like chloramphenicol, florfenicol is a broad spectrum antibiotic that has activity against many bacteria. It acts by binding to the 50S ribosome, thereby inhibiting bacterial protein synthesis.

Uses/Indications - The drug is approved for use in cattle only (in the USA) for the treatment of bovine respiratory disease (BRD) associated with *Pasteurella haemolytica, Pasteurella multocida* and *Haemophilus somnus.*

Because florfenicol has activity against a wide range of microorganisms (e.g., Mycoplasma), it may be useful for treating other infections in cattle (or other species) as well, but specific data supporting these uses is presently lacking.

Pharmacokinetics - After IM injection, approximately 79% of the dose is bioavailable. The drug appears to be well distributed throughout the body, including achievement of therapeutic levels in the CSF. In cattle, only about 13% is bound to serum proteins. Mean serum half life is 18 hours, but wide interpatient variation exists.

Contraindications/Precautions/Reproductive Safety - No contraindications are listed in the package insert, but see residue warnings (below). Safety or effects when used in breeding cattle, during pregnancy or during lactation are unknown and the manufacturer states that the drug is not for use in cattle of breeding age.

Caution: Do not give this drug IV.

Adverse Effects/Warnings - Noted transient adverse reactions in cattle include anorexia, decreased water consumption or diarrhea. Injection site reactions can occur that may result in trim loss. Reactions may be more severe if injected at sites other than the neck.

Overdosage - In toxicology studies where feeder calves were injected with up to 10X of the recommended dosage, the adverse effects noted above were seen, plus increased serum enzymes were noted. These effects were generally transient in nature. Long term (43 day) standard dosage studies showed a transient decrease in feed consumption, but no long-term negative effects were noted.

Drug Interactions - No specific drug interactions for florfenicol were located, but the drug may behave similarly to chloramphenicol. If so, florfenicol could antagonize the bactericidal activity of the **penicillins** or **aminoglycosides**. This antagonism has not been demonstrated *in vivo*, and these drug combinations have been used successfully many times clinically. Other antibiotics that bind to the 50S ribosomal subunit of susceptible bacteria (**erythromycin, clindamycin, lincomycin, tylosin**, etc.) may potentially antagonize the activity of chloramphenicol or vice versa, but the clinical significance of this potential interaction has not been determined. For other drug interactions that florfenicol may share with chloramphenicol, see that monograph or refer to other drug information resources.

Doses -
  Cattle:
    For treatment of BRD:
      a) 20 mg/kg IM (in neck muscle only); repeat in 48 hours. Alternatively, a single 40 mg/kg SubQ dose (in neck) may be used. Note: 20 mg/kg equates to 3 ml of the injection per 100 lb. of body weight. Do not exceed 10 ml per injection site. (*Nuflor*® Package Insert—Schering Plough)

Monitoring Parameters -1) Clinical efficacy 2) Injection site reactions

Client Information - Residue Warnings: Slaughter withdrawal is 28 days post injection if using the IM route; 38 days after the SubQ route. Not to be used in female dairy cattle 20 months of age or older. A withdrawal period has not been established in preruminating calves. Do not use in calves to be processed for veal.

Dosage Forms/Preparations/FDA Approval Status -
  Veterinary-Approved Products:
    Florfenicol Injection 300 mg/ml in 100 ml, 250 ml and 500 ml multi-dose vials; NuFlor® (Schering-Plough); (Rx). Approved for use in cattle; see residue warnings above.
  Human-Approved Products: None

FLUCONAZOLE

Chemistry - A synthetic triazole antifungal agent, fluconazole occurs as a white crystalline powder. It is slightly soluble (8 mg/ml) in water.

Storage/Stability/Compatibility - Fluconazole tablets should be stored at temperatures less than 30°C in tight containers. Fluconazole injection should be stored at temperatures from 5-30°C (5-25°C for the *Viaflex*® bags); avoid freezing. Do not add additives to the injection.

Pharmacology - Fluconazole is a fungistatic triazole compound. Triazole-derivative agents, like the imidazoles (clotrimazole, ketoconazole, etc.), presumably act by altering the cellular membranes of susceptible fungi, thereby increasing membrane permeability and allowing leakage of cellular contents and impaired uptake of purine and pyrimidine precursors. Fluconazole has efficacy against a variety of pathogenic fungi including yeasts and dermatophytes. *In vivo* studies using laboratory models have shown that fluconazole has fungistatic activity against some strains of *Candida, Cryptococcus, Histoplasma* and *Blastomyces. In vivo* studies of efficacy against *Aspergillus* strains have been conflicting.

Uses/Indications - Fluconazole may have use in veterinary medicine in the treatment of systemic mycoses, including cryptococcal meningitis, blastomycosis, and histoplasmosis. It may also be useful for superficial candidiasis or dermatophytosis. Because of the drug's unique pharmacokinetic qualities it is probably more useful in treating CNS infections than other azole derivatives. Fluconazole does not have appreciable effects (unlike ketoconazole) on hormone synthesis and may have fewer side effects than ketoconazole in small animals.

Pharmacokinetics - Fluconazole is rapidly and nearly completely absorbed (90%) after oral administration. It has low protein binding and is widely distributed throughout the body and has good penetration into the CSF, eye, and peritoneal fluid. Fluconazole is eliminated primarily via the kidneys and achieves high concentrations in the urine. In humans, fluconazole's serum half life is about 30 hours in patients with normal renal function. Patients with impaired renal function may have half-lives extended significantly and dosage adjustment may be required.

Contraindications/Precautions/Reproductive Safety - Fluconazole should not be used in patients hypersensitive to it or other azole antifungal agents and in patients with hepatic impairment only when the potential benefits outweigh the risks. Because fluconazole is eliminated primarily by the kidneys, fluconazole doses or dosing intervals may need to be adjusted in patients with renal impairment.

Safety during pregnancy has not been established and it is not recommended to be used in pregnant animals unless the benefits outweigh the risks.

Adverse Effects/Warnings - At the time of writing there is limited experience with this drug in domestic animals. Thus far, it appears to be safe to use in dogs. In humans, the side effects have been generally limited to occasional GI effects (vomiting, diarrhea, anorexia/nausea), and headache. Rarely, increased liver enzymes and hepatic toxicity, exfoliative skin disorders, and thrombocytopenia have been reported.

Overdosage/Acute Toxicity - There is very limited information on the acute toxicity of fluconazole. Rats and mice survived doses of 1 g/kg, but died within several days after receiving 1-2 g/kg. Rats and mice receiving very high dosages demonstrated respiratory depression, salivation, lacrimation, urinary incontinence, and cyanosis. If a massive overdose occurs, consider gut emptying and give supportive therapy as required. Fluconazole may be removed by hemodialysis or peritoneal dialysis.

Drug Interactions - Lab animal studies have shown that fluconazole used concomitantly with **amphotericin B** may have additive activity against *Candida*, indifferent effects on *Cryptococcus* and the effects may be antagonistic against *Aspergillus*. The clinical importance of these findings is not yet clear.

Fluconazole may cause increased prothrombin times in patients receiving **warfarin** or other coumarin anticoagulants. **Rifampin** may enhance the rate of metabolism of fluconazole; fluconazole dosage adjustment may be required. Fluconazole may increase the serum levels of **oral antidiabetic agents** (*e.g.,* chlorpropamide, glipizide, etc.) which may result in hypoglycemia.

Fluconazole may decrease the metabolism of **phenytoin or cyclosporin**. Veterinary significance is unclear.

Fluconazole may increase the risks of cardiovascular effects occurring if used concomitantly with either **terfenadine or astemizole**. If fluconazole is required, it is best to switch to another antihistamine.

Doses -
  Dogs:
      a) For susceptible fungal infections: 2.5 - 5 mg/kg PO once daily for 8-12 weeks (Forney and Allen 1992)

  Cats:
      For Cryptococcus, urinary tract or CNS mycoses: 2.5 - 10 mg/kg PO q12h (Wolf 1994)
      For cryptococcosis: 50 mg PO twice daily. Treatment should continue for 1 month beyond resolution of clinical signs. (Legendre 1995)

  Birds:
      As an alternate treatment of aspergillosis:
      a) 5 - 10 mg/kg PO once daily for up to 6 weeks, with or after amphotericin B. (Oglesbee and Bishop 1994a)

Monitoring Parameters - 1) Clinical Efficacy; 2) With long-term therapy, occasional liver function tests are recommended

Client Information - Compliance with treatment recommendations must be stressed. Have clients report any potential adverse effects. Fluconazole therapy may be prolonged (several weeks to months) and an average dosage in a cat (50 mg *bid*) may cost approximately $18/day.

Dosage Forms/Preparations/FDA Approval Status/Withholding Times -
   Veterinary-Approved Products: None
   Human-Approved Products:

   Fluconazole Oral Tablets 50 mg, 100 mg, 150 mg, 200 mg; *Diflucan®* (Roerig); (Rx)

   Fluconazole Powder for oral suspension: 10 mg/ml (when reconstituted) in 350 mg and 40 mg/ml (when reconstituted) in 1400 mg; *Diflucan®* (Roerig) (Rx)

   Fluconazole Injection: 2 mg/ml in 100 or 200 ml bottles or Viaflex Plus (available with sodium chloride or dextrose diluents); *Diflucan®* (Roerig) (Rx)

FLUCYTOSINE

Chemistry - A fluorinated pyrimidine antifungal agent, flucytosine occurs as a white to off-white, crystalline powder that is odorless or has a slight odor with pK_as of 2.9 and 10.71. It is sparingly soluble in water and slightly soluble in alcohol. Flucytosine may also be known as 5-fluorocytosine or 5-FC.

Storage/Stability/Compatibility - Store flucytosine capsules in tight, light-resistant containers at temperatures less than 40°C, and preferably at room temperature (15-30°C). The commercially available capsules are assigned an expiration date of 5 years from the date of manufacture.

Pharmacology - Flucytosine penetrates fungal cells where it is deaminated by cytosine deaminase to fluorouracil. Fluorouracil acts as an antimetabolite by competing with uracil, thereby interfering with pyrimidine metabolism and eventually RNA and protein synthesis. It is also thought that flucytosine is converted to fluorodeoxyuredylic acid that inhibits thmidylate synthesis and ultimately DNA synthesis.
   In human cells, cytosine deaminase is apparently not present or only has minimal activity. Rats apparently metabolize some of the drug to fluorouracil, which may explain the teratogenic effects seen in this species. It is unclear how much cytosine deaminase activity dog and cat cells possess.

Uses/Indications - Flucytosine is principally active against strains of *Cryptococcus* and *Candida*. When used alone, resistance can develop quite rapidly to flucytosine, particularly with *Cryptococcus*. Some cases of subcutaneous and systemic chromoblastosis may also respond to flucytosine.

Pharmacokinetics - Flucytosine is well absorbed after oral administration. The rate, but not extent of absorption will be decreased if given with food.
   Flucytosine is distributed widely throughout the body. CSF concentrations may be 60-100% of those found in the serum. In healthy humans, the volume of distribution is about 0.7 L/kg. Only about 2-4% of the drug is bound to plasma proteins. It is unknown if flucytosine is distributed into milk.
   Absorbed flucytosine is excreted basically unchanged in the urine via glomerular filtration. In humans, the half-life is about 3-6 hours in patients with normal renal function, but may be significantly prolonged in patients with renal dysfunction.

Contraindications/Precautions/Reproductive Safety - Flucytosine is contraindicated in patients hypersensitive to it.
   Flucytosine should be used with extreme caution in patients with renal impairment. Some clinicians recommend monitoring serum flucytosine levels in these patients and adjusting dosage (or dosing interval) to maintain serum levels at less than 100 micrograms/ml. One clinician (Macy 1987), recommends dividing the flucytosine dose by the serum creatinine level if azotemia develops.
   Use flucytosine with extreme caution in patients with preexisting bone marrow depression, hematologic diseases, or receiving other bone marrow suppressant drugs. Flucytosine should also be used cautiously (with enhanced monitoring) in patients with hepatic disease.
   Flucytosine has caused teratogenic effects in rats. It should be used in pregnant animals when the benefits of therapy outweigh the risks.

Adverse Effects/Warnings - Adverse effects that may be seen with flucytosine include bone marrow depression (anemia, leukopenia, thrombocytopenia), GI disturbances (nausea, vomiting, diarrhea), cutaneous eruption and rash, oral ulceration and increased levels of hepatic enzymes. Reports of aberrant behavior and seizures in a cat without concurrent CNS infection have also been noted after flucytosine use.

Overdosage/Acute Toxicity - No specifics regarding flucytosine overdosage was located. It is suggested that a substantial overdose be handled with gut emptying, charcoal and cathartic administration unless contraindicated.

Drug Interactions - When used with **amphotericin B**, synergism against Cryptococcus and Candida has been demonstrated *in vitro*. Toxicity of flucytosine may be enhanced however, secondary to amphotericin-caused diminished renal function and flucytosine accumulation. If clinically significant renal toxicity develops, flucytosine dosage may need to be adjusted.

Drug/Laboratory Interactions - When determining **serum creatinine** using the *Ektachem*® analyzer, false elevations in levels may be noted if patients are also taking flucytosine.

Doses -
 Dogs:
 For cryptococcosis:
 a) 25 - 50 mg/kg *qid* PO for a minimum of 6 weeks; with amphotericin B (0.5 mg/kg IV 3 times weekly for a minimum of 4-5 weeks until a cumulative dose of 4 mg/kg attained—see amphotericin B monograph for more information). (Noxon 1989)
 b) Flucytosine 150 - 175 mg/kg PO divided *tid-qid* with amphotericin B 0.15 - 0.4 mg/kg IV 3 times a week. When a total dose of amphotericin B reaches 4 - 6 mg/kg start maintenance dosage of amphotericin B at 0.15 - 0.25 mg/kg IV once a month with flucytosine at dosage above or with ketoconazole at 10 mg/kg PO once daily or divided *bid*. (Greene, O'Neal, and Barsanti 1984)

 For candiduria:
 a) To treat aggressively: After correcting identifiable predisposing factors, alkalinize urine to pH of >7.5 with oral sodium bicarbonate. Then give flucytosine at 67 mg/kg PO q8h. Reduce dose if patient has renal failure. (Polzin and Osborne 1985)

 Cats:
 For cryptococcosis:
 a) As an alternate to ketoconazole therapy: Flucytosine 200 mg/kg/day PO divided q6h with amphotericin B (0.25 mg/kg in 30 ml D5W given IV over 15 minutes q48h—See amphotericin B monograph for more information.). Continue therapy for 3-4 weeks after clinical signs have resolved and no organisms can be recovered. (Legendre 1989)
 b) 25 - 50 mg/kg *qid* PO for a minimum of 4-6 weeks; with amphotericin B (0.25 mg/kg IV 3 times weekly for a minimum of 3-4 weeks—see amphotericin B monograph for more information). (Noxon 1989)
 c) Flucytosine 125 - 250 mg/day PO divided *tid-qid* with amphotericin B 0.15 - 0.4 mg/kg IV 3 times a week. When a total dose of amphotericin B reaches 4 - 6 mg/kg start maintenance dosage of amphotericin B at 0.15 - 0.25 mg/kg IV once a month with flucytosine at dosage above or with ketoconazole at 10 mg/kg PO once daily or divided *bid*. (Greene, O'Neal, and Barsanti 1984)

 Birds:
 For susceptible fungal infections:
 a) In Psittacines: 250 mg/kg *bid* as a gavage. May be used for extended periods of time for aspergillosis. May cause bone marrow toxicity; periodic hematologic assessment is recommended.
 In raptors: 18 - 30 mg/kg q6h as a gavage.
 In Psittacines and Mynahs: 100 - 250 mg/lb in feed for flock treatment of severe aspergillosis or Candida (especially respiratory Candida). Apply to favorite food mix or mixed with mash. (Clubb 1986)

Monitoring Parameters -
 1) Renal function (at least twice weekly if also receiving amphotericin B)
 2) CBC with platelets
 3) Hepatic enzymes at least monthly

Client Information - Clients should report any symptoms associated with hematologic toxicity (abnormal bleeding, bruising, etc.). Prolonged treatment times, as well as costs of medication and associated monitoring, require substantial client commitment.

Dosage Forms/Preparations/FDA Approval Status -
 Veterinary-Approved Products: None

 Human-Approved Products:
 Flucytosine 250 mg, 500 mg Capsules; *Ancobon*® (Roche); (Rx)

FLUDROCORTISONE ACETATE

Chemistry - A synthetic glucocorticoid with significant mineralocorticoid activity, fludrocortisone acetate occurs as hygroscopic, fine, white to pale yellow powder or crystals. It is odorless or practically odorless and has a melting point of approximately 225°C. Fludrocortisone is insoluble in water and slightly soluble in alcohol.

Fludrocortisone acetate may also be known as fluohydrisone acetate, fluohydrocortisone acetate, 9alpha-fluorohydrocortisone acetate, or by the trade name *Florinef®* *Acetate* (SquibbMark).

Storage/Stability/Compatibility - Fludrocortisone acetate tablets should be stored at room temperature (15-30°C) in well-closed containers; avoid excessive heat. The drug is relatively stable in light and air.

Pharmacology - Fludrocortisone acetate is a potent corticosteroid that possesses both glucocorticoid and mineralocorticoid activity. It is approximately 10-15 times as potent a glucocorticoid agent as hydrocortisone, but is a much more potent mineralocorticoid (125 times that of hydrocortisone). It is only used clinically for its mineralocorticoid effects.

The site of action of mineralocorticoids is at the renal distal tubule where it increases the absorption of sodium. Mineralocorticoids also enhance potassium and hydrogen ion excretion.

Uses/Indications - Fludrocortisone is used in small animal medicine for the treatment of adrenocortical insufficiency (Addison's disease). It has also been suggested to be used as adjunctive therapy in hyperkalemia.

Additionally in humans, fludrocortisone has been used in salt-losing congenital adrenogenital syndrome and in patients with severe postural hypotension.

Pharmacokinetics - Fludrocortisone is well absorbed from the GI with peak levels occurring in approximately 1.7 hours in humans. Also in humans, plasma half-life is about 3.5 hours, but biologic activity persists for 18-36 hours.

Contraindications/Precautions - Fludrocortisone is contraindicated in patients known to be hypersensitive to it.

Fludrocortisone may be excreted in clinically significant quantities in milk. Puppies or kittens of mothers receiving fludrocortisone should receive milk replacer after colostrum is consumed.

Adverse Effects/Warnings - Adverse effects of fludrocortisone are generally a result of excessive dosage (see Overdosage below) or if withdrawal is too rapid. Since fludrocortisone also possesses glucocorticoid activity, it theoretically could cause the adverse effects associated with those compounds. (See the section on the glucocorticoids following this monograph for more information.)

Some dogs or cats may require additional supplementation with a glucocorticoid agent on an ongoing basis. All animals with hypoadrenocorticism should receive additional glucocorticoids (2-10 times basal) during periods of stress or acute illness.

Overdosage - Overdosage may cause hypertension, edema and hypokalemia. Electrolytes should be aggressively monitored and potassium may need to be supplemented. Patients should have the drug discontinued until symptoms and signs associated with overdosage have resolved and then restart drug at a lower dosage.

Drug Interactions - Patients may develop hypokalemia if fludrocortisone is administered concomitantly with **amphotericin B** or **potassium-depleting diuretics** (*e.g.,* thiazides, furosemide). As **diuretics** can cause a loss of sodium, they may counteract the effects fludrocortisone.

Potentially, fludrocortisone could increase the **insulin** requirements of diabetic patients or reduce **salicylate** blood levels. The clinical significance of these potential interactions with fludrocortisone have not been defined.

Doses -
  Dogs:
    For hypoadrenocorticism:
      a) Maintenance therapy: Initial dosage of 0.1 - 0.3 mg PO daily, either as a single dose or divided. Monitor serum sodium and potassium values every 1-2 weeks and adjust dosage by 0.05 - 0.1 mg per day. Once electrolytes have stabilized, monitor BUN, creatinine, and electrolytes every 3-4 months. Many patients require gradual increase in dosage over the first 6-18 months of therapy. Average long-term maintenance dosage is approximately 0.1 mg per 5 kg of body weight. Adjunctive therapy with oral sodium chloride supplementation (1 - 5 grams per day PO) may also be useful. (Schrader 1986)

      b) For maintenance: Usually 0.05 mg/kg divided *bid* daily; 20 kg dog usually requires 2 - 4 tablets daily. Only 50% of dogs receiving fludrocortisone require supplemental glucocorticoids chronically. Oral salt supplementation may lessen the amount of fludrocortisone required. (Feldman and Nelson 1987a)

   c) For chronic or subacute therapy: Begin at 0.1 mg PO daily for small dogs to 0.5 mg PO daily for large dogs; adjust based on serial electrolytes. Also give glucocorticoid supplementation (prednisone/- prednisolone 0.2 - 0.4 mg/kg/day) and IV fluid therapy if required (see reference for more information). (Feldman, Schrader, and Twedt 1988)

For adjunctive therapy of hyperkalemia:
   a) 0.1 - 1.0 mg per day PO; may induce iatrogenic hyperadrenocorticism. (Wheeler 1986)

Cats:
For maintenance therapy of hypoadrenocorticism:
   a) Once stabilized, 0.1 mg per day PO. Monitor serum electrolytes every 1-2 weeks initially and adjust dosage as necessary. For additional glucocorticoid supplementation, give either oral prednisolone or prednisone at 1.25 mg per day or monthly injections of methylprednisolone acetate 10 mg IM monthly. (Greco and Peterson 1989), (Peterson and Randolph 1989)

Monitoring Parameters -
   1) Serum electrolytes, BUN, creatinine; initially every 1-2 weeks, then every 3-4 months once stabilized
   2) Weight, PE for edema

Client Information - Clients should be familiar with the symptoms associated with both hypoadrenocorticism (*e.g.,* weakness, depression, anorexia, vomiting, diarrhea, etc.) and fludrocortisone overdosage (*e.g.,* edema) and report these to the veterinarian immediately.

Dosage Forms/Preparations/FDA Approval Status/Withholding Times -
  Veterinary-Approved Products: None
  Human-Approved Products:
   Fludrocortisone Acetate Tablets 0.1 mg; *Florinef®️ Acetate* (Apothecon); (Rx)

FLUMAZENIL

Chemistry - A benzodiazepine antagonist, flumazenil is a 1,4-imidazobenzodiazepine derivative.

Storage/Stability/Compatibility - Flumazenil is compatible with lactated Ringer's, D5W, or normal saline solutions. Once drawn into a syringe or mixed with the above solutions, discard after 24 hours.

Pharmacology - Flumazenil is a competitive blocker of benzodiazepines at benzodiazepine receptors in the CNS. It antagonizes the sedative and amnestic qualities of benzodiazepines.

Uses/Indications - Flumazenil may be useful for the reversal of benzodiazepine effects after either therapeutic use or overdoses. Flumazenil may be of benefit in the treatment of encephalopathy in patients with chronic intractable portosystemic encephalopathy. More studies are required for this potential indication however.

Pharmacokinetics - Flumazenil is administered by rapid IV injection. It is rapidly distributed and also rapidly metabolized in the liver. In humans, the average half life is about one hour.

Contraindications/Precautions/Reproductive Safety - Flumazenil is contraindicated in patients hypersensitive to it or other benzodiazepines or in patients with where benzodiazepines are being used to treat a potentially life-threatening condition (*e.g.*, status epilepticus, increased CSF pressure). It should also not be used in patients with a serious tricyclic antidepressant overdose. Flumazenil should not be used, or used with extreme caution, in patients with mixed overdoses where benzodiazepine reversal may lead to seizures or other complications.

 Flumazenil has caused some teratogenic effects in lab animals after very high dosages. Use during pregnancy only when necessary.

Adverse Effects/Warnings - In some human patients, flumazenil use has been associated with seizures. These patients usually have a long history of benzodiazepine use or are showing signs of serious tricyclic antidepressant toxicity. Adverse effects reported in humans include injection site reactions, vomiting, cutaneus vasodilatation, vertigo, ataxia and blurred vision. Deaths have been associated with its use in humans having serious underlying diseases.

Overdosage/Acute Toxicity - Large IV overdoses have rarely caused symptoms in otherwise healthy humans. Seizures, if precipitated have been treated with barbiturates benzodiazepines and phenytoin, usually with prompt responses.

Drug Interactions - Flumazenil does not alter benzodiazepine pharmacokinetics. Effects of **long-acting benzodiazepines** may recur after flumazenil's effects subside.

Doses -
Dogs, Cats:
As an antagonist for benzodiazepines:
a) 2 - 5 mg/kg IV (**Note**: this reference states the dose in mg/kg, but this may in fact be a "typo" and the dose may actually be: 2 - 5 mg IV (total dose); use with caution) (Bednarski 1992)
b) 0.1 mg/kg IV (Ilkiw 1992)

Monitoring Parameters - 1) Efficacy; 2) Monitor for seizures in susceptible patients

Client Information - Flumazenil should only be used in a controlled environment by clinically-experienced professionals.

Dosage Forms/Preparations/FDA Approval Status/Withholding Times -
Veterinary-Approved Products: None
Human-Approved Products:
Flumazenil Injection (for IV use) 0.1 mg/ml in 5 and 10 ml vials; *Romazicon*® (Hoffman-LaRoche) (Rx)

FLUMETHASONE

Note: For more information refer to the monograph: Glucocorticoids, General Information.

Chemistry - Flumethasone occurs as an odorless, white to creamy white, crystalline powder. Its chemical name is 6alpha,9alpha-difluoro-16alpha methylprednisolone.

Pharmacokinetics - No information was located for this agent.

Contraindications/Precautions - Flumethasone is contraindicated during the last trimester of pregnancy. Refer to the General Statement on the glucocorticoids for more information.

Doses -
Dogs:
For labeled indications (musculoskeletal conditions due to inflammation..., certain acute and chronic dermatoses ... when given orally, and also for allergic states or shock when given intravenously). Treat and adjust dosage on an individual basis:
a) Orally: 0.0625 - 0.25 mg daily in divided doses. Dosage is dependent on size of animal, stage and severity of disease.
Parenterally: 0.0625 - 0.25 mg IV, IM, SQ daily; may repeat.
Intra-articularly: 0.166 - 1 mg
Intra-lesionally: 0.125 - 1 mg (Package insert; *Flucort*®—Syntex)
b) 0.06 - 0.25 mg IV, IM, SQ, or PO once daily. (Kirk 1989)

Cats:
For labeled indications (certain acute and chronic dermatoses...). Treat and adjust dosage on an individual basis:
a) Orally: 0.03125 - 0.125 mg daily in divided doses.
Parenterally: 0.03125 - 0.125 mg IV, IM, or SQ. If necessary, may repeat. (Package insert; *Flucort*®—Syntex)
b) 0.03 - 0.125 mg IV, IM, SQ, or PO once daily. (Kirk 1989)

Horses:
For labeled indications (musculoskeletal conditions due to inflammation, where permanent changes do not exist..., and also for allergic states such as hives, urticaria and insect bites):
a) 1.25 - 2.5 mg daily by IV, IM or intra-articular injection. If necessary, the dose may be repeated. (Package insert; *Flucort*®—Syntex)
b) 1.0 - 2.5 mg/450 kg IV or IM (Robinson 1987)

Dosage Forms/Preparations/Approval Status/Withdrawal Times-
Veterinary-Approved Products: None
Flumethasone Tablets 0.0625 mg; *Flucort*® *Tablets* (Fort Dodge); (Rx) Approved for use in dogs and cats. Note: may not presently be available.

Flumethasone Injection 0.5 mg/ml in 100 ml vials; *Flucort*® *Solution* (Fort Dodge); (Rx) Approved for use in dogs, cats, and horses.
Human-Approved Products: None

FLUNIXIN MEGLUMINE

Chemistry - Flunixin meglumine, a nonsteroidal anti-inflammatory agent that is a highly substituted derivative of nicotinic acid, is unique structurally when compared to other NSAIDs. The chemical name for flunixin is 3-pyridine-carboxylic acid.

Storage/Stability/Compatibility - All flunixin products should be stored between 2-30°C (36-86°F). It has been recommended that flunixin meglumine injection not be mixed with other drugs because of unknown compatibilities.

Pharmacology - Flunixin is a very potent inhibitor of cyclooxygenase and like other NSAIDs, it exhibits analgesic, anti-inflammatory and antipyrexic activity. Flunixin does not appreciably alter GI motility in horses and may improve hemodynamics in animals with septic shock.

Pharmacokinetics - In the horse, flunixin is rapidly absorbed following oral administration with an average bioavailability of 80% and peak serum levels in 30 minutes. The onset of action is generally within 2 hours; peak response occurs between 12-16 hours and the duration of action lasts up to 36 hours. It is unknown how extensively flunixin is bound to plasma proteins or where it distributes in the body. It is unclear if the drug is extensively metabolized and exactly how the drug is removed from the body. Serum half-lives have been determined in horses ≈ 1.6 hours, dogs ≈ 3.7 hours; cattle ≈ 8.1 hours. Flunixin is detectable in equine urine for at least 48 hrs. after a dose.

Uses/Indications - In the United States, flunixin meglumine is approved for use in horses and cattle. However, it is approved for use in dogs in other countries. The approved indications for its use in the horse are for the alleviation of inflammation and pain associated with musculoskeletal disorders and alleviation of visceral pain associated with colic in the horse. In cattle it is approved for the control of pyrexia associated with bovine respiratory disease and endotoxemia, and for the control of inflammation in endotoxemia.

Flunixin has been touted for many other indications in various species, including: Horses: foal diarrheas, shock, colitis, respiratory disease, post-race treatment, and pre- and post ophthalmic and general surgery; Dogs: disk problems, arthritis, heat stroke, diarrhea, shock, ophthalmic inflammatory conditions, pre- and post ophthalmic and general surgery, and treatment of parvovirus infection; Cattle: acute respiratory disease, acute coliform mastitis with endotoxic shock, pain (downer cow), and calf diarrheas; Swine: agalactia/hypogalactia, lameness, and piglet diarrhea. It should be noted that the evidence supporting some of these indications is equivocal and flunixin may not be appropriate for every case.

Contraindications/Precautions - The only contraindication the manufacturer lists for flunixin's use in horses is for patients with a history of hypersensitivity reactions to it. It is suggested, however, that flunixin be used cautiously in animals with preexisting GI ulcers, renal, hepatic or hematologic diseases. When using to treat colic, flunixin may mask the behavioral and cardiopulmonary signs associated with endotoxemia or intestinal devitalization and must be used with caution.

In cattle, the drug is contraindicated in animals who have shown prior hypersensitivity reactions to it and is not recommended to be used in breeding bulls (lack of reproductive safety data).

Although reports of teratogenicity, effects on breeding performance, or gestation length have not been noted, flunixin should be used cautiously in pregnant animals.

Flunixin is usually considered to be contraindicated in cats, but some clinicians may use it short term (see doses).

Adverse Effects/Warnings - In horses following IM injection, reports of localized swelling, induration, stiffness, and sweating have been reported. Do not inject intra-arterially as it may cause CNS stimulation (hysteria), ataxia, hyperventilation, and muscle weakness. Symptoms are transient and generally do not require any treatment. Flunixin appears to be a relatively safe agent for use in the horse, but the potential does exist for GI intolerance, hypoproteinemia, and hematologic abnormalities to occur. Flunixin is not to be used in horses intended for food.

In horses and cattle, rare anaphylactic-like reactions have been reported, primarily after rapid IV administration.

In dogs, GI distress is the most likely adverse reaction. Symptoms may include, vomiting, diarrhea, and ulceration with very high doses or chronic use. There have been anecdotal reports of flunixin causing renal shutdown in dogs when used at higher dosages pre-operatively.

Overdosage - No clinical case reports of flunixin overdoses were discovered. It is suggested that acute overdosage be handled by using established protocols of emptying the gut (if oral ingestion and practical or possible) and treating the patient supportively.

Drug Interactions - Drug/drug interactions have not been appreciably studied for flunixin, but if it follows other NSAIDs it should be used cautiously with highly protein bound drugs such as **phenytoin, valproic acid, oral anticoagulants**, other **anti-inflammatory agents, salicylates, sulfonamides**, and the **sulfonylurea antidiabetic agents.**

Additionally, use flunixin cautiously with **warfarin, methotrexate**, and **aspirin** or other ulcerigenic agents. Flunixin could theoretically reduce the saluretic and diuretic effects of **furosemide**. Use with caution in patients with severe cardiac failure.

Doses -
Dogs:
a) 0.5 - 2.2 mg/kg IM or IV one time only (Jenkins 1987)
b) 1 mg/kg IM or IV once a day for no longer than 3 days (Davis 1985b)
c) For ocular indications: 0.25 mg/kg IV once daily for no more than 5 days at a time. May also be used preoperatively by injecting IV 30 minutes before ocular surgery. May dilute 1:9 (flunixin: sterile water) in syringe to administer accurately to very small animals. (Wyman 1986)
d) For ocular disease: 0.5 mg/kg IV *bid* for 1-2 treatments;
For acute gastric dilatation: 1 mg/kg IV once;
For GI tract obstruction: 0.5 mg/kg IV once to twice daily for 3 treatments (Morgan 1988)
e) For surgical pain: 1 mg/kg IV, subQ or IM initially once; 1 mg/kg subsequent daily doses
For pyrexia: 0.25 mg/kg IV, subQ or IM once, may be repeated in 12-24 hours if needed
For ophtho procedures: 0.25 - 1 mg/kgIV, IM or SubQ once, may be repeated in 12-24 hours if needed (Johnson 1996)

Cats:
As an antiinflammatory/analgesic:
For surgical pain: 0.25 mg/kg subQ once; once, may be repeated in 12-24 hours if needed
For pyrexia: 0.25 mg/kg IV, subQ or IM once, may be repeated in 12-24 hours if needed (Johnson 1996)

Rabbits/Rodents:
a) Rabbits: 1.1 mg/kg SubQ or IM q12h
Rodents: 2.5 mg/kg SubQ or IM q12h (Huerkamp 1995)

Cattle:
a) For labeled indications: 1.1 - 2.2 mg/kg (1 -2 mls per 100 lbs. BW) given slow IV either once a day as a single dose or divided into two doses q12h for up to 3 days. Avoid rapid IV administration. (Package Insert; *Banamine*® — Schering).
b) For treatment of radial nerve injury: 250 - 500 mg IV or IM *bid*, may need only one treatment; taper and discontinue usually after 2-3 days. (Rebhun 1986)
c) For aseptic lameness in cattle: 1.1 mg/kg, must be administered within 24 hrs after onset of symptoms to be effective. (Berg 1986)
d) 2.2 mg/kg then 1.1 mg/kg q8h IV (Jenkins 1987)

Horses:
a) Injectable: 1.1 mg/kg IV or IM once daily for up to 5 days. For colic cases, use IV route and may redose when necessary.
Oral Paste: 1.1 mg/kg PO (see markings on syringe—calibrated in 250 lb. weight increments) once daily. One syringe will treat a 1000 lb. horse for 3 days. Do not exceed 5 days of consecutive therapy.
Oral Granules: 1.1 mg/kg PO once daily. One packet will treat 500lbs of body weight. May apply on feed. Do not exceed 5 consecutive days of therapy. (Package Inserts - Schering Animal Health for *Banamine*®)
b) 1.1 mg/kg IM or IV q12h to treat moderate to severe pain. (Clark and Becht 1987)
c) 1.1 mg/kg IM or IV; duration of effect averages 4-36 hrs depending upon cause and severity of abdominal pain. (Muir 1987)

Birds:
a) 1 - 10 mg/kg IM. May be indicated for pain, shock and trauma. True analgesic effects unknown in avian species, but has no detrimental respiratory effects. Vomiting and straining to defecate may occur after administration. (Wheler 1993)

Monitoring Parameters -
1) Analgesic/anti-inflammatory/antipyrexic effects
2) GI effects in dogs
3) CBC's, occult blood in feces with chronic use in horses

Client Information - If injecting IM, do not inject into neck muscles.

Dosage Forms/Preparations/FDA Approval Status/Withholding Times -
Veterinary-Approved Products: Flunixin is approved only for use in horses not intended for food; for beef cattle and non-lactating dairy cattle. Slaughter withdrawal time in cattle = 4 days.

Flunixin Meglumine for Injection 50 mg/ml; in 50 and 100 ml vials; *Banamine*® (Schering); (Rx)

Flunixin Meglumine Oral Paste 1500 mg/syringe; 30 gram syringe containing 1500 mg flunixin in boxes of 6; *Banamine*® (Schering); (Rx)

Flunixin Meglumine Oral Granules 250 mg: 10 gram sachets, each sachet contains 250 mg flunixin in boxes of 50. 500 mg: 20 g sachets, each sachet contains 500 mg flunixin in boxes of 25; *Banamine*® (Schering); (Rx)

Flunixin may also be known as *Finadyne*®.

Human-Approved Products: None

5-Fluorocytosine - see Flucytosine

FLUOXETINE HCL

Chemistry - A member of the phenylpropylamine-derivative antidepressant group, fluoxetine differs both structurally and pharmacologically from either the tricyclic or monoamine oxidase inhibitor antidepressants. Fluoxetine HCl occurs as a white to off-white crystalline solid. Approximately 50 mg is soluble in 1 ml of water.

Storage/Stability/Compatibility - Capsules should be stored in well-closed containers. The oral liquid should be stored in tight, light-resistant containers. Both products should be stored at room temperature.

Pharmacology - Fluoxetine is a highly selective inhibitor of the reuptake of serotonin in the CNS thereby potentiating the pharmacologic activity of serotonin. Fluoxetine apparently has little effect on other neurotransmitters (*e.g.*, dopamine or norepinephrine).

Uses/Indications - While there has been considerable interest and lay press coverage of the use of fluoxetine in dogs, there is a general lack of scientific information available on its usefulness. The drug purportedly may have efficacy in treating stereotypic and obsessive-compulsive behaviors as well as phobic disorders, however much more experience and study is necessary before it or the other serotonin inhibitors can be routinely recommended..

Pharmacokinetics - Fluoxetine is apparently well absorbed after oral administration. In a study done in beagles, approximately 70% of an oral dose reached the systemic circulation. The presence of food altered the rate, but not the extent of absorption. The oral capsules and oral liquid apparently are bioequivalent.

Fluoxetine and its principal metabolite, norfluoxetine (active) are apparently distributed throughout the body with highest levels found in the lungs and the liver. CNS concentrations are detected within one hour of dosing. In humans, fluoxetine is approximately 95% bound to plasma proteins. Fluoxetine crosses the placenta in rats, but it is unknown if it does so in other species. Fluoxetine enters maternal milk in concentrations about 20-30% of those found in the plasma.

Fluoxetine is primarily metabolized in the liver to a variety of metabolites, including norfluoxetine, which is active. Both fluoxetine and norfluoxetine are eliminated slowly. In humans, the elimination half of fluoxetine is about 2-3 days and norfluoxetine, about 7-9 days. Wide interpatient variation does occur however. Renal impairment does not apparently affect elimination rates substantially, but liver impairment will decrease clearance rates.

Contraindications/Precautions/Reproductive Safety - Fluoxetine is considered to be contraindicated in patients with known hypersensitivity to it, as well as those receiving monoamine oxidase inhibitors (see Drug Interactions below). It should be used with caution in patients with diabetes mellitus as it may alter blood glucose. Its effect on patients with seizure disorders is not known (some overdose patients have developed seizures), so use with caution in these patients. Dosages may need to be reduced in patients with severe hepatic impairment.

Fluoxetine's safety during pregnancy has not been established. Preliminary studies done in rats demonstrated no overt teratogenic effects. The drug is excreted into milk (20-30% of plasma levels) so caution is advised in nursing patients.

Adverse Effects/Warnings - The adverse effect profile in dogs has not been well established. In humans, potential adverse effects are extensive and diverse, but most those most commonly noted include anxiety, nervousness, insomnia, drowsiness, fatigue, dizziness, anorexia, nausea, diarrhea and sweating. About 15% of human patients discontinue treatment due to adverse effects.

Overdosage/Acute Toxicity - The LD$_{50}$ for rats is 452 mg/kg. Five of six dogs given an oral "toxic" dose developed seizures that immediately stopped after giving IV diazepam. The dog having the lowest plasma level of fluoxetine that developed seizures, had a level twice that expected of a human taking 80 mg day (highest recommended dose).

Treatment of fluoxetine overdoses consist of symptomatic and supportive therapy. Gut emptying techniques should be employed when warranted and otherwise not contraindicated. Diazepam should be used to treat seizures.

Drug Interactions - Fluoxetine is highly bound to plasma proteins and could potentially displace **other highly bound drugs** (*e.g.*, warfarin, phenylbutazone, digitoxin, etc). Clinical significance is not clear.

Fluoxetine may enhance the effects of the following psychometric agents: **diazepam** (increased half life), **haloperidol** (increased extrapyramidal effects), **lithium** (increased lithium levels), **L-tryptophan** (CNS stimulation, GI distress), **tricyclic antidepressants** (increased tricyclic side effects), and **buspirone** (increased anxiety).

Preliminary studies indicate that the use of fluoxetine and **monoamine oxidase inhibitors** may cause significant morbidity. It is recommended in human medicine to discontinue the use of fluoxetine at least 5 weeks before beginning monoamine oxidase inhibitors and discontinuing monoamine oxidase inhibitors at least two weeks before beginning fluoxetine.

Doses -
  Dogs:
    For the adjunctive treatment of behavior disorders (see Indications above):
        a) 1 mg/kg PO once daily (Marder 1991)

Monitoring Parameters - 1) Efficacy; 2) Adverse Effects; including appetite (weight)

Client Information - Because there has not been widespread use of fluoxetine in dogs and its adverse effect profile and efficacy have not been yet determined, clients should be briefed on the "investigational" nature of this compound and advised to report any abnormal findings immediately.

Dosage Forms/Preparations/FDA Approval Status/Withholding Times -
  Veterinary-Approved Products: None
  Human-Approved Products:
    Fluoxetine HCl Pulvules/Capsules: 10 mg, 20 mg; *Prozac*® (Dista; Lilly); (Rx)
    Fluoxetine HCl Oral Liquid: 20 mg/5 ml in 120 mls; *Prozac*® (Dista; Lilly) (Rx)

FLUPROSTENOL SODIUM

Chemistry - A synthetic analogue of prostaglandin F_{2alpha}, fluprostenol sodium occurs as a white or almost white hygroscopic powder that is soluble in water and alcohol. The drug's potency is expressed in terms of fluprostenol; 52.4 micrograms of fluprostenol sodium is equivalent to 50 micrograms of fluprostenol.

Storage/Stability/Compatibility - Fluprostenol should be stored in airtight containers and protected from light. The manufacturer recommends discarding any unused product after opening the vial.

Pharmacology - Fluprostenol exhibits pharmacologic effects similar to those of the other agents in this class. Effects on the female reproductive system include stimulation of myometrial activity, relaxation of the cervix, inhibition of steroidogenesis by corpora lutea, and potential lysing of corpora lutea. Fluprostenol reportedly has less smooth muscle stimulant activity and, therefore, may be safer to use to induce parturition in the mare.

Uses/Indications - The labeled indications for fluprostenol are to synchronize estrus for breeding management and for postpartum breeding. Suggested therapeutic uses by the manufacturer include: induction of luteolysis following early fetal death and resorption; termination of persistent diestrus; termination of pseudopregnancy; termination of lactational anestrus; establishing estrous cycles in barren/maiden mares; and to determine if a mare is cycling.

The drug has also been used as an induction agent for parturition and as an abortifacient.

Pharmacokinetics - No information was located for this agent.

Contraindications/Precautions - Fluprostenol should not be used in pregnant mares unless parturition induction or abortion is desired. It should also not be used in mares with acute or subacute disorders of the GI tract or respiratory disease.

The manufacturer states that mares receiving non-steroidal antiinflammatory drugs should not receive fluprostenol, as this drug can inhibit the synthesis and release of prostaglandins. The clinical significance of such an interaction is in doubt, however.

The manufacturer recommends conducting a through breeding exam prior to the use of this drug.

Adverse Effects/Warnings - In horses, sweating, increased respiration, mild abdominal discomfort, uneasiness and defecation may be seen after fluprostenol injection. Adverse effects are more likely at doses above those recommended by the manufacturer.

See the warnings regarding the handling of the agent under Client Information below.

Overdosage - No specific information was located. It would be expected that mild overdoses would result in the adverse effects listed above (sweating, diarrhea, increased respiratory rate). The animal should be treated supportively if necessary.

Drug Interactions - Other **oxytocic agents'** activity may be enhanced by fluprostenol. Reduced effect of fluprostenol would be expected with concomitant administration of a **progestin**.

Doses -

Horses:

Manufacturer's suggested dosage for all labeled indications (see above or package insert):

     a)   0.55 micrograms/kg (average dose 250 micrograms or 5 ml) IM

To induce parturition in the mare:

     a)   2.2 micrograms/kg (0.0022 mg/kg) IM; delivery generally occurs in about 4 hours (Carleton and Threlfall 1986)

     b)   Pony mares 250 micrograms IM, full-sized mares 1000 micrograms IM. First stage of labor ensues in 30 minutes, onset of second stage labor occurs in about 1/2 -3 hours. Duration of second stage labor varies from about 5-35 minutes. Author recommends further studies before recommending procedure. (Hillman 1987)

As an abortifacient:

     a)   Prior to the 12th day of pregnancy: 250 micrograms IM (Lofstedt 1986)

     b)   Prior to day 35 of gestation: 250 micrograms IM one time; after day 35: 250 micrograms IM daily for 3-5 days are required. (Squires and McKinnon 1987)

For estrus synchronization in normally cycling mares:

     a)   Two injection method: On day 1 give 250 micrograms (*Note: The text from this reference reads: 0.250 micrograms; it is believed that this is an error as the manufacturer's recommended dose is approximately 250 micrograms*) and again on day 16. Most (60%) mares will begin estrus 4 days after the second injection and about 90% will show estrous behavior by the 6th day after the second injection. Breed using AI every second day during estrus or inseminated at predetermined times without estrus detection. Alternatively, an IM injection of HCG (2500-3300 Units) can be added on the first or second day (usually day 21) of estrus to hasten ovulation. Breed using AI on days 20, 22, 24, and 26. This may be of more benefit when used early in the breeding season. (Bristol 1987)

Client Information - Fluprostenol should only be used by individuals familiar with its use and precautions. Pregnant women, asthmatics or other persons with bronchial diseases should handle this product with extreme caution. Any accidental exposure to skin should be washed off immediately using soap and water.

Dosage Forms/Preparations/FDA Approval Status/Withholding Times -

Veterinary-Approved Products:

Fluprostenol sodium for Injection, equivalent to 50 micrograms/ml fluprostenol in 5 ml vials; *Equimate*® (Bayer); (Rx) Approved for use in horses. It is not for use in horses intended for food.

Human-Approved Products: None

FOLLICLE STIMULATING HORMONE-PITUITARY (FSH-P)

Chemistry - Follicle stimulating hormone-pituitary (FSH-P) is available commercially as a lyophilized powder. It is obtained from the pituitary glands of food producing animals. Reportedly, FSH-P may also have small amounts of luteinizing hormone present.

One mg of FSH-P = 1 Armour Unit. One Armour Unit, however, can contain from 9.4 - 14.2 International Units (IU) of FSH. When using to induce estrus in the bitch, one clinician (Barton and Wolf 1988) recommends contacting the manufacturer to determine how many IU of FSH are contained per Armour Unit in the lot number of the product obtained.

Storage/Stability/Compatibility - FSH-P should be stored at room temperature; protect from light, heat and moisture.

After reconstituting, the manufacturer (Schering) recommends disposing of any unused drug, but it has been reported that it is relatively stable in the frozen state after reconstitution.

Pharmacology - FSH is produced by the anterior pituitary gland by the same cells that produce luteinizing hormone (LH). Its actions include stimulation of follicular growth and estrogen production in the female, and spermatogenesis in the male.

Uses/Indications - Although labeled for "use in cattle, horses, swine, sheep and dogs as a supplemental source of FSH when there is a general deficiency", its primary use in veterinary medicine has been to induce follicular growth for the purposes of superovulation and out-of-season breeding.

Pharmacokinetics - No specific information was located.

Contraindications/Precautions - FSH should not be used in animals with preexisting endometrial hyperplasia or follicular cysts.

Adverse Effects/Warnings - Cystic endometrial hyperplasia, undesired superovulation and follicular cysts are all potential adverse effects with FSH therapy. High dosages and prolonged treatment increase the likelihood of these effects developing.

Although not reported, hypersensitivity reactions are potentially possible with this product.

Overdosage - No specific information was located; refer to Adverse effects section above.

Doses -

Dogs:
For induction of estrus:
a) 20 IU/kg SQ (must convert Armour Units to IU; contact manufacturer to determine potency of lot number) for 10 days. Proestrus usually occurs between days 7-10 and lasts 2-3 days. Give human chorionic gonadotropin (HCG) 500 IU SQ on days 10 and 11; breed on days 12, 14, and 16. (Barton and Wolf 1988)

For labeled indications (FSH deficiency):
a) 5 -15 mg IV, IM or SQ (Package Insert; *F.S.H.-P.* —Schering)

Cats:
To induce estrus in anestrus queens:
a) FSH: 2 mg IM daily for up to 5 days until estrus observed, then give hCG on first and second day of estrus. (Kraemer and Bowen 1986)

To stimulate follicle maturation and estrous behavior in cats:
a) FSH-P 2 mg IM once daily for 5 days, may reduce dosage to 0.5 or 1 mg on the 2nd-5th day. Do not use longer than 5 days. Discontinue as soon as female is sexually receptive and mates. Most queens are in estrus within 5-6 days after treatment has begun and will remain sexually receptive for approximately 6 days. If female fails to exhibit estrual behavior with 7 days after last injection, may repeat treatment regimen in 5-6 weeks. (Wildt 1986)

Cattle:
For induction of superovulation:
a) For induction of superovulation: Reconsitute as directed on label, then inject 1.6 ml IM twice a day for 3 days. At the fifth injection give a lutalyzing dose of prostaglandin per manufacturer's directions to induce estrus. Breed 4 - 22 hours after onset of estrus. (Package Insert; Super-OV®—AUSA Int.)
b) If estrus = day 0, institute treatment between days 8-14 (usually day 10). Two methods used; method 1 is simpler, but may be less desirable.
Method 1: Give FSH 5 mg IM or SQ twice daily beginning on day 10 through day 13. Perform AI during the PM of days 14 and AM and PM of day 15.
Method 2: Give FSH 5 mg AM and PM on day 10; 4 mg AM and PM on day 11; 3 mg AM and PM on day 12; 2 mg AM and PM on day 13. Perform AI during the PM of days 14 and AM and PM of day 15. (Mapletoff 1986)

For labeled indications (FSH deficiency):
a) 10 - 50 mg IV, IM or SQ (Package Insert; *F.S.H.-P.* —Schering)

Horses:
For labeled indications (FSH deficiency):
a) 10 - 50 mg IV, IM or SQ (Package Insert; *F.S.H.-P.* —Schering)

Swine:
For labeled indications (FSH deficiency):
a) 5 - 25 mg IV, IM or SQ (Package Insert; *F.S.H.-P.* —Schering)

Sheep:
For labeled indications (FSH deficiency):
a) 5 - 25 mg IV, IM or SQ (Package Insert; *F.S.H.-P.* —Schering)

Rabbits:
For induction of superovulation:
a) FSH: 0.5 mg injected *bid* for days, followed by LH: 1.5 mg/kg IV or hCG: 30 - 50 IU, 12-24 hours after last FSH dose. Will produce 40-60 ovulations. (Kraemer and Bowen 1986)

Dosage Forms/Preparations/FDA Approval Status/Withholding Times -
Veterinary-Approved Products: Note: The ongoing availability of FSH-P products has been reported to be an issue; these products may or may not be avialable in the marketplace. Check with suppliers for more information.

Follicle Stimulating Hormone-Pituitary (FSH-P) lyophilized powder for reconstitution and injection. Each vial contains 50 mg Armour Standard and is packaged with one 10 ml vial of diluent (sodium chloride injection).; *F.S.H.-P.* (Schering) (Rx) Approved for use in cattle, horses, swine, sheep, and dogs.

Follicle Stimulating Hormone   Each vial contains 75 mg NIH-FSH-S1 Standard and is packaged with one 10 ml vial of buffered diluent .; Super-OV® (AUSA Int.) (Rx) Approved for use in cattle. No milk or meat withdrawal periods are required when used as directed.

Human-Approved Products: None

FOMEPIZOLE
4-METHYLPYRAZOLE

Chemistry - A synthetic alcohol dehydrogenase inhibitor, fomepizole is commonly called 4-methylpyrazole (4-MP).

Storage/Stability/Compatibility - Commercially available solutions should be stored at room temperature. The concentrate for injection may solidify at temperatures less than 25°C. Should this occur, resolubolize by running warm water over the vial. Solidification or resolubolization does not affect drug potency or stability. Store reconstituted vial at room temperature and discard after 72 hours. Reconstituted solutions may be further diluted in D5W or normal saline for IV infusion.

Pharmacology - Ethylene glycol itself is only mildly toxic in dogs, but when it is metabolized to glycoaldehyde, glycolate, glyoxalic acid and oxalic acids the resultant metabolic acidosis and renal tubular necrosis can be fatal. Fomepizole is a competitive inhibitor of alcohol dehydrogenase, the primary enzyme that converts ethylene glycol into glycoaldehyde and other toxic metabolites. This allows ethylene glycol to be excreted primarily unchanged in the urine decreasing the morbidity and mortality associated with ethylene glycol ingestion.

Uses/Indications - Fomepizole is used for the treatment of known or suspected ethylene glycol toxicity in dogs (and humans).

Pharmacokinetics - Fomepizole is excreted primarily by the kidneys and apparently exhibits a dose-dependent accumulation of the drug over time. Therefore, a reduction in subsequent doses can safely occur.

Contraindications/Precaution/Reproductive Safety- There are no labeled contraindications to fomepizole's use. Fomepizole does not appear to be effective for treating ethylene glycol toxicity in cats.

Fomepizole's safe use during pregnancy, lactation or in breeding animals has not been established. However, because of the morbidity and mortality associated with ethylene glycol toxicity, the benefits of fomepizole should generally outweigh its risks.

Adverse Effects/Warnings - Giving concentrated drug rapidly intravenously may cause vein irritation and phlebosclerosis. Dilute as directed in the commercially available kit.

One dog during clinical trials was reported to develop anaphylaxis.

Use of fomepizole alone without adequate monitoring and adjunctive supportive care (e.g., correction of acid/base, fluid, electrolyte imbalances) may lead to therapeutic failure. If animal presents within 1-2 hours post ingestion, consider inducing vomiting and/or gastric lavage with activated charcoal to prevent further absorption.

Overdosage - Overdosage may cause significant CNS depression. No specific treatment is recommended.

Drug Interactions - Both fomepizole and **ethanol** may inhibit the elimination of the other, prolonging serum half lives and enhancing CNS depression (especially caused by ethanol). Clinical significance (positive or negative) is unclear at this time.

Doses -
  Dogs: For treatment of ethylene glycol toxicity:
    a) Initially load at 20 mg/kg IV; at 12 hours post initial dose give 15 mg/kg IV; at 24 hours post initial dose give another 15 mg/kg IV and at 36 hours after initial dose give 5 mg/kg; may give additional 5 mg/kg doses as necessary (animal has not recovered or has additional ethylene glycol in blood). (Package Insert — *Antizol-Vet®*)

Monitoring Parameters - 1) Ethylene glycol blood levels (mostly important to document diagnosis if necessary and to determine if therapy can be discontinued after 36 hours of Tx.) 2) Blood gases and serum electrolytes 3) Hydration status 4) Renal function tests (*e.g.*, Urine output and urinalysis; BUN or serum creatinine)

Client Information - Clients should be informed that treatment of serious ethylene glycol toxicity is an "intensive care" admission and that appropriate monitoring and therapy can be quite expensive, particularly when fomepizole is used in large dogs. Because time is of the essence in this therapy, clients will need to make an informed decision rapidly. Dogs treated within 8 hours post ingestion have a significantly better prognosis than those treated after 10-12 hours post ingestion

Dosage Forms/Preparations/FDA Approval Status -
  Veterinary-Approved Products:
    Fomepizole 1.5 g Kit for Injection; *Antizol-Vet*® (Orphan Medical); (Rx) Approved for use in dogs.
    Preparation: If drug has solidified run warm water over vial; Add entire contents to 30 ml vial of 0.9% NaCl (in kit), mix well. Resultant solution is: 50 mg/ml
    Note: At recommended doses 1 kit will treat a 26 kg dog (up to 58 lb.); larger dogs will require additional kits
  Human-Approved Products:
    Fomepizole 1 g/ml for Injection (must be diluted); *Antizol*® (Orphan Medical); (Rx)

FURAZOLIDONE

Chemistry - A synthetic nitrofuran-derivative antibacterial/antiprotozoal, furazolidone occurs as a bitter-tasting, yellow, crystalline powder. It is practically insoluble in water.

Storage/Stability/Compatibility - Store protected from light in tight containers. Do not expose the suspension to excessive heat.

Pharmacology - Furazolidone interferes with susceptible bacterial enzyme systems. Its mechanism against susceptible protozoa is not well determined. Furazolidone has activity against *Giardia, Vibrio cholerae, Trichomonas,* Coccidia and many strains of *E. Coli, Enterobacter, Campylobacter, Salmonella* and *Shigella*. Not all strains are sensitive, but resistance is usually limited and develops slowly. Furazolidone also inhibits monoamine oxidase.

Uses/Indications - Furazolidone is usually a drug of second choice in small animals to treat enteric infections caused by the organisms listed above.

Pharmacokinetics - Conflicting information on furazolidone's absorption characteristics are published. As colored metabolites are found in the urine, it is clearly absorbed to some extent. Because furazolidone is used to treat enteric infections, absorption becomes important only when discussing adverse reactions and drug interaction issues. Furazolidone is reported to be distributed into the CSF. Absorbed furazolidone is rapidly metabolized in the liver and the majority of absorbed drug is eliminated in the urine.

Contraindications/Precautions/Reproductive Safety - Furazolidone is contraindicated in patients hypersensitive to it.
  While the safe use of furazolidone during pregnancy has not been established, neither have there been any teratogenic problems reported for the drug. It is unknown if furazolidone enters maternal milk.

Adverse Effects/Warnings - Adverse effects noted with furazolidone are usually minimal. Anorexia, vomiting, cramping and diarrhea may occasionally occur. Some human patients are reported to be hypersensitive to the drug. Because furazolidone also inhibits monoamine oxidase, it may potentially interact with several other drugs and foods (see Drug Interactions below). The clinical significance of these interactions is unclear, particularly in light of the drug's poor absorptive characteristics.

Overdosage/Acute Toxicity - No information was located; but moderate overdoses are unlikely to cause significant toxicity. Gut emptying may be considered for large overdoses.

Drug Interactions - Because furazolidone inhibits monoamine oxidase, its use concurrently with **buspirone, sympathomimetic amines (phenylpropanolamine, ephedrine, etc.), tricyclic antidepressants, other monamine oxidase inhibitors, and fish or poultry** (high tyramine content) is not recommended because dangerous hypertension could occur. **Alcohol** used concurrently with furazolidone may cause a disulfiram-like reaction.

Laboratory Considerations - Furazolidone may cause a false-positive urine glucose determination when using the cupric sulfate solution test (*e.g., Clinitest*®).

Doses -
  Dogs:
      a) For amebic colitis: 2.2 mg/kg PO q8h for 7 days; For coccidiosis: 8 - 20 mg/kg PO for one week (Sherding and Johnson 1994a)
  Cats:
      a) For treatment of *Giardia*: 4 mg/kg PO twice daily (q12h) for 7 -10 day; if re-treatment is required, elevated dosages or lengthened treatment regimens may provide better results. (Reinemeyer 1992)

   b) For amebic colitis: 2.2 mg/kg PO q8h for 7 days; For coccidiosis: 8 - 20 mg/kg PO for one week; for Giardia: 4 mg/kg PO q12h for 5 days (Sherding and Johnson 1994a)

Horses:
   a) 4 mg/kg PO *tid* (Robinson 1992)

Monitoring Parameters - Efficacy (stool exams for parasitic infections)

Client Information - Furazolidone may discolor urine to a dark yellow to brown color; this is not significant. Have clients report prolonged or serious GI effects.

Dosage Forms/Preparations/FDA Approval Status/Withholding Times -
  Veterinary-Approved Products: None
  Human-Approved Products:

  Furazolidone Oral Liquid 3.34 mg/ml (50 mg/15 ml) in 60 ml and pint bottles; *Furoxone*® (Procter & Gamble Pharm);(Rx)

  Furazolidone Oral Tablets 100 mg; *Furoxone*® (Procter & Gamble Pharm); (Rx)

FUROSEMIDE

Chemistry - A loop diuretic related structurally to the sulfonamides, furosemide occurs as an odorless, practically tasteless, white to slightly yellow, fine, crystalline powder. Furosemide has a melting point between 203° - 205° with decomposition, and a pK_a of 3.9. It is practically insoluble in water, sparingly soluble in alcohol and freely soluble in alkaline hydroxides. The injectable product has its pH adjusted to 8 - 9.3 with sodium hydroxide. Furosemide may also be known as frusemide.

Storage/Stability/Compatibility - Furosemide tablets should be stored in light-resistant, well-closed containers. The oral solution should be stored at room temperature and protected from light and freezing. Furosemide injection should be stored at room temperature. A precipitate may form if the injection is refrigerated, but will resolubolize when warmed without alteration in potency. The human injection (10 mg/ml) should not be used if it is a yellow-color. The veterinary injection (50 mg/ml) normally has a slight yellow color. Furosemide is unstable at an acid pH, but is very stable under alkaline conditions.

  Furosemide injection (10 mg/ml) is reportedly **compatible** with all commonly used intravenous solutions and the following drugs: amikacin sulfate, cimetidine HCl, kanamycin sulfate, tobramycin sulfate and verapamil.

  It is reportedly **incompatible** with the following agents: ascorbic acid solutions, dobutamine HCl, epinephrine, gentamicin sulfate, netilmicin sulfate and tetraclyines. It should generally not be mixed with antihistamines, local anesthetics, alkaloids, hypnotics, or opiates.

Pharmacology - Furosemide reduces the absorption of electrolytes in the ascending section of the loop of Henle, decreases the reabsorption of both sodium and chloride and increases the excretion of potassium in the distal renal tubule, and directly effects electrolyte transport in the proximal tubule. The exact mechanisms of furosemide's effects have not been established. It has no effect on carbonic anhydrase nor does it antagonize aldosterone.

  Furosemide increases renal excretion of water, sodium, potassium, chloride, calcium, magnesium, hydrogen, ammonium, and bicarbonate. It causes some renal venodilation and transiently increases glomerular filtration rates (GFR). Renal blood flow is increased and decreased peripheral resistance may occur. Furosemide can cause hyperglycemia, but to a lesser extent than the thiazides.

Uses/Indications - Furosemide is used for its diuretic activity in all species. It is used in small animals for the treatment of congestive cardiomyopathy, pulmonary edema, hypercalcuric nephropathy, uremia, as adjunctive therapy in hyperkalemia and, occasionally, as an antihypertensive agent. In cattle, it is approved for use for the treatment of post-parturient udder edema. It has been used to help prevent or reduce epistaxis (exercise-induced pulmonary hemorrhage; EIPH) in race horses.

Pharmacokinetics - The pharmacokinetics of furosemide have been studied in a limited fashion in domestic animals. In dogs, the oral bioavailability is approximately 77% and the elimination half-life approximately 1 - 1.5 hours.

  In humans, furosemide is 60-75% absorbed following oral administration. The diuretic effect takes place within 5 minutes after IV administration and within one hour after oral dosing. Peak effects occur approximately 30 minutes after IV dosing, and 1-2 hours after oral dosing. The drug is approximately 95% bound to plasma proteins in both azotemic and normal patients. The serum half-life is about 2 hours, but is prolonged in patients with renal failure, uremia, CHF, and in neonates.

Contraindications/Precautions - Furosemide is contraindicated in patients with anuria or who are hypersensitive to the drug. The manufacturer states that the drug should be discontinued in patients with progressive renal disease if increasing azotemia and oliguria occur during therapy.

Furosemide should be used with caution in patients with preexisting electrolyte or water balance abnormalities, impaired hepatic function (may precipitate hepatic coma) and diabetes mellitus. Patients with conditions that may lead to electrolyte or water balance abnormalities (*e.g.*, vomiting, diarrhea, etc.) should be monitored carefully. Patients hypersensitive to sulfonamides may also be hypersensitive to furosemide (not documented in veterinary species).

Adverse Effects/Warnings - Furosemide may induce fluid and electrolyte abnormalities. Patients should be monitored for hydration status and electrolyte imbalances (especially potassium, calcium and sodium). Other potential adverse effects include ototoxicity (especially in cats with high dose IV therapy), gastrointestinal disturbances, hematologic effects (anemia, leukopenia), weakness and restlessness.

Overdosage - The LD$_{50}$ in dogs after oral administration is > 1000 mg/kg and after IV injection > 300 mg/kg. Chronic overdosing at 10 mg/kg for six months in dogs led to development of calcification and scarring of the renal parenchyma.

Acute overdosage may cause electrolyte and water balance problems, CNS effects (lethargy to coma and seizures) and cardiovascular collapse.

Treatment consists of emptying the gut after recent oral ingestion, using standard protocols. Avoid giving concomitant cathartics as they may exacerbate the fluid and electrolyte imbalances that can occur. Aggressively monitor and treat electrolyte and water balance abnormalities supportively. Additionally, monitor respiratory, CNS, and cardiovascular status. Treat supportively and symptomatically if necessary.

Drug Interactions - Pharmacologic effects of **theophylline** may be enhanced when given with furosemide.

Ototoxicity and nephrotoxicity associated with the **aminoglycoside antibiotics** may be increased when furosemide is also used.

If used concomitantly with **corticosteroids, corticotropin or amphotericin B,** furosemide may increase the chance of hypokalemia development. Furosemide-induced hypokalemia may increase chances of **digitalis** toxicity.

Patients on **aspirin** therapy may need dosage adjustment as furosemide competes for renal excretory sites.

Furosemide may inhibit the muscle relaxation qualities of **tubocurarine**, but increase the effects of **succinylcholine**.

Enhanced effects may occur if furosemide is used concomitantly with **other diuretics**.

The uricosuric effects of **probenecid** or **sulfinpyrazone** may be inhibited by furosemide.

Furosemide may alter the requirements of **insulin** or other anti-diabetic agents in diabetic patients.

Doses -
Dogs, Cats:
As a general diuretic:
   a) 2.2 - 4.4 mg/kg (lower dose suggested for cats) once or twice daily at 6-8 hour intervals PO, IV or IM (Package Insert; Lasix® - Hoechst)

For cardiogenic or pulmonary edema:
   a) 2 - 4 mg/kg PO for chronic therapy (may increase up to 8 mg/kg IV for acute short term situations); dosage frequency may be from once every 2-3 days to every 6 hours for oral administration and as frequently as every hour for IV administration. (Kittleson 1985)
   b) 2 - 4 mg/kg IV, IM, PO *bid-tid* (Morgan 1988)
   c) For Cats: 0.5 - 1 mg/kg IV, IM, SQ q8h - every other day.; may switch to oral therapy when stabilized (Bonagura 1989)

For hypercalcemia/hypercalcuric nephropathy:
   a) Patient should be well hydrated before therapy. Give 5 mg/kg bolus IV, then begin 5 mg/kg/hr infusion. Maintain hydration status and electrolyte balance with normal saline with KCl added. Furosemide generally only reduces serum calcium levels by only 3 mg/dl. (Polzin and Osborne 1985)
   b) For moderate hypercalcemia (14-16 mg/dl): Start infusion of normal saline, give furosemide at 5 mg/kg IV once to twice daily. If dehydrated, alternate saline with LRS. Also give glucocorticoids. (Weller 1988)

For acute renal failure/uremia:
   a) After replacing fluid deficit, give furosemide at 2 mg/kg IV. If no diuresis within 1 hour, repeat dose at 4 mg/kg IV. If no response within 1 hour, give another dose at 6

mg/kg IV. The use of low dose dopamine as adjunctive therapy is often recommended; see dopamine monograph. (Polzin and Osborne 1985)
    b) 5 - 20 mg/kg IV *prn* (Morgan 1988)

To promote diuresis in hyperkalemic states:
    a) 2 mg/kg IV; attempted if mannitol is ineffective after one hour (Seeler and Thurmon 1985)

As a diuretic for the treatment of ascites:
    a) 1 - 2 mg/kg PO, SQ once to twice daily (Morgan 1988)

As an antihypertensive:
    a) 1- 2 mg/kg PO *bid* (Morgan 1988)

Cattle:
    a) 500 mg once daily or 250 mg twice daily; 2 grams PO once daily. Treatment not to exceed 48 hours post-partum (for udder edema). Package Insert; *Lasix*® - Hoechst)
    b) 2.2 - 4.4 mg/kg IV q12h (Howard 1986)

Horses:
As a diuretic:
    a) 0.25 - 1.0 mg/kg IV (Muir and McGuirk 1987)
    b) 1 mg/kg IV (Robinson 1987)

For epistaxis prevention:
    a) 0.3 - 0.6 mg/kg 60-90 minutes prior to race. (Robinson 1987) (Note: Refer to state guidelines for use of furosemide in racing animals)

Birds:
As a diuretic:
    a) 0.05 mg/300 gm IM *bid* (Note: Lories are very sensitive to this agent and can be easily overdosed) (Clubb 1986)

Reptiles:
    a) For most species: 5 mg/kg IV or IM as needed. (Gauvin 1993)

Monitoring Parameters -
    1) Serum electrolytes, BUN, creatinine, glucose
    2) Hydration status
    3) Blood pressure, if indicated
    4) Symptoms of edema, patient weight, if indicated
    5) Evaluation of ototoxity, particularly with prolonged therapy or in cats

Client Information - Clients should contact veterinarian if symptoms of water or electrolyte imbalance occur. Symptoms such as excessive thirst, lethargy, lassitude, restlessness, oliguria, GI distress or tachycardia may indicate electrolyte or water balance problems.

Dosage Forms/Preparations/FDA Approval Status/Withholding Times -
Veterinary-Approved Products:

Furosemide Tablets 12.5 mg, 50 mg ; *Lasix*® (Hoechst); Generic; (Rx) Approved for use in dogs and cats.

Furosemide Oral Solution: 10 mg/ml in 60 ml btls; *Lasix*® (Hoechst) (Rx) Approved for use in dogs.

Furosemide 2 gram boluses; *Lasix*® (Hoechst); (Rx) Approved for use in cattle. A 48 hour withdrawal time has been assigned for both milk and slaughter for cattle.

Furosemide 50 mg/ml (5%) for Injection in 50 ml vials; *Lasix*® (Hoechst), *Diuride*® (Anthony), Generic (Rx) Approved for use in dogs, cats, horses not intended for food, and cattle. Milk withdrawal time = 48 hours; slaughter withdrawal = 48 hours.

Human-Approved Products:

Furosemide Tablets 20 mg, 40 mg, 80 mg; *Lasix*® (Hoechst Marion Roussel); Generic (Rx)

Furosemide Oral Solution: 8 mg/ml in 5, 10, & 500 ml btls; 10 mg/ml in 60 ml & 120 ml bottles; *Lasix*® (Hoechst Marion Roussel); Generic (Rx)

Furosemide 10 mg/ml for Injection in 2, 4, & 10 ml amps, vials and syringes; *Lasix*® (Hoechst Marion Roussel); Generic (Rx)

GENTAMICIN SULFATE

Chemistry - An aminoglycoside obtained from cultures of *Micromonaspora purpurea*, gentamicin sulfate occurs as a white to buff powder that is soluble in water and insoluble in alcohol. The commercial product is actually a combination of gentamicin sulfate C_1, C_2 and C_3, but all these compounds apparently have similar antimicrobial activities. Commercially available injections have a pH from 3 - 5.5.

Storage/Stability/Compatibility - Gentamicin sulfate for injection and the oral solution should be stored at room temperature (15-30°C); freezing or temperatures above 40°C should be avoided. The soluble powder should be stored from 2-30°C. Do not store or offer medicated drinking water in rusty containers or the drug may be destroyed.

While the manufacturer does not recommend that gentamicin be mixed with other drugs, it is reportedly **compatible** and stable in all commonly used intravenous solutions and with the following drugs: bleomycin sulfate, cefoxitin sodium, cimetidine HCl, clindamycin phosphate, methicillin sodium, metronidazole (with and without sodium bicarbonate), penicillin G sodium and verapamil HCl.

The following drugs or solutions are reportedly **incompatible** or only compatible in specific situations with gentamicin: amphotericin B, ampicillin sodium, carbenicillin disodium, cefamandole naftate, cephalothin sodium, cephapirin sodium, dopamine HCl, furosemide, and heparin sodium. Compatibility is dependent upon factors such as pH, concentration, temperature and diluents used. It is suggested to consult specialized references for more specific information (*e.g., Handbook on Injectable Drugs* by Trissel; see bibliography).

In vitro inactivation of aminoglycoside antibiotics by beta-lactam antibiotics is well documented. Gentamicin is very susceptible to this effect and it is usually recommended to avoid mixing these compounds together. Refer to the Drug Interaction section in the amikacin sulfate monograph for more information.

Pharmacology - Gentamicin has a mechanism of action and spectrum of activity (primarily gram negative aerobes) similar to the other aminoglycosides. This information is outlined in more detail in the amikacin monograph. Gentamicin resistance by certain bacteria, principally *Klebsiella*, *E. coli* and *Pseudomonas aeruginosa* is a continuing concern for many areas. However, most strains of gentamicin-resistant bacteria of these species remain susceptible to amikacin.

Uses/Indications - The inherent toxicity of the aminoglycosides limit their systemic (parenteral) use to the treatment of serious gram negative infections when there is either a documented lack of susceptibility to other less toxic antibiotics or when the clinical situation dictates immediate treatment of a presumed gram negative infection before culture and susceptibility results are reported.

Various gentamicin products are approved for parenteral use in dogs, cats, chickens, turkeys and swine. Although routinely used parenterally in horses, gentamicin is only approved for intrauterine infusion in that species. Oral products are approved for gastrointestinal infections in swine and turkeys. For more information refer to the Dosage section below.

Pharmacokinetics - Gentamicin, like the other aminoglycosides is not appreciably absorbed after oral or intrauterine administration, but is absorbed from topical administration (not skin or urinary bladder) when used in irrigations during surgical procedures. Patients receiving oral aminoglycosides with hemorrhagic or necrotic enteritises may absorb appreciable quantities of the drug. After IM administration to dogs and cats, peak levels occur from 1/2 to 1 hour later. Subcutaneous injection results in slightly delayed peak levels and with more variability than after IM injection. Bioavailability from extravascular injection (IM or SQ) is greater than 90%.

After absorption, aminoglycosides are distributed primarily in the extracellular fluid. They are found in ascitic, pleural, pericardial, peritoneal, synovial and abscess fluids and high levels are found in sputum, bronchial secretions and bile. Aminoglycosides are minimally protein bound (<20%, streptomycin 35%) to plasma proteins. Aminoglycosides do not readily cross the blood-brain barrier or penetrate ocular tissue. CSF levels are unpredictable and range from 0-50% of those found in the serum. Therapeutic levels are found in bone, heart, gallbladder and lung tissues after parenteral dosing. Aminoglycosides tend to accumulate in certain tissues, such as the inner ear and kidneys, which may help explain their toxicity. Volumes of distribution have been reported to be 0.15-0.3 L/kg in adult cats and dogs, and 0.26-0.58 L/kg in horses. Volumes of distribution may be significantly larger in neonates and juvenile animals due to their higher extracellular fluid fractions. Aminoglycosides cross the placenta. Fetal concentrations range from 15-50% of those found in maternal serum.

Elimination of aminoglycosides after parenteral administration occurs almost entirely by glomerular filtration. The elimination half-lives for gentamicin have been reported to be 1.82-3.25 hours in horses, 2.2-2.7 hours in calves, 2.4 hours in sheep, 1.8 hours in cows, 1.9 hours in swine, 1 hour in rabbits, and 0.5-1.5 hours in dogs and cats. Patients with decreased renal function can have significantly prolonged half-lives. In humans with normal renal function, elimination rates can be highly variable with the aminoglycoside antibiotics.

Contraindications/Precautions/Reproductive Safety - Aminoglycosides are contraindicated in patients who are hypersensitive to them. Because these drugs are often the only effective agents in severe gram-negative infections there are no other absolute contraindications to their use.

However, they should be used with extreme caution in patients with preexisting renal disease with concomitant monitoring and dosage interval adjustments made. Other risk factors for the development of toxicity include age (both neonatal and geriatric patients), fever, sepsis and dehydration.

Because aminoglycosides can cause irreversible ototoxicity, they should be used with caution in "working" dogs (*e.g.*, "seeing-eye", herding, dogs for the hearing impaired, etc.).

Aminoglycosides should be used with caution in patients with neuromuscular disorders (*e.g.*, myasthenia gravis) due to their neuromuscular blocking activity.

Because aminoglycosides are eliminated primarily through renal mechanisms, they should be used cautiously, preferably with serum monitoring and dosage adjustment in neonatal or geriatric animals.

Aminoglycosides are generally considered contraindicated in rabbits as they adversely affect the GI flora balance in these animals.

Aminoglycosides can cross the placenta and while rare, may cause 8th cranial nerve toxicity or nephrotoxicity in fetuses. Because the drug should only be used in serious infections, the benefits of therapy may exceed the potential risks.

Adverse Effects/Warnings - The aminoglycosides are infamous for their nephrotoxic and ototoxic effects. The nephrotoxic (tubular necrosis) mechanisms of these drugs are not completely understood, but are probably related to interference with phospholipid metabolism in the lysosomes of proximal renal tubular cells, resulting in leakage of proteolytic enzymes into the cytoplasm. Nephrotoxicity is usually manifested by increases in BUN, creatinine, nonprotein nitrogen in the serum and decreases in urine specific gravity and creatinine clearance. Proteinuria and cells or casts may also be seen in the urine. Nephrotoxicity is usually reversible once the drug is discontinued. While gentamicin may be more nephrotoxic than the other aminoglycosides, the incidences of nephrotoxicity with all of these agents require equal caution and monitoring.

Ototoxicity (8th cranial nerve toxicity) of the aminoglycosides can be manifested by either auditory and/or vestibular symptoms and may be irreversible. Vestibular symptoms are more frequent with streptomycin, gentamicin, or tobramycin. Auditory symptoms are more frequent with amikacin, neomycin, or kanamycin, but either forms can occur with any of the drugs. Cats are apparently very sensitive to the vestibular effects of the aminoglycosides.

The aminoglycosides can also cause neuromuscular blockade, facial edema, pain/inflammation at injection site, peripheral neuropathy and hypersensitivity reactions. Rarely, GI symptoms, hematologic and hepatic effects have been reported.

Overdosage/Acute Toxicity - Should an inadvertant overdosage be administered, three treatments have been recommended. Hemodialysis is very effective in reducing serum levels of the drug, but is not a viable option for most veterinary patients. Peritoneal dialysis also will reduce serum levels, but is much less efficacious. Complexation of drug with either carbenicillin or ticarcillin (12-20 g/day in humans) is reportedly nearly as effective as hemodialysis.

Drug Interactions - Aminoglycosides should be used with caution with other nephrotoxic, ototoxic, and neurotoxic drugs. These include **amphotericin B, other aminoglycosides, acyclovir, bacitracin** (parenteral use), **cisplatin, methoxyflurane, polymyxin B**, or **vancomycin**.

The concurrent use of aminoglycosides with **cephalosporins** is controversial. Potentially, cephalosporins could cause additive nephrotoxicity when used with aminoglycosides, but this interaction has only been well documented with cephaloridine (no longer marketed) and cephalothin.

Concurrent use with loop (**furosemide, ethacrynic acid**) or osmotic diuretics (**mannitol, urea**) may increase the nephrotoxic or ototoxic potential of the aminoglycosides.

Concomitant use with **general anesthetics** or **neuromuscular blocking agents** could potentiate neuromuscular blockade.

Synergism against *Pseudomonas aeruginosa* and *enterococci* may occur with beta-**lactam antibiotics** and the aminoglycosides. This effect is apparently not predictable and its clinical usefulness is in question.

Drug/Laboratory Interactions - Gentamicin **serum concentrations** may be falsely decreased if the patient is also receiving beta-lactam antibiotics and the serum is stored prior analysis. It is recommended that if assay is delayed, samples be frozen and if possible, drawn at times when the beta-lactam antibiotic is at a trough.

Doses -Note: There is significant interpatient variability with regards to aminoglycoside pharmacokinetic parameters. To insure therapeutic levels and to minimize the risks for toxicity development, it is recommended to consider monitoring serum levels for this drug.

For small animals, one pair of authors (Aronson and Aucoin 1989) make the following recommendations with regard to minimizing risks of toxicity yet maximizing efficacy:
   1) Dose according to animal size. The larger the animal, the smaller the dose (on a mg/kg basis).

2) The more risk factors (age, fever, sepsis, renal disease, dehydration) the smaller the dose.
3) In old patients or those suspected of renal disease, increase dosing interval from q8h to q16-24h.
4) Determine serum creatinine prior to therapy and adjust by changes in level even if it remains in "normal range".
5) Monitor urine for changes in sediment (*e.g.,* casts) or concentrating ability. Not very useful in patients with UTI.
6) Therapeutic drug monitoring is recommended when possible.

Dogs:
For susceptible infections:
　a) 2.2 - 4.4 mg/kg IV (only if acute sepsis) or IM q8h; see recommendations above for dosage/interval adjustment. (Aronson and Aucoin 1989)
　b) 2 - 4 mg/kg IV, IM or SubQ q8h (avoid use or reduce dosage in patients with renal failure; recommend therapeutic drug monitoring, particularly in young animals) (Vaden and Papich 1995)

Cats:
For susceptible infections:
　a) 2.2 - 4.4 mg/kg IV (only if acute sepsis) or IM q8h; see recommendations above for dosage/interval adjustment. (Aronson and Aucoin 1989)
　b) 2 - 4 mg/kg IV, IM or SubQ q8h (avoid use or reduce dosage in patients with renal failure; recommend therapeutic drug monitoring, particularly in young animals) (Vaden and Papich 1995)
　c) 3 mg/kg IV, SQ q8h (Jernigan et al. 1988)

Pocket Pets/Rodents:
For empiric antibiotic therapy:
　a) 5 mg/kg once daily IM or SubQ (Oglesbee 1995)

Cattle:
For susceptible infections:
　a) 4.4 - 6.6 mg/kg/day IM divided *tid* (Upson 1988)
　b) Intramammary: 100-150 mg q12h (Schultz 1986)
　c) 2.2 mg/kg q12h (McConnell and Hughey 1987)
　d) 5 mg/kg IM q8h (Haddad et al. 1987)

Horses:
For susceptible infections:
　a) 1 - 3 mg/kg IM *qid* (Robinson 1987)
　b) For gram negative respiratory infections: 2.2 mg/kg IM or IV 4 times a day in mature horses and 3 times a day in foals. (Beech 1987a)
　c) In foals: 2 - 3 mg/kg IV q12h; use lower dose in premature foals or those less than 7 days of age. Monitor serum levels if possible. (Caprile and Short 1987)
　d) For prophylaxis (with penicillin G) for surgical colic: 2.2. mg/kg *tid* IV. (Stover 1987)
　e) 2.2 mg/kg IV q6h; animals must be well hydrated. (Sweeney et al. 1988)
　f) 2 - 4 mg/kg IM q8-12h (Baggot and Prescott 1987)
　g) 4.4 mg/kg IV q12h (Duran 1992)
　h) There is increased interest in giving gentamicin once daily at an initial dosage of 6.6 mg/kg preferably as an IV infusion over one hour. Therapeutic drug monitoring would be beneficial. Watch for futher references documenting the safety and efficacy of this dosing method. (Plumb)

Swine:
For susceptible infections:
　a) For colibacillosis in neonates: 5 mg PO or IM once (Label directions; *Garacin® Pig Pump and Piglet Injection*—Schering)
　b) For weanling and other swine:
　　Colibacillosis: 1.1 mg/kg/day in drinking water (concentration of 25 mg/gallon) for 3 days.
　　Swine dysentery (*Treponema hyodysenteriae*): 2.2 mg/kg/day in drinking water (concentration of 50 mg/gallon) for 3 days. (Label directions; *Garacin® Soluble Powder & Oral Solution*—Schering)

Birds:

For susceptible infections:

a) For Pheasants and Cranes: 5 mg/kg IM *tid* for 5-10 days. For Quail, African Grey Parrots: 10 mg/kg IM *tid*. Blue and Gold McCaws: 10 mg/kg IM *bid*. Once or twice daily dosing may be effective in less serious infections. (Clubb 1986)

b) For gut sterilization/gut infections: 40 mg/kg PO 1-3 times a day for 2-3 days. (Clubb 1986)

c) For pneumonia (with carbenicillin or tylosin given IM): 5 - 10 mg/kg intratracheally once daily. (Clubb 1986)

Reptiles:

For susceptible infections:

a) For bacterial gastritis in snakes: gentamicin 2.5 mg/kg IM every 72 hours with oral neomycin 15 mg/kg plus oral live lactobacillus. (Burke 1986)

b) For bacterial shell diseases in turtles: 5 - 10 mg/kg daily in water turtles, every other day in land turtles and tortoises for 7-10 days. Used commonly with a beta-lactam antibiotic. Recommend beginning therapy with 20 ml/kg fluid injection. Maintain hydration and monitor uric acid levels when possible. (Rosskopf 1986)

Monitoring Parameters (parenteral use)-

1) Efficacy (cultures, clinical signs and symptoms associated with infection).

2) Renal toxicity; baseline urinalysis, serum creatinine/BUN. Casts in the urine are often the initial sign of impending nephrotoxicity. Frequency of monitoring during therapy is controversial. It can be said that daily urinalyses early in the course of treatment is not too often nor are daily creatinines once casts are seen or increases noted in serum creatinine levels.

3) Gross monitoring of vestibular or auditory toxicity is recommended.

4) Serum levels, if possible; see the reference by Aronson and Aucoin for more information.

Client Information - With appropriate training, owners may give subcutaneous injections at home, but routine monitoring of therapy for efficacy and toxicity must still be done. Clients should also understand that the potential exists for severe toxicity (nephrotoxicity, ototoxicity) developing from this medication.

Dosage Forms/Preparations/FDA Approval Status/Withholding Times -
Veterinary-Approved Products:

Gentamicin Sulfate Injection 50 mg/ml & 100 mg/ml (horses only) in 50 ml & 100 ml vials ; *Gentocin*® (Schering);*Ultragex*® *100* (Anthony); Generic (Rx) Approved for use in dogs, cats, and horses (not for food).

Gentamicin Sulfate Injection 5 mg/ml in 250 ml vials; *Garacin*® *Piglet Injection* (Schering); (OTC) Approved for use in swine. Slaughter withdrawal = 40 days.

Gentamicin Sulfate Oral Solution 50 mg/ml in 80 ml bottles; *Garacin*® *Oral Solution* (Schering); (OTC) Approved for use in swine. Slaughter withdrawal = 3 days.

Gentamicin Sulfate Oral Solution 4.35 mg/ml in 115 ml pump bottles (1 pump delivers approximately 5 mg); *Garacin*® *Pig Pump Oral Solution* (Schering); (OTC) Approved for use in swine. Slaughter withdrawal = 14 days.

Gentamicin Sulfate Soluble Powder 2 g gentamicin/30 grams of powder in 360 gram jar or 2 g gentamicin in 120 gram packets; *Garacin*® *Soluble Powder* (Schering); (OTC) Approved for use in swine. Slaughter withdrawal = 10 days.

Veterinary-approved injections for chickens and turkeys plus a water additive for egg dipping are available. Ophthalmic, otic and topical preparations are also available with veterinary labeling.

Human-Approved Products (partial listing):

Gentamicin Sulfate Injection 40 mg/ml & 10 mg/ml as sulfate and 2 mg/ml as sulfate in 2 & 20 ml vials and 1.5 & 2 ml cartridge-needle units/disp. syringes and 2 ml amps; *Garamycin*® (Schering); *Jenamicin*® (Hauck); *Pediatric Gentamicin Sulfate*® (Elkins-Sinn; *Garamycin Pediatric*® (Schering); *Garamycin Intrathecal*® (Schering); generic, (Rx)

Topical, otic and ophthalmic labeled products are also available.

GLEPTOFERRON

Chemistry - Gleptoferron, a macromolecular complex of ferric hydroxide and dextran glucoheptonic acid, is available commercially as an aqueous colloidial solution. Each ml contains 200 mg of elemental iron.

Storage/Stability/Compatibility - Gleptoferron injection should be stored at temperatures less than 25°C (77°F).

Pharmacology - Refer to the information in the ferrous sulfate monograph for more information.

Uses/Indications - Gleptoferron is indicated for the prevention and treatment of baby pig anemia due to iron deficiency.

Pharmacokinetics - No information located.

Contraindications/Precautions/Reproductive Safety - None noted.

Adverse Effects/Warnings - The manufacturer states that, occasionally, pigs may show a reaction characterized by prostration and muscular weakness. In extreme cases, death may occur.

Overdosage/Acute Toxicity - No information located on this product, refer to the iron dextran monograph for more information.

Drug Interactions, **Drug/Laboratory Interactions** - None are listed, but it is suggested to refer to the iron dextran monograph for more information.

Doses -
  Swine:
      a) For prevention or iron deficiency anemia in baby pigs: 1 ml (200 mg) IM per pig on or before 3 days of age.
      For treatment of iron deficiency anemia in baby pigs: 1 ml (200 mg) IM per pig as soon as signs of deficiency appear. (Label directions; *Gleptosil®*—Schering)

Client Information - Very specific instructions on how and where to use this product are listed in the package instructions; for more information refer to them.

Dosage Forms/Preparations/FDA Approval Status/Withholding Times -
  Veterinary-Approved Products:

    Gleptoferron Injection 200 mg elemental iron per ml in 100 ml collapsible vials; *Gleptosil®* (Fisons); (OTC) Approved for use in baby pigs. No slaughter w'drawal time required.

GLIPIZIDE

Chemistry - A sulfonylurea antidiabetic agent, glipizide (also known as glydiazinamide) occurs as a whitish powder. It is practically insoluble in water and has pK_a of 5.9.

Storage/Stability/Compatibility - Tablets should be stored in tight, light-resistant containers at room temperature.

Pharmacology - Sulfonylureas lower blood glucose concentrations in both diabetic and non-diabetics. The exact mechanism of action is not known, but these agents are thought to exert the effect primarily by stimulating the Beta cells in the pancreas to secrete additional endogenous insulin. Extrapancreatic effects include enhanced tissue sensitivity of circulating insulin. Ongoing use of the sulfonylureas appear to also enhance peripheral sensitivity to insulin and reduce the production of hepatic basal glucose. The mechanisms causing these effects are yet to be fully explained, however.

Uses/Indications - Glipizide may be of benefit in treating cats with type II diabetes. It potentially may be useful in treating canine patients with type II or III diabetes as well, but some pharmacologists state that by the time dogs present with hyperglycemia, they are absolutely or relatively insulinopenic and glipizide would probably be ineffective.

Pharmacokinetics - Glipizide is rapidly and practically completely absorbed after oral administration. The absolute bioavailability reported in humans ranges from 80-100%. Food will alter the rate but not the extent of absorption. Glipizide is very highly bound to plasma proteins. It is primarily biotransformed in the liver to inactive metabolites which are then excreted by the kidneys. In humans, half life is about 2-4 hours. Effects on insulin levels in cats tend to be short-lived. Effects peak in about 15 minutes and return to baseline after about 60 minutes.

Contraindications/Precautions/Reproductive Safety - Oral antidiabetic agents are considered contraindicated with the following conditions: severe burns, severe trauma, severe infection, diabetic coma or other hypoglycemic conditions, major surgery, ketosis, ketoacidosis or other significant acidotic conditions. Glipizide should only be used when its potential benefits outweigh its risks during untreated adrenal or pituitary insufficiency; thyroid, renal or hepatic function impairment; prolonged vomiting; high fever; malnourishment or debilitated condition is present.

  Some patients with type II or type III diabetes may have their disease complicated by the production of excessive amounts of cortisol or growth hormone which may antagonize insulin's effects. These causes should be ruled out before initiating oral antidiabetic therapy.

  Safe use during pregnancy has not been established. Glipizide was found to be mildly fetotoxic in rats when given at doses at 5-50 mg/kg. However, no other teratogenic effects were noted. Use in pregnancy only when benefits outweigh potential risks. It is unknown if glipizide enters milk.

Adverse Effects/Warnings - Experience with glipizide is limited in veterinary medicine. Some cats receiving this drug have reportedly developed hypoglycemia, vomiting, icterus and increased ALT (SGPT) levels. Should toxicity develop, reinstitution of drug therapy may be attempted at a lower dosage after sign/symptom resolution.

Other adverse effects that are possible (noted in humans) include: allergic skin reactions, bone marrow suppression, or cholestatic jaundice.

Glipizide does not appear to be effective in cats demonstrating insulin resistance.

Overdosage/Acute Toxicity - Oral LD_{50}'s are greater than 4 g/kg in all animal species tested. Profound hypoglycemia is the greatest concern after an overdose. Gut emptying protocols should be employed when warranted. Because of its shorter half life than chlorpropamide, prolonged hypoglycemia is less likely with glipizide, but blood glucose monitoring and treatment with parenteral glucose may be required for several days. Massive overdoses may also require additional monitoring (blood gases, serum electrolytes) and supportive therapy.

Drug Interactions - A disulfiram-like reaction (anorexia, nausea, vomiting) has been reported in humans who have ingested **alcohol** within 48-72 hours of receiving glipizide.

The following drugs may displace glipizide, or be displaced by glipizide from plasma proteins, thereby causing enhanced pharmacologic effects of the two drugs involved: **chloramphenicol, furazolidone, non-steroidal anti-inflammatory agents, salicylates, sulfonamides, warfarin**.

beta **adrenergic blocking agents** (*e.g.*, **propranolol**) may affect diabetes (mellitus) control.

Glipizide may prolong the duration of action of **barbiturates**. **Probenecid** or **monamine oxidase inhibitors** may increase the hypoglycemic effects of glipizide.

Thiazide diuretics may exacerbate diabetes mellitus.

Cimetidine may potentiate the hypoglycemic effects of glipizide.

Doses -
Cats:
For diabetes mellitus:
   a) In obese, non-ketotic cats: 0.25 - 0.5 mg/kg twice daily (Nichols 1992)
   b) For nonketotic, relatively healthy (on PE) cats whose owners refuse to administer insulin: 2.5 mg PO twice daily with food (with increased fiber content). If vomiting, icterus and euglycemia have not occurred, dosage is increased to 5 mg PO twice daily and continued for as long as the cat is stable. Dosage may need to be adjusted downward should hypoglycemia or toxicity occur. (Nelson and Feldman 1995)
   c) 5 mg/cat PO q8-12h, with correction of obesity and dietary therapy (Nelson 1994)

Monitoring Parameters - Weekly exams during first month of therapy, including PE, body weight, urine glucose/ketones and several blood glucose exams. In addition, adverse effects (vomiting, icterus), and occassional liver enzymes and CBC.

Client Information - Clients should be informed on symptoms to watch for that would indicated either hypoglycemia or hyperglycemia and be instructed to report these to the veterinarian. Compliance with dosing regimen should also be stressed.

Dosage Forms/Preparations/FDA Approval Status/Withholding Times -
Veterinary-Approved Products: None
Human-Approved Products:
Glipizide Oral Tablets 5 mg, 10 mg; *Glucotrol*® (Pfizer) (Rx); generic (Rx)
Glipizide Extended Release Tablets: 5 mg, 10 mg; *Glucotrol XL*® (Pfizer) (Rx)

GLUCOCORTICOID AGENTS, GENERAL INFORMATION

Glucocorticoid Comparison Table

DRUG	EQUIV. ANTI-INFLAMMA-TORY DOSE (mg)	RELATIVE ANTI-INFLAMMA-TORY POTENCY	RELATIVE MINERALO-CORTICOID ACTIVITY	PLASMA HALF-LIFE DOGS (min) [Humans]	DURATION OF ACTION AFTER ORAL/IV [IM] ADMIN.
Hydrocortisone (Cortisol)	20	1	1-2	52-57 [90]	<12 hrs
Betamethasone Sod. Succ./ Sod. Phos.	0.6	25	0	?[300+]	>48 hrs
Dexamethasone Sod. Succ./ Sod. Phos.	0.75	30	0	119-136 [200-300+]	>48 hrs
Flumethasone	1.5	15-30	?	?	
Isoflupredone		17			
Methylpred-nisolone	4	5	0	91 [200]	12-36 hrs
Prednisolone	5	4	1	69-197 [115-212]	12-36 hrs
Prednisone	5	4	1	[60]	12-36 hrs
Triamcinolone Acetonide	4	5	0	[200+]	12-36 hrs [weeks]

Pharmacology - Glucocorticoids have effects on virtually every cell type and system in mammals. An overview of the effects of these agents follows:

Cardiovascular System: Glucocorticoids can reduce capillary permeability and enhance vasoconstriction. A relatively clinically insignificant positive inotropic effect can occur after glucocorticoid administration. Increased blood pressure can result from both the drugs' vasoconstrictive properties and increased blood volume that may be produced.

Cells: Glucocorticoids inhibit fibroblast proliferation, macrophage response to migration inhibiting factor, sensitization of lymphocytes and the cellular response to mediators of inflammation. Glucocorticoids stabilize lysosomal membranes.

CNS/Autonomic Nervous System: Glucocorticoids can lower seizure threshold, alter mood and behavior, diminish the response to pyrogens, stimulate appetite and maintain alpha rhythm. Glucocorticoids are necessary for normal adrenergic receptor sensitivity.

Endocrine System: When animals are not stressed, glucocorticoids will suppress the release of ACTH from the anterior pituitary, thereby reducing or preventing the release of endogenous corticosteroids. Stress factors (*e.g.*, renal disease, liver disease, diabetes) may sometimes nullify the suppressing aspects of exogenously administered steroids. Release of thyroid-stimulating hormone (TSH), follicle-stimulating hormone (FSH), prolactin and luteinizing hormone (LH) may all be reduced when glucocorticoids are administered at pharmacological doses. Conversion of thyroxine (T_4) to triiodothyronine (T_3) may be reduced by glucocorticoids and plasma levels of parathyroid hormone increased. Glucocorticoids may inhibit osteoblast function. Vasopressin (ADH) activity is reduced at the renal tubules and diuresis may occur. Glucocorticoids inhibit insulin binding to insulin-receptors and the post-receptor effects of insulin.

Hematopoietic System: Glucocorticoids can increase the numbers of circulating platelets, neutrophils and red blood cells, but platelet aggregation is inhibited. Decreased amounts of lymphocytes (peripheral), monocytes and eosinophils are seen as glucocorticoids can sequester these cells into the lungs and spleen and prompt decreased release from the bone marrow. Removal of old red blood cells is diminished. Glucocorticoids can cause involution of lymphoid tissue.

GI Tract and Hepatic System: Glucocorticoids increase the secretion of gastric acid, pepsin and trypsin. They alter the structure of mucin and decrease mucosal cell proliferation. Iron salts and calcium absorption are decreased while fat absorption is increased. Hepatic changes can include increased fat and glycogen deposits within hepatocytes, increased serum levels of alanine aminotransferase (ALT) and gamma-glutamyl transpeptidase (GGT). Significant increases can be seen in serum alkaline phosphatase levels. Glucocorticoids can cause minor increases in BSP (bromosulfophthalein) retention time.

Immune System (also see Cells and Hematopoietic System): Glucocorticoids can decrease circulating levels of T-lymphocytes; inhibit lymphokines; inhibit neutrophil, macrophage, and monocyte migration; reduce production of interferon; inhibit phagocytosis and chemotaxis; antigen processing; and diminish intracellular killing. Specific acquired immunity is affected less than nonspecific immune responses. Glucocorticoids can also antagonize the complement cascade and mask the clinical signs of infection. Mast cells are decreased in number and histamine synthesis is suppressed. Many of these effects only occur at high or very high doses and there are species differences in response.

Metabolic effects: Glucocorticoids stimulate gluconeogenesis. Lipogenesis is enhanced in certain areas of the body (*e.g.,* abdomen) and adipose tissue can be redistributed away from the extremities to the trunk. Fatty acids are mobilized from tissues and their oxidation is increased. Plasma levels of triglycerides, cholesterol and glycerol are increased. Protein is mobilized from most areas of the body (not the liver).

Musculoskeletal: Glucocorticoids may cause muscular weakness (also caused if there is a lack of glucocorticoids), atrophy, and osteoporosis. Bone growth can be inhibited via growth hormone and somatomedin inhibition, increased calcium excretion and inhibition of vitamin D activation. Resorption of bone can be enhanced. Fibrocartilage growth is also inhibited.

Ophthalmic: Prolonged corticosteroid use (both systemic or topically to the eye) can cause increased intraocular pressure and glaucoma, cataracts and exophthalmos.

Reproductive Tract, Pregnancy, & Lactation: Glucocorticoids are probably necessary for normal fetal development. They may be required for adequate surfactant production, myelin, retinal, pancreas and mammary development. Excessive dosages early in pregnancy may lead to teratogenic effects. In horses and ruminants, exogenous steroid administration may induce parturition when administered in the latter stages of pregnancy. Glucocorticoids unbound to plasma proteins will enter milk. High dosages or prolonged administration to mothers may potentially inhibit the growth of nursing newborns.

Renal, Fluid, & Electrolytes: Glucocorticoids can increase potassium and calcium excretion; sodium and chloride reabsorption and extracellular fluid volume. Hypokalemia and/or hypocalcemia occur rarely. Diuresis may occur following glucocorticoid administration.

Skin: Thinning of dermal tissue and skin atrophy can be seen with glucocorticoid therapy. Hair follicles can become distended and alopecia may occur.

Uses/Indications - Glucocorticoids have been used in attempt to treat practically every malady that afflicts man or animal. Among some of the uses for glucocorticoids are: endocrine (adrenal insufficiency), rheumatic (arthritis), collagen diseases (systemic lupus), allergic states, respiratory diseases (asthma), dermatologic diseases (pemphigus, allergic dermatoses), hematologic (thrombocytopenias, autoimmune hemolytic anemias), neoplasias, nervous system (increased CSF pressure), GI (ulcerative colitis exacerbations) and renal (nephrotic syndrome). Some glucocorticoids are used topically in the eye and skin for various conditions or are injected intra-articularly or intra-lesionally. The above listing is certainly not complete. For specific dosages and indications refer to the Doses section for each glucocorticoid drug monograph.

Contraindications/Precautions - Systemic use of glucocorticoids are generally considered to be contraindicated in systemic fungal infections (unless used for replacement therapy in Addison's), when administered IM in patient's with idiopathic thrombocytopenia and in patient's hypersensitive to a particular compound. Use of sustained-release injectable glucocorticoids are considered to be contraindicated for chronic corticosteroid therapy of systemic diseases.

Animals who have received glucocorticoids systemically other than with "burst" therapy, should be tapered off the drugs. Patients who have received the drugs chronically should be tapered off slowly as endogenous ACTH and corticosteroid function may return slowly. Should the animal undergo a "stressor" (*e.g.,* surgery, trauma, illness, etc.) during the tapering process or until normal adrenal and pituitary function resume, additional glucocorticoids should be administered.

Corticosteroid therapy may induce parturition in large animal species during the latter stages of pregnancy.

Adverse Effects/Warnings - Adverse effects are generally associated with long-term administration of these drugs, especially if given at high dosages or not on an alternate day regimen. Effects generally are manifested as symptoms of hyperadrenocorticism. When administered to young, growing animals, glucocorticoids can retard growth. Many of the potential effects, adverse and otherwise, are outlined above in the Pharmacology section.

In dogs, polydipsia (PD), polyphagia (PP) and polyuria (PU), may all be seen with short-term "burst" therapy as well as with alternate-day maintenance therapy on days when the drug is given. Adverse effects in dogs can include dull, dry haircoat, weight gain, panting, vomiting, diarrhea, elevated liver enzymes, pancreatitis, GI ulceration, lipidemias, activation or worsening of diabetes mellitus, muscle wasting and behavioral changes (depression, lethargy, viciousness). Discontin-uation of the drug may be necessary; changing to an alternate steroid may also alleviate the problem. With the exception of PU/PD/PP, adverse effects associated with antiinflammatory therapy are relatively uncommon. Adverse effects associated with immunosuppressive doses are more common and potentially more severe.

Cats generally require higher dosages than dogs for clinical effect, but tend to develop fewer adverse effects. Occasionally, polydipsia, polyuria, polyphagia with weight gain, diarrhea, or depression can be seen. Long-term, high dose therapy can lead to "Cushinoid" effects, however.

Administration of dexamethasone or triamcinolone may play a role in the development of laminitis in horses.

Overdosage - Glucocorticoids when given short-term are unlikely to cause harmful effects, even in massive dosages. One incidence of a dog developing acute CNS effects after accidental ingestion of glucocorticoids has been reported. Should symptoms occur, use supportive treatment if required.

Chronic usage of glucocorticoids can lead to serious adverse effects. Refer to Adverse Effects above for more information.

Drug Interactions - **Amphotericin B** or potassium-depleting diuretics (**furosemide, thiazides**) when administered concomitantly with glucocorticoids may cause hypokalemia. When these drugs are used concurrently with **digitalis glycosides**, an increased chance of digitalis toxicity may occur should hypokalemia develop. Diligent monitoring of potassium and digitalis glycoside levels are recommended.

Glucocorticoids may reduce **salicylate** blood levels.

Insulin requirements may increase in patients taking glucocorticoids. **Phenytoin, phenobarbital, rifampin** may increase the metabolism of glucocorticoids.

Concomitant administration of glucocorticoids and **cyclosporin** may increase the blood levels of each, by mutually inhibiting the hepatic metabolism of each other. The clinical significance of this interaction is not clear. Glucocorticoids may also inhibit the hepatic metabolism of **cyclophosphamide**. Dosage adjustments may be required.

The hepatic metabolism of **methylprednisolone** may be inhibited by **erythromycin**.

Mitotane may alter the metabolism of steroids; higher than usual doses of steroids may be necessary to treat mitotane-induced adrenal insufficiency.

Patients taking corticosteroids at immunosuppressive dosages should generally not receive **live attenuated-virus vaccines** as virus replication may be augmented. A diminished immune response may occur after **vaccine, toxoid, or bactrin** administration in patients receiving glucocorticoids.

Administration of **ulcerogenic drugs** (*e.g.,* **non-steroidal antiinflammatory drugs**) with glucocorticoids may increase the risk of gastrointestinal ulceration.

The effects of **hydrocortisone**, and possibly other glucocorticoids, may be potentiated by concomitant administration with **estrogens**.

In patients with myasthenia gravis, concomitant glucocorticoid and **anticholinesterase agent** (*e.g.,* pyridostigmine, neostigmine, etc.) administration may lead to profound muscle weakness. If possible, discontinue anticholinesterase medication at least 24 hours prior to corticosteroid administration.

Drug/Laboratory Interactions - Glucocorticoids may increase **serum cholesterol** and **urine glucose** levels. Glucocorticoids may decrease **serum potassium**.

Glucocorticoids can suppress the release of thyroid stimulating hormone (TSH) and reduce T_3 & T_4 values. Thyroid gland atrophy has been reported after chronic glucocorticoid administration. Uptake of I^{131} by the thyroid may be decreased by glucocorticoids.

Reactions to **skin tests** may be suppressed by glucocorticoids.

False-negative results the **nitroblue tetrazolium test** for systemic bacterial infections may be induced by glucocorticoids.

Monitoring Parameters - Monitoring of glucocorticoid therapy is dependent on its reason for use, dosage, agent used (amount of mineralocorticoid activity), dosage schedule (daily versus alternate day therapy), duration of therapy, and the animal's age and condition.The following list may not be appropriate or complete for all animals; use clinical assessment and judgement should adverse effects be noted:

    1) Weight, appetite, signs of edema
    2) Serum and/or urine electrolytes
    3) Total plasma proteins, albumin
    4) Blood glucose
    5) Growth and development in young animals
    7) ACTH stimulation test if necessary

Client Information - Clients should carefully follow the dosage instructions and should not discontinue the drug abruptly without consulting with veterinarian beforehand. Clients should be briefed on the potential adverse effects that can be seen with these drugs and instructed to contact the veterinarian should these effects become severe or progress.

GLYCERINE, ORAL

Chemistry - A trihydric alcohol, glycerin occurs as clear, sweet-tasting, syrupy, hygroscopic liquid that has a characteristic odor. It is miscible with water and alcohol, but not miscible in oils. Glycerin solutions are neutral to litmus. Glycerin may also be known as glycerol.

Storage/Stability/Compatibility - Glycerin oral solution should be stored in tight containers at room temperature; protect from freezing.

Pharmacology - Glycerin in therapeutic oral doses increases the osmotic pressure of plasma so that water from extracellular spaces is drawn into the blood. This can decrease intraocular pressure (IOP). The amount of decrease in IOP is dependent upon the dose of glycerin, and the cause and extent of increased IOP. Glycerin also decreases extracellular water content from other tissues and can cause dehydration and decreased CSF pressure.

Uses/Indications - Oral glycerin is used primarily for the short-term reduction of IOP in small animals with acute glaucoma. It may also be considered for use to reduce increased CSF pressure.
   The IOP-lowering effect of glycerin may be more variable than with mannitol, but since it may be given orally, it may be more advantageous to use in certain cases.

Pharmacokinetics - Glycerin is rapidly absorbed from the GI tract; peak serum levels generally occur within 90 minutes and maximum decreases in IOP usually occur within an hour of dosing and usually persist for up to 8 hours. Glycerin is distributed throughout the blood and is primarily metabolized by the liver. About 10% of the drug is excreted unchanged in the urine. Serum half-life in humans is about 30-45 minutes.

Contraindications/Precautions/Reproductive Safety - Glycerin is contraindicated in patients hypersensitive to it. It is also contraindicated in patients with anuria (well established), severely dehydrated, severely cardiac decompensated, or with frank or impending acute pulmonary edema.
   Glycerin should be used with caution in animals with hypovolemia, cardiac disease, or diabetes. Acute urinary retention should be avoided during the preoperative period.
   The safety of this drug in pregnant animals is unknown; use only when potential benefits outweigh the risks of therapy.

Adverse Effects/Warnings - Vomiting after dosing is the most common adverse effect seen with glycerin use. In humans, headache, nausea, thirst and diarrhea have also been reported.

Overdosage/Acute Toxicity - No specific information was located, but cardiac arrhythmias, non-ketotic hyperosmolar coma, severe dehydration have been reported with the drug.

Drug Interactions - Concomitant administration of **carbonic anhydrase inhibitors** (*e.g.,* **acetozolamide, dichlorphenamide) or topical miotic agents** may prolong the IOP-reducing effects of glycerin.

Doses -
   Dogs & Cats:
      For acute glaucoma:
         a) 1 - 2 ml/kg (of 50% solution), may repeat in 8 hours if necessary; withhold water for 30-60 minutes after administration. (Brooks 1986), (Brooks 1990)
         b) Dog: 0.6 ml/kg (percentage not specified) PO for 1-2 treatments. (Morgan 1988)

Monitoring Parameters -
   1) IOP
   2) Urine output
   3) Hydration status

Dosage Forms/Preparations/FDA Approval Status/Withholding Times -
   Veterinary-Approved Products: None
   Human-Approved Products:
      Glycerin Oral Liquid 50% (0.6 grams of glycerin per ml) in 220 ml bottles; *Osmoglyn®* (Alcon); (Rx)

Glycerin is also available in a topical ophthalmic solution and as suppositories or liquid for rectal laxative use.

Glyceryl Guaiacolate; GG - see Guaifenesin

GLYCOPYRROLATE

Chemistry - A synthetic quaternary ammonium antimuscarinic agent, glycopyrrolate occurs as a bitter-tasting, practically odorless, white, crystalline powder with a melting range of 193 - 198°C. One gram is soluble in 20 ml of water; 30 ml of alcohol. The commercially available injection is adjusted to a pH of 2-3 and contains 0.9% benzyl alcohol as a preservative. Glycopyrrolate may also be known as glycopyrronium bromide.

Storage/Stability/Compatibility - Glycopyrrolate tablets should be stored in tight containers and both the injection and tablets should be stored at room temperature (15-30°C).

Glycopyrrolate is stable under ordinary conditions of light and temperature. It is most stable in solution at an acidic pH and undergoes ester hydrolysis at pH's above 6.

Glycopyrrolate injection is physically **stable** in the following IV solutions: D5W, D5/half normal saline, Ringer's injection, and normal saline. Glycopyrrolate may be administered via the tubing of an IV running lactated Ringer's, but rapid hydrolysis will occur if it is added to an IV bag of LRS. The following drugs are reportedly physically **compatible** with glycopyrrolate: atropine sulfate, benzquinamide, chlorpromazine HCl, codeine phosphate, diphenhydramine HCl, droperidol, droperidol/fentanyl, hydromorphone, hydroxyzine HCl, lidocaine HCl, meperidine HCl, meperidine HCl/promethazine HCl, morphine sulfate, neostigmine methylsulfate, oxymorphone HCl, procaine HCl, prochlorperazine HCl, promazine HCl, promethazine HCl, pyridostigmine Br, scopolamine HBr, trimethobenzamide HCl.

The following drugs are reportedly **incompatible** with glycopyrrolate: chloramphenicol sodium succinate, dexamethasone sodium phosphate, diazepam, dimenhydrinate, methohexital sodium, methylprednisolone sodium succinate, pentazocine lactate, pentobarbital sodium, secobarbital sodium, sodium bicarbonate, and thiopental sodium. Other alkaline drugs (*e.g.,* thiamylal) would also be expected to be incompatible with glycopyrrolate. Compatibility is dependent upon factors such as pH, concentration, temperature, and diluents used and it is suggested to consult specialized references for more specific information.

Pharmacology - An antimuscarinic with similar actions as atropine, glycopyrrolate is a quaternary ammonium compound and, unlike atropine, does not cross appreciably into the CNS. It, therefore, should not exhibit the same extent of CNS adverse effects that atropine possesses. For further information, refer to the atropine monograph.

Uses/Indications - Glycopyrrolate injection is approved for use in dogs and cats. The FDA approved indication for these species is as a preanesthetic anticholinergic agent. The drug is also used to treat sinus bradycardia, sinoatrial arrest, incomplete AV block where anticholinergic therapy may be beneficial. When cholinergic agents such as neostigmine or pyridostigmine are used to reverse neuromuscular blockade due to non-depolarizing muscle relaxants, glycopyrrolate may administered simultaneously to prevent the peripheral muscarinic effects of the cholinergic agent.

Pharmacokinetics - Quaternary anticholinergic agents are not completely absorbed after oral administration, but quantitative data reporting the rate and extent of absorption of glycopyrrolate is not available. In dogs, following IV administration, the onset of action is generally within one minute. After IM or SQ administration, peak effects occur approximately 30-45 minutes post injection. The vagolytic effects persist for 2-3 hours and the antisialagogue (reduced salivation) effects persist for up to 7 hours. After oral administration, the anticholinergic effects of glycopyrrolate may persist for 8-12 hours.

Little information is available regarding the distributory aspects of glycopyrrolate. Being a quaternary ammonium compound, glycopyrrolate is completely ionized. Therefore, it has poor lipid solubility and does not readily penetrate into the CNS or eye. Glycopyrrolate crosses the placenta only marginally; it is unknown if it is excreted into milk.

Glycopyrrolate is eliminated rapidly from the serum after IV administration and virtually no drug remains in the serum 30 minutes to 3 hours after dosing. Only a small amount is metabolized and the majority is eliminated unchanged in the feces and urine.

Contraindications/Precautions - The manufacturer (Robins) of the veterinary product lists contraindications to glycopyrrolate's use in dogs and cats in animals hypersensitive to it and that it should not be used in pregnant animals. However, it would be prudent to refer to the recommendations listed in the atropine monograph regarding contraindications and precautions.

Adverse Effects/Warnings - With the exceptions of rare CNS adverse effects and being slightly less arrhythmogenic, glycopyrrolate can be expected to have a similar adverse effect profile as atropine. The manufacturer of the veterinary product (Robins) lists only mydriasis, tachycardia, and xerostomia as adverse effects in dogs and cats at the doses they recommend. For more information refer to the atropine monograph.

Overdosage - In dogs, the LD_{50} for glycopyrrolate is reported to be 25 mg/kg IV. Doses of 2 mg/kg IV daily for 5 days per week for 4 weeks demonstrated no signs of toxicity. In the cat, the LD_{50} after IM injection is 283 mg/kg. Because of its quaternary structure, it would be expected that minimal CNS effects would occur after an overdose of glycopyrrolate when compared to atropine. See the information listed in the atropine monograph for more information.

Drug Interactions - Glycopyrrolate would be expected to have a similar drug interaction profile as atropine. The following drugs may enhance the activity of glycopyrrolate and its derivatives: **antihistamines, procainamide, quinidine, meperidine, benzodiazepines, phenothiazines.**

The following drugs may potentiate the adverse effects of glycopyrrolate and its derivatives: **primidone, disopyramide, nitrates, long-term corticosteroid use** (may increase intraocular pressure).

Glycopyrrolate and its derivatives may enhance the actions of **nitrofurantoin, thiazide diuretics, sympathomimetics.**

Glycopyrrolate and its derivatives may antagonize the actions of **metoclopramide.**

Doses -
Dogs:
As an adjunct to anesthesia:
a) 0.011 mg/kg IV, IM, or SQ (Package Insert - *Robinul*®-*V*, Robins)
b) 0.01 - 0.02 mg/kg SQ or IM (Bellah 1988)

For adjunctive therapy of bradyarrhythmias:
a) 0.011 mg/kg IV or IM (Russell and Rush 1995)

To reduce hypersialism:
a) 0.01 mg/kg SQ *prn* (Krahwinkel 1988)

Cats:
As an adjunct to anesthesia:
a) 0.011 mg/kg IM, for maximum effect give 15 minutes prior to anesthetic administration (Package Insert - *Robinul*®-*V*, Robins)

For bradyarrhythmias:
a) 0.005 - 0.01 mg/kg IV or IM, 0.01 - 0.02 mg/kg SQ (Tilley and Miller 1986)

Rabbits/Rodents:
As adjunct to anesthesia: 0.01 - 0.02 mg/kg SubQ as need (Huerkamp 1995)

Horses:
For treatment of bradyarrhythmias due to increased parasympathetic tone:
a) 0.005 mg/kg IV (Muir and McGuirk 1987a)

As a bronchodilator:
a) Initially, 2 -3 mg IM *bid-tid* for a 450 kg animal (Beech 1987)

Monitoring Parameters - Dependent on route of administration, dose, and reason for use. See the atropine monograph for more information.

Client Information - Parenteral glycopyrrolate administration is best performed by professional staff and where adequate cardiac monitoring is available. If animal is receiving glycopyrrolate tablets, allow animal free access to water and encourage drinking if dry mouth is a problem

Dosage Forms/Preparations/FDA Approval Status/Withholding Times -
Veterinary-Approved Products:
Glycopyrrolate for Injection 0.2 mg/ml in 20 ml vials; *Robinul*®-*V* (Veterinary - 20 ml vial only); (Fort Dodge) (Rx) Approved for use in dogs and cats.

Human-Approved Products:
Glycopyrrolate Tablets 1 mg & 2 mg; *Robinul*® & *Robinul Forte*® (2 mg) (Robins); Generic; (Rx)

Glycopyrrolate for Injection 0.2 mg/ml in 1, 2, 5, & 20 ml vials; *Robinul*® (Robins); Generic; (Rx)

GONADORELIN

Chemistry - A hormone produced by the hypothalamus, gonadorelin is obtained either from natural sources or is synthetically produced. It is a decapeptide that occurs as white or faintly yellowish-white powder. One gram is soluble in 25 ml of water or in 50 ml of methyl alcohol. 50 mcg of gonadorelin acetate is approximately equivalent to 31 units. The commercially available product in the United States (*Cystorelin*®—Ceva) is the diacetate decahydrate salt. It is available as the hydrochloride elsewhere.

Gonadorelin has many synonyms, including: gonadotrophin-releasing hormone (GnRH), LH/FSH-RH, LH-RH, LH/FSH-RF, LH-RF, gonadoliberin, and luliberin.

Storage/Stability/Compatibility - The manufacturers recommend storing gonadorelin in the refrigerator (2-8°C). There is very little information available on the stability and compatibility of gonadorelin. Because bacterial contamination can inactivate the product, it has been recommended that multi-dose vials be used completely as rapidly as possible.

Pharmacology - Gonadorelin stimulates the production and the release of FSH and LH from the anterior pituitary. Secretion of endogenous GnRH from the hypothalamus is thought to be controlled by several factors, including circulating sex hormones.

Gonadorelin causes a surge-like release of FSH and LH after a single injection. In cows and ewes, this can induce ovulation, but not in estrus mares. A constant infusion of gonadorelin will initially stimulate LH and FSH release, but after a period of time, levels will return to baseline.

Uses/Indications - Gonadorelin (*Cystorelin*®—Ceva; *Factrel*®—Fort Dodge) is indicated (approved) for the treatment of ovarian follicular cysts in dairy cattle. Additionally, gonadorelin has been used in cattle to reduce the time interval from calving to first ovulation and to increase the number of ovulations within the first 3 months after calving. This may be particularly important in increasing fertility in cows with retained placenta.

In dogs, gonadorelin has been used experimentally to help diagnose reproductive disorders or to identify intact animals versus castrated ones by maximally stimulating FSH and LH production. It has also been used experimentally in dogs to induce estrus through pulsatile dosing. While apparently effective, specialized administration equipment is required for this method.

Gonadorelin has been used in cats as an alternate therapy to FSH or hCG to induce estrus in cats with prolonged anestrus.

In Europe, a synthetic analogue buserelin, has been used in horses to stimulate cyclic estrus. Its efficacy is poor when compared to an artificial light program, however.

In human medicine, gonadorelin has been used for the diagnosis of hypothalamic-pituitary dysfunction, cryptorchidism and depression secondary to prolonged severe stress.

Pharmacokinetics - After intravenous injection in pigs, gonadorelin is rapidly distributed to extracellular fluid, with a distribution half-life of about 2 minutes. The elimination half-life of gonadorelin is approximately 13 minutes in the pig.

After intravenous injection in humans, gonadorelin reportedly has a plasma half-life of only a few minutes. Within one hour, approximately half the dose is excreted in the urine as metabolites.

Contraindications/Precautions - None noted.

Adverse Effects/Warnings - No reported adverse reactions were located for this agent. Synthetically prepared gonadorelin should not cause any hypersensitivity reactions. This may not be the case with pituitary-obtained LH preparations or hCG.

Overdosage - In doses of up to 120 micrograms/kg, no untoward effects were noted in several species of test animals. Gonadorelin is unlikely to cause significant adverse effects after inadvertent overdosage.

Drug Interactions - None noted.

Doses -
  Dogs:
      GnRH challenge to test pituitary sufficiency or testicular steroidogenesis:
        a) 125 - 250 ng/kg (refer to reference for more information) (Amann 1986)
      To aid in the descent of cryptorchid testes:
        a) 50 - 100 micrograms SQ or IV; if no response give additional dose in 4-6 days (Cox 1986)
  Cats:
      To stimulate ovulation after mating:
        a) 25 micrograms IM after mating (Morgan 1988)
  Cattle:
      To treat of ovarian cysts in cattle:
        a) 100 micrograms IM or IV (Package Insert; *Cystorelin*®—Ceva)
        b) 100 micrograms IM per cow (Package insert; *Factrel*®—Fort Dodge)
  Sheep & Goats:
      To induce ovulation outside of the breeding season in the doe:
        a) 100 micrograms injected daily for 4-5 days (Smith 1986b)

Dosage Forms/Preparations/FDA Approval Status/Withholding Times -
  Veterinary-Approved Products:
      Gonadorelin (diacetate tetrahydrate) for Injection 50 micrograms/ml, 2 ml single-use or 10 ml multi-dose vials; *Cystorelin*® (Rhone Merieux); *Fertagyl*® (Intervet); (Rx) Approved for use in dairy cattle. There are no withdrawal times required for either milk or slaughter.

      Gonadorelin HCl Solution for Injection 50 mcg/ml in 2 ml single-use, and 20 ml multi-dose vials; *Factrel*® (Fort Dodge); (Rx) Approved for use in cattle. No withdrawal period required.

Human-Approved Products:
Gonadorelin Acetate Powder for Injection (lyophilized) 0.8 and 3.2 mg in 10 ml vials; *Lutrepulse*® (Ferring) (Rx)

Gonadorelin HCl Powder for Injection 100 mcg/vial, 500 mcg/vial; *Factrel*® (Wyeth-Ayerst); (Rx)

GRISEOFULVIN (MICROSIZE)
GRISEOFULVIN (ULTRAMICROSIZE)

Chemistry - A fugistatic antibiotic produced by species of Penicillium (primarily *P. griseoful- vum*), griseofulvin occurs as an odorless or nearly odorless, bitter tasting, white to creamy white powder. It is very slightly soluble in water and sparingly soluble in alcohol.

Two forms of the drug are available commercially. Microsize griseofulvin contains particles with a predominant size of 4 μm in diameter, while the ultramicrosize form particle size averages less than 1 μm in diameter.

Storage/Stability/Compatibility - Although griseofulvin is relatively thermostable, products should be stored at less than 40°C, preferably at 15-30°C. Griseofulvin suspension should be stored in tight, light-resistant containers. Microsize tablets and capsules should be stored in tight containers; the ultramicrosize tablets should be stored in well-closed containers.

Pharmacology - Griseofulvin acts on susceptible fungi by disrupting the structure of the cell's mitotic spindle, thereby arresting the metaphase of cell division. Griseofulvin has activity against species of *Trichophyton*, *Microsporum* and *Epidermophyton*. Only new hair or nail growth is resistant to infection. It has no antibacterial activity, and is not clinically useful against other pathogenic fungi.

Uses/Indications - In veterinary species, griseofulvin is approved for use in dogs and cats to treat dermatophytic fungal (see above) infections of the skin, hair and claws, and to treat ringworm (caused by *T. equinum* and *M. gypseum*) in horses. It has also been used in laboratory animals and ruminants for the same indications.

Pharmacokinetics - The microsized form of the drug is absorbed variably (25-70%); dietary fat will enhance absorption. The ultramicrosize form of the drug may be nearly 100% absorbed. Generally, the ultramicrosize form is absorbed 1.5 times as well as the microsized form for a given patient.

Griseofulvin is concentrated in skin, hair, nails, fat, skeletal muscle and the liver, and can be found in the stratum corneum within 4 hours of dosing.

Griseofulvin is metabolized by the liver via oxidative demethylation and glucuronidation to 6-desmethylgriseofulvin which is not active. In humans, the half-life is 9-24 hours. A serum half-life of 47 minutes has been reported for dogs. Less than 1% of the drug is excreted unchanged in the urine.

Contraindications/Precautions/Reproductive Safety - Griseofulvin is contraindicated in patients hypersensitive to it or with hepatocellular failure.

Because kittens may be overly sensitive to the adverse effects associated with griseofulvin, they should be monitored carefully if treatment is instituted.

Griseofulvin is a known teratogen in cats. Dosages of 35 mg/kg given to cats during the first trimester caused cleft palate, and other skeletal and brain malformations in kittens. Griseofulvin may also inhibit spermatogenesis. Because dermatophytic infections are not generally life-threatening and alternative therapies are available, use of the drug should be considered contraindicated during pregnancy.

Adverse Effects/Warnings - Griseofulvin can cause anorexia, vomiting, diarrhea, anemia, neutropenia, leukopenia, depression, ataxia, hepatotoxicity or dermatitis/photosensitivity. With the exception of GI symptoms, adverse effects are uncommon at usual doses. Cats, particularly kittens, may be more susceptible to adverse effects than other species. This could be due to this species' propensity to more slowly form glucuronide conjugates and thus metabolize the drug at a slower rate than either dogs or humans.

Overdosage/Acute Toxicity - No specifics regarding griseofulvin overdosage or acute toxicity was located. It is suggested that significant overdoses be handled with gut emptying, charcoal and cathartic administration unless contraindicated. Contact a poison control center for more information.

Horses have received 100 mg/kg PO for 20 days without apparent ill effect.

Drug Interactions - **Phenobarbital** (and other barbiturates) has been implicated in causing decreased griseofulvin blood concentrations, presumably by inducing hepatic microsomal enzymes and/or reducing absorption. If phenobarbital and griseofulvin are given concurrently, griseofulvin dosage adjustment may be necessary.

Coumarin (*e.g.,* warfarin) **anticoagulants** may have their anticoagulant activity reduced by griseofulvin; anticoagulant adjustment may be required.

Griseofulvin may potentiate the effects of **alcohol**.

Doses -
Note: all doses are for microsize preparations unless otherwise indicated.

Dogs:
For susceptible dermatophytic infections:
a) Microsize: 50 mg/kg/day divided q8-12h PO; Ultramicrosize: 25 mg/kg/day divided q8-12h PO. Give following a fatty meal or administration of corn oil. Continue until no clinical evidence of disease remains (6-8 weeks). (Schultz 1986)
b) Microsize: 20 - 50 mg/kg in divided doses with fat divided *bid* for 4-6 weeks for *M. canis*; and until cultures are negative for *Trichophyton*.
Ultramicrosize: 5 - 10 mg/kg PO once daily. Duration as above. (Foil 1986)

Cats:
For susceptible dermatophytic infections:
a) Microsize: 50 mg/kg/day divided q8-12h PO; Ultramicrosize: 25 mg/kg/day divided q8-12h PO. Give following a fatty meal or administration of corn oil. Continue until no clinical evidence of disease remains (6-8 weeks). (Schultz 1986)
b) For feline *M. canis*: After total body clip, griseofulvin 80 - 130 mg/kg PO once daily with a fatty meal or 2.5 - 5 ml of corn oil. Re-clip after one month and continue treatment until signs of infection have disappeared and cultures are negative. (Thoday 1986)
c) Microsize: 20 - 50 mg/kg in divided doses with fat divided *bid* for 4-6 weeks for *M. canis*, and until cultures are negative for *Trichophyton*.
Ultramicrosize: 5 - 10 mg/kg PO once daily. Duration as above. (Foil 1986)

Cattle (and other ruminants):
For susceptible dermatophytic infections:
a) Ultramicrosize: 10 - 20 mg/kg PO once daily for 1-2 weeks. 100 mg/kg PO given twice (or more) 1 week apart may also be effective. Not approved for use in food animals and can be very expensive. (Pier 1986)
b) 20 mg/kg PO once daily for 6 weeks. (Howard 1986)

Horses:
For susceptible dermatophytic infections:
a) 10 mg/kg PO once daily (Robinson 1987)
b) 10 mg/kg PO (in feed) daily for 7 days (Brumbaugh 1987)

Swine:
For susceptible dermatophytic infections:
a) 20 mg/kg PO once daily for 6 weeks. (Howard 1986)

Monitoring Parameters -
1) Clinical efficacy; culture
2) Adverse effects
3) CBC q2-3 weeks during therapy
4) Liver enzymes (if indicated)

Client Information - Clients should be instructed in procedures used to prevent reinfection (destruction of old bedding, disinfection, periodic reexaminations, hair clipping, etc.) and the importance of compliance with the dosage regimen. Should animal develop adverse effects other than mild GI disturbances, they should contact their veterinarian.

Dosage Forms/Preparations/FDA Approval Status/Withholding Times -
Veterinary-Approved Products:
Griseofulvin (Microsize) Powder 2.5 g griseofulvin in 15 g sachets
Fulvicin-U/F® Powder (Schering-Plough); (Rx) Approved for use in horses.

Griseofulvin (Microsize) Tablets 250 mg, 500 mg (scored); *Fulvicin-U/F® Tablets* (Schering-Plough); (Rx) Approved for use in dogs and cats.

Human-Approved Products:
Griseofulvin (Microsize) Capsules 250 mg; *Grisactin®* (Wyeth-Ayerst); (Rx)

Griseofulvin (Microsize) Tablets 250 mg, 500 mg; *Fulvicin-U/F®* (Schering); *Grifulvin V®* (Ortho); *Grisactin 500®* (Wyeth-Ayerst); (Rx)

Griseofulvin (Microsize) Oral Suspension 125 mg/5 ml in 120 ml; *Grifulvin V®* (Ortho Derm); (Rx)

Griseofulvin (Ultramicrosize) Tablets 125 mg, 165 mg, 250 mg, 330 mg; *Fulvicin P/G®* (Schering); *Grisactin Ultra®* (Wyeth-Ayerst); *Gris-PEG®* (Allergan Herbert); generic. (Rx)

GUAIFENESIN

Chemistry - Formerly known as glyceryl guaiacolate, guaifenesin occurs as a white to slightly gray, crystalline powder which may have a characteristic odor. It is nonhygroscopic and melts between 78° - 82°C. One gram is soluble in 15 ml of water and it is soluble in alcohol, propylene glycol and glycerin. Guaifenesin may also be known as glyceryl guaiacolate, GG, or guaiphenesin.

Storage/Stability/Compatibility - Guaifenesin is stable in light and heat (less than melting point). It should be stored in well closed containers.

When dissolved into aqueous solutions, guaifenesin may slightly precipitate out of solution when the temperature is less than 22°C (72°F). Slight warming and agitation generally resolubilizes the drug. A microwave oven has been suggested for heating and dissolving the drug. It is recommended that the solution be prepared freshly before use, but a 10% solution (in sterile water) may apparently be stored safely at room temperature for up to one week with only slight precipitation occurring.

Guaifenesin is physically **compatible** with sterile water or D5W. It is also reportedly compatible with ketamine, pentobarbital, thiamylal, thiopental, and xylazine.

Pharmacology - While the exact mechanism of action for the muscle relaxant effects are not known, it is believed that guaifenesin acts centrally by depressing or blocking nerve impulse transmission at the internuncial neuron level of the subcortical areas of the brain, brainstem and spinal cord. It relaxes both the laryngeal and pharyngeal muscles, thus allowing easier intubation. Guaifenesin also has mild intrinsic analgesic and sedative qualities.

Guaifenesin causes an excitement-free induction and recovery from anesthesia in horses. It produces relaxation of skeletal muscles, but does not affect diaphragmatic function and has little, if any, effects on respiratory function at usual doses. Possible effects on the cardiovascular system include transient mild decreases in blood pressure and increases in cardiac rate. Gastrointestinal motility may be increased, but generally no adversity is seen with this.

Guaifenesin potentiates the activity of preanesthetic and anesthetic agents.

Uses/Indications - In veterinary medicine, guaifenesin is used to induce muscle relaxation and restraint as an adjunct to anesthesia for short procedures (30-60 minutes) in large and small animal species.

In human medicine, guaifenesin has long been touted as an oral expectorant, but definitive proof of its efficacy is lacking.

Pharmacokinetics - The pharmacokinetics of guaifenesin have not been thoroughly studied in most species. When administered alone to horses IV, recumbency usually occurs within 2 minutes and light (not surgical level) restraint persists for about 6 minutes. Muscle relaxation reportedly persists for 10-20 minutes after a single dose.

Guaifenesin is conjugated in the liver and excreted into the urine. A gender difference in the elimination half-life of guaifenesin in ponies has been demonstrated, with males having a $t_{1/2}$ of approximately 85 minutes, and females a $t_{1/2}$ of about 60 minutes. Guaifenesin reportedly crosses the placenta, but adverse effects in newborns of mothers who received guaifenesin have not been described.

Contraindications/Precautions - The manufacturer states that the use of physostigmine is contraindicated with guaifenesin (see Drug Interactions).

Adverse Effects/Warnings - At usual doses, side effects are transient and generally minor. A mild decrease in blood pressure and increase in cardiac rate can be seen. Thrombophlebitis has been reported after IV injection, and perivascular administration may cause some tissue reaction. Hemolysis may occur in solutions containing greater than a 5% concentration of guaifenesin, but some sources state this is insignificant at even a 15% concentration.

Overdosage - The margin of safety is reportedly 3 times the usual dose. Symptoms of apneustic breathing, nystagmus, hypotension, and contradictory muscle rigidity are associated with toxic levels of the drug. No specific antidote is available. It is suggested that treatment be supportive until the drug is cleared to sub-toxic levels.

Drug Interactions - Drug interactions with guaifenesin are not well studied. The manufacturer (Robins) states that **physostigmine** is contraindicated in horses receiving guaifenesin, but does not elucidate on the actual interaction. It may be logical to assume that other anticholinesterase agents (neostigmine, pyridostigmine, edrophonium) may also be contraindicated.

Doses -
Dogs:
- a) Guaifenesin only: 44 - 88 mg/kg IV; or guaifenesin 33 - 88 mg/kg IV with 2.2 - 6.6 mg/kg thiamylal or 1.1 mg/kg ketamine (Muir)
- b) 110 mg/kg IV for muscle relaxation during certain toxicoses (*e.g.,* strychnine) or tetanus (Morgan 1988), (Bailey 1986a)
- c) For chemical restraint for ventilatory support: Combination of guaifenesin 50 mg/ml, ketamine 1 mg/ml, & xylazine 0.25 mg/ml; give 0.55 ml bolus initially followed by 2.2 ml/kg/hr thereafter (Pascoe 1986)

Cattle:
- a) Guaifenesin only: 66 - 132 mg/kg IV; or guaifenesin 44 - 88 mg/kg IV with 2.2 - 6.6 mg/kg thiamylal or 0.66 - 1.1 mg/kg ketamine (Muir)
- b) 55 - 110 mg/kg IV (Mandsager 1988)

Horses:
- a) 110 mg/kg IV, give first 1/3-1/2 of dose until horse falls gently, then give remainder unless respiratory or cardiovascular effects are observed. (Package Insert, *Guailaxin*® - Robins)
- b) Guaifenesin only: 66 - 132 mg/kg IV; or guaifenesin 44 - 88 mg/kg IV with 2.2 - 6.6 mg/kg thiamylal (Muir)
- c) 55 - 110 mg/kg IV (Mandsager 1988)
- d) For anesthesia: 100 mg/kg IV combined with barbiturate in 5% dextrose. As an expectorant: 3 mg/kg PO (Robinson 1987)

Swine:
- a) Guaifenesin only: 44 - 88 mg/kg IV; or guaifenesin 33 - 88 mg/kg IV with 2.2 - 6.6 mg/kg thiamylal or 1.1 mg/kg ketamine (Muir)

Goats:
- a) Guaifenesin only: 66 - 132 mg/kg IV; or guaifenesin 44 - 88 mg/kg IV with 0.66 - 1.1 mg/kg ketamine (Muir)

Monitoring Parameters -
1) Level of muscle relaxation
2) Cardiac and respiratory rate

Dosage Forms/Preparations/FDA Approval Status/Withholding Times -
Veterinary-Approved Products:
Guaifenesin Sterile Powder for Injection 50 gram for reconstitution in 4 oz and 32 oz containers; *Guailaxin*® (Fort Dodge), *Gecolate*® (Summit Hill); (Rx) Approved for use in horses.

Guaifenesin Injection 50mg/ml 1000ml; *Gecolate*® (Summit Hill); generic (Phoenix); (Rx) Approved for use in horses.

Human-Approved Products: No parenteral preparations are approved. There are many OTC oral expectorant/cough preparations on the market.

HALOTHANE

Chemistry - An inhalant general anesthetic agent, halothane occurs as a colorless, nonflammable, heavy liquid. It has a characteristic odor resembling chloroform and sweet, burning taste. Halothane is slightly soluble in water and miscible with alcohol. At 20°C, halothane's specific gravity is 1.872-1.877 and vapor pressure is 243 mm Hg.

Storage/Stability/Compatibility - Store halothane below 40°C in a tight, light-resistant container. Halothane stability is maintained by the addition of thymol and ammonia. The thymol does not vaporize so it may accumulate in the vaporizer causing a yellow discoloration. Do not use discolored solutions. Discolored vaporizer and wick may be cleaned with diethyl ether (all ether must be removed before reuse).

In the presence of moisture, halothane vapor can react with aluminum, brass and lead (not copper). Rubber and some plastics are soluble in halothane leading to their rapid deterioration.

Pharmacology - While the precise mechanism that inhalant anesthetics exert their general anesthetic effect is not precisely known, they may interfere with functioning of nerve cells in the brain by acting at the lipid matrix of the membrane. Some key pharmacologic effects noted with halothane include: CNS depression, depression of body temperature regulating centers, increased cerebral blood flow, respiratory depression (pronounced in ruminants), hypotension, vasodilatation, and myocardial depression.

Minimal Alveolar Concentration (MAC; %) in oxygen reported for halothane in various species: Dog = 0.76; Cat = 0.82; Horse = 0.88; Human = 0.76. Several factors may alter MAC (acid/base status, temperature, other CNS depressants on board, age, ongoing acute disease, etc.).

Uses/Indications - Halothane remains a useful general anesthetic in veterinary medicine due to its relative safety, potency, controllability, non-flammability, and comparative low cost.

Pharmacokinetics - Halothane is rapidly absorbed through the lungs. About 12% of absorbed drug is metabolized by the liver to trifluoroacetic acid (only small amounts), chlorine and bromine radicals which are excreted in the urine. The bulk of the absorbed drug is re-excreted by the lungs and eliminated with expired air. Halothane is distributed into milk.

Contraindications/Precautions/Reproductive Safety - Halothane is contraindicated in patients with a history or predilection towards malignant hyperthermia or significant hepatotoxicity after previous halothane exposure (see Adverse Reactions below). It should be used with caution (benefits vs. risks) in patients with hepatic function impairment, cardiac arrhythmias, increased CSF or head injury, myasthenia gravis, or pheochromocytoma (cardiac arrhythmias due to catecholamines).

Some animal studies have shown that halothane may be teratogenic; use only when benefits outweigh potential risks.

Adverse Effects/Warnings - Hypotension may occur and is considered to be dosage related. A malignant hyperthermia-stress syndrome has been reported in pigs, horses, dogs and cats. Halothane may cause cardiac depression and dysrhythmias. Halothane-induced hypotension may be treated by volume expansion and dobutamine. Lidocaine has been used to treat or prevent halothane-induced cardiac dysrhythmias.

In humans, jaundice and a postanesthetic fatal liver necrosis has been reported rarely. The incidence of this effect in veterinary species is not known. However, halothane should be considered contraindicated for future use if unexplained fever, jaundice or other symptoms associated with hepatotoxicity occur.

Drug Interactions - **Acetaminophen** is not recommended to be used for post-operative analgesia in animals who have received halothane anesthesia.

Because halothane sensitizes the myocardium to the effects of sympathomimetics, especially catecholamines, severe ventricular arrhythmias may result. Drugs included are: **dopamine, epinephrine, norepinephrine, ephedrine, metaraminol, etc.** If these drugs are needed, they should be used with caution and in significantly reduced dosages with intensive monitoring.

Non-depolarizing neuromuscular blocking agents, systemic aminoglycosides, systemic lincomycins should be used with caution with halogenated anesthetic agents as additive neuromuscular blockade may occur.

Reportedly, **d-tubocurarine** may cause significant hypotension if used with halothane.

Concomitant administration of **succinylcholine** with inhalation anesthetics (halothane, cyclopropane, nitrous oxide, diethyl ether) may induce increased incidences of cardiac effects (bradycardia, arrhythmias, sinus arrest and apnea) and in susceptible patients, malignant hyperthermia.

Laboratory Considerations - Halothane may transiently increase values of **liver function tests.**

Doses -

Dogs/Cats: (Note: Concentrations are dependent upon fresh gas flow rate; the lower the flow rate, the higher the concentration required.
- a) 3% (induction); 0.5 - 1.5% (maintenance) (Papich 1992)
- b) 0.5 - 3.5%, inhaled (Hubbell 1994)

Pocket Pets:
- a) Using a non-rebreathing system: Induction: 2 - 4%, maintenance: 0.25 - 2% (Anderson 1994)

Horses:
- a) For draft horses: Following induction, the largest ET tube that will comfortably fit (20 - 40 mm) should be placed and cuff inflated. In an oxygen-enriched semi-closed large animal circle system 4-5% of halothane is administered initially and is reduced as indicated by physical monitoring of neural reflexes and cardiopulmonary parameters. The goal should be the lowest concentration inhalant anesthetic that provides adequate surgical anesthesia and restraint. Most draft horses can be maintained on 2.5 - 3% halothane. (See reference for more information on monitoring and use.) (Geiser 1992)

Monitoring Parameters - 1) Respiratory and ventilatory status; 2) Cardiac rate/rhythm; blood pressure (particularly with "at risk" patients); 3) Level of anesthesia

Dosage Forms/Preparations/FDA Approval Status/Withholding Times -
Veterinary-Approved Products:
Halothane, USP (with thymol 0.01% and ammonia 0.00025%) in 250 ml bottles; (Fort Dodge); (Rx)

Human-Approved Products:

Halothane in 125 & 250 ml bottles; *Halothane*® (Abbott) (Rx), *Fluothane*® (Wyeth-Ayerst) (Rx)

HCG - see Chorionic Gonadotropin

HEMOGLOBIN GLUTAMER-200 (BOVINE) OXYGLOBIN®

Chemistry - Oxyglobin® is a sterile, clear, dark purple solution containing 13 g/dL purified, polymerized hemoglobin of bovine origin in a modified lactated Ringer's solution. It has an osmolality of 300 mOsm/kg and a pH of 7.8. Less than 5% of the hemoglobin are as unstabilized tetramers, and approximately 50% have a molecular weight between 65 and 130 kD, with no more than 10% having a molecular weight >500 kD. The product contains less than the detectable level of 3.5 μg/ml free-glutaraldehyde and 0.05 EU/mL endotoxin.

Storage/Stability/Compatibility - The product remains stable at room temperature or refrigerated (2°-30°C) for 2 years. Do not freeze. It must remain in its overwrap during storage; once removed, it should be used within 24 hours. The foil overwrap serves as an oxygen barrier, protecting the hemoglobin from conversion to methemoglobin.

The manufacturer states that Oxyglobin® is compatible with any other IV fluid, but should not be mixed with other solutions or medications in the bag. Other intravenous solutions and medications may be administered via a separate site and line, however,

Pharmacology - The bovine hemoglobin in the product is polymerized into larger molecules to increase safety, efficacy and intravascular persistence, and is shipped in a deoxygenated state and becomes oxygenated once circulated through the lungs. Oxyglobin® releases oxygen to tissue in a mechanism similarly to endogenous hemoglobin. Oxyglobin® thereby increases plasma and total hemoglobin concentrations and increases systemic oxygen content.

Oxyglobin® also has colloidal properties similar to dextran 70 and hetastarch.

Uses/Indications - Oxyglobin® is indicated for the treatment of dogs with anemia, regardless of the cause of anemia (hemolysis, blood loss, or ineffective erythropoiesis). From a prognostic standpoint, the drug should be more valuable in dog's with regenerative anemias (versus nonregenerative anemias).

Pharmacokinetics - In dogs receiving 15 ml/kg, peak plasma hemoglobin concentrations increased approximately 2.5 g/dL; at 30 ml/kg, approximately 4 mg/dl. Duration of effect continues for at least 24 hours. The plasma half-life in dogs at present labeled dosages is approximately 30-40 hours and Oxyglobin® can be detected in the plasma for 5-7 days after a single dose.

As with endogenous hemoglobin, Oxyglobin® is metabolized and eliminated by the reticuloendothelial system. Small amounts of unstabilized hemoglobin (<5%) may be excreted through the kidneys, causing discoloration (red) of the urine.

Contraindications/Precautions/Reproductive Safety - As safe use of Oxyglobin® has not been tested for the following conditions and plasma expanders are generally contraindicated in them, the product is labeled as contraindicated in dogs with advanced cardiac disease (i.e., congestive heart failure) or otherwise severely impaired cardiac function or renal impairment with oliguria or anuria. The safety and efficacy of Oxyglobin® has not been evaluated in dogs with DIC, thrombocytopenia with active bleeding, hemoglobinemia and hemoglobinuria, or autoagglutination.

Administration of any foreign protein has the potential to cause immunologic reactions; while low levels of IgG antibodies have been detected after multiple dosages, no anaphylactic reactions have been reported thus far. If an immediate hypersensitivity reaction occurs, infusion should be immediately discontinued and appropriate treatment administered. If a delayed type of hypersensitivity reaction occurs, immunosuppressant therapy is recommended.

Safe use in breeding dogs and pregnant or lactating bitches has not been determined.

Adverse Effects/Warnings - The package insert lists the following frequency of adverse reactions that occurred in greater than 4% of dogs treated with Oxyglobin® (**Note**: first figure is % of dogs treated; in parentheses: % treated having hemolytic anemia): Discolored mucous membranes 69% (47%); discolored sclera (yellow, red, brown) 56% (48%); discolored urine (orange, red, brown) 52% (41%); discolored skin (yellow) 12% (83%); increased central venous pressure (CVP) 33% (47%); ventricular arrhythmias (AV block, tachycardia, ventricular premature contractions) 15% (78%); ecchymoses/petechiae 8% (50%); bradycardia 6% (67%); vomiting 35% (72%); diarrhea 15% (50%); anorexia 8% (25%); tachypnea 15% (50%); dyspnea 14% (71%); pulmonary edema 12% (67%); harsh lung sounds/crackles 8% (50%); pleural effusion 6%

(67%); fever 17% (40%); death/euthanasia 15% (63%); peripheral edema 8% (25%); hemoglobinuria 6% (67%); dehydration 6% (33%).

Adverse reactions occurring in 4% of the dogs treated with Oxyglobin® included: coughing, disseminated intravascular coagulopathy, melena, nasal discharge/crusts (red), peritoneal effusion, respiratory arrest, and weight loss (5-7% body weight). Adverse reactions occurring in less than 2% of the dogs treated with Oxyglobin® included: abdominal discomfort on palpation, acidosis, cardiac arrest, cardiovascular volume overload (by echocardiography), collapse, cystitis, dark stool, discolored soft stool (red-brown) and tongue (purple), focal hyperemic areas on gums, forelimb cellulitis/lameness, hematemesis or hemoptysis (unable to differentiate), hypernatremia, hypotension, hypoxemia, lack of neurologic responses, left forebrain signs, nystagmus, pancreatitis, pendulous abdomen, polyuria, pulmonary thromboembolism, ptosis, reddened pinnae with papules/head shaking, reduction in heart rate, thrombocytopenia (worsening), and venous thrombosis.

Small amounts of unstabilized hemoglobin (<5%) may be excreted through the kidneys, resulting in transient discoloration (red) of the urine following the infusion. This discoloration of the urine should not be interpreted as due to intravascular hemolysis and has no effect on renal function.

Increases in aspartate aminotransferase (AST) and alanine aminotransferase (ALT) not associated with histopathologic changes in the liver, increase in serum total protein, and hemoglobinuria may also be seen.

Overdosage - The clinical signs associated with Oxyglobin® administered at 1, 2, and 3 times the recommended dose twice, 3 days apart include yellow-orange discoloration of skin, ear canals, pinnae, mucous membranes (gums), and sclera, red-dark-green-black discoloration of feces, brown-black discoloration of urine, red spotting of skin and/or lips (less common finding), decreased appetite and thirst, vomiting, diarrhea, and decreased skin elasticity. The frequency and/or intensity of these signs increased with repeated dose and with increasing dose. Healthy dogs administered 3X overdoses twice, all survived.

Overdosage or an excessively rapid administration rate (i.e., > 10 ml/kg/hr) may result in circulatory overload.

Drug Interactions/Drug Lab Interactions - Other than concerns with compatibility (noted above), no specific drug interactions have been noted.

The presence of Oxyglobin® in serum may cause artifactual increases or decreases in the results of **serum chemistry tests**, depending on the type of analyzer and reagents used. Refer to the actual package insert for specific information.

There is reportedly no interference with hematology tests, but due to the dilutional effects of Oxyglobin®, **PCV** and **RBC count** are not accurate measures of the degree of anemia for 24 hours following administration. Prothrombin time (PT) and activated partial thromboplastin time (aPTT) determined using methods that are mechanical, magnetic and light scattering are accurate, but optical methods are not reliable while Oxyglobin® is present.

Urine **dipstick measurements** (i.e., pH, glucose, ketones, protein) are inaccurate while gross discoloration of the urine is present.

Doses -
  Dogs: For labeled indications:
    a) One-time dose of 30 ml/kg IV at a rate of up to 10 mL/kg/hr.
       May be warmed to 37°C prior to administration. Blood transfusions are not contraindicated in dogs which receive Oxyglobin® nor is Oxyglobin® contraindicated in dogs which have previously received a blood transfusion. There is no need for typing or crossmatching before use. Should be administered using aseptic technique via a standard intravenous infusion set and catheter through a central or peripheral vein at a rate of 10 mL/kg/hr. Do not administer with other fluids or drugs via the same infusion set. Do not add medications or other solutions to the bag. Do not combine the contents of more than one bag. (Package Insert; Oxyglobin®—Biopure)

Monitoring Parameters - 1) Hgb; clinical signs of adequate tissue oxygenation; 2) Signs of circulatory overload (CVP); 3) Other adverse effects (see above)

Client Information - Clients should be informed of the cost/risk/benefit profile for this agent before use.

Dosage Forms/Preparations/FDA Approval Status -
  Veterinary-Approved Products: None

    Hemoglobin Glutamer-200 (bovine) in 125 ml ready to use infusion bags; *Oxyglobin®* (Biopure); (Rx). Approved for use in dogs.

HEPARIN SODIUM
HEPARIN CALCIUM

Chemistry - Heparin is an anionic, heterogeneous sulfated glycosaminoglycan molecule with an average molecular weight of 12,000 that is found naturally in mast cells. It is available commercially as either sodium or calcium salts and is obtained from either porcine intestinal mucosa (both calcium and sodium salts) or from bovine lung tissue (sodium salt only). Heparin sodium and calcium occur as white or pale-colored, amorphous, hygroscopic powders having a faint odor. Both are soluble in water and practically insoluble in alcohol; the commercial injections have a pH of 5-7.5. Heparin potency is expressed in terms of USP Heparin units and values are obtained by comparing against a standard reference from the USP. The USP requires that potencies be not less than 120 units/mg on a dried basis for heparin derived from lung tissue, and 140 units/mg when derived from all other tissue sources.

Storage/Stability/Compatibility - Heparin solutions should be stored at room temperature (15-30°C) and not frozen. Avoid excessive exposure to heat.

Heparin sodium is reportedly **compatible** with the following intravenous solutions and drugs: amino acids 4.25%-dextrose 25%, dextrose-Ringer's combinations, dextrose-lactated Ringer's solutions, fat emulsion 10%, Ringer's injection, Normosol R, aminophylline, amphotericin B w/ or w/o hydrocortisone sodium phosphate, ascorbic acid injection, bleomycin sulfate, calcium gluconate, cephapirin sodium, chloramphenicol sodium succinate, clindamycin phosphate, dimenhydrinate, dopamine HCl, erythromycin gluceptate, isoproterenol HCl, lidocaine HCl, methylprednisolone sodium succinate, metronidazole with sodium succinate, nafcillin sodium, norepinephrine bitartrate, potassium chloride, prednisolone sodium succinate, promazine HCl, sodium bicarbonate, verapamil HCl and vitamin B-complex w/ or w/o vitamin C.

Heparin **compatibility information conflicts** or is dependent on diluent or concentration factors with the following drugs or solutions: dextrose-saline combinations, dextrose in water, lactated Ringer's injection, saline solutions, ampicillin sodium, cephalothin sodium, dobutamine HCl, hydrocortisone sodium succinate, methicillin sodium, oxytetracycline HCl, penicillin G sodium/potassium, and tetracycline HCl. Compatibility is dependent upon factors such as pH, concentration, temperature and diluents used. It is suggested to consult specialized references for more specific information (*e.g., Handbook on Injectable Drugs* by Trissel; see bibliography).

Heparin sodium is reported **incompatible** with the following solutions or drugs: sodium lactate 1/6 M, amikacin sulfate, chlorpromazine HCl, codeine phosphate, cytarabine, daunorubicin HCl, diazepam, doxorubicin HCl, droperidol HCl w/ & w/o fentanyl citrate, erythromycin lactobionate, gentamicin sulfate, hyaluronidase, kanamycin sulfate, levorphanol bitartrate, meperidine HCl, methadone HCl, morphine sulfate, pentazocine lactate, phenytoin sodium, polymyxin B sulfate, streptomycin sulfate and vancomycin HCl.

Pharmacology - Heparin acts on coagulation factors in both the intrinsic and extrinsic coagulation pathways. Low concentrations of heparin when combined with antithrombin III inactivate factor X_a and prevent the conversion of prothrombin to thrombin. In higher doses, heparin inactivates thrombin, blocks the conversion of fibrinogen to fibrin and when combined with antithrombin III inactivates factors IX, X, XI, XII. By inhibiting the activation of factor XIII (fibrin stabilizing factor), heparin also prevents the formation of stable fibrin clots. While heparin will inhibit the reactions that lead to clotting, it does not significantly change the concentrations of clotting factors. Heparin does not lyse clots, but can prevent the growth of existing clots.

Heparin also causes increased release of lipoprotein lipase, thereby increasing the clearance of circulating lipids and increasing plasma levels of free fatty acids.

Uses/Indications - Heparin's primary uses in small animal medicine include treatment of Disseminated Intravascular Coagulation (DIC), and treatment of thromboembolic disease. In horses, it has also been used in the treatment of DIC and as prophylactic therapy for laminitis (unproven efficacy).

Pharmacokinetics - Heparin is not absorbed by the gut if administered orally and must be given parenterally to be effective. Anticoagulant activity begins immediately after direct IV bolus injection, but may take up to one hour after deep SQ injection. When heparin is given by continuous IV infusion, an initial bolus must be administered for full anticoagulant activity to begin.

Heparin is extensively protein bound, primarily to fibrinogen, low-density lipoproteins and globulins. It does not appreciably cross the placenta or enter milk.

Heparin's metabolic fate is not completely understood. The drug is apparently partially metabolized by the liver and also inactivated by the reticuloendothelial system. Serum half-lives in humans average 1-2 hours.

Contraindications/Precautions/Reproductive Safety - Heparin is contraindicated in patients hypersensitive to it, have severe thrombocytopenia or uncontrollable bleeding (caused by something other than DIC). One author (Green 1989) states that with DIC "heparin should not be given to actively bleeding patients that have severe factor depletion and thrombocytopenia, as fatal hemorrhage may result."

Do not administer IM, as heparin may cause hematoma formation. Hematomas, pain, and irritation may also occur after deep SQ dosing.

While heparin does not cross the placenta and is generally felt to be the anticoagulant of choice during pregnancy, its safe use in pregnancy has not been firmly established and pregnancy outcomes may be unfavorable. It should be used cautiously and only when clearly necessary.

Adverse Effects/Warnings - Bleeding and thrombocytopenia are the most common adverse effects associated with heparin therapy. Because heparin is derived from bovine or porcine tissues, hypersensitivity reactions may be possible. Less commonly encountered adverse effects that have been reported in animals and/or humans include vasospastic reactions (after several days of therapy), osteoporosis and diminished renal function (after long-term, high-dose therapy), rebound hyperlipidemia, hyperkalemia, alopecia, suppressed aldosterone synthesis and priapism.

Overdosage/Acute Toxicity - Overdosage of heparin is associated with bleeding. Symptoms that could be seen before frank bleeding occurs may be manifested by hematuria, tarry stools, petechiae, bruising, etc. Protamine can reverse heparin's effects; see the Protamine monograph for more information.

Drug Interactions - Use heparin with caution with other drugs that can cause changes in coagulation status or platelet function (*e.g.,* **aspirin, phenylbutazone, dipyridamole, warfarin**, etc.); more intensive monitoring may be indicated.

Heparin may antagonize the actions of **corticosteroids, insulin or ACTH**.

Heparin may increase plasma levels of **diazepam**.

Antihistamines, intravenous nitroglycerin, propylene glycol, digoxin, and **tetracyclines** may partially counteract the actions of heparin.

Drug/Laboratory Interactions - Unless heparin is administered by continuous infusion, it can alter **prothrombin time (PT)** which can be misleading in patients also receiving a coumarin or an indandione anticoagulant.

Heparin can interfere with the results of the **BSP** (sulfobromophthaelein, bromosulfophthalein) test by changing the color intensity of the dye and shifting the absorption peak from 580 nm to 595 nm.

Heparin can cause falsely elevated values of **serum thyroxine** if using competitive protein binding methods of determination. Radioimmunoassay (RIA) and protein bound iodine methods are apparently unaffected by heparin.

When heparin is used as an anticoagulant *in vitro* (*e.g.,* in blood collection containers), **white cell counts** should be performed within 2 hours of collection. Do not use heparinized blood for **platelet counts, erythrocyte sedimentation rates, erythrocyte fragmentation tests,** or for any tests involving **complement or isoagglutinins**. Errors in **blood gas determinations** for CO_2 pressure, bicarbonate concentration or base excess may occur if heparin encompasses 10% or more of the blood sample.

Doses - Doses of heparin are controversial; dosage ranges and methods may vary widely depending on the clinician/author. Refer to the actual references for these doses for more complete information.

Dogs & Cats:

For adjunctive treatment of DIC: Note: Heparin therapy may be only one aspect of successful treatment of DIC. Alleviation of the precipitating cause, administration of fluids, blood, aspirin, and diligent monitoring of coagulation tests (APTT, PT), fibrin degradation products, and fibrinogen may all be important factors in the treatment of DIC.

a) 75 Units/kg SQ *tid* (Wingfield and Van Pelt 1989)

b) Add 5,000 U of heparin/500 ml warmed whole blood 30 minutes before transfusion. Alternatively, give 10 - 150 U/kg SQ q12h. Heparin must be tapered over 48 hours or a "rebound effect" may occur. (Feldman 1985)

c) After pH has been corrected and perfusion maximized, transfuse heparinized whole fresh blood or plasma (75 U/kg heparin) one time. Then begin mini-dose heparin therapy at 5 - 10 U/kg/hour by continuous IV infusion or 75 U/kg SQ q8h. Continue without interruption until DIC has completely disappeared. With these doses, bleeding risk is negligible and APTT monitoring not necessary, although thrombocytopenia may develop. (Slappendel 1989)

d) Before administering heparin, provide sufficient fresh whole blood to maintain platelet counts above 30,000/µl and fibrinogen levels over 50 mg/dl. Then give heparin at 50 - 100 U/kg SQ q6h. Alternatively, dose heparin sufficiently to increase APTT to 1.5-2 times normal (may be more effective in patients susceptible to thromboembolization). (Green 1989)

For adjunctive treatment of thromboembolic disease:
   a) Dogs: 500 Units/kg q8h SQ
   Cats: 250-375 U/kg q8h SQ; adjust dose frequently by monitoring APTT to 1.5-2.5 times normal (control). (Roudebush 1985)
   b) For feline aortic thromboembolism: 220 U/kg IV, followed by 66 U/kg SQ 3 hours later and then give SQ 4 times daily. Adjust SQ heparin dose so that clotting time is 2-2.5 times normal. (Harpster 1986)
   c) For arterial thromboembolism; pulmonary thromboembolism: Initially, 200 U/kg IV, then 50 - 10 U/kg SQ *tid-qid*. Adjust dose to prolong PTT or ACT to 2-2.5 times normal. (Harpster 1988), (Bauer 1988)
   d) For feline thromboembolic disease associated with cardiomyopathy: Initially, heparin at 1000 U IV, then 50 U/kg SQ 3 hours later and repeated at 6-8 hour intervals. Adjust dose to prolong clotting time to 2-2.5 times pretreatment baseline index value. (Fox 1989)
   e) For canine arterial thrombosis and thromboembolism: Keep dog in a quiet and warm place; give analgesics if necessary. Give heparin initially at 220 U/kg IV. Correct dehydration and dilute blood by administering electrolyte solutions. Dextran products may be helpful. Follow-up doses of heparin should be started low and increased until APTT is 2-2.5 times normal. After 3-5 days of therapy, gradually reduce heparin over 48-72 hours while dog is put on oral anticoagulant therapy (see warfarin monograph). (Suter 1989)

To prevent clots forming when performing closed chest lavage with pyothorax:
   a) Add 1000 U of heparin per liter of lavage fluid (warm normal saline). This fluid is instilled at 20 ml/kg *bid* for 5-7 days. Antibiotics (often penicillin) or enzymes (*e.g.,* streptokinase) may also be added to fluid. (Berkwitt and Berzon 1988)

For adjunctive therapy of acute complicated or severe pancreatitis in dogs:
   a) 50 - 75 U/kg SQ *bid-tid*; may reduce thromboembolic tendencies, but efficacy is unknown and heparin is not indicated in all cases. (Bunch 1988)

For detection of lipoprotein lipase activity (heparin stimulation test):
   a) Measure serum lipids just before and 15 minutes after heparin at 100 U/kg IV. Lack of increase in lipolytic activity is suggestive of lipoprotein lipase deficiency. (Kay, Kruth, and Twedt 1988)

For adjunctive therapy of severe thermal burns:
   a) 100 - 200 U/kg IV for 1-4 doses; routine use is of questionable value. Select patients based on individual considerations. (Morgan 1988)

Horses:
   For adjunctive treatment of DIC: Note: Heparin therapy may be only one aspect of successful treatment of DIC. Alleviation of the precipitating cause, administration of fluids, blood, aspirin, and diligent monitoring of coagulation tests (APTT, PT), fibrin degradation products, and fibrinogen may all be important factors in the treatment of DIC.
   a) 80 - 100 U/kg IV q4-6h (may be added to fluids and given as a slow drip). Low grade DIC may be treated with 25 - 40 U/kg SQ 2-3 times a day. (Byars 1987)

As adjunctive therapy in endotoxic shock:
   a) 40 Units/kg IV or SQ 2-3 times a day may prevent the development of microthrombi; additional studies required to confirm positive benefits. (Semrad and Moore 1987)

Monitoring Parameters - Note: The frequency of monitoring is controversial and is dependent on several factors, including heparin dose, patient's condition, concomitant problems, etc. Because of the high incidence of hemorrhage associated with heparin use, frequent monitoring of APTT is essential early in therapy (particularly using higher dosages) and in critically ill animals.
   1) While whole blood clotting time (WBCT), partial thromboplastin time (PTT) and activated partial thromboplastin times (APTT) may all be used to monitor therapy, APTT is most often recommended.
   2) Platelet counts and hematocrit (PCV) should be done periodically
   3) Occult blood in stool and urine; other observations for bleeding
   4) Clinical efficacy

Client Information - Because of the intense monitoring necessary with heparin's use and the serious nature of the disease states in which it is used, this drug should be utilized only by professionals familiar with it and, preferably, in an inpatient setting.

Dosage Forms/Preparations/FDA Approval Status/Withholding Times -
Veterinary-Approved Products: None located.

Human-Approved Products:
Heparin Sodium Injection 1000 U/ml, 2000 U/ml, 2500 U/ml, 5000 U/ml, 10,000 U/ml, 20,000 U/ml, 40,000 U/ml in 0.5, 1, 2, 4, 5, 10, and 30 ml amps and multi-dose vials (depending on concentration and manufacturer).

Also available for heparin sodium are pre-filled syringes in various concentrations and amounts, and premixed in normal saline and half-normal saline in 250 ml, 500 ml and 1000 ml containers.

HETACILLIN POTASSIUM

For general information on the penicillins, including adverse effects, contraindications, overdosage, drug interactions and monitoring parameters, refer to the monograph: Penicillins, General Information..

Chemistry - An aminopenicillin, hetacillin potassium occurs as a white to light buff crystalline powder that is freely soluble in water and soluble in alcohol. Hetacillin is rapidly converted into ampicillin *in vivo*. 1.1 g of the potassium salt is approximately equivalent to 1 gram of the base and 900 mg of ampicillin.

Storage/Stability/Compatibility - Hetacillin tablets should be stored in airtight containers.

Pharmacology - Because hetacillin is rapidly converted into ampicillin after administration, it shares identical mechanisms of action and spectrums of activity with ampicillin. For more information, refer to the ampicillin monograph.

Uses/Indications - Hetacillin is approved for oral use in dogs in cats and when oral ampicillin therapy may be indicated. It is also approved in an intramammary syringe formulation to treat mastitis in lactating dairy cattle caused by ampicillin-susceptible organisms.

Pharmacokinetics (specific) - Hetacillin is rapidly hydrolyzed *in vivo* to ampicillin, and therefore reportedly possesses identical pharmacokinetic parameters as ampicillin. For further information refer to the ampicillin monograph.

Doses -
Dogs:
    For susceptible infections:
      a) 11 - 22 mg/kg PO *bid*, up to 44 mg/kg PO *bid* for stubborn UTI's. (Package insert; *Hetacin®-K*—Fort Dodge)
      b) 10 - 20 mg/kg PO q8h (Kirk 1989)
      c) 20 mg/kg PO *tid* (Morgan 1988)

Cats:
    For susceptible infections:
      a) 50 mg PO *bid* (Package insert; *Hetacin®-K*—Fort Dodge)
      b) 10 - 20 mg/kg PO q8h (Kirk 1989)
      c) 10 - 15 mg/kg PO *tid* (Morgan 1988)

Cattle:
    For susceptible infections:
      a) For mastitis: Infuse entire contents of one syringe into each affected quarter. Repeat at 24 hour intervals until a maximum of 3 treatments are given. If definite improvement not noted after 48 hours after treatment, further investigate causal organism. (Package insert; *Hetacin®-K*—Fort Dodge)

Client Information - Unless otherwise directed by veterinarian, give oral medication 1-2 hours prior to feeding animal.

Dosage Forms/Preparations/FDA Approval Status/Withholding Times -
Veterinary-Approved Products:
Hetacillin Potassium Tablets: Equivalent to 50 mg, 100 mg, and 200 mg of ampicillin activity in bottles of 100 & 500; *Hetacin®-K* (Fort Dodge); (Rx) Approved for use in dogs and cats.

Hetacillin Potassium for Intramammary Infusion: equivalent to 62.5 mg of ampicillin activity per 10 ml syringe; *Hetacin®-K* (Fort Dodge); (Rx) Approved for use in lactating dairy cattle. Slaughter withdrawal = 10 days; Milk withdrawal = 72 hours.

Human-Approved Products: None

HETASTARCH

Chemistry - A synthetic polymer derived from a waxy starch, hetastarch is composed primarily of amylopectin. To avoid degradation by serum amylase, hydroxyethyl ether groups are added to the glucose units. It has an average molecular weight of 450,000, but ranges in size from about MW 10,000 - 1,000,000. Hetastarch occurs as a white powder. It is very soluble in water and insoluble in alcohol. Hetastarch may also be known as hydroxyethyl starch or HES.

The commercially available colloidal solution appears as a clear, pale yellow to amber solution. In 500 ml of the commercial preparation containing hetastarch 6% and 0.9% sodium chloride, there are 77 mEq of sodium and chloride. It has an osmolality of 310 mOsm/L and a pH of about 5.5.

Storage/Stability/Compatibility - Hetastarch 6% in 0.9% NaCl should be stored at temperatures less than 40°C; freezing should be avoided. Exposure to temperature extremes may result in formation of a crystalline precipitate or a color change to a turbid deep brown. Should this occur, do not use.

Pharmacology - Hetastarch acts as a plasma volume expander by increasing the oncotic pressure within the intravascular space similarly to either dextran or albumin. Maximum volume expansion occurs within a few minutes of the completion of infusion. Duration of effect is variable, but may persist for 24 hours or more. When added to whole blood in humans, hetastarch causes an increase in erythrocyte sedimentation rate.

Uses/Indications - In hypovolemic patients where total protein is less than 3.5 g/dl and crystalloid therapy is likely to reduce this level further, colloid therapy (plasma, dextran or hetastarch) should be considered as part of intravascular volume restoration. It is often used when colloid therapy is required and blood products are unavailable or when time is of the essence and the wait for cross-matching is unacceptable. Because of the expense, hetastarch is generally used only in small animals.

Pharmacokinetics - Lower molecular weight molecules (less than 50,000) are rapidly excreted by the kidneys, larger molecules are slowly degraded enzymatically to a size where they then can be excreted. About 40% of a dose is excreted in the first 24 hours after infusion. After about 2 weeks, practically all the drug is excreted.

Contraindications/Precautions/Reproductive Safety - In humans, hetastarch is contraindicated in patients with severe heart failure, severe bleeding disorders and patients in oliguric or anuric renal failure.

Because of the danger of volume overload, use of hetastarch for the treatment of of shock not accompanied by hypovolemia may be hazardous. As it has no oxygen carrying capacity, hetastarch is not a replacement for whole blood or red blood cells.

Because of its effect on platelets, hetastarch should be used with caution in patients with thrombocytopenia and it should be used with extreme caution in patients undergoing CNS surgery. Because of its effects on indirect serum bilirubin levels, hetastarch should be used with caution in patients with liver disease.

Because of the threat of volume overload, hetastarch should be used in caution in patients with renal dysfunction, congestive heart failure or pulmonary edema.

Hetastarch's safety during pregnancy has not been established, but no untoward effects have apparently been reported thus far.

Adverse Effects/Warnings - Hetastarch can affect platelet function and clotting tests can be transiently prolonged. It is less antigenic than dextran, but can cause sensitivity reactions and interfere with antigen-antibody testing. Anaphylactic reactions and coagulopathies are considered to occur rarely, however.

When given via rapid infusion to cats, hetastarch may cause signs of nausea and vomiting. If administered over 15-30 minutes, these signs are eliminated. At recommended dosages, hetastarch may cause minor changes in clotting times and platelet counts due to direct (precipitation of factor VIII) and dilutional causes. Clinically these effects are usually insignificant, but patients with preexisting coagulapathies may be predisposed to further bleeding.

In humans, increases in serum indirect bilirubins have occurred occasionally in humans. No effect on other liver function tests were noted and the increases subsided over several days. Serum amylase levels may be falsely elevated for several days after hetastarch is administered. While clinically insignificant, the changes may preclude using serum amylase to diagnosis or monitor patients with acute pancreatitis.

Circulatory overload leading to pulmonary edema is possible, particularly when large dosages are administered to patients with diminished renal function. Do not give intramuscularly as bleeding, bruising, or hematomas may occur.

Overdosage - Overdosage could result in volume overload in susceptible patients. Dose and monitor fluid status carefully.

Drug Interactions - Hetastarch apparently has no drug interactions that are clinically significant.

Doses -

Dogs/Cats: For use as a plasma volume expander in shock:

    Note: Rate of administration is determined by individual patient requirements (i.e., blood volume, indication, and patient response); adequate monitoring for successful treatment of shock is mandatory. The following dosages are NOT "Give and forget"; they should be used as general guidelines for treatment.

    a) Dogs: 20 ml/kg/day IV
        Cats: 10 - 15 ml/kg IV (Morgan 1997)

    b) Dog: 16 ml/kg (range 10 - 20 ml/kg/day; use rapid IV infusion for shock therapy) (Papich 1995)

    c) Up to 30 ml/kg/day (Haskins 1992)

Monitoring Parameters - Other than the regular monitoring performed in patients that would require volume expansion therapy, there is no inordinate monitoring required specific to hetastarch therapy.

Client Information - As hetastarch is used in an in-patient setting only, the two factors to consider when communicating with clients are the drug's cost and the reasons for using colloid therapy.

Dosage Forms/Preparations/FDA Approval Status -

Veterinary-Approved Products: None

Human-Approved Products:

    Hetastarch 6% in 0.9% sodium chloride, in 500 ml IV infusion bottle; *Hespan*® (DuPont); (Rx)

HYALURONATE SODIUM
SODIUM HYALURONATE

Chemistry - Hyaluronate sodium (HS) is the sodium salt of hyaluronic acid which is a naturally occurring high-viscosity mucopolysaccharide.

Storage/Stability/Compatibility - Store at room temperature or refrigerate depending on the product used—check label; do not freeze. Protect from light.

Pharmacology - Hyaluronate sodium (HS) is found naturally in the connective tissue of both man and animals and is identical chemically regardless of species. Highest concentrations found naturally are in the synovial fluid, vitreous of the eye and umbilical cord. Surfaces of articular cartilage are covered with a thin layer of a protein-hyaluronate complex, hyaluronate is also found in synovial fluid, and the cartilage matrix. The net effects in joints are: a cushioning effect, reduction of protein and cellular influx into the joint and a lubricating effect. Hyaluronate also has a direct antiinflammatory effect in joints by scavenging free radicals and suppressing prostaglandins.

Uses/Indications - HS is useful in the treatment of synovitis not associated with severe degenerative joint disease. It may be helpful to treat secondary synovitis in conditions where full thickness cartilage loss exists.

    The choice of a high molecular weigh product (MW >1 x 10^6) versus a low molecular weight one is quite controversial. One author (Nixon 1992) states that "...low molecular weight products (which tend to be less expensive) can be equally efficacious in ameliorating signs of joint disease. When synovial adhesions and pannus are to be avoided (as in most surgeries for carpal and fetlock fracture fragment removal), higher molecular weight preparations are recommended because they inhibit proliferation of synovial fibroblasts."

Pharmacokinetics - No specific information located.

Contraindications/Precautions/Reproductive Safety - No contraindications to HS's use are noted on the label. HS should not be used as a substitute for adequate diagnosis; radiographic examinations should be performed to rule out serious fractures. Do not perform intra-articular injections through skin that has been recently fired or blistered, or that has excessive scurf and counterirritants on it.

    While HS would unlikely cause problems, safe use in breeding animals has not been established and most manufacturers caution against its use in these animals.

Adverse Effects/Warnings - Some patients may develop local reactions manifested by heat, swelling and/or effusion. Effects generally subside within 24-48 hours; some animals may require up to 96 hours for resolution. No treatment for this effect is recommended. When used in combination with other drugs, incidence of flares may actually be higher. No systemic adverse effects have been noted.

Overdosage/Acute Toxicity - Acute toxicology studies performed in horses have demonstrated no systemic toxicity associated with overdoses.

Drug Interactions/Laboratory Considerations - None noted.

Doses -

Horses: Because of the differences in the commercially products see each individual product's label for specific dosing information.

Dogs:

For the adjunctive treatment of synovitis (rather than the presence of a damaged articular cartilage):

a) Using a high molecular weight compound: 3 - 5 mg intra-articularly using sterile technique at weekly intervals. Long term effects are not achieved. (Bloomberg 1992)

Client Information - HS should be administered by a veterinarian only using aseptic technique.

Dosage Forms/Preparations/FDA Approval Status/Withholding Times -

Veterinary-Approved Products:

Hyaluronate Sodium (average MW of 500,000 - 730,000) 20 mg/ml in 2 ml disposable syringes; *Hyalovet*® (Fort Dodge); (Rx)

Hyaluronate Sodium Injection *Legend*® (Bayer) (Rx); 2 ml vial for IA administration; 4 ml vials for IV administration. Approved for use in horses.

Also available *Hyvisc*® (Boehringer Ingelheim) (Rx)

Hyaluronate Sodium 10 mg/ml (MW 3.5×10^6) in 2 ml disposable syringes; *Hylartin*® (Pharmacia & Upjohn); (Rx)

All the above products are approved for use in horses. Not for use in horses intended for food.

HYDRALAZINE HCL

Chemistry - A phthalazine-derivative antihypertensive/vasodilating agent, hydralazine HCl occurs as an odorless, white to off-white crystalline powder with a melting point between 270 - 280°C and a pK_a of 7.3. One gram is soluble in approximately 25 ml of water or 500 ml of alcohol. The commercially available injection has a pH of 3.4 - 4. Hydralazine may also be known as Hydrallazine.

Storage/Stability/Compatibility - Hydralazine tablets should be stored in tight, light resistant containers at room temperature. The injectable product should be stored at room temperature; avoid refrigeration or freezing.

When mixed with most infusion solutions a color change can occur which does not necessarily indicate a loss in potency (if occured over 8-12 hours).

Hydralazine is reported to be **compatible** with the following infusion solutions/drugs: dextrose-Ringer's combinations, dextrose-saline combinations, Ringer's injection, lactated Ringer's injection, sodium chloride solutions, and dobutamine HCl.

Hydralazine is reported to be **incompatible** with 10% dextrose or fructose and is reported to be incompatible with the following drugs: aminophylline, ampicillin sodium, chlorothiazide sodium, edetate calcium disodium, hydrocortisone sodium succinate, mephentermine sulfate, methohexital sodium, phenobarbital sodium, verapamil HCl. Compatibility is dependent upon factors such as pH, concentration, temperature, and diluents used and it is suggested to consult specialized references for more specific information.

Pharmacology - Hydralazine has direct action on vascular smooth muscle and reduces peripheral resistance and blood pressure. It is believed that hydralazine acts by altering cellular calcium metabolism in smooth muscle, thereby interfering with calcium movements and preventing the initiation and maintenance of the contractile state. Hydralazine has more effect on arterioles than on veins.

In patients with CHF, hydralazine significantly increases cardiac output and decreases systemic vascular resistance. Cardiac rate may be slightly increased or unchanged, while blood pressure, pulmonary venous pressure, and right atrial pressure may be decreased or unchanged.

When used to treat hypertensive patients (without CHF), increased heart rate, cardiac output and stroke volume can be noted. The renin-angiotensin system can be activated with a resultant increase in sodium and water retention if not given with diuretics or sympathetic blocking drugs. Parenteral hydralazine administration can cause respiratory stimulation.

Uses/Indications - Primary use of hydralazine at the present time in veterinary medicine is as an afterload reducer for the adjunctive treatment in CHF in small animals, particularly if mitral valve insufficiency is the primary cause. It is also used to treat systemic hypertension.

Pharmacokinetics - In dogs, hydralazine is rapidly absorbed after oral administration with an onset of action within one hour and peak effects at 3-5 hours. There is a high first-pass effect after oral administration. The presence of food may enhance the bioavailability of hydralazine tablets.

Hydralazine is widely distributed in body tissues. In humans, approximately 85% of the drug in the blood is bound to plasma proteins. Hydralazine crosses the placenta and very small amounts are excreted into the milk.

Hydralazine is extensively metabolized in the liver and approximately 15% is excreted unchanged in the urine. The half-life in humans is usually 2-4 hours, but may be as long as 8 hours. The pharmacokinetic parameters for this drug in veterinary species was not located, but the duration of action of hydralazine in dogs after oral administration is reportedly 11-13 hours.

Contraindications/Precautions - Hydralazine is contraindicated in patients hypersensitive to it and in those with coronary artery disease. The drug is listed as contraindicated in human patients with mitral valvular rheumatic disease, but it has been recommended to be used in small animal patients with mitral valve insufficiency. It is recommended not to use the drug in patients with hypovolemia or preexisting hypotension.

Hydralazine should be used with caution in patients with severe renal disease or intracerebral bleeding. In humans, a syndrome resembling systemic lupus erythematosis (SLE) has been documented after hydralazine use. While this syndrome has not been documented in veterinary patients, the drug should be used with caution in patients with preexisting autoimmune diseases.

Adverse Effects/Warnings - The most prevalent adverse effects seen in small animals include: hypotension, tachycardia, sodium/water retention (if not given concurrently with a diuretic), and GI distress (vomiting, diarrhea). Initially, transient weakness and lethargy can be seen, but usually resolve in 3-4 days. Other adverse effects documented in humans which could occur, include an SLE-like syndrome, lacrimation, conjunctivitis, peripheral neuritis, blood dyscrasias, urinary retention, constipation and hypersensitivity reactions.

Tachycardias may be treated with concomitant digitalis treatment or a beta-blocker (Caution: beta-blockers may reduce cardiac performance).

Overdosage - Overdoses may be characterized by severe hypotension, tachycardia or other arrhythmias, skin flushing, and myocardial ischemia. Cardiovascular system support is the primary treatment modality. Evacuate gastric contents and administer activated charcoal using standard precautionary measures if the ingestion was recent and if cardiovascular status has been stabilized. Treat shock using volume expanders without using pressor agents if possible. If a pressor agent is required to maintain blood pressure, the use of a minimally arrhythmogenic agent (*e.g.,* phenylephrine or methoxamine) is recommended. Digitalis agents may be required. Monitor blood pressure and renal function diligently.

Drug Interactions - **Sympathomimetics** (*e.g.,* phenylpropanolamine) may cause additive tachycardia.

Hydralazine may enhance the oral absorption of **propranolol** (or other beta-blockers). Other **antihypertensive agents** may cause additive hypotension. The pressor response to **epinephrine** may be reduced by hydralazine.

Doses - Because of the sodium/water retention associated with this drug it should be given concurrently with a diuretic. Many clinicians recommend adding a venous dilating agent (*e.g.,* nitroglycerin ointment) to also reduce preload.

Dogs:

For adjunctive therapy in treatment of heart failure:
a) Get initial baseline monitoring parameters. Initial dose of 1 mg/kg PO. Measure blood pressure in 1 hour and blood gas in 3 hours, or reevaluate clinical signs from 5 hours to 1 day later. If mean blood pressure has decreased by 15-20 mmHg or is < 70 mmHg; or if venous pO2 was <35 mmHg and is now > 35 mmHg; if mucous membrane color has improved dramatically and pulmonary edema is decreased, the titration is complete and give 1 mg q12h. If the 1 mg/kg dose was ineffective, give another 1 mg/kg if the last dose given was less than 8 hours previous; if greater than 12 hours ago, give 2 mg/kg. Evaluate as above. If still no response, increase dose to 3 mg/kg. Maintenance dosing can be given at 12 hour intervals. (Kittleson 1985b)
b) 1-3 mg/kg PO *bid* (Morgan 1988)

For treatment of systemic hypertension:
a) 0.5 - 2.0 mg/kg PO *bid-tid* (Morgan 1988)

For acute arterial embolism:
a) 1 - 2 mg/kg PO, IM *bid* (Morgan 1988)

Cats:
  For adjunctive therapy in treatment of heart failure:
    a) See (a) above (For adjunctive therapy in treatment of heart failure in dogs:), but start
       titration at 2.5 mg (total dose) and if necessary, increase up to 10 mg. (Kittleson
       1985b)
  For treatment of systemic hypertension:
    a) 2.5 mg PO *bid* (Morgan 1988)
    For acute arterial embolism:
    a) 2.5 mg PO *bid* (Morgan 1988)
Monitoring Parameters -
    1) Baseline thoracic radiographs
    2) Mucous membrane color
    3) Serum electrolytes
    4) If possible, arterial blood pressure and venous PO_2
    5) Because blood dyscrasias are a possibility, an occasional CBC should be considered.
Client Information - Compliance with directions is necessary to maximize the benefits from this
drug. If possible, give medication with food. Notify veterinarian if patient's condition deterio-
rates or if the animal becomes lethargic or depressed.
Dosage Forms/Preparations/FDA Approval Status/Withholding Times -
  Veterinary-Approved Products: None
  Human-Approved Products:
    Hydralazine HCl Tablets 10 mg, 25 mg, 50 mg, 100 mg; *Apresoline®* (Ciba); Generic; (Rx)

    Hydralazine 20 mg/ml in 1 ml amps or vials; *Apresoline®* (Ciba); Generic (Rx)

HYDROCHLOROTHIAZIDE

For information on **Pharmacology, Uses/Indications, Contraindications-/Precautions,
Adverse Effects/Warnings, Overdosage, Drug Interactions, and Monitoring Parameters;**
see the Chlorothiazide monograph.

Chemistry - Hydrochlorothiazide occurs as a practically odorless, slightly bitter-tasting, white,
or practically white, crystalline powder with pK_as of 7.9 and 9.2. It is slightly soluble in water
and soluble in alcohol.

Storage/Stability/Compatibility - Hydrochlorothiazide oral solution and tablets should be
stored at room temperature in well-closed containers. Avoid freezing the oral solution and the
injectable product.

Pharmacokinetics - The pharmacokinetics of the thiazides have apparently not been studied in
domestic animals. In humans, hydrochlorothiazide is about 65 to 75% absorbed after oral administration. The onset of diuretic activity occurs in 2 hours; peaks at 4 - 6 hours. The serum half-life
is approximately 5.6 - 14.8 hours and the duration of activity is 6-12 hours. The drug is apparently not metabolized and is excreted unchanged into the urine. Like all thiazides, the antihypertensive effects of hydrochlorothiazide may take several days to occur.

Doses -
  Dogs:
    For treatment of nephrogenic diabetes insipidus:
      a) 0.5 - 1.0 mg/kg PO *bid* (Morgan 1988)
      b) 2.5 - 5.0 mg/kg PO *bid* (Nichols 1989)
    For treatment of systemic hypertension:
      a) 2 - 4 mg/kg PO q12-24h with dietary salt restriction (Cowgill and Kallet 1986)
    For treatment of recurrent calcium oxalate uroliths with renal hypercalcuria:
      a) 2 mg/kg q12h PO. Note: Do not use in patients with absorptive (intestinal) hypercal-
          curia as hypercalcemia may result (Polzin and Osborne 1985)
    As a diuretic:
      a) 2 - 4 mg/kg PO once to twice daily (Morgan 1988)
    For treatment of hypoglycemia (with diazoxide):
      a) 2 - 4 mg/kg PO *bid* (Morgan 1988)
  Cattle:
    For udder edema:
      a) 125 - 250 mg IV or IM once or twice a day; may continue for several days if neces-
          sary. Consider switching to oral chlorothiazide after initial dose. (Package Insert -
          Hydrozide® Injection; MSD)

Client Information - Clients should contact veterinarian if symptoms of water or electrolyte imbalance occur. Symptoms such as excessive thirst, lethargy, lassitude, restlessness, oliguria, GI distress or tachycardia may indicate electrolyte or water balance problem.

Dosage Forms/Preparations/FDA Approval Status/Withholding Times -
   Veterinary-Approved Products:
   Hydrochlorothiazide Veterinary Injection 25 mg/ml, 50 ml vial; *Hydrozide*® Injection (Rhone Merieux); (Rx) Approved for use in cattle. There is a 72 hour milk-witholding time for lactating dairy cattle; no meat witholding time is listed.

   Human-Approved Products:
   Hydrochlorothiazide Tablets 25 mg, 50 mg, 100 mg; *HydroDiuril*® (Merck); Generic (Rx)

   Hydrochlorothiazide Oral Solution 10 mg/ml in 500 ml bottles; Generic (Rx)

Fixed dose combinations of hydrochlorothiazide with: hydralazine, amiloride, propranolol, triamterene, captopril, reserpine, enalapril, guanethidine, metoprolol, spironolactone, timolol, methyldopa or labetolol are also available.

HYDROCODONE BITARTRATE

Chemistry - A phenanthrene-derivative opiate agonist, hydrocodone bitartrate occurs as fine, white crystals or crystalline powder. One gram is soluble in about 16 mls of water; it is slightly soluble in alcohol. This compound may also be known as dihydrocodeinone bitartrate.

Storage/Stability/Compatibility - Products should be protected from light.

Pharmacology - While hydrocodone exhibits the characteristics of other opiate agonists (see the monographs on opiates in the CNS section), it tends to have a slightly greater antitussive effect than codeine (on a weight basis). The mechanism of this effect is thought to be as a result of direct suppression of the cough reflex on the cough center in the medulla. Hydrocodone also tends to have a drying effect on respiratory mucosa and the viscosity of respiratory secretions may be increased. The addition of homatropine MBr (in *Hycodan*® and others) may enhance this effect. Hydrocodone may also be more sedating than codeine, but not more constipating.

Uses/Indications - Used principally in canine medicine as an antitussive for cough secondary to conditions such as collapsing trachea, bronchitis, or canine upper respiratory infection complex (C-URI, "kennel cough", canine infectious tracheobronchitis). Its use is generally reserved for harsh, dry, non-productive coughs.

Pharmacokinetics - In humans, hydrocodone is well absorbed after oral administration, and has a serum half-life of about 3.8 hours. Antitussive effect usually lasts 4-6 hours in adults.
   There does not appear to be any pharmacokinetic data published in dogs. The antitussive action generally persists for 6-12 hours.

Contraindications/Precautions - Hydrocodone is contraindicated in cases where the patient is hypersensitive to narcotic analgesics and in patients taking monoamine oxidase inhibitors (MAOIs). It is also contraindicated in patients with diarrhea caused by a toxic ingestion until the toxin is eliminated from the GI tract. All opiates should be used with caution in patients with hypothyroidism, severe renal insufficiency, adrenocortical insufficiency (Addison's), and in geriatric or severely debilitated patients.
   Hydrocodone should be used with caution in patients with head injuries or increased intracranial pressure and acute abdominal conditions as it may obscure the diagnosis or clinical course of these conditions. It should be used with extreme caution in patients suffering from respiratory diseases when respiratory secretions are increased or when liquids are nebulized into the respiratory tract.

Adverse Effects/Warnings - Side effects that may be encountered with hydrocodone therapy in dogs include: sedation, constipation (with chronic therapy), vomiting or other GI disturbances.
   Hydrocodone may mask the symptoms (cough) of respiratory disease and should not take the place of appropriate specific treatments for the underlying cause of coughs.

Overdosage - The initial concern with a very large overdose of *Hycodan*® (or equivalent) would be the CNS, cardiovascular and respiratory depression secondary to the opiate effects. If the ingestion was recent, emptying the gut using standard protocols should be performed and treatment with naloxone instituted as necessary. The homatropine ingredient may give rise to anticholinergic effects which may complicate the clinical picture, but its relatively low toxicity may not require any treatment. For further information on handling opiate or anticholinergic overdoses, refer to the meperidine and atropine monographs, respectively.

Drug Interactions - Other **CNS depressants** (*e.g.,* anesthetic agents, antihistamines, phenothiazines, barbiturates, tranquilizers, alcohol, etc.) may cause increased CNS or respiratory depression when used with hydrocodone.

Doses -
Dogs:

a) 2.5 - 10 mg (hydrocodone) PO q6-12h, not to exceed 0.5 - 1.0 mg/kg (Roudebush 1985)

b) For collapsing trachea: 0.25 mg/kg PO *bid-qid* (Prueter 1988b)

c) For adjunctive treatment of bacterial bronchitis: 0.22 mg/kg PO *bid-qid* (Bauer 1988)

d) For persistent, dry, hacking cough in canine upper respiratory infection complex: 0.22 mg/kg PO *bid-qid* (Allen 1988)

Monitoring Parameters - Clinical efficacy and adverse effects

Dosage Forms/Preparations/FDA Approval Status/Withholding Times -
Veterinary-Approved Products: None
Human-Approved Products:

Hydrocodone is available commercially only in combination products approved for human use.

Hydrocodone Bitartrate 5 mg, Homatropine MBr 1.5 mg Tablets; *Hycodan*® Tablets (Du Pont); *Tussigon*® Tablets (Daniels); (Rx)

Hydrocodone Bitartrate 5 mg, Homatropine MBr 1.5 mg (per 5 ml) Oral Liquid; in pints and gallons; *Hycodan*® Syrup (Du Pont); *Hydropane*® Syrup (Halsey); *Mycodone*® Syrup (My-K); *Codan*® Syrup (Warner Chilcott); *Hydrotropine*® Syrup (Rugby); Generic Hydrocodone Syrup; (Rx)

The products listed above are the ones most commonly used in small animal medicine. Other oral tablets and liquids with hydrocodone are available in combination with decongestants (pseudoephedrine, phenylephrine, or phenylpropanolamine), antihistamines (chlorpheniramine), analgesics (acetominophen or aspirin) or expectorants (guaifenesin). All commercially available products containing hydrocodone are **Class-III** controlled substances.

HYDROCORTISONE
HYDROCORTISONE ACETATE
HYDROCORTISONE CYPIONATE
HYDROCORTISONE SODIUM PHOSPHATE
HYDROCORTISONE SODIUM SUCCINATE

Note: For more information refer to the monograph: Glucocorticoids, General Information.

Chemistry - Also known as compound F or cortisol, hydrocortisone is secreted by the adrenal gland. Hydrocortisone occurs as an odorless, white to practically white, crystalline powder. It is very slightly soluble in water and sparingly soluble in alcohol. Hydrocortisone is administered orally.

Hydrocortisone acetate occurs as an odorless, white to practically white, crystalline powder. It is insoluble in water and slightly soluble in alcohol. Hydrocortisone acetate is administered via intra-articular, intrabursal, intralesional, intrasynovial or soft tissue injection.

Hydrocortisone cypionate occurs as an odorless or with a slight odor, white to practically white, crystalline powder. It is insoluble in water and soluble in alcohol. It is administered orally.

Hydrocortisone sodium phosphate occurs as an odorless or practically odorless, hygroscopic, white to light yellow powder. It is freely soluble in water and slightly soluble in alcohol. Hydrocortisone sodium phosphate may be administered via IM, SQ, or IV routes.

Hydrocortisone sodium succinate occurs as an odorless, white to nearly white, hygroscopic, amorphous solid. It is very soluble in both water and alcohol. Hydrocortisone sodium succinate injection is administered via IM or IV routes.

Storage/Stability/Compatibility - Hydrocortisone tablets should be stored in well-closed containers. The cypionate oral suspension should be stored in tight, light resistant containers. All products should be stored at room temperature (15-30°C); avoid freezing the suspensions or solutions. After reconstituting solutions, only use products that are clear. Discard unused solutions after 3 days.

Hydrocortisone sodium phosphate solution for injection is reportedly **compatible** with the following solutions and drugs: 10% fat emulsion, amikacin sulfate, amphotericin B (with or without heparin sodium), bleomycin sulfate, cephapirin sodium, metaraminol bitartrate, sodium bicarbonate, and verapamil HCl.

Hydrocortisone sodium succinate is reportedly **compatible** with the following solutions and drugs: dextrose-Ringer's injection combinations, dextrose-Ringer's lactate injection combinations, dextrose-saline combinations, dextrose injections, Ringer's injection, lactated Ringer's injection, sodium chloride injections, amikacin sulfate, aminophylline, amphotericin B (limited quantities), calcium chloride/gluconate, cephalothin sodium (not in combination with aminophylline), cephapirin sodium, chloramphenicol sodium succinate, clindamycin phosphate, corticotropin, daunorubicin HCl, dopamine HCl, erythromycin gluceptate, erythromycin lactobionate, lidocaine HCl, mephentermine sulfate, metronidazole with sodium bicarbonate, netilmicin sodium, penicillin G potassium/sodium, piperacillin sodium, polymyxin B sulfate, potassium chloride, prochlorperazine edisylate, sodium bicarbonate, thiopental sodium, vancomycin HCl, verapamil HCl and vitamin B-complex with C.

Hydrocortisone sodium succinate is reportedly **incompatible** with the following solutions and drugs: ampicillin sodium, bleomycin sulfate, colistemethate sodium, diphenhydrinate, diphenhydramine HCl, doxorubicin HCl, ephedrine sulfate, heparin sodium, hydralazine HCl, metaraminol bitartrate, methicillin sodium, nafcillin sodium, oxytetracycline HCl, pentobarbital sodium, phenobarbital sodium, promethazine HCl, secobarbital sodium and tetracycline HCl. Compatibility is dependent upon factors such as pH, concentration, temperature and diluents used. It is suggested to consult specialized references for more specific information (*e.g., Handbook on Injectable Drugs* by Trissel; see bibliography).

Doses -
Dogs:
For glucocorticoid (antiinflammatory) activity:
- a) 5 mg/kg PO every 12 hours; 5 mg/kg (salt not specified) IV or IM once daily. (Jenkins 1985)
- b) 4.4 mg/kg PO q12h (Kirk 1989)

For adjunctive therapy for various forms of shock:
- a) Hydrocortisone sodium succinate: 150 mg/kg IV (Kemppainen 1986)
- b) Hydrocortisone sodium succinate: 50 mg/kg IV (Kirk 1989)

For glucocorticoid "coverage" in animals who have iatrogenic secondary adrenocortical insufficiency and/or HPA suppression:
- a) Animals exhibiting mild to moderate signs of glucocorticoid deficiency: 0.2 - 0.5 mg/kg PO every day.
  For animals with HPA suppression undergoing a "stress" factor: Hydrocortisone sodium succinate 4 - 5 mg/kg just before and after stressful events (*e.g.,* major surgery). Continue with lower dosages until at least 3rd post-operative day. Access to a water-soluble form of glucocorticoid should be available should animal "collapse". (Kemppainen 1986)

For adrenalectomy in patients with hyperadrenocorticism:
- a) Soluble salt of hydrocortisone 4 -5 mg/kg IV either 1 hour prior to surgery or at the time of anesthesia induction. May also be added to IV fluids and infused during surgery. Repeat dosage at end of procedure; may give IM or IV. Glucocorticoid supplementation must be maintained using an oral product (initially predniso(lo)ne 0.5 mg/kg *bid*, cortisone acetate 2.5 mg/kg *bid*, or dexamethasone 0.1 mg/kg once daily). Slowly taper to maintenance levels (predniso(lo)ne 0.2 mg/kg once a day, or cortisone acetate 0.5 mg/kg *bid*) over 7-10 days. Should complications develop during the taper, reinitiate doses at 5 times maintenance. Most dogs can stop exogenous steroid therapy in about 2 months (based on an ACTH stimulation test). (Peterson 1986)

Cats:
For glucocorticoid (antiinflammatory) activity:
- a) 5 mg/kg PO, IV or IM every 12 hours (Davis 1985)
- b) 4.4 mg/kg PO q12h (Kirk 1989)

For adjunctive therapy for various forms of shock:
- a) Hydrocortisone sodium succinate: 150 mg/kg IV (Kemppainen 1986)
- b) Hydrocortisone sodium succinate: 50 mg/kg IV (Kirk 1989)

Cattle:
For adjunctive treatment of photosensitization reactions:
- a) 100 - 600 mg (salt not specified) in 1000 ml of 10% dextrose saline IV or SQ. (Black 1986)

Horses:
As a glucocorticoid:
- a) Hydrocortisone sodium succinate: 1 - 4 mg/kg as an IV infusion (Robinson 1987)

Dosage Forms/Preparations/Approval Status/Withdrawal Times-
There are no known veterinary-approved products containing hydrocortisone (or its salts) for systemic use. There are a variety of hydrocortisone veterinary products for topical use. A 10 ppb tolerance has been established for hydrocortisone (as the succinate or acetate) in milk.

Human-Approved Products (all require a prescription):

Hydrocortisone oral tablets 5 mg, 10 mg, 20 mg; *Cortef®* (Upjohn), *Hydrocortone®* (MSD),*Hydrocortisone®* (Major) generic

Hydrocortisone acetate Injection; 25 mg/ml, 50 mg/ml in 5 & 10 ml vials; *Hydrocortone® Acetate* (MSD); generic (Rx)

Hydrocortisone cypionate oral suspension 2 mg/ml hydrocortisone in 120 ml;*Cortef®* (Upjohn)

Hydrocortisone sodium phosphate Injection 50 mg/ml in 2 & 10 ml vials; *Hydrocortone® Phosphate* (MSD)

Hydrocortisone sodium succinate injection; 100 mg/vial, 250 mg/vial, 500 mg/vial, 1000 mg/vial; *Solu-Cortef®* (Upjohn), *A-hydroCort®* (Abbott)

There are many OTC and Rx topical and anorectal products available in a variety of dosage forms.

HYDROXYUREA

Chemistry - Structurally similar to urea and acetohydroxamic acid, hydroxyurea occurs as white, crystalline powder that is freely soluble in water. It is moisture labile.

Storage/Stability/Compatibility - Capsules should be stored in tight containers at room temperature. Avoid excessive heat.

Pharmacology - While the exact mechanism of action for hydroxyurea has not been determined, it appears to interfere DNA synthesis without interfering with RNA or protein synthesis. It apparently inhibits thymidine incorporation into DNS and may also directly damage DNA. It is an S-phase inhibitor, but may also arrest cells at the G_1-S border.

Hydroxyurea also inhibits urease, but is less potent than acetohydroxamic acid. Hydroxyurea can also stimulate production of fetal hemoglobin.

Uses/Indications - Hydroxyurea may be useful n the treatment of polycythemia vera, mastocytomas, and leukemias in dogs and cats. It potentially may be of benefit in the treatment of feline hypereosinophilic syndrome.

Pharmacokinetics - Hydroxyurea is well absorbed after oral administration and crosses the blood-brain barrier. Approximately 50% of an absorbed dose is excreted unchanged in the urine and about 50% is metabolized in the liver and then excreted in the urine.

Contraindications/Precautions/Reproductive Safety - Risk versus benefit should be considered before using hydroxyurea with the following conditions: anemia, bone marrow depression, history of urate stones, current infection, impaired renal function, or in patients who have received previous chemotherapy or radiotherapy.

Hydroxyurea is a teratogen. Use only during pregnancy when the benefits to the mother outweigh the risks to the offspring. Hydroxyurea can suppress gonadal function; arrest of spermatogenesis has been noted in dogs. Although hydroxyurea distribution into milk has not been documented, nursing puppies or kittens should receive milk replacer when the bitch or queen is receiving hydroxyurea.

Adverse Effects/Warnings - Potential adverse effects include GI effects (anorexia, vomiting, diarrhea), stomatitis, sloughing of nails, alopecia, and dysuria. The most serious adverse effect associated with hydroxyurea is bone marrow depression (anemia, thrombocytopenia, leukopenia). If these occur, it is recommended to halt therapy until values return to normal.

Overdosage/Acute Toxicity - No specific information located. Because of the potential toxicity of the drug, overdoses should be treated aggressively with gut emptying protocols employed when possible. For further information, refer to an animal poison center.

Drug Interactions - **Other bone marrow depressant drugs** (*e.g., other neoplastics, chloramphenicol, flucytosine, amphotericin B or colchicine*) may cause additive myelosuppression when used with hydroxyurea.

Laboratory Considerations - Hydroxyurea may raise serum **uric acid** levels. Drugs such as allopurinol may be required to control hyperuricemia.

Doses -

  Dogs:

    For polycythemia vera; chronic granulocytic leukemia:

      a) 50 mg/kg 3 times per week (Jacobs, Lumsden et al. 1992)

      b) For polycythemia vera: 30 mg/kg once daily for one week, then 15 mg/kg once daily until remission; then taper to lowest effective frequency by monitoring hematocrit. (Raskin 1994)

Cats:
For polycythemia vera; chronic granulocytic leukemia:
   a) 25 mg/kg 3 times per week (Jacobs, Lumsden et al. 1992)
   b) For polycythemia vera: 30 mg/kg once daily for one week, then 15 mg/kg once daily until remission; then taper to lowest effective frequency by monitoring hematocrit. Cats must be monitored more frequently than dogs as they have a greater risk of developing bone marrow toxicity. (Raskin 1994)

Monitoring Parameters - 1) CBC with platelets at least every 1-2 weeks until stable; then every 3 months; 2) BUN/Serum Creatinine; initially before starting treatment and then every 3-4 months

Dosage Forms/Preparations/FDA Approval Status/Withholding Times -
   Veterinary-Approved Products: None
   Human-Approved Products:
   Hydroxyurea Oral Capsules 500 mg; *Hydrea*® (Immunex); (Rx)

HYDROXYZINE HCL
HYDROXYZINE PAMOATE

Chemistry - A piperazine-derivative antihistamine, hydroxyzine HCl occurs as a white, odorless powder. It is very soluble in water and freely soluble in alcohol. Hydroxyzine pamoate occurs as a light yellow, practically odorless powder. It is practically insoluble in water or alcohol.

Storage/Stability/Compatibility - Hydroxyzine oral products should be stored at room temperature in tight, light-resistant containers. Avoid freezing all liquid products.

The HCl injection has been reported to be compatible with the following drugs when mixed in syringes: atropine sulfate, benzquinamide HCl, butorphanol tartrate, chlorpromazine HCl, cimetidine HCl, codeine phosphate, diphenhydramine HCl, doxapram HCl, droperidol, fentanyl citrate, glycopyrrolate, hydromorphone HCl, lidocaine HCl, meperidine HCl, methotrimeprazine, metoclopramide HCl, midazolam HCl, morphine sulfate, oxymorphone HCl, pentazocine lactate, procaine HCl, prochlorperazine edisylate, promazine HCl, promethazine HCl, and scopolamine HBr. Compatibility is dependent upon factors such as pH, concentration, temperature and diluents used. It is suggested to consult specialized references (*e.g., Handbook on Injectable Drugs* by Trissel; see bibliography) for more specific information.

Pharmacology - Like other H_1-receptor antihistamines, hydroxyzine acts by competing with histamine for sites on H_1-receptor sites on effector cells. Antihistamines do not block histamine release, but can antagonize its effects. In addition to its antihistaminic effects, hydroxyzine possesses anticholinergic, sedative, tranquilizing, antispasmodic, local anesthetic, mild bronchodilative, and antiemetic activities.

Uses/Indications - Hydroxyzine is used principally for its antihistaminic, antipruritic and sedative/tranquilization qualities, often in atopic patients.

Pharmacokinetics - Hydroxyzine is rapidly and well absorbed after oral administration. Effects generally persist for 6-8 hours in dogs and up to 12 hours in cats. Hydroxyzine is apparently metabolized in liver.

Contraindications/Precautions/Reproductive Safety - Hydroxyzine is contraindicated in patients hypersensitive to it. It should be used with caution in patients with prostatic hypertrophy, bladder neck obstruction, severe cardiac failure, angle-closure glaucoma, or pyeloduodenal obstruction.

At doses substantially greater than used therapeutically, hydroxyzine has been shown to be teratogenic in lab animals. Use during pregnancy (particularly during the first trimester) only when the benefits outweigh the risks. It is unknown if hydroxyzine enters maternal milk.

Adverse Effects/Warnings - The most likely adverse effect associated with hydroxyzine is sedation. In dogs, this is usually mild and transient. Occasionally antihistamines can cause a hyperexcitability reaction. Dogs have reportedly developed fine rapid tremors, whole body tremors and rarely, seizures while taking this drug. Safe dosages have not been established for cats.

Overdosage/Acute Toxicity - There is limited information available. There are no specific antidotes available. Overdoses would be expected to cause increased sedation and perhaps, hypotension. Gut emptying protocols should be considered with large or unknown quantity overdoses. Supportive and symptomatic treatment is recommended if necessary.

Drug Interactions - Additive CNS depression may be seen if combining hydroxyzine with other **CNS depressant medications**, such as barbiturates, tranquilizers, etc. Additive anticholinergic effects may occur when hydroxyzine is used concomitantly with other **anticholinergic agents**. Hydroxyzine may inhibit or reverse the vasopressor effects of **epinephrine**. Use norepinephrine or metaraminol instead.

Laboratory Considerations - False increases have been reported in **17-hydroxycorticosteroid urine** values after hydroxyzine use. Because antihistamines can decrease the wheal and flair response to **skin allergen testing**, antihistamines should be discontinued from 3-7 days (depending on the antihistamine used and the reference) before intradermal skin tests.

Doses -
Dogs:
    a) For pruritus: 2.2 mg/kg PO *tid* (q8h) (Gershwin 1992), (Paradis and Scott 1992)
    b) For atopy: 2.2 mg/kg PO q8-12h (White 1994)
    c) For flea allergy dermatitis: 2 mg/kg q8h PO (Griffen 1994)
    d) As an antihistamine: 2.2 mg/kg PO *tid* (Bevier 1990)

Horses:
    a) 0.5 - 1 mg/kg IM or PO *bid* (Robinson 1992)
    b) Using the pamoate salt: 0.67 mg/kg PO twice daily (Duran 1992)

Birds:
    a) For pruritus associated with allergies, feather picking or self-mutilation: 2 mg/kg q8h PO or 1.5 - 2 mg per 4 oz of drinking water daily; adjust dose to minimize drowsiness and maximize effect. (Hillyer 1994)

Monitoring Parameters - Efficacy and Adverse Effects

Client Information - May cause drowsiness and impede working dogs' abilities.

Dosage Forms/Preparations/FDA Approval Status/Withholding Times -
Veterinary-Approved Products: None
Human-Approved Products:

Hydroxyzine HCl Oral Tablets 10 mg, 25 mg, 50 mg, 100 mg; *Atarax®* (Roerig), *Anxanil®* (film coated tabs) (Econo Med), generic; (Rx)

Hydroxyzine HCl Oral Solution 10 mg/5 ml; *Atarax®* (Roerig), generic; (Rx)

Hydroxyzine HCl Injection (for IM use only) 25 mg/ml in 2 ml syringes & 1 and 10 ml vials & 50 mg/ml in 2 ml amps, 1 & 2 ml syringes & 1, 2 and 10 ml vials *Vistaril®* (Roerig) is the most commonly known trade name, there are several others including generically labeled products available; (Rx)

Hydroxyzine Pamoate Oral Capsules (equivalent to hydroxyzine HCl) 25 mg, 50 mg, 100 mg; *Vistaril®* (Pfizer), generic; (Rx)

Hydroxyzine Pamoate Oral Suspension (equivalent to hydroxyzine HCl) 25 mg/5 ml; *Vistaril®* (Pfizer); (Rx)

IMIDACLOPRID

Chemistry/Storage/Stability/Compatibility - Imidacloprid is a chloronicotinyl nitroguanidine insecticidal agent synthesized from the nitromethylene class of compounds. Its chemical formula is 1-[(6-Chloro-3-pyridinyl) methyl] - N-nitro-2-imidazolidinimine. The commercially available product should be stored in a cool, dry area.

Pharmacology - Imidacloprid's mechanism of action as an insecticide is to act on nicotinic acetylcholine receptors on the postsynaptic membrane causing CNS impairment and death. Certain insect species are more sensitive to these agents than are mammalian receptors. This is a different mechanism of action than other insecticidal agents (organophosphates, pyrethrins, carbamates, insect growth regulators (IGR's) and insect development inhibitors (IDI's). The manufacturer states that imidacloprid is non-teratogenic, non-hypersensitizing, non-mutagenic, non-allergenic, non-carcinogenic and non-photosensitizing. Imidacloprid does not have activity against ascarids.

Uses/Indications - Imidacloprid topical solution is indicated for the treatment of adult and larval stage fleas in dogs and cats.

Pharmacokinetics - The manufacturer states that when applied topically the compound is not absorbed into the bloodstream or internal organs.

Contraindications/Precautions/Reproductive Safety - The manufacturer lists the following contraindications to the compound: do not use on debilitated, aged, pregnant, or nursing animals and do not use on kittens or puppies less than 4 months of age. However, other information provided by the manufacturer states that the compound is safe to use in puppies as young as 7 weeks old and kittens as young as 8 weeks old and can be safely used in geriatric dogs and cats.

  While the manufacturer states that the drug is not teratogenic, it also states not to use on pregnant animals. Use during pregnancy only when the benefits outweigh the potential risks of therapy.

Adverse Effects/Warnings - When used as directed, no adverse effects were noted. Because the drug is bitter tasting, oral contact may cause excessive salivation. Do not get product in eyes. If eye contact occurs (human or animal), flush well with ophthalmic irrigation solution or water.

Human exposure: While gloving is not required, avoid contact with skin, and wash hands with soap and water after handling. Keep out of reach of children and do not contaminate feed or food.

Overdosage - Limited data are available, but animals administered up to 5X overdoses topically, did not demonstrate overt adverse effects.

Drug Interactions - None were noted. The manufacturer states that the compound has been shown to be compatible with fenthion, lufenuron, milbemycin, praziquantel, pyrantel pamoate and febantel.

Doses - Note: Refer to the package information for specific instructions on application of imidacloprid products.

Dogs/Cats:

As an adulticide/larvicide for fleas: Apply as directed once monthly; do not re-treat more often than once weekly. (Package instructions—*Advantage®*; Bayer)

Monitoring Parameters - Efficacy

Client Information - Apply as directed in the product instructions. Human exposure: While gloving is not required, avoid contact with skin, and wash hands with soap and water after handling. Keep out of reach of children and do not contaminate feed or food. While swimming, bathing, and rain do not apparently significantly affect the duration of action, repeated shampooing may require additional treatment(s) before the monthly dosing interval is completed. Do not reapply more often than once weekly for these animals. Dispose of unused contents and containers as directed.

Dosage Forms/Preparations/EPA Approval Status -

Veterinary-Approved Products:

Imidacloprid Topical Solution 9.1% available in cards of 4 tubes in 0.4 ml (Cats/Kittens under 9 lb.; orange), 0.8 ml (Cats/Kittens over 9 lb.; purple), 0.4 ml (Dogs/Puppies under 10 lb.; green), 1 ml (Dogs/Puppies 11 - 20 lb.; turquoise), 2.5 ml (Dogs/Puppies 21 - 55 lb.; maroon), 4 ml (Dogs/Puppies over 55 lb.; blue); *Advantage®* (Bayer); (OTC) Approved for use in dogs and cats.

Human-Approved Products: None

IMIDOCARB DIPROPINATE

Chemistry/Storage/Stability/Compatibility - Imidocarb dipropinate is a diamidine of the carbanalide series of antiprotozoal compounds. The injection should be stored between 2°-25°C (36°-77°F) and protected from light.

Pharmacology - Imidocarb is thought to act by combining with nucleic acids of DNA in susceptible organisms, causing the DNA to unwind and denature. This damage to DNA is believed to inhibit cellular repair and replication.

Uses/Indications - Imidocarb is approved for use to treat *Babesia canis* infections (babesiosis) in dogs, but the drug may also be efficacious against *Ehrlichia canis* in this species. Imidocarb may also be of benefit in treating Babesia and related parasitic diseases in a variety of domestic and exotic animals.

Imidocarb appears to be more effective against *B. canis* than *B. gibsoni*.

Pharmacokinetics - No specific information was located for this drug.

Contraindications/Precautions/Reproductive Safety - Do not use imidocarb in patients exposed to cholinesterase-inhibiting drugs, pesticides or chemicals.

Safety in puppies, pregnant, lactating or breeding animals has not been established; manufacturer states to consider risk versus benefit before treating dogs with impaired lung, hepatic or renal function.

Adverse Effects/Warnings - Most common reported adverse effects in dogs include pain during injection and mild cholinergic signs (salivation, nasal drip and brief episodes of vomiting). Less common reported effects include panting, diarrhea, injection site inflammation (rarely ulceration) and restlessness. Imidocarb has reportedly caused an increase incidence of tumor formation in rats.

Do **not** administer intravenously.

Overdosage - Dogs receiving a dosage of 9.9 mg/kg (1.5X labeled dose) showed signs of liver injury (slightly increased liver enzymes), pain and swelling at the injection site, and vomiting. Overdoses or chronic toxicity may present with cholinergic signs (vomiting, weakness, lethargy, salivation) or adverse changes in liver, kidney, lung or intestinal function. Treatment with atropine may be useful to treat cholinergic signs associated with imidocarb.

Drug Interactions - See <u>Contraindications</u> above.

Doses -
  Dogs:
> For treatment of babesiosis: 6.6 mg/kg IM or SubQ; repeat dose in 2 weeks (Package Insert; *Imizol®*—Schering)

  Sheep:
> For treatment of babesiosis: 1.2 mg/kg IM; repeat in 10-14 days (McHardy, Woolon et al. 1986)

Monitoring Parameters - Efficacy and adverse effect profile

Dosage Forms/Preparations/FDA Approval Status -
  Veterinary-Approved Products:
  Imidocarb Dipropinate for IM or SQ Injection 120 mg/ml in 10 ml multi-dose vials; *Imizol®*—Schering (Rx); Approved for use in dogs.

  Human-Approved Products: None

IMIPENEM-CILASTATIN SODIUM

Chemistry - Imipenem monohydrate is a carbapenem antibiotic that occurs as white or off-white, non-hygroscopic, crystalline compound. At room temperature, 11 mg are soluble in 1 ml of water. Cilastatin sodium, an inhibitor of dehydropeptidase I (DHP I), occurs as an off-white to yellowish, hygroscopic, amorphous compound. More than 2 grams are soluble in 1 ml of water.

The commercially available injections are available in a 1:1 fixed dose ratio. The solutions are clear to yellowish in color. pH after reconstitution ranges from 6.5 to 7.5. These products also have sodium bicarbonate added as a buffer. The suspensions for IM use are white to light tan in color.

Storage/Stability/Compatibility - Commercially available sterile powders for injection should be stored at room temperature (<30°C). After reconstitution with 100 ml of sterile normal saline, the solution is stable for 10 hours at room temperature and 48 hours when refrigerated. If other diluents are used, stability times may be reduced (see package insert or *Trissell*). Do not freeze solutions. The manufacturer does not recommend admixing with other drugs.

After reconstitution the sterile powder for suspension with 1% lidocaine HCl injection, the suspension should be used within one hour.

Pharmacology - This fixed combination of a carbapenem antibiotic (imipenem) and an inhibitor (cilastatin) of dehydropeptidase I (DHP I) has a very broad spectrum of activity. Imipenem is considered to be generally a bactericidal agent, but may be static against some bacteria. It has an affinity and binds to most penicillin-binding protein sites, thereby inhibiting bacterial cell wall synthesis.

Imipenem has activity against a wide variety of bacteria, including Gram-positive aerobic cocci (including some bacteriostatic activity against enterococci), Gram-positive aerobic bacilli (including static activity against *Listeria*), Gram-negative aerobic bacteria (H*aemophilus*, *Enterobacteriaceae*, many strains of *Pseudomonas aeruginosa*), and anaerobes (including some strains of *Bacteroides*).

Cilastatin inhibits the metabolism of imipenem by DHP 1 on the brush borders of renal tubular cells. This serves two functions: it allows higher urine levels and may also protect against proximal renal tubular necrosis that can occur when imipenem is used alone.

Uses/Indications - Imipenem may be useful in equine or small animal medicine to treat serious infections when other less expensive antibiotics are ineffective or have unacceptable adverse effect profiles.

Pharmacokinetics - Neither drug is absorbed appreciably from the GI tract and therefore they are given parenterally. Bioavailability after IM injection is approximately 95% for imipenem and 75% for cilastatin. Imipenem is distributed widely throughout the body, with the exception of the CSF. Imipenem crosses the placenta and is distributed into milk. When given with cilastatin, imipenem is eliminated by both renal and non-renal mechanisms. Approximately 75% of a dose is excreted in the urine and about 25% is excreted by unknown non-renal mechanisms. Half lives in patients with normal renal function range from 1-3 hours on average.

Contraindications/Precautions/Reproductive Safety - The potential risks versus benefits should be carefully weighed before using imipenem/cilastatin in patients hypersensitive to it or other beta-lactam antibiotics (*e.g.*, penicillins, cephalosporins as partial cross-reactivity may occur), in patients with renal function impairment (dosages may need to be reduced or time between doses lengthened), or in patients with CNS disorders (*e.g.*, seizures, head trauma) as CNS adverse effects may be more likely to occur.

While no teratogenic effects have been noted in animal studies, safe use during pregnancy has not been firmly established. While imipenem enters milk, no adverse effects attributable to it have been noted in nursing offspring.

Adverse Effects/Warnings - Potential adverse effects include: GI effects (vomiting, anorexia, diarrhea), CNS toxicity (seizures, tremors), hypersensitivity (pruritus, fever to anaphylaxis) and infusion reactions (thrombophlebitis; too rapid IV infusions may cause GI toxicity or other untoward effects).

Rarely, transient increases in renal (BUN or serum creatinine values) or hepatic (AST/ALT/Alk Phosphatase) function tests may be noted, as well as hypotension or tachycardias.

Overdosage/Acute Toxicity - Little information is available. The LD$_{50}$ of imipenem:cilastatin in a1:1 ratio in mice and rats is approximately 1 g/kg/day. Acute overdoses should be handled by halting therapy and treating supportively and symptomatically.

Drug Interactions - There apparently is no therapeutic benefit in adding **probenecid** to prolong the half lives of imipenem/cilastatin (does not appreciably affect imipenem excretion).

Additive effects or synergy may result when **aminoglycosides** are added to imipenem/cilastatin therapy, particularly against *Enterococcus, Staph. aureus, and Listeria monocytogenes*. There is apparently neither synergy nor antagonism when used in combination against Enterobacteriaceae, including *Pseudomonas aeruginosa*.

Antagonism may occur when used in combination with **other** beta **lactam antibiotics** against several Enterobacteriaceae (including many strains of *Pseudomonas aeruginosa* and some strains of *Klebsiella, Enterobacter, Serratia, Enterobacter, Citrobacter* and *Morganella*. The clinical importance of this interaction is unclear, but at present it is not recommended to use imipenem in conjunction with other beta lactam antibiotics.

Synergy may occur against *Nocardia asteroides* when used in combination with **trimethoprim/sulfa**.

Chloramphenicol may antagonize the antibacterial effects of imipenem.

Laboratory Considerations - When using Kirby-Bauer disk diffusion procedures for testing susceptibility, a specific 10 micrograms imipenem disk should be used. An inhibition zone of 16 mm or more indicates susceptibility; 14-15 mm, intermediate; and 13 mm or less, resistant.

When using a dilution susceptibility procedure, an organism with a MIC of 4 micrograms/ml or less is considered susceptible; 8 micrograms /ml moderately susceptible; and 16 micrograms/ml or greater, resistant.

Imipenem may cause a **false-positive urine glucose determination** when using the cupric sulfate solution test (*e.g.*, *Clinitest*®).

Doses -
  Dogs/Cats:
    For susceptible infections:
      a) 2 - 5 mg/kg IV q6-8h (avoid or reduce dose in animals with severe renal failure) (Vaden and Papich 1995)
      b) 2 - 5 mg/kg every 8 hours (tid) (Lappin 1997)
  Horses:
    For susceptible infections: 15 mg/kg IV (over a 20 minute period) q 4- 6 hours (Walker 1992)

Monitoring Parameters - 1) Efficacy; 2) Adverse effects (including renal and hepatic function tests if treatment is prolonged or patient's renal or hepatic function are in question)

Client Information - Imipenem/cilastatin should be administered in an inpatient setting. Clients should be informed of the cost of using this medication.

Dosage Forms/Preparations/FDA Approval Status/Withholding Times -
  Veterinary-Approved Products: None
  Human-Approved Products:
    Imipenem:Cilastatin Parenteral for Injection for IV infusion: 250 mg:250 mg (with 10 mg sodium bicarbonate), 500 mg:500 mg (with 20 mg sodium bicarbonate); *Primaxin*® *I.V.* (Merck); (Rx)

    Imipenem:Cilastatin Suspension for IM Injection: 500 mg:500 mg, 750 mg:750 mg; *Primaxin*® *I.M.* (Merck); (Rx)

IMIPRAMINE HCL
IMIPRAMINE PAMOATE

Chemistry - A tricyclic antidepressant agent, imipramine is available commercially in either the hydrochloride or pamoate salts. Imipramine HCl occurs as an odorless or practically odorless, white to off-white crystalline powder that is freely soluble in water or alcohol. Imipramine pamoate occurs as a fine yellow powder that is practically insoluble water, but soluble in alcohol. The HCl injection has a pH of 4-5.

Storage/Stability/Compatibility - Imipramine HCl tablets and the pamoate capsules should be stored in tight, light resistant containers, preferably at room temperature. The HCl injection should be stored at temperatures less than 40°C and freezing should be avoided. Expiration dates for oral HCL products are from 3-5 years after manufacture and for the pamoate, 3 years following manufacture.

   Imipramine HCl will turn yellow to reddish on exposure. Slight discoloration will not affect potency, but marked changes in color are associated with a loss of potency. If small crystals are noted in the injection solution, they may be resolubolized by immersing the ampule in hot water and agitating.

Pharmacology - Imipramine and its active metabolite, desipramine, have a complicated pharmacologic profile. From a slightly oversimplified viewpoint, they have 3 main characteristics: blockage of the amine pump, thereby increasing neurotransmitter levels (principally serotonin, but also norepinephrine), sedation, and central and peripheral anticholinergic activity. While not completely understood, the antienuretic activity of imipramine is thought to be related to its anticholinergic effects. In animals, tricyclic antidepressants are similar to the actions of phenothiazines in altering avoidance behaviors.

Uses/Indications - In dogs, imipramine has been used to treat cataplexy and urinary incontinence. In horses, imipramine has been used to treat narcolepsy and ejaculatory dysfunction.

Pharmacokinetics - Imipramine is rapidly absorbed from both the GI tract and from parenteral injection sites. Peak levels occur within 1-2 hours after oral dosing. Imipramine and desipramine enter the CNS and maternal milk in levels equal to that found in maternal serum. The drug is metabolized in the liver to several metabolites, including desipramine, which is active. In humans the terminal half life is approximately 8-16 hours.

Contraindications/Precautions/Reproductive Safety - These agents are contraindicated if prior sensitivity has been noted with any other tricyclic. Concomitant use with monoamine oxidase inhibitors is generally contraindicated. Isolated reports of limb reduction abnormalities have been noted; restrict use to pregnant animals when the benefits clearly outweigh the risks.

Adverse Effects/Warnings - While there is little experience with this drug in domestic animals, the most predominant adverse effects seen with the tricyclics are related to their sedating and anticholinergic properties. However, adverse effects can run the entire gamut of systems, including hematologic (bone marrow suppression), GI (diarrhea, vomiting), endocrine, etc. Refer to other human references for additional information.

Overdosage/Acute Toxicity - Overdosage with tricyclics can be life-threatening (arrhythmias, cardiorespiratory collapse). Because the toxicities and therapies for treatment are complicated and controversial, it is recommended to contact a poison control center for further information in any potential overdose situation.

Drug Interactions - Because of additive effects, use imipramine cautiously with other agents with **anticholinergic** or **CNS depressant** (including barbiturates and phenothiazines) effects. Tricyclic antidepressants used with antithyroid agents may increase the potential risk of agranulocytosis. **Cimetidine** may inhibit tricyclic antidepressant metabolism and increase the risk of toxicity. Use in combination with **sympathomimetic agents** may increase the risk of cardiac effects (arrhythmias, hypertension, hyperpyrexia). Concomitant use with **monoamine oxidase inhibitors** is generally contraindicated.

Laboratory Considerations - Tricyclics can widen QRS complexes, prolong PR intervals and invert or flatten T-waves on **ECG**. Tricyclics may alter (increase or decrease) **blood glucose** levels.

Doses -
  Dogs:
      a) For urethral incompetence: 5 - 15 mg PO q12h (Labato 1994)
      b) For cataplexy: 0.5 - 1 mg/kg *tid* PO; titrate dose based on clinical effect. (Fenner 1994)
      c) For adjunctive treatment of separation anxiety or other tricyclic antidepressant-responsive behavior disorders: 2.2 - 4.4 mg/kg PO once to twice daily. (Marder 1991)

Cats:
   a)   For urethral incompetence: 2.5 - 5 mg PO q12h (Labato 1994)

Monitoring Parameters - 1) Efficacy; 2) Adverse Effects

Client Information - All tricyclics should be dispensed in child-resistant packaging and kept well away from children or pets. Inform clients that several weeks may be required before efficacy is noted and to continue dosing as prescribed.

Dosage Forms/Preparations/FDA Approval Status/Withholding Times -
   Veterinary-Approved Products: None
   Human-Approved Products:
   Imipramine HCl Tablets 10 mg, 25 mg, 50 mg; *Tofranil*® (Geigy), Generic; (Rx)

   Imipramine HCl Injection 12.5 mg/ml in 2 ml amps; *Tofranil*® (Geigy); (Rx)

   Imipramine Pamoate Capsules 75 mg, 100 mg, 125 mg, 150 mg; *Tofranil*®-*PM* (Geigy); (Rx)

Innovar-Vet® **- see Fentanyl/Droperidol**

INSULIN INJECTION, REGULAR
INSULIN, ISOPHANE SUSPENSION (NPH)
INSULIN, PROTAMINE ZINC SUSPENSION (PZI)
INSULIN, ZINC SUSPENSION, EXTENDED (ULTRALENTE)

Note: Insulin preparations available to the practitioner are in a constant state of change. It is highly recommended to review current references or sources of information pertaining to insulin therapy for dogs and cats, to maximize efficacy of therapy and reduce chances of errors.

Chemistry - Insulin is a 2 chained hormone linked by disulfide linkages secreted by the beta cells of the pancreatic islets. It has an approximate molecular weight of 6000 daltons. Insulin is measured in Units/ml; one International Unit (IU) is equivalent to 0.04167 mg of the 4th International Standard (a mixture containing 52% beef insulin and 48% pork insulin). There are species variations of insulin, with different amino acids found at positions 8, 9, & 10 of the A chain and position 30 of the B chain. Dog and cat insulin are thought to more closely resemble porcine insulin, rather than beef insulin. There are two basic purity grades of insulin available from bovine and porcine sources. Single-peak insulins contain not more than 25 parts per million (ppm) of proinsulin. Purified insulins contain not more than 10 parts per million (ppm) of proinsulin.

   Regular insulin, also known as crystalline zinc insulin or unmodified insulin, is obtained for commercial uses from the pancreases of pigs and/or cattle at slaughter. The insulin is prepared by precipitating the insulin with zinc chloride, forming zinc insulin crystals. The commercially available solutions have a pH of 7 - 7.8.

   Isophane insulin, more commonly known as **NPH insulin**, occurs as a sterile suspension of zinc insulin crystals and protamine zinc in buffered water for injection. It is a cloudy or milky suspension with a pH of 7.1-7.4. NPH insulin is an abbreviation for neutral protamine Hagedorn insulin.

   Protamine zinc insulin (PZI) occurs as a sterile suspension of insulin modified by the addition of protamine sulfate and zinc chloride in buffered water for injection. It is cloudy or milky suspension with a pH of 7.1-7.4.

Storage/Stability/Compatibility - **Regular insulin** is recommended by the manufacturers to be stored in the original container at refrigerated temperatures (2 - 8°C), but the new neutral formulations have been demonstrated to be stable at room temperature for 24-30 months. Temperature extremes should be avoided; do not freeze. Do not use regular insulin that is turbid, discolored or has an alteration in viscosity. Regular insulin has been shown to adsorb to the surface of IV bottles/bags and tubing. This may be of greater importance when concentrations of less than 100 IU/liter are used intravenously. Flushing the IV set before administering may allow a more consistent delivery of insulin to the patient. Since IV insulin is given to effect and patients are closely monitored, the problem may be overstated. Difficulties in determining subsequent SQ doses using the quantities of insulin required during intravenous therapy may occur, however.

   Regular insulin is reportedly **compatible** with following drugs/solutions: normal saline, TPN solutions (4% amino acids, 25% dextrose with electrolytes & vitamins; must occasionally shake bag to prevent separation), bretylium tosylate, cimetidine HCl, lidocaine HCl, oxytetracycline HCl and verapamil HCl. Regular insulin may also be mixed with other insulin products (*e.g.*, NPH, PZI, etc.).

   Regular insulin is reportedly **incompatible** with the following drugs/solutions: aminophylline, amobarbital sodium, chlorothiazide sodium, dobutamine HCl, nitrofurantoin sodium, pentobarbital sodium, phenobarbital sodium, phenytoin sodium, secobarbital sodium, sodium bicarbonate, sulfisoxizole sodium, and thiopental sodium. Compatibility is dependent upon factors such as pH, concentration, temperature and diluents used. It is suggested to consult specialized references for more specific information (*e.g., Handbook on Injectable Drugs* by Trissel; see bibliography).

NPH insulin and **Protamine zinc insulin (PZI)** should be stored in a manner similar to that of regular insulin (see above). Freezing may cause improper resuspension of the particles with resultant improper dosing; do not use if solution is clear or if the particles appear clumped or granular.

Pharmacology - Insulin is responsible for the proper usage of glucose and other metabolic fuels by cells in the normal metabolic processes. After binding to specific receptors of target cells, the insulin-receptor complex is thought to activate a membrane protease that catalyzes a peptide mediator(s) that affects certain intracellular enzymes.

Insulin affects primarily liver, muscle and adipose tissues. In the liver, insulin decreases glycogenolysis, gluconeogenesis, ketogenesis, and increases glycogen synthesis and fatty acid synthesis. In muscle, insulin decreases protein catabolism and amino acid output, and increases amino acid uptake, protein synthesis and glycogen synthesis. In adipose tissue, insulin decreases lipolysis and increases glycerol and fatty acid synthesis.

Uses/Indications - Insulin preparations have been used for the adjunctive treatment of diabetic ketoacidosis, uncomplicated diabetes mellitus and as adjunctive therapy in treating hyperkalemia. Insulin treatment in veterinary species has been primarily in dogs and cats. Experience in using insulin in large animals is rather limited.

Pharmacokinetics - In dogs and cats, regular insulin's effects are continuous when infused at low dosages intravenously, but effects tend to cease immediately when the infusion is stopped. After IM or IV bolus injection, the duration of action is only 2-4 hours. After subcutaneous injection, regular insulin's actions may persist for 4-6 hours.

In dogs, PZI insulin may take from 1-4 hours for onset of action to take place. The effects of PZI peak between 5-20 hours after dosing and persist for up to 30 hours. The majority of dogs receiving PZI injections can be adequately controlled with once daily administration. The onset of effect after SQ injection of NPH insulin may be immediate or take up to 3 hours. NPH peaks generally 2-10 hours after injection and its effects may persist for up to 24 hours. Most dogs require twice daily injections for optimal control, however.

In cats, PZI insulin will begin to lower blood glucose in about 1-3 hours and has its peak effects in 4-10 hours after injection. The duration of action of PZI in cats may be from 12-30 hours. Because of the variability of PZI's duration in cats, some animals may require twice daily injections for optimal control. NPH insulin peaks sooner (1.5-6 hours) and has a shorter duration of action (4-10 hours) than PZI. Nearly all cats will require twice daily administration of NPH for good control.

Contraindications/Precautions - Because there are no alternatives for insulin when it is used for diabetic indications, there are no absolute contraindications to its use. If animals develop hypersensitivity (local or otherwise) or should insulin resistance develop, a change in type or species of insulin should be tried. Insulin derived from swine is closest in structure to canine insulin and is thought to be closer to feline insulin, than is insulin derived from bovine sources.

Do not inject insulin at the same site day after day or lipodystrophic reactions can occur.

Adverse Effects/Warnings - Adverse effects of insulin therapy can include, hypoglycemia (see overdosage below), insulin-induced hyperglycemia ("Somogyi effect"), insulin antagonism/resistance, rapid insulin metabolism, and local reactions to the "foreign" proteins.

Overdosage - Overdosage of insulin can lead to various degrees of hypoglycemia. Symptoms may include weakness, shaking, head tilting, lethargy, ataxia, seizures and coma. Prolonged hypoglycemia can result in permanent brain damage or death.

Mild hypoglycemia may be treated by offering the animal its usual food. More serious symptoms should be treated with oral dextrose solutions (*e.g., Karo*® syrup) rubbed on the oral mucosa or by intravenous injections of 50% dextrose solutions. Should the animal be convulsing, fluids should not be forced orally nor fingers placed in the animal's mouth. Once the animal's hypoglycemia is alleviated, it should be closely monitored (both by physical observation and serial blood glucose levels) to prevent a recurrence of hypoglycemia (especially with the slower absorbed products) and also to prevent hyperglycemia from developing. Future insulin dosages or feeding habits should be adjusted to prevent further occurrences of hypoglycemia.

Drug Interactions - The following drugs may potentiate the hypoglycemic activity of insulin: **alcohol, anabolic steroids** (*e.g.,* **stanozolol, boldenone, etc.**), beta-**adrenergic blockers (e.g propranolol), monoamine oxidase inhibitors, guanethidine, phenylbutazone, sulfinpyrazone, tetracycline, aspirin or other salicylates.**

The following drugs may decrease the hypoglycemic activity of insulin: **glucocorticoids, dextrothyroxine, dobutamine, epinephrine, estrogen/progesterone combinations, furosemide and thiazide diuretics.** Thyroid hormones can also elevate blood glucose levels in diabetic patients when **thyroid hormone** therapy is first initiated.

Because insulin can alter serum potassium levels, patients receiving concomitant **cardiac glycoside** (*e.g.,* **digoxin**) therapy should be closely monitored. This is especially true in patients also receiving concurrent **diuretic therapy.**

Doses -
Note: The reader is strongly encouraged to refer to the original referenced materials for the doses below, for more thorough discussions on the treatment of diabetes.

Dogs:
For adjunctive therapy (must also correct dehydration, electrolyte & acid/base imbalances, identify and treat precipitating factors (*e.g.,* infection), and provide a carbohydrate substrate when necessary) for diabetic ketoacidosis:
   a) Regular insulin: Loading dose of 0.2 U/kg IM, repeat IM doses of 0.1 U/kg hourly until blood glucose drops below 250 mg/dl. Monitor blood glucoses every hour. Attempt to reduce blood glucose by 50 - 100 mg/dl/hr. When blood glucose reaches 250 mg/dl, begin concomitant IV dextrose 5% and maintain fluid therapy. Then regular insulin 0.5 U/kg IM (or SQ if hydration is normal) q4-6h.
   Insulin may be diluted with normal saline, sterile water or special diluent (not available commercially; obtained from Eli Lilly Co.) if necessary. Once animal is eating, alert, not receiving IV fluids, and relatively stable, may switch to either PZI or NPH insulin using the protocol listed under "Insulin treatment for uncomplicated diabetes mellitus", below. (Nelson and Feldman 1988)
   b) Low dose regular insulin infusion method: Add 1 Unit of regular insulin for each 100 ml of IV fluid. Administer at a rate so that animal receives between 0.5 - 1 Unit per hour or 0.025 - 0.05 Units/kg/hour. Use the lowest dose in small dogs.
   Low dose IM method: Initially, 2 Units of regular insulin for dogs less than 10 kg and 0.25 Units/kg for dogs over 10 kg of body weight. Thereafter, 1 Unit IM every hour for dogs <10 kg and 0.1 Unit/kg IM every hour for dogs >10 kg.
   With either method blood glucose should be monitored hourly and the insulin dosages outlined above stopped when blood glucose is between 200-250 mg/dl. Then, either infuse glucose and insulin to promote ketone utilization or convert to conventional therapy.
   To promote ketone utilization infuse glucose (2 - 3 mg/kg/min) and regular insulin (about 0.035 U/kg/hr) until animal is eating without vomiting. Alternatively, begin conventional therapy by following the guidelines outlined below: "Insulin treatment of uncomplicated diabetes mellitus". (Schall 1985)
Insulin treatment of uncomplicated diabetes mellitus:
   a) Begin NPH at 1 Unit/kg for smaller dogs (<15 kg) and 0.5 Units/kg for larger dogs (>25 kg). Determine blood glucose once or twice an afternoon for the first 2-3 days of treatment to determine if dose is too high. Animal should preferably be hospitalized during the this period. Begin dietary therapy at this time; multiple (3-4) small meals throughout the day, beginning with the insulin dose is best. After this initial equilibration period, serial blood glucose measurements (every 1-2 hours) should be taken over the course of the day. Adjust feeding times, frequency of insulin administration, insulin dosage, insulin type (PZI, if once daily NPH doesn't adequately cover and twice a day NPH is not feasible) so that the lowest blood glucose level occurs about 10-12 hours after injection with a range of 80-120 mg/dl. At no time should the blood glucose get below 80 mg/dl. The highest acceptable blood glucose is 180 - 200 mg/dl 24 hours post-injection. (Nelson and Feldman 1986)
   b) Begin PZI at 1 Unit/kg body weight once daily, usually in the morning. Initially, monitor urine glucose (at home) every AM. If there is deviation from the desired 100 - 250 mg/dl urine glucose, increase/decrease insulin by 5-10% accordingly. Feed 1/2 of daily ration in the morning and the remainder in the late afternoon or evening. If the animal refuses food in the AM, give only 1/2 the scheduled dose.
   Alternatively, use NPH at same dosage as PZI, but most animals will require twice daily injections to obtain adequate 24 hour control. (Schall 1985)
For adjunctive treatment of hyperkalemia:
   a) Regular insulin 5 Units/kg/hr IV combined with glucose at 2 grams per Unit of insulin given. Onset of action approximately 30 minutes and effects may last for several hours. (Senior 1989)
   b) For hyperkalemia associated with hypoadrenocorticism: Regular insulin IV bolus at 0.5 Units/kg. Follow with 1.0 - 1.5 grams of dextrose per unit of insulin administered.

Dextrose should be added to IV fluids and administered over 4-6 hours. (Feldman, Schrader, and Twedt 1988)

Cats: Because at the present time PZI insulin is unavailable, most veterinarians are substituting ultralente insulin initially on a unit for unit basis, although some recommend reducing insulin dose by 25%, particularly when switching to r-DNA human ultralente. Animals should be carefully monitored during this intial phase ideally with glucose-response curves, but at a minimum for signs of hyper- or hypoglycemia.

For adjunctive therapy (must also correct dehydration, electrolyte & acid/base imbalances, identify and treat precipitating factors (*e.g.*, infection), and provide a carbohydrate substrate when necessary) for diabetic ketoacidosis:

a) Regular insulin: Loading dose of 0.2 U/kg IM, repeat IM doses of 0.1 U/kg hourly until blood glucose drops below 250 mg/dl. When blood glucose reaches 250 mg/dl, begin concomitant IV dextrose 2.5 - 5% and maintain fluid therapy until cat can begin eating. Then regular insulin 0.5 U/kg SQ q6h; adjust in increments of 0.5 - 1 units to maintain blood glucose between 100-250 mg/dl.

Insulin may be diluted 1:10 with normal saline or special diluent (not available commercially; obtained from Eli Lilly Co.) if necessary. Monitor blood glucose frequently (every 1-2 hours until patient stabilizes). Once cat is eating and relatively stable, may switch to either PZI or NPH insulin using the protocol listed under "Insulin treatment for uncomplicated diabetes mellitus". (Peterson and Randolph 1989)

Insulin treatment of uncomplicated diabetes mellitus:

a) Patients on NPH insulin should receive doses every 12 hours. PZI insulin may be used once daily. Begin at 0.25 - 0.5 U/kg/day and slowly increase dose as needed. Feed one-half of daily caloric allotment at the time the morning injection is given (both NPH & PZI) and the other half 12 hours later (with 2nd NPH injection, if used). If diluted with sterile water or isotonic saline when using very low dosages, discard unused insulin after 2 months.

During first 1-2 weeks of therapy the owner should monitor urine glucose and ketone levels 1-2 times per day, if possible. Dosage should be adjusted by 0.5 - 1 Unit increments every 3-4 days if necessary (based on serial urine glucose, clinical symptomatology). Dosage should not be adjusted based on a single urine glucose value. Frequent blood glucose measurements (over the course of day, preferable at 1-2 week intervals until stable) are a better method of monitoring therapy and adjusting dosage. (Peterson and Randolph 1989)

b) Begin PZI at 0.5 Unit/kg body weight once daily, usually in the morning. Initially, monitor urine glucose (at home) every AM. If there is deviation from the desired 100 - 250 mg/dl urine glucose, increase/decrease insulin by 5-10% accordingly. Feed 1/2 of daily ration in the morning and the remainder in the late afternoon or evening. If the animal refuses food in the AM, give only 1/2 the scheduled dose.

Alternatively, use NPH at same dosage as PZI, but most animals will require twice daily injections of NPH to obtain adequate 24 hour control. (Schall 1985)

For adjunctive treatment of hyperkalemia:

a) Regular insulin 0.5 Units/kg IV combined with glucose at 2 grams per Unit of insulin given. Onset of action is approximately 30 minutes and effects may last for several hours. (Senior 1989)

b) For hyperkalemia associated with hypoadrenocorticism: Regular insulin IV bolus at 0.5 Units/kg. Follow with 1.0 - 1.5 grams of dextrose per unit of insulin administered. Dextrose should be added to IV fluids and administered over 4-6 hours. (Feldman, Schrader, and Twedt 1988)

Cattle:

For hyperglycemia:

a) Adult cow:150 - 200 Units SQ every 36 hours (*type of insulin not specified; PZI?*). (Howard 1986)

Horses:

For diabetes mellitus:

a) True diabetes mellitus rarely occurs in horses. Most cases are a result of pituitary tumors that cause hyperglycemia secondary to excessive ACTH or Growth Hormone. A case is cited where an animal received 0.5 - 1.0 Unit/kg of PZI insulin and the hyperglycemia was controlled. Patients with hyperglycemia secondary to a pituitary tumor are apparently insulin-resistant. (Merritt 1987)

b) PZI insulin 0.15 U/kg IM or SQ *bid* (Robinson 1987)

Birds:

For diabetes mellitus:

a) NPH (U-40) insulin: 0.002 - 0.1 Units IM. Insulin should be diluted 1:1000 yielding a concentration of 0.04 Units/ml. At this concentration, initially give 0.05 ml/30 grams body weight IM. Adjust dosage by monitoring urine glucose. When urine glucose reaches 1+, recheck blood glucose. Generally takes 1-2 weeks to regulate the dosage. (Stunkard 1984)

b) If urine glucose exceeds 0.5 per cent, check serum glucose. If it is > 1000 mg/dl, begin empiric insulin therapy. If serum glucose levels are between 600 - 1000 mg/dl; repeat test in 24 hours and start insulin if repeat test is the same or elevated.

Dilute 0.3 ml of insulin (U-40) with 2.7 ml of lactated Ringer's for larger birds, yielding a solution containing 4 Units/ml. For smaller birds, further dilute 0.1 ml (0.4 Units) of this solution with an additional 0.9 ml of lactated Ringer's to yield a 0.04 Units/0.1 ml solution. Diluted insulin may be stored in the refrigerator for 3-4 months.

Dosages of insulin are extremely variable. Smaller birds generally require more insulin per gram of body weight than larger birds. Reported dosages for budgerigars range from 0.000067 - 0.00333 Units per gram of body weight. Bird should have free access to food. Twice a day therapy is recommended with monitoring of droppings to maintain a slightly positive glucose level in the urine. (Lothrop et al. 1986)

Monitoring Parameters - 1) Blood glucose; 2) Patient weight, appetite, fluid intake/output; 3) Blood, urine ketones (if warranted); 4) Glycosylated hemoglobin (if available and warranted)

Client Information - Keep insulin products away from temperature extremes. If stored in the refrigerator, allow to come to room temperature in syringe before injecting.

Clients must be instructed in proper techniques for withdrawing insulin into the syringe, including rolling the vial, not shaking before withdrawing into syringe, and to use the proper syringe size with insulin concentration (*e.g.,* don't use U-40 insulin with U-100 syringes). Proper injection techniques should be taught and practiced with the client before the animal's discharge. The symptoms of hypoglycemia should be thoroughly reviewed with the owner. A written protocol outlining monitoring procedures and treatment steps for hypoglycemia should be also be sent home with the owner.

Dosage Forms/Preparations/FDA Approval Status/Withholding Times - All products except 500 U/ml insulin are available without prescription.

Veterinary-Approved Products: None

Human-Approved Products (partial listing):

Insulin Injection, Regular

From pork sources; 100 Units/ml
Regular Insulin (Novo-Nordisk)
Regular Purified Pork insulin (Novo-Nordisk); *Pork Regular Iletin II* (Lilly)

Human (either rDNA or semi-synthetic) insulin:
Humulin® R (Lilly); *Novolin® R* (Novo-Nordisk), *Velosulin® Human* (Novo-Nordisk)

Insulin, Isophane Suspension (NPH)

From beef sources; 100 Units/ml
Insulin, NPH (Novo-Nordisk)

From pork sources (purified); 100 Units/ml
Iletin® II, NPH Purified Pork (Lilly), *NPH-N®* (Novo-Nordisk)

Human (either rDNA or semi-synthetic) insulin:
Humulin® N, (Lilly); *Novolin® N* (Novo-Nordisk),

Insulin, Zinc Suspension, Extended (Ultralente)

From rDNA Human sources; 100 Units/ml
Humulin® U Ultralente (Lilly)

Other insulins that are commercially available, but have not been used extensively in veterinary patients, include: Insulin Zinc (Lente), and fixed dose combination products containing regular insulin and isophane insulin (NPH).

INTERFERON ALFA-2A, HUMAN RECOMBINANT

Chemistry - Prepared from genetically engineered cultures of *E. coli* with genes from human leukocytes, interferon alfa-2a is commercially available as a sterile solution or sterile powder. Human interferon alfa is a complex protein that contains 165 or 166 amino acids.

Storage/Stability/Compatibility - Commercially available products should be stored in the refrigerator; do not freeze the accompanying diluent. Do not expose solutions to room temperature for longer than 24 hours. Do not vigorously shake solutions.

An article proposing using this product in cats for the treatment of FeLV states that after dilution of 3 million IU in one liter of sterile saline the resultant solution remains active for years if frozen or for months if refrigerated. However, data corroborating this is apparently not available.

Pharmacology - The pharmacologic effects of the interferons are widespread and complex. Suffice it to say, that interferon alfa has antiviral, antiproliferative and immunomodulating effects. Its antiproliferative and antiviral activities are thought to be due to its effects on the synthesis of RNA, DNA, and cellular proteins (oncogenes included). The mechanisms for its antineoplastic activities are not well understood, but are probably related these effects as well.

Uses/Indications - Thus far, interferon alfa use in veterinary medicine has primarily been centered around its oral administration in cats to treat non-neoplastic FeLV disease. However, studies published at this point have not been controlled and the usefulness of these agents after oral administration is in question. Potentially, interferons may be useful in treating a variety of conditions (neoplastic disease, some viral infections) in veterinary species, but toxicities and high drug costs may limit their usefulness.

Oral interferon may also be of benefit in the treatment of ocular herpes infection, but controlled studies need to be performed.

Pharmacokinetics - Interferon alfa is poorly absorbed after oral administration as it is degraded by proteolytic enzymes and studies have not detected measurable levels in the systemic circulation. However, there may be some absorption via upper GI mucosa.

Interferon alfa is widely distributed throughout the body, although it does not penetrate into the CNS well. It is unknown if it crosses the placenta. Interferon alfa is freely filtered by the glomeruli, but is absorbed by the renal tubules where it is metabolized by brush border or lysosomes. Hepatic metabolism is of minor importance. The plasma half life in cats has been reported as 2.9 hours.

Contraindications/Precautions/Reproductive Safety - When used parenterally, consider the risks versus benefits in patients with preexisting autoimmune disease, severe cardiac disease, pulmonary disease, "brittle" diabetes, Herpes infections, hypersensitivity to the drug, or CNS disorders.

Safety during pregnancy has not been established; high parenteral doses in monkeys did not cause teratogenic effects, but did increase abortifacient activity.

Adverse Effects/Warnings - When used orally in cats, adverse effects have apparently not yet been noted. When used systemically in humans, adverse effects have included anemia, leukopenias, thrombocytopenia, hepatotoxicity, neurotoxicity, changes in taste sensation, anorexia, nausea, vomiting, diarrhea, dizziness, "flu-like" syndrome, transient hypotension, skin rashes and dry mouth. Except for the "flu-like "syndrome most adverse effects are dose related and may vary depending on the condition treated.

Overdosage/Acute Toxicity - No information located. Determine dosages carefully.

Drug Interactions - Additive or synergistic antiviral effects may occur when interferon alfa is used in conjunction with **zidovudine** (AZT) or **acyclovir**. This effect does not appear to occur with **vidarabine**, although increased toxicities may occur. The veterinary significance of these potential interactions are unclear.

Doses -
  Dogs:
    As an appetite stimulant:
      a) 1 IU per 10 pounds of body weight PO every other week. Efficacy is not proven. (Kemp 1992)
  Cats:
    For treatment of non-neoplastic FeLV-associated disease:
      a) 30 IU/cat (1 ml) given PO once daily for 7 days on a one-week-on, one-week-off schedule until clinically normal. Most cats remain FeLV positive. If clinical signs resume, may reinstitute therapy.
      b) 0.5 - 5 U/kg/day PO (Barta 1992)
    For treatment of ocular herpes lesions (see indications above):
      a) 10 units orally once daily for seven days, discontinue treatment for seven days, and then treat for seven days. Needs more research to determine efficacy. (Olivero 1994)
    Preparation of solution: Using the 3 million IU vial (see below), dilute the entire contents into a 1 L bag of sterile normal saline; mix well. Resulting solution contains approximately 3,000 IU/ml. Divide into aliquots of either 1 or 10 ml and freeze. By diluting further 100 fold (1 ml of 3000 IU/ml solution with 100 ml of sterile saline, or 10 ml

with 1000 ml of sterile saline) a 30 IU/ml solution will result. Authors state that the frozen solution will remain stable for "years" and the final diluted solution 30 IU/ml will remain stable for several months when refrigerated. Refreezing unused portions of 30 IU/ml solution is not recommended.

Client Information - Oral use in cats: Owners should be made aware of the "investigational" nature of this compound and understand that efficacy and safety have not necessarily been established.

Dosage Forms/Preparations/FDA Approval Status/Withholding Times -
   Veterinary-Approved Products: None
   Human-Approved Products:
      Interferon Alfa-2a (recombinant DNA origin) for Parenteral Injection, 3 million I.U./ml (1 ml vial), 6 million I.U./ml (3 ml vial), 36 million I.U./ml (1 ml vial); Powder for Injection 6 million I.U./ml when reconstituted (3 ml vial); *Roferon-A*® (Roche); (Rx)

IPECAC SYRUP

Chemistry - Ipecac syrup is prepared from powdered ipecac which is derived from the roots and rhizomes of certain plants. Ipecac has two active alkaloids, emetine and cephaeline. Each ml of Ipecac syrup contains 70 mg of powdered ipecac (1.23 - 1.57 mg of the ether soluble alkaloids). Ipecac syrup has a characteristic odor and occurs as a clear, to amber colored hydroalcoholic syrup. Ipecac syrup may also be known as syrup of ipecac or ipecacuanha syrup.

Storage/Stability/Compatibility - Store ipecac syrup in tight containers at temperatures less than 25°C. Although ipecac syrup may be effective for several years after the labeled expiration date, delayed emetic action or lack of efficacy have also been reported with the use of expired product and expired product cannot be recommended for use if alternatives exist.

Pharmacology - The major alkaloids of ipecac, emetine and cephaeline are believed to cause the major pharmacologic actions of the drug. Ipecac acts both locally by irritating the gastric mucosa and centrally by stimulating the chemoreceptor trigger zone. The medullary centers must be responsive for emesis to occur, however. Contents of both the stomach and upper intestinal tract may be evacuated by ipecac.

Uses/Indications - Ipecac is used to induce vomiting in dogs and cats after ingestions of certain toxic compounds or drugs in overdose quantities.

Pharmacokinetics - Little is known regarding the pharmacokinetics of ipecac or its alkaloids. The amount of absorbed tends to be highly interpatient variable. When administered to dogs or cats, vomiting usually occurs within 10-30 minutes.

Contraindications/Precautions/Reproductive Safety - Emetics can be an important aspect in the treatment of orally ingested toxins, but must not be used injudiciously. Emetics should not be used in rodents or rabbits, because they are either unable to vomit or do not have stomach walls strong enough to tolerate the act of emesis. Emetics are also contraindicated in patients that are: hypoxic, dyspneic, in shock, lack normal pharyngeal reflexes, seizuring, comatose, severely CNS depressed or where CNS function is deteriorating, or extremely physically weak. Emetics should also be withheld in patients who have previously vomited repeatedly. Emetics are contraindicated in patients who have ingested strong acids, alkalies, other caustic agents because of the risks of additional esophogeal or gastric injury with emesis. Because of the risks of aspiration, emetics are usually contraindicated after petroleum distillate ingestion, but may be employed when the risks of toxicity of the compound are greater than the risks of aspiration. Use of emetics after ingestion of strychnine or other CNS stimulants may precipitate seizures.

Emetics generally do not remove more than 80% of the material in the stomach (usually 40-60%) and successful induction of emesis does not signal the end of appropriate monitoring or therapy. Because of the drug's potential cardiotoxic effects, use with caution in animals with pre-existing severe cardiac dysfunction.

Adverse Effects/Warnings - At recommended doses, ipecac rarely exhibits toxic effects, but can induce lacrimation, salivation, and an increase in bronchial secretions. In humans, ipecac has rarely caused protracted vomiting, diarrhea and lethargy.

If after a second ipecac dose emesis does not occur, many clinicians recommend performing gastric lavage because of the potential for ipecac-induced cardiotoxicity and also to remove the ingested toxicant.

Warning: Do not confuse ipecac syrup with ipecac fluidextract which is about 14 times more potent than ipecac syrup and could cause cardiotoxicity and death if used at ipecac syrup dosages. Ipecac fluidextract is no longer commercially available in the United States.

Overdosage/Acute Toxicity - Overdoses of ipecac may result in serious cardiotoxicity with resulting arrhythmias, hypotension or fatal myocarditis. No specific antidotal therapy is available, but activated charcoal may be given to help adsorb any unabsorbed ipecac; supportive therapy may also be employed.

Drug Interactions - While **activated charcoal** will adsorb ipecac syrup and several veterinary references state that ipecac should not be used when charcoal therapy is contemplated, ipecac may be given initially followed by activated charcoal after vomiting has occurred.

Do not administer with **milk, dairy products, or carbonated beverages** as ipecac efficacy may be diminished.

Doses -
  Dogs:
    To induce emesis:
    a) 1 - 2.5 ml/kg PO; if animal has a nearly empty stomach, give 5 ml/kg of water immediately after ipecac. (Beasley and Dorman 1990)
    b) 1 - 2 ml/kg PO (Riviere 1985)
    c) 1 - 2 ml/kg PO; do not exceed 15 ml total per dog; repeat in 20 minutes if emesis does not occur. If emesis does not occur after second dose, perform gastric lavage to recover ipecac. (Bailey 1989)

  Cats:
    To induce emesis:
    a) 3.3 ml/kg PO; because cats find ipecac syrup objectionable, a diluted 50:50 solution in water (total volume 6.6 ml/kg) via stomach or nasogastric tube may be preferable. (Beasley and Dorman 1990)
    b) 1 - 2 teaspoonsful (5 - 10 ml) PO; may require second dose, but if not effective, institute gastric lavage. (Reid and Oehme 1989)
    c) 1 - 2 ml/kg PO; repeat in 20 minutes if emesis does not occur. If emesis does not occur after second dose, perform gastric lavage to recover ipecac. (Bailey 1989)

Monitoring Parameters -
  1) Cardiac function (rate/rhythm, blood pressure) should monitored in susceptible animals and if animal does not vomit after ipecac
  2) Vomitus should be quantitated, examined for contents and saved for possible later analysis

Client Information - If clients are instructed to use this agent at home or in transit to professional help, they should be instructed to save any vomitus for analysis if necessary.

Dosage Forms/Preparations/FDA Approval Status/Withholding Times -
  Veterinary-Approved Products: None
  Human-Approved Products:
  Ipecac Oral Syrup in 15 ml, 30 ml ; Generic: (OTC & Rx)

IRON DEXTRAN

Chemistry - Iron dextran is a complex of ferric oxyhydroxide and low molecular weight partially hydrolyzed dextran derivative. The commercially available injection occurs as a dark brown, slightly viscous liquid that is completely miscible with water or normal saline and has a pH of 5.2 - 6.5.

Storage/Stability/Compatibility - Iron dextran injection should be stored at room temperature (15-30°C); avoid freezing. Iron dextran injection is reportedly **incompatible** with oxytetracycline HCl and sulfadiazine sodium.

Pharmacology - Iron is necessary for myoglobin and hemoglobin in the transport and utilization of oxygen. While neither stimulating erythropoiesis nor correcting hemoglobin abnormalities not caused by iron deficiency, iron administration does correct both physical symptoms and decreased hemoglobin levels secondary to iron deficiency.

Ionized iron is also a component in the enzymes cytochrome oxidase, succinic dehydrogenase, and xanthine oxidase.

Uses/Indications - Iron dextran is used in the treatment and prophylaxis of iron deficiency anemias, primarily in neonatal food-producing animals.

Pharmacokinetics - After IM injection, iron dextran is slowly absorbed primarily via the lymphatic system. About 60% of the drug is absorbed within 3 days of injection and up to 90% of the dose is absorbed after 1-3 weeks. The remaining drug may be absorbed slowly over several months.

After absorption, the reticuloendothelial cells of the liver, spleen and bone marrow gradually clear the drug from the plasma. The iron is cleaved from the dextran component and the dextran is then metabolized or excreted. The iron is immediately bound to protein elements to form either hemosiderin, ferritin or transferrin. Iron crosses the placenta, but in what form is unknown. Only traces of iron are excreted in milk.

Iron is not readily eliminated from the body. Iron liberated by the destruction of hemoglobin is reused by the body and only small amounts are lost by the body via hair and nail growth, normal skin desquamation and GI tract sloughing. Accumulation can result with repeated dosing as only trace amounts of iron are eliminated in the feces, bile or urine.

Contraindications/Precautions/Reproductive Safety - Iron dextran is contraindicated in patients with known hypersensitivity to it, or with any anemia other than iron deficiency anemia. It is also not to be used in patients with acute renal infections, and should not be used in conjunction with oral iron supplements.

High dosages may cause increased incidences of teratogenicity and embryotoxicity. Use only when clearly necessary at recommended doses in pregnant animals.

Adverse Effects/Warnings - The manufacturers of iron dextran injection for use in pigs state that occasionally pigs may react after injection with iron dextran, characterized by prostration and muscular weakness. Rarely, death may result as a result of an anaphylactoid reaction. Iron dextran used in pigs born of vitamin E/selenium-deficient sows may demonstrate nausea, vomiting and sudden death within 1 hour of injection. Iron dextran injected IM in pigs after 4 weeks of age may cause muscle tissue staining.

Large SQ doses have been associated with the development of sarcomas in laboratory animals (rabbits, mice, rats, and hamsters).

Overdosage/Acute Toxicity - Depending on the size of the dose, inadvertent overdose injections may require chelation therapy. For more information, refer to the Ferrous Sulfate monograph for information on using deferoxamine and other treatments for iron toxicity.

Drug Interactions - Because **chloramphenicol** may delay the response to iron administration, avoid using chloramphenicol in patients with iron deficiency anemia.

Drug/Laboratory Interactions - Large doses of injectable iron may discolor the serum brown which can cause falsely elevated serum **bilirubin** values and falsely decreased serum **calcium** values. After large doses of iron dextran, **serum iron** values may not be meaningful for up to 3 weeks.

Doses -
  Dogs:
    For iron deficiency anemia:
      a) Iron dextran 10 - 20 mg/kg once, followed by oral therapy with ferrous sulfate (see ferrous sulfate monograph). (Weiser 1989b)

  Cats:
    For iron deficiency anemia:
      a) For prevention of transient neonatal iron deficiency anemia: 50 mg iron dextran injection at 18 days of age. (Weiser 1989a)

  Swine:
      a) For prevention or iron deficiency anemia in baby pigs (1-3 days of age): 100 - 150 mg of elemental iron IM per pig.
        For treatment of iron deficiency anemia in baby pigs: 100 - 200 mg of elemental iron IM per pig. May repeat in 10-14 days. (Label directions; *Ferrextran-100*®—Fort Dodge)

  Birds:
    For iron deficiency anemia or following hemorrhage:
      a) 10 mg/kg IM; repeat in 7-10 days if PCV fails to return to normal. (Clubb 1986)
      b) 10 mg/kg IM; repeat weekly. (McDonald 1989)

Monitoring Parameters -
    1) If indicated: CBC, RBC indices
    2) Adverse reactions

Client Information - In pigs, inject IM in the back of the ham.

Dosage Forms/Preparations/FDA Approval Status/Withholding Times -
  Veterinary-Approved Products:
    Iron Dextran Injection 100 mg of elemental iron/ml and 200 mg of elemental iron/ml in 100 ml vials; *Armedexan*® (Schering), *Ferrextran*® *100* (Fort Dodge), *Imposil*® (Fisons), generic; (OTC) Approved for use in swine. No slaughter withdrawal time required.

  Human-Approved Products:
    Iron Dextran Injection 50 mg of elemental iron/ml in 2 ml amps/single dose vials and 10 ml vials; *InFeD*® (Schein);*DexFerrum*® (American Regent) (Rx)

ISOFLURANE

Chemistry - An inhalant general anesthetic agent, isoflurane occurs as a colorless, non-flammable, stable liquid. It has a characteristic mildly pungent musty, ethereal odor. At 20°C, isoflurane's specific gravity is 1.496 and vapor pressure is 238 mm Hg.

Storage/Stability/Compatibility - Isoflurane should be stored at room temperature; it is relatively unaffected by exposure to light, but should be stored in a tight, light-resistant container. Isoflurane does not attack aluminum, brass, tin, iron or copper.

Pharmacology - While the precise mechanism that inhalent anesthetics exert their general anesthetic effects is not precisely known, they may interfere with functioning of nerve cells in the brain by acting at the lipid matrix of the membrane. Some key pharmacologic effects noted with isoflurane include: CNS depression, depression of body temperature regulating centers, increased cerebral blood flow, respiratory depression, hypotension, vasodilatation, and myocardial depression (less so than with halothane) and muscular relaxation.

Minimal Alveolar Concentration (MAC; %) in oxygen reported for isoflurane in various species: Dog = 1.5; Cat = 1.2; Horse = 1.31; Human = 1.2. Several factors may alter MAC (acid/base status, temperature, other CNS depressants on board, age, ongoing acute disease, etc.).

Uses/Indications - Isoflurane is an inhalant anesthetic that has some distinct advantages over either halothane or methoxyflurane due to its lessened myocardial depressant and catecholamine sensitizing effects, and the ability to use it safely in patients with either hepatic or renal disease. Isoflurane's higher cost than either methoxyflurane or halothane is a disadvantage.

Horses may recover more rapidly than with halothane, but be more susceptible to anesthetic associated-myopathy.

Pharmacokinetics - Isoflurane is rapidly absorbed from the alveoli. It is rapidly distributed into the CNS and crosses the placenta. The vast majority of the drug is eliminated via the lungs; only about 0.17% is metabolized in liver and only very small amounts of inorganic fluoride is formed.

Contraindications/Precautions/Reproductive Safety - Isoflurane is contraindicated in patients with a history or predilection towards malignant hyperthermia. It should be used with caution (benefits vs. risks) in patients with increased CSF or head injury, or myasthenia gravis.

Some animal studies have indicated that isoflurane may be fetotoxic. Use during pregnancy with caution.

Adverse Effects/Warnings - Hypotension (secondary to vasodilation, not cardiodepression) may occur and is considered to be dose related. Dose-dependent respiratory depression, and GI effects (nausea, vomiting, ileus) have been reported. While cardiodepression generally is minimal at doses causing surgical planes of anesthesia, it may occur. Arrhythmias have also rarely been reported.

Drug Interactions - While isoflurane sensitizes the myocardium to the effects of sympathomimetics less so than halothane, arrhythmias may still result. Drugs included are: **dopamine, epinephrine, norepinephrine, ephedrine, metaraminol, etc.** Caution and monitoring is advised.

Non-depolarizing neuromuscular blocking agents, systemic aminoglycosides, systemic lincomycins should be used with caution with halogenated anesthetic agents as additive neuromuscular blockade may occur.

Concomitant administration of **succinylcholine** with inhalation anesthetics may induce increased incidences of cardiac effects (bradycardia, arrhythmias, sinus arrest and apnea) and in susceptible patients, malignant hyperthermia as well.

Doses -

Dogs/Cats: (Note: Concentrations are dependent upon fresh gas flow rate; the lower the flow rate, the higher the concentration required.)

    a) 5% induction; 1.5 - 2.5% maintenance (Papich 1992)

    b) 0.5 - 3 %, inhaled (Hubbell 1994)

Pocket Pets:

    a) Using a non-rebreathing system: Induction: 2 - 3%, maintenance: 0.25 - 2% (Anderson 1994)

Reptiles:

    a) Give 5% isoflurane and oxygen in a clear plastic bag or induction chamber. Fill chamber with gas and seal. Induction time may take 30 - 60 minutes, but can be shortened to 15 - 30 minutes with increased depth of anesthesia if animal is injected with 10-20 mg/kg of ketamine (SubQ or IM). Patient should be kept warm by placing on a water blanket. Surgical anesthesia can be determined by the loss of righting reflex. After induction, use either a mask, ET tube, or leave head in chamber. Maintenance levels are 3-5% (if isoflurane used alone). If apnea occurs during or after anesthesia, discontinue gas anesthetic and apply gentle manual ventilation 2 - 4 times per minute with small doses of doxapram IV. Normal respiration generally resumes in 3-5 minutes. Righting reflex generally recovers in an hour, but animal may be tranquilized for 24 hours. (Gillespie 1994)

Birds:

    a)   Small birds can be anesthetized safely in 15-30 seconds at 4% (Ludders 1992)

Monitoring Parameters - 1) Respiratory and ventilatory status; 2) Cardiac rate/rhythm; blood pressure (particularly with "at risk" patients; 3) Level of anesthesia

Dosage Forms/Preparations/FDA Approval Status/Withholding Times -

Veterinary-Approved Products:

Isoflurane in 100 ml bottles; *Aerrane*® (Anaquest; *Isovet*® (Schering) (Rx) Approved for use in dogs and cats.; *IsoFlo*® (Abbott) (Rx); Approved for dogs and horses.

Human-Approved Products:

Isoflurane in 100 ml bottles; *Isoflurane*®(Abbott), *Forane*® (Anaquest); (Rx)

ISOPROPAMIDE IODIDE

Also see the Prochlorperazine monograph for information on the product *Darbazine*®.

Chemistry - A synthetic quaternary ammonium anticholinergic agent, isopropamide iodide occurs as a bitter-tasting, odorless, white to pale yellow, crystalline powder. It has a melting point of 183° and is sparingly soluble in water at 25° (freely soluble at 100°) and soluble in alcohol. One mg of isopropamide is equivalent to 1.36 mg of isopropamide iodide.

Storage/Stability/Compatibility - Store isopropamide tablets in well-closed, light-resistant containers.

Pharmacology - An antimuscarinic with actions similar to atropine, isopropamide is a quaternary ammonium compound, however, and does not cross appreciably into the CNS. It, therefore, should not exhibit the same extent of CNS adverse effects that atropine possesses. For further information, refer to the atropine monograph.

Uses/Indications - Isopropamide is used in small animal medicine for its antiemetic, antidiarrheal and anticholinergic antiarrhythmic effects. It is often used in a fixed-dose combination with prochlorperazine for the treatment of vomiting and/or diarrhea.

Pharmacokinetics - Quaternary anticholinergic agents are not completely absorbed after oral administration, but quantitative data reporting the rate and extent of absorption of isopropamide is not available. After oral administration, the anticholinergic effects of isopropamide may persist for 8-12 hours.

Little information is available regarding the distributory aspects of isopropamide. Being a quaternary ammonium compound, isopropamide is completely ionized. Therefore, it has poor lipid solubility and does not readily penetrate into the CNS or eye. It is unknown if it is excreted into milk or crosses the placenta.

Isopropamide is excreted in the urine as both unchanged drug and metabolites. Much of the drug is eliminated unchanged in the feces because of its poor absorption.

Contraindications/Precautions - Isopropamide should be considered contraindicated if the patient has a history of hypersensitivity to anticholinergic drugs, tachycardias secondary to thyrotoxicosis or cardiac insufficiency, myocardial ischemia, unstable cardiac status during acute hemorrhage, GI obstructive disease, paralytic ileus, severe ulcerative colitis, obstructive uropathy or myasthenia gravis (unless used to reverse adverse muscarinic effects secondary to therapy).

Antimuscarinic agents should be used with extreme caution in patients with known or suspected GI infections. Atropine or other antimuscarinic agents can decrease GI motility and prolong retention of the causative agent(s) or toxin(s) resulting in prolonged symptoms. Antimuscarinic agents must also be used with extreme caution in patients with autonomic neuropathy.

Antimuscarinic agents should be used with caution in patients with hepatic disease, renal disease, hyperthyroidism, hypertension, CHF, tachyarrhythmias, prostatic hypertrophy, esophogeal reflux, and geriatric or pediatric patients.

Adverse Effects/Warnings - With the exception of fewer effects on the eye and the CNS, isopropamide can be expected to have a similar adverse reaction profile as atropine (dry mouth, dry eyes, urinary hesitancy, tachycardia, constipation, etc.). High doses may lead to the development of ileus in susceptible animals. For more information refer to the atropine monograph.

Overdosage - Because of its quaternary structure, it would be expected that minimal CNS effects would occur after an overdose of isopropamide when compared to atropine. See the information listed in the atropine monograph for more information.

If a recent oral ingestion, emptying of gut contents and administration of activated charcoal and saline cathartics may be warranted. Treat symptoms supportively and symptomatically. Do not use phenothiazines as they may contribute to the anticholinergic effects. Fluid therapy and standard treatments for shock may be instituted.

The use of physostigmine is controversial and should probably be reserved for cases where the patient exhibits either extreme agitation and is at risk of injuring themselves or others, or for cases where supraventricular tachycardias and sinus tachycardias are severe or life-threatening. The usual dose for physostigmine (human) is 2 mg IV slowly (for average sized adult); if no response may repeat every 20 minutes until reversal of toxic antimuscarinic effects or cholinergic effects takes place. The human pediatric dose is 0.02 mg/kg slow IV (repeat q10 minutes as above) and may be a reasonable choice for treatment of small animals. Physostigmine adverse effects (bronchoconstriction, bradycardia, seizures) may be treated with small doses of IV atropine.

Drug Interactions - The following drugs may enhance the activity of isopropamide and its derivatives: **antihistamines, procainamide, quinidine, meperidine, benzodiazepines, phenothiazines**.

The following drugs may potentiate the adverse effects of isopropamide and its derivatives: **primidone, disopyramide, nitrates, long-term corticosteroid use** (may increase intraocular pressure).

Isopropamide and its derivatives may enhance the actions of **nitrofurantoin, thiazide diuretics, sympathomimetics**.

Isopropamide and its derivatives may antagonize the actions of **metoclopramide**.

Drug/Laboratory Interactions - Isopropamide iodide may alter **thyroid function tests** (due to the iodine component) and will suppress iodine[131] uptake. It is recommended that the drug be discontinued one week prior to testing or treatment.

Doses -
Dogs:
Isopropamide:
   As an antiemetic/antidiarrheal:
      a)   0.2 - 1.0 mg/kg PO q12h (DeNovo 1986)

   For sinus bradycardia, incomplete AV block, etc.:
      a)   2.5 - 5.0 mg PO *bid-tid* (Tilley and Miller 1986)
      b)   0.2 - 0.4 mg/kg PO *bid-tid* (Moses 1988)

Prochlorperazine/Isopropamide (*Darbazine®*)
      a)   As an antiemetic/antidiarrheal: 0.14 - 0.22 mg/kg SQ *bid* (Morgan 1988)
      b)   As an antiemetic: 0.5 - 0.8 mg/kg IM or SQ q12h (DeNovo 1986)
      c)   Injectable:
           Weighing:
              up to 4 pounds = 0.25 ml;
              5 - 14 lb = 0.5 - 1 ml;
              15 - 30 lb = 2 - 3 ml;
              30 - 45 lb = 3 - 4 ml;
              45 - 60 lb = 4 - 5 ml;
              over 60 lb = 6 ml
           Oral: *Darbazine®* #1: Weighing 2 - 7 kg: 1 capsule q12h PO; Weighing 7 - 14 kg: 2 capsules q12h PO.
           Darbazine® #3: Weighing over 14 kg: 1 capsule q12h PO (Package Insert, *Darbazine®* - SKB Labs)

Cats:
Isopropamide:
   As an antiemetic/antidiarrheal:
      a)   0.2 - 1.0 mg/kg PO q12h (DeNovo 1986)

Prochlorperazine/Isopropamide (*Darbazine®*)
      a)   As an antiemetic: 0.5 - 0.8 mg/kg IM or SQ q12h (DeNovo 1986)
      b)   Injectable: Up to 4 pounds = 0.25 ml; 5 - 14 lbs = 0.5 - 1 ml (Package Insert, *Darbazine®* - SKB Labs)

Monitoring Parameters - Dependent of reason for use
      1) Clinical efficacy
      2) Heart rate and rhythm if indicated
      3) Adverse effects

Client Information - Dry mouth may be relieved by applying small amounts of water to animal's tongue for 10-15 minutes. Protracted vomiting and diarrhea can be serious; contact veterinarian if symptoms are not alleviated.

Isopropamide has been approved for use in humans by the FDA, but has not been approved for use in veterinary patients. It is a prescription (legend) drug.

Dosage Forms/Preparations/FDA Approval Status/Withholding Times -
  Veterinary-Approved Products: No single agent products are approved. The following products are approved for use in dogs and cats (injection only) and require a prescription.

Prochlorperazine dimaleate/Isopropamide iodide sustained-release capsules; *Darbazine*® #1 (Pfizer): 3.33 mg prochlorperazine, 1.67 mg isopropamide; *Darbazine*® #3 (Pfizer): 10 mg prochlorperazine, 5 mg isopropamide

Prochlorperazine edisylate/Isopropamide iodide Injection; *Darbazine*® (Pfizer): 6 mg/ml prochlorperazine, 0.38 mg/ml isopropamide iodide

  Human-Approved Products: None

ISOPROTERENOL HCL

Chemistry - Also called isoprenaline HCl, isoproterenol HCl is a synthetic beta adrenergic agent that occurs as a white to practically white, crystalline powder that is freely soluble in water and sparingly soluble in alcohol. The pH of the commercially available injection is 3.5 - 4.5.

Storage/Stability/Compatibility - Store isoproterenol preparations in tight, light-resistant containers. It is stable indefinitely at room temperature. Isoproterenol salts will darken with time, upon exposure to air, light, or heat. Sulfites or sulfur dioxide may be added to preparations as an antioxidant. Solutions may become pink or brownish-pink if exposed to air, alkalies or metals. Do not use solutions that are discolored or contain a precipitate. If isoproterenol is mixed with other drugs or fluids that results in a solution with a pH greater than 6, it is recommended that it be used immediately.

Isoproterenol for injection is reported to be **compatible** with all commonly used IV solutions (except 5% sodium bicarbonate), and the following drugs: calcium chloride/gluceptate, cephalothin sodium, cimetidine HCl, dobutamine HCl, heparin sodium, magnesium sulfate, multivitamin infusion, netilmicin sulfate, oxytetracycline HCl, potassium chloride, succinylcholine chloride, tetracycline HCl, verapamil HCl, and vitamin B complex w/C.

It is reported to be **incompatible** with: aminophylline or sodium bicarbonate. Compatibility is dependent upon factors such as pH, concentration, temperature, and diluents used and it is suggested to consult specialized references for more specific information.

Pharmacology - Isoproterenol is a synthetic beta$_1$ and beta$_2$ adrenergic agonist that has no appreciable alpha activity at therapeutic doses. It is thought that isoproterenol's adrenergic activity is a result of stimulating cyclic-AMP production. Its primary actions are increased inotropism and chronotropism, relaxation of bronchial smooth muscle and peripheral vasodilitation. Isoproterenol may also increase perfusion to skeletal muscle (at the expense of vital organs in shock). Isoproterenol will also inhibit the antigen-mediated release of histamine and slow releasing substance of anaphylaxis (SRS-A).

Hemodynamic effects noted include decreased total peripheral resistance, increased cardiac output, increased venous return to the heart and increased rate of discharge by cardiac pacemakers.

Uses/Indications - Isoproterenol is primarily used in veterinary medicine in the treatment of acute bronchial constriction, cardiac arrhythmias (complete AV block) and occasionally as adjunctive therapy in shock or heart failure (limited use because of increases in heart rate and ventricular arrhythmogenicity).

Pharmacokinetics - Isoproterenol is rapidly inactivated by the GI tract and metabolized by the liver after oral administration. Sublingual administration is not reliably absorbed and effects may take up to 30 minutes to be seen. Intravenous administration result in immediate effects, but only persist for a few minutes after discontinuation.

It is unknown if isoproterenol is distributed into milk. The pharmacologic actions of isoproterenol are ended primarily through tissue uptake. Isoproterenol is metabolized in the liver and other tissues by catechol-*O*-methyltransferase (COMT) to a weakly active metabolite.

Contraindications/Precautions - Isoproterenol is contraindicated in patients that have tachycardias or AV block caused by cardiac glycoside intoxication. It is also contraindicated in ventricular arrhythmias that do not require increased inotropic activity.

Use isoproterenol with caution in patients with coronary insufficiency, hyperthyroidism, renal disease, hypertension or diabetes. Isoproterenol is not a substitute for adequate fluid replacement in shock.

Adverse Effects/Warnings - Isoproterenol can cause tachycardia, anxiety, tremors, excitability, headache, weakness and vomiting. Because of isoproterenol's short duration of action, adverse effects are usually transient and do not require cessation of therapy, but may require lowering the dose or infusion rate. Isoproterenol is considered to be more arrhythmogenic than either dopamine or dobutamine, so it is rarely used in the treatment of heart failure.

Overdosage - In addition to the symptoms listed in the adverse effects section, high doses may cause an initial hypertension, followed by hypotension as well as tachycardias and other arrhythmias. Besides halting or reducing the drug, treatment is considered to be supportive. Should tachycardias persist, a beta blocker could be considered for treatment (if patient does not have a bronchospastic disease).

Drug Interactions - Do not use with other **sympathomimetic amines** (*e.g.,* **epinephrine**) because of additive effects and toxicity.

Propranolol (or other beta-blockers) may antagonize isoproterenol's cardiac, bronchodilating, and vasodilating effects by blocking the beta effects of isoproterenol. Beta blockers may be administered to treat the tachycardia associated with isoproterenol use, but should not be given to patients with bronchospastic disease.

When isoproterenol is used with drugs that sensitize the myocardium (**halothane, digoxin**) monitor for signs of arrhythmias.

Hypertension may result if isoproterenol is used with **oxytocic agents**. When isoproterenol is used with **potassium depleting diuretics** (*e.g.,* **furosemide**) or other drugs that affect cardiac rhythm, there is an increased chance of arrhythmias occurring.

Although not unequivocally established, there is some evidence that isoproterenol used concomitantly with **theophylline** may induce increased cardiotoxic effects.

Doses - Note: Because of the cardiostimulatory properties of isoproterenol, its parenteral use in human medicine for the treatment of bronchospasm has been largely supplanted by other more beta$_2$ specific drugs (*e.g.,* terbutaline) and administration methods (nebulization). Use with care.

Dogs:
For sinoatrial arrest, sinus bradycardia, complete AV block:
a) 0.4 mg in 250 ml D$_5$W drip slowly to effect; or Isuprel® Glossets 5 - 10 mg sublingually or rectally q 4-6h (Tilley and Miller 1986)
b) 0.04 - 0.08 micrograms/kg/min IV infusion; or 0.1 - 0.2 mg IM, SQ q4h; or 0.4 mg in 250 ml D$_5$W IV slowly (Morgan 1988)

For bronchodilitation:
a) 0.1 - 0.2 mg q6h IM or SQ (Papich 1986)

Cats:
For sinoatrial arrest, sinus bradycardia, complete AV block:
a) 0.4 mg in 250 ml D$_5$W drip slowly to effect (Tilley and Miller 1986))

For feline asthma:
a) 0.2 mg in 100 ml of D$_5$W and give IV to effect *tid*; or 0.004 - 0.006 mg IM q30 minutes *prn* (Morgan 1988)

Horses:
For short-term bronchodilitation:
a) Dilute 0.2 mg in 50 ml of saline and administer 0.4 micrograms/kg as an IV infusion, monitor heart rate continuously and discontinue when heart rate doubles. Effects may only last for an hour. (Derksen 1987)

Monitoring Parameters -
1) Cardiac rate/rhythm
2) Respiratory rate/auscultation during anaphylaxis
3) Urine flow if possible
4) Blood pressure, and blood gases if indicated and if possible

Client Information - Isoproterenol for injection should be used only by trained personnel in a setting where adequate monitoring can be performed.

Dosage Forms/Preparations/FDA Approval Status/Withholding Times -
Veterinary-Approved Products: None
Human-Approved Products:
Isoproterenol for Injection 1:5000 solution (0.2 mg/ml) in 1 & 5 ml amps; *Isuprel*® (Winthrop Pharm.); Generic; (Rx)

Isoproterenol sublingual or rectal Glossets 10 mg, 15 mg; *Isuprel*® *Glossets* (Winthrop); (Rx)

Isoproterenol is also available in aerosol or solution form for oral inhalation.

ISOTRETINOIN

Chemistry - A synthetic retinoid, isotretinoin occurs as a yellow-orange to orange, crystalline powder. It is insoluble in both water and alcohol. Commercially, it is available in soft gelatin capsules as a suspension in soybean oil.

Storage/Stability/Compatibility - Capsules should be stored at room temperature in tight, light resistant containers. The drug is photosensitive and will degrade with light exposure. Expiration dates of 2 years are assigned after manufacture.

Pharmacology - A retinoid, isotretinoin's major pharmacologic effects appear to be regulation of epithelial cell proliferation and differentiation. It also affects monocyte and lymphocyte function which can cause changes in cellular immune responses. The effects on skin include reduction of sebaceous gland size and activity, reducing sebum production. It also has anti-keratinization and anti-inflammatory activity. It may indirectly reduce bacterial populations in sebaceous pores.

Uses/Indications - Isotretinoin may be useful in treating a variety of dermatologic-related conditions, including canine lamellar ichthyosis, cutaneus T-cell lymphoma, intracutaneous cornifying epitheliomas, multiple epidermal inclusion cysts, comedo syndrome in Schnauzers, and sebaceous adenitis seen in standard poodles.

Pharmacokinetics - Isotretinoin is rapidly absorbed from the gut once the capsule disintegrates and the drug is dispersed in the GI contents. This may require up to 2 hours after dosing. Animal studies have shown that only about 25% of dose reaches the systemic circulation, but food or milk may increase this amount. Isotretinoin is distributed into many tissues, but is not stored in the liver (unlike vitamin A). It crosses the placenta and is highly bound to plasma proteins. It is unknown if it enters milk. Isotretinoin is metabolized in the liver and is excreted in the urine and feces. IN humans, terminal half life is about 10-20 hours.

Contraindications/Precautions/Reproductive Safety - Isotretinoin should only be used when the potential benefits outweigh the risks when the following conditions exist: hypertriglyceridemia or sensitivity to isotretinoin.

Isotretinoin is a known teratogen. Major anomalies have been reported in children of women taking the medication. It should also be considered to be absolutely contraindicated in pregnant veterinary patients. At this time, it is not recommended to be used in nursing mothers. Isotretinoin also appears to inhibit spermatogenesis.

Adverse Effects/Warnings -Although at the present time veterinary experience with this medication is minimal, there appears to be a low incidence of adverse effects, particularly in dogs. Potential adverse effects include: GI effects (anorexia, vomiting, abdominal distention), CNS effects (lassitude, hyperactivity, collapse), pruritus, erythema of feet and mucocutaneous junctions, polydipsia, keratoconjunctivitis (KCS), swollen tongue.

Incidence of adverse effects may be higher in cats. Effects reported include: blepharospasm, periocular crusting, erythema, diarrhea and especially weight loss secondary to anorexia. If cats develop adverse effects, the time between doses may be prolonged (e.g., Every other week give every other day) to reduce the total dose given.

Overdosage/Acute Toxicity - There appears to be very limited information on overdoses with this agent. Because of the drug's potential adverse effects, gut emptying should be considered with acute overdoses when warranted.

Drug Interactions - Isotretinoin used with **other retinoids** (etretinate, tretinoin, or vitamin A) may cause additive toxic effects. Use with **tetracyclines** may increase the potential for the occurrence of pseudotumor cerebri (cerebral edema and increased CSF pressure).

Laboratory Considerations - Increases in **serum triglyceride and cholesterol** levels may be noted which can be associated with corneal lipid deposits. **Platelets** may be increased. **ALT (SGOT), AST (SGPT) and LDH** levels may be increased.

Doses -
Dogs:
For sebaceous adenitis when more conservative treatments have failed:
a) 1 mg/kg PO q12h for one month; if improvement is noted reduce dose to 1 mg/kg PO once daily> long term goal is to treat with either 1 mg/kg PO every other day or 0.5 mg/kg once daily. (Rosser 1992)

For treatment of Schnauzer comedo syndrome: 1 mg/kg once daily or divided q12h PO.

For sebaceous adenitis in poodles; granulomatous sebaceous adenitis in viszlas: 1 - 2 mg/kg once daily or divided q12h PO.

For epitheliotrophic lymphoma, cutaneous lymphoma: 2 mg/kg once daily or divided q12h PO. (Power and Ihrke 1995)

Cats:
> For feline acne:
>> a) 5 mg/kg PO once daily (Hall and Campbell 1994)
>> b) 10 mg per cat once daily PO (Power and Ihrke 1995)
>
> For epitheliotrophic lymphoma, cutaneous lymphoma: 10 mg/cat once daily PO. (Power and Ihrke 1995)

Monitoring Parameters - See Lab Considerations and Adverse Effects. 1) Efficacy 2) Liver function tests (baseline and if symptoms appear) 3) Dogs: Schirmer Tear tests (monthly—especially in older dogs) 4) Cats: Weight.

Client Information - Isotretinoin should be handled by pregnant females in the household with extreme care, if at all. Veterinarians must take the personal responsibility to educate clients of the potential risk of ingestion by pregnant females.

   Milk or high fat foods will increase the absorption of etretinate. To reduce variability of absorption, either have clients consistently give with meals or not. Long term therapy can be quite expensive.

Dosage Forms/Preparations/FDA Approval Status/Withholding Times -
  Veterinary-Approved Products: None
  Human-Approved Products:
    Isotretinoin Oral Capsules 10 mg, 20 mg, 40 mg; *Accutane*® (Roche); (Rx)

ISOXSUPRINE HCL

Chemistry - A peripheral vasodilating agent, isoxsuprine occurs as an odorless, bitter-tasting, white, crystalline powder with a melting point of about 200°C. It is slightly soluble in water and sparingly soluble in alcohol.

Storage/Stability/Compatibility - Tablets should be stored in tight containers at room temperature (15-30°C).

Pharmacology - Isoxsuprine causes direct vascular smooth muscle relaxation primarily in skeletal muscle. While it stimulates beta-adrenergic receptors it is believed that this action is not required for vasodilitation to occur. In horses with navicular disease, it has been demonstrated that isoxsuprine will raise distal limb temperatures significantly. Isoxsuprine will also relax uterine smooth muscle and may have positive inotropic and chronotropic effects on the heart. At high doses, isoxsuprine can decrease blood viscosity and reduce platelet aggregation.

Uses/Indications - Isoxsuprine is used in veterinary medicine principally for the treatment of navicular disease in horses. It has been used in humans for the treatment of cerebral vascular insufficiency, dysmenorrhea, and premature labor, but efficacies are unproven for these indications.

Pharmacokinetics - In humans, isoxsuprine is almost completely absorbed from the GI tract, but in one study that looked at the cardiovascular and pharmacokinetic effects of isoxsuprine in horses (Mathews and et 1986), bioavailability was low after oral administration, probably due to a high first-pass effect. After oral dosing of 0.6 mg/kg, the drug was non-detectable in the plasma and no cardiac changes were detected. This study did not evaluate cardiovascular effects in horses with navicular disease, nor did it attempt to measure changes in distal limb blood flow. After IV administration in horses, the elimination half-life is between 2.5 - 3 hours.

Contraindications/Precautions - Isoxsuprine should not be administered to animals immediately post-partum or in the presence of arterial bleeding.

Adverse Effects/Warnings - After parenteral administration, horses may show symptoms of CNS stimulation (uneasiness, hyperexcitability, nose-rubbing) or sweating. Adverse effects are unlikely after oral administration, but hypotension, tachycardia, and GI effects are possible.

Overdosage - Serious toxicity is unlikely in horses after an inadvertent oral overdose, but symptoms listed in the Adverse Effects section could be seen. Treat symptoms if necessary. CNS hyperexcitability could be treated with diazepam, and hypotension with fluids.

Drug Interactions - No clinically significant drug interactions have been reported for this agent.

Doses -   .
  Horses:
> For treatment of navicular disease:
>> a) 0.6 - 0.66 mg/kg *bid* PO X 21 days; then once daily for 14 days; then once every other day for 7 days. (Note: 0.66 mg/kg is fifteen 20 mg tabs for a 1000 lb. horse)
>> For refractory cases: regimen may be repeated at 1.32 mg/kg. If no improvement seen after 6 week course then discontinue. (Forney and Allen 1984)

Monitoring Parameters -
  1) Clinical efficacy

2) Adverse effects (tachycardia, GI disturbances, CNS stimulation)

Client Information - To be maximally effective, doses must be given routinely as directed. Tablets may be crushed and made into a slurry/suspension/paste by adding corn syrup, cherry syrup, etc., just before administration.

Dosage Forms/Preparations/FDA Approval Status/Withholding Times -
  Veterinary-Approved Products: None
  Human-Approved Products:
    Isoxsuprine HCl Tablets 10 mg, 20 mg; *Vasodilan®* (Mead Johnson), *Voxsuprine®* (Major), Generic; (Rx)

ITRACONAZOLE

Chemistry - A synthetic triazole antifungal, itraconazole is structurally related to fluconazole. It has a molecular weight of 706 and a pKa of 3.7.

Pharmacology - Itraconazole is a fungistatic triazole compound. Triazole-derivative agents, like the imidazoles (clotrimazole, ketoconazole, etc.), presumably act by altering the cellular membranes of susceptible fungi, thereby increasing membrane permeability and allowing leakage of cellular contents and impaired uptake of purine and pyrimidine precursors. Itraconazole has efficacy against a variety of pathogenic fungi, including yeasts and dermatophytes. *In vivo* studies using laboratory models have shown that itraconazole has fungistatic activity against many strains of *Candida, Aspergillus, Cryptococcus, Histoplasma, Blastomyces* and *Trypanosoma cruzi*.

Uses/Indications - Itraconazole may have use in veterinary medicine in the treatment of systemic mycoses, including aspergillosis, cryptococcal meningitis, blastomycosis, and histoplasmosis. It may also be useful for superficial candidiasis or dermatophytosis. Itraconazole does not have appreciable effects (unlike ketoconazole) on hormone synthesis and may have fewer side effects than ketoconazole in small animals.

In horses, itraconazole may be useful in the treatment of sporotrichosis and *Coccidioides immitis* osteomyelitis.

Pharmacokinetics - Itraconazole absorption is highly dependent on gastric pH and presence of food. When given on an empty stomach bioavailability may only be 50% or less, with food it may approach 100%.

Itraconazole has very high protein binding and is widely distributed throughout the body, particularly to tissues high in lipids (drug is highly lipophilic). Skin, female reproductive tract and pus all have concentrations greater than found in the serum. Only minimal concentration are found in the CSF, aqueous humor and saliva, however.

Itraconazole is metabolized by the liver to many different metabolites, including to hydroxyitraconazole which is active. In humans, itraconazole's serum half life ranges from 21-64 hours. Elimination may be a saturable process.

Contraindications/Precautions/Reproductive Safety - Itraconazole should be used in patients hypersensitive to it or other azole antifungal agents, in patients with hepatic impairment, or achlorhydria (or hypochlorhydria) only when the potential benefits outweigh the risks.

In laboratory animals, itraconazole has caused dose-related maternotoxicity, fetotoxicity and teratogenicity at high dosages (5-20 times labeled). As safety has not been established, use only when the benefits outweigh the potential risks. Itraconazole does enter maternal milk, significance is unknown.

Adverse Effects/Warnings - In dogs, hepatic toxicity appears to be the most significant adverse effect. Approximately 10% of dogs recieving 10 mg/kg/day and 5% of dogs recieving 5 mg/kg/day develop hepatic toxicosis serious enough to discontinue (at least temporarily) treatment. Hepatic injury is determined by an increased ALT activity. Anorexia is often the symptomatic marker for toxicity and usually occurs in the second moth of treatment. Some dogs given itraconazole at the higher dosage rate (10 mg/kg/day) may develop ulcerative skin lesions/vasculitis and limb edema that may require dosage reduction.

In cats, adverse effects appear to be dose related. GI effects (anorexia, weight loss, vomiting), hepatotoxicity (increased ALT, jaundice) and depression and have been noted. Should adverse effects occur and ALT is elevated, the drug should be discontinued. Once ALT levels return to normal and other adverse effects have diminished, and if necessary, the drug may be restarted at a lower dosage or longer dosing interval with intense monitoring.

Overdosage/Acute Toxicity - There is very limited information on the acute toxicity of itraconazole. Giving oral antacids may help reduce absorption. If a large overdose occurs, consider gut emptying and give supportive therapy as required. Itraconazole is not removed by dialysis.

In chronic toxicity studies, dogs receiving 40 mg/kg PO daily for 3 months demonstrated no overt toxicity.

Drug Interactions - Itraconazole requires an acidic environment for maximal absorption, therefore **antacids**, **Histamine2-blockers (cimetidine, ranitidine, etc)** or **didanosine** will cause marked reduction in absorption of itraconazole. Didanosine must not be taken concurrently with itraconazole, the others (noted above), if required, should be given two hours after itraconazole dose.

Itraconazole may cause increased prothrombin times in patients receiving **warfarin** or other coumarin anticoagulants. **Rifampin** may enhance the rate of metabolism of itraconazole; itraconazole dosage adjustment may be required.

Itraconazole may decrease the metabolism of **phenytoin or cyclosporine**. Veterinary significance is unclear.

Itraconazole may increase the risks of cardiovascular effects occurring if used concomitantly with either **terfenadine or astemizole**. If itraconazole is required, it is best to switch to another antihistamine.

Itraconazole may increase serum **digoxin** concentrations; monitor serum digoxin levels.

Itraconazole may increase the serum levels of **oral antidiabetic agents** (*e.g.,* chlorpropamide, glipizide, etc.) which may result in hypoglycemia.

Elevated concentrations of **cisapride** with resultant ventricular arrhythmias may result if coadministered with ketoconazole, itraconazole, IV miconazole or troleandomycin. At present, the manufacturer states that cisapride should not be used with these drugs.

Laboratory Considerations - Itraconazole may cause **hypokalemia** or increases in **liver function tests** in a small percentage of patients.

Doses -
Dogs:
For systemic mycoses:
a) 5 mg/kg PO once or twice daily; consider adding amphotericin in rapidly progressive, life threatening infections. (Sherding and Johnson 1994b);
b) 5 mg/kg PO once to twice daily; author usually recommends higher dsoage rate and reduce if toxicity develops (Legendre 1995)

Cats:
For susceptible systemic mycoses:
a) 5 mg/kg PO once to twice daily; author usually recommends higher dsoage rate and reduce if toxicity develops. Cats will eat the pellets (found within the capsules) if placed into food (Legendre 1995)

For generalized dermatophytosis:
a) 10 mg/kg PO once daily (Medleau and Moriello 1992)

For systemic mycoses:
a) 5 mg/kg PO once or twice daily; consider adding amphotericin in rapidly progressive, life threatening infections. (Sherding and Johnson 1994b)

For systemic mycoses, generalized dermatophytosis, dematiaceous fungi:
a) 5 - 10 mg/kg PO q12-24h (Wolf 1994)

Horses:
For aspergillosis:
a) 3 mg/kg twice a day (Legendre 1993)

A method to prepare an itraconazole suspension has been provided by the manufacturer with the following caveats: 1) No bioavailability data available; 2) Use only if no other alternative.

Empty 24 (twenty four) 100 mg capsules into a glass mortar. Add 4 to 5 ml of 95% ethyl alcohol USP and let stand 3 to 4 minutes to soften. Grind to a heavy paste; this will leave a powder when the alcohol dries. Slowly triturate with 15 ml of simple syrup. Transfer to a 60 ml amber bottle and continue to rinse mortar with simple syrup to get 60 ml. Shake Well and Refrigerate. Discard after 35 days. Janssen Corp.: 1-800-526-7736

Monitoring Parameters - 1) Clinical Efficacy; 2) With long-term therapy, routine liver function tests are recommended (monthly ALT) 3) Appetite 4) Physical asssessment for ulcerative skin lesions in dogs

Client Information - Compliance with treatment recommendations must be stressed. Have clients report any potential adverse effects. Give with food.

Dosage Forms/Preparations/FDA Approval Status/Withholding Times -
Veterinary-Approved Products: None
Human-Approved Products:
Itraconazole Oral Capsules 100 mg; *Sporanox*® (Janssen); (Rx)

IVERMECTIN

Chemistry - An avermectin anthelmintic, ivermectin occurs as an off-white to yellowish powder. It is very poorly soluble in water (4 micrograms/ml), but is soluble in propylene glycol, polyethylene glycol, and vegetable oils.

Storage/Stability/Compatibility - Ivermectin is photolabile in solution; protect from light. Unless otherwise specified by the manufacturer, store ivermectin products at room temperature (15-30°C).

Ivermectin 1% oral solution (equine tube wormer product) is stable at 1:20 and 1:40 dilutions with water for 72 hours when stored in a tight container, at room temperature and protected from light.

Pharmacology - Ivermectin enhances the release of gamma amino butyric acid (GABA) at presynaptic neurons. GABA acts as an inhibitory neurotransmitter and blocks the post-synaptic stimulation of the adjacent neuron in nematodes or the muscle fiber in arthropods. By stimulating the release of GABA, ivermectin causes paralysis of the parasite and eventual death. As liver flukes and tapeworms do not use GABA as a peripheral nerve transmitter, ivermectin is ineffective against these parasites.

Uses/Indications - Ivermectin is approved in **horses** for the control of: large strongyles (adult) (*Strongylus vulgaris, S. edentatus, S. equinus, Triodontophorus spp.*), small strongyles, pinworms (adults and 4th stage larva), ascarids (adults), hairworms (adults), large-mouth stomach worms (adults), neck threadworms (microfilaria), bots (oral and gastric stages), lungworms (adults and 4th stage larva), intestinal threadworms (adults) and summer sores (cutaneous 3rd stage larva) secondary to *Hebronema* or *Draschia Spp.*.

In **cattle**, ivermectin is approved for use in the control of: gastrointestinal roundworms (adults and 4th stage larva), lungworms (adults and 4th stage larva), cattle grubs (parasitic stages), sucking lice, and mites (scabies). For a listing of individual species covered, refer to the product information.

In **swine**, ivermectin is approved for use to treat GI roundworms, lungworms, lice, and mange mites. For a listing of individual species covered, refer to the product information.

In **reindeer**, ivermectin is approved for use in the control of: warbles.

In **American Bison**, ivermectin is approved for use in the control of: grubs.

In **dogs**, ivermectin is approved only for use as a preventative for heartworm. It is also been used as a microfilaricide, ectoparasiticide and endoparasiticide.

Pharmacokinetics - In simple-stomached animals, ivermectin is up to 95% absorbed after oral administration. Ruminants only absorb 1/4 - 1/3 of a dose due to inactivation of the drug in the rumen. While there is greater bioavailability after SQ administration, absorption after oral dosing is more rapid than SQ. It has been reported that ivermectin's bioavailability is lower in cats than in dogs, necessitating a higher dosage for prophylaxis of heartworm in this species.

Ivermectin is well distributed to most tissues, but does not readily penetrate into the CSF, thereby minimizing its toxicity. Collie-Breed dogs apparently allow more ivermectin into the CNS than other breeds/species.

Ivermectin has a long terminal half-life in most species (see table below). It is metabolized in the liver via oxidative pathways and is primarily excreted in the feces. Less than 5% of the drug (as parent compound or metabolites) is excreted in the urine.

Pharmacokinetic parameters of ivermectin have been reported for various species:

Species	Bioavailability (F)	Volume of Distribution (Vd) (L/kg)	T 1/2 (terminal) (in days)	Total Body Clearance (L/kg/day)
Cattle		0.45 - 2.4	2 - 3	0.79
Dogs	.95	2.4	2	
Swine		4	0.5	
Sheep	1.0 intra-abomasal .251 intra-ruminal	4.6	2 - 7	

Contraindications/Precautions/Reproductive Safety - The manufacturer recommends that ivermectin not be used in foals less than 4 months old, as safety of the drug in animals this young has not been firmly established. However, foals less than 30 days of age have tolerated doses as high as 1 mg/kg without symptoms of toxicity.

Ivermectin is not recommended for use in puppies less than 6 weeks old. Most clinicians feel that ivermectin should not be used in Collies or Collie-mix breeds at the doses specified for treating microfilaria or other parasites unless alternative therapies are unavailable. After receiving heartworm prophylaxis doses, the manufacturer recommends observing Collie-breeds for at least 8 hours after administration.

Because milk withdrawal times have not been established, the drug is not approved for use in lactating dairy animals or females of breeding age.

The injectable products for use in cattle and swine should be given subcutaneously only; do not give IM or IV.

Ivermectin is considered to be safe to use during pregnancy. Reproductive studies performed in dogs, horses, cattle and swine have not demonstrated adverse effects to fetuses. Reproductive performance in male animals is also apparently unaltered.

Adverse Effects/Warnings - In horses, swelling and pruritis at the ventral mid-line can be seen approximately 24 hours after ivermectin administration due to a hypersensitivity reaction to dead *Onchocerca spp.* microfilaria. The reaction is preventable by administering a glucocorticoid just prior to, and for 1-2 days after ivermectin. If untreated, swelling usually subsides within 7 to 10 days and pruritis will resolve within 3 weeks.

Dogs may exhibit a shock-like reaction when ivermectin is used as a microfilaricide, presumably due to a reaction associated with the dying microfilaria.

When used to treat *Hypoderma bovis* larva (Cattle grubs) in cattle, ivermectin can induce serious adverse effects by killing the larva when they are in vital areas. Larva killed in the vertebral canal can cause paralysis and staggering. Larva killed around the gullet can induce salivation and bloat. These effects can be avoided by treating for grubs immediately after the Heal fly (Warble fly) season or after the stages of grub development where these areas would be affected. Cattle may also experience discomfort or transient swelling at the injection site. Using a maximum of 10 ml at any one injection site can help minimize these effects.

In birds, death, lethargy or anorexia may be seen. Orange-cheeked Waxbill Finches and budgerigars may be more sensitive to ivermectin than other species.

For additional information refer to the Overdosage/Acute Toxicity section below.

Overdosage/Acute Toxicity - In horses, doses of 1.8 mg/kg (9X recommended dose) PO did not produce symptoms of toxicity, but doses of 2 mg/kg caused symptoms of visual impairment, depression and ataxia.

In cattle, toxic effects generally do not appear until dosages of 30X those recommended are injected. At 8 mg/kg, cattle showed symptoms of ataxia, listless, and occasionally death.

Sheep showed symptoms of ataxia and depression at ivermectin doses of 4 mg/kg.

Swine showed symptoms of toxicosis (lethargy, ataxia, tremors, lateral recumbency, and mydriasis) at doses of 30 mg/kg. Neonatal pigs may be more susceptible to ivermectin overdosages, presumably due to a more permeable blood-brain barrier. Accurate dosing practices are recommended.

In dogs, symptoms of acute toxicity rarely occur at single dosages of 2 mg/kg (2000 micrograms/kg) or less. At 2.5 mg/kg mydriasis occurs, and at 5 mg/kg tremors occur. At doses of 10 mg/kg, severe tremors and ataxia are seen. Deaths occurred when dosages exceeded 40 mg/kg, but the LD$_{50}$ is 80 mg/kg. Dogs (Beagles) receiving 0.5 mg/kg PO for 14 weeks developed no signs of toxicity, but at 1 - 2 mg/kg for the same time period, developed mydriasis and had some weight decreases. Half of the dogs receiving 2 mg/kg/day for 14 weeks developed symptoms of depression, tremors, ataxia, anorexia, and dehydration.

The Collie breed appears to be more sensitive to the toxic effects of ivermectin than other canine breeds. This may be due to a more permeable blood-brain barrier to the drug or drug accumulation in the CNS of this breed. At the dosage recommended for heart worm prophylaxis, it is generally believed that the drug is safe to use in Collies.

Dogs who receive an overdosage of ivermectin or develop signs of acute toxicity (CNS effects, GI, cardiovascular) should receive supportive and symptomatic therapy. Emptying the gut should be considered for recent massive oral ingestions in dogs or cats. For more information on ivermectin toxicity in dogs, refer to the following reference: Paul, A., and W. Tranquilli. 1989. Ivermectin. In Current Veterinary Therapy X: Small Animal Practice. Edited by R. W. Kirk. 140-142. Philadelphia: WB Saunders.

Acute toxic symptoms in cats will appear within 10 hours of ingestion. Symptoms may include agitation, vocalization, anorexia, mydriasis, rear limb paresis, tremors, and disorientation. Blindness, head-pressing, wall-climbing, absence of oculomotor menace reflex, and a slow and incomplete response to pupillary light may also be seen. Neurologic symptoms usually diminish over several days and most animals completely recover within 2-4 weeks. Symptomatic and supportive care are recommended.

Drug Interactions - None were located.

Drug/Laboratory Interactions - When used at microfilaricide dosages, ivermectin may yield false-negative results in animals with **occult heartworm** infection.

Doses -
  Dogs:
    As a preventative for heartworm:
      a) 0.006 mg/kg PO once monthly (Hribernik 1989)
      b) 0.003 - 0.006 mg/kg PO once monthly (Knight 1988)
      c) Minimum dosage of 5.98 micrograms/kg (0.00598 mg/kg) PO per month (Rawlings and Calvert 1989)
      d) Minimum dosage of 6 micrograms/kg (0.006 mg/kg) PO per month. Three tablet sizes are available: For dogs up to 25 lbs (68 micrograms); 26-50 lbs (136 micrograms); and 51-100 lbs (272 micrograms). Dogs weighing more than 100 lbs. should receive additional drug so that the minimum dosage is covered. (Package insert; *Heartgard 30®*—MSD)

    As a microfilaricide:
      a) 3-4 weeks after aldulticide therapy, admit to hospital and administer 0.05 mg/kg (Dilute 10 mg/ml solution (*Ivomec®*) to a 1:10 solution with propylene glycol). Monitor for symptoms of toxicity (depression, mydriasis, ataxia, vomiting, diarrhea, and shock) throughout the day. If adverse effects are severe (usually less than 5% of the time), treat with fluids and corticosteroids. If no adverse effects are noted, animal may be sent home to return in 3 weeks for microfilaricide concentration test. If negative at that time, begin prophylaxis therapy. If positive, recheck in one week. If 4 weeks after therapy microfilaria persist, reevaluate for adult heartworms. *See the complete reference for more information.* (Hribernik 1989)
      b) 50 - 200 micrograms/kg (0.05 - 0.2 mg/kg) as a single dose; contraindicated in collies. (Knight 1988)
      c) 4 weeks after aldulticide therapy, give 50 micrograms/kg PO (dilute as in "a" above) in the morning. Monitor for adverse effects throughout the day; if no serious effects, may discharge in late afternoon. Do not use in Collies or Collie-Mix breeds. (Rawlings and Calvert 1989)

    As an ectoparasiticide (miticide):
      a) For treatment of *Sarcoptes scabiei* or *Otodectes cynotis* infestations: 300 micrograms/kg (0.3 mg/kg) SQ or PO; repeat in 14 days. (Paradis 1989)

    As an endoparasiticide:
      a) For treatment of parasitic lung disease (*Capillaria spp.*): 0.2 mg/kg PO once. (Bauer 1988)
      b) For roundworms, hooks, or whips: 200 micrograms/kg PO once. DO not use in Collies. (Upson 1988)
      c) For *Oslerus osleri:* 0.4 mg/kg SubQ once (Reinemeyer 1995)
      d) For *Eucoleus boehmi*: 0.2 mg/kg PO once (Reinemeyer 1995)
      e) For *Pneumonyssoides caninum*: 0.2 mg/kg SubQ once (Reinemeyer 1995)

  Cats:
    As a preventative for heartworm:
      a) Minimum effective dosage: 0.024 mg/kg (24 micrograms/kg) PO every 30-45 days. (Note: also controls hookworms at this dosage.) (Knight 1995)

    For *Aelurostrongylus abstrusus:*
      a) 0.4 mg/kg SubQ once (Reinemeyer 1995)

  Cattle:
    For susceptible parasites:
      a) 200 micrograms/kg SQ. Doses greater than 10 ml should be given at two separate sites. (Paul 1986)
      b) For psoroptic mange: 200 mg/kg IM (Note: Reference was written before approval of the SQ labeled bovine product); isolate from other cattle for at least 5 days after treatment. (Mullowney 1986)
      c) 200 micrograms/kg (0.2 mg/kg) SQ under the loose skin in front of or behind the shoulder. (Product Information; *Ivomec® Inj. for Cattle 1%*—MSD)

  Horses:
    For susceptible parasites:
      a) 200 micrograms/kg (0.2 mg/kg) PO using oral paste or oral liquid. (Product Information; *Eqvalan®*—MSD)
      b) 0.2 mg/kg PO; 0.2 mg/kg PO at 4 day intervals for lice and mange. (Robinson 1987)
      c) As a larvacidal for arterial stages of *S. vulgaris*: 0.2 mg/kg once. (Herd 1987)

Swine:
For susceptible parasites:
    a) 300 micrograms/kg (0.3 mg/kg) SQ in the neck immediately behind the ear. (Product Information; *Ivomec*® *Inj. for Swine 1%*—MSD)
    b) For general control of endo- and ectoparasites in potbellied pigs: 300 micrograms/kg SubQ or IM once for internal parasites and repeated in 10-14 days for external parasites (only partially effective against whipworms—see fenbendazole) (Braun 1995)

Sheep:
For susceptible parasites:
    a) 200 micrograms/kg for nasal bot infection. (Bennett 1986)
    b) 200 micrograms/kg SQ for one dose (goats also). (Upson 1988)

Llamas:
For susceptible parasites:
    a) 0.2 mg/kg PO or SQ for one dose (Cheney and Allen 1989), (Fowler 1989)

Birds:
For susceptible parasites:
    a) For ascarids, *Capillaria* and other intestinal worms, *Knemidocoptes pilae* (scaly face and leg mites): Dilute to a 2 mg/ml concentration. After diluting product, use immediately.
       Most birds: Inject 220 micrograms/kg IM.
       Parakeets: 0.02 mg/30 g (2000 micrograms/30 gram) IM.
       Amazon: 0.1 mg IM
       Macaw: 0.2 mg IM
       Finches: 0.02 mg (Stunkard 1984)
    b) For ascarids, coccidia and other intestinal nematodes, *Oxysipura*, gapeworms, *Knemidocoptes pilae* (scaly face and leg mites): Dilute bovine preparation (10 mg/ml) 1:4 with propylene glycol.
       For most species: 200 micrograms/kg IM or orally; repeat in 10-14 days.
       Budgerigars: 0.01 ml of diluted product (see above) IM or PO (Clubb 1986)
    c) 200 micrograms/kg (0.2 mg/kg) SQ; dilute using propylene glycol. (Sikarskie 1986)

Reptiles:
For most nematodes, ectoparasites:
    a) For lizards, snakes, and alligators: 0.2 mg/kg (200 μg/kg) IM, SubQ, or PO once; repeat in 2 weeks. Note: Ivermectin is toxic to chelonians. (Gauvin 1993)

Monitoring Parameters -
    1) Clinical efficacy
    2) Adverse effects/toxicity (see Adverse Effects and Overdosage Sections)

Client Information - When using large animal products the manufacturer recommends not eating or smoking and to wash hands after use. Avoid contact with eyes. Dispose of unused products and containers by incineration or in approved-landfills. Ivermectin may adversely affect fish or other water-borne organisms if disposed in water.
    Contact veterinarian if any treated animal exhibits symptoms of toxicity (see Adverse effects and Overdosage sections above).

Dosage Forms/Preparations/FDA Approval Status/Withholding Times -
Veterinary Approved Products -
Ivermectin for Injection 10 mg/ml (1%) in 50 ml, 200 ml, 500 ml and 1000 ml bottles
Ivomec® *1% Injection for Cattle* (MSD-AgVet); (OTC) Approved for use in nonlactating dairy cattle, beef cattle and reindeer. Slaughter withdrawal = 35 days (cattle); 56 days (reindeer and bison)

Ivermectin for Injection 10 mg/ml (1%) & Clorsulon 100 mg/ml; *Ivomec*® *Plus Injection* (MSD-AgVet); (OTC) Approved for use in cattle.

Ivermectin Oral Paste 0.153% (1.53 mg/gram) in 10.4 oz tubes; *Ivomec*® *Cattle Paste 0.153%* (MSD-AgVet); (OTC) Approved for use in nonlactating dairy cattle, and beef cattle. Slaughter withdrawal = 24 days

Ivermectin for Injection 10 mg/ml (1%) in 50 ml, 200 ml, 500 ml bottles; *Ivomec*® *1% Injection for Swine* (MSD-AgVet); (OTC) Approved for use in swine. Slaughter withdrawal = 18 days

Ivermectin for Injection 2.7 mg/ml (0.27%) in 200 ml bottles; *Ivomec*® *0.27% Injection for Feeder and Grower Pigs* (MSD-AgVet); (OTC) Approved for use in swine. Slaughter withdrawal = 18 days

Ivermectin Oral Paste 1.87% (18.7 mg/gram) in 6.08 g syringes; *Eqvalan*® *Paste* 1.87% (MSD-AgVet), *Zimectrin*® *Paste* (Farnam); (OTC) Approved for use in horses (not intended for food purposes).

Ivermectin Liquid 1% (10 mg/ml) in 50 ml and 100 ml btls (for tube administration; **not** for injection);*Eqvalan*® *Liquid* for Horses (MSD-AgVet); (Rx) Approved for use in horses (not intended for food purposes).

Ivermectin Oral Tablets 68 micrograms, 136 micrograms, 272 micrograms (Plain or Chewable) in 6 or 9 packs; *Heartgard 30*® (MSD-AgVet) (Rx) Approved for use in dogs.

Ivermectin/Pyrantel Oral Tablets 68 mcg/57 mg, 136 mcg/114mg, 272 mcg/228 mg) in packs; *Heartgard 30*® *Chewables Plus*(MSD-AgVet) (Rx) Approved for use in dogs.

KAOLIN/PECTIN

Chemistry - Kaolin is a naturally occurring hydrated aluminum silicate which is powdered and refined for pharmaceutical use. Kaolin is a white/light, odorless, almost tasteless powder that is practically insoluble in water.

Pectin is a carbohydrate polymer consisting primarily of partially methoxylated polygalacturonic acids. Pectin is a course or fine, yellowish-white, almost odorless with a mucilagenous flavor. It is obtained from the inner rind of citrus fruits or from apple pomace. One gram of pectin is soluble in 20 ml of water and forms a viscous, colloidal solution.

In the United States, the two compounds generally are used together in an oral suspension formulation in most proprietary products.

Storage/Stability/Compatibility - Kaolin/pectin should be stored in airtight containers; protect from freezing. It is incompatible with alkalis, heavy metals, salicylic acid, tannic acid or strong alcohol.

Pharmacology - Kaolin/pectin is thought to posses adsorbent and protective qualities. Presumably, bacteria and toxins are adsorbed in the gut and the coating action of the suspension may protect inflamed GI mucosa. The pectin component, by forming galcturonic acid, has been demonstrated to decrease pH in the intestinal lumen.

In one study in children with acute nonspecific diarrhea, stool fluidity was decreased, but stool frequency, water content and weight remained unchanged. No studies documenting the clinical efficacy of this combination in either human or veterinary species were located.

Uses/Indications - Although its efficacy is in question, kaolin/pectin is used primarily in veterinary medicine as an oral anti-diarrheal agent. It has also been used as an adsorbent agent following the ingestion of certain toxins. Administration may be difficult due to the large volumes that may be necessary to give orally.

Pharmacokinetics - Neither kaolin nor pectin are absorbed after oral administration. Up to 90% of the pectin administered may be decomposed in the gut.

Contraindications/Precautions - There are no absolute contraindications to kaolin/pectin therapy, but it should not be relied on to control severe diarrheas. Kaolin/pectin should also not replace adequate fluid/electrolyte monitoring or replacement therapy in severe or chronic diarrheas.

Adverse Effects/Warnings - At usual doses, kaolin/pectin generally have no adverse effects. Constipation may occur, but is usually transient and associated with high dosages. High doses in debilitated patients or in very old or young patients may rarely cause fecal impaction to occur. In rats, kaolin/pectin has been demonstrated to increase fecal sodium loss in diarrhea.

In humans, kaolin/pectin is only recommended to be used in patients less than 3 years of age or for longer than 48 hours under the direct supervision of a physician.

Overdosage - Overdosage is unlikely to cause any serious effects, but constipation requiring treatment may occur.

Drug Interactions - Kaolin/pectin may inhibit the oral absorption of **lincomycin**. If both drugs are to be used, administer kaolin/pectin at least 2 hours before or 3-4 hours after the lincomycin dose.

Some evidence exists that kaolin/pectin may impair the oral absorption of **digoxin**. While the clinical significance of this potential interaction is unknown, it is recommended to separate the dosages as outlined above for lincomycin.

Doses -
 Dogs:
   For diarrhea:
      a) 1 - 2 ml/kg PO q4-6h (Davis 1985a)
      b) 1 - 2 ml/kg PO *qid* (Johnson 1984)
      c) 1 - 2 ml/kg PO q2-6h (Kirk 1986)

For enterotoxins secondary to garbage ingestion:
   a) 2 - 5 ml/kg PO q1-6 hours (Coppock and Mostrom 1986)
   b) 10 - 15 grams of kaolin/kg PO *qid* (Grauer and Hjelle 1988a)

Cats:
   For diarrhea:
   a) 1 - 2 ml/kg PO q4-6h (Davis 1985a)
   b) 1 - 2 ml/kg PO *qid* (Johnson 1984)
   c) 1 - 2 ml/kg PO q2-6h (Kirk 1986)

Cattle:
   a) Adult: 4 - 10 fl. oz. PO; Calves: 2 - 3 fl. oz PO; repeat every 2-4 hours or as indicated
       until condition improves. If no improvement in 48 hours additional treatment is indi-
       cated. (Label Directions, Kao-Forte®—Vet-A-Mix)

Horses:
   For diarrhea:
   a) 2 - 4 quarts PO per 450 kg body weight *bid* (Robinson 1987)
   b) 1 oz. per 8 kg body weight PO 3-4 times a day (Clark and Becht 1987)
   c) Foals: 3 - 4 oz PO q6-8h (authors believe that bismuth subsalicylate is superior)
       (Martens and Scrutchfield 1982)

Swine:
   a) 1/2 - 2 fl. oz PO; repeat every 2-4 hours or as indicated until condition improves. If no
       improvement in 48 hours additional treatment is indicated. (Label Directions, Kao-
       Forte®—Vet-A-Mix)

Sheep:
   a) 3 - 4 oz PO q2-3h (McConnell and Hughey 1987)

Birds:
   a) Canary or parakeet: 1 drop PO *bid* or 1 & 1/2 dropperful in 2/3 oz. drinking water.
       Medium-sized birds: 0.5 ml PO
       Large birds: 1 ml PO 1 to 4 times a day (Stunkard 1984)
   b) 2 ml/kg PO *bid-qid* (Clubb 1986)

Monitoring Parameters -
   1) Clinical efficacy
   2) Fluid & electrolyte status in severe diarrhea

Client Information - Shake well before using. If diarrhea persists, contact veterinarian. If animal
appears listless or develops a high fever, contact veterinarian.

Dosage Forms/Preparations/FDA Approval Status/Withholding Times - There are variety of
kaolin/pectin products available without prescription. Several products are labeled for veterinary
use; their approval status is not known. Many products that formerly contained kaolin (e.g.,
Kaopectate®) no longer contain any kaolin, but use attapulgite as the adsorbent.

KETAMINE HCL

Chemistry - A congener of phencyclidine, ketamine HCl occurs as white, crystalline powder. It
has a melting point of 258-261°C., a characteristic odor, and will precipitate as the free base at
high pH. One gram is soluble in 5 ml of water, and 14 ml of alcohol. The pH of the commercially
available injections are between 3.5-5.5.

Storage/Stability/Compatibility - Ketamine may be mixed with sterile water for injection,
D_5W, and normal saline for diluent purposes. Ketamine is compatible with xylazine in the same
syringe. Do not mix ketamine with barbiturates or diazepam in the same syringe or IV bag as
precipitation may occur.

Pharmacology - Ketamine is a rapid acting general anesthetic that also has significant analgesic
activity and a lack of cardiopulmonary depressant effects. It is thought to induce both anesthesia
and amnesia by functionally disrupting the CNS through over stimulating the CNS or inducing a
cataleptic state. Ketamine inhibits GABA, and also may block serotonin, norepinephrine, and
dopamine in the CNS. The thalamoneocortical system is depressed while the limbic system is
activated. It induces anesthetic stages I & II, but not stage III. In cats, it causes a slight hypothermic effect as body temperatures decrease on average by 1.6°C after therapeutic doses.
   Effects on muscle tone are described as being variable, but ketamine generally either causes no
changes in muscle tone or increased tone. Ketamine does not abrogate the pinnal and pedal reflexes, nor the photic, corneal, laryngeal or pharyngeal reflexes.
   Ketamine's effects on the cardiovascular system include increased cardiac output, heart rate,
mean aortic pressure, pulmonary artery pressure, and central venous pressure. Its effects on total
peripheral resistance are described as being variable. Cardiovascular effects are secondary to in-

creased sympathetic tone; ketamine has negative inotropic effects if the sympathetic system is blocked,

Ketamine does not cause significant respiratory depression at usual doses, but at higher doses it can cause respiratory rates to decrease. In humans with asthma, ketamine causes decreased airway resistance.

Uses/Indications - Ketamine has been approved for use in humans, sub-human primates and cats, although it has been used in many other species (see dosage section). The approved indications for cats include, "for restraint, or as the sole anesthetic agent for diagnostic, or minor, brief, surgical procedures that do not require skeletal muscle relaxation.... and in subhuman primates for restraint." (Package Insert; *Ketaset*® - Bristol).

Pharmacokinetics - After IM injection in the cat, peak levels occur in approximately 10 minutes. Ketamine is distributed into all body tissues rapidly, with highest levels found in the brain, liver, lung, and fat. Plasma protein binding is approximately 50% in the horse, 53% in the dogs, and 37-53% in the cat.

The drug is metabolized in the liver principally by demethylation and hydroxylation and these metabolites along with unchanged ketamine are eliminated in the urine. Ketamine will induce hepatic microsomal enzymes, but there appears to be little clinical significance associated with this effect. The elimination half-life in the cat, calf, and horse is approximately 1 hour, in humans it is 2-3 hours. Like the thiobarbiturates, the redistribution of ketamine out of the CNS is more of a factor in determining duration of anesthesia than is the elimination half-life.

By increasing the dose, the duration of anesthesia will increase, but not the intensity.

Contraindications/Precautions - Ketamine is contraindicated in patients who have exhibited prior hypersensitivity reactions to it and in animals to be used for human consumption. Its use in patients with significant hypertension, heart failure, and arterial aneurysms could be hazardous. The manufacturer warns against its use in hepatic or renal insufficiency, but in humans with renal insufficiency the duration of action has been demonstrated not to be prolonged. Because ketamine does not give good muscle relaxation, it is contraindicated when used alone for major surgery.

Ketamine can cause increases in CSF pressure and it should not be used in cases with elevated pressures or when head trauma has occurred. Because of its supposed epileptogenic potential, it should generally not be used (unless very cautiously) in animals with preexisting seizure disorders. As myelography can induce seizures, ketamine should be used cautiously in animals undergoing this procedure.

Ketamine is considered to be relatively contraindicated when increased intra-ocular pressure or open globe injuries exist, and for procedures involving the pharynx, larynx, or trachea. Animals who have lost significant amounts of blood, may require significantly reduced ketamine dosages.

While ketamine has been used safely in humans with malignant hyperthermia, its use in animals susceptible to this is controversial. Hyperthyroid human patients (and those receiving exogenous thyroid replacement) may be susceptible to developing severe hypertension and tachycardia when given ketamine. The veterinary significance of this potential problem is unknown.

Cat's eyes remain open after receiving ketamine, and should be protected from injury plus an ophthalmic lubricant (*e.g., Lacrilube*®) should be applied to prevent excessive drying of the cornea.

To minimize the incidences of emergence reactions, it is recommended to minimize exposure to handling or loud noises during the recovery period. The monitoring of vital signs should still be performed during the recovery phase, however.

Because ketamine can increase blood pressure, careful control of hemorrhaging post-surgery (*e.g.,* declawing) should be accomplished. It is not essential to withhold food or water prior to surgery, but in elective procedures it is recommended to withhold food for 6 hours prior to surgery.

Adverse Effects/Warnings - In approved species the following adverse reactions are listed by the manufacturer: "respiratory depression....following high doses, emesis, vocalization, erratic and prolonged recovery, dyspnea, spastic jerking movements, convulsions, muscular tremors, hypertonicity, opisthotonos and cardiac arrest. In the cat, myoclonic jerking and/or tonic/clonic convulsions can be controlled by ultrashort-acting barbiturates or acepromazine. These latter drugs must be given intravenously, cautiously, and slowly, to effect (approximately 1/6 to 1/4 the normal dose may be required)." (Package Insert; *Ketaset*® - Bristol)

Seizures have been reported to occur in up to 20% of cats that receive ketamine at therapeutic dosages. Diazepam is suggested to be been used for treatment if necessary.

Pain after IM injection may occur.

To reduce the incidence of hypersalivation and other autonomic signs, atropine or glycopyrrolate is often administered.

Overdosage - Ketamine is considered to have a wide therapeutic index (approximately 5 times greater when compared to pentobarbital). When given in excessive doses or too rapidly, significant respiratory depression may occur. Treatment using mechanically assisted respiratory support is recommended versus the use of analeptic agents. In cats, yohimbine with 4-aminopyridine has been suggested to be used as a partial antagonist.

Drug Interactions - **Narcotics**, **barbiturates**, or **diazepam** may prolong the recovery time after ketamine anesthesia. When used with **halothane**, ketamine recovery rates may be prolonged and the cardiac stimulatory effects of ketamine may be inhibited. Close monitoring of cardiac status is recommended when using ketamine with halothane. **Chloramphenicol** (parenteral) may prolong the anesthetic actions of ketamine.

Thyroid hormones when given concomitantly with ketamine have induced hypertension and tachycardia in humans. Beta-blockers (*e.g.*, propranolol) may be of benefit in treating these effects.

Neuromuscular blockers (*e.g.*, succinylcholine and tubocurarine) may cause enhanced or prolonged respiratory depression.

Doses -

Dogs: Note: Ketamine/xylazine has induced cardiac arrhythmias, pulmonary edema, and respiratory depression in dogs. This combination should be used with caution.
   a) Diazepam 0.5 mg/kg IV, then ketamine 10 mg/kg IV to induce general anesthesia (Booth 1988a)
   b) Midazolam 0.066 - 0.22 mg/kg IM or IV, then ketamine 6.6 - 11 mg/kg IM (Mandsager 1988)
   c) Xylazine 2.2 mg/kg IM, in 10 minutes give ketamine 11 mg/kg IM. Dogs weighing more than 22.7 kg (50 lbs.) reduce dose of both drugs by approx. 25%. (Booth 1988a)
   d) Atropine (0.044 mg/kg) IM, in 15 minutes give xylazine (1.1 mg/kg) IM, 5 minutes later give ketamine (22 mg/kg) IM (Booth 1988a)

Cats:
   Most clinicians recommend giving atropine or glycopyrrolate before use to decrease hypersalivation.
   a) 11 mg/kg IM for restraint; 22 - 33 mg/kg for diagnostic or minor surgical procedures not requiring skeletal muscle relaxation. (Package Insert; *Ketaset®* - Bristol)
   b) 2 - 4 mg/kg IV or 11 - 33 mg/kg IM (Davis 1985b)
   c) Restraint: 0.1 ml (10 mg) IV.
      Anesthesia: 22 - 33 mg/kg IM or 2.2 - 4.4 mg/kg IV (with atropine) (Morgan 1988)
   d) Sedation, restraint: 6.6 - 11 mg/kg IM
      Anesthetic: 17.6 - 26.4 mg/kg IM
      Induction (following sedation): 4.4 - 11 mg/kg IV (Mandsager 1988)
   e) Restraint: 11 mg/kg IM
      Anesthesia: 22 - 33 mg/kg IM; 2.2 - 4.4 mg/kg IV (Kirk 1986)

Rabbits/Rodents/Pocket Pets:
   a) Rabbits: 35 mg/kg SubQ or IM once (in combination with xylazine, useful for minimally invasive procedures lasting less than 30-45 minutes)
      Rats/Mice: 87 mg/kg IP once (in combo with xylazine)
      Guinea pig: 60 mg/kg IP once (in combo with xylazine)
      Hamsters: 200 mg/kg IP once (in combo with xylazine) (Huerkamp 1995)

Cattle:
   a) Premedicate with atropine and xylazine, then ketamine 2.0 mg/kg IV bolus (Thurmon and Benson 1986)
   b) After sedation, 2.2 mg/kg IV (Mandsager 1988)

Horses: Note: Always used after heavy premedication with a sedative.
   a) Initially give xylazine 1.1 mg/kg IV and wait for full sedative effect (4-8 minutes); then give ketamine 2.2 - 2.75 mg/kg IV only (the higher dose may be necessary for ponies, young "high-strung" Arabians, Hackneys, and Thoroughbreds) as a bolus. Do not administer to an "excited" horse. If surgery time requires additional anesthesia, 1/3-1/2 of the original xylazine/ketamine doses may be given IV. For procedures where better muscle relaxation is required, use guaifenesin-thiobarbiturate. Do not disturb horse until fully recovered. (Thurmon and Benson 1987)
   b) For foals and ponies: Add 500 mg ketamine and 250 mg xylazine to 500 ml of 5% guaifenesin solution. For induction, give 1.1 ml/kg IV rapidly. Anesthesia may be maintained by constant IV infusion of 2-3 ml/kg/hr. Lower doses for foals, higher doses for ponies. (Thurmon and Benson 1987)
   c) For induction of surgical colic patients: Use guaifenesin to effect, than 1.6 - 2.2 mg/kg ketamine (Mandsager 1988)

    d) 200 mg bolus (in a 454 kg horse) intra-operatively to reduce movement with light general anesthesia (Mandsager 1988)

Swine:
    a) Give atropine, then ketamine at 11 mg/kg IM. To prolong anesthesia and increase analgesia give additional ketamine 2 - 4 mg/kg IV. Local anesthetics injected at the surgical site (*e.g.,* 2% lidocaine) may enhance analgesia. (Thurmon and Benson 1986)
    b) Ketamine (22 mg/kg) combined with acepromazine (1.1 mg/kg) IM (Swindle 1985)
    c) 4.4 mg/kg IM or IV after sedation (Mandsager 1988)

Sheep:
    a) Premedicate with atropine (0.22 mg/kg) and acepromazine (0.55 mg/kg; then ketamine 22 mg/kg IM. To extend anesthetic time, may give ketamine intermittently IV at 2 - 4 mg/kg. (Thurmon and Benson 1986)
    b) 2 mg/kg IV for induction, then 4 ml/minute constant infusion of ketamine in a concentration of 2 mg/ml in D5W. (Thurmon and Benson 1986)

Goats:
    a) Give atropine 0.4 mg/kg, followed by xylazine 0.22 mg/kg IM 20-25 minutes later. Approximately 10 minutes after xylazine give ketamine 11 mg/kg IM. To extend anesthesia give ketamine 2 - 4 mg/kg IV (shorter extension) or 6 mg/kg (longer extension). (Thurmon and Benson 1986)

Reptiles:
    a) 20 - 60 mg/kg IM (McConnell and Hughey 1987)

Sub-Human Primates:
    a) Doses vary with regard to individual species; refer to package insert for *Ketaset®*.

Birds:
    a) Birds weighing:
        < 100 grams (canaries, finches, budgies): 0.1 - 0.2 mg/gm IM
        250 - 500 grams (parrots, pigeons): 0.05 - 0.1 mg/gm IM
        500 gms - 3 kg (chickens, owls, hawks): 0.02 - 0.1 mg/gm IM
        > 3 kg (ducks, geese, swans): 0.02 - 0.05 mg/gm IM (Booth 1988a)
    b) In combination with xyalzine: Ketamine 10 - 30 mg/kg IM; Xyalzine 2 - 6 mg/kg IM; birds less than 250 g require a higher dosae than birds weighing greater than 250 g. Xylazine is not recommended to be used in debilitated birds because of its cardiodepressant effects.
        In combination with diazepam: Ketamine 10 - 50 mg/kg IM; Diazepam 0.5 - 2 mg/kg IM or IV; doses can be halved for IV use.
        In combination with acepromazine: Ketamine 25 - 50 mg/kg IM; Acepromazine 0.5 - 1 mg/kg IM. (Wheler 1993)

Exotics:
    An excellent list of dosages can be found on page 264 of Veterinary Pharmacology and Therapeutics, 6th Ed., Booth, NH & McDonald, LE, Eds.; 1988; Iowa State University Press; Ames, Iowa.

Monitoring Parameters -
    1) Level of anesthesia/analgesia
    2) Respiratory function; cardiovascular status (rate, rhythm, BP if possible)
    3) Monitor eyes to prevent drying or injury
    4) Body temperature

Client Information - Should only be administered by individuals familiar with its use.

Dosage Forms/Preparations/FDA Approval Status/Withholding Times -
Veterinary-Approved Products:
    Ketamine HCl for Injection 100 mg/ml in 10 ml vials; *Ketaset®* (Fort Dodge); *Vetalar®* (Fort Dodge); *VetaKet®* (Lloyd) (Rx) Approved for use in cats and sub-human primates.

Human-Approved Products:
    Ketamine HCl for Injection 10 mg/ml in 20, 25, and 50 ml vials; 50 mg/ml in 10 ml vials; 100 mg/ml in 5 ml vials; *Ketalar®* (Parke-Davis); (Rx)

KETOCONAZOLE

Chemistry - An imidazole antifungal agent, ketoconazole occurs as a white to slightly beige powder with pK_as of 2.9 and 6.5. It is practically insoluble in water.

Storage/Stability/Compatibility - Ketoconazole tablets should be stored at room temperature in well-closed containers.

Pharmacology - At usual doses and serum concentrations, ketoconazole is fungistatic against susceptible fungi. At higher concentrations for prolonged periods of time or against very susceptible organisms, ketoconazole may be fungicidal. It is believed that ketoconazole increases cellular membrane permeability and causes secondary metabolic effects and growth inhibition. The exact mechanism for these effects have not been determined, but may be due to ketoconazole interfering with ergosterol synthesis. The fungicidal action of ketoconazole may be due to a direct effect on cell membranes.

Ketoconazole has activity against most pathogenic fungi, including Blastomyces, Coccidiodes, Cryptococcus, Histoplasma, Microsporum and Trichophyton. Higher levels are necessary to treat most strains of Aspergillus and Sporothrix. Resistance to ketoconazole has been documented for some strains of *Candida albicans.*

Ketoconazole also has *in vitro* activity against *Staphylococcus aureas* and *epidermidis*, Nocardia, enterococci, and herpes simplex virus types 1 & 2. The clinical implications of this activity are unknown.

Ketoconazole also has endocrine effects as steroid synthesis is directly inhibited by blocking several P-450 enzyme systems. Measurable reductions in testosterone or cortisol synthesis can occur at dosages used for antifungal therapy, but higher dosages are generally required to reduce levels of testosterone or cortisol to be clinically useful in the treatment of prostatic carcinoma or hyperadrenocorticism. Effects on mineralocorticoids are negligible.

Uses/Indications - Because of its comparative lack of toxicity when compared to amphotericin B, oral administration and relatively good efficacy, ketoconazole is used to treat several fungal infections in dogs, cats and other small species. See the Dosage section or Pharmacology section for specifics. Although newer antifungal agents (fluconazole, itraconazole) have advantages over ketoconazole–usually less toxicity and/or enhanced efficacy–ketoconazole is significantly less expensive.

Ketoconazole is also used clinically for the medical treatment of hyperadrenocorticism in dogs (and sometimes cats).

Pharmacokinetics - Although it is reported that ketoconazole is well absorbed after oral administration, oral bioavailability of ketoconazole tablets in dogs is highly variable. One study (Baxter et al. 1986) in six normal dogs, found bioavailabilities ranging from 0.04-0.89 (4-89%) after 400 mg (19.5 - 25.2 mg/kg) were administered to fasted dogs. Peak serum concentrations occur between 1 and 4.25 hours after dosing and peak serum levels in the 6 dogs studied ranged from 1.1 - 45.6 micrograms/ml. This wide interpatient variation may have significant clinical implications from both a toxicity and efficacy standpoint, particularly since ketoconazole is often used in life-threatening infections and assays for measuring serum levels are not readily available.

Ketoconazole absorption is enhanced in an acidic environment and should not be administered (at the same time) with H_2 blockers or antacids (see Drug Interactions below). Whether to administer ketoconazole with meals or during a fasted state to maximize absorption is controversial. The manufacturer recommends giving with food in human patients. Dogs or cats who develop anorexia/vomiting during therapy may benefit from administration with meals.

After absorption, ketoconazole is distributed into the bile, cerumen, saliva, urine, synovial fluid and CSF. CSF levels are generally less than 10% of those found in the serum, but may be increased if the meninges are inflamed. High levels of the drug are found in the liver, adrenals and pituitary gland, while more moderate levels are found in the kidneys, lungs, bladder, bone marrow and myocardium. At usual doses (10 mg/kg), attained levels are probably inadequate in the brain, testis and eyes to treat most infections; higher dosages are required. Ketoconazole is 84-99% bound to plasma proteins and crosses the placenta (at least in rats). The drug is found in bitch's milk.

Ketoconazole is metabolized extensively by the liver into several inactive metabolites. These metabolites are excreted primarily into the feces via the bile. About 13% of a given dose is excreted into the urine and only 2-4% of the drug is excreted unchanged in the urine. Half-life in dogs is about 1-6 hours (avg. 2.7 hours).

Contraindications/Precautions/Reproductive Safety - Ketoconazole is contraindicated in patients with know hypersensitivity to it. It should be used with caution in patients with hepatic disease or thrombocytopenia.

Ketoconazole is a known teratogen and embryotoxin in rats. There have been reports of mummified fetuses and stillbirths in dogs who have been treated. Ketoconazole should not be considered absolutely contraindicated in pregnant animals, however, as it is often used in potentially life-threatening infections. The benefits of therapy should be weighed against the potential risks.

Ketoconazole may cause infertility in male dogs by decreasing testosterone synthesis. Testosterone production rebounds once the drug is discontinued.

Adverse Effects/Warnings - Gastrointestinal symptoms of anorexia, vomiting, and/or diarrhea are the most common adverse effects seen with ketoconazole therapy. Anorexia may be minimized by dividing the dose and/or giving with meals. Hepatic toxicity consisting of cholangiohepatitis and increased liver enzymes has been reported with ketoconazole, and may be either idiosyncratic in nature or a dose-related phenomenon. Cats may be more prone to developing hepatoxicity than dogs. Thrombocytopenia has also been reported with ketoconazole therapy, but is rarely encountered. A reversible lightening of haircoat may also occur in patients treated with ketoconazole.

Ketoconazole has a transient dose-related suppressant effect on gonadal and adrenal steroid synthesis. Doses as low as 10 mg/kg depressed serum testosterone levels in dogs within 3-4 hours after dosing, but levels returned to normal within 10 hours. Doses of 30 mg/kg/day have been demonstrated to suppress serum cortisol levels in dogs with hyperadrenocorticism (see Dosages section). Dogs undergoing high dose antifungal therapy may need additional glucocorticoid support during periods of acute stress.

Overdosage/Acute Toxicity - No reports of acute toxicity associated with overdosage were located. The oral LD$_{50}$ in dogs after oral administration is >500 mg/kg. Should an acute overdose occur, the manufacturer recommends employing supportive measures, including gastric lavage with sodium bicarbonate.

Drug Interactions - Antacids, anticholinergics (propantheline, etc.) H$_2$ blockers (*e.g.,* **cimetidine, ranitidine**) increase stomach pH and may inhibit the absorption of ketoconazole. If these agents must be used with ketoconazole, they should be given 2 hours after the ketoconazole dose.

Mitotane and ketoconazole are not recommended to be used together to treat hyperadrenocorticism as the adrenolytic effects of mitotane may be inhibited by ketoconazole's inhibition of cytochrome P450 enzymes.

Ketoconazole may increase the anticoagulant effects of **warfarin**. Prothrombin times should be monitored and dosage adjustments made as required.

Phenytoin and ketoconazole may alter the metabolism of each other. Phenytoin levels and ketoconazole efficacy/toxicity should be monitored. Ketoconazole alters the disposition and extends the duration of activity of **methylprednisolone.**

Elevated concentrations of **cisapride** with resultant ventricular arrhythmias may result if coadministered with ketoconazole, itraconazole, IV miconazole or troleandomycin. At present, the manufacturer states that cisapride should not be used with these drugs.

Ketoconazole may decrease serum **theophylline** concentrations in some patients; theophylline levels should be monitored.

Ethanol may interact with ketoconazole and produce a disulfiram-like reaction (vomiting).

Rifampin may decrease the serum levels of ketoconazole if administered together. If these drugs must be used together, ketoconazole dosages may need to be adjusted.

Ketoconazole may exhibit synergism with **acyclovir** against herpes simplex viruses.

Cyclosporin blood levels may be increased by ketoconazole.

Because ketoconazole can cause hepatoxicity, it should be used cautiously with **other hepatotoxic agents**.

Doses - (Note: Clinical antifungal effects may require 10-14 days of therapy)
Dogs:
For coccidioidomycosis:
a) For the systemic form of the disease: 5 - 10 mg/kg PO *bid*; For the CNS form: 15 - 20 mg/kg PO *bid*. Treatment should persist for a minimum of 3-6 months. Animals with boney lesions or relapses after discontinuing therapy, give lifelong therapy at 5 mg/kg PO every other day. (Macy 1988)

For blastomycosis:
a) 10 mg/kg PO *bid* (15 - 20 mg/kg PO *bid* if CNS involvement) for at least 3 months with amphotericin B: initially at 0.25 - 0.5 mg/kg every other day IV. If tolerated, increase dose to 1 mg/kg until 4-5 mg/kg total dose is administered. See amphotericin B monograph for more information. (Macy 1988)
b) Ketoconazole 20 mg/kg/day PO once daily or divided *bid*; 40 mg/kg divided *bid* for ocular or CNS involvement (for at least 2-3 months or until remission then start maintenance) with amphotericin B 0.15 - 0.5 mg/kg IV 3 times a week. When a total dose of amphotericin B reaches 4 - 6 mg/kg start maintenance dosage of amphotericin B at 0.15 - 0.25 mg/kg IV once a month or use ketoconazole at 10 mg/kg PO either once daily, divided *bid* or ketoconazole at 2.5 - 5 mg/kg PO once daily. If CNS/ocular involvement, use ketoconazole at 20 - 40 mg/kg PO divided *bid*. (Greene, O'Neal, and Barsanti 1984)

For histoplasmosis:
a) 10 mg/kg PO once a day or twice a day for at least 3 months. Treat at least 30 days after complete resolution of clinical disease. If patient relapses, retreat as above then put on maintenance 5 mg/kg PO every other day indefinitely. For acute cases: use

with amphotericin B (see blastomycosis recommendation by same author above). (Macy 1988)

   b) Ketoconazole 10 - 20 mg/day PO once daily or divided *bid* (for at least 2-3 months or until remission then start maintenance) with amphotericin B at 0.15 - 0.5 mg/kg IV 3 times a week. When a total dose of amphotericin B reaches 2 - 4 mg/kg start maintenance dosage of amphotericin B at 0.15 - 0.25 mg/kg IV once a month or use ketoconazole at 10 mg/kg PO either once daily, divided *bid* or at 2.5 - 5 mg/kg PO once daily. (Greene, O'Neal, and Barsanti 1984)

For aspergillosis:
   a) 20 mg/kg PO for at least 6 weeks; may require long-term/maintenance therapy. (Macy 1988)

For cryptococcosis:
   a) Amphotericin B 0.15 - 0.4 mg/kg IV 3 times a week with flucytosine 150 - 175 mg/kg PO divided *tid-qid*. When a total dose of amphotericin B reaches 4 - 6 mg/kg start maintenance dosage of amphotericin B at 0.15 - 0.25 mg/kg IV once a month with flucytosine at dosage above or with **ketoconazole** at 10 mg/kg PO once daily or divided *bid*. (Greene, O'Neal, and Barsanti 1984)

For fungal myocarditis:
   a) 10 mg/kg PO *tid* (Ogburn 1988)

For Candidal stomatitis (systemic therapy):
   a) 10 mg/kg PO q8h until lesions resolve. (McKeever 1986)

For *Malassezia* dermatitis:
   a) 5 - 10 mg/kg PO twice a day for 30 days. Often used with therapeutic shampoos containing selenium disulfide, miconazole, ketoconazole or chlorhexidine. Underlying conditions must be identified and remedied or condition will recur. (Noxon 1997)

For treatment of hyperadrenocorticism:
   a) 30 mg/kg PO once daily or divided *bid*. (Feldman 1989)
   b) Initially, 10 mg/kg q12h for 7-10 days; monitor water consumption, appetite, and activity. Discontinue drug for 24-48 hours if adverse reactions occur. Reevaluate ACTH stimulation test at end of 7-10 days. If response is inadequate, increase dose to 15 mg/kg q12h and repeat ACTH in 7-10 days. Once controlled, continue dosage long-term. (Bruyette and Feldman 1988)

Cats:
For coccidioidomycosis:
   a) For the systemic form of the disease: 5 - 10 mg/kg PO *bid*; For the CNS form: 15 - 20 mg/kg PO *bid*. Treatment should persist for a minimum of 3-6 months. Animals with boney lesions or relapses after discontinuing therapy, give lifelong therapy at 5 mg/kg PO every other day. (Macy 1988)
   b) Very rare in the cat. Ketoconazole at 10 mg/kg PO once or twice a day (adjusted as necessary). Long term therapy (>6 months) likely to be necessary. (Legendre 1989)

For blastomycosis:
   a) 10 mg/kg PO *bid* (15 - 20 mg/kg PO *bid* if CNS involvement) for at least 3 months with amphotericin B: initially at 0.25 - 0.5 mg/kg every other day IV. If tolerated, increase dose to 1 mg/kg until 4-5 mg/kg total dose is administered. See amphotericin B monograph for more information. (Macy 1988)
   b) 10 mg/kg q12h PO (for at least 60 days) with amphotericin B: 0.25 mg/kg in 30 ml D5W IV over 15 minutes q48h. Continue amphotericin B therapy until a cumulative dose of 4 mg/kg is given or until BUN > 50 mg/dl. If renal toxicity does not develop, may increase dose to 0.5 mg/kg of amphotericin B. (Legendre 1989)
   c) Ketoconazole 10 mg/day PO once daily or divided *bid* (for at least 2-3 months or until remission, then start maintenance) with amphotericin B 0.15 - 0.5 mg/kg IV 3 times a week. When a total dose of amphotericin B reaches 4 - 6 mg/kg start maintenance dosage of amphotericin B at 0.15 - 0.25 mg/kg IV once a month or use ketoconazole at 10 mg/kg PO either once daily, divided *bid* or ketoconazole at 2.5 - 5 mg/kg PO once daily. If CNS/ocular involvement, use ketoconazole at 20 - 40 mg/kg PO divided *bid*. (Greene, O'Neal, and Barsanti 1984)

For histoplasmosis:
   a) 10 mg/kg PO once a day or twice a day for at least 3 months. Treat at least 30 days after complete resolution of clinical disease. If patient relapses, retreat as above then put on maintenance 5 mg/kg PO every other day indefinitely. For acute cases: use with amphotericin B (see blastomycosis recommendation by same author). (Macy 1988)

b) 10 mg/kg PO q12h with amphotericin B at 0.25 mg/kg in 30 ml D_5W IV over 15 minutes q48h. Continue Amphotericin B therapy for 4-8 weeks or until BUN > 50 mg/dl. If BUN increases greater than 50 mg/dl, continue ketoconazole alone. Ketoconazole is used long-term (at least 6 months of duration). Despite aggressive therapy prognosis is poor. (Legendre 1989)

c) Ketoconazole 10 mg/day PO once daily or divided *bid* (for at least 2-3 months or until remission then start maintenance) with amphotericin B 0.15 - 0.5 mg/kg IV 3 times a week. When a total dose of amphotericin B reaches 2 - 4 mg/kg start maintenance dosage of amphotericin B at 0.15 - 0.25 mg/kg IV once a month or use ketoconazole at 10 mg/kg PO either once daily, divided *bid* or at 2.5 - 5 mg/kg PO once daily. (Greene, O'Neal, and Barsanti 1984)

For cryptococcosis:
a) 10 mg/kg PO once a day or twice a day for 3 months or for at least 30 days after clinical disease has resolved. (Macy 1988)

b) 10 mg/kg *bid*. Very useful for this condition in cats, but at this dosage can produce anorexia and debility. (Legendre 1995)

c) Amphotericin B 0.15 - 0.4 mg/kg IV 3 times a week with flucytosine 125 - 250 mg/day PO divided *tid-qid*. When a total dose of amphotericin B reaches 4 - 6 mg/kg start maintenance dosage of amphotericin B at 0.15 - 0.25 mg/kg IV once a month with flucytosine at dosage above or with ketoconazole at 10 mg/kg PO once daily or divided *bid*. (Greene, O'Neal, and Barsanti 1984)

For aspergillosis:
a) 20 mg/kg PO for at least 6 weeks; may require long-term/maintenance therapy. (Macy 1988)

b) 10 mg/kg PO q12h. (Legendre 1989)

For treatment of hyperadrenocorticism:
a) 10 mg/kg PO *bid*. Only 2 patients treated. One died 7 days later of thrombocytopenia; other patient had an excellent response for 6 months. (Feldman 1989)

Horses:
For susceptible fungal infections:
a) 10 mg/kg PO daily (McConnell and Hughey 1987)

Birds:
For susceptible fungal infections:
a) For severe refractory candidiasis in Psittacines: 5 - 10 mg/kg as a gavage *bid* for 14 days. For local effect in crop dissolve 1/4 tablet (50 mg) in 0.2 ml of 1 N hydrochloric acid and add 0.8 ml of water. Solution turns pale pink when dissolved. Add mixture to food for gavage.
To add to water for most species: 200 mg/L for 7-14 days. As drug is not water soluble at neutral pH, dissolve in acid prior to adding to water (see above).
To add to feed for most species: 10 - 20 mg/kg for 7-14 days. Add to favorite food or add to mash. (Clubb 1986)

b) For Candida infections of the oropharyngeal area: 10 - 15 mg/kg PO *bid* for 10-14 days. (Flammer 1986)

Reptiles:
For susceptible infections:
a) For most species:15 - 30 mg/kg PO once daily for 2-4 weeks. (Gauvin 1993)

For fungal shell diseases in turtles/tortoises:
a) 25 mg/kg PO once a day for 2-4 weeks (Rosskopf 1986)

Monitoring Parameters -
1) Liver enzymes with chronic therapy (at least every 2 months; some clinicians say monthly)
2) CBC with platelets
3) Efficacy and other adverse effects

Client Information - If animal develops gastrointestinal symptoms divide dose and administer with meals. Long-term therapy with adequate dosing compliance is usually necessary for successful results; clients must be committed for both the financial and dosing burdens associated with therapy.

Dosage Forms/Preparations/FDA Approval Status/Withholding Times -
Veterinary-Approved Products: None

Human-Approved Products:
Ketoconazole 200 mg Tablets (scored); *Nizoral*® (Janssen); (Rx)

KETOPROFEN

Chemistry - A propionic acid derivative nonsteroidal anti-inflammatory agent, ketoprofen occurs as an off white to white, fine to granular powder. It is practically insoluble in water, but freely soluble in alcohol at 20°C. Ketoprofen has a pK_a of 5.9 in a 3:1 methanol:water solution.

Storage/Stability/Compatibility - Ketoprofen oral capsules should be stored at room temperature in tight, light resistant containers. The veterinary injection should be stored at room temperature. Compatibility studies with injectable ketoprofen and other compounds have apparently not been published.

Pharmacology - Ketoprofen exhibits actions similar to that of other nonsteroidal antiinflammatory agents in that it possesses antipyretic, analgesic and antiinflammatory activity. Its purported mechanism of action is the inhibition of cyclooxygenase catalysis of arachidonic acid to prostaglandin precursors (endoperoxides), thereby inhibiting the synthesis of prostaglandins in tissues. Ketoprofen purportedly has inhibitory activity on lipoxygenase, whereas flunixin reportedly does not at therapeutic doses.

Uses/Indications - Ketoprofen is labeled for use in horses for the alleviation of inflammation and pain associated with musculoskeletal disorders. Like flunixin (and other NSAIDs), ketoprofen potentially has many other uses in a variety of species and conditions; however well controlled studies for these uses are generally unavailable.

Pharmacokinetics - In species studied (rats, dog, man), ketoprofen is rapidly and nearly completely absorbed after oral administration. The presence of food or milk decreases oral absorption. Oral absorption characteristics in horses was not located. It has been reported that when comparing IV vs. IM injections in horses, the areas under the curve are relatively equivalent.

While distribution characteristics are not well described, the drug does enter synovial fluid and is highly bound to plasma proteins (99% in humans, and approximately 93% in horses). In horses, the manufacturer reports that the onset of activity is within 2 hours and peak effects 12 hours post dose.

Ketoprofen is eliminated via the kidneys both as a conjugated metabolite and unchanged drug. The elimination half life in horses is approximately 1.5 hours.

Contraindications/Precautions/Reproductive Safety - While the manufacturer states that there are no contraindications to the drug's use (other than previous hypersensitivity to ketoprofen), it should be used only when the potential benefits outweigh the risks in cases where GI ulceration or bleeding is evident or in patients with significant renal or hepatic impairment. Ketoprofen may mask the signs and symptoms (inflammation, hyperpyrexia) of infection. Because ketoprofen is highly protein bound, patients with hypoproteinemia may have increased levels of free drug, thereby increasing the risks for toxicity.

The manufacturer cautions against ketoprofen's use in breeding animals, because effects on fertility, pregnancy or fetal health have not been established in horses. However, rat and mice studies have not demonstrated increased teratogenicity or embryotoxicity. Rabbits receiving twice the human dose exhibited increased embryotoxicity, but not teratogenicity. Because nonsteroidal antiinflammatory agents inhibit prostaglandin synthesis, adversely affecting neonatal cardiovascular systems (premature closure of patent ductus), ketoprofen should not be used late in pregnancy. Studies in male rats demonstrated no changes in fertility.

It is presently unknown whether ketoprofen enters equine milk. Ketoprofen does enter canine milk.

Adverse Effects/Warnings - Because ketoprofen is a relatively new agent, its adverse effect profile in horses has not been clearly elucidated. Preliminary studies and reports indicate that ketoprofen appears relatively safe to use in horses and may have a lower incidence of adverse effects than either phenylbutazone or flunixin. Potentially, gastric mucosal damage and GI ulceration, renal crest necrosis, and mild hepatitis may occur.

Do not administer intra-arterially and avoid SubQ injections. While not labeled for IM use in horses, it reportedly is effective and may only cause occasional inflammation at the injection site.

Overdosage/Acute Toxicity - Horses given ketoprofen at doses up to 11 mg/kg administered IV once daily for 15 days exhibited no signs of toxicity. Severe laminitis was observed in a horse given 33 mg/kg/day (15X over labeled dosage) for 5 days. Anorexia, depression, icterus, and abdominal swelling was noted in horses given 55 mg/kg/day (25X labeled dose) for 5 days. Upon necropsy, gastritis, nephritis and hepatitis were diagnosed in this group.

Humans have survived oral ingestions of up to 5 grams. The LD_{50} in dogs after oral ingestion has been reported to be 2000 mg/kg. General drug removal and supportive measures have been recommended in cases of oral overdosage.

Drug Interactions - Because ketoprofen is highly bound to plasma proteins, it can displace or be displaced by other highly protein bound drugs, including **warfarin, phenylbutazone, etc.**

Because ketoprofen may inhibit platelet aggregation and also cause gastrointestinal ulceration, when used with other drugs that alter hemostasis (*e.g.*, **heparin, warfarin, etc**.) and/or cause gastrointestinal erosion (*e.g.*, **aspirin, flunixin, phenylbutazone, corticosteroids, etc**.), increased likelihood of bleeding or ulceration may occur.

Ketoprofen and **probenecid** are not recommended to be used together. Probenecid reduces renal clearance of ketoprofen and also reduces its protein binding; thereby increasing the risk of toxicity.

NSAIDs (including ketoprofen) may potentially significantly reduce the excretion of **methotrexate** and cause toxicity.

Laboratory Considerations - Ketoprofen may cause falsely elevated **blood glucose values** when using the glucose oxidase and peroxidase method using ABTS as a chromogen; falsely elevated **serum bilirubin** values when using DMSO as a reagent; falsely elevated **serum iron** concentrations using the Ramsey method, or falsely decreased **serum iron** concentrations when using bathophenanthroline disulfonate as a reagent.

Doses -
  Dogs:
      As an antiinflammatory/analgesic:
      a) For surgical pain: 2 mg/kg IV, subQ or IM initially once; 1 mg/kg subsequent daily doses
        For chronic pain: 2 mg/kg PO initially, then 1 mg/kg PO daily (Johnson 1996)

  Cats:
      As an antiinflammatory/analgesic:
      a) For surgical pain: 2 mg/kg subQ initially once; 1 mg/kg subsequent daily doses
        For chronic pain: 2 mg/kg PO initially, then 1 mg/kg PO daily (Johnson 1996)
  Horses:
      For labeled indications: 2.2 mg/kg (1 ml/100 lbs) IV once daily for up to 5 days. (Package insert - *Ketofen*®)

Monitoring Parameters - 1) Efficacy; 2) Adverse Effects (in humans, occasional liver function tests are recommended with long term therapy)

Dosage Forms/Preparations/FDA Approval Status/Withholding Times -
Veterinary-Approved Products:
    Ketoprofen Injection 100 mg/ml in 50 ml and 100 ml multi-dose vials; *Ketofen*® (Fort Dodge); (Rx) Approved for use in horses not intended for food.

Human-Approved Products:
    Ketoprofen Oral Capsules 25 mg, 50 mg, 75 mg;*Orudis*® (Wyeth-Ayerst), generic; (Rx)
    Ketoprofen 12.5 mg Tablets *Orudis KT*® (Whitehall-Robins) (OTC);*Actron Caplets*® (Bayer) (OTC)
    Ketoprofen Extended Release 100 mg, 150 mg, 200 mg Capsules *Oruvail*® (Wyeth-Ayerst) (Rx)

L-Asparaginase - see Asparaginase

L-Thyroxine - see Levothyroxine

Lactated Ringer's—see the appendix section on intravenous fluids

LACTULOSE

Chemistry - A synthetic derivative of lactose, lactulose is a disaccharide containing one molecule of galactose and one molecule of fructose. It occurs as a white powder that is very slightly soluble in alcohol and very soluble in water. The commercially available solutions are viscous, sweet liquids with an adjusted pH of 3-7.

Storage/Stability/Compatibility - Lactulose syrup should be stored in tight containers, preferably at room temperature; avoid freezing. If exposed to heat or light, darkening or cloudiness of the solution may occur, but apparently does not affect drug potency.

Pharmacology - Lactulose is a disaccharide (galactose/fructose) that is not hydrolyzable by mammalian and, probably, avian gut enzymes. Upon reaching the colon, lactulose is metabolized by the resident bacteria resulting in the formation of low molecular weight acids (lactic, formic, acetic) and CO_2. These acids have a dual effect; they increase osmotic pressure drawing water into the bowel causing a laxative effect and also acidify colonic contents. The acidification causes ammonia NH_3 (ammonia) to migrate from the blood into the colon where it is trapped as $[NH_4]^+$ (ammonium ion) and expelled with the feces.

Uses/Indications - The primary use of lactulose in veterinary medicine is to reduce ammonia blood levels in the prevention and treatment of hepatic encephalopathy (portal-systemic encephalopathy; PSE) in small animals and pet birds. It is also used as a laxative in small animals.

Pharmacokinetics - In humans, less than 3% of an oral dose of lactulose in absorbed (in the small intestine). The absorbed drug is not metabolized and is excreted unchanged in the urine within 24 hours.

Contraindications/Precautions - Lactulose syrup contains some free lactose and galactose, and may alter the insulin requirements in diabetic patients. In patients with preexisting fluid and electrolyte imbalances, lactulose may exacerbate these conditions if it causes diarrhea; use cautiously.

Adverse Effects/Warnings - Symptoms of flatulence, gastric distention, cramping, etc. are not uncommon early in therapy, but generally abate with time. Diarrhea and dehydration are symptoms of overdosage; dosage should be reduced.

Cats dislike the taste of lactulose and administration may be difficult.

Overdosage - Excessive doses may cause flatulence, diarrhea, cramping and dehydration. Replace fluids and electrolytes if necessary.

Drug Interactions - Do not use lactulose with **other laxatives** as the loose stools that are formed can be falsely attributed to the lactulose with resultant inadequate therapy for hepatic encephalopathy.

Theoretically, orally administered **antibiotics** (*e.g., **neomycin***) could eliminate the bacteria responsible for metabolizing lactulose, thereby reducing its efficacy. However some data suggests that synergy may occur when lactulose is used with an oral antibiotic (*e.g., neomycin*) for the treatment of hepatic encephalopathy. Enhanced monitoring of lactulose efficacy is probably warranted in cases where an oral antibiotic is added to the therapy.

Oral antacids (non-adsorbable) may reduce the colonic acidification effects (efficacy) of lactulose.

Doses -
Dogs:
For hepatic encephalopathy:
a) 15 - 30 ml PO *qid*; adjust the dosage to produce 2-3 soft stools per day (Cornelius and Bjorling 1988)
b) 30 - 45 mls PO q8h (Kirk 1986)
c) 5 - 15 ml PO *tid*; adjust dose to induce 2-3 soft stools per day; reduce dosage if diarrhea develops. In certain cases, neomycin with lactulose may be superior to either drug alone. (Hardy 1985)

For constipation:
a) 1 ml per 4.5 kg of body weight PO q8h initially, then adjust *prn* (Kirk 1986)

Cats:
For hepatic encephalopathy:
a) 0.25 - 1 ml PO; individualize dosage until semi-formed stools are produced. (Center, Hornbuckle, and Scavelli 1986)

For constipation:
a) 1 ml per 4.5 kg of body weight PO q8h initially, then adjust *prn* (Kirk 1986)
b) 0.5 ml/kg q8-12h PO (Sherding 1989)

Birds:
For hepatic encephalopathy; to stimulate appetite, improve intestinal flora:
a) Cockatiel: 0.03 ml PO *bid-tid*; Amazon: 0.1 ml PO *bid-tid*. Reduce dosage if diarrhea develops. May be used for weeks. (Clubb 1986)

Monitoring Parameters -
1) Clinical efficacy (2-3 soft stools per day) when used for PSE
2) In long-term use (months) or in patients with preexisting fluid/electrolyte problems, serum electrolytes should be monitored.

Client Information - Contact veterinarian if diarrhea develops. Also contact veterinarian when lactulose is used for hepatic encephalopathy if symptoms worsen or less than 2-3 soft stools are produced per day.

Dosage Forms/Preparations/FDA Approval Status/Withholding Times -
Veterinary-Approved Products: None
Human-Approved Products:
Lactulose 666 mg/ml (10 grams/15 ml); [containing (per ml): < 147 mg galactose, < 80 mg lactose, and ≤80 mg other sugars] in 237, 240, 473, 480, 946, 960, 1920 ml, gal and UD 30

ml; *Chronulac*® or *Cephulac*® (Merrill Dow), *Constilac*® or *Cholac*® (Alra), *Constulose*® or *Enulose*® (Barre), Generic; (Rx)

Note: Two separate products (trade names) are marketed by the same company; one product is marketed as a laxative and one product is marketed for hepatic encephalopathy.

LEVAMISOLE

Chemistry - The *levo*-isomer of *dl*-tetramisole, levamisole has a greater safety margin than does the racemic mixture. It is available commercially in two salts, a phosphate and a hydrochloride. Levamisole hydrochloride occurs as a white to pale cream colored, odorless or nearly odorless, crystalline powder. One gram is soluble in 2 ml of water.

Storage/Stability/Compatibility - Levamisole hydrochloride products should be stored at room temperature (15-30°C), unless otherwise instructed by the manufacturer; avoid temperatures greater than 40°C. Levamisole phosphate injection should be stored at temperatures at or below 21°C (70°F); refrigeration is recommended and freezing should be avoided.
Levamisole tablets should not be crushed nor suspensions made from them.

Pharmacology - Levamisole stimulates the parasympathetic and sympathetic ganglia in susceptible worms. At higher levels, levamisole interferes with nematode carbohydrate metabolism by blocking fumarate reduction and succinate oxidation. The net effect is a paralyzing effect on the worm which is then expelled alive. Levamisole's effects are considered to be nicotine-like in action.
Levamisole's mechanism of action for its immunostimulating effects are not well understood. It is believed it restores cell-mediated immune function in peripheral T-lymphocytes and stimulates phagocytosis by monocytes. Its immune stimulating effects appear to be more pronounced in animals that are immune-compromised.

Uses/Indications - Depending on the product licensed, levamisole is indicated for the treatment of many nematodes in cattle, sheep & goats, swine, poultry. In sheep and cattle, levamisole has relatively good activity against abomasal nematodes, small intestinal nematodes (not particularly good against *Strongyloides spp.*), large intestinal nematodes (not *Trichuris spp.*), and lungworms. Adult forms of species that are usually covered by levamisole, include: *Haemonchus spp., Trichostrongylus spp., Osteragia spp., Cooperia spp., Nematodirus spp., Bunostomum spp., Oesophagostomum spp., Chabertia spp.,* and *Dictyocaulus vivapurus.* Levamisole is less effective against the immature forms of these parasites and is generally ineffective in cattle (but not sheep) against arrested larval forms. Resistance of parasites to levamisole is a growing concern.
In swine, levamisole is indicated for the treatment of *Ascaris suum, Oesophagostomum spp., Strongyloides, Stephanurus,* and *Metastrongylus.*
Levamisole has been used in dogs as a microfilaricide to treat *Dirofilaria immitis* infection. It has also garnered much interest as an immunostimulant in the adjunctive therapy of various neoplasms.
Because of its narrow margin for safety and limited efficacy against many equine parasites, levamisole is not generally used in horses.

Pharmacokinetics - Levamisole is absorbed from the gut after oral dosing and through the skin after dermal application, although bioavailabilities are variable. It is reportedly distributed throughout the body. Levamisole is primarily metabolized with less than 6% excreted unchanged in the urine. Plasma elimination half-lives have been determined for several veterinary species: Cattle 4-6 hours; Dogs 1.8-4 hours; and Swine 3.5-6.8 hours. Metabolites are excreted in both the urine (primarily) and feces.

Contraindications/Precautions - Levamisole is contraindicated in lactating animals (not approved). It should be used cautiously, if at all, in animals that are severely debilitated, or have significant renal or hepatic impairment. Use cautiously or, preferably, delay use in cattle that are stressed due to vaccination, dehorning or castration.
There is no information regarding the safety of this drug in pregnant animals. Although levamisole is considered relatively safe to use in large animals that are pregnant, use only if the potential benefits outweigh the risks.

Adverse Effects/Warnings - Adverse effects that may seen in cattle can include muzzle-foaming or hypersalivation, excitement or trembling, lip-licking and head shaking. These effects are generally noted with higher than recommended doses or if levamisole is used concomitantly with organophosphates. Symptoms generally subside within 2 hours. When injecting into cattle, swelling may occur at the injection site. This will usually abate in 7-14 days, but may be objectionable in animals that are close to slaughter.
In sheep, levamisole may cause a transient excitability in some animals after dosing. In goats, levamisole may cause depression, hyperesthesia and salivation. Injecting levamisole SQ in goats apparently causes a stinging sensation.

In swine, levamisole may cause salivation or muzzle foaming. Swine infected with lungworms may develop coughing or vomiting.

Adverse effects that may seen in dogs include GI disturbances (usually vomiting, diarrhea), neurotoxicity (panting, shaking, agitation or other behavioral changes), agranulocytosis, dyspnea, pulmonary edema, immune-mediated skin eruptions (erythroedema, erythema multiforme, toxic epidermal necrolysis) and lethargy.

Adverse effects seen in cats include hypersalivation, excitement, mydriasis and vomiting.

Overdosage/Toxicity - Symptoms of levamisole toxicity often mimic those of organophosphate toxicity. Symptoms may include hypersalivation, hyperesthesias and irritability, clonic seizures, CNS depression, dyspnea, defecation, urination, and collapse. These effects are best treated by supportive means, as animals generally recover within hours of dosing. Acute levamisole over-dosage can result in death due to respiratory failure. Should respiratory failure occur, artificial ventilation with oxygen should be instituted until recovery takes place. Cardiac arrhythmias may also be seen. If the ingestion was oral, emptying the gut and/or administering charcoal with cathartics may be indicated.

Levamisole is considered to be more dangerous when administered parenterally than when given orally or topically. Intravenous administration is particularly hazardous, and is never recommended.

In pet birds (cockatoos, budgerigars, Mynah birds, parrots, etc.), 40 mg/kg has been reported as a toxic dose when administered SQ. IM injections may cause more severe toxicity. Depression, ataxia, leg and wing paralysis, mydriasis, regurgitation, and death may be seen after a toxic dose in birds.

Drug Interactions - Other **nicotine-like compounds** (*e.g.,* **pyrantel, morantel, diethylcarbamazine), or cholinesterase-inhibitor drugs** (*e.g.,* **organophosphates, neostigmine)** could theoretically enhance the toxic effects of levamisole; use together with caution.

Levamisole may enhance the immune-reaction and efficacy to **Brucella vaccines**.

Fatalities have been reported after concomitant levamisole and **chloramphenicol** administration; avoid using these agents together.

Doses -
Dogs:
  As an immune stimulant:
    a) For recurrent cutaneous infections: 2.2 mg/kg PO every other day, with appropriate antimicrobial therapy. (Rosenkrantz 1989)
    b) 0.5 - 2 mg/kg PO 3 times a week. (Kirk 1989)
    c) For adjunctive therapy in dogs with chronic pyoderma: 0.5 - 1.5 mg/kg PO 2-3 times a week (efficacy not established). (Lorenz 1984)
    d) For adjunctive therapy in dogs with chronic pyoderma: 2.2 mg/kg PO every other day (may only be efficacious in 10% of cases). (Ihrke 1986)
    e) For adjunctive therapy in aspergillosis/penicillinosis: 2 - 5 mg/kg PO every other day. (Prueter 1988)

  As a microfilaricide:
    a) 10 mg/kg PO once a day for 6-10 days. (Kirk 1989)
    b) 11 mg/kg PO for 6-12 days. Examine blood on 6th day of treatment; discontinue therapy when microfilaria negative. May cause neurologic signs, vomiting, behavioral changes, or possibly death. If treatment is prolonged (>15 days), there is increased likelihood of toxicity. (Todd, Paul, and DiPietro 1985)
    c) If dithiazanine is ineffective: 11 mg/kg PO after a small meal for 7 days. Examine blood, and if microfilaria still are present, may continue for another 5 days. (Kittleson 1985)
    d) 11 mg/kg PO for 6-12 days. Examine for microfilaria within 7-10 days and at weekly intervals until eliminated or treatment is halted. Retching and vomiting are common. Avoid giving on an empty stomach or immediately after drinking water. A "conditioning" dose of 5 mg/kg PO once a day may be necessary. Stop therapy if abnormal behavior or ataxia develops. (Knight 1988)

  For the treatment of lungworms:
    a) For *Crenosoma vulpis*: 8 mg/kg once. (Todd, Paul, and DiPietro 1985)
    b) For *Capillaria*: 7-12 mg/kg once daily PO for 3-7 days.
       For *Filaroides osleri*: 7-12 mg/kg once daily PO for 20-45 days. (Roudebush 1985)
    c) 7.5 mg/kg PO *bid* or 25 mg/kg PO every other day for 10 days. (Bauer 1988)
    e) For *Capillaria aerophilia*: 10 mg/kg PO once daily for 5 days; repeat in 9 days (Reinemeyer 1995)

Cats:
For the treatment of lungworms:
a) 20 - 40 mg/kg PO every other day for 5-6 treatments (Kirk 1989)
b) For *Aelurostrongylus abstrusus*: 100 mg PO daily every other day for 5 treatments; give atropine (0.5 mg SQ, 15 minutes before administering); or 15 mg/kg PO every other day for 3 treatments, then 3 days later: 30 mg/kg PO, then 2 days later: 60 mg/kg.
For *Capillaria aerophilia*: 4.4 mg/kg SQ for 2 days, then 8.8 mg/kg once 2 weeks later; or 5 mg/kg PO once daily for 5 days, followed by 9 days of no therapy, repeat two times. (Todd, Paul, and DiPietro 1985)
c) 25 mg/kg every other day for 10-14 days. (Roudebush 1985)
d) For *Capillaria aerophilia*: 10 mg/kg PO once daily for 5 days; repeat in 9 days (Reinemeyer 1995)

For treatment of *Ollulanus tricuspis*:
a) 5 mg/kg SQ (Todd, Paul, and DiPietro 1985)

As a microfilaricide:
a) 10 mg/kg PO for 7 days. (Dillon 1986)

As an immune-stimulant:
a) For adjunctive therapy of feline plasma-cell gingivitis/pharyngitis: 25 mg PO every other day for 3 doses. (DeNovo, Potter, and Woolfson 1988)

Cattle:
For treatment of susceptible nematodes (also refer to specific label directions for approved products):
a) For removal of mature and immature *Dictyocaulus vivapurus*: 5.5 - 11 mg/kg PO, either given in feed or as a drench or oral bolus. May also be administered SQ at 3.3 - 8 mg/kg. (Bennett 1986)
b) 7.5 mg/kg PO (Brander, Pugh, and Bywater 1982)

Llamas:
For treatment of susceptible nematodes:
a) 5 - 8 mg/kg IM, or PO (Fowler 1989)
b) 5 - 8 mg/kg PO or SQ for 1 day (Cheney and Allen 1989)

Swine:
For treatment of susceptible nematodes (also refer to specific label directions for approved products):
a) For removal of mature and immature *Metastrongylus:* 8 mg/kg PO in feed or water. (Bennett 1986)
b) 8 mg/kg PO in feed or water. (Howard 1986)
c) 7.5 mg/kg PO (Brander, Pugh, and Bywater 1982)

Sheep & Goats:
For treatment of susceptible nematodes (also refer to specific label directions for approved products):
a) For removal of mature and immature *Dictyocaulus vivapurus*: 8 mg/kg PO. (Bennett 1986)
b) 7.5 mg/kg PO (Brander, Pugh, and Bywater 1982)

Birds:
a) Using 13.65% injectable:
For intestinal nematodes: 5-15 ml/gallon of drinking water for 1-3 days; repeat in 10 days. If birds refuse to drink, withhold water prior to treating.
For gavage in Australian Parakeets (or desert species that refuse to drink water): 15 mg/kg; repeat in 10 days.
For parenteral use: 4 - 8 mg/kg IM or SQ; repeat in 10-14 days. May cause vomiting, ataxia, or death. Do not use in debilitated birds.
For immunostimulation: 0.3 ml/gallon of water for several weeks.
As a parenteral immunostimulant: 2 mg/kg IM or SQ. 3 doses at 14 day intervals. (Clubb 1986)
b) As a nebulized immunostimulant: 1 ml (of 13.65% levamisole phosphate) in 15 ml saline. (Spink 1986)
c) For *Capillaria* infections: 15 - 30 mg/kg orally as a single bolus or through a crop tube; or 2.25 mg/gallon of drinking water for 4-5 days. Repeat treatment in 10-14 days. (Flammer 1986)
d) Poultry: 18 - 36 mg/kg PO (Brander, Pugh, and Bywater 1982)

Monitoring Parameters -
1) Clinical efficacy
2) Adverse effects/toxicity observation

Client Information - Levamisole is not approved to be used in dairy animals of breeding age. Follow directions on the product label unless otherwise directed by veterinarian. Animals that are severely parasitized or in conditions with constant helminth exposure should be retreated 2-4 weeks after initial treatment. Do not administer injectable products IV. Report serious adverse effects to veterinarian.

Dosage Forms/Preparations/FDA Approval Status/Withdrawal Times -
In cattle, sheep, and swine a level of 0.1 ppm has been established for negligible residues in edible tissues.

Veterinary-Approved Products:
Dosage Forms/Preparations/FDA Approval Status/Withdrawal Times -
In cattle, sheep, and swine a level of 0.1 ppm has been established for negligible residues in edible tissues.

Veterinary-Approved Products:
Levamisole Phosphate Injection 136.5 mg/ml (13.65%)

Levasole® *Injectable Solution* (Schering Plough); *Tramisol*® *Injectable* (Cyanamid). (OTC) Approved for use in beef cattle and non-lactating dairy cattle. Slaughter withdrawal=7 days.

Levamisole HCl Soluble Powder for Oral Use

Levasole® *Soluble Drench Powder* 11.7 grams/packet (Schering Plough); (OTC) Approved for use in sheep. Slaughter withdrawal=3 days.

Levasole® *Soluble Pig Wormer* 18.15 grams/packet (Schering Plough); (OTC) Approved for use in swine. Slaughter withdrawal=9 days.

Levasole® *Soluble Drench Powder* 46.8 grams/packet (Schering Plough); (OTC) Approved for use in beef cattle, non-lactating dairy cattle, and sheep. Slaughter withdrawal=2 days (cattle); 3 days (sheep).

Tramisol® *Soluble Drench Powder, Tramisol Drench* 46.8 grams/packet (American Cyanamid). (OTC) Approved for use in beef cattle, non-lactating dairy cattle, and sheep. Slaughter withdrawal=2 days (cattle); 3 days (sheep).

Ripercol® *L* 9.075 grams (American Cyanamid). (OTC) Approved for use in swine. Slaughter withdrawal=3 days.

Levamisole Oral Feed Mixes

Tramisol® *Hog Wormer* (American Cyanamid) Each 2.05 oz packet contains levamisole resinate equivalent to 45.5 grams levamisole. (OTC) Approved for use in swine. Slaughter withdrawal=3 days.

Medicated Feed Premix 50% (American Cyanamid) 227 g levamisole HCl/lb. (OTC) Approved for use in non-lactating dairy and beef cattle and swine. Slaughter withdrawal=2 days (cattle); 3 days (swine).

Levamisole HCl Oral Pastes/Gels

Levasole® *Gel* 11.5% (115 mg/gram) (Schering Plough) 237.4 g cartridge. Each cartridge will deliver 27.3 g of levamisole HCl. (OTC) Approved for use in beef cattle, and non-lactating dairy cattle. Slaughter withdrawal=6 days.

Tramisol® *Gel* 11.5% (115 mg/gram) (American Cyanamid). (OTC) Approved for use in beef cattle, and non-lactating dairy cattle, and swine. Slaughter withdrawal=6 days (cattle); 11 days (swine).

Levamisole HCl Oral Tablets/Boluses; 184 mg bolus: *Levasole*® *Sheep Wormer Bolus* (Schering Plough); *Tramisole*® *Sheep Wormer* (Cyanamid); *Ripercol*® *L Wormer Oblets* (American Cyanamid). (OTC) Approved for use in sheep. Slaughter withdrawal=3 days.

2.19 gram bolus: *Levasole*® *Cattle Wormer Bolus* (Schering Plough); *Ripercol*® *L Bolus* (Cyanamid); (OTC) Approved for use in beef and non-lactating dairy cattle. Slaughter withdrawal=2 days.

Levamisole Topical (Pour-On) 200 mg/ml; *Totalon*® (Schering); *Tramisol*® *Pour On* (American Cyanamid). (OTC) Approved for use on beef and non-lactating dairy cattle. Slaughter withdrawal=9 days.

Human-Approved Products:
Levamisol HCl Tablets: 50 mg levamisole base; *Ergamisol*® (Janssen) (Rx)

LEVOTHYROXINE SODIUM

Chemistry - Prepared synthetically for commercial use, levothyroxine sodium is the *levo* isomer of thyroxine which is the primary secretion of the thyroid gland. It occurs as an odorless, light yellow to buff-colored, tasteless, hygroscopic powder that is very slightly soluble in water and slightly soluble in alcohol. The commercially available powders for injection also contain mannitol.

Levothyroxine sodium may also be known as sodium levothyroxine, thyroxine sodium, L-thyroxine sodium, T4, or T4 thyroxine sodium. 100 micrograms of levothyroxine is approximately equivalent to 65 mg (1 grain) of dessicated thyroid.

Storage/Stability/Compatibility - Levothyroxine sodium preparations should be stored at room temperature in tight, light-resistant containers. The injectable product should be reconstituted immediately before use; unused injection should be discarded after reconstituting. Do not mix levothyroxine sodium injection with other drugs or IV fluids.

Pharmacology - Thyroid hormones affect the rate of many physiologic processes including: fat, protein and carbohydrate metabolism, increasing protein synthesis, increasing gluconeogenesis and promoting mobilization and utilization of glycogen stores. Thyroid hormones also increase oxygen consumption, body temperature, heart rate and cardiac output, blood volume, enzyme system activity, and growth and maturity. Thyroid hormone is particularly important for adequate development of the central nervous system. While the exact mechanisms how thyroid hormones exert their effects are not well understood, it is known that thyroid hormones (primarily triiodothyronine) act at the cellular level.

In humans, triiodothyronine (T3) is the primary hormone responsible for activity. Approximately 80% of T3 found in the peripheral tissues is derived from thyroxine (T4) which is the principle hormone released by the thyroid.

Uses/Indications - Levothyroxine sodium is indicated for the treatment of hypothyroidism in all species.

Pharmacokinetics - In dogs, peak plasma concentrations after oral dosing reportedly occur 4-12 hours after administration and the serum half-life is approximately 12-16 hours. There is wide variability from animal to animal, however.

Contraindications/Precautions - Levothyroxine (and other replacement thyroid hormones) are contraindicated in patients with acute myocardial infarction, thyrotoxicosis or untreated adrenal insufficiency. It should be used with caution, and at a lower initial dosage, in patients with concurrent hypoadrenocorticism (treated), cardiac disease, diabetes, or in those who are aged.

Adverse Effects/Warnings - When administered at an appropriate dose to patients requiring thyroid hormone replacement, there should not be any adverse effects associated with therapy. For adverse effects associated with overdosage, see below.

Overdosage - Chronic overdosage will produce symptoms of hyperthyroidism, including tachycardia, polyphagia, PU/PD, excitability, nervousness and excessive panting. Dosage should be reduced and/or temporarily withheld until symptoms subside. Some (10%?) cats may exhibit symptoms of "apathetic" (listlessness, anorexia, etc.) hyperthyroidism.

Acute massive overdosage can produce symptoms resembling thyroid storm. After oral ingestion, treatment to reduce absorption of drug should be accomplished using standard protocols (emetics or gastric lavage, cathartics, charcoal) unless contraindicated by the patient's condition. Treatment is supportive and symptomatic. Oxygen, artificial ventilation, cardiac glycosides, beta blockers (*e.g.,* propranolol), fluids, dextrose and antipyrexic agents have all been suggested for use if necessary.

Drug Interactions - Levothyroxine increases the actions of **epinephrine, norepinephrine** and other catecholamines and sympathomimetics.

Thyroid hormones increase the catabolism of vitamin K-dependent clotting factors which may increase the anticoagulation effects in patients on **warfarin**.

In diabetic patients, the addition of thyroid hormones may alter **insulin** requirements; monitor carefully during initiation of therapy.

Estrogens may increase thyroid requirements by increasing TBg. Therapeutic effects of **digoxin or digitoxin** may be decreased by thyroid hormones.

Ketamine may cause tachycardia and hypertension when used in patients receiving thyroid hormones.

Drug/Laboratory Interactions - The following drugs (in humans) that may be used in veterinary species may have effects on thyroid function tests; evaluate results accordingly:

Effects on serum **T4**: aminoglutethimide↓, anabolic steroids/androgens↓, antithyroid drugs (PTU, methimazole)↓, asparaginase↓, barbiturates↓, corticosteroids↓, danazol↓, diazepam↓, estrogens↑ (Note: estrogens may have no effect on canine T3 or T4 concentrations), fluorouracil↑, heparin↓, insulin↑, lithium carbonate↓, mitotane (*o,p*-DDD)↓, nitroprusside↓, phenylbutazone↓, phenytoin↓, propranolol↑, salicylates (large doses)↓, & sulfonylureas↓.

Effects on serum **T3**: antithyroid drugs (PTU, methimazole)↓, barbiturates↓, corticosteroids↓, estrogens↑, fluorouracil↑, heparin↓, lithium carbonate↓, phenytoin↓, propranolol↓, salicylates (large doses)↓, & thiazides↑.

Effects on **T3 uptake resin**: anabolic steroids/androgens↑, antithyroid drugs (PTU, methimazole)↓, asparaginase↑, corticosteroids↑, danazol↑, estrogens↓, fluorouracil↓, heparin↑, lithium carbonate↓, phenylbutazone↑, & salicylates (large doses)↑.

Effects on serum **TSH**: aminoglutethimide↑, antithyroid drugs (PTU, methimazole)↑, corticosteroids↓, danazol↓, & lithium carbonate↑.

Effects on **Free Thyroxine Index (FTI)**: antithyroid drugs (PTU, methimazole)↓, barbiturates↓, corticosteroids↓, heparin↑, lithium carbonate↓, & phenylbutazone↓.

Doses -
 Dogs:
   For hypothyroidism:
     a) Use a trade name product initially, with a starting dosage of 20 micrograms/kg body weight PO q12h. Some dogs may only require once a day dosing, but initially, all dogs should receive twice daily dosing. After clinical symptoms have resolved, once daily dosing may be attempted. Dogs who have concomitant cardiac problems should receive 5 micrograms/kg twice daily; may increase dosage gradually over 3-4 weeks. (Nelson 1989b)
     b) Initiate treatment at 22 micrograms/kg PO twice daily (0.1 mg/10 lbs body weight *bid*); reevaluate dosage after monitoring clinical response and serum levels after 4-8 weeks.
       If clinical response is satisfactory and T4 is elevated (≥ 60 nmol/L) may reduce dosage to 22 micrograms/kg once daily. If clinical response is not satisfactory, either reevaluate the need for T4 supplementaion or increase the dose. Daily dosage of 20 - 40 micrograms/day appears to be adequate for most dogs. (Refsal and Nachreiner 1995)
     c) 0.02 - 0.04 mg/kg daily, or perhaps more logically: 0.5 mg/m^2 daily. Many dogs may only need once daily dosing, but some will require twice daily doses. In patients with hypoadrenocorticism, cardiac disease, diabetes, or those who are aged, it is recommended to start low (0.1 mg/m^2 *bid*), and increase dosage by 20-25% increments over 4-8 weeks. In hypoadrenal dogs, start glucocorticoid supplementation before thyroid replacement. All patients should have therapy assessed after 6-12 weeks using clinical or laboratory criteria. (Ferguson 1986)
 Cats:
   For hypothyroidism:
     a) Initially, 10 - 20 micrograms/kg per day; adjust dosage on basis of clinical response and post-dose serum thyroxine level. (Peterson and Randolph 1989)
     b) Initially, 0.05 - 0.1 mg once daily. Wait a minimum of 4-6 weeks to assess cat's clinical response to treatment. Then obtain a serum T4 level prior to, and 6-8 hours after, dosing. Increase or decrease dose and/or dosing frequency after reviewing these values and clinical response. If levothyroxine is ineffective, may try liothyronine. (Feldman and Nelson 1987d)
 Horses:
   For hypothyroidism:
     a) 10 mg in 70 ml of corn syrup once daily. Monitor T4 levels one week after initiation of therapy. Obtain one blood sample just before administration and on sample 2-3 hours after dosing. (Chen and Li 1987)

Birds:

For hypothyroidism:

a) One 0.1 mg tablet in 30 ml - 120 ml of water daily; stir water and offer for 15 minutes and remove. Use high dose for budgerigars and low dose for water drinkers. Used for respiratory clicking, vomiting in budgerigars and thyroid responsive problems. (Clubb 1986)

Reptiles:

a) For hypthyroidism in tortoises: 0.02 mg/kg PO every other day. (Gauvin 1993)

Monitoring Parameters -

1) Serum thyroid hormone concentrations (T_4/T_3). Monitoring before therapy is begun can help confirm diagnosis. After therapy is started wait at least 5-10 days before measuring T_4, one month may be better, especially if dosage is ineffective or symptoms of thyrotoxicosis develop. Serum levels should be drawn before the dose and 6-8 hours after. Dosage should be reduced if serum thyroxine levels exceed 100 ng/ml or symptoms of thyrotoxicosis develop.

Client Information - Clients should be instructed in the importance of compliance with therapy as prescribed. Also, review the symptoms that can be seen with too much thyroid supplementation (see Overdosage section above).

Dosage Forms/Preparations/FDA Approval Status - All levothyroxine products require a prescription. There have been bioavailability differences between products reported. It is recommended to use a reputable product and not to change brands indiscriminately.

Veterinary-Approved Products -

Levothyroxine Sodium Tablets 0.1 mg, 0.2 mg, 0.3 mg, 0.4 mg, 0.5 mg, 0.6 mg, 0.7 mg, 0.8 mg; *Soloxine®* (Daniels), *Thyro-Tabs ®* (Vet-A-Mix); *Thyrozine Tablets®* (Anthony) (Rx) Approved for use in dogs.

Levothyroxine Sodium Tablets Chewable (Veterinary) 0.2 mg, 0.5 mg, 0.8 mg; *Thyro-Form®* (Vet-A-Mix) (Rx) — Approved for use in dogs.

Levothyroxine Sodium Tablets Chewable (Veterinary) 0.1 mg, 0.2 mg, 0.3 mg, 0.4 mg, 0.5 mg, 0.6 mg, 0.7 mg, 0.8 mg; *HESKA Chewable Thyroid Supplement for Dogs* (Heska); Approved for use in dogs (Rx)

Levothyroxine Sodium Powder (Veterinary) 0.22% (1 gram of T_4 in 454 grams of powder): One level teaspoonful contains 12 mg of T_4. Available in 1 lb. and 10 lb. containers.; *Thyro-L®* (Vet-A-Mix) (Rx) — Approved for use in horses.

Human-Approved Products -

Levothyroxine Sodium Tablets 0.025 mg, 0.05 mg, 0.075 mg, 0.088 mg, 0.1 mg, 0.112 mg, 0.125 mg, 0.137 mg, 0.15 mg, 0.175 mg, 0.2 mg, 0.3 mg; *Synthroid®* (Knoll), *Levothroid®* (Forest); *Levo-T®* (Lederle); Levoxyl® (Daniels); *Eltroxin®* (Roberts); generic, (Rx)

Levothyroxine Powder for Injection 200 micrograms per vial, 500 micrograms/vial in 6 ml and 10 ml vials; *Synthroid®* (Knoll), *Levothroid®* (Forest); *Levoxine®* (Daniels), generic (Rx)

LIDOCAINE HCL

Chemistry - A potent local anesthetic and antiarrhythmic agent, lidocaine HCl occurs as a white, odorless, slightly bitter tasting, crystalline powder with a melting point between 74° - 79°C and a pK_a of 7.86. It is very soluble in water and alcohol. The pH of the commercial injection is adjusted to 5 - 7, and the pH of the commercially available infusion in dextrose 5% is adjusted to 3.5 - 6.

Lidocaine is also known as lignocaine HCl.

Storage/Stability/Compatibility - Lidocaine for injection should be stored at temperatures less than 40°C and preferably between 15-30°C; avoid freezing.

Lidocaine is **compatible** with most commonly used IV infusion solutions, including D5W, lactated Ringer's, saline, and combinations of these. It is also reportedly physically compatible with: aminophylline, bretylium tosylate, calcium chloride/glucceptate/gluconate, carbenicillin disodium, chloramphenicol sodium succinate, chlorothiazide sodium, cimetidine HCl, dexamethasone sodium phosphate, digoxin, diphenhydramine HCl, dobutamine HCl, ephedrine sulfate, erythromycin lactobionate, glycopyrrolate, heparin sodium, hydrocortisone sodium succinate, hydroxyzine HCl, insulin (regular), mephentermine sulfate, metaraminol bitartrate, methicillin sodium, metoclopramide HCl, nitrofurantoin sodium, oxytetracycline HCl, penicillin G potassium, pentobarbital sodium, phenylephrine HCl, potassium chloride, procainamide HCl, prochlorperazine edisylate, promazine HCl, sodium bicarbonate, sodium lactate, tetracycline HCl, verapamil HCl, and Vitamin B-Complex w/C.

Lidocaine **may not be compatible** with dopamine, epinephrine, isoproterenol or norepinephrine as these require low pH's for stability. Lidocaine is reportedly **incompatible** with: ampicillin sodium, cefazolin sodium, methohexital sodium, or phenytoin sodium. Compatibility is dependent upon factors such as pH, concentration, temperature, and diluents used and it is suggested to consult specialized references for more specific information.

Pharmacology - Lidocaine is considered to be a class IB (membrane-stabilizing) antidysrhythmic agent. It is thought that lidocaine acts by combining with fast sodium channels when inactive which inhibits recovery after repolarization. Class IB agents demonstrate rapid rates of attachment and dissociation to sodium channels. At therapeutic levels, lidocaine causes phase 4 diastolic depolarization attenuation, decreased automaticity, and either a decrease or no change in membrane responsiveness and excitability. These effects will occur at serum levels that will not inhibit the automaticity of the SA node, and will have little effect on AV node conduction or His-Purkinje conduction.

Uses/Indications - Besides its use as a local and topical anesthetic agent, lidocaine is used to treat ventricular arrhythmias, principally ventricular tachycardia and ventricular premature complexes in all species. Cats tend to be rather sensitive to the drug and some clinicans feel that it should not be used in this species as an antiarrhythmic.

Pharmacokinetics - Lidocaine is not effective orally as it has a high first-pass effect. If very high oral doses are given, toxic symptoms occur (due to active metabolites?) before therapeutic levels can be reached. Following a therapeutic IV bolus dose, the onset of action is generally within 2 minutes and has a duration of action of 10-20 minutes. If a constant infusion is begun without an initial IV bolus it may take up to an hour for therapeutic levels to be reached. IM injections may be given every 1.5 hours in the dog, but because monitoring and adjusting dosages are difficult, it should be reserved for cases where IV infusions are not possible.

After injection, the drug is rapidly redistributed from the plasma into highly perfused organs (kidney, liver, lungs, heart) and is distributed widely throughout body tissues. It has a high affinity for fat and adipose tissue and is bound to plasma proteins, primarily $alpha_1$-acid glycoprotein. It has been reported that lidocaine binding to this protein is highly variable and concentration dependent in the dog and may be higher in dogs with inflammatory disease. Lidocaine is distributed into milk. The apparent volume of distribution (V_d) has been reported to be 4.5 L/kg in the dog.

Lidocaine is rapidly metabolized in the liver to active metabolites (MEGX and GX). The terminal half-life of lidocaine in humans is 1.5-2 hours and has been reported to be 0.9 hours in the dog. The half-lives of lidocaine and MEGX may be prolonged in patients with cardiac failure or hepatic disease. Less than 10% of a parenteral dose is excreted unchanged in the urine.

Contraindications/Precautions - Cats tend to be more sensitive to the CNS effects of lidocaine; use with caution. Lidocaine is contraindicated in patients with known hypersensitivity to the amide-class local anesthetics, a severe degree of SA, AV or intraventricular heart block (if not being artificially paced), or Adams-Stokes syndrome. The use of lidocaine in patients with Wolff-Parkinson-White (WPW) syndrome is controversial. Some manufacturers state its use is contraindicated, but several physicians have used the drug in people.

Lidocaine should be used with caution in patients with liver disease, congestive heart failure, shock, hypovolemia, severe respiratory depression, or marked hypoxia. It should be also be used with caution in patients with bradycardia or incomplete heart block having VPC's, unless the heart rate is first accelerated. Patients susceptible to developing malignant hyperthermia should receive lidocaine with intensified monitoring.

Adverse Effects/Warnings - At usual doses and if the serum level remains within the proposed therapeutic range (1 - 5 micrograms/ml), serious adverse reactions are quite rare. The most common adverse effects reported are dose related (serum level) and mild. CNS signs include drowsiness, depression, ataxia, muscle tremors, etc. Nausea and vomiting may occur, but are usually transient. Adverse cardiac effects generally only occur at high plasma concentrations and are usually associated with PR and QRS interval prolongation and QT interval shortening. Lidocaine may increase ventricular rates if used in patients with atrial fibrillation. If an IV bolus is given too rapidly, hypotension may occur.

Be certain **not** to use the product which contains **epinephrine** intravenously.

Overdosage - In dogs, if serum levels of >8 micrograms/ml are attained, toxicity may result. Symptoms may include ataxia, nystagmus, depression, seizures, bradycardia, hypotension and, at very high levels, circulatory collapse. Because lidocaine is rapidly metabolized, cessation of therapy or reduction in infusion rates with monitoring may be all that is required for minor symptoms. Seizures or excitement may be treated with diazepam, or a short or ultrashort acting barbiturate. Longer acting barbiturates (e.g., pentobarbital) should be avoided. Should circulatory depression occur, treat with fluids, pressor agents and if necessary, begin CPR.

Drug Interactions - Lidocaine levels or effects may be increased by concomitant administration of **cimetidine** or **propranolol**.

Other antiarrhythmics such as **procainamide, quinidine, propranolol, phenytoin** administered with lidocaine may cause additive or antagonistic cardiac effects and toxicity may be enhanced. **Phenytoin** when given IV with lidocaine may cause increased cardiac depression.

Large doses of lidocaine may prolong **succinylcholine**-induced apnea.

Laboratory Interactions - Lidocaine may cause increased **creatine kinase levels (CK)**.

Doses -
   Dogs:
   a) Initially, IV bolus of 2 - 4 mg/kg given slowly; then begin constant IV infusion of 25 - 80 micrograms/kg/min (Moses 1988)
   b) 4 mg/kg bolus STAT, then begin 50 micrograms/kg/min constant infusion. If no effect repeat 4 mg/kg bolus or if effect is lost give another 2 mg/kg bolus during infusion equilibration period. Adjust infusion rate from 25 - 100 micrograms/kg/min to control arrhythmias and minimize toxicity.
       Alternatively, give 6 mg/kg IM ever 1.5 hours; results may be more variable and management more difficult. (Wilcke 1985)
   c) 2 - 3 mg/kg slow IV, may repeat several times at 10-15 minute intervals; maximum of 8 mg/kg over 10 minutes. Begin constant rate infusion (may be required for 1-3 days). (Tilley and Miller 1986)

   Cats: Caution: Cats are reportedly very sensitive to the CNS effects of lidocaine, monitor carefully and treat seizures with diazepam.
   a) Initially, IV bolus of 0.25 - 0.75 mg/kg given slowly; then begin constant IV infusion of 10 - 40 micrograms/kg/min (Moses 1988)
   b) 0.5 mg/kg slow IV (Miller 1985)

   Horses:
   a) Initially IV bolus of 1 - 1.5 mg/kg. Will generally distinguish between ventricular tachyarrhythmias (effective) and supraventricular tachyarrhythmias (no effect). To maintain effect, a constant IV infusion will be required. (Hilwig 1987)

Monitoring Parameters -
   1) ECG
   2) Symptoms of toxicity (see Adverse Effects and Overdosage)
   3) If available and indicated, serum levels may be monitored. Therapeutic levels are considered to range from 1 - 6 micrograms/ml.

Client Information - This drug should only be used by professionals familiar with its use and in a setting where adequate patient monitoring can be performed.

Dosage Forms/Preparations/FDA Approval Status/Withholding Times -Lidocaine is approved for use in veterinary medicine (dogs, cats, horses, and cattle) as an injectable anesthetic, but it is not approved for use as an antiarrhythmic agent. Information regarding its use in food-producing species is conflicting. It is a prescription (Rx) drug.

   Lidocaine HCl for Injection
      1% (10 mg/ml) in 5 ml (50mg) and 10 ml (100 mg) syringes
      2% (20 mg/ml) in 5 ml single use vials and syringes (preservative free)
      2% (20 mg/ml) in 100 ml multi-use vials; Veterinary (contains preservatives)

To prepare IV infusion solution using the veterinary 2% solution add 1 gram (50 ml of 2% solution to 1 liter of D_5W or other compatible solution, this will give an approximate concentration of 1 mg/ml (1000 micrograms/ml). When using a mini-drip (60 drops/ml) IV set, each drop will contain approximately 17 micrograms. In small dogs and cats, a less concentrated solution may be used for greater dosage accuracy. When preparing solution be certain that you are **not using** the lidocaine product that also contains **epinephrine**.

Lidocaine (human approved) is also available in 4%, 10%, and 20% preservative free solutions for IV admixture, for direct IM administration, and premixed with D_5W for IV infusion in concentrations of 2 mg/ml, 4 mg/ml, and 5 mg/ml.

Also known as lignocaine HCl. A common trade name is *Xylocaine*® (Astra).

LINCOMYCIN HCL

Chemistry - An antibiotic obtained from cultures of *Streptomyces lincolnensis*, lincomycin is available commercially as the monohydrate hydrochloride. It occurs as a white to off-white, crystalline powder that is freely soluble in water. The powder may have a faint odor and has a

pK_a of 7.6. The commercially available injection has a pH of 3-5.5 and occurs as a clear to slightly yellow solution.

Storage/Stability/Compatibility - Lincomycin capsules, tablets and soluble powder should be stored at room temperature (15-30°C) in tight containers. Lincomycin injectable products should be stored at room temperature; avoid freezing.

Lincomycin HCl for injection is reportedly **compatible** for at least 24 hours in the following IV infusion solutions and drugs: D_5W, D_5W in sodium chloride 0.9%, $D_{10}W$, sodium chloride 0.9%, Ringer's injection, amikacin sulfate, cephalothin sodium, chloramphenicol sodium succinate, cimetidine HCl, cytarabine, heparin sodium, penicillin G potassium/sodium (4 hours only), polymyxin B sulfate, tetracycline HCl, and vitamin B-complex with C.

Drugs that are reportedly **incompatible** with lincomycin, data conflicts, or compatibility is concentration and/or time dependent include: ampicillin sodium, carbenicillin disodium, methicillin sodium and phenytoin sodium. Compatibility is dependent upon factors such as pH, concentration, temperature and diluents used. It is suggested to consult specialized references for more specific information (*e.g., Handbook on Injectable Drugs* by Trissel; see bibliography).

Pharmacology - The lincosamide antibiotics lincomycin and clindamycin, share mechanisms of action and have similar spectrums of activity although lincomycin is usually less active against susceptible organisms. Complete cross-resistance occurs between the two drugs; at least partial cross-resistance occurs between the lincosamides and erythromycin. They may act as bacteriostatic or bactericidal agents, depending on the concentration of the drug at the infection site and the susceptibility of the organism. The lincosamides are believed to act by binding to the 50S ribosomal subunit of susceptible bacteria, thereby inhibiting peptide bond formation.

Most aerobic gram positive cocci are susceptible to the lincosamides (*Strep. faecalis* is not), including Staphylococcus and Streptococci. Other organisms that are generally susceptible include: *Corynebacterium diphtheriae, Nocardia asteroides, Erysepelothrix,* and *Mycoplasma sp..* Anaerobic bacteria that may be susceptible to the lincomycin include: *Clostridium perfringens. C. tetani* (not *C. difficile*), *Bacteroides* (including many strains of *B. fragilis*), *Fusobacterium, Peptostreptococcus, Actinomyces,* and *Peptococcus.*

Uses/Indications - Lincomycin has dosage forms approved for use in dogs, cats, swine, and in combination with other agents for chickens. Because clindamycin is generally better absorbed, more active, and probably less toxic, it has largely supplanted the use of lincomycin for oral and injectable therapy in small animals. Lincomycin is more economical however, and is still used by many clinicians. For further information refer to the Pharmacology or Doses sections.

Pharmacokinetics - The pharmacokinetics of lincomycin have apparently not been extensively studied in veterinary species. Unless otherwise noted, the following information applies to humans. The drug is rapidly absorbed from the gut, but only about 30-40% of the total dose is absorbed. Food both decreases the extent and the rate of absorption. Peak serum levels are attained about 2-4 hour after oral dosing. IM administration gives peak levels about double those reached after oral dosing, and peak at about 30 minutes post injection.

Lincomycin is distributed into most tissues. Therapeutic levels are achieved in bone, synovial fluid, bile, pleural fluid, peritoneal fluid, skin and heart muscle. CNS levels may reach 40% of those in the serum if meninges are inflamed. Lincomycin is bound from 57-72% to plasma proteins, depending on the drug's concentration. The drug crosses the placenta and also can be distributed into milk at concentrations equal to those found in the plasma.

Lincomycin is partially metabolized in the liver. Unchanged drug and metabolites are excreted in the urine, feces and bile. Half-lives can be prolonged in patients with renal or hepatic dysfunction. The elimination half-life of lincomycin is reportedly 3-4 hours in small animals.

Contraindications/Precautions/Reproductive Safety - Although there have been case reports of parenteral administration of lincosamides to horses, cattle and sheep, the lincosamides are considered to be contraindicated for use in rabbits, hamsters, guinea pigs, horses and ruminants because of serious gastrointestinal effects that may occur, including death.

Lincomycin is contraindicated in patients with known hypersensitivity to it or having a preexisting monilial infection.

Lincomycin crosses the placenta and cord blood concentrations are approximately 25% of those found in maternal serum. Safe use during pregnancy has not been established, but neither has the drug been implicated in causing teratogenic effects.

Because lincomycin is distributed into milk, nursing puppies or kittens of mothers taking lincomycin may develop diarrhea.

Adverse Effects/Warnings - Adverse effects reported in dogs and cats include gastroenteritis (emesis, loose stools, and infrequently bloody diarrhea in dogs). IM injections reportedly cause pain at the injection site. Rapid intravenous administration can cause hypotension and cardiopulmonary arrest.

Swine may also develop gastrointestinal disturbances while taking the medication.

Overdosage/Acute Toxicity - There is little information available regarding overdoses of this drug. In dogs, oral doses of up to 300 mg/kg/day for up to one year or parenterally at 60 mg/kg/day apparently did not result in toxicity.

Drug Interactions - Kaolin (found in several over-the-counter antidiarrheal preparations) has been shown to reduce the absorption of lincomycin by up to 90% if both are given concurrently. If both drugs are necessary, separate doses by at least 2 hours. Because lincomycin has been associated with severe diarrheas in several species, the need for an antidiarrheal product may indicate impending toxicity. Clindamycin absorption does not appear to be significantly altered by kaolin.

Lincomycin possesses intrinsic neuromuscular blocking activity and should be used cautiously with other **neuromuscular blocking agents**.

Drug/Laboratory Interactions - Slight increases in **liver function tests** (AST, ALT, Alk. Phosph.) may occur. There is apparently not any clinical significance associated with these increases.

Doses -
Dogs:
    For susceptible infections:
        a) 22 - 33 mg/kg PO q12h (Aronson and Aucoin 1989)
        b) 15 mg/kg PO q8h; 10 mg/kg IV or IM q12h (Kirk 1989)
        c) 15 - 25 mg/kg PO q12h (Papich 1988)
        d) For mastitis: 15 mg/kg PO *tid* for 21 days;
           For *Staph.* infections: 10 - 15 mg/kg PO *tid* (Morgan 1988)

Cats:
    For susceptible infections:
        a) 22 - 33 mg/kg PO q12h (Aronson and Aucoin 1989)
        b) 15 mg/kg PO q8h; 10 mg/kg IV or IM q12h (Kirk 1989)
        c) 15 - 25 mg/kg PO q12h (Papich 1988)
        d) For mastitis: 15 mg/kg PO *tid* for 21 days;
           For *Staph.* infections: 10 - 15 mg/kg PO *tid* (Morgan 1988)

Swine:
    For susceptible infections:
        a) 10 mg/kg IM q24h (Jenkins 1987b)
        2) 11 mg/kg IM once daily for 3-7 days; or added to drinking water at a rate of 250 mg/gallon (average of 8.36 mg/kg/day). (Label directions; *Lincocin*®—Upjohn)

Monitoring Parameters -
    1) Clinical efficacy
    2) Adverse effects; particularly severe diarrheas

Client Information - Clients should be instructed to report the incidence of severe, protracted or bloody diarrhea to the veterinarian.

Dosage Forms/Preparations/FDA Approval Status/Withholding Times -
Veterinary-Approved Products:
    Lincomycin Oral Tablets 100 mg, 200 mg, 500 mg
        Lincocin® (Upjohn); (Rx) Approved for use in dogs and cats.
    Lincomycin Oral Solution 50 mg/ml in 20 ml dropper bottles.
        Lincocin® *Aquadrops* (Upjohn); (Rx) Approved for use in dogs and cats.
    Lincomycin Sterile Injection 100 mg/ml in 20 ml vials.
        Lincocin® (Upjohn); (Rx) Approved for use in dogs and cats.
    Lincomycin Sterile Injection 25 mg/ml in 100 ml vials, 50 mg/ml in 50 ml vials, and 100 mg/ml in 50 ml vials.
        Veterinary Lincocin® (Upjohn); (OTC) Approved for use in swine. Slaughter withdrawal = 48 hours.
    Lincomycin 40 gram (16 grams of lincomycin) packets for addition to 64 gallons of drinking water.
        Lincocin® *Soluble Powder* (Upjohn); (OTC) Approved for use in swine. Slaughter withdrawal = 6 days.
    There are also several lincomycin combination feed/water additive products for use in swine and/or poultry.

Human-Approved Products:
    Lincomycin Oral Capsules 250 mg, 500 mg; *Lincocin*® (Upjohn); (Rx)
    Lincomycin Injection 300 mg/ml in 2 and 10 ml vials; *Lincocin*® (Upjohn); (Rx)

LIOTHYRONINE SODIUM

Chemistry - A synthetically prepared sodium salt of the naturally occurring hormone T3, liothyronine sodium occurs as an odorless, light tan crystalline powder. It is very slightly soluble in water and slightly soluble in alcohol. Each 25 micrograms of liothyronine is approximately equivalent to 60-65 mg (1 grain) of thyroglobulin or dessicated thyroid and 100 micrograms or less of levothyroxine.

Liothyronine sodium may also be known as T3, T3 thyronine sodium, L-triiodothyronine, or Sodium L-triiodothyronine.

Storage/Stability/Compatibility - Liothyronine tablets should be stored at room temperature (15-30°C) in tight containers.

Pharmacology, Contraindications/Precautions, Adverse Effects/Warnings, Drug Interactions, Drug/Laboratory Interactions, & Overdosage - Refer to the previous monograph (Levothyroxine Sodium) for information on liothyronine.

Uses/Indications - Because of its shorter duration of action, liothyronine is generally not considered to be the drug of first choice in treating hypothyroidism. Infrequently, animals not responding to levothyroxine may respond to liothyronine.

Pharmacokinetics - In dogs, peak plasma levels of liothyronine occur 2-5 hours after oral dosing. The plasma half-life is approximately 5-6 hours. In contrast to levothyroxine, it is believed that liothyronine is nearly completely absorbed by dogs and absorption is not as affected by stomach contents, intestinal flora changes, etc.

Doses -
  Dogs:
    For hypothyroidism:
      a) Initially, 4 - 6 micrograms/kg PO q8h. Some dogs may require less frequent dosing. (Nelson 1989b)
      b) 4.4 micrograms/kg PO q8h (Mulnix 1985)
      c) 4 - 6 micrograms/kg PO *tid*, or possibly twice a day. (Ferguson 1986)
  Cats:
    For hypothyroidism:
      a) Initially, 4.4 micrograms/kg PO 2-3 times a day. (Feldman and Nelson 1987d)

Monitoring Parameters - Similar to levothyroxine, but T4 levels will remain low. When monitoring T3 levels, draw serum just prior to dosing and again 2-4 hours after administering the drug.

Client Information - Clients should be instructed in the importance of compliance with therapy as prescribed. Also, review the symptoms that can be seen with too much thyroid supplementation (see Overdosage section in the levothyroxine monograph).

Dosage Forms/Preparations/FDA Approval Status/Withholding Times -
  Veterinary-Approved Products:
  Liothyronine Sodium Tablets (Veterinary) 60 micrograms, 120 micrograms in bottles of 500; *Cytobin*® (Pfizer); (Rx) Approved for use in dogs.
  Human-Approved Products:
  Liothyronine Sodium Tablets 5 micrograms, 25 micrograms, 50 micrograms; *Cytomel*® (SK-Beecham); Generic; (Rx)

  Liothyronine Sodium Injection: 10 mcg/ml in 1 ml vials *Tiostat*® (SK-Beecham) (Rx)

LOMUSTINE (CCNU)

Chemistry - A nitrosourea derivative alkylating agent, lomustine occurs as a yellow powder that is practically insoluble in water and soluble in alcohol.

Storage/Stability/Compatibility - Store capsules in well-closed containers at room temperature. Expiration dates of two years are assigned after manufacture.

Pharmacology - While lomustine's mechanism of action is not totally understood, it is believed it acts as an alkylating agent. However, other mechanisms such as carbamoylation and cellular protein modification may be involved. The net effects are of DNA and RNA synthesis inhibition. Lomustine is cell cycle-phase nonspecific.

Uses/Indications - Lomustine may be useful in the adjunctive treatment of CNS neoplasms in dogs. It potentially could be of benefit in the adjunctive therapy of other neoplastic diseases in small animals as well.

Pharmacokinetics - Lomustine is absorbed rapidly and extensively from the GI tract and some absorption occurs after topical administration. Lomustine or its active metabolites are widely distributed in the body. While lomustine is not detected in the CSF, its active metabolites are detected in substantial concentrations. Lomustine is metabolized extensively in the liver to both active and inactive metabolites which are then eliminated primarily in the urine. Lomustine half life in humans is very short (about 15 minutes), but its biologic activity is significantly longer due to the longer elimination times of active metabolites.

Contraindications/Precautions/Reproductive Safety - Lomustine should be used only when its potential benefits outweigh its risks with the following conditions: anemia, bone marrow depression, pulmonary function impairment, current infection, impaired renal function, sensitivity to lomustine or patients who have received previous chemotherapy or radiotherapy.

Lomustine is a teratogen in lab animals. Use only during pregnancy when the benefits to the mother outweigh the risks to the offspring. Lomustine can suppress gonadal function. Lomustine and its metabolites have been detected in maternal milk, nursing puppies or kittens should receive milk replacer when the bitch or queen is receiving lomustine.

Adverse Effects/Warnings - Potential adverse effects include GI effects (anorexia, vomiting, diarrhea), stomatitis, alopecia, and rarely, hepatotoxicity and pulmonary infiltrates or fibrosis. The most serious adverse effect likely is bone marrow depression (anemia, thrombocytopenia, leukopenia). Nadirs in dogs generally occur about 1-3 weeks after treatment has begun.

Cross-resistance may occur between lomustine and carmustine.

Overdosage/Acute Toxicity - No specific information located. Because of the potential toxicity of the drug, overdoses should be treated aggressively with gut emptying protocols employed when possible. For further information, refer to an animal poison center.

Drug Interactions - The principal concern with lomustine is with its concurrent use with other drugs that are also myelosuppressive, including many of the **other antineoplastics and other bone marrow depressant drugs (*e.g.*, chloramphenicol, flucytosine, amphotericin B, or colchicine)**. Bone marrow depression may be additive. Use with other **immunosuppressant drugs (*e.g.*, azathioprine, cyclophosphamide, corticosteroids)** may increase the risk of infection. **Live virus vaccines** should be used with caution if at all during lomustine therapy.

Doses -
  Dogs:
    For the treatment of brain neoplasms:
      a) Initially, 60 mg/m^2 PO; if toxicity is minimal the dosage is increased slowly to 80 mg/m^2. Treatments given every 5-8 weeks. CBC done every week between treatments. (Fulton 1991)

    For the treatment of canine mast cell sarcoma: See the protocol in the appendix.

Monitoring Parameters - 1) CBC with platelets at least every 1-2 weeks until stable; then every 3 months; 2) Liver function tests; initially before starting treatment and then every 3-4 months

Dosage Forms/Preparations/FDA Approval Status/Withholding Times -
  Veterinary-Approved Products: None
  Human-Approved Products:
    Lomustine Capsules 10 mg, 40 mg, 100 mg; Dose Pack (two 100 mg capsules, two 40 mg capsules & two 10 mg capsules) *CeeNu*® (Bristol-Myers Oncology); (Rx)

Loperamide - see Opiate Antidiarrheals

LUFENURON

Chemistry/Storage/Stability/Compatibility - A benzoylphenylurea derivative, lufenuron is classified as an insect development inhibitor. The drug is considered to be lipophilic. The commercially available tablets and suspension should be stored at room temperature (15-30°C). The manufacturer states that intermittent exposure or exposure less than 48 hours to temperatures outside of storage recommendations for the tablets or suspension should not affect potency. Lufenuron tablets are assigned a 4 year expiration date after manufacture; the suspension, 3 years after manufacture; and Sentinel® tablets 3 years after manufacture. Opened pouches of the suspension are not recommended to be stored until the following dosing cycle.

Pharmacology - Lufenuron acts by inhibiting chitin synthesis, polymerization and deposition in fleas, thereby preventing eggs from developing into adults. The exact mechanism for this action was not noted. Lufenuron does not kill adult fleas.

Uses/Indications - Lufenuron is approved for use in dogs and cats 6 weeks of age and older for the control of flea populations. The combination product of lufenuron and milbemycin (Sentinel®) is indicated for use in puppies and dogs 4 weeks and older for prevention and control flea populations, prevention of heartworm disease, control of adult hookworms, and the removal and control of adult roundworms and whipworms.

Pharmacokinetics - Approximately 40% of an oral dose is absorbed with the remainder eliminated in the feces. To maximize oral absorption, the manufacturer recommends to administer in conjunction with or immediately after (within 30 minutes) a full meal. The drug is absorbed in the small intestine and stored in lipose tissue which acts as depot reservoir to slowly redistribute the drug back into the circulation. While the drug concentrates in the milk of lactating animals, it apparently does not cause ill effects in nursing animals.

After cats receive the injectable product, 2 -3 weeks are required before blood levels attain effective concentrations. Cats require a substantially higher oral dosage per kg than do dogs for equivalent efficacy. The drug is apparently not metabolized, but excreted unchanged into the bile and eliminated in the feces.

Contraindications/Precautions/Reproductive Safety - No listed contraindications are noted.

The oral lufenuron products are considered to be safe to use in pregnant, breeding or lactating animals; safety of the injectable product in reproducing cats has not been formally established at this time.

Adverse Effects/Warnings - Adverse effects reported in dogs and cats after oral lufenuron include: vomiting, lethargy/depression, pruritus/urticaria, diarrhea, dyspnea, anorexia and reddened skin. The manufacturer reports that the adverse reaction rate is less than 5 animals in one million doses.

After receiving the injectable product, a small lump at the injection site has been noted in some cats. A few weeks may be required for this to dissipate.

Overdosage - Growing puppies were dosed at levels up to 30X for 10 months without overt effect on growth or viability noted. Cats receiving oral dosages of up to 17X apparently were unaffected.

Drug Interactions - Limited data available; the manufacturer states that when used with a variety of adulticides, vaccines, antibiotics, anthelminthics and steroids no adverse effects or interactions were noted in either dogs or cats.

Doses -

Dogs:

> For control of flea populations: Lufenuron 10 mg/kg PO once monthly. See dosage form recommendations below. (Package Insert—*Program*®; Novartis)

> For control of fleas, heartworm prevention, hookworm, ascarid or whipworms: Lufenuron/Milbemycin (Sentinel®) at 10 mg/kg lufenuron/0.5 mg/kg milbemycin PO once monthly. See dosage form recommendations below. (Package Insert—*Program*®; Novartis)

Cats:

> For control of flea populations: Lufenuron 30 mg/kg PO once monthly or 10 mg/kg SubQ once every 6 months. See dosage form recommendations below. (Package Insert—*Program*®; Novartis)

Monitoring Parameters - Efficacy

Client Information - Must be used every 30 days to maximize efficacy. All animals in a household should be treated. If animal vomits within 2 hours after dosing, the drug should be re-dosed. If a dose is missed, re-dose and then resume a monthly dosage regimen (dogs receiving the lufenuron/milbemycin product should be tested in 6 months or more for heartworm exposure with an antigen test). Do not split tablets.

Dosage Forms/Preparations/FDA Approval Status -

Veterinary-Approved Products:

> Lufenuron Oral Tablets in six tablet cards or strips: 45 mg (for dogs up to 10 lb..,—brown), 90 mg (for dogs 11 to 20 lb..,—red), 204.9 mg (for dogs 21 to 45 lb..,—yellow), 409.8 mg (for dogs 46 to 90 lb..,—white); *Program*® (Novartis) (Rx). Approved for use in dogs.

> Lufenuron Oral Suspension in six tube packs: 135 mg (for cats up to 10 lb..,—orange), 270 mg (for cats 11 to 20 lb..,—green); *Program*® (Novartis) (Rx). Approved for use in cats.

> Lufenuron 6 Month Injectable for Cats 100 mg/ml in 10 syringe packages: 0.4 ml (40 mg) prefilled syringe (for cats up to 8.8 lb..), 0.8 ml (80 mg) prefilled syringe (for cats 8.9 - 17.6 lb..); *Program*® *6 Month Injectable* (Novartis) (Rx). Approved for use in cats.

> Milbemycin/Lufenuron Oral Tablets in six tablet cards: 2.3 mg/46 mg (for dogs 2 to 10 lb..,—brown), 5.75 mg/115 mg (for dogs 11 to 25 lb..,—green), 11.5 mg/230 mg (for dogs 26 to 50 lb..,—yellow), 23 mg/460 mg (for dogs 51 to 100 lb..,—white); *Sentinel*® *Flavor Tabs* (Novartis) (Rx). Approved for use in dogs.

Lysodren® **- see Mitotane**

Magnesium containing Laxatives - see Saline/Hyperosmotic Laxatives

Magnesium containing Antacids - see Antacids, Oral

MAGNESIUM
MAGNESIUM SULFATE, PARENTERAL

For information on the use of oral magnesium hydroxide, refer to the monograph for Oral Antacids in the GI section. Magnesium oxide and oral magnesium sulfate are also detailed in the monograph for Saline/Hyperosmotic laxatives in the GI section

Chemistry - Magnesium sulfate occurs as small, usually needle-like, colorless crystals with a cool, saline, bitter taste. It is freely soluble in water and sparingly soluble in alcohol. Magnesium sulfate injection has a pH of 5.5-7. One gram of magnesium sulfate hexahydrate contains 8.1 mEq of magnesium. Magnesium sulfate is also known as Epsom salts.

Storage/Stability/Compatibility - Magnesium sulfate for injection should be stored at room temperature (15-30°C); avoid freezing. Refrigeration may result in precipitation or crystallization.

Magnesium sulfate is reportedly **compatible** with the following intravenous solutions and drugs: dextrose 5%, calcium gluconate, cephalothin sodium, chloramphenicol sodium succinate, cisplatin, hydrocortisone sodium succinate, isoproterenol HCl, methyldopate HCl, metoclopramide HCl (in syringes), norepinephrine bitartrate, penicillin G potassium, potassium phosphate, and verapamil HCl. Additionally, at Y-sites: acyclovir sodium, amikacin sulfate, ampicillin sodium, carbenicillin disodium, cefamandole naftate, cefazolin sodium, cefoperazone sodium, ceforanide, cefotaxime sodium, cefoxitin sodium, cephalothin sodium, cephapirin sodium, clindamycin phosphate, doxycycline phosphate, erythromycin lactobionate, esmolol HCl, gentamicin sulfate, heparin sodium, kanamycin sulfate, labetolol HCl, metronidazole (RTU), moxalactam disodium, nafcillin sodium, oxacillin sodium, piperacillin sodium, potassium chloride, tetracycline HCl, ticarcillin disodium, tobramycin sulfate, trimethoprim/sulfamethoxasole, vancomycin HCl, and vitamin B-complex with C.

Magnesium sulfate is reportedly **incompatible** with alkali hydroxides, alkali carbonates, salicylates and many metals, including the following solutions or drugs: fat emulsion 10 %, calcium gluceptate, dobutamine HCl, polymyxin B sulfate, procaine HCl, and sodium bicarbonate. Compatibility is dependent upon factors such as pH, concentration, temperature and diluents used. It is suggested to consult specialized references for more specific information (*e.g., Handbook on Injectable Drugs* by Trissel; see bibliography).

Pharmacology - Magnesium is used as a cofactor in a variety of enzyme systems and plays a role in muscular excitement and neurochemical transmission.

Uses/Indications - Parenteral magnesium sulfate is used as a source of magnesium in magnesium deficient states (hypomagnesemia), for adjunctive therapy of malignant hyperthermia in swine, and also as an anticonvulsant.

Pharmacokinetics - IV magnesium results in immediate effects, IM administration may require about 1 hour for effect. Magnesium is about 30-35% bound to proteins and the remainder exists as free ions. It is excreted by the kidneys at a rate proportional to the serum concentration and glomerular filtration.

Contraindications/Precautions - Parenteral magnesium is contraindicated in patients with myocardial damage or heart block. Magnesium should be given with caution to patients with impaired renal function. Patients receiving parenteral magnesium should be observed and monitored carefully to avoid hypermagnesemia.

Adverse Effects/Warnings - Magnesium sulfate (parenteral) adverse effects are generally the result of magnesium overdosage and may include drowsiness or other CNS depressant effects, muscular weakness, bradycardia, hypotension, respiratory depression and increased Q-T intervals on ECG. Very high magnesium levels may cause neuromuscular blocking activity and eventually cardiac arrest.

Overdosage/Acute Toxicity - See Adverse Effects above. Treatment of hypermagnesemia is dependent on the serum magnesium level and any associated clinical effects. Ventilatory support and administration of intravenous calcium may be required for severe hypermagnesemia.

Drug Interactions - When parenteral magnesium sulfate is used with **other CNS depressant agents** (*e.g.,* **barbiturates, general anesthetics**) additive CNS depression may occur.

Parenteral magnesium sulfate with **nondepolarizing neuromuscular blocking agents** has caused excessive neuromuscular blockade.

Because serious conduction disturbances can occur, parenteral magnesium should be used with extreme caution with **digitalis cardioglycosides**.

Concurrent use of **calcium salts** may negate the effects of parenteral magnesium.

Doses -
   Dogs & Cats:
   For hypomagnesemia:
   a) Magnesium sulfate 25% solution: Dose is dependent on magnitude of intoxication, but usually ranges from 5 - 15 ml IM or IV over 1-2 hours; have calcium gluconate available should magnesium intoxication occur. (Seeler and Thurmon 1985)
   b) 0.75 - 1 mEq/kg/day administered by a constant rate infusion in D5W. Concentrate should be diluted to at least 20%. . A lower dose of 0.3 - 0.5 mEq/kg/day may be used for an additional 3-5 days as complete repletion occurs slowly. If needed for life-threatening ventricluar arrhythmias: 0.15 - 0.3 mEq/kg may be administered over 5 - 15 minutes. (Holland and Chastain 1995)

   Ruminants:
   For hypomagnesemia (grass and other magnesium-related tetanies):
   a) Cattle: Magnesium sulfate 20-50%: 200 ml SQ, followed by a slow IV infusion of 500 ml of a calcium/magnesium solution (Calcium borogluconate 23%; MgCl2 6%). (Phillips 1988a)
   b) Cattle: 350 ml (250 ml of 25% calcium borogluconate and 100 ml of 10% of magnesium sulfate) by slow IV. If not a proprietary mixture, give calcium first. Relapses occur frequently after IV therapy, and 350 ml SQ of magnesium sulfate 20% may give more sustained magnesium levels. Alternating calcium and magnesium may prevent adverse effects. Continue control measures for 4-7 days to prevent relapse.
   Sheep and Goats: 50 - 100 ml of above solution (calcium/magnesium).
   For whole milk tetany in calves 2-4 months of age: Magnesium sulfate 10% 100 ml; followed by oral magnesium oxide at daily doses of 1 gram PO (0-5 weeks old), 2 gram PO (5-10 weeks old), and 3 grams PO (10-15 weeks old). (Merrall and West 1986)

   Swine:
   For adjunctive therapy of malignant hyperthermia syndrome:
   a) Magnesium sulfate 50%: Incremental doses of 1 gram injected slowly IV until heart rate and muscle tone are reduced. Use calcium if magnesium-related cardiac arrest occur. (Booth 1988)

Monitoring Parameters -
   1) Serum magnesium
   2) Physical signs and symptoms associated with hypomagnesemia
   3) Serum calcium if indicated

Dosage Forms/Preparations/FDA Approval Status/Withholding Times -
   Veterinary-Approved Products: There are no parenteral magnesium-only products approved for veterinary medicine. There are, however, several proprietary magnesium-containing products available that may also include calcium, phosphorus, potassium and/or dextrose; refer to the individual product's labeling for specific dosage information. Trade names for these products include: *Norcalciphos®*—Pfizer, *Cal-Dextro® Special,* & *#2,*—Fort Dodge, and *CMPK®,* & *Cal-Phos® #2*—(TechAmerica). They are legend (Rx) drugs.

   Human-Approved Products:
   Magnesium Sulfate Injection 10% (0.8 mEq/ml), 12.5% (1 mEq/ml), & 50% (4 mEq/ml) in 2, 5, 10, 20 & 50 ml amps, vials and/or syringes; Generic; (Rx)

MANNITOL

Chemistry - An osmotic diuretic, mannitol occurs as an odorless, sweet-tasting, white, crystalline powder with a melting range of 165° - 168° and a pK_a of 3.4. One gram is soluble in about 5.5 ml of water (at 25°) and it is very slightly soluble in alcohol. The commercially available injectable products have approximate pH's of 4.5 - 7.

Storage/Stability/Compatibility - Mannitol solutions are stable but are recommended to be stored at room temperature; avoid freezing.

Crystallization may occur at low temperatures in concentrations greater than 15% (see procedure for resolubolization in Dosage Forms/Preparations section). Alternatively, heated storage chambers (35° - 50°C) have been suggested to assure that soluble product is available at all times. Microwaving glass ampules/vials has been suggested, but explosions have been documented and this procedure cannot be recommended. Supersaturated solutions of mannitol in PVC bags may show a white floccullant precipitate that will tend to reoccur even after heating.

Drugs reported to be **compatible** with mannitol include: amikacin sulfate, bretylium tosylate, cefamandole naftate, cefoxitin sodium, cimetidine HCl, dopamine HCl, gentamicin sulfate, metoclopramide HCl, netilmicin sulfate, tobramycin sulfate, and verapamil HCl.

Mannitol should not be added to whole blood products to be used for transfusion. Sodium or potassium chloride can cause mannitol to precipitate out of solution when mannitol concentrations are 20% or greater. Mannitol may be incompatible with strongly acidic or alkaline solutions.

Mannitol is reportedly stable when mixed with cisplatin for a short period of time, but advanced premixing of the drugs should be avoided because of a complex that may form between the two drugs.

Pharmacology - After intravenous administration, mannitol is freely filtered at the glomerulus and poorly reabsorbed in the tubule. The increased osmotic pressure prevents water from being reabsorbed at the tubule. To be effective, there must be sufficient renal blood flow and filtration for mannitol to reach the tubules. Although water is proportionately excreted at a higher rate, sodium, other electrolytes, uric acid and urea excretions are also enhanced.

Mannitol may have a nephro-protective effect by preventing the concentration of nephrotoxins from accumulating in the tubular fluid. Additionally, it may increase renal blood flow and glomerular filtration by causing renal arteriole dilatation, decreased vascular resistance and decreased blood viscosity.

Mannitol does not appreciably enter the eye or the CNS, but can decrease intraocular and CSF pressure through its osmotic effects. Rebound increases in CSF pressures may occur after the drug is discontinued.

Uses/Indications - Mannitol is used to promote diuresis in acute oliguric renal failure, reduce intraocular and intracerebral pressures, enhance urinary excretion of some toxins (*e.g.,* aspirin, some barbiturates, bromides, ethylene glycol) and, in conjunction with other diuretics to rapidly reduce edema or ascites when appropriate (see Contraindications-/Precautions below). In humans, it is also used as an irrigating solution during transurethral prostatic resections.

Pharmacokinetics - Although long believed to be unabsorbed from the GI, up to 17% of an oral dose is excreted unchanged in the urine after oral dosing in humans. After intravenous dosing, mannitol is distributed to the extracellular compartment and does not penetrate the eye. Unless the patient has received very high doses, is acidotic, or there is loss of integrity of the blood-brain barrier, it does not cross into the CNS.

Only 7-10% of mannitol is metabolized, the remainder is excreted unchanged in the urine. The elimination half-life of mannitol is approximately 100 minutes in adult humans. Half-lives in cattle and sheep are reported to be between 40-60 minutes.

Contraindications/Precautions - Mannitol is contraindicated in patients with anuria secondary to renal disease, severe dehydration, intracranial bleeding (unless during craniotomy), severe pulmonary congestion or pulmonary edema.

Mannitol therapy should be stopped if progressive heart failure, pulmonary congestion, progressive renal failure or damage (including increasing oliguria and azotemia) develop after mannitol therapy is instituted.

Do not administer more than a test dose of mannitol until determining whether the patient has some renal function and urine output. Adequate fluid replacement must be administered to dehydrated animals before mannitol therapy is begun. Do not give mannitol with whole blood products, unless at least 20 mEq/l of sodium chloride is added to the solution or pseudo-agglutination may result.

Adverse Effects/Warnings - Fluid and electrolyte imbalances are the most severe adverse effects generally encountered during mannitol therapy. Adequate monitoring and support are imperative.

Other adverse effects that may be encountered include GI (nausea, vomiting), cardiovascular (pulmonary edema, CHF, tachycardia), and CNS effects (dizziness, headache, etc.).

Overdosage - Inadvertent overdosage can cause excessive excretion of sodium, potassium and chloride. If urine output is inadequate, water intoxication or pulmonary edema may occur. Treat by halting mannitol administration and monitoring and correcting electrolyte and fluid imbalances. Hemodialysis is effective in clearing mannitol.

Drug Interactions - Mannitol can increase the renal elimination of **lithium**.

Drug/Laboratory Interactions - Mannitol can interfere with blood inorganic **phosphorus** concentrations and blood **ethylene glycol** determinations.

Doses -
Dogs, Cats:
   For treatment of oliguric renal failure:
      a) After correcting fluid, electrolyte, acid/base balance and determining that the patient is not anuric: Mannitol (20 - 25% solution) 0.25 - 0.5 gm/kg IV over 15-20 minutes.

If diuresis occurs, may repeat q4-6 hours or administered as a constant infusion (8 - 10% solution) for first 12-24 hours of therapy. Note: This method is a secondary choice of therapy; furosemide with dopamine is therapy of first choice.) (Polzin and Osborne 1985)

   b) After rehydration, give mannitol 0.5 gm/kg IV slowly; repeat dose at 15 minute intervals up to 1.5 gm/kg total. Urine production should begin with 15 minutes; monitor carefully for dehydration and give fluids as necessary to maintain balance. (Breitschwerdt 1988)

For treatment of acute glaucoma: (Note: See also the monographs for acetazolamide and glycerin)

   a) 1 - 2 gm/kg IV over 15-20 minute period; withhold water for 30-60 minutes after administration (Brooks 1986)

   b) 1 - 3 gm/kg IV of a 20 -25% solution. Withhold water for first few hours after dosing. May repeat 2-4 times in the first 48 hours; monitor animal for signs of dehydration. (Vestre 1985)

For adjunctive treatment of increased CSF pressure:

   a) 1.5 gm/kg IV once (Fenner 1986)

To measure glomerular filtration rate in dogs:

   a) 1.1 - 2.2 grams/kg IV slowly over 15-30 minutes (McConnell and Hughey 1987)

Cattle, Swine, Sheep, Goats:
For adjunctive treatment of cerebral edema:

   a) 1 - 3 gm/kg IV (usually with steroids and/or DMSO) (Dill 1986)

As a diuretic for oliguric renal failure:

   a) 1 - 2 gm/kg (5-10 ml of 20% solution) IV after rehydration; monitor urine flow and fluid balance (Osweiler 1986)

Horses:

   a) 0.25 - 2.0 gm/kg as a 20% solution by slow IV infusion (Schultz 1986)

Monitoring Parameters -
   a) Serum electrolytes, osmolality
   b) BUN, serum creatinine
   c) Urine output
   d) Central venous pressure, if possible
   e) Lung auscultation

Client Information - Mannitol should be administered by professional staff in a setting where adequate monitoring can occur.

Dosage Forms/Preparations/FDA Approval Status/Withholding Times -
  Veterinary-Approved Products:

Mannitol for Injection 180 mg/ml in 100 ml vials; *Mannitol Injection*® (Anthony) (Rx); Approved for use in dogs

  Human-Approved Products:
Mannitol for Injection
   5% (50 mg/ml; 275 mOsm/l) in 1000 ml
   10% (100 mg/ml; 550 mOsm/l) in 500 and 1000 ml
   15% (150 mg/ml; 825 mOsm/l) in 500 ml
   20% (200 mg/ml; 1100 mOsm/l) in 250 and 500 ml
   25% (250 mg/ml; 1375 mOsm/l) in 50 ml vials & syringes (12.5 grams/vial)

Note: Mannitol may tend to crystallize in concentrations of 15% or more when exposed to low temperatures. Resolubolization of the crystals can be accomplished by heating the bottle in hot (up to 80°C) water. Cool to body temperature before administering. An in-line IV filter is recommended when administering concentrated mannitol solutions.

MECHLORETHAMINE HCL

Chemistry - A bifunctional alkylating agent, mechlorethamine occurs as a hygroscopic, white, crystalline powder that is very soluble in water. After reconstitution with sterile water or sterile saline, the resultant solution is clear and has a pH of 3-5.

Storage/Stability/Compatibility - Store the powder for injection at room temperature. Mechlorethamine is highly unstable in neutral or alkaline aqueous solutions and rapidly degrades. While more stable in an acidic environment, the drug should be administered immediately after preparation. Mechlorethamine may also be known as nitrogen mustard, mustine or HN_2.

Pharmacology - Mechlorethamine is an alkylating agent, thereby interfering with DNA replication, RNA transcription, and protein synthesis. It is cell cycle-phase nonspecific.

With intracavitary administration, mechlorethamine causes sclerosing and an inflammatory response on serous membranes, thereby causing adherence of serosal surfaces.

Uses/Indications - In small animals, mechlorethamine may be useful for the adjunctive treatment of lymphoreticular neoplasms or with intracavitary administration, for treating pleural and peritoneal effusions.

Pharmacokinetics - Because mechlorethamine is so irritating to tissues it must be given IV for systemic use. It is incompletely absorbed after intracavitary administration. After injection, mechlorethamine is rapidly (within minutes) inactivated.

Contraindications/Precautions/Reproductive Safety - Mechlorethamine should be used only when its potential benefits outweigh its risks with the following conditions: anemia, bone marrow depression, tumor cell infiltration into bone marrow, current infection, sensitivity to mechlorethamine or patients who have received previous chemotherapy or radiotherapy.

Mechlorethamine is a teratogen in lab animals. Use only during pregnancy when the benefits to the mother outweigh the risks to the offspring. Mechlorethamine can suppress gonadal function. While it is unknown whether mechlorethamine enters maternal milk, nursing puppies or kittens should receive milk replacer when the bitch or queen is receiving mechlorethamine.

Adverse Effects/Warnings - Bone marrow depression, GI effects (vomiting, nausea) are quite common and can be serious and therapy halting. Ototoxicity may occur with either high dosages or regional perfusions. Other potential effects include alopecia, hyperuricemia, hepatotoxicity, peripheral neuropathy and GI ulcers.

Because severe tissue sloughing may occur; avoid extravasation.

Overdosage/Acute Toxicity - Because of the toxic potential of this agent, overdoses must be avoided. Determine dosages carefully.

Drug Interactions - Use extreme caution when used concurrently with other drugs that are also myelosuppressive, including many of the **other antineoplastics and other bone marrow depressant drugs (*e.g.*, chloramphenicol, flucytosine, amphotericin B, or colchicine)**. Bone marrow depression may be additive. Use with other **immunosuppressant drugs (*e.g.*, azathioprine, cyclophosphamide, corticosteroids**) may increase the risk of infection. **Live virus vaccines** should be used with caution if at all during therapy.

Laboratory Considerations - Mechlorethamine may raise serum **uric acid** levels. Drugs such as allopurinol may be required to control hyperuricemia.

Doses -
  Dogs:
    For the adjunctive treatment of lymphoreticular neoplasms or with intracavitary administration for treating pleural and peritoneal effusions:
      a) 5 mg/m^2 IV or intracavitary; repeat prn. (Jacobs, Lumsden et al. 1992)

Monitoring Parameters - 1) CBC with platelets at least every 1-2 weeks until stable; then every 3 months; 2) Liver function tests; initially before starting treatment and then every 3-4 months; 3) Injection site for signs of extravasation

Dosage Forms/Preparations/FDA Approval Status/Withholding Times -
  Veterinary-Approved Products: None
  Human-Approved Products:
    Mechlorethamine Powder for Injection 10 mg; *Mustargen*® (Merck); (Rx)

MECLIZINE HCL

Chemistry - Meclizine HCl is a piperazine derivative antiemetic antihistamine.

Storage/Stability/Compatibility - Meclizine products should be stored at room temperature in well-closed containers.

Pharmacology - Meclizine is a piperazine antihistamine and beside its antihistamine activity, it also possesses antiemetic, CNS depressant, antiemetic, antispasmodic and local anesthetic effects. The exact mechanism of action for its antiemetic and anti-motion-sickness effects are not completely understood, but it is thought they are as a result of the drug's central anticholinergic and CNS depressant activity. The antiemetic effect is probably mediated through the chemoreceptor trigger zone (CTZ).

Uses/Indications - Meclizine is principally used in small animals as an antiemetic and for the treatment and prevention of motion sickness.

Pharmacokinetics - Very little information is available. Meclizine is metabolized in the liver and has a serum half life of about 6 hours.

Contraindications/Precautions/Reproductive Safety - Meclizine is contraindicated in patients hypersensitive to it. It should be used with caution in patients with prostatic hypertrophy, bladder neck obstruction, severe cardiac failure, angle-closure glaucoma or pyeloduodenal obstruction. Meclizine is considered to be teratogenic in animals. Cleft palates have been noted in rats at 25-50 times higher than labeled dosages. It should be used during pregnancy only when the potential benefits outweigh the risks. It is unknown if it enters maternal milk and its anticholinergic activity may potentially inhibit lactation.

Adverse Effects/Warnings - The usual adverse effect noted with meclizine is sedation; less frequently anticholinergic effects may be noted (dry mucous membranes, eyes, tachycardia, etc.). Contradictory CNS stimulation has also been reported.

Overdosage/Acute Toxicity - Moderate overdosage may result in drowsiness alternating with hyperexcitability. Massive overdosages may result in profound CNS depression, hallucinations, seizures and other anticholinergic effects (tachycardia, urinary retention, etc.). Treatment is considered symptomatic and supportive. Consider gut emptying when patients present soon after ingestion. Avoid respiratory depressant medications.

Drug Interactions - Use with **other CNS depressants** may cause additive sedation. Other **anticholinergic drugs** may cause additive anticholinergic effects.

Laboratory Considerations - Because these drugs are antihistamines, they may affect the results of **skin tests using allergen extracts**. Do not use within 3-7 days before testing.

Doses -
Dogs:
    a) 25 mg per dog PO once daily, for motion sickness: give one hour before traveling. (Papich 1992)
    b) As an antihistamine: 25 mg PO once daily (Bevier 1990)

Cats:
    a) 12.5 mg per cat PO once daily. (Papich 1992)
    b) 6.25 mg/5 kg of body weight PO (Day 1993)

Monitoring Parameters - 1) Efficacy; 2) Adverse Effects

Client Information - When using for motion sickness prevention, instruct client to give medication 30 - 60 minutes before travel.

Dosage Forms/Preparations/FDA Approval Status/Withholding Times -
Veterinary-Approved Products: None
Human-Approved Products:

Meclizine HCl Tablets 12.5 mg, 25 mg, 50 mg; *Antivert*® (Roerig) (Rx), *Antrizine*® (Major) (Rx); *Antivert/25*® (Roerig) (Rx), *Dramamine II*® (Upjohn) (OTC); *Ru-Vert-M*® (Solvay) (Rx); *Bonine*® (Leeming) (OTC); *Dizmiss*® (JMI Canton) (OTC); *Antivert/50*® (Roerig) (Rx); generic; (Rx). Note: 25 mg chewable tablets may be labeled OTC.

Meclizine Oral Capsules 25 mg, 30 mg; *Meni-D*® (Seatrace); (Rx); *Vergon*® (Marnel) (OTC)

MECLOFENAMIC ACID

Chemistry - An anthranilic acid derivative (fenamate), meclofenamic acid is a white, crystalline powder that is practically insoluble in water. The sodium salt of meclofenamic acid is available commercially for human use. It is freely soluble in water.

Storage/Stability/Compatibility - Should be stored in tight, light-resistant packaging at temperatures below 30°C (86°F).

Pharmacology - Meclofenamic acid exhibits pharmacologic actions similar to those of aspirin. It is a potent inhibitor of cyclooxygenase, thereby inhibiting the release of prostaglandins. Like aspirin, meclofenamic acid (sodium salt administered IV) has been demonstrated to reduce the cardiovascular and respiratory effects of experimentally induced anaphylaxis in ponies and calves by its antagonistic effects at high concentrations on histamine, kinins, and prostaglandins.

It also has a transient effect on platelet aggregation, but unlike aspirin, does not appear to affect bleeding times.

Pharmacokinetics - Meclofenamic acid is reported to be well absorbed following oral administration, with measurable plasma levels being reached in 30 minutes and peak levels in 1-4 hours.

In studies done with monkeys, highest meclofenamic acid levels were detected in the plasma, liver, and kidneys. Lower levels were detected in skeletal muscle, fat, spleen, heart, and brain. At plasma levels of 1 micrograms/ml, the drug was 99.8% bound to albumin. It rapidly crosses the placenta, but it is unknown whether it is distributed into milk.

The plasma half-life has been reported to range from 1-8 hours in horses. Therapeutic efficacy does not seem to be closely related with blood levels, however, as the onset of action may take 36-96 hours and significant efficacy may be seen for days following a dose.

Meclofenamic acid is metabolized in the liver primarily by oxidation to an active hydroxymethyl metabolite which may be further oxidized to an inactive metabolite (carboxyl). In humans, meclofenamic acid and its metabolites are then excreted by the kidneys (approx. 70% within 7 days) or eliminated with the feces (20-30%). In horses, meclofenamic acid can be detected in the urine for at least 96 hours following the final dose.

Uses/Indications - Meclofenamic acid is used clinically in dogs for the symptomatic relief of symptoms associated with chronic inflammatory disease of the musculoskeletal system; often in an attempt to improve mobility in animals with hip dysplasia or chronic osteoarthritis.

In horses, it is indicated for the "oral treatment of acute or chronic inflammatory diseases involving the musculoskeletal system..." (Package Insert; *Arquel*®—Parke-Davis). Meclofenamic acid has also been used for the treatment of laminitis, with varying degrees of success.

Contraindications/Precautions - The manufacturer states that meclofenamic acid is contraindicated in animals with "active gastrointestinal, hepatic or renal diseases" (Package Insert; *Arquel*®—Parke-Davis). Additionally, meclofenamic acid is contraindicated in patients demonstrating previous hypersensitivity reactions to it or salicylates. It is relatively contraindicated in patients with active or historical hemorrhagic disorders, or bronchospastic disease. Because meclofenamic acid is highly bound to plasma proteins, patients with hypoproteinemia may require lower dosages to prevent symptoms of toxicity.

Meclofenamic acid has been shown to delay parturition in some species and therefore should be avoided during the last stages of pregnancy. It has caused teratogenic effects (minor skeletal abnormalities, delayed ossification) in rodents. Some preliminary studies have shown no effects with regard to either mare or stallion reproductive performance and no gross defects were seen in foals born to mares who received meclofenamic acid during pregnancy. It should, nevertheless, be used in pregnancy only when the potential benefits outweigh the potential risks of therapy.

Adverse Effects/Warnings - Adverse reactions are reported to be fairly uncommon in horses. However, hematologic changes (decreased hematocrit/PCV) and GI effects (buccal erosions, diarrhea, colic, anorexia, changes in stool consistency) have been reported. The diarrheal and colic reactions may be more likely in horses that have a heavy infestation of bots (*Gasterophilus* sp.) With chronic therapy, decreases in plasma protein concentrations may occur.

In dogs, vomiting, decreased hemoglobin, leukocytosis, tarry stools, and small intestinal ulcers have all been reported following therapy at usual effective doses. Clients should be counseled with regard to these potential adverse effects and instructed to monitor their animal carefully for symptoms associated with them.

In humans, NSAIDs have caused hepatotoxicity and it is recommended that human patients receiving chronic meclofenamate sodium therapy undergo occasional liver function tests. Although it does not appear that this adverse reaction is of major concern in either dogs or horses, the potential for hepatotoxicity does exist.

Overdosage - There is very limited information regarding acute overdoses of this drug in humans and no information was located regarding overdoses in domestic animals. Following an acute, massive overdose in humans, generalized CNS stimulation initially occurs, with seizures possible. After this initial phase, acute renal failure may occur with secondary azotemia and anuria.

Treatment should follow standard overdose procedures (empty gut following oral ingestion, etc.). Supportive treatment should be instituted as necessary and IV diazepam used to help control seizures. Because meclofenamic acid may cause renal effects, monitor electrolyte and fluid balance carefully and manage renal failure using established guidelines.

Drug Interactions - Because meclofenamic acid is highly bound to plasma proteins and may displace other highly bound drugs, increased serum levels and duration of actions of **phenytoin, valproic acid, oral anticoagulants**, other **anti-inflammatory agents, salicylates, sulfonamides**, and the **sulfonylurea antidiabetic agents** can occur. If meclofenamic acid is used concurrently with **warfarin**, enhanced hypoprothrombinemic effects may transpire.

When **aspirin** is used concurrently with meclofenamic acid, plasma levels of meclofenamic acid may decrease as well as a likelihood of increased GI adverse effects (blood loss) developing. Concomitant administration of aspirin with meclofenamic acid is not recommended.

Doses -
　Dogs:
　　　a) 1.1 mg/kg PO daily for 5-7 days (Booth 1988a)
　　　b) 1.1 mg/kg PO daily for 5-7 days, if therapeutic results are obtained, hold dose until signs exacerbate and then give 1.1 mg/kg every 3rd day for 7 days. If still efficacious, give dose every 4th day. Then every 5th day, etc. until signs recur. Then drop back to

the dosing interval where symptomatic relief is obtained until next dose. (McConnell and Hughey 1987)

   c) 1.1 mg/kg PO daily; at the same time each day and after a full meal (Wallace 1988)

Note: 1/4 teaspoonful of the granules contains approximately 55 mg meclofenamic acid. Alternatively, an oral solution may be prepared by adding a 500 mg (10 gram) packet to 120 ml of water. One ml of this solution will contain approximately 4.1 mg of meclofenamic acid. At the doses listed above one ml will treat a 10 pound dog. (McConnell and Hughey 1987)

Horses:

   a) 2.2 mg/kg PO once daily for 5-7 days, this equates to two 500 mg packets per 454 kg (1000 lb.) animal daily. If treatment is desired past the 7 days recommended, decrease the dosage and increase the dosing interval to obtain the lowest effective dose. The package contents may be added to the daily grain feed ration, a moist feed with molasses added will help to prevent separation of the granules from the feed. (Package Insert; *Arquel*®, Parke-Davis, 1981)

   b) 2.2 mg/kg PO q12h (Jenkins 1987)

Monitoring Parameters -

   1) Analgesic/anti-inflammatory efficacy

   2) GI: appetite, feces (occult blood, diarrhea)

   3) PCV (packed cell volume), hematocrit if indicated or on chronic therapy

   4) WBC's if indicated or on chronic therapy

Client Information/FDA Approval Status - Notify veterinarian if symptoms of GI distress (anorexia, vomiting in dogs, diarrhea, black feces or blood in stool) occur or if the animal becomes depressed.

   Meclofenamic acid is approved for use in dogs (see note below regarding available dosage forms) and horses (not intended for food). Meclofenamic acid is a veterinary prescription (legend) drug.

Dosage Forms/Preparations -

Veterinary-Approved Products:

   Meclofenamic acid 5% granules in 10 gram packets (500 mg meclofenamic acid/10 gram packet) & scored 10 mg & 20 mg tablets; *Arquel*® (Fort Dodge)

MEDETOMIDINE HCL

Chemistry/Storage/Stability/Compatibility - An alpha2-adrenergic agonist, medetomidine occurs as a white or almost white crystalline substance. It is soluble in water. While the compound exists as two stereoisomers, only the D-isomer is active.

   The commercially available injection should be stored at room temperature (15-30°C) and protected from freezing.

Pharmacology - An alpha adrenergic receptor, medetomidine has an alpha2:alpha1 selectivity factor of 1620, and when compared to xylazine is reportedly 10X more specific for alpha2 receptors versus alpha1 receptors. The pharmacologic effects of medetomidine include: depression of CNS (sedation), GI (decreased secretions, varying affects on intestinal muscle tone) and endocrine functions, peripheral and cardiac vasoconstriction, bradycardia, respiratory depression, diuresis, hypothermia, analgesia, muscle relaxation, blanched or cyanotic mucous membranes and anxiolytic effects. Effects on blood pressure are variable.

Uses/Indications - Medetomidine is labeled for use as a sedative and analgesic in dogs over 12 weeks of age to facilitate clinical examinations and procedures, minor surgical procedures not requiring muscle relaxation, and minor dental procedures not requiring intubation. The manufacturer recommends the IV route of administration for dental procedures.

   Medetomidine has also been used in cats, primarily in Europe. But there is apparently much less data available to evaluate its use; caution is advised.

Pharmacokinetics - After IV or IM injection, onset of effect is rapid (5 mins. for IV; 10-15 mins. for IM). After subQ injection, responses are unreliable and this method of administration cannot be recommended. The drug is absorbed via the oral mucosa when administered sublingually in dogs, but efficacy at a given dose may be less than IM dosing.

Contraindications/Precautions/Reproductive Safety - The label states that medetomidine is contraindicated in dogs having the following conditions: cardiac disease, respiratory disorders, liver or kidney diseases, shock, severe debilitation, or dogs stressed due to heat, cold or fatigue.

   Dogs that are extremely agitated or excited may have a decreased response to medetomidine, the manufacturer suggests allowing these dogs to rest quietly before administration of the drug.

Dogs not responding to medetomidine should not be re-dosed. Use in very young or older dogs should be done with caution.

The drug is not recommended to be used in pregnant dogs or those used for breeding purposes as safety data for use during pregnancy is insufficient; therefore use only when the benefits clearly outweigh the drug's benefits.

Adverse Effects/Warnings - The adverse effects reported with medetomidine are basically an extension of its pharmacologic effects including bradycardia, occasional AV blocks, decreased respiration, hypothermia, urination, vomiting, hyperglycemia, and pain on injection (IM). Rare effects have also been reported, including prolonged sedation, paradoxical excitation, hypersensitivity, apnea and death from circulatory failure.

Overdosage - Single doses of up to 5X (IV) and 10X (IM) were tolerated in dogs, but adverse effects can occur (see above). Death has occurred rarely in dogs (1 in 40,000) receiving 2X doses.

Because of the potential of additional adverse effects occurring (heart block, PVC's or tachycardia), treatment of medetomidine-induced bradycardia with anticholinergic agents (atropine or glycopyrrolate) is often not recommended. Atipamezole is probably a safer choice to treat any medetomidine-induced effect.

Drug Interactions - Note: Before attempting combination therapy with medetomidine, it is strongly advised to access references from veterinary anesthesiologists familiar with the use of this product.

When **propofol** is used after medetomidine, hypoxemia may occur. Dosage adjustments may be required along with adequate monitoring. Enhancement of sedation and analgesia may occur when medetomidine is used concurrently with **fentanyl**, **butorphanol** or **meperidine**, but adverse effects may be pronounced as well. Reduced dosages and monitoring is advised if contemplating combination therapy. The use of **atropine** or **glycopyrrolate** to prevent or treat medetomidine-caused bradycardia is controversial as tachycardia and hypertension may result.

Doses -

Dogs:

For sedation/analgesia:

a) 750 mcg (0.75 mg)/m^2 body surface area IV or 1000 mcg (1 mg)/m^2 body surface area IM. Allow to rest quietly for 15 minutes after injection. Practically, the following dosing table may used:

IV Dosing Weight in lb.	Injection Volume in mls	IM Dosing Weight in lbs.
3-4	0.1	-
5-7	0.15	4-5
8-11	0.2	6-7
12-15	0.25	8-9
16-21	0.3	10-14
22-31	0.4	51-20
32-43	0.5	21-27
44-55	0.6	28-35
56-68	0.7	36-44
69-82	0.8	45-53
83-97	0.9	54-63
98-121	1	64-78
122-156	1.2	79-101
157-194	1.4	102-126
195+	1.6	127-165
-	2	166+

(Package Insert; Domitor®—Pfizer)

b) 10 - 40 mcg/kg IM; higher doses do not cause greater sedation, but increase the duration of effect (McGrath and Ko 1997a)

Cats: Caution not approved for this species.

For sedation/analgesia:

a) 40 - 80 mcg/kg IM; higher doses do not cause greater sedation, but increase the duration of effect (McGrath and Ko 1997a)

Monitoring Parameters - Level of sedation and analgesia; heart rate; body temperature. Additionally, heart rhythm, blood pressure, respiration rate and pulse oximetry should be considered, particularly in higher risk patients if the drug is to be used.

Client Information - This drug should be administered and monitored by veterinary professionals only. Clients should be made aware of the potential adverse effects associated with its use, particularly in dogs at risk (older, preexisting conditions).

Dosage Forms/Preparations/FDA Approval Status -
   Veterinary-Approved Products:
      Medetomidine HCl for Injection 1 mg/ml in 10 ml multidose vials; *Domitor*® (Pfizer); (Rx) Approved for use in dogs.

MEDIUM CHAIN TRIGLYCERIDES (MCT OIL)

Chemistry - MCT Oil is a lipid fraction of coconut oil consisting principally of the triglycerides C_8 (approx. 67%) and C_{10} (approx. 23%) saturated fatty acids. Each 15 ml contains 115 kcal (7.67 kcal/ml).

Storage/Stability/Compatibility - Unless otherwise noted by the manufacturer, store at room temperature in glass bottles.

Pharmacology - Medium chain triglycerides (MCT) are more readily hydrolyzed than conventional food fat. They also require less bile acids for digestion, are not dependent for chylomicron formation or lymphatic transport and are transported by the portal vein. Medium chain triglycerides are not a source for essential fatty acids.

Uses/Indications - MCT is used to offset the caloric reduction when long-chain triglycerides found in dietary fat are restricted, usually in chronic infiltrative diseases of the small intestine or when there is fat malabsorption of any cause.

Pharmacokinetics - No specific information located, see pharmacology above.

Contraindications/Precautions/Reproductive Safety - MCT oil should be used with caution in patients with significant hepatic disease (*e.g.*, portacaval shunts, cirrhosis, etc.). Because medium chain triglycerides are rapidly absorbed via the portal vein and their hepatic clearance is impaired, significantly high systemic blood and CSF levels of medium chain fatty acids can occur, thereby precipitating or exacerbating hepatic coma.

Although, no reproductive safety data was located, MCT oil would not likely cause problems.

Adverse Effects/Warnings - Adverse effects seen with MCT oil in small animals include, unpalatability, bloating, flatulence, and diarrhea. These may be transient and minimized by starting doses at the low end of the spectrum and then gradually increasing the dose. Fat soluble vitamin supplementation (Vitamins A, D, E, & K) by using a commercial feline or canine vitamin-mineral supplement has been recommended.

Overdosage/Acute Toxicity - Overdosage would likely exacerbate the GI adverse effects noted above. Treat severe diarrhea supportively if necessary.

Drug Interactions - None listed, but MCT oil could theoretically affect absorption of drugs that are dependent on fat (*e.g.,* griseofulvin, fat soluble vitamins, etc.).

Doses -
   Dogs:
      To offset the caloric reduction when long-chain triglycerides found in dietary fat are restricted:
      a)   1 - 2 ml/kg in daily ration of food (Sherding 1986)
      b)   Begin with one teaspoonful per meal added to food and slowly increase to a maximal tolerated dose, not to exceed 30 ml/lb of food. (Zimmer 1986)

Monitoring Parameters - 1) Adverse Effects/Efficacy (weight, stool consistency)

Client Information - Because of the unpalatability of the oil, it should be mixed with small quantities of food before offering to the patient.

Dosage Forms/Preparations/FDA Approval Status/Withholding Times -
   Veterinary-Approved Products: None
   Human-Approved Products:
      Medium Chain Triglycerides in quart bottles; *MCT*® *Oil* (Mead Johnson); (OTC)

MEDROXYPROGESTERONE ACETATE

Chemistry - A synthetic progestin, medroxyprogesterone acetate (MPA) occurs as an odorless, white to off-white, crystalline powder. It is insoluble in water and sparingly soluble in alcohol. It has a melting range of 200°-210°C. Medroxyprogesterone acetate may also be known as MPA, MAP, acetoxymethylprogesterone or methylacetoxyprogesterone.

Storage/Stability/Compatibility - Medroxyprogesterone acetate suspensions for injection should be stored at room temperature (15-30°C); avoid freezing and temperatures above 40°C. MPA tablets should be stored in well-closed containers at room temperature.

Pharmacology - Progestins are primarily produced endogenously by the corpus luteum. They transform proliferative endometrium to secretory endometrium, enhance myometrium hypertrophy and inhibit spontaneous uterine contraction. Progestins have a dose-dependent inhibitory effect on the secretion of pituitary gonadotropins and can have an anti-insulin effect. Medroxyprogesterone has exhibited a pronounced adrenocorticoid effect in animals (species not listed) and can suppress ACTH and cortisol release. MPA is anti-estrogenic and will also decrease plasma testosterone levels in male humans and dogs.

MPA has antineoplastic activity against endometrial carcinoma and renal carcinoma (efficacy in doubt) in human patients. The mechanism for this activity is not known.

Uses/Indications - In cats, MPA has been used when either castration is ineffective or undesirable to treat sexually dimorphic behavior problems such as roaming, inter-male aggressive behaviors, spraying, mounting, etc. MPA has also been used as a tranquilizing agent to treat syndromes such as feline psychogenic dermatitis and alopecia, but treatment with "true" tranquilizing agents may be preferable.

In humans, parenteral MPA has been used as a long-acting contraceptive in females, to decrease sexually deviant behavior in males and as an antineoplastic agent for some carcinomas (see Pharmacology section above). Oral MPA is used in human females to treat secondary amenorrhea and to treat abnormal uterine bleeding secondary to hormone imbalances.

Pharmacokinetics - No specific pharmacokinetic parameters in veterinary species were located for this drug. It has been reported (Beaver 1989) that injectable MPA has an approximate duration of action of 30 days when used to treat behavior disorders in cats. When administered IM to women, MPA has contraceptive activity for at least 3 months.

Contraindications/Precautions - Progestagen therapy can cause serious adverse effects (see below). Safer alternative treatments should be considered when possible, otherwise, weigh the potential risks versus benefits before instituting therapy. Many clinicians believe that progestagens are grossly overused.

Because this drug can suppress adrenal function, exogenous steroids may need to be administered if the patient is stressed (*e.g.,* surgery, trauma).

Adverse Effects/Warnings - If MPA is administered subcutaneously, permanent local alopecia, atrophy and depigmentation may occur. If injecting SQ, it is recommended to use the inguinal area to avoid these manifestations. Adverse reactions that are possible in dogs and cats include increased appetite and/or thirst, depression, lethargy, personality changes, adrenocortical depression, mammary changes (including enlargement, milk production, and neoplasms), diabetes mellitus, pyometra and temporary inhibition of spermatogenesis. In dogs, acromegaly and increased growth hormone levels have been seen when used in patients with diabetes mellitus.

Overdosage - No reports or information was located on inadvertent overdosage with this agent. Refer to the Adverse effects section above.

Drug Interactions - None reported. A potential interaction exists with **Rifampin**, which may decrease progestin activity if administered concomitantly. This is presumably due to microsomal enzyme induction with resultant increase in progestin metabolism. The clinical significance of this potential interaction is unknown.

Drug/Laboratory Interactions - In humans, progestins in combination with estrogens (*e.g.,* oral contraceptives) have been demonstrated to increase **thyroxine-binding globulin (TBG)** with resultant increases in total circulating thyroid hormone. Decreased **T3 resin uptake** also occurs, but free T4 levels are unaltered. **Liver function tests** may also be altered.

The manufacturer recommends **notifying the pathologist** of patient medroxyprogesterone exposure when submitting relevant specimens.

Doses -
  Dogs:
    For progestin-responsive dermatitis:
      a) 20 mg/kg IM; may repeat in 3-6 months if needed (Kunkle 1986)
    For adjunctive treatment of aggressive behaviors:
      a) 10 mg/kg IM or SQ (see Adverse effects above) as necessary; works best when combined with behavior modification. To treat inter-male aggression: as above, but do not exceed 3 treatments per year. (Voith and Marder 1988a)
  Cats:
    To treat behavioral disorders:
      a) Male cats: 100 mg IM initially, then reduce dosage by 1/3 - 1/2 and administer q30 days. Female cats: As above, but use 50 mg IM (Beaver 1989)

    b) 10 - 20 mg/kg SQ; may repeat as necessary up to 3 injections per year maximum (Voith and Marder 1988b)

For feline psychogenic alopecia and dermatitis:
    a) 75 - 150 mg IM or SQ (see Adverse effects above); repeat as necessary, but never more often than every 2-3 months. (Walton 1986)

For progestagen-responsive dermatitis:
    a) 50 - 100 mg IM may repeat in 3-6 months if needed (Kunkle 1986)

To treat recurrent abortion secondary to progesterone-deficiency:
    a) 1 - 2 mg/kg IM once weekly, stop treatment 7-10 days prior to parturition (Barton and Wolf 1988)

To alleviate signs of estrus and mating activity:
    a) 5 mg PO once daily for up to 5 days will alleviate signs within 24 hours. Parenteral MPA at 25 - 100 mg will inhibit estrus from 2-4 months. (Wildt 1986)
    b) 25 mg injected every 6 months to postpone estrus (Henik, Olson, and Rosychuk 1985)
For long-term reproductive control:
    a) 2.5 - 5 mg PO once weekly (Henik, Olson, and Rosychuk 1985)

Birds:
As an antipruritic and to suppress ovulation:
    a) 0.025 - 1 ml (3 mg/100 grams body weight) IM once every 4-6 weeks. May cause obesity, fatty liver, polydipsia/polyuria and lethargy if used repeatedly. (Clubb 1986)

Monitoring Parameters -
    1) Weight
    2) Blood glucose (draw baseline before therapy)
    3) Mammary gland development
    4) Adrenocortical function
    5) Efficacy

Dosage Forms/Preparations/FDA Approval Status/Withholding Times -
  Veterinary-Approved Products: None
  Human-Approved Products:
    Medroxyprogesterone Acetate Oral Tablets (scored): 2.5 mg, 5 mg, 10 mg; *Provera*® (Upjohn) (Rx), *Amen*® (Carnrick); (Rx); *Cycrin*® (ESI Pharma) (Rx); *Curretab*® (Solvay Pharm) (Rx); generic (Rx)

    Medroxyprogesterone Acetate Injection: 150 mg/ml in 1 ml vials, 400 mg/ml in 2.5 and 10 ml vials and 1 ml U-ject; *Depo-Provera*® (Upjohn) (Rx)

MEGESTROL ACETATE

Chemistry - A synthetic progestin, megestrol acetate (MA) occurs as an essentially odorless, tasteless, white to creamy white, crystalline powder that is insoluble in water, sparingly soluble in alcohol, and slightly soluble in fixed oils. It has a melting range of 213°-219°C over a 3° range and a specific rotation of +8° to +12°.

Storage/Stability/Compatibility - Megestrol acetate tablets should be stored in well-closed containers at a temperature of less than 40°C. The tablets may be crushed and administered with food. The veterinary manufacturer recommends storing the tablets from 2°-30°C (36°-86°F).

Pharmacology - Megestrol acetate possess the pharmacologic actions expected of the other progestationals discussed (*e.g.,* medroxyprogesterone acetate). It has significant anti-estrogen and glucocorticoid activity (with resultant adrenal suppression). It does not have anabolic nor masculinizing effects on the developing fetus.

Uses/Indications - Megestrol acetate (*Ovaban*®—Schering) is approved by FDA for use in dogs only for the postponement of estrus and the alleviation of false pregnancy in the dog. It is used clinically in the United States and elsewhere for many dermatologic and behavior-related conditions, primarily in the cat. See the Dosage section for specific indications and dosages for both dogs and cats.
  Megestrol acetate is indicated in humans for the palliative treatment of advanced carcinoma of the breast or endometrium.

Pharmacokinetics - Megestrol acetate is well absorbed from the GI tract and appears to be metabolized completely in the liver to conjugates and free steroids.
  The half-life of megestrol acetate is reported to be 8 days in the dog.

Contraindications/Precautions - Megestrol acetate is contraindicated in pregnant animals or in animals with uterine disease, diabetes mellitus or mammary neoplasias. It has been recommended that MA not be used in dogs prior to their first estrous cycle or for anestrus therapy in dogs with abnormal cycles. The manufacturer (Schering) recommends that should estrus occur within 30 days of cessation of MA therapy, mating be prevented.

For estrus control, the manufacturer recommends that drug must be given for the full treatment regimen to be effective and that MA should not be given for more than two consecutive treatments.

In humans, megestrol acetate is to be used with caution in patients with thrombophlebitis and is contraindicated as a test for pregnancy.

Adverse Effects/Warnings - In cats, megestrol acetate can induce a profound adrenocortical suppression, adrenal atrophy, and an iatrogenic "Addison's" syndrome can develop at "standard" dosages (2.5 - 5.0 mg every other day) within 1 - 2 weeks. Once the drug has been discontinued, serum cortisol levels (both resting and ACTH-stimulated) will return to normal levels within a few weeks. Clinical symptoms of adrenocortical insufficiency (*e.g.,* vomiting, lethargy) are uncommon, but exogenous steroid support should be considered if the animal is stressed (surgery, trauma, etc.). Cats may develop a transient diabetes mellitus while receiving MA. Polydipsia/polyuria, personality changes, increased weight, endometritis, cystic endometrial hyperplasia, mammary hypertrophy and neoplasias may also occur. Increased appetite and weight gain is not consistently seen, but MA is occasionally used as an appetite stimulant. Rarely, megestrol acetate can cause hepatotoxicity in cats.

Limited clinical studies have suggested that megestrol acetate may cause less cystic endometrial hyperplasia than other progestational agents, but cautious use and vigilant monitoring is still warranted.

In dogs, increased appetite and weight gain, lethargy, change in behavior or hair color, mucometra, endometritis, cystic endometrial hyperplasia, mammary enlargement and neoplasia, acromegaly, adrenocortical suppression or lactation (rare) may occur.

Overdosage/Toxicology Studies - No information was located regarding acute overdosage of megestrol acetate. In humans, dosages of up to 800 mg/day caused no observable adverse reactions.

Toxicity studies performed in dogs at dosages of 0.1 - 0.25 mg/kg/day PO for 36 months yielded no gross abnormalities in the study population. Histologically, cystic endometrial hyperplasia was noted at 36 months, but resolved when therapy was discontinued. At dosages of 0.5 mg/kg/day PO for 5 months, a reversible uterine hyperplasia was seen in treated dogs. Dosages of 2 mg/kg/day demonstrated early cystic endometritis in biopsies done on dogs at 64 days.

No effects were noted in either the bitch or litter when pregnant dogs received 0.25 mg/kg/day for 32 days during the first half of pregnancy. Reduced litter sizes and puppy survival were detected when the dose was given during the last half of pregnancy. Fetal hypospadias are possible if progestational agents are administered during pregnancy.

Drug Interactions - None reported. A potential interaction exists with **Rifampin**, which may decrease progestin activity if administered concomitantly. This is presumably due to microsomal enzyme induction with resultant increase in progestin metabolism. The clinical significance of this potential interaction is unknown.

Concurrent **corticosteroid** use (long-term) may exacerbate adrenocortical suppression and diabetes mellitus.

Doses -
Dogs:
    For estrus control:
        a) To halt cycle in proestrus: 2.2 mg/kg once daily for 8 days starting during the first 3 days of proestrus. While the timing of the next cycle is variable, it may be prolonged with 2.2 mg/kg/day for 4 days, then 0.55 mg/kg/day for 16-20 days.
            To postpone an anticipated cycle: 0.55 mg/kg/day for 32 days, beginning at least 7 days prior to proestrus (Burke 1985)
        b) For suppression during proestrus (first 3 days): 2.2 mg/kg once daily for 8 days (92% efficacy). Bitch must be controlled until behavioral signs of estrus disappear. If mating occurs during first 3 days of therapy, stop treatment and consider mismating therapy. There is a an increased likelihood of pyometra developing if progestins are used concomitantly with estrogens. If mating occurs after 3 or more days of therapy continue at a dosage rate of 3-4 mg/kg PO.
            To delay an anticipated heat during anestrus: 0.55 mg/kg PO for 32 days initiated 7 days prior to proestrus. Recommend doing vaginal cytology prior to therapy. If no erythrocytes are seen, initiate therapy if cycle time frame is appropriate. If erythrocytes are seen, delay therapy until proestrus therapy can be instituted. Do not repeat therapy more often than once every 6 months. (Woody 1988)
    For pseudocyesis (false pregnancy):
        a) 0.5 mg/kg PO once daily for 8 days (Barton and Wolf 1988)

To prevent vaginal hyperplasia development:
  a) 2.2 mg/kg PO for 7 days early in proestrus (Wykes 1986)

For treatment of severe galactorrhea:
  a) 0.55 mg/kg PO once daily for 7 days (Olson and Olson 1986)

For adjunctive treatment of aggressive or unacceptable masculine behavior:
  a) 1.1 - 2.2 mg/kg PO once daily for 2 weeks, then 0.5 - 1.1 mg/kg once daily for 2 weeks. Should be used with behavior modification. (Voith and Marder 1988a)

Cats:

For suppression of estrus:
  a) If in behavioral estrus, signs may be inhibited by giving 5 mg/day PO until estrus stops (generally within 3-5 days), then 2.5 - 5.0 mg PO once weekly for 10 weeks. Postponement of estrus (if started during diestrus): 2.5 mg PO daily for 8 weeks. Postponement of estrus (if started during anestrus): 2.5 mg PO once weekly for up to 18 months. Recommend allowing cat to have a cycle (unmedicated) before beginning another treatment cycle. (Woody 1988)
  b) If started in diestrus: 2.5 mg per day PO for up to 2 months.
      If started in anestrus: 2.5 mg per week for up to 18 months.
      For prevention of estrus: 5 mg daily PO for 3 days as soon as behavioral signs of estrus are seen; next estrus period will occur in approximately 4 weeks. (Romatowski 1989) (derived from package inserts; *Ovarid®*—Glaxovet)

For treatment of idiopathic feline miliary dermatitis:
  a) 2.5 - 5 mg once every other day, followed by weekly maintenance dosages. May be necessary to treat for animal's lifetime. Reserve use for severe cases; explain risks to owner and do not exceed 2.5 mg per week during maintenance phase. (Kwochka 1986)

As an alternative treatment for immune-mediated skin diseases:
  a) 2.5 - 5.0 mg PO once daily for 10 days, then every other day (Giger and Werner 1988)

For adjunctive therapy of eosinophilic granulomas:
  a) 0.5 mg/kg PO once daily for 2 weeks, then twice weekly *prn* (Coppoc 1988)

For eosinophilic ulcers:
  a) Alone or in combination with methylprednisolone acetate (*Depo-Medrol®*): 5 - 10 mg PO every other day for 10-14 doses, then every 2 weeks *prn* (DeNovo, Potter, and Woolfson 1988)

For eosinophilic keratitis (feline proliferative keratitis):
  a) 0.5 mg/kg PO daily until a response is noted, then reduce dose to 1.25 mg PO 2-3 times weekly as required. (Nelson 1986)

For feline plasma cell gingivitis:
  a) 2.5 mg PO once daily for 10 days, then once every other day for 5 treatments, then *prn* (Morgan 1988)

As a secondary therapy (thyroid hormone replacement first choice) for treatment of feline endocrine alopecia (FEA):
  a) 5 mg PO every second to third day initially, then 2.5 mg PO once to twice weekly (Thoday 1986)

For feline psychogenic alopecia and dermatitis:
  a) 2.5 - 5 mg every other day initially, then taper to the lowest maintenance dosage possible, given weekly *prn*. (Walton 1986)

For adjunctive therapy (with urine acidification, increased urine crystalloid solubility, and antispasmodics if required) for persistent hematuria and urethritis in a non-obstructed cat:
  a) 2.5 - 5 mg PO once daily to every other day (with prednisone: 2.5 - 5.0 mg PO daily). (Lage, Polzin, and Zenoble 1988)

For urine marking, intraspecies aggression, anxiety:
  a) 5 mg PO once daily for 5-7 days, then once weekly (Morgan 1988)
  b) 2 mg/kg/day for 5 days, then 1 mg/kg/day for 5 days, then 0.5 mg/kg/day for 5 days. (Romatowski 1989) (derived from package inserts; *Ovarid®*—Glaxovet)

Monitoring Parameters -
  1) Weight
  2) Blood glucose (draw baseline before therapy)
  3) Mammary gland development & appearance
  4) Adrenocortical function
  5) Efficacy

Client Information - The client should fully understand the potential risks of therapy (see Adverse effects above) before starting therapy and should report changes in mammary glands or other symptoms of adverse reactions (*e.g.,* PU/PD, extreme lethargy, behavior changes, etc.) to the veterinarian.

Dosage Forms/Preparations/FDA Approval Status/Withholding Times -
  Veterinary-Approved Products:
   Megestrol Acetate Oral Tablets 5 mg, 20 mg; available in bottles of 100 & 250 tablets and in 30 foil strips of 8 and packaged in cartons of 240 tablets; *Ovaban®* (Schering); (Rx) Approved for use in dogs only.

  Human-Approved Products:
   Megestrol Acetate Oral Tablets 20 mg, 40 mg; *Megace®* (Bristol-Myers Oncology);*Generic* (Rx)

MELARSOMINE

Chemistry/Storage/Stability/Compatibility - An organic arsenical compound, melarsomine dihydrochloride has a molecular weight of 501 and is freely soluble in water. The unreconstituted powder should be stored upright at room temperature. Once reconstituted, the solution should be kept in the original container and kept refrigerated for up to 24 hours. Do not freeze. Do not mix with any other drug.

Pharmacology - While melarsomine is an arsenical compound, its exact mechanism of action is not known. Both laboratory and field studies have demonstrated that melarsomine is 90-99% effective in killing adult and L5 larvae of D. *immitis* in dogs at recommended dosages.

Uses/Indications - Melarsomine is indicated for the treatment of stabilized class I, II and III heartworm disease caused by immature (4 month old, stage L5) to mature adult infections of *D. immitis* in dogs. When compared with thiacetarsamide, melarsomine appears to be more efficacious, less irritating to tissues and does not cause hepatic necrosis.

Pharmacokinetics - The drug is reportedly rapidly absorbed after IM injection. The time to peak plasma concentration is about 11 minutes after IM injection. The apparent volume of distribution is about 0.7 l/kg. Terminal half life is approximately 3 hours.

Contraindications/Precautions/Reproductive Safety - Melarsomine is contraindicated in dogs with class IV (very severe) heartworm disease. Class IV is having caval syndrome (heartworms present in venae cavae and right atrium). Melarsomine is reportedly very toxic to cats and its use cannot be recommend for this species at this time.
  Safety has not been established for use in pregnant, lactating or breeding dogs. Risks versus potential benefits of therapy should be weighed before use.

Adverse Effects/Warnings - Approximately 1/3 of dogs show signs of injection site reactions (pain, swelling, tenderness, reluctance to move) after receiving melarsomine. Most of these signs resolve within weeks, but rarely severe injection reactions can occur. Firm nodules at the injection site can persist indefinitely. SubQ or IV injections must be avoided.
  Other reactions reported in 5% or more dogs treated include: coughing/gagging (22% incidence; average day of onset after treatment = 10); depression/lethargy (15% incidence; average day of onset after treatment = 5); anorexia/inappetence (13% incidence; average day of onset after treatment = 5); fever (7%); lung congestion (6%); vomiting (5%). There is significant interpatient variance in both the date of onset and duration for the above effects.
  Animals not exhibiting adverse effects after the first dose or course of therapy may demonstrate them after the second dose or course of therapy.
  A plethora of other adverse effects in dogs have been noted for melarsomine with reported incidences less than 3%; some of these however are serious. Refer to the package insert for specifics.
  Do NOT give IV or SubQ; significant toxicity or tissue damage may occur. Administer only deep IM as directed (lumbar epaxial muscles (L3-L5). Do not administer at any other site.
  While all dogs with heartworm disease are at risk for post-treatment pulmonary thromboembolism, those with severe pulmonary artery disease are at increased risk for post treatment morbidity and mortality. Dogs should be exercise restricted after treatment.
  Wash hands after use or wear gloves. Avoid contact with animal's eyes; if exposed wash with copious amounts of water. Avoid human exposure. If human exposure occurs, contact a physician.

Overdosage - There is low margin of safety with melarsomine dosages. A 3X dose (7.5 mg/kg) in healthy dogs have demonstrated respiratory inflammation and distress, excessive salivation, restlessness, panting, vomiting, edema, tremors, lethargy, ataxia, cyanosis, stupor and death. Signs of diarrhea, excessive salivation, restlessness, panting, vomiting and fever have been noted in infected dogs who have received inadvertent overdoses (2X).

Treatment with dimercaprol (BAL in Oil) may be considered to treat melarsomine overdoses. Clinical efficacy of melarsomine may be reduced, however.

Drug Interactions - The manufacturer reports that during clinical field trials, melarsomine was given to dogs receiving anti-inflammatory agents, antibiotics, insecticides, heartworm prophylactic medications and various other drugs commonly used to stabilize and support dogs with heartworm disease and that no adverse drug interactions were noted. However, drugs that have similar adverse effects (e.g., depression caused by CNS depressants, etc) may cause additive adverse effects or increase their incidence when used with melarsomine.

Doses -
NOTE: Because of the low margin of safety; calculate dosages very carefully. Do not confuse mg/lb with mg/kg!

Dogs:
> For treatment of heartworm disease:
>> After diagnosis, determine the class (stage) of the disease. Note: The manufacturer provides worksheets that assist in the classification and treatment regime determination. It is highly recommended to use these treatment records to avoid confusion and document therapy.
>> Class I: 2.5 mg/kg deep IM as directed (lumbar epaxial muscles (L3-L5) twice 24 hours apart and rest. Use alternating sides with each administration. In 4 months, the regimen may be repeated.
>> Class II: 2.5 mg/kg deep IM as directed (lumbar epaxial muscles (L3-L5) twice 24 hours apart and rest; give symptomatic treatment as required. Use alternating sides with each administration. In 4 months, the regimen may be repeated.
>> Class III: 2.5 mg/kg deep IM as directed (lumbar epaxial muscles (L3-L5). Strict rest and give all necessary systemic treatment. One month later, give 2.5 mg/kg deep IM as directed (lumbar epaxial muscles (L3-L5) twice 24 hours apart.
>> Note: Recommended needle size for dogs 10kg or less = 23 gauge 1 inch; 10 kg or more body weight = 22 gauge 1.5 inch. (Package Insert; *Immiticide®*—Merial)

Monitoring Parameters/Client Information - Clinical efficacy and adverse effects. Because of the seriousness of the disease and the potential for morbidity and mortality associated with the treatment, clients should give informed consent before electing to treat.

Dosage Forms/Preparations/FDA Approval Status -
> **Veterinary-Approved Products**:
>> Melarsomine Dihydrochloride Powder for Injection 50 mg/vial; *Immiticide®* (Merial); (Rx) Approved for use in dogs.
>> Reconstitute with 2 ml of the diluent provided (sterile water for injection) with a resultant concentration of 25 mg/ml. Once reconstituted, the solution should be kept in the original container and kept refrigerated for up to 24 hours. Do not freeze.
> **Human-Approved Products**: None

MELPHALAN

Chemistry - A nitrogen mustard derivative, melphalan occurs as an off-white to buff-colored powder that is practically insoluble in water. Melphalan is also known as L-PAM, L-Phenylalanine Mustard, or L-Sarcolysin.

Storage/Stability/Compatibility - Store melphalan tablets in well-closed, light-resistant, glass containers at room temperature.

Pharmacology - Melphalan is a bifunctional alkylating agent and interferes with RNA transcription and DNA replication, thereby disrupting nucleic acid function. Because it is bifunctional, it has affect on both dividing and resting cells.

Uses/Indications - Melphalan may be useful in the treatment of a variety of neoplastic diseases, including ovarian carcinoma, multiple myeloma, lymphoreticular neoplasms, osteosarcoma, and mammary or pulmonary neoplasms.

Pharmacokinetics - Melphalan absorption is variable and often incomplete. It is distributed throughout the body water, but it is unknown whether it crosses the placenta, blood brain barrier or enters maternal milk. Melphalan is eliminated principally by hydrolysis in the plasma. In humans, terminal half lives average about 90 minutes.

Contraindications/Precautions/Reproductive Safety - Melphalan should be used only when its potential benefits outweigh its risks with the following conditions: anemia, bone marrow depression, current infection, impaired renal function, tumor cell infiltration of bone marrow, sensitivity to melphalan or patients who have received previous chemotherapy or radiotherapy.

Safe use of melphalan during pregnancy has not been established and other alkylating agents are known teratogens. Use only during pregnancy when the benefits to the mother outweigh the risks to the offspring. Melphalan can suppress gonadal function. While it is unknown whether melphalan enters maternal milk, nursing puppies or kittens should receive milk replacer when the bitch or queen is receiving melphalan.

Adverse Effects/Warnings - Potential adverse effects include GI effects (anorexia, vomiting, diarrhea), and pulmonary infiltrates or fibrosis. The most serious adverse effect likely with melphalan is bone marrow depression (anemia, thrombocytopenia, leukopenia).

Overdosage/Acute Toxicity - Because of the toxic potential of this agent, overdoses must be avoided. Determine dosages carefully.

Drug Interactions - Use extreme caution when using concurrently with other drugs that are also myelosuppressive, including many of the **other antineoplastics and other bone marrow depressant drugs (*e.g.*, chloramphenicol, flucytosine, amphotericin B, or colchicine)**. Bone marrow depression may be additive. Use with other **immunosuppressant drugs (*e.g.*, azathioprine, cyclophosphamide, corticosteroids)** may increase the risk of infection. **Live virus vaccines** should be used with caution, if at all during therapy.

Anecdotal reports of melphalan causing increased nephrotoxicity associated with systemic **cyclosporin** use and severe hemorrhagic necrotic enterocolitis associated with **nalidixic acid** in human pediatric patients have been noted.

Laboratory Considerations - Melphalan may raise serum **uric acid** levels. Drugs such as allopurinol may be required to control hyperuricemia.

Doses -
Dogs:
For adjunctive treatment of ovarian carcinoma, multiply myeloma, lymphoreticular neoplasms, osteosarcoma, and mammary or pulmonary neoplasms:
a) 2 - 4 mg/m^2 PO every 48 hours (every other day). 1.5 mg/m^2 PO every 24 hours (once daily) for 7 - 10 days. (Jacobs, Lumsden et al. 1992)

For multiple myeloma:
a) 2 - 4 mg/m^2 PO q 24- 48h (Gilson and Page 1994)
b) 0.1 mg/kg PO daily for 10 days then every other day (Vail and Ogilvie 1994)

For anal sac or apocrine gland adenocarcinomas:
a) 2 mg/m^2 PO once daily for one week, then every other day (Peterson and Couto 1994b)

Cats:
For adjunctive treatment of FIP:
a) Predniso(lo)ne 4 mg/kg PO once daily with melphalan 2 mg/m^2 (or about 1/4 of a 2 mg tablet) once every 48 hours. (Weiss 1994)

For chronic lymphocytic leukemia:
a) 2 mg/m^2 PO every other day with or without prednisone at 20 mg/m^2 PO every other day. (Peterson and Couto 1994a)

Monitoring Parameters - 1) CBC with platelets at least every 1-2 weeks until stable

Client Information - Clients must understand the importance of both administering melphalan as directed and to report immediately any signs associated with toxicity (*e.g.*, abnormal bleeding, bruising, urination, depression, infection, shortness of breath, etc.).

Dosage Forms/Preparations/FDA Approval Status/Withholding Times -
Veterinary-Approved Products: None
Human-Approved Products:
Melphalan Oral Tablets 2 mg; *Alkeran*® (Glaxo Wellcome); (Rx)

Melphalan Powder for injection: 50 mg in single use vials with 10 ml vial of sterile diulent; *Alkeran*® (Glaxo Wellcome) (Rx)

MEPERIDINE HCL

Chemistry - A synthetic opiate analgesic, meperidine HCl is a fine, white, crystalline, odorless powder that is very soluble in water, sparingly soluble in ether and soluble in alcohol. It has a pK$_a$ of 7.7 - 8.15 and a melting range of 186 - 189°. The pH of the commercially available injectable preparation is between 3.5 and 6. Meperidine may also be known as: Pethidine HCl; Dolantin, Dolantol, Eudolat, or Isonipecaine.

Storage/Stability/Compatibility - Meperidine is stable at room temperature. Avoid freezing the injectable solution and protect from light during storage. Meperidine has not exhibited significant sorption to PVC IV bags or tubing in studies to date.

Meperidine is reported to be physically **compatible** with the following fluids and drugs: sodium chloride 0.45 & 0.9%, Ringer's injection, lactated Ringers injection, dextrose 2.5, 5 & 10% for injection, dextrose/ saline combinations, dextrose/Ringers lactated solutions, atropine, benzquinamide, butorphanol, chlorpromazine, dimenhydrinate, diphenhydramine HCl, dobutamine, droperidol, fentanyl citrate, glycopyrrolate, metoclopramide, pentazocine lactate, promazine HCl, succinylcholine and verpamil HCl.

Meperidine is reported to be physically **incompatible** with the following agents: aminophylline, amobarbital sodium, heparin sodium, hydrocortisone sodium succinate, methicillin, methylprednisolone sodium succinate, morphine sulfate, nitrofurantoin sodium, oxytetracycline HCl, pentobarbital sodium, phenobarbital sodium, phenytoin sodium, sodium iodide, tetracycline HCl, thiopental sodium and thiamylal sodium.

Pharmacology - Refer to the monograph: Narcotic (opiate) Analgesic Agonists, Pharmacology of, for more information.

Meperidine is primarily a *Mu* agonist. It is approximately 1/8th as potent as morphine, but produces equivalent respiratory depression at equi-analgesic doses as morphine. Like morphine, it can cause histamine release. It does not have antitussive activity at doses lower than those causing analgesia. Meperidine is the only used opioid that has vagolytic and negative inotropic properties at clinically used doses. One study in ponies demonstrated changes in jejunal activity after meperidine administration, but no effects on transit time or colonic electrical activity were noted.

Pharmacokinetics - Although generally well absorbed orally, a marked first-pass effect limits the oral effectiveness of these agents (codeine and oxycodone are exceptions). After injection by IM or subcutaneous routes the peak analgesic effects occur between 30 minutes and one hour, with the IM route having a slightly faster onset. Duration of action is variable with effects generally lasting from 1-6 hours in most species. In dogs and cats a duration of action of only 1-2 hours is generally seen at clinically used doses. The drug is metabolized primarily in the liver (mostly hydrolysis with some conjugation) and approximately 5% is excreted unchanged in the urine.

Uses/Indications - Although no product is licensed in the United States for veterinary use, this agent has been used as an analgesic in several different species. It has been used as sedative/analgesic in small animals for both post-operative pain and for medical conditions such as acute pancreatitis and thermal burns. It is occasionally used in equine medicine in the treatment of colic and in other large animal species for pain control.

Contraindications/Precautions - All opiates should be used with caution in patients with hypothyroidism, severe renal insufficiency, adrenocortical insufficiency (Addison's disease), and in geriatric or severely debilitated patients. Meperidine is contraindicated in cases where the patient is hypersensitive to narcotic analgesics, or in patients taking monamine oxidase inhibitors (MAOIs). It is also contraindicated in patients with diarrhea caused by a toxic ingestion until the toxin is eliminated from the GI tract.

Meperidine should be used with caution in patients with head injuries or increased intracranial pressure and acute abdominal conditions (*e.g.,* colic) as it may obscure the diagnosis or clinical course of these conditions. It should be used with extreme caution in patients suffering from respiratory disease or from acute respiratory dysfunction (*e.g.,* pulmonary edema secondary to smoke inhalation).

Opiate analgesics are also contraindicated in patients who have been stung by the scorpion species *Centruroides sculpturatus* Ewing and *C. gertschi* Stahnke as they may potentiate these venoms.

Adverse Effects/Warnings - Meperidine may be irritating when administered subcutaneously and must be given very slowly IV or it may cause severe hypotension. At usual doses, the primary concern is the effect the opioids have on respiratory function. Decreased tidal volume, depressed cough reflex and the drying of respiratory secretions may all have a detrimental effect on a susceptible patient. Bronchoconstriction following IV doses has been noted in dogs. The CNS depressant effects of the these drugs may encumber the abilities of working animals. Gastrointestinal effects may include: nausea, vomiting, and decreased intestinal persitalsis. In dogs, meperidine causes mydriasis (unlike morphine). If given orally, the drug may be irritating to the buccal mucosa and cause salivation; this is of particular concern in cats. Chronic administration can lead to physical dependence.

In horses undergoing general anesthesia, meperidine has been associated with a reaction that manifests as tachycardia with PVC's, profuse sweating, and hyperpnea.

Overdosage - Overdosage may produce profound respiratory and/or CNS depression in most species. Other effects can include cardiovascular collapse, hypothermia, and skeletal muscle hypotonia. Some species (especially cats) may demonstrate CNS excitability (hyperreflexia, tremors) and seizures at doses greater than 20 mg/kg. Naloxone is the agent of choice in treating respiratory depression. In massive overdoses, naloxone doses may need to be repeated, and animals should be closely observed as naloxone's effects may diminish before subtoxic levels of meperidine are attained. Mechanical respiratory support should also be considered in cases of severe respiratory depression.

Pentobarbital has been suggested as a treatment for CNS excitement and seizures in cats. Caution must be used as barbiturates and narcotics can have additive effects on respiratory depression.

Drug Interactions - Other **CNS depressants** (*e.g.,* anesthetic agents, antihis tamines, phenothiazines, barbiturates, tranquilizers, alcohol, etc.) may cause increased CNS or respiratory depression when used with meperidine.

Meperidine is contraindicated in patients receiving **monamine oxidase (MOA) inhibitors** (rarely used in veterinary medicine) for at least 14 days after receiving MOA inhibitors in humans. Some human patients have exhibited signs of opiate overdose after receiving therapeutic doses of meperidine while on these agents.

Laboratory Interactions- Plasma **amylase** and **lipase** values may be increased for up to 24 hours following administration of opiate analgesics as they may increase biliary tract pressure.

Doses -
   Dogs: Analgesic duration in dogs usually lasts 45 minutes to 1 hour. Drug may also be given IV, but SLOWLY.
   a) Analgesic for acute pancreatitis: 5 - 10 mg/kg IM (Morgan 1988)
   b) Analgesic for burns: 3 - 5 mg/kg IM prn (Morgan 1988)
   c) Sedative: 5 - 10 mg/kg IM (Morgan 1988)
   d) Preanesthetic: 2.5 - 6.5 mg/kg (Booth 1988a)

   Cats:
   a) Analgesic: 2 - 10 mg/kg IM or SC q2h prn (Jenkins 1987)
   b) Sedative: 1 - 4 mg/kg IM (Morgan 1988)
   c) Preanesthetic: 2.2 - 4.4 mg/kg (Booth 1988a)

   Rabbits/Rodents:
   a) Analgesic (patient administered moderate pain relief): 0.2 mg/ml of drinking water (Huerkamp 1995)

   Cattle:
   As an analgesic:
   a) 3.3 - 4.4 mg/kg SC or IM (Jenkins 1987)
   b) 500 mg IM (Booth 1988a)
   c) 150 - 200 mg/100 lbs IM or SC (or slow IV) (McConnell and Hughey 1987)

   Horses:
   As an analgesic:
   a) 2.2 - 4 mg/kg IM or 0.2-0.4 mg/kg IV (may cause excitement) (Robinson 1987)
   b) 2 - 4 mg/kg IM or IV (may cause excitement and hypotension with IV use) (Jenkins 1987)
   c) 500 mg IV (slowly, CNS excitement may occur) or 1000 mg IM (Booth 1988a)
   d) 0.2 - 0.4 mg/kg IV (Muir 1987)
Note: Narcotics (meperidine included) may cause CNS excitement in the horse. Some recommend pretreatment with acepromazine (0.02 - 0.04 mg/kg IV), or xylazine (0.3 - 0.5 mg/kg IV) to reduce the behavioral changes these drugs can cause.
Warning: Narcotic analgesics can mask the behavioral and cardiovascular symptoms associated with mild colic.

   Swine:
   a) As a restraining agent: Given alone does not give much restraint in large animals. Has been used in combination with promazine (2 mg/kg IM) and atropine (0.07-0.09 mg/kg IM) at a dose of 1-2 mg/kg IM as a preanesthetic 45-60 minutes before barbiturate/inhalant anesthesia. All the above should be given in separate sites. (Booth 1988a)
   b) Analgesic: 2 mg/kg IM q4h IM prn (Jenkins 1987)

   Sheep & Goats:
   a) As an analgesic: Up to 200 mg total dose IM (Jenkins 1987)

Monitoring Parameters -1) Respiratory rate/depth; 2) CNS level of depression/excitation; 3) Blood pressure if possible and indicated (especially with IV use); 4) Analgesic activity

Client Information - Oral dosage forms may cause mouth irritation. When given parenterally, this agent should be used in an inpatient setting or with direct professional supervision.

Dosage Forms/Preparations/FDA Approval Status/Withholding Times -
   Veterinary-Approved Products: None
   Human-Approved Products:
      Meperidine HCl for Injection: 50 mg/ml in 30 ml multi-dose vials (MDV); 100 mg/ml in 20
      ml MDV; 10 mg/ml in 5 & 10 ml single-dose vial & 30 ml vials for IV infusion only; 25
      mg, 50 mg, 75 mg & 100 mg in 1 ml amps and vials, 1 ml fill in 2 ml Tubex, 0.5 ml Uni-
      Nest amps, 0.5 ml Uni-Amps and 2 ml Carpuject
      Meperidine HCl for oral use: 50 mg, 100 mg tablets, 10 mg/ml oral syrup in 500 ml and pt.

A common trade name is: *Demerol HCl®* (Winthrop-Breon)

Note: Meperidine is listed as a **Class-II** controlled substance and all products require a prescription. Very accurate record keeping is required as to use and disposition of stock.

MEPHENYTOIN

Chemistry - A hydantoin anticonvulsant, mephenytoin occurs a white, crystalline powder. It is
very slightly soluble in water. Mephenytoin is also known as methoin, methylphenylhydantoin or
phenantoin.

Storage/Stability/Compatibility - Store mephenytoin tablets in well-closed containers at room
temperature.

Pharmacology - The anticonvulsant actions of mephenytoin and nirvanol are thought to mirror
those of other hydantoin agents. By promoting sodium efflux from neurons it inhibits the spread
of seizure activity in the motor cortex. It is believed that excessive stimulation or environmental
changes can alter the sodium gradient which may lower the threshold for seizure spread.
Hydantoins tend to stabilize this threshold and limit seizure propagation from epileptogenic foci.
   Mephenytoin reportedly has some antiarrhythmic activity similar to that of phenytoin.

Pharmacokinetics - Mephenytoin is absorbed from the GI tract. In humans, the onset of action
is about 30 minutes and duration of effect from 24-48 hours. Distribution characteristics have not
been described. It is metabolized in the liver to an active metabolite, nirvanol, that has a very
prolonged half life, giving the drug its long duration of action in humans and reasonable duration
of effect in canines. It is also metabolized to a toxic compound, 5,5-ethylphenylhydantoin, that
may explain its increase hematopoietic toxicity.

Uses/Indications - Mephenytoin is a second or third line anticonvulsant in dogs, who have not
responded to phenobarbital and bromides. Its efficacy results from the long half life of its active
metabolite, nirvanol.

Contraindications/Precautions/Reproductive Safety - Mephenytoin is contraindicated in patients known to be hypersensitive to it or other hydantoins. Risk/benefit should be weighed if patient has preexisting blood dyscrasias or hepatic disease. Safe use of this drug has not been established during pregnancy or lactation.

Adverse Effects/Warnings - Adverse effects noted in dogs, include dose related (blood level related) sedation and ataxia. Experience with this agent in dogs is very limited and the preceding
adverse effects may not be complete. In humans, dermatitis, lymphadenopathy, blood dyscrasias,
hepatotoxicity, and fever have been reported. Mephenytoin causes a greater incidence of blood
dyscrasias, or sedation in humans than does phenytoin (DPH).

Overdosage/Acute Toxicity - Symptoms of overdosage may include sedation, anorexia, and
ataxia at lower levels, and coma, hypotension and respiratory depression at higher levels. Severe
intoxications should be handled supportively.

Drug Interactions - **Note**: the following interactions are from the human literature and are for
the compound, phenytoin. Because of the significant differences in pharmacokinetics in dogs,
their applicability to mephenytoin are in question. They are included here as a caution. This list
includes only agents used commonly in small animal medicine, many more agents have been
implicated in the human literature. The following agents may increase the effects of phenytoin:
**allopurinol, cimetidine, chloramphenicol, diazepam, ethanol, isoniazid, phenylbutazone,
sulfonamides, trimethoprim, valproic acid, salicylates, and chlorpheniramine**.
   The following agents may decrease the pharmacologic activity of phenytoin: **barbiturates, diazoxide, folic acid, theophylline, antacids, antineoplastics, calcium (dietary and gluconate),
enteral feedings, nitrofurantoin, and pyridoxine**.
   Phenytoin may decrease the pharmacologic activity of the following agents: **corticosteroids,
disopyramide, doxycycline, estrogens, quinidine, dopamine, and furosemide**.
   Phenytoin may decrease the analgesic properties of **meperidine**, but enhance its toxic effects.
The toxicity of **lithium** may be enhanced. The pharmacologic effects of **primidone** may be altered. Some data suggest that additive hepatotoxicity may result if phenytoin is used with either
primidone or **phenobarbital**. Weigh the potential risks versus the benefits before adding

phenytoin to either of these drugs in dogs. **Pyridoxine (Vitamin B6)** may reduce the serum levels of phenytoin.

Doses -
  Dogs:
  a) For adjunctive therapy of refractory seizures (not controlled with Phenobarbital or primidone and potassium bromide): Initially, 10 mg/kg PO every 8 hours; increase dosage to achieve a nirvanol (active metabolite) blood level of 25 - 40 micrograms/ml. Steady state is reached in about 6 days. (Schwartz-Porsche 1992)
  b) As a second-line agent when first line drugs are not effective: 10 mg/kg *tid*. Therapeutic blood levels as above. (Neer 1994)

Monitoring Parameters - 1) Level of seizure control; sedation/ataxia; 2) CBC with platelets on a regular basis; 3) Serum drug levels until therapeutic levels attained, then if signs of toxicity or lack of seizure control occur

Client Information - Notify veterinarian if dog becomes anorexic, lethargic, ataxic, has abnormal bleeding/bruising, or if seizures are not adequately controlled. The importance of regular dosing is imperative for successful therapy.

Dosage Forms/Preparations/FDA Approval Status/Withholding Times -
  Veterinary-Approved Products: None
  Human-Approved Products:
  Mephenytoin Oral Tablets 100 mg; *Mesantoin*® (Sandoz); (Rx)

MERCAPTOPURINE

Chemistry - A purine analog, mercaptopurine occurs as a slightly yellow, crystalline powder. It is insoluble in water and has a pKa of 7.6. Mercaptopurine may also be known as 6-mercaptopurine or 6-MP.

Storage/Stability/Compatibility - Mercaptopurine tablets should be stored at room temperature in well-closed containers.

Pharmacology - Intracellularly, mercaptopurine is converted into a ribonucleotide which acts as a purine antagonist, thereby inhibiting RNA and DNA synthesis. Mercaptopurine also acts as an immunosuppressant, primarily inhibiting humoral immunity.

Uses/Indications - Veterinary uses of mercaptopurine include adjunctive therapy of lymphosarcoma, acute leukemias, and severe rheumatoid arthritis. It may have potential benefit in treating other autoimmune conditions (*e.g.*, unresponsive ulcerative colitis) as well.

Pharmacokinetics - Absorption after oral dosing is variable and incomplete. Absorbed drug and its metabolites are distributed throughout the total body water. The drug crosses the blood-brain barrier, but not in levels significant enough to treat CNS neoplasms. It is unknown whether mercaptopurine enters milk.

Via the enzyme, xanthine oxidase, mercaptopurine is rapidly metabolized in the liver to 6-thiouric acid, which along with the parent compound and other metabolites are principally excreted in the urine.

Contraindications/Precautions/Reproductive Safety - Mercaptopurine is contraindicated in patients hypersensitive to it. The drug should be used cautiously (risk versus benefit) in patients with hepatic dysfunction, bone marrow depression, infection, renal function impairment (adjust dosage) or have a history of urate urinary stones.

Mercaptopurine is mutagenic and teratogenic and is not recommended for use during pregnancy. Use of milk replacer is recommended for nursing bitches or queens.

Adverse Effects/Warnings - At usual doses, GI effects (nausea, anorexia, vomiting, diarrhea) are most likely seen in small animals. However, bone marrow suppression, hepatotoxicity, pancreatitis, GI (including oral) ulceration, and dermatologic reactions are potentially possible.

Overdosage/Acute Toxicity - Toxicity may present acutely (GI effects) or be delayed (bone marrow depression, hepatotoxicity, gastroenteritis). It is suggested to use standard protocols to empty the GI tract if ingestion was recent and to treat supportively.

Drug Interactions - The hepatic metabolism of mercaptopurine may be decreased by concomitant administration of **allopurinol**. In humans, it is recommended to reduce the mercaptopurine dose to 1/4-1/3 usual if both drugs are to used together.

Use extreme caution when used concurrently with other drugs that are also myelosuppressive, including many of the **other antineoplastics and other bone marrow depressant drugs** (*e.g.*, **chloramphenicol, flucytosine, amphotericin B, or colchicine**). Bone marrow depression may be additive. In humans, enhanced bone marrow depression has occurred when used concomitantly with **trimethoprim/sulfa**. Use with other **immunosuppressant drugs** (*e.g.*, **azathioprine,**

cyclophosphamide, corticosteroids) may increase the risk of infection. **Live virus vaccines** should be used with caution, if at all during therapy.

Mercaptopurine should be used cautiously with other drugs that can cause hepatotoxicity (*e.g.,* halothane, ketoconazole, valproic acid, phenobarbital, primidone, etc.). In humans, one study demonstrated increased hepatotoxicity when mercaptopurine was used in conjunction with **doxorubicin.**

Laboratory Considerations - Mercaptopurine may give falsely elevated serum glucose and uric acid values when using a **SMA (sequential multiple analyzer) 12/60.**

Doses -
  Dogs:
    For treatment of immune-mediated diseases or acute lymphocytic and granulocytic leukemias:
      a) 50 mg/m^2 PO once daily (q24h) to effect, then every other day (q48h) or as needed. (Jacobs, Lumsden et al. 1992)

Monitoring Parameters - 1) Hemograms (including platelets) should be monitored closely; initially every 1-2 weeks and every 1-2 months once on maintenance therapy. It is recommended by some clinicians that if the WBC count drops to between 5,000-7,000 cells/mm^3 the dose be reduced by 25%. If WBC count drops below 5,000 cells/mm^3 treatment should be discontinued until leukopenia resolves; 2)Liver function tests; serum amylase, if indicated; 3) Efficacy

Client Information - Clients must be briefed on the possibilities of severe toxicity developing from this drug, including drug-related neoplasms or mortality. Clients should contact veterinarian should the animal exhibit symptoms of abnormal bleeding, bruising, anorexia, vomiting or infection.

Although, no special precautions are necessary with handling intact tablets, it is recommended to wash hands after administering the drug.

Dosage Forms/Preparations/FDA Approval Status/Withholding Times -
  Veterinary-Approved Products: None
  Human-Approved Products:
    Mercaptopurine Oral Tablets 50 mg; *Purinethol*® (Glaxo Wellcome); (Rx)

METHENAMINE MANDELATE
METHENAMINE HIPPURATE

Chemistry - Methenamine is chemically unrelated to other anti-infective agents. It is commercially available in two salts, methenamine mandelate and methenamine hippurate. Methenamine mandelate occurs as a white, crystalline powder and contains approximately 48% methenamine and 52% mandelic acid. It is very soluble in water. Methenamine hippurate occurs as a white, crystalline powder with a sour taste and contains approximately 44% methenamine and 56% hippuric acid. It is freely soluble in water.

Storage/Stability/Compatibility - Commercially available methenamine products should be stored at room temperature. As methenamine is hydrolyzed by acids to formaldehyde and ammonia, do not mix with acidic vehicles before administering. Methenamine is also incompatible with most alkaloids and metallic salts (*e.g.,* ferric, mercuric or silver salts). Ammonium salts or alkalis will darken methenamine.

Pharmacology - In an acidic urinary environment, methenamine is converted to formaldehyde. Formaldehyde is a non-specific antibacterial agent that exerts a bactericidal effect. It has activity on a variety of bacteria, including both gram positive (*Staphylococcus aureus, S. epidermidis, Enterococcus*) and gram negative organisms (*E. Coli, Enterobacter, Klebsiella, Proteus,* and *Pseudomonas aeruginosa*). Reportedly, methenamine also has activity against fungal urinary tract infections.

Mandelic acid or hippuric acid are added primarily to help acidify the urine, but they also have some non-specific antibacterial activity. Bacterial resistance to formaldehyde, mandelic acid or hippuric acid does not usually occur.

Uses/Indications - Methenamine is used as an antimicrobial agent for the treatment and prophylaxis of recurrent urinary tract infection.

Pharmacokinetics - Human data: While methenamine and it salts are well absorbed from the GI tract, up to 30% of a dose may be hydrolyzed by gastric acid to ammonia and formaldehyde. With enteric-coated tablets the amount hydrolyzed in the gut is reduced. While absorbed, plasma concentrations of both formaldehyde and methenamine are very low and have negligible systemic antibacterial activity. Methenamine does cross the placenta and is distributed into milk.

Within 24 hours, 70-90% of a dose is excreted unchanged into the urine. In an acidic urine, conversion to ammonia and formaldehyde takes place, maximal hydrolysis occurs at urine pH's of 5.5 or less. Peak formaldehyde concentrations occur in the urine at about 2 hour post-dose (3-8 hours with enteric-coated tablets)

Contraindications/Precautions/Reproductive Safety - Methenamine and its salts are contraindicated in patients known to be hypersensitive to it, with renal insufficiency, severe hepatic impairment (due to ammonia production) or severe dehydration.

While methenamine crosses the placenta and lab animal studies have not demonstrated any teratogenic effects, it should be used with caution during pregnancy. Methenamine enters milk and can potentially cause adverse effects; its use in nursing mothers should be carefully considered.

Adverse Effects/Warnings - The most likely adverse effect noted is gastrointestinal upset, with nausea, vomiting, and anorexia predominant. Some patients may dysuria probably secondary to irritation secondary to high formaldehyde concentrations. Lipoid pneumonitis has been reported in some humans receiving prolonged therapy with the suspension.

Because methenamine requires an acid urine to be beneficial, urine pH should be kept at or below 5.5. Some urea-splitting bacteria (*e.g.*, *Proteus* and some strains of *Staphylococci*, *Enterobacter* and *Pseudomonas*) may increase urine pH. Addition of a urinary acidification program may be required using dietary modification and acidifying drugs (*e.g.*, ascorbic acid, methionine, sodium biphosphate, ammonium chloride).

Overdosage/Acute Toxicity - Dogs have received single IV dosages of up to 600 mg/kg of methenamine hippurate without overt toxic effects. Large oral overdoses should be handled using established gut emptying protocols, maintaining hydration status and supporting as required.

Drug Interactions - Use of **urinary alkalinizing drugs** (*e.g.*, **calcium or magnesium containing antacids, carbonic anhydrase inhibitors, citrates, sodium bicarbonate, thiazide diuretics**) may reduce the efficacy of the methenamine.

Use of methenamine with **sulfamethiazole** is not recommended. An insoluble precipitate may form.

Laboratory Considerations - Urinary values of the following compounds may be falsely elevated: **catecholamines, vanilmandelic acid (VMA), 17-hydrocorticosteroid**. Falsely decreased urinary values of **estriol** or **5-HIAA** may occur.

Doses -
  Dogs:
    a) Methenamine hippurate: 500 mg PO q12h; Methenamine mandelate: 10 - 20 mg/kg PO q8-12h (Papich 1992)

  Cats:
    a) Methenamine hippurate: 250 mg PO q12h (Papich 1992)

Monitoring Parameters - 1) Urine pH; 2) Efficacy

Client Information - Give after meals if GI distress occurs; encourage compliance.

Dosage Forms/Preparations/FDA Approval Status/Withholding Times -
  Veterinary-Approved Products: None
  Human-Approved Products:

  Methenamine Mandelate Oral Tablets enteric coated 500 mg, 1 g; *Mandelamine*® (Parke-Davis), Generic; (Rx)

  Methenamine Mandelate Oral Suspension 50 mg/ml in 480 ml *Mandelamine*® (Parke-Davis), Generic; (Rx)

  Methenamine Hippurate Oral Tablets 1 g; *Hiprex*® (Hoechst Marion Roussel); *Urex*® (3M Pharmaceuticals); (Rx)

METHIMAZOLE

Chemistry - A thioimidazole-derivative antithyroid drug, methimazole occurs as a white to pale buff crystalline powder, having a faint characteristic odor and a melting point of 144 -147°C. It is freely soluble (1 gram in 5 ml) in water or alcohol.

Storage/Stability/Compatibility - Methimazole tablets should be stored in well-closed, light-resistant containers at room temperature.

Pharmacology - Methimazole interferes with iodine incorporation into tyrosyl residues of thyroglobulin, thereby inhibiting the synthesis of thyroid hormones. It also inhibits iodinated tyrosyl residues from coupling to form iodothyronine. Methimazole has no effect on the release or activity of thyroid hormones already formed or in the general circulation.

Uses/Indications - Methimazole is considered by most clinicians to be the agent of choice when using drugs to treat feline hyperthyroidism. Propylthiouracil has significantly higher incidences of adverse reactions when compared to methimazole.

Pharmacokinetics - Information on the pharmacokinetics of methimazole in cats is available (Trepanier, Peterson, and Aucoin 1989). These researchers reported that in normal cats, the bioavailability of the drug is highly variable (45-98%), as is the volume of distribution (0.12 - 0.84 L/kg). After oral dosing, the plasma elimination half-life ranges from 2.3 - 10.2 hours. There is usually a 1-3 week lag time between starting the drug and significant reductions in serum T_4.

Methimazole apparently concentrates in thyroid tissue.

Contraindications/Precautions - Methimazole is contraindicated in patients who are hypersensitive to it. It should be used very cautiously in patients with a history of or concurrent hematologic abnormalities, liver disease or autoimmune disease.

Adverse Effects/Warnings - Approximately 15-20% of cats treated with methimazole develop adverse effects. In a study of 262 cats receiving methimazole (Peterson, Kintzer, and Hurvitz 1988), the following adverse effects (% incidence) were reported: anorexia (11.1%), vomiting (10.7%), lethargy (8.8%), excoriations (2.3%), bleeding (2.3%), hepatopathy (1.5%), thrombocytopenia (2.7%), agranulocytosis (1.5%), leukopenia (4.7%), eosinophilia (11.3%), lymphocytosis (7.2%), positive ANA (21.8%), positive direct antiglobulin test (1.9%). Clinical symptoms were noted in 18.3% of the cats. The gastrointestinal adverse effects generally developed within the first month of treatment and usually resolved even with continued therapy.

High levels of methimazole cross the placenta and may induce hypothyroidism in kittens born of queens receiving the drug. Levels higher than those found in plasma are found in human breast milk. It is suggested that kittens be placed on a milk replacer after receiving colostrum from mothers on methimazole.

Overdosage - Acute toxicity that may be seen with overdosage include those that are listed above under Adverse Effects. Agranulocytosis, hepatopathy, and thrombocytopenias are perhaps the most serious effects that may be seen. Treatment consists of following standard protocols in handling an oral ingestion (empty stomach if not contraindicated, administer charcoal, etc.) and to treat symptomatically and supportively.

Drug Interactions - Apparently no significant drug interactions have been reported for this drug.

Doses -

  Cats:

   For hyperthyroidism:
   a) Initially, 5 mg (**not** 5 mg/kg) PO q8h. Recheck serum thyroxine in 3 weeks, if little or no decrease, increase dose by 5 mg every 3 weeks until appropriate response occurs. During first 3 months of therapy, examine cat every 3 weeks to monitor both efficacy and adverse effects. Cats receiving long-term therapy should be monitored every 3-6 months. Use lowest effective dose. Some cats may only require once daily administration. (Meric 1989)
   b) Initially, 10 - 15 mg/day divided every 8-12 hours PO (depending on the severity of hyperthyroidism). If little or no decrease in T_4 occurs, gradually increase dose in 5 mg increments. Exclude poor owner compliance or difficulty in administering before increasing dose. If drug is being used as a pre-operative treatment, may perform thyroidectomy when T_4 decreases to low or normal levels. When used for long-term treatment, if T_4 levels fall to low or low-normal values, may decrease dose by 2.5 - 5 mg until lowest effective dosage is reached. Some cats may tolerate once daily dosing. (Peterson, Kintzer, and Hurvitz 1988)
   c) Initially 5 mg *tid*, many cats maintain an euthyroid state at 5 - 7.5 mg *bid*. (Feldman and Nelson 1987b)

Monitoring Parameters -

  During first 3 months of therapy (baseline values and every 2-3 weeks):
   1) CBC, platelet count
   2) Serum T_4
   3) If indicated by symptomatology: liver function tests, ANA

  After stabilized (at least 3 months of therapy):
   1) T_4 at 3 - 6 month intervals
   2) Other diagnostic tests as dictated by adverse effects

Client Information - It must be stressed to owners that this drug will decrease excessive thyroid hormones, but does not cure the condition and that compliance with the treatment regimen is necessary for success.

Dosage Forms/Preparations/FDA Approval Status/Withholding Times -

  Veterinary-Approved Products: None

  Human-Approved Products:

   Methimazole Tablets (scored) 5 mg, 10 mg; *Tapazole*® (Lilly); (Rx)

METHIONINE
DL-METHIONINE

Chemistry - A sulfur-containing amino acid, methionine occurs as a white, crystalline powder with a characteristic odor. One gram is soluble in about 30 ml of water and it is very slightly soluble in alcohol. 74.6 mg is equivalent to 1 mEq of methionine.

Storage/Stability/Compatibility - Methionine should be stored at room temperature.

Pharmacology - Methione has several pharmacologic effects. It is an essential amino acid (*l*-form) and nutrient, a lipotrope (prevents or corrects fatty liver in choline deficiency), and a urine acidifier. Two molecules of methionine can be converted to 1 molecule of cysteine. Methionine supplies both sulfahydryl and methyl groups to the liver for metabolic processes. Choline is formed when methionine supplies a methyl group to ethanolamine. After methionine is metabolized, sulfate is excreted in the urine as sulfuric acid, thereby acidifying it.

Uses/Indications - In small animals, methionine has been used primarily for its urine acidification effects in the treatment and prevention of certain types (*e.g.,* struvite) of stone formation and to reduce ammoniacal urine odor. In food animals, it has been used as a nutritional supplement in swine and poultry feed and in the treatment of ketosis in cattle. It also has been touted as a treatment for laminitis in horses and cattle (purportedly provides a disulfide bond substrate to maintain the hoof-pedal bone bond), but definitive studies demonstrating its effectiveness for this indication are lacking.

The drug is used in humans to reduce urine ammonia (pH) and odor.

Pharmacokinetics - No information is available on the pharmacokinetics of this agent in veterinary species or humans.

Contraindications/Precautions - Methionine (in therapeutic doses) is considered to be contraindicated in patients with renal failure or pancreatic disease. If used in patients with frank hepatic insufficiency, methionine can cause increased production of mercaptan-like compounds and intensify the symptoms of hepatic dementia or coma. Methionine should not be given to animals with preexisting acidosis or urate calculi. It is not recommended to be used in kittens.

Adverse Effects/Warnings - At usual doses, gastrointestinal distress can occur; give with food to alleviate this effect and to enhance efficacy. Methionine may cause Heinz-body hemolytic anemia in cats. See Overdosage (below) for other potential adverse effects.

Overdosage - Methionine may be toxic to kittens who consume other cats' food in which methionine has been added. When methionine was administered at a dose of 2 grams orally per day to mature cats, anorexia, methemoglobinemia, Heinz body formation (with resultant hemolytic anemia), ataxia and cyanosis were noted. No specific information was located on the treatment of methionine overdosage.

Drug Interactions - Urine acidification may increase the renal excretion of **quinidine**.

The **aminoglycosides** (*e.g.,* gentamicin) and **erythromycin** are more effective in an alkaline medium; urine acidification may diminish these drugs effectiveness in treating bacterial urinary tract infections.

Doses -

Dogs:
For urine acidification:
   a) In struvite dissolution therapy if diet and antimicrobials do not result in acid urine: 0.2 - 1.0 grams PO q8h (Lage, Polzin, and Zenoble 1988), (Kirk 1986)

Cats:
For urine acidification:
   a) 1000 - 1500 mg per day given in the food once daily (if diet and antimicrobials do not reduce pH) (Lewis, Morris, and Hand 1987)
   b) 0.2 -1.0 grams PO once daily (Lage, Polzin, and Zenoble 1988)

Cattle:
   a) 20 - 30 grams PO (Jenkins 1988)

Horses:
   a) 22 mg/kg PO once daily for one week; then 11 mg/kg PO once daily for 1 week; then 5.5 mg/kg PO once daily for one week. (Robinson 1987)
   b) 12.5 grams IV in one liter saline/dextrose solution (may be effective in *Senecio*-induced liver damage. (Rossoff 1974)

Monitoring Parameters -
   1) Urine pH (Urine pH's of ≤6.5 have been recommended as goals of therapy)
   2) Blood pH if symptoms of toxicity are present
   3) CBC in cats exhibiting symptoms of toxicity

Client Information - Give with meals or mixed in food, unless otherwise instructed by veterinarian.

Dosage Forms/Preparations/FDA Approval Status/Withholding Times -

Veterinary-Approved Products: Methionine is approved for use in dogs, cats, and horses in pharmaceutical dosage forms. Products labeled as nutritionals may be approved for use in other species. Depending on the product, methionine may be available without prescription.

Methionine Tablets 200 mg & 500 mg; *Ammonil*® (Daniels), *Odor-Trol*® (Miles), *Methio-Tabs*® (Vet-A-Mix) (Rx) Approved for use in cats and dogs

Methionine Tablets Chewable 500 mg; *Methio-Form*® (Vet-A-Mix) Approved for use in dogs

Methionine Powder, Granules, Pellets (concentration varies with product); Trade Names/Products include: *Methio-Vet*® Pellets (Vet-A-Mix) (OTC); Bio-Meth® (Vet-A-Mix) Approved for use in horses.

Human-Approved Products:

Methionine Capsules 200 mg, 500 mg; Tablets 500 mg; Liquid 75 mg/5 ml; May be available generically labeled or tradenames may include: *Pedameth*® (Forest), *Uracid*® (Wesley), *Uranap*® (Vortech). Depending product, is either an OTC or Rx item.

METHOCARBAMOL

Chemistry - A centrally acting muscle relaxant related structurally to guaifenesin, methocarbamol occurs as a fine, white powder with a characteristic odor. In water, it has a solubility 25 mg/ml. The pH of commercial injection is approximately 4-5.

Storage/Stability/Compatibility - Methocarbamol tablets should be stored at room temperature in tight containers; the injection should be stored at room temperature and not frozen. Solutions prepared for IV infusion should not be refrigerated as a precipitate may form. Because a haze or precipitate may form, all diluted intravenous solutions should be physically inspected before administration.

Pharmacology - Methocarbamol's exact mechanism of causing skeletal muscle relaxation is unknown. It is thought to work centrally, perhaps by general depressant effects. It has no direct relaxant effects on striated muscle, nerve fibers, or the motor endplate. It will not directly relax contracted skeletal muscles. The drug has a secondary sedative effect.

Uses/Indications - In dogs and cats, methocarbamol is indicated (FDA approved) "as adjunctive therapy of acute inflammatory and traumatic conditions of the skeletal muscle and to reduce muscular spasms." In horses, intravenous use is indicated (FDA approved) "as adjunctive therapy of acute inflammatory and traumatic conditions of the skeletal muscle to reduce muscular spasms, and effect striated muscle relaxation." (Package insert; *Robaxin*® -*V* - Robins)

Pharmacokinetics - Limited pharmacokinetic data is available in veterinary species. In humans, methocarbamol ha an onset of action of about 30 minutes after oral administration. Peak levels occur approximately 2 hours after dosing. Serum half-life is about 1-2 hours. The drug is metabolized and the inactive metabolites are excreted into the urine and the feces (small amounts).

In horses, plasma clearances appear to be dose dependent after IV administration (Muir, Sams, and Ashcraft 1984), lower clearances were measured after higher doses were given. The serum half-life of methocarbamol in the horse is approximately 60-70 minutes. Guaifenesin is a minor metabolite of methocarbamol, but because of very low concentrations, it probably has no clinical effect in the horse.

Contraindications/Precautions - Because the injectable product contains polyethylene glycol 300, the manufacturer lists known or suspected renal pathology as a contraindication to injectable methocarbamol therapy. Polyethylene glycol 300 has been noted to increase preexisting acidosis and urea retention in humans with renal impairment.

Methocarbamol should be used with caution during pregnancy as studies demonstrating its safety during pregnancy are lacking. Methocarbamol should not be used in patients hypersensitive to it or in animals to be used for food purposes.

Do not administer subcutaneously and avoid extravasation. Do not exceed 2 ml per minute when injecting IV in dogs and cats.

Adverse Effects/Warnings - Side effects can include sedation, salivation, emesis, lethargy, weakness and ataxia in dogs and cats. Sedation and ataxia are possible in horses. Because of its CNS depressant effects, methocarbamol may impair the abilities of working animals.

Overdosage - Overdosage is generally characterized by CNS depressant effects (loss of righting reflex, prostration). Excessive doses in dogs and cats may be represented by emesis, salivation, weakness and ataxia. If the overdose is after oral administration, emptying the gut may be indicated if the overdose was recent. Do not induce emesis if the patient's continued consciousness is not assured. Other symptoms should be treated if severe and in a supportive manner.

Drug Interactions - Because methocarbamol is a CNS depressant, additive depression may occur when given with other **CNS depressant agents**.

One patient (human) with myasthenia gravis and taking **pyridostigmine**, developed severe weakness after receiving methocarbamol.

Doses -
Dogs:
  a) Injectable: For relief of moderate conditions: 44 mg/kg IV; For controlling severe effects of strychnine and tetanus: 55 - 220 mg/kg IV, do not exceed 330 mg/kg/day. Administer half the estimated dose rapidly, then wait until animal starts to relax and continue administration to effect.
  Tablets: Initially, 132 mg/kg/day PO divided q8h-q12h, then 61-132 mg/kg divided q8-12h. If no response in 5 days, discontinue. (Package insert; *Robaxin®-V* —Robins)
  b) For muscle relaxation for intervertebral disk disease: 15 - 20 mg/kg PO *tid*.
  For muscle relaxation for certain toxicosis (*e.g.,* strychnine, metalaldehyde, tetanus): 150 mg/kg IV (Morgan 1988)
  c) For strychnine/brucine poisoning:Average first dose is 149 mg/kg IV, repeat half dose as needed (Bailey 1986a)

Cats:
  a) Injectable: For relief of moderate conditions: 44 mg/kg IV; For controlling severe effects of strychnine and tetanus: 55 - 220 mg/kg IV, do not exceed 330 mg/kg/day. Administer half the estimated dose rapidly, then wait until animal starts to relax and continue administration to effect.
  Tablets: Initially, 132 mg/kg/day PO divided q8h-q12h, then 61 - 132 mg/kg divided q8-12h. If no response in 5 days, discontinue. (Package insert, *Robaxin®-V* —Robins)

Cattle:
  For treatment of CNS hyperactivity:
  a) 110 mg/kg IV (Bailey 1986b)

Horses:
  a) For moderate conditions: 4.4 - 22 mg/kg IV to effect; for severe conditions: 22 - 55 mg/kg IV (Package insert, *Robaxin®-V —* Robins)
  b) 15 - 25 mg/kg IV by slow infusion (Robinson 1987)
  c) To give orally: Use 2-3 times the recommended IV dose. (Cunningham, Fisher et al. 1992)

Monitoring Parameters -
  1) Level of muscle relaxation/sedation

Client Information - Animal's urine color may darken, but need not be of concern.

Dosage Forms/Preparations/FDA Approval Status/Withholding Times -
Veterinary-Approved Products:
  Methocarbamol Tablets 500 mg; *Robaxin®-V* (Fort Dodge); (Rx) Approved for use in dogs and cats.

  Methocarbamol Injection 100 mg/ml in vials of 20 ml and 100 ml; *Robaxin®-V* (Fort Dodge); (Rx) Approved for use in dogs, cats, and horses not intended for food.

Human-Approved Products:
  Methocarbamol Tablets 500 mg, 750 mg; *Robaxin®* (Robins); *Robaxin-750®* (Robins); Generic (Rx)

  Methocarbamol Injection 100 mg/ml in 10 ml vials; *Robaxin®* (Robins); generic (Rx)

METHOTREXATE
METHOTREXATE SODIUM

Chemistry - A folic acid antagonist, methotrexate is available commercially as the sodium salt. It occurs as a yellow powder that is soluble in water. Methotrexate sodium injection has a pH of 7.5-9. Methotrexate may also be known as Amethoptrin or MTX.

Storage/Stability/Compatibility - Methotrexate sodium tablets should be stored at room temperature (15-30°C) in well-closed containers and protected from light. The injection and powder for injection should be stored at room temperature (15-30°C) and protected from light.

Methotrexate sodium is reportedly **compatible** with the following intravenous solutions and drugs: Amino acids 4.25%/dextrose 25%, D5W, sodium bicarbonate 0.05 M, cephalothin sodium, cytarabine, 6-mercaptopurine sodium, sodium bicarbonate, and vincristine sulfate. In syringes, methotrexate is compatible with: bleomycin sulfate, cyclophosphamide, doxorubicin HCl, fluorouracil, furosemide, leucovorin calcium, mitomycin, vinblastine sulfate, and vincristine sulfate.

Methotrexate sodium **compatibility information conflicts** or is dependent on diluent or concentration factors with the following drugs or solutions: heparin sodium and metoclopramide HCl. Compatibility is dependent upon factors such as pH, concentration, temperature and diluents used. It is suggested to consult specialized references for more specific information (*e.g., Handbook on Injectable Drugs* by Trissel; see bibliography).

Methotrexate sodium is reportedly **incompatible** with the following solutions or drugs: bleomycin sulfate (as an IV additive only; compatible in syringes and Y-lines), fluorouracil (as an IV additive only; compatible in syringes and Y-lines), prednisolone sodium phosphate, droperidol and ranitidine HCl.

Pharmacology - An S-phase specific antimetabolite antineoplastic agent, methotrexate competitively inhibits folic acid reductase, thereby inhibiting the reduction of dihydrofolate to tetrahydrofolate and affecting production of purines and pyrimidines. Rapidly proliferating cells (*e.g.,* neoplasms, bone marrow, GI tract epithelium, fetal cells, etc.) are most sensitive to the drug's effects.

Dihydrofolate reductase has a much greater affinity for methotrexate than either folic acid or dihydrofolic acid and coadministration of folic acid will not reduce methotrexate's effects. Leucovorin calcium, a derivative of tetrahydrofolic acid, can block the effects of methotrexate.

Methotrexate also has immunosuppressive activity, possibly due to its effects on lymphocyte replication. Tumor cells have been noted to develop resistance to methotrexate which may be due to decreased cellular uptake of the drug.

Uses/Indications - Indicated for lymphomas and some solid tumors in dogs and cats (see the Doses section and the recommended treatment protocol references at the end of this section). In human medicine, methotrexate is also being used to treat refractory rheumatoid arthritis and severe psoriasis.

Pharmacokinetics - Methotrexate is well absorbed from the GI tract after oral administration of dosages <30 mg/m^2 with a bioavailability of about 60%. In humans, peak levels occur within 4 hours after oral dosing, and between 30 minutes and 2 hours after IM injection.

Methotrexate is widely distributed in the body and is actively transported across cell membranes. Highest concentrations are found in the kidneys, spleen, gallbladder, liver and skin. When given orally or parenterally, methotrexate does not reach therapeutic levels in the CSF. When given intrathecally, methotrexate attains therapeutic levels in the CSF and also passes into the systemic circulation. Methotrexate is about 50% bound to plasma proteins and crosses the placenta.

Methotrexate is excreted almost entirely by the kidneys via both glomerular filtration and active transport. Serum half-lives are less than 10 hours and generally between 2-4 hours.

Contraindications/Precautions/Reproductive Safety - Methotrexate is contraindicated in patients with preexisting bone marrow depression, severe hepatic or renal insufficiency, or hypersensitive to the drug. It should be used with caution in patients who are susceptible to, or who have preexisting signs or symptoms associated with, the adverse reactions associated with this drug.

When administering MTX, either wear gloves or immediately wash hands after handling. Gloves are particularly important if handling split, broken or crushed tablets. Preparation of intravenous solutions should ideally be performed in a vertical laminar flow hood.

Methotrexate is teratogenic, embryotoxic and may affect spermatogenesis in male animals.

Adverse Effects/Warnings - In dogs and cats, gastrointestinal side effects are most prevalent with diarrhea, nausea, and vomiting seen. Higher dosages may lead to listlessness, GI toxicity (ulcers, mucosal sloughing, stomatitis), hematopoietic toxicity (nadir at 4-6 days), hepatopathy, renal tubular necrosis, alopecia, depigmentation, pulmonary infiltrates and fibrosis. CNS toxicity (encephalopathy) may be noted if methotrexate is given intrathecally. Rarely, anaphylaxis may be seen.

Overdosage/Acute Toxicity - Acute overdosage in dogs is associated with exacerbations of the adverse effects outlined above, particularly myelosuppression and acute renal failure. Acute tubular necrosis is secondary to drug precipitation in the tubules. In dogs, the maximally tolerated dose is reported to be 0.12 mg/kg q24h for 5 days.

Treatment of acute oral overdoses include, emptying the gut and preventing absorption using standard protocols if the ingestion is recent. Additionally, oral neomycin has been suggested to help prevent absorption of MTX from the intestine. In order to minimize renal damage, forced alkaline diuresis should be considered. Urine pH should be maintained between 7.5 and 8 by the addition of 0.5 -1 mEq/kg of sodium bicarbonate per 500 ml of IV fluid.

Leucovorin calcium is specific therapy for methotrexate overdoses. It should be given as soon as possible, preferably within the first hour and definitely within 48 hours. Doses of leucovorin required are dependent on the MTX serum concentration. Humans having serum concentrations greater than 5×10^{-7} M at 48 hours are likely to develop severe toxicity. Leucovorin in doses ranging from 25-200 mg/m^2 every 6 hours doses is given until serum levels fall below 1×10^{-8} M. Dogs treated with leucovorin at 15 mg/m^2 every 3 hours IV for 8 doses, then IM q6h for 8 doses were able to tolerate MTX doses as high as 3 g/m^2 (O'Keefe and Harris 1990). Another dose of 3 mg/m^2 for leucovorin in dogs has also been suggested (Coppoc 1988).

Drug Interactions - Highly protein-bound drugs such as **salicylates, sulfonamides, phenytoin, phenylbutazone, oral anticoagulants, tetracycline and chloramphenicol** may displace MTX or be displaced by MTX from plasma proteins with resultant increased blood levels and toxicity of both drugs.

In humans, severe hematologic and GI toxicity has resulted in patients receiving both MTX and **non-steroidal antiinflammatory agents**. Therefore, it is recommended not to use agents such as **flunixin, naproxen, or meclofenamic acid** in dogs also on MTX.

Salicylates or probenicid may inhibit the tubular secretion of MTX and increase its half life.

It has been suggested that **folic acid supplements** can inhibit the response to MTX, but this has neither been confirmed nor refuted.

Pyrimethamine, a similar folic acid antagonist, may increase MTX toxicity and should not be given to patients receiving MTX.

Oral **neomycin** may decrease the absorption of oral methotrexate if given concomitantly.

Drug/Laboratory Interactions - Methotrexate may interfere with the microbiologic assay for **folic acid**.

Doses - Dosages of methotrexate sodium are expressed in terms of methotrexate as are the dosage forms. For more information, refer to the protocol references found in the appendix or other protocols found in other small animal medicine texts.

Dogs:

For susceptible neoplastic diseases (usually as part of a multi-drug protocol):

a) 2.5 mg/m^2 PO daily (Rosenthal 1985)

b) For malignant lymphoma: 5 mg/m^2 on days 1 and 5 of a weekly maintenance schedule. (Coppoc 1988)

c) 2.5 mg/m^2 PO 2-3 times weekly; 0.3 - 0.8 mg/m^2 IV every 7 days. (O'Keefe and Harris 1990)

d) "High dose therapy": 5 - 10 mg/m^2 PO, IV, IM or intrathecally followed 2-4 hours later with leucovorin at 3 mg/m^2.

"Normal dose therapy": 2.5 mg/m^2 once daily. Adjust dosage/frequency according to toxicity. (Thompson 1989a)

e) For lymphoma (as part of protocol—see reference): 0.5 mg/kg IV (maximum dose 25 mg) on day 14. (Matus 1989)

f) 2.5 mg/m^2 PO daily. (MacEwen and Rosenthal 1989)

g) In combination with other antineoplastics (per protocol) 5 mg/m^2 PO twice weekly or 0.8 mg/kg IV every 21 days; alternatively 2.5 mg/m^2 PO daily. (USPC 1990)

Cats:

For susceptible neoplastic diseases (usually as part of a multi-drug protocol):

a) 2.5 mg/m^2 PO 2-3 times weekly; 0.3 - 0.8 mg/m^2 IV every 7 days. (O'Keefe and Harris 1990)

b) For lymphoma (as part of protocol—see reference): 0.8 mg/kg IV on day 14 with 5 mg prednisone *bid* PO. (Matus 1989)

c) For lymphosarcoma: 2.5 - 5 mg/m^2 PO 2 - 3 times per week.

For carcinomas and some sarcomas: 10 - 15 mg/m^2 every 1-3 weeks. (Couto 1989b)

d) In combination with other antineoplastics (per protocol) 5 mg/m^2 PO twice weekly. (USPC 1990)

Monitoring Parameters - 1. Efficacy; 2. Toxicity: a) Monitor for clinical signs and symptoms of GI irritation and ulceration. b) Complete blood counts (with platelets) should be performed weekly early in therapy and eventually every 4-6 weeks when stabilized. If WBC is < 4000/mm^3 or platelet count is <100,000/mm^3 therapy should be discontinued. c) Baseline renal function tests. Continue to monitor if abnormal. d) Baseline hepatic function tests. Monitor liver enzymes on a regular basis during therapy.

Client Information - Clients must be briefed on the possibilities of severe toxicity developing from this drug, including drug-related mortality. Clients should contact the veterinarian should the patient exhibit any symptoms of profound depression, abnormal bleeding (including bloody diarrhea) and/or bruising.

Wear gloves when administering tablets (particularly if crushed or split); if gloves are not used, wash hands thoroughly after handling tablets.

Dosage Forms/Preparations/FDA Approval Status/Withholding Times -
  Veterinary-Approved Products: None
  Human-Approved Products:

    Methotrexate Sodium Oral Tablets (scored) 2.5 mg; *Methotrexate*® (Immunex), *Rheumatrex*® & *Rheumatrex Dose Pack*® (Lederle) (Rx)

    Methotrexate Sodium Injection 2.5 mg/ml in 2 ml vials and 25 mg/ml in 2, 4, 8, & 10 ml vials; *Methotrexate* (Lederle), generic; (Rx). Also available in preservative-free 25 mg/ml formulations: *Folex*®*PFS* (Adria), *Methotrexate LPF*® (Lederle); (Rx)

    Methotrexate Powder for Injection in 20 mg/vial, 50 mg/vial, and 1 g vials for reconstitution; (Rx)

METHOXYFLURANE

Chemistry - An inhalant general anesthetic agent, methoxyflurane occurs as a clear, mobile liquid. It has a characteristic fruity odor. Methoxyflurane is very slightly soluble in water and miscible with alcohol or olive oil. At 20°C, methoxyflurane's specific gravity is 1.420-1.425.

Storage/Stability/Compatibility - Store at room temperature in tight, light-resistant containers. Protect from freezing. Methoxyflurane is very soluble in rubber and soda lime. Avoid contact with polyvinyl chloride (PVC) plastics as they can be extracted by methoxyflurane.

Methoxyflurane contains an antioxidant (BHT) which may accumulate in the vaporizer causing a yellow to brown discoloration. Do not use discolored solutions. Discolored vaporizer and wick may be cleaned with diethyl ether (all ether must be removed before reuse).

Pharmacology - While the precise mechanism that inhalent anesthetics exert their general anesthetic effects is not precisely known, they may interfere with functioning of nerve cells in the brain by acting at the lipid matrix of the membrane. Some key pharmacologic effects noted with methoxyflurane include: CNS depression, depression of body temperature regulating centers, increased cerebral blood flow, respiratory depression, hypotension, vasodilatation, and myocardial depression (less so than with halothane) and muscular relaxation.

Uses/Indications - Methoxyflurane's is used as an inhalent anesthetic. Its use is apparently diminishing due to its potential for causing nephrotoxicity, slow onset of action (a short-acting barbiturate is often used as an induction agent), and prolonged recovery time. However, it does produce some muscle relaxation and analgesia, even at relatively low concentrations.

Pharmacokinetics - Methoxyflurane is rapidly absorbed from the alveoli, but it has a comparatively slow onset of activity. It is rapidly distributed into the CNS and crosses the placenta. Approximately 35% of a dose is eliminated via the lungs and approximately 50% is metabolized in the liver; substantial amounts of inorganic fluoride is formed which are excreted by the kidneys.

Minimal Alveolar Concentration (MAC; %) in oxygen reported for methoxyflurane in various species: Dog = 0.23; Cat = 0.23; Horse = 0.22; Human = 0.16. Several factors may alter MAC (acid/base status, temperature, other CNS depressants on board, age, ongoing acute disease, etc.).

Contraindications/Precautions/Reproductive Safety - Methoxyflurane should be used cautiously, if at all, in patients with preexisting renal or hepatic disease. It should be used with caution (benefits vs. risks) in patients with increased CSF or head injury, or myasthenia gravis.

Studies are not definitive, but methoxyflurane may cause teratogenic effects; other inhalent anesthetic agents may be safer alternatives. If methoxyflurane is used during delivery or C-section, oxygen may need to be given to newborns after delivery.

Adverse Effects/Warnings - The most concerning adverse effect associated with methoxyflurane is its potential for causing nephrotoxicity, particularly with prolonged procedures in patients predisposed to nephrotoxicity.

While methoxyflurane potentially may cause hepatotoxicity, this apparently occurs rarely and may be associated with hypoxic episodes. Nevertheless, it should be used with caution in patients with preexisting hepatic dysfunction.

Overdosage/Acute Toxicity - Overdosage or acute toxicities may cause circulatory depression and hypotension, cardiac arrhythmias, bradycardia, prolonged respiratory depression, emergence delirium, or malignant hyperthermic crises.

Drug Interactions - Because of methoxyflurane's potential for causing nephrotoxicity, it should not be used concurrently with **other nephrotoxic drugs** (*e.g.*, aminoglycosides, amphotericin B, cisplatin, NSAIDS, penicillamine, rifampin, tetracycline).

While methoxyflurane sensitizes the myocardium to the effects of sympathomimetics less so than halothane, arrhythmias may still result. Drugs included are: **dopamine, epinephrine, norepinephrine, ephedrine, metaraminol, etc.** Caution and monitoring is advised.

Non-depolarizing neuromuscular blocking agents, systemic aminoglycosides, systemic lincomycins should be used with caution with halogenated anesthetic agents as additive neuromuscular blockade may occur.

Concomitant administration of **succinylcholine** with inhalation anesthetics may induce increased incidences of cardiac effects (bradycardia, arrhythmias, sinus arrest and apnea) and in susceptible patients, malignant hyperthermia as well.

Doses -
  Dogs/Cats:
    a) 3% (induction); 0.5 - 1.5% (maintenance) (Papich 1992)
  Ruminants & Swine:
    a) Induction 1%; maintenance 0.5% (Howard 1993)

Monitoring Parameters - 1) Respiratory and ventilatory status; 2) Cardiac rate/rhythm; blood pressure (particularly with "at risk" patients; 3) Level of anesthesia; 4) Renal function tests, if patient's post-operative urine output is excessive or markedly reduced

Dosage Forms/Preparations/FDA Approval Status/Withholding Times -
  Veterinary-Approved Products:
    Methoxyflurane in 120 ml bottles; *Metofane*® (Schering); (Rx)
  Human-Approved Products:
    Methoxyflurane in 15 ml and 125 ml bottles; *Penthrane*® (Abbott); (Rx)

METHYLENE BLUE

Chemistry - A thiazine dye, methylene blue occurs as dark green crystals or crystalline powder that has a bronze-like luster. It may have a slight odor and is soluble in water and sparingly soluble in alcohol. When dissolved, a dark blue solution results. Commercially available methylene blue injection (human-labeled) has a pH from 3-4.5.

Storage/Stability/Compatibility - Unless otherwise instructed by the manufacturer, store methylene blue at room temperature. Methylene blue is reportedly incompatible with caustic alkalies, dichromates, iodides, and oxidizing or reducing agents.

Pharmacology - Methylene blue is rapidly converted to leucomethylene blue in tissues. This compound serves as a reducing agent which helps to convert methemoglobin (Fe^{+++}) to hemoglobin (Fe^{++}). Methylene blue is an oxidating agent, and if high doses (species dependent) are administered may actually cause methemoglobinemia.

Uses/Indications - Methylene blue is used primarily for treating methemoglobinemia secondary to oxidative agents (nitrates, chlorates) in ruminants. It is also employed occasionally as adjunctive or alternative therapy for cyanide toxicity.

Intra-operative methylene blue is also being used to preferentially stain islet-cell tumors of the pancreas in dogs in order to aid in their surgical removal or in determining the animal's prognosis.

Pharmacokinetics - Methylene blue is absorbed from the GI tract, but is usually administered parenterally in veterinary medicine. It is excreted in the urine and bile, primarily in the colorless form, but some unchanged drug may be also excreted.

Contraindications/Precautions/Reproductive Safety - Methylene blue is contraindicated in patients with renal insufficiency; hypersensitive to methylene blue; or as a intraspinal (intrathecal) injection. Because cats may develop Heinz body anemia and methemoglobinemia secondary to methylene blue, it is considered contraindicated in this species by most clinicians. Methylene blue is considered to be relatively ineffective in reducing methemoglobin in horses.

Safe use of this agent during pregnancy has not been demonstrated.

Adverse Effects/Warnings - The greatest concern with methylene blue therapy is the development of Heinz body anemia or other red cell morphological changes, methemoglobinemia, and decreased red cell lifespans. Cats tend to be very sensitive to these effects and the drug is usually considered to be contraindicated in them, but dogs and horses can also develop these effects at relatively low dosages.

When injected SQ or if extravasation occurs during IV administration, necrotic abscesses may develop.

Overdosage/Acute Toxicity - The LD_{50} for IV administered 3% methylene blue is approximately 43 mg/kg in sheep.

Drug Interactions; Drug/Laboratory Interactions - None located.

Doses -
  Dogs:
    To preferentially stain islet-cell tumors of the pancreas:
      a) 3 mg/kg in 250 ml sterile normal saline and administered IV over 30-40 minutes intraoperatively. Initial tumor staining requires approximately 20 minutes after infusion has begun and is maximal at about 25-35 minutes after infusion is started. Tumors generally appear to be a reddish-violet in color versus a dusky blue (background staining). (Fingeroth and Smeak 1988)

  Ruminants:
    Note: Methylene blue can be obtained from various chemical supply houses, but there has been some concern raised that the FDA will not allow it to be used in food animals as it is a susepected carcinogen. It is recommended to contact the FDA before treating for guidance when contemplating using this compound.
    For methemoglobin-producing toxins (nitrites, nitrates, chlorates):
      a) Cattle: 8.8 mg/kg by slow IV using a maximum of a 1% solution; repeat if necessary. To prevent hypotension during nitrite poisoning, give a sympathomimetic drug such as epinephrine or ephedrine. (Bailey 1986b)
      b) Cattle: 4.4 mg/kg IV in a 2-4% solution. (Ruhr and Osweiler 1986)
      c) Cattle, sheep: 8.8. mg/kg slow IV as a 1% solution in normal saline; may repeat carefully in 15-30 minutes if response is not satisfactory. Other species should use 4.4 mg/kg dosage rate (as above). (Hatch 1988b)
    For cyanide toxicity:
      a) 4 - 6 g IV per 454 kg (1000 lb.) of body weight. (Oehme 1986b)

Monitoring Parameters -
    1) Methemoglobinemia
    2) Red cell morphology, red cell indices, hematocrit, hemoglobin

Client Information - Because of the potential toxicity of this agent and the seriousness of methemoglobin-related intoxications, this drug should be used with close professional supervision only. Methylene blue may be very staining to clothing or skin. Removal may be accomplished using hypochlorite solutions (bleach).

Dosage Forms/Preparations/FDA Approval Status/Withholding Times -
  Veterinary-Approved Products: None.

  Human-Approved Products:
  Methylene Blue Injection 10 mg/ml in 1 ml and 10 ml amps; Generic; (Rx)

  Methylene Blue Tablets 65 mg *Methblue 65*® (Manne Co);*Urolene Blue*® (Star) (Rx)

  Methylene Blue, U.S.P. powder may be available from chemical supply houses.

METHYLPREDNISOLONE
METHYLPREDNISOLONE ACETATE
METHYLPREDNISOLONE SODIUM SUCCINATE

Note: For more information refer to the monograph: Glucocorticoids, General Information or to the manufacturer's product information.

Chemistry - Also known as 6-alpha-methylprednislone, methylprednisolone is a synthetically produced glucocorticoid. Both the free alcohol and the acetate ester occur as odorless, white or practically white, crystalline powder. They are practically insoluble in water and sparingly soluble in alcohol.

Methylprednisolone sodium succinate occurs as an odorless, white or nearly white, hygroscopic, amorphous solid. It is very soluble in both water and alcohol.

Storage/Stability/Compatibility - Commercially available products of methylprednisolone should be stored at room temperature (15-30°C); avoid freezing the acetate injection. After reconstituting the sodium succinate injection, store at room temperature and use within 48 hours; only use solutions that are clear.

Methylprednisolone sodium succinate injection is reportedly **compatible** with the following fluids and drugs: amino acids 4.25%/dextrose 25%, amphotericin B (limited amounts), chloramphenicol sodium succinate, cimetidine HCl, clindamycin phosphate, dopamine HCl, heparin sodium, metoclopramide, norepinephrine bitartrate, penicillin G potassium, sodium iodide/aminophylline, and verapamil.

The following drugs and fluids have either been reported to be **incompatible** with methylprednisolone sodium succinate, **compatible dependent upon concentration, or data conflicts**: D5/half normal saline, D5 normal saline (80 mg/l reported compatible), D5W (up to 5 grams/L reported compatible), Lactated Ringer's (up to 80 mg/L reported compatible), normal saline (data conflicts; some reports of up to 60 grams/liter compatible), calcium gluconate, cephalothin sodium (up to 500 mg/L in D5W or NS compatible), glycopyrrolate, insulin, metaraminol bitartrate, nafcillin sodium, penicillin G sodium and tetracycline HCl. Compatibility is dependent upon factors such as pH, concentration, temperature and diluents used. It is suggested to consult specialized references for more specific information (*e.g., Handbook on Injectable Drugs* by Trissel; see bibliography).

Contraindications/Precautions - The manufacturer (Upjohn Veterinary) states that the drug (tablets) should not be used in dogs or cats "in viral infections, ...animals with arrested tuberculosis, peptic ulcer, acute psychoses, corneal ulcer, and Cushinoid syndrome. The presence of diabetes, osteoporosis, chronic psychotic reactions, predisposition to thrombophlebitis, hypertension, CHF, renal insufficiency, and active tuberculosis necessitates carefully controlled use."

The injectable acetate product is contraindicated as outlined above when used systemically. When injected intrasynovially, intratendinously, or by other local means, it is contraindicated in the "presence of acute local infections."

Doses -

Dogs:

As an antiinflammatory agent:
  a) Initially 1 - 2 mg/kg/day divided *bid-tid* for 5 to 10 days. After clinical signs are suppressed, consolidate dose (1 - 2 mg/kg/day) and give at 7-10 AM once a day for 1 week. Then reduce dose to 0.5 - 1 mg/kg/day for 5-7 days. Convert to alternate day dosing by giving 1 -2 mg/kg on alternate mornings. Reduce dosage by 1/2 each week until a minimally effective dose is reached. (Kemppainen 1986)
  b) Methylprednisolone: 1 mg/kg PO q8h; methylprednisolone acetate: 1 mg/kg IM every 14 days. (Jenkins 1985)
  c) Methylprednisolone acetate: 1.1 mg/kg SQ or IM; effects (for dermatologic indications) generally last for 1-3 weeks. (Scott 1982)
  d) For labeled uses:
     Oral:
     Dogs weighing 5 -15 lbs: 2 mg
     Dogs weighing 15 - 40 lbs: 2 - 4 mg
     Dogs weighing 40 - 80 lbs: 4 - 8 mg;
     These total daily doses should be divided and given 6 - 10 hours apart.
     Intramuscularly: 2 - 120 mg IM (average 20 mg); depending on breed (size), severity of condition, and response. May repeat at weekly intervals or in accordance with the severity of the condition and the response. (Package insert; *Depo-Medrol®*—Upjohn) The manufacturer has specific directions for use of the drug intrasynovially. It is recommended to refer directly to the package insert for more information.

As an immunosuppressant:
  a) Pulse therapy to induce remission or control of autoimmune skin diseases: Methylprednisolone sodium succinate 11 mg/kg in 250 ml D5W infused IV over 1 hour for 3 consecutive days. Cimetidine 4 mg/kg PO q8h may also be given to reduce GI implications. After day 3, begin oral prednisone maintenance at 1.1 mg/kg q24-48h. Azathioprine can also be added during maintenance phase. (White, Stewart, and Bernstein 1987)

For adjunctive medical therapy of spinal cord trauma:
  a) Methylprednisolone sodium succinate: Initially, 30 mg/kg IV; 2 hours later give 15 mg/kg IV. Then give 10 mg/kg IV or SQ 4 times a day for 24-36 hours. Reduce dosage gradually over next 7 days. Cimetidine may be helpful in preventing hemorrhagic gastroenteritis associated with high dose glucocorticoids. (Schunk 1988a)

For adjunctive therapy for various forms of shock:
  a) Methylprednisolone sodium succinate: 30 - 35 mg/kg IV (Kemppainen 1986)

For intralesional (sub-lesional) use:
  a) A sufficient volume of 20 mg/ml methylprednisolone acetate is used to undermine the lesion (10-40 mg total dose). (Scott 1982)

Cats:

As an antiinflammatory agent:
  a) Methylprednisolone acetate: 5.5 mg/kg SQ or IM (average sized cat = 20 mg); effects (for dermatologic indications) generally last for 1 week to 6 months. (Scott 1982)

    b) For labeled uses:
        Oral:
        Cats weighing 5 -15 lbs: 2 mg
        Cats weighing >15 lbs: 2 - 4 mg
        These total daily doses should be divided and given 6 - 10 hours apart.
        Intramuscularly: up to 20 mg (average 10 mg) IM; depending on breed (size), severity
        of condition, and response. May repeat at weekly intervals or in accordance with the
        severity of the condition and the response. (Package insert; *Depo-Medrol*®—Upjohn)

For eosinophilic ulcer:
    a) Methylprednisolone acetate 20 mg SQ every 2 weeks for 2-3 doses. If chronic case,
        maintenance therapy may be required at 20 mg SQ *prn*. May also consider adding
        megestrol acetate. (DeNovo, Potter, and Woolfson 1988)

As alternate adjunctive therapy for feline plasma cell gingivitis-pharyngitis:
    a) Methylprednisolone acetate 10 - 20 mg SQ *prn*. May also consider adding megestrol
        acetate. (DeNovo, Potter, and Woolfson 1988)

As an antiinflammatory for the adjunctive treatment of feline asthma:
    a) Methylprednisolone acetate: 2 mg/kg (dosage interval or route not specified) (Papich
        1986)
    b) Methylprednisolone acetate: 1 - 2 mg/kg IM (dosage interval not specified) (Noone
        1986)

For adjunctive therapy of flea allergy:
    a) Methylprednisolone acetate: 5 mg/kg SQ; generally will keep animal comfortable for
        3-6 weeks. Do not use more often than every 2 months. (Kwochka 1986)

For adjunctive treatment of idiopathic feline miliary dermatoses:
    a) Methylprednisolone acetate: 5 mg/kg SQ; if favorable response is noted, may repeat
        same dosage two times at 2-3 week intervals. Thereafter, do not use more often than
        every 2 months. (Kwochka 1986)

For adjunctive treatment of pulmonary edema secondary to blood transfusion reactions:
    a) 30 mg/kg repeated every 6 hours (route not specified) (Auer and Bell 1986)

For intralesional (sub-lesional) use:
    a) A sufficient volume of 20 mg/ml methylprednisolone acetate is used to undermine the
        lesion (10-40 mg total dose). (Scott 1982)

Horses:
As an antiinflammatory (glucocorticoid effects):
    a) Methylprednisolone: 0.5 mg/kg PO; Methylprednisolone sodium succinate: 0.5 mg/kg
        IV or IM (Robinson 1987)
    b) For labeled uses: Methylprednisolone acetate 200 mg IM repeated as necessary
        (Package insert; *Depo-Medrol*®—Upjohn) The manufacturer has specific directions
        for use of the drug intrasynovially. It is recommended to refer directly to the package
        insert for more information.

For shock:
    a) Methylprednisolone sodium succinate: 10 - 20 mg/kg IV (Robinson 1987)

Dosage Forms/Preparations/Approval Status/Withdrawal Times-
Veterinary-Approved Products: A 10 ppb tolerance has been established for methylpred-
nisolone in milk.
    Methylprednisolone Tablets 1 mg, 2 mg
        Medrol® (Upjohn), generic; (Rx) Approved for use in dogs and cats.
    Methylprednisolone Acetate Injection 20 mg/ml, 40 mg/ml
        Depo-Medrol® (Upjohn), generic; (Rx) Approved for use in dogs, cats and horses.
Human-Approved Products:
    Methylprednisolone Tablets 2 mg, 4 mg, 8 mg, 16 mg, 24 mg, 32 mg; *Medrol*® (Upjohn),
        generic; (Rx)
    Methylprednisolone Acetate for Injection 20 mg/ml, 40 mg/ml, 80 mg/ml in 1, 5 & 10 ml
        vials; *Depo-Medrol*® (Upjohn) many other trade names and generically-labeled products are
        available; (Rx)
    Methylprednisolone Sodium Succinate Powder for Injection: 40 mg/vial; 125 mg/vial; 500
        mg/vial; 1000 mg/vial (62.5 mg/ml after reconstitution), 2000 mg/vial; *Solu-Medrol*®
        (Upjohn), *A-methaPred*® (Abbott), generic; (Rx)

4-Methylpyrazole—see Fomepizole

METOCLOPRAMIDE HCL

Chemistry - A derivative of para-aminobenzoic acid, metoclopramide HCl occurs as an odorless, white, crystalline powder with pK_as of 0.6 and 9.3. One gram is approximately soluble in 0.7 ml of water or 3 ml of alcohol. The injectable product has a pH of 3-6.5.

Storage/Stability/Compatibility - Metoclopramide is photosensitive and must be stored in light resistant containers. All metoclopramide products should be stored at room temperature. Metoclopramide tablets should be kept in tight containers.

The injection is reportedly **stable** in solutions of a pH range of 2-9 and with the following IV solutions: D_5W, 0.9% sodium chloride, D5-1/2 normal saline, Ringer's, and lactated Ringer's injection.

The following drugs have been stated to be **compatible** with metoclopramide for at least 24 hours: aminophylline, ascorbic acid, atropine sulfate, benztropine mesylate, chlorpromazine HCl, cimetidine HCl, clindamycin phosphate, cyclophosphamide, cytarabine, dexamethasone sodium phosphate, dimenhydrinate, diphenhydramine HCl, doxorubicin HCl, droperidol, fentanyl citrate, heparin sodium, hydrocortisone sodium phosphate, hydroxyzine HCl, insulin (regular), lidocaine HCl, magnesium sulfate, mannitol, meperidine HCl, methylprednisolone sodium succinate, morphine sulfate, multivitamin infusion (MVI), pentazocine lactate, potassium acetate/chloride/phosphate, prochlorperazine edisylate, TPN solution (25% dextrose w/4.25% *Travasol*® w/ or w/o electrolytes), verapamil and vitamin B-complex w/vitamin C.

Metoclopramide is reported to be **incompatible** with the following drugs: ampicillin sodium, calcium gluconate, cephalothin sodium, chloramphenicol sodium succinate, cisplatin, erythromycin lactobionate, methotrexate sodium, penicillin G potassium, sodium bicarbonate, and tetracycline. Compatibility is dependent upon factors such as pH, concentration, temperature and diluents used. It is suggested to consult specialized references for more specific information (*e.g.*, *Handbook on Injectable Drugs* by Trissel; see bibliography).

Pharmacology - The primary pharmacologic effects of metoclopramide are associated with the GI tract and the CNS. In the GI tract, metoclopramide stimulates motility of the upper GI without stimulating gastric, pancreatic or biliary secretions. While the exact mechanisms for these actions are unknown, it appears that metoclopramide sensitizes upper GI smooth muscle to the effects of acetylcholine. Intact vagal innervation is not necessary for enhanced motility, but anticholinergic drugs will negate metoclopramide's effects. Gastrointestinal effects seen include increased tone and amplitude of gastric contractions, relaxed pyloric sphincter, and increased duodenal and jejunal peristalsis. Gastric emptying and intestinal transit times can be significantly reduced. There is little or no effect on colon motility. Additionally, metoclopramide will increase lower esophageal sphincter pressure and prevent or reduce gastroesophageal reflux. The above actions evidently give metoclopramide its local antiemetic effects.

In the CNS, metoclopramide apparently antagonizes dopamine at the receptor sites. This action can explain its sedative, central anti-emetic (blocks dopamine in the chemo-receptor trigger zone), extrapyramidal, and prolactin secretion stimulation effects.

Uses/Indications - Metoclopramide has been used in veterinary species for both its GI stimulatory and antiemetic properties. It has been used clinically for gastric stasis disorders, gastroesophageal reflux, to allow intubation of the small intestine, as a general antiemetic (for parvovirus, uremic gastritis, etc.) and as an antiemetic to prevent or treat chemotherapy induced vomiting.

Pharmacokinetics - Metoclopramide is absorbed well after oral administration, but a significant first-pass effect in some human patients may reduce systemic bioavailability to 30%. There apparently is a great deal of interpatient variation with this effect. Bioavailability after intramuscular administration has been measured to be 74-96%. After oral dosing, peak plasma levels generally occur within 2 hours.

The drug is well distributed in the body and enters the CNS. Metoclopramide is only weakly bound to 13-22% of plasma proteins. The drug also crosses the placenta and enters the milk in concentrations approximately twice those of the plasma.

Metoclopramide is primarily excreted in the urine in humans. Approximately 20-25% of the drug is excreted unchanged in the urine. The majority of the rest of the drug is metabolized to glucuronidated or sulfated conjugate forms and then excreted in the urine. Approximately 5% is excreted in the feces. The half-life of metoclopramide in the dog has been reported to be approximately 90 minutes.

Contraindications/Precautions - Metoclopramide is contraindicated in patients with GI hemorrhage, obstruction or perforation and in those hypersensitive to it. It is relatively contraindicated in patients with seizure disorders. In patients with pheochromocytoma, metoclopramide may induce a hypertensive crisis.

Adverse Effects/Warnings - In dogs, the most common (although infrequent) adverse reactions seen are changes in mentition and behavior. Cats may exhibit signs of frenzied behavior or disorientation. Both species can develop constipation while taking this medication.

In adult horses, IV metoclopramide administration has been associated with the development of severe CNS effects. Alternating periods of sedation and excitement, behavioral changes and abdominal pain have been noted. These effects are less common in foals. Because of the incidence of adverse effects one group of authors (Clark and Becht 1987) does not at the present time recommend its use in adult horses.

Other adverse effects that have been reported in humans and are potentially plausible in animals include extrapyramidal effects, nausea, diarrhea, transient hypertension and elevated prolactin levels.

Overdosage - The oral LD_{50} doses of metoclopramide in mice, rats, and rabbits are 465 mg/kg, 760 mg/kg and 870 mg/kg, respectively. Because of the high dosages required for lethality, it is unlikely an oral overdose will cause death in a veterinary patient. Likely symptoms of overdosage include sedation, ataxia, agitation, extrapyramidal effects, nausea, vomiting and constipation.

There is no specific antidotal therapy for metoclopramide intoxication. If an oral ingestion was recent, the stomach should be emptied using standard protocols. Anticholinergic agents (diphenhydramine, benztropine, etc.) that enter the CNS may be helpful in controlling extrapyramidal effects. Peritoneal dialysis or hemodialysis is thought not to be effective in enhancing the removal of the drug.

Drug Interactions - **Atropine** (and related anticholinergic compounds) and **narcotic analgesics** may negate the GI motility effects of metoclopramide.

The GI stimulatory effects of metoclopramide may affect the absorption of many drugs. Drugs that dissolve, disintegrate and/or are absorbed in the stomach (*e.g.,* **digoxin**) may be absorbed less. Due to its small particle size, *Lanoxin*® brand of digoxin is apparently unaffected by metoclopramide administration. Metoclopramide may enhance absorption of drugs that are absorbed primarily in the small intestine (*e.g.,* **cimetidine, tetracycline, aspirin, & diazepam**). Metoclopramide may accelerate **food absorption** and thereby alter **insulin** doses and/or timing of insulin effects.

Phenothiazines (*e.g.,* acepromazine, chlorpromazine, etc.) and **butyrephenones** (*e.g.,* droperidol, azaperone) may potentiate the extrapyramidal effects of metoclopramide. The CNS effects of metoclopramide may be enhanced by other **sedatives, tranquilizers** and **narcotics.**

Doses -
Dogs:
As an antiemetic:
- a) 0.2 - 0.4 mg/kg q6h PO, SubQ or IM; or 1-2 mg/kg/day as a continuous IV infusion (Washabau and Elie 1995)
- b) 0.2 - 0.4 mg/kg SQ *tid* or as a continuous IV infusion at 0.01 - 0.02 mg/kg/hour (Chiapella 1988)
- c) For bilious vomiting syndrome: 0.2 - 0.4 mg/kg PO once daily given late in the evening (Hall and Twedt 1988)
- d) 1 - 2 mg/kg every 24 hours as a slow IV for severe emesis (DeNovo 1986)
- e) To help prevent vomiting in patients with laryngeal paralysis and resultant tracheostomy: 0.05 mg/kg SQ or slowly IV before small feedings (O'Brien, 1986)

For disorders of gastric motility:
- a) 0.2 - 0.4 mg/kg PO *tid* given 30 minutes before meals (Hall and Twedt 1988)
- b) 0.2 - 0.5 mg/kg PO or SQ q8h; give 30 minutes prior to meals and at bedtime for gastro-motility disorders and esophageal reflux (DeNovo 1986)
- c) 0.2 - 0.4 mg/kg PO q6-8h (Burrows 1983)

For esophageal reflux:
- a) 0.5 mg/kg PO q8h (Jones 1985)
- b) 0.2 - 0.5 mg/kg PO or SQ q8h; give 30 minutes prior to meals and at bedtime for gastro-motility disorders and esophageal reflux (DeNovo 1986)
- c) 0.2 mg/kg PO *tid* (with cimetidine or ranitidine, weight restriction, and high protein - low fat diet) (Watrous 1988)

Cats:
- a) 0.2 - 0.5 mg/kg PO, SQ q8h; give 30 minutes prior to meals and at bedtime for gastro-motility disorders and esophageal reflux (DeNovo 1986)
- b) 0.2 - 0.4 mg/kg PO q6-8h (Burrows 1983)

Horses:
To stimulate the gastrointestinal tract in foals:
- a) 0.02 - 0.1 mg/kg IM or IV 3 - 4 times a day (Clark and Becht 1987)

Monitoring Parameters -
   1) Clinical efficacy and adverse effects

Client Information - Contact veterinarian if animal develops symptoms of involuntary movement of eyes, face, or limbs, or develops a rigid posture.

Dosage Forms/Preparations/FDA Approval Status/Withholding Times -
  Veterinary-Approved Products: None
  Human-Approved Products: All doses expressed in terms of metoclopramide base.

    Metoclopramide HCl Tablets 5 mg, 10 mg; *Reglan*® (Robins); *Clopra*® (Quantum); *Maxolon*® (Beecham); *Octamide*® (Adria); *Reclomide*® (Major); Generic; (Rx)

    Metoclopramide HCl Oral Solution (syrup) 1 mg/ml in pints, unit-dose (10 ml); *Reglan*® (Robins), Generic; (Rx)

    Metoclopramide HCl Injection 5 mg/ml in 2 & 10 ml amps, and 2, 10, 30, 50 & 100 ml vials (some contain preservatives, some are preservative free and labeled for single-use only); *Reglan*® (Robins); *Metoclopramide HCl*® (Quad); Generic; (Rx)

METOPROLOL TARTRATE
METOPROLOL SUCCINATE

Chemistry - A beta1 specific adrenergic blocker, metoprolol tartrate occurs as a white, crystalline powder having a bitter taste. It is very soluble in water. Metoprolol succinate occurs as a white, crystalline powder and is freely soluble in water.

Storage/Stability/Compatibility - Store all products protected from light. Store tablets in tight, light-resistant containers at room temperature. Avoid freezing the injection.

Pharmacology - Metoprolol is a relatively specific beta1 blocker. At higher dosages this specificity may be lost and beta2 blockade can occur. Metoprolol does not possess any intrinsic sympathomimetic activity like pindolol nor does it possess membrane stabilizing activity like pindolol or propranolol. Cardiovascular effects secondary to metoprolol's negative inotropic and chronotropic actions include: decreased sinus heart rate, slowed AV conduction, diminished cardiac output at rest and during exercise, decreased myocardial oxygen demand, reduced blood pressure, and inhibition of isoproterenol-induced tachycardia.

Uses/Indications - Because metoprolol is relatively safe to use in animals with bronchospastic disease, it is often chosen over propranolol. It may be effective in supraventricular tachyarrhythmias, premature ventricular contractions (PVC's, VPC's), systemic hypertension and in treating cats with hypertrophic cardiomyopathy.

Pharmacokinetics - Metoprolol tartrate is rapidly and nearly completely absorbed from the GI tract, but it has a relatively high first pass effect (50%) so systemic bioavailability is reduced. The drug has very low protein binding characteristics (5-15%) and is distributed well into most tissues. Metoprolol crosses the blood-brain barrier and CSF levels are about 78% of those found in the serum. It crosses the placenta and levels in milk are higher (3-4X) than those found in plasma. Metoprolol is primarily biotransformed in the liver; unchanged drug and metabolites are then principally excreted in the urine. Reported half lives in various species: Dogs: 1.6 hours; Cats: 1.3 hours; Humans 3-4 hours.

Contraindications/Precautions/Reproductive Safety - Metoprolol is contraindicated in patients with overt heart failure, hypersensitivity to this class of agents, greater than first degree heart block, or sinus bradycardia. Non-specific beta-blockers are generally contraindicated in patients with CHF unless secondary to a tachyarrhythmia responsive to beta-blocker therapy. They are also relatively contraindicated in patients with bronchospastic lung disease.

  Metoprolol should be used cautiously in patients with significant hepatic insufficiency. It should also be used cautiously in patients with sinus node dysfunction.

  Metoprolol (at high dosages) can mask the symptoms associated with hypoglycemia. It can also cause hypoglycemia or hyperglycemia and, therefore, should be used cautiously in labile diabetic patients.

  Metoprolol can mask the symptoms associated with thyrotoxicosis, but it may be used clinically to treat the symptoms associated with this condition.

  Safe use during pregnancy has not been established, but adverse effects to fetuses have apparently not been documented.

Adverse Effects/Warnings - It is reported that adverse effects most commonly occur in geriatric animals or those that have acute decompensating heart disease. Adverse effects considered to be clinically relevant include: bradycardia, lethargy and depression, impaired AV conduction, CHF or worsening of heart failure, hypotension, hypoglycemia, and bronchoconstriction (less so with beta1 specific drugs like metoprolol). Syncope and diarrhea have also been reported in canine patients with beta blockers.

Exacerbation of symptoms have been reported following abrupt cessation of beta-blockers in humans. It is recommended to withdraw therapy gradually in patients who have been receiving the drug chronically.

Overdosage - There is limited information available on metoprolol overdosage. Humans have apparently survived dosages of up to 5 grams. The most predominant symptoms expected would be extensions of the drug's pharmacologic effects: hypotension, bradycardia, bronchospasm, cardiac failure and potentially hypoglycemia.

If overdose is secondary to a recent oral ingestion, emptying the gut and charcoal administration may be considered. Monitor ECG, blood glucose, potassium, and, if possible, blood pressure. Treatment of the cardiovascular effects are symptomatic. Use fluids, and pressor agents to treat hypotension. Bradycardia may be treated with atropine. If atropine fails, isoproterenol given cautiously has been recommended. Use of a transvenous pacemaker may be necessary. Cardiac failure can be treated with a digitalis glycosides, diuretics, and oxygen. Glucagon (5-10 mg IV - Human dose) may increase heart rate and blood pressure and reduce the cardiodepressant effects of metoprolol.

Drug Interactions - Sympathomimetics (metaproterenol, terbutaline, beta effects of epinephrine, phenylpropanolamine, etc.) may have their actions blocked by metoprolol and they may, in turn, reduce the efficacy of metoprolol. Additive myocardial depression may occur with the concurrent use of metoprolol and myocardial depressant **anesthetic agents**. **Phenothiazines** given with metoprolol may exhibit enhanced hypotensive effects. **Furosemide and hydralazine** or other hypotensive producing drugs may increase the hypotensive effects of metoprolol. Metoprolol may prolong the hypoglycemic effects of **insulin** therapy. Concurrent use of beta blockers with **calcium channel blockers** (or other negative inotropics should be done with caution; particularly in patients with preexisting cardiomyopathy or CHF.

Doses -
  Dogs:
    As an oral beta blocker:
      a) 5 - 50 mg (total dose) two to three times a day; initial dose should be low followed by individual dosage titration. (Ware 1992)
      b) 5 - 60 mg (total dose) PO q8h (Papich 1992)
      c) As adjunctive therapy (with a class I drug) for ventricular arrhythmias in patients who have responded adequately to shock: 0.2 - 0.4 mg/kg PO q12h (Russell and Rush 1995)

  Cats:
    As an oral beta blocker:
      a) 2 - 15 mg (total dose) PO q8h (Papich 1992)

Monitoring Parameters - 1) Cardiac function, pulse rate, ECG if necessary, BP if indicated; 2) Toxicity (see Adverse Effects/Overdosage)

Client Information - To be effective, the animal must receive all doses as prescribed. Notify veterinarian if animal becomes lethargic or becomes exercise intolerant, has shortness of breath or cough, or develops a change in behavior or attitude.

Dosage Forms/Preparations/FDA Approval Status/Withholding Times -
  Veterinary-Approved Products: None
  Human-Approved Products:

  Metoprolol Tartrate Oral Tablets 50 mg, 100 mg; *Lopressor*® (Geigy); generic (Rx)

  Metoprolol Succinate Extended Release Tablets equivalent to metoprolol tartrate: 50 mg, 100 mg, 200 mg; *Toprol XL*® (Astra); (Rx)

  Metoprolol Tartrate Injection 1 mg/ml in 5 ml amps; *Lopressor*® (Geigy); Generic (Rx)

METRONIDAZOLE

Chemistry - A synthetic, nitroimidazole antibacterial and antiprotozoal agent, metronidazole occurs as white to pale yellow crystalline powder or crystals with a pK_a of 2.6. It is sparingly soluble in water or alcohol. Metronidazole base is commercially available as tablets or solution for IV injection and metronidazole HCl is available as injectable powder for reconstitution. The hydrochloride is very soluble in water.

Storage/Stability/Compatibility - Metronidazole tablets and HCl powder for injection should be stored at temperatures less than 30°C and protected from light. The injection should be protected from light and freezing and stored at room temperature.

Specific recommendations on the reconstitution, dilution, and neutralization of metronidazole HCl powder for injection are detailed in the package insert of the drug and should be referred to if this product is used. Do not use aluminum hub needles to reconstitute or transfer this drug as a reddish-brown discoloration may result in the solution.

The following drugs and solutions are reportedly **compatible** with metronidazole ready-to-use solutions for injection: amikacin sulfate, aminophylline, carbenicillin disodium, cefazolin sodium, cefotaxime sodium, cefoxitin sodium, cefuroxime sodium, cephalothin sodium, chloramphenicol sodium succinate, clindamycin phosphate, disopyramide phosphate, gentamicin sulfate, heparin sodium, hydrocortisone sodium succinate, hydromorphone HCl, magnesium sulfate, meperidine HCl, morphine sulfate, moxalactam disodium, multielectrolyte concentrate, multivitamins, netilmicin sulfate, penicillin G sodium, and tobramycin sulfate.

The following drugs and solutions are reportedly **incompatible** (or compatibility data conflicts) with metronidazole ready-to-use solutions for injection: aztreonam, cefamandole naftate and dopamine HCl.

Pharmacology - Metronidazole is bactericidal against susceptible bacteria. Its exact mechanism of action is not completely understood, but it is taken up by anaerobic organisms where it is reduced to an unidentified polar compound. It is believed that this compound is responsible for the drug's antimicrobial activity by disrupting DNA and nucleic acid synthesis in the bacteria.

Metronidazole has activity against most obligate anaerobes including *Bacteroides sp.* (including *B. fragilis*), *Fusobacterium*, *Veillonella*, *Clostridium sp.*, peptococcus, and peptostreptococcus. *Actinomyces* is frequently resistant to metronidazole.

Metronidazole is also trichomonacidal and amebicidal in action and acts as a direct amebicide. Its mechanism of action for its antiprotozoal activity is not understood. It has therapeutic activity against *Entamoeba histolytica*, *Trichomonas*, *Giardia*, and *Balantidium coli*. It acts primarily against the trophozoite forms of *Entamoeba* rather than encysted forms.

Uses/Indications - Although there are no veterinary-approved metronidazole products, the drug has been used extensively in the treatment of *Giardia* in both dogs and cats. It is also used clinically in small animals for the treatment of other parasites (*Trichomonas* and *Balantidium coli*) as well as treating both enteric and systemic anaerobic infections.

In horses, metronidazole has been used clinically for the treatment of anaerobic infections.

Pharmacokinetics - Metronidazole is relatively well absorbed after oral administration. The oral bioavailability in dogs is high, but interpatient variable with ranges from 50-100% reported. The oral bioavailability of the drug in horses averages about 80% (range 57-100%). If given with food, absorption is enhanced in dogs, but delayed in humans. Peak levels occur about one hour after dosing.

Metronidazole is rather lipophilic and is rapidly and widely distributed after absorption. It is distributed to most body tissues and fluids, including to bone, abscesses, the CNS, and seminal fluid. It is less than 20% bound to plasma proteins in humans.

Metronidazole is primarily metabolized in the liver via several pathways. Both the metabolites and unchanged drug are eliminated in the urine and feces. Elimination half-lives of metronidazole in patients with normal renal and hepatic function in various species are reported as: humans 6-8 hours, dogs 4-5 hours, and horses 2.9-4.3 hours.

Contraindications/Precautions/Reproductive Safety - Metronidazole is contraindicated in animals hypersensitive to the drug or nitroimidazole derivatives. It has also been recommended not to use the drug in severely debilitated, pregnant or nursing animals. Metronidazole should be used with caution in animals with hepatic dysfunction.

Metronidazole has been implicated as being a teratogen in some laboratory animal studies, but no information is available for dogs and cats. Unless the benefits to the mother outweigh the risks to the fetuses, it should not be used during pregnancy, particularly during the first 3 weeks of gestation.

Adverse Effects/Warnings - Adverse effects reported in dogs include neurologic disorders, lethargy, weakness, neutropenias, hepatotoxicity, hematuria, anorexia, nausea, vomiting and diarrhea.

Neurologic toxicity may be manifested after acute high dosages or, more likely, with chronic moderate to high-dose therapy. Symptoms reported are described below in the Overdosage section.

Overdosage/Acute Toxicity - Signs of intoxication associated with metronidazole in dogs and cats, include anorexia and/or vomiting, depression, mydriasis, nystagmus, ataxia, head-tilt, deficits of proprioception, joint knuckling, disorientation, tremors, seizures, bradycardia, rigidity and stiffness. These effects may be seen with either acute overdoses or in some animals with chronic therapy when using "recommended" doses.

Acute overdoses should be handled by attempting to limit the absorption of the drug using standard protocols. Extreme caution should be used before attempting to induce vomiting in patients demonstrating CNS effects or aspiration may result. If acute toxicity is seen after chronic therapy, the drug should be discontinued and the patient treated supportively and symptomatically. Neurologic symptoms may require several days before showing signs of resolving.

Drug Interactions - Metronidazole may prolong the PT in patients taking **warfarin** or other coumarin anticoagulants. Avoid concurrent use if possible; otherwise, intensify monitoring.

Phenobarbital or phenytoin may increase the metabolism of metronidazole, thereby decreasing blood levels.

Cimetidine may decrease the metabolism of metronidazole and increase the likelihood of dose-related side effects occurring.

Alcohol may induce a disulfiram-like (nausea, vomiting, cramps, etc.) reaction when given with metronidazole.

Drug/Laboratory Interactions - Metronidazole causes falsely decreased readings of **AST** (SGOT) and **ALT** (SGPT) when determined using methods measuring decreases in ultraviolet absorbance when NADH is reduced to NAD.

Doses -
  Dogs:
    For treatment of *Giardia*:
      a) 44 mg/kg PO initially, then 22 mg/kg PO q8h for 5 days. (Todd, Paul, and DiPietro 1985)
      b) 50 mg/kg PO per day for 5 days. (Jones 1985)
      c) 25 - 65 mg/kg PO once daily for 5 days. (Longhofer 1988)
      d) 30 - 60 mg/kg PO once daily for 5-7 days (also for trichomoniasis) (Chiapella 1988)
      e) 25 mg/kg PO *bid* (Aronson and Aucoin 1989)
    For anaerobic infections:
      a) For anaerobic bacterial meningitis: 25 - 50 mg/kg PO q12h. (Schunk 1988)
      b) For suppurative cholangitis: 25 - 30 mg/kg PO *bid*; may be used with chloramphenicol. Therapy may be necessary for 4-6 weeks. (Cornelius and Bjorling 1988)
      c) 30 mg/kg/day PO divided q6-8h. (Dow 1989)
      d) 44 mg/kg PO q12h (Aronson and Aucoin 1989)
    For adjunctive therapy of plasmacytic/lymphocytic enteritis:
      a) 30 - 60 mg/kg PO once daily. (Chiapella 1988)
      b) 10 mg/kg PO *tid* for 2-4 weeks. (Magne 1989)
    For adjunctive therapy of plasmacytic/lymphocytic colitis:
      a) 10 - 30 mg/kg PO q8-24h for 2-4 weeks in refractory cases. (Leib, Hay, and Roth 1989)
      b) For ulcerative colitis in dogs refractory to other therapies (*e.g.*, sulfasalazine, immunosuppressants, diet, etc.): 10 - 15 mg/kg once to twice a day; discontinue after 2 weeks if response is inadequate. (DeNovo 1988)
    For amebiasis, balatidiasis:
      a) 60 mg/kg PO once daily for 5 days (DeNovo 1988)
    For adjunctive therapy of hepatic encephalopathy:
      a) 20 mg/kg PO q8h (Hardy 1989)
  Cats:
    For treatment of *Giardia*:
      a) 10 - 25 mg/kg PO once daily for 5 days. (Longhofer 1988)
      b) 8 - 10 mg/kg PO *bid* for 10 days (also for trichomoniasis) (Chiapella 1988)
    For anaerobic infections:
      a) For adjunctive therapy of plasmacytic/lymphocytic enteritis: 10 mg/kg PO once daily. (Chiapella 1988)
      b) For adjunctive therapy of hepatic lipidoses: 25 - 30 mg/kg PO *bid* for 2-3 weeks (unproven, but may be of benefit) (Cornelius and Bjorling 1988)
  Horses:
    For susceptible anaerobic infections:
      a) 15 - 25 mg/kg PO q6h (Sweeney et al. 1986)
      b) 20 - 25 mg/kg PO q12h as crushed tablets in an aqueous suspension. (Baggot, Wilson, and Hietela 1988)
  Birds:
    For susceptible infections (anaerobes):
      a) 50 mg/kg PO once daily for 5 days (Bauck and Hoefer 1993)
  Reptiles:
      a) For anaerobic infections in most species:150 mg/kg PO once; repeat in one week.

For amoeba and flagellates in most species: 100 - 275 mg/kg PO once; repeat in 1-2 weeks. In *Drymarchon* spp., *Lampropeltis pyromelana*, & *lampropeltis zonata*: 40 mg/kg PO once; repeat in 2 weeks (Gauvin 1993)

Monitoring Parameters -
1) Clinical efficacy
2) Adverse effects (clients should report any neurologic symptomatology)

Client Information - Report any neurologic symptoms to veterinarian (see Overdose section).

Dosage Forms/Preparations/FDA Approval Status/Withholding Times -
Veterinary-Approved Products: None

Human-Approved Products:

Metronidazole Tablets 250 mg, 500 mg; Capsules 375 mg; *Flagyl*® (Searle); *Metric 21*® (Fielding); *Protostat*® (Ortho); *Flagyl 375*® (Searle); generic; (Rx)

Metronidazole HCl Powder for Injection 500 mg/vial; *Flagyl*®*IV* (Searle); (Rx)

Metronidazole 500 mg/100 ml injection (ready to use); *Flagyl*®*I.V.* (Searle); *Metro*®*I.V.* (McGaw); *Metronidazole Redi-Infusion*® (Elkins-Sinn); *Metronidazole*® (Abbott); (Rx)

MEXILETINE HCL

Chemistry - A class IB antiarrhythmic, mexiletine HCl occurs as a white or almost white, odorless, crystalline powder. It is freely soluble in water.

Storage/Stability/Compatibility - Mexiletine capsules should be stored in tight containers at room temperature.

Pharmacology - Mexiletine is similar to lidocaine in its mechanism of antiarrhythmic activity. It inhibits the inward sodium current (fast sodium channel), thereby reducing the rate of rise of the action potential, Phase O. In the Purkinje fibers, automaticity is decreased, action potential is shortened, and to a lesser extent, effective refractory period is decreased. Usually conduction is unaffected, but may be slowed in patients with preexisting conduction abnormalities. Mexiletine is considered a class IB antiarrhythmic agent.

Uses/Indications - Mexiletine may be useful to treat some ventricular arrhythmias, including PVC's and ventricular tachycardia in small animals

Pharmacokinetics - Mexiletine is relatively well absorbed from the gut and has a low first-pass effect. In humans, it is moderately bound to plasma proteins (60-75%), metabolized in the liver to inactive metabolites with an elimination half-life of about 10-12 hours. Half lives may be significantly increased in patients with moderate to severe hepatic disease, or in those having severely reduced cardiac outputs. Half lives may be slightly prolonged in patients with severe renal disease or after acute myocardial infarction.

Contraindications/Precautions/Reproductive Safety - Mexiletine should be used with extreme caution if at all, in patients with pre-existing 2nd or 3rd degree AV block (without pacemaker), or in patients with cardiogenic shock. It should be used when the following medical conditions exist only when the benefits of therapy outweigh the risks: severe congestive heart failure or acute myocardial infarction, hepatic function impairment, hypotension, intraventricular conduction abnormalities or sinus node function impairment, seizure disorder, or sensitivity to the drug.

Lab animal studies have not demonstrated teratogenicity. Because mexiletine is secreted into maternal milk, it has been recommended to use milk replacer if the mother is taking the drug.

Adverse Effects/Warnings - The most likely adverse effect noted in animals is GI distress, including vomiting. Giving with meals may alleviate this. Potentially (reported in humans) CNS effects (trembling, unsteadiness, dizziness), shortness of breath, PVC's and chest pain could occur. Rarely, seizures, agranulocytosis, and thrombocytopenia have been reported in humans.

Overdosage/Acute Toxicity - Toxicity associated with overdosage may be significant. Case reports in humans have noted that CNS signs always preceded cardiovascular signs. Treatment should consist of GI tract emptying protocols when indicated, acidification of the urine to enhance urinary excretion, and supportive therapy. Atropine may be useful if hypotension or bradycardia occur.

Drug Interactions - **Urinary acidifying drugs** (*e.g.*, methionine, ammonium chloride, potassium or sodium phosphates) may accelerate the renal excretion of mexiletine. **Urinary alkalinizing drugs** (*e.g.*, citrates, bicarb, carbonic anhydrase inhibitors) may reduce the urinary excretion of mexiletine.

Drugs that induce hepatic enzymes (*e.g.*, phenobarbital, griseofulvin, primidone, rifampin, tolbutamide) may accelerate the metabolism of mexiletine. **Theophylline** (**aminophylline**) metabolism may be reduced by mexiletine, thereby leading to theophylline toxicity. **Cimetidine** may increase or decrease mexiletine blood levels.

Aluminum-magnesium containing antacids or **opiates** may slow the absorption of mexiletine. **Metoclopramide** may accelerate the absorption of mexiletine.

Laboratory Considerations - Some human patients (1-3%) have had **AST** values increase by as much as three times or more above the upper limit of normal. This is reportedly a transient effect and asymptomatic.

Doses -
   Dogs:
      For treating or assisting in treatment of ventricular arrhythmias:
      a)   4 - 8 mg/kg PO *tid* (Hamlin 1992)
      b)   5 - 8 mg/kg PO q8-12h (Muir and Bonagura 1994)
      c)   4 - 10 mg/kg PO *tid* (Lunney and Ettinger 1991)

Monitoring Parameters - 1) In humans, therapeutic plasma concentrations are: 0.5 - 2.0 micrograms/ml. Toxicity may be noted at therapeutic levels; 2) ECG; 3) Adverse Effects

Client Information - Instruct to give with food, if animal develops anorexia or vomiting. Reinforce compliance with prescribed therapy.

Dosage Forms/Preparations/FDA Approval Status/Withholding Times -
   Veterinary-Approved Products: None
   Human-Approved Products:
      Mexiletine Oral Capsules 150 mg, 200 mg, 250 mg; *Mexitil*® (Boehringer Ingelheim); generic; (Rx)

MIBOLERONE

Chemistry - A non-progestational, androgenic, anabolic, antigonadotropic, 19-nor-steroid, mibolerone occurs as a white, crystalline solid. Mibolerone may also be known as dimethyl-nortestosterone.

Storage/Stability/Compatibility - The manufacturer (Upjohn) states that the compound in *Cheque*® *Drops* is stable under ordinary conditions and temperatures.

Pharmacology - Mibolerone acts by blocking the release of lutenizing hormone (LH) from the anterior pituitary via a negative feedback mechanism. Because of the lack of LH, follicles will develop to a certain point, but will not mature and hence no ovulation or corpus luteum development occurs. The net result is a suppression of the estrous cycle if the drug is given prior to (as much as 30 days) the onset of proestrus. After discontinuation of the drug, the next estrus may occur within 7-200 days (avg. 70 days).

Uses/Indications - *Cheque*® *Drops* are labeled as indicated "for estrous (heat) prevention in adult female dogs not intended primarily for breeding purposes." In clinical trials it was 90% effective in suppressing estrus.

   Although not approved, mibolerone at dosages of 50 micrograms per day will prevent estrus in the cat, but its use is generally not recommended because of the very narrow therapeutic index of the drug in this species (see the Adverse effects and Overdosage sections for more information).

Pharmacokinetics - Mibolerone is reported to be well absorbed from the intestine after oral administration and is rapidly metabolized in the liver to over 10 separate metabolites. Excretion is apparently equally divided between the urine and feces.

Contraindications/Precautions - Mibolerone is contraindicated in female dogs with perianal adenoma, perianal adenocarcinoma or other androgen-dependent neoplasias. It is also contraindicated in patients with ongoing or a history of, liver or kidney disease. The manufacturer also recommends not using the drug in Bedlington Terriers.

   Mibolerone should not be used in pregnant bitches. Masculinization of the female fetuses will occur. Alterations seen may include, changes in vagina patency, multiple urethral openings in the vagina, a phallus-like structure instead of a clitoris, formation of testes-like structures, and fluid accumulation in the vagina and uterus. Because it may inhibit lactation, it should not be used in nursing bitches.

   The manufacturer recommends discontinuing the product after 24 months of use. It should not be used to try to attempt to abbreviate an estrous period or in bitches prior to their first estrous period.

Adverse Effects/Warnings - Immature females may be more prone to develop adverse reactions than more mature females. In prepuberal females, mibolerone can induce premature epiphyseal closure, clitoral enlargement, and vaginitis. Adverse effects that may be seen in the adult bitch, include mild clitoral hypertrophy (may be partially reversible), vulvovaginitis, increased body odor, abnormal behavior, urinary incontinence, voice deepening, riding behavior, enhanced symptoms of seborrhea oleosa, epiphora (tearing), hepatic changes (intranuclear hyaline bodies) and increased kidney weight (without pathology). Although reported, overt hepatic dysfunction would be considered to occur rarely in dogs. With the exception of residual mild clitoral hypertrophy, adverse effects will generally resolve after discontinuation of therapy.

In the cat, dosages of 60 micrograms/day have caused hepatic dysfunction and 120 micrograms/day have caused death. Other adverse effects that have been noted in cats, include clitoral hypertrophy, thyroid dysfunction, os clitorides formation, cervical dermis thickening, and pancreatic dysfunction.

Overdosage/Toxicology Studies - Many toxicology studies have been performed in dogs. The drug did not cause death in doses up to 30,000 micrograms/kg/day when administered to beagles for 28 days. For a more detailed discussion of the toxicology of the drug, the reader is referred to the package insert for *Cheque® Drops*.

In the cat, dosages of as low as 120 micrograms/day have resulted in fatalities.

Drug Interactions - Increased seizure activity has been reported in a dog after receiving mibolerone who was previously controlled on **phenytoin**. Mibolerone should generally not be used concurrently with **progestins or estrogen** agents.

Drug/Laboratory Interactions - Mibolerone has been reported to cause **thyroid dysfunction in cats**.

Doses -
Dogs:
For suppression of estrus (treatment must begin at least 30 days prior to proestrus):
a) Bitches weighing:
0.5-11 kg: 30 micrograms (0.3 ml) PO per day
12-22 kg: 60 micrograms (0.6 ml) PO per day
23-45 kg: 120 micrograms (1.2 ml) PO per day
>45 kg: 180 micrograms (1.8 ml) PO per day
German shepherds or German shepherd crosses: 180 micrograms (1.8 ml) PO per day; regardless of weight (Package Insert; *Cheque® Drops*—Upjohn)
b) As above, but should dog come into estrus after receiving the drug for 30 or more days. Stop drug and determine that the dog is not pregnant before resuming therapy. If owner compliance has been determined, increase dosage by 20-50%. (Woody 1988), (Burke 1985)

For psuedocyesis (false pregnancy):
a) Use 10 times the dosage listed above for suppression of estrus PO once daily for 5 days (Barton and Wolf 1988)
b) 16 micrograms/kg PO once daily for 5 days (Concannon 1986)

For treatment of severe galactorrhea:
a) 8 - 18 micrograms/kg PO once a day for 5 days. Once discontinued, prolactin may surge and galactorrhea resume. (Olson and Olson 1986)

Cats: **WARNING**: Because of the very low margin of safety with this drug in cats, it cannot be recommended for use in this species.

Monitoring Parameters -
1) Symptoms of estrus
2) Liver function tests (baseline, annual, or *prn*)
3) Physical examination of genitalia

Client Information - It must be stressed to owners that compliance with dosage and administration directions are crucial for this agent to be effective.

Dosage Forms/Preparations/FDA Approval Status/Withholding Times -
Veterinary-Approved Products:
Mibolerone Oral Drops 100 micrograms/ml in 55 ml dropper bottles; *Cheque® Drops* (Upjohn); (Rx) Approved for use in dogs only.

Human-Approved Products: None

MIDAZOLAM HCL

Chemistry - An imidazobenzodiazepine, midazolam occurs as a white to light yellow crystalline powder with a pK_a of 6.15. Midazolam HCl's aqueous solubility is pH dependent. At 25°C and a pH of 3.4, 10.3 mg are soluble in 1 ml of water. The pH of the commercially prepared injection is approximately 3.

Storage/Stability/Compatibility - It is recommended to store midazolam injection at room temperature (15°-30°C) and protect from light. After being frozen for 3 days and allowed to thaw at room temperature, the injectable product was physically stable. Midazolam is stable at a pH from 3-3.6.

Midazolam is reportedly **compatible** when mixed with the following products: D5W, normal saline, lactated Ringer's, atropine sulfate, fentanyl citrate, glycopyrrolate, hydroxyzine HCl, ketamine HCl, meperidine HCl, morphine sulfate, nalbuphine HCl, promethazine HCl, sufantanil citrate, and scopolamine Hbr. Compatibility is dependent upon factors such as pH, concentration, temperature, and diluents used and it is suggested to consult specialized references for more specific information.

Pharmacology - Midazolam exhibits similar pharmacologic actions as other benzodiazepines (refer to the diazepam monograph for more information). Its unique solubility characteristics (water soluble injection but lipid soluble at body pH) give it a very rapid onset of action after injection.

Uses/Indications - In humans, midazolam has been suggested to be used as a premedicant before surgery, and when combined with potent analgesic/anesthetic drugs (*e.g.,* ketamine or fentanyl), as a conscious sedative. In humans, midazolam reduces the incidences of "dreamlike" emergence reactions and increases in blood pressure and cardiac rate that ketamine causes.

When compared to the thiobarbiturate induction agents (*e.g.,* thiamylal, thiopental), midazolam has less cardiopulmonary depressant effects, is water soluble, can be mixed with several other agents, and does not tend to accumulate in the body after repeated doses. There is much interest in using the drug alone as an induction agent. Several veterinary anesthesiologists are studying the clinical applications of this agent in veterinary medicine and additional information regarding its use should be forthcoming.

Pharmacokinetics - Following IM injection, midazolam is rapidly and nearly completely (91%) absorbed. Although no oral products are being marketed, midazolam is well absorbed after oral administration, but because of a rapid first-pass effect, bioavailibilities suffer (31-72%). The onset of action following IV administration is very rapid due to the high lipophilicity of the agent. In humans, the loss of the lash reflex or counting occurs within 30-97 seconds of administration.

The drug is highly protein bound (94-97%) and rapidly crosses the blood-brain barrier. Because only unbound drug will cross into the CNS, changes in plasma protein concentrations and resultant protein binding may significantly alter the response to a given dose.

Midazolam is metabolized in the liver, principally by microsomal oxidation. An active metabolite (alpha-hydroxymidazolam) is formed, but because of its very short half-life and lower pharmacologic activity, it probably has negligible clinical effects. The serum half-life and duration of activity of midazolam in humans is considerably shorter than that of diazepam. Elimination half-lives measured in humans average approximately 2 hours (vs. approx. 30 hrs for diazepam).

Contraindications/Precautions - The manufacturer lists the following contraindications for use in humans: hypersensitivity to benzodiazepines, or acute narrow-angle glaucoma. Additionally, intra-carotid artery injections must be avoided.

Use cautiously in patients with hepatic or renal disease and in debilitated or geriatric patients. Patients with congestive heart failure may eliminate the drug more slowly. The drug should be administered to patients in coma, shock or having significant respiratory depression very cautiously.

Although midazolam has not been demonstrated to cause fetal abnormalities, in humans other benzodiazepines have been implicated in causing congenital abnormalities if administered during the first trimester of pregnancy. Infants born of mothers receiving large doses of benzodiazepines shortly before delivery have been reported to suffer from apnea, impaired metabolic response to cold stress, difficulty in feeding, hyperbilirubinemia, hypotonia, etc. Withdrawal symptoms have occurred in infants whose mothers chronically took benzodiazepines during pregnancy. The veterinary significance of these effects is unclear, but the use of these agents during the first trimester of pregnancy should only occur when the benefits clearly outweigh the risks associated with their use. It is unknown if midazolam is distributed into milk, but other benzodiazepines and their metabolites are distributed into milk and may cause CNS effects in nursing neonates.

Adverse Effects/Warnings - Few adverse effects have been reported in human patients receiving midazolam. Most frequently effects on respiratory rate, cardiac rate and blood pressure have been reported. Respiratory depression has been reported in patients who have received narcotics or have COPD. The following adverse effects have been reported in more than 1%, but less than 5% of patients receiving midazolam: pain on injection, local irritation, headache, nausea, vomiting, and hiccups.

The principle concern in veterinary patients is the possibility of respiratory depression occurring.

Overdosage - Very limited information is currently available. The IV LD_{50} in mice has been reported to be 86 mg/kg. It is suggested that accidental overdoses be managed in a supportive manner, similar to diazepam.

Drug Interactions - Use with **barbiturates or other CNS depressants** may increase the risk of respiratory depression occurring. **Narcotics** (including Innovar®) may increase the hypnotic effects of midazolam and hypotension has been reported when used with **meperidine**. Midazolam may decrease the dosages required for **inhalation anesthetics or thiopental**.

Doses -
   Dogs:
      As a preoperative agent: 0.066 - 0.22 mg/kg IM or IV (Mandsager 1988)
   Cats:
      As a preoperative agent: 0.066 - 0.22 mg/kg IM or IV (Mandsager 1988)
   Rabbits/Rodents/Pocket Pets:
      Rabbits: As a tranquilizer (to increase relaxation of lightly anesthetized animals and permit ET intubation): 1 mg/kg IV prn.
      Rodents: 5 mg/kg IV (in combination with fentanyl/droperidol or fentanyl-fluanisone for neuroleptanesthesia) (Huerkamp 1995)
   Horses:
      As a preoperative agent: 0.011 - 0.0.44 mg/kg IV (Mandsager 1988)

Monitoring Parameters -
      1) Level of sedation
      2) Respiratory and cardiac signs

Client Information - This agent should be used in an inpatient setting only or with direct professional supervision where cardiorespiratory support services are available.

Dosage Forms/Preparations -
   Veterinary-Approved Products: None
   Human-Approved Products:
      Midazolam HCl for Injection 1mg/ml in 2, 5, & 10 ml vials; 5 mg/ml in 1, 2, 5, & 10 ml vials, 2 ml syringes; *Versed*® (Roche); (Rx)

      Midazolam is a Class-IV controlled substance.

MILBEMYCIN OXIME

Note: For information on the combination product with lufenuron (*Sentinel*®), see the lufenuron monograph

Chemistry - Milbemycin oxime consists of approximately 80% of the A4 derivatives and 20% of the A3 derivatives of 5-didehydromilbemycin. Milbemycin is considered to be a macrolide antibiotic structurally.

Storage/Stability - Store milbemycin oxime tablets at room temperature.

Pharmacology - Milbemycin is thought to act by disrupting the transmission of the neurotransmitter gamma amino butyric acid (GABA) in invertebrates.

Uses/Indications - Milbemycin tablets are labeled as a once-a-month heartworm preventative (*Dirofilaria immitis*.) and for hookworm control (*Ancylostoma caninum*). It also has activity against a variety of other parasites, including roundworms (*Toxocara canis*), *Trichuris vulpis*, and for demodicosis. In cats, milbemycin has been used successfully to prevent larval infection of *Dirofilaria immitis*.

Pharmacokinetics - No specific information was located. At labeled doses, milbemycin is considered effective for at least 45 days after infection by *D. immitis* larva.

Contraindications/Precautions/Reproductive Safety - Because some dogs with a high number of circulating microfilaria will develop a transient, shock-like syndrome after receiving milbemycin, the manufacturer recommends testing for preexisting heartworm infections.

   Studies in pregnant dogs at daily doses 3X those labeled showed no adverse effects to offspring or bitch. Milbemycin does enter maternal milk; at standard doses, no adverse effects have been noted in nursing puppies.

Adverse Effects/Warnings - At labeled doses, adverse effects appear to be negligible in microfilaria-free dogs, including Collie breeds (see Overdosage below). There have been unconfirmed reports of an increased incidence of seizure disorders or other neurologic signs seen in dogs receiving milbemycin, but a causal relationship has not been documented at the time of this writing.

   When replacing diethylcarbamazine as a heartworm preventative, milbemycin should be administered within 30 days of discontinuing DEC.

   Eight week old puppies receiving 2.5 mg/kg (5X label) for 3 consecutive days showed no symptoms after the first day, but after the second or third consecutive dose showed some ataxia and trembling. The manufacturer states that at labeled doses the drug is safe to use in puppies as young as 8 weeks old.

Overdosage/Acute Toxicity - Beagles have tolerated a single oral dose of 200 mg/kg (200 times monthly rate). Rough-coated collies have tolerated doses of 10 mg/kg (20 times labeled) without adversity; doses of 12.5 mg/kg (25X label) caused ataxia, pyrexia, and periodic recumbency.

Drug Interactions - No interactions were noted. The manufacturer states that the drug was used safely during testing in dogs receiving other frequently used veterinary products, including vaccines, anthelmintics, antibiotics, steroids, flea collars, shampoos and dips.

Doses -
  Dogs:
    For prevention of heartworm:
      a) 0.5 - 0.99 mg/kg PO once monthly (also controls hookworm, roundworm and whipworm infestations) (Calvert 1994)

    For microfilaricide chemotherapy:
      a) In adulticide -pretreated dogs: Use preventative/prophylaxis dosage; repeat in 2 weeks if necessary. If heartworm transmission season has started, continue monthly prohylaxis. (Knight 1995)

    For treatment of generalized demodicosis:
      a) 0.5 - 1 mg/kg PO once daily for at least 90 days (Miller 1992)
      b) 1 mg/kg PO daily for one month past the point of negative skin scrapings. (Mundell 1994)

  Cats:
    For prevention of heartworm:
      a) 0.5 - 0.99 mg/kg PO once monthly (Miller 1994)

Client Information - Review importance of compliance with therapy and to be certain that the dose was consumed.

Dosage Forms/Preparations/FDA Approval Status -
  Veterinary-Approved Products:
    Milbemycin Oxime Oral Tablets 2.3 mg, 5.75 mg, 11.50 mg, 23 mg; *Interceptor®*; *Safeheart®* (Novartis); (Rx) Approved for use in dogs.

    Milbemycin/Lufenuron Oral Tablets in six tablet cards: 2.3 mg/46 mg (for dogs 2 to 10 lbs.,—brown), 5.75 mg/115 mg (for dogs 11 to 25 lbs.,—green), 11.5 mg/230 mg (for dogs 26 to 50 lbs.,—yellow), 23 mg/460 mg (for dogs 51 to 100 lbs.,—white); (Rx) *Sentinel®* (Novartis). Approved for use in dogs.

  Human-Approved Products: None

MINERAL OIL
WHITE PETROLATUM

Chemistry - Mineral Oil, also known as liquid petrolatum, liquid paraffin or white mineral oil occurs as a tasteless, odorless (when cold), transparent, colorless, oily liquid that is insoluble in both water and alcohol. It is a mixture of complex hydrocarbons and is derived from crude petroleum. For pharmaceutical purposes, heavy mineral oil is recommended over light mineral oil, as it is believed to have a lesser tendency to be absorbed in the gut or aspirated after oral administration.

White petrolatum, also known as white petroleum jelly or white soft paraffin occurs as a white or faintly yellow unctious mass. It is insoluble in water and almost insoluble in alcohol. White petrolatum differs from petrolatum only in that it is further refined to remove more of the yellow color.

Storage/Stability/Compatibility - Petrolatum products should be stored at temperatures less than 30°C.

Pharmacology - Mineral oil and petrolatum act as a laxatives by lubricating fecal material and the intestinal mucosa. They also reduce reabsorption of water from the GI tract, thereby increasing fecal bulk and decreasing intestinal transit time.

Uses/Indications - Mineral oil is commonly used in horses to treat constipation and fecal impactions. It is also employed as a laxative in other species as well, but used less frequently. Mineral oil has been administered after ingesting lipid-soluble toxins (*e.g.,* kerosene, metaldehyde) to retard the absorption of these toxins through its laxative and solubility properties.

Petrolatum containing products (*e.g., Felaxin®, Laxatone®, Kat-A-Lax®*, etc.) may be used in dogs and cats as a laxative or to prevent/reduce "hair-balls" in cats.

Pharmacokinetics - It has been reported that after oral administration, emulsions of mineral oil may be up to 60% absorbed, but most reports state that mineral oil preparations are only minimally absorbed from the gut.

Contraindications/Precautions - No specific contraindications were noted with regard to veterinary patients. In humans, mineral oil (orally administered) is considered to be contraindicated in patients less than 6 yrs. old, debilitated or pregnant patients, and in patients with hiatal hernia, dysphagia, esophogeal or gastric retention. Use caution when administering by tube to avoid aspiration, especially in debilitated or recalcitrant animals. To avoid aspiration in small animals, orally administered mineral oil should not be attempted when there is an increased risk of vomiting, regurgitation or other preexisting swallowing difficulty.

Adverse Effects/Warnings - When used on a short-term basis and at recommended doses, mineral oil or petrolatum should cause minimal adverse effects. The most serious effect that could be encountered is aspiration of the oil with resultant lipid pneumonitis. This can be prevented by using the drug in appropriate cases and when "tubing" to ascertain that the tube is in the stomach and to administer the oil at a reasonable rate.

Granulomatous reactions have occurred in the liver, spleen and mesenteric lymph nodes when significant quantities of mineral oil are absorbed from the gut. Oil leakage from the anus may occur and be of concern in animals with rectal lesions or in house pets. Long-term administration of mineral oil/petrolatum may lead to decreased absorption of fat-soluble vitamins (A, D, E, & K). No reports were found documenting clinically significant hypovitaminosis in cats receiving long-term petrolatum therapy, however.

Overdosage - No specific information was located regarding overdoses of mineral oil; but it would be expected that with the exception of aspiration, the effects would be self-limiting. See adverse effects section for more information.

Drug Interactions - Theoretically, mineral oil should not be given with **docusate** (**DSS**) as enhanced absorption of the mineral oil could occur. However, this does not appear to be of significant clinical concern with large animals.

Chronic administration of mineral oil may affect **Vitamin K and other fat soluble vitamin** absorption. It has been recommended to administer mineral oil products between meals to minimize this problem.

Doses -
  Dogs:
    As a laxative:
      a) 2 - 60 mls PO (Jenkins 1988), (Kirk 1989)
      b) 5 - 30 mls PO (Davis 1985a)
      c) 5 - 25 mls PO (Burrows 1986)
  Cats: See specific label directions for "Cat Laxative" Products
    As a laxative:
      a) 2 - 10 mls PO (Jenkins 1988), (Kirk 1989)
      b) 2 - 6 mls PO (Davis 1985a)
      c) 5 ml per day with food (Sherding 1989)
  Cattle: Administer via stomach tube
    As a laxative:
      a) 1 - 4 liters (Howard 1986)
      b) Adults: 0.5 - 2 liters ; Calves: 60 - 120 mls (Jenkins 1988)
    For adjunctive treatment of metaldehyde poisoning:
      a) 8 ml/kg; may be used with a saline cathartic (Smith 1986)
    For adjunctive treatment of nitrate poisoning:
      a) 1 liter per 400 kg body weight (Ruhr and Osweiler 1986)
  Horses: Administer via stomach tube
    As a laxative:
      a) For large colon impactions: 2 - 4 quarts q12-24 hours, may take up to 5 gallons. Mix 1 - 2 quarts of warm water with the oil to ease administration and give more fluid to the horse. Pumping in at a moderate speed is desirable over gravity flow. (Sellers and Lowe 1987)
      b) Adults: 2 - 4 liters, may be repeated daily; Foals: 240 mls (Clark and Becht 1987)
      c) Adults: 0.5 - 2 liters; Foals: 60 - 120 mls (Jenkins 1988)
  Swine: Administer via stomach tube
    As a laxative:
      a) 50 - 100 mls (Howard 1986)

Sheep & Goats: Administer via stomach tube
> As a laxative:
> > a) 100 - 500 mls (Howard 1986)

Birds:
> As a laxative and to aid in the removal of lead from the gizzard.
> > a) 1 - 3 drops per 30 grams of body weight or 5 ml/kg PO once. Repeat as necessary. Give via tube or slowly to avoid aspiration. (Clubb 1986)

Monitoring Parameters -
> 1) Clinical efficacy
> 2) If possibility of aspiration: auscultate, radiograph if necessary

Client Information - Follow veterinarian's instructions or label directions for "cat laxative" products. Do not increase dosage or prolong treatment beyond veterinarian's recommendations.

Dosage Forms/Preparations/FDA Approval Status/Withholding Times - These products and preparations are available without a prescription (OTC).

> **Veterinary-Approved Products**: Mineral oil products have not been formally approved for use in food animals.

Petrolatum Oral Preparations
> Products may vary in actual composition; some contain liquid petrolatum in place of white petrolatum. Trade names include: *Felaxin®* (Schering), *Kat-A-Lax®* (P/M; Mallinckrodt), *Laxatone®* (Evsco), *Kit-Tonne®* (Miles), *Lax 'aire®* (Beecham)

Human-Approved Products:
> Mineral Oil, Heavy in pints, quarts, gallons and drums
>
> Mineral Oil, Extra Heavy in pints, quarts, gallons and drums
>
> Mineral Oil Emulsions
>
> There are several products available that are emulsions of mineral oil and may be more palatable for oral administration. Because of expense and with no increase in efficacy they are used only in small animals. They may be dosed as described above, factoring in the actual percentage of mineral oil in the preparation used. Trade names include: *Agoral® Plain* (Parke-Davis), *Kondremul® Plain* (Fisons), and *Milkinol®* (Kremers-Urban).

MISOPROSTOL

Chemistry - A synthetic prostaglandin E_1 analog, misoprostol occurs as a yellow, viscous liquid having a musty odor.

Storage/Stability/Compatibility - Misoprostol tablets should be stored in well-closed containers at room temperature. After manufacture, misoprostol has an expiration date of 18 months.

Pharmacology - Misoprostol has two main pharmacologic effects that make it a potentially useful agent. By a direct action on parietal cells it inhibits basal and nocturnal gastric acid secretion as well as gastric acid secretion that is stimulated by food, pentagastrin or histamine. Pepsin secretion is decreased under basal conditions, but not when stimulated by histamine.

Misoprostol also has a cytoprotective effect on gastric mucosa. Probably by increasing production of gastric mucosa and bicarbonate, increasing turnover and blood supply of gastric mucosal cells, misoprostol enhances mucosal defense mechanisms and enhances healing in response to acid-related injuries.

Other pharmacologic effects of misoprostol include, increased amplitude and frequency of uterine contractions, stimulate uterine bleeding, and causing total or partial expulsion of uterine contents in pregnant animals.

Uses/Indications - Misoprostol may be useful as primary or adjunctive therapy in treating or preventing gastric ulceration, especially when caused or aggravated by non-steroidal antiinflammatory drugs (NSAIDS). Misoprostol may be efficacious in reducing or reversing cyclosporin-induced nephrotoxicity. More data is needed to confirm this effect.

Pharmacokinetics - Approximately 88% of an oral dose of misoprostol is rapidly absorbed from the GI tract, but a significant amount is metabolized via the first-pass effect. The presence of food and antacids will delay the absorption of the drug. Misoprostol is rapidly de-esterified to misoprostol acid which is the primary active metabolite. Misoprostol and misoprostol acid are thought be equal in their effects on gastric mucosa. Both misoprostol and the acid metabolite are fairly well bound to plasma proteins (approximately 90% bound). It is not believed that misoprostol enters maternal milk, but it is unknown whether the acid enters milk.

Misoprostol acid is further biotransformed via oxidative mechanisms to pharmacologically inactive metabolites. These metabolites, the free acid and small amounts of unchanged drug are principally excreted into the urine. In humans, the serum half life of misoprostol is about 30 minutes and its duration of pharmacological effect is about 3-6 hours.

Contraindications/Precautions/Reproductive Safety - Misoprostol is contraindicated during pregnancy due to its abortifacient activity. It is not recommended to be used in nursing mothers as it potentially could cause significant diarrhea in the nursing offspring.

It should be used in patients with the following conditions only when its potential benefits outweigh the risks: Sensitivity to prostaglandins or prostaglandin analogs; patients with cerebral or coronary vascular disease (although not reported with misoprostol, some prostaglandins and prostaglandin analogs have precipitated seizures in epileptic human patients, and have caused hypotension which may adversely affect these patients).

Adverse Effects/Warnings - The most prevalent adverse effect seen with misoprostol is GI distress, usually manifested by diarrhea, abdominal pain, vomiting and flatulence. Adverse effects are often transient and resolve over several days or may be minimized by dosage adjustment or giving doses with food. Potentially, uterine contractions and vaginal bleeding could occur in female dogs.

Overdosage/Acute Toxicity - There is limited information available. Overdoses in laboratory animals have produced diarrhea, GI lesions, emesis, tremors, focal cardiac, hepatic or renal tubular necrosis, seizures and hypotension. Overdoses should be treated seriously and standard gut emptying techniques employed when applicable. Resultant toxicity should be treated symptomatically and supportively.

Drug Interactions - **Magnesium-containing antacids** may aggravate misoprostol-induced diarrhea. If an antacid is required and aluminum-only antacid may be a better choice. **Antacids and food** do reduce the rate of absorption and may reduce the systemic availability, but probably do not affect therapeutic efficacy.

Doses -
  Dogs:
    For the prevention and treatment of GI ulcers:
    a) 1 - 3 micrograms/kg PO q6-8h (Davenport 1992)
    b) 2 - 5 micrograms/kg PO q8h (Matz 1995)
    c) 3 - 5 micrograms/kg PO q6h (Johnson, Sherding et al. 1994)

Monitoring Parameters - Efficacy and adverse effects

Client Information - Caution pregnant women to handle the drug with caution. If diarrhea or other GI adverse effects become severe or persist, reduce dose or give with food or aluminum antacids to alleviate. Severe diarrhoeas may require supportive therapy.

Dosage Forms/Preparations/FDA Approval Status/Withholding Times -
  Veterinary-Approved Products: None
  Human-Approved Products:
    Misoprostol Oral Tablets 100 micrograms, 200 micrograms; *Cytotec*® (Searle); (Rx)

MITOTANE
O, P' - DDD

Chemistry - Mitotane, also commonly known in veterinary medicine as *o,p'*-DDD, is structurally related to the infamous insecticide, chlorophenothane (DDT). It occurs as a white, crystalline powder with a slightly aromatic odor. It is practically insoluble in water and soluble in alcohol.

Storage/Stability/Compatibility - Mitotane tablets should be stored at room temperature (15-30°C), in tight, light resistant containers.

Pharmacology - While mitotane is considered to be an adrenal cytotoxic agent, it apparently can also inhibit adrenocortical function without causing cell destruction. The exact mechanisms of action for these effects are not clearly understood.

In dogs with pituitary-dependent hyperadrenocorticism (PDH), mitotane has been demonstrated to cause severe, progressive necrosis of the zona fasiculata and zona reticularis. These effects occur quite rapidly (within days of starting therapy). It has been stated that mitotane spares the zona glomerulosa and therefore aldosterone synthesis is unaffected. This is only partially true, as the zona glomerulosa may also be affected by mitotane therapy, but it is uncommon for clinically significant effects on aldosterone production to be noted with therapy.

Uses/Indications - In veterinary medicine, mitotane is used primarily for the medical treatment of pituitary-dependent hyperadrenocorticism (PDH), principally in the dog. It has also been used for the palliative treatment of adrenal carcinoma in humans and dogs.

Pharmacokinetics - In dogs, the systemic bioavailability of mitonane is poor. Oral absorption can be enhanced by giving the drug with food. In humans, approximately 40% of an oral dose of mitotane is absorbed after dosing, with peak serum levels occuring about 3-5 hours after a single dose. Distribution of the drug occurs to virtually all tissues in the body. The drug is stored in the fat and does not accumulate in the adrenal glands. A small amount may enter the CSF. It is unknown if the drug crosses the placenta or is distributed into milk.

Mitotane has a very long plasma half-life in humans, with values ranging from 18-159 days being reported. Serum half-lives may increase in a given patient with continued dosing, perhaps due to a depot effect from adipose tissue releasing the drug. The drug is metabolized in the liver and is excreted as metabolites in the urine and bile. Approximately 15% of an oral dose is excreted in the bile, and 10% in the urine within 24 hours of dosing.

Contraindications/Precautions - Mitotane is contraindicated in patients known to be hypersensitive to it. As it is unknown whether mitotane crosses the placenta, it should be used in pregnant bitches cautiously. As it is also unknown if the drug enters into milk, it's suggested that puppies be given milk replacer after receiving colostrum if the mother is receiving mitotane.

Patients with concurrent diabetes mellitus may have rapidly changing insulin requirements during the initial treatment period. These animals should be closely monitored until they are clinically stable.

Dogs with preexisting renal or hepatic disease should receive the drug with caution and with more intense monitoring.

Some clinicians recommend giving prednisolone at 0.2 mg/kg/day during the initial treatment period (0.4 mg/kg/day to diabetic dogs) to reduce the potential for side effects from acute endogenous steroid withdrawal. Other clinicians have argued that routinely administering steroids masks the clinical markers that signify when the endpoint of therapy has been reached and must be withdrawn 2-3 days before ACTH stimulation tests can be done. Since in adequately observed patients, adverse effects requiring glucocorticoid therapy may only be necessary in 5% of patients, the benefits of routine glucocorticoid administration may not be warranted.

Adverse Effects/Warnings - Most common adverse effects seen with initial therapy in dogs include lethargy, ataxia, weakness, anorexia, vomiting, and/or diarrhea. Adverse effects are commonly associated with plasma cortisol levels of less than 1 micrograms/dl or a too rapid decrease of plasma cortisol levels into the normal range. Adverse effects may also be more commonly seen in dogs weighing less than 5 kg, which may be due to the inability to accurately dose. The incidence of one or more of these effects is approximately 25% and they are usually mild. If adverse effects are noted, it is recommended to temporarily halt mitotane therapy and supplement with glucocorticoids. Owners should be provided with a small supply of predniso(lo)ne tablets to initiate treatment. Should the symptoms persist 3 hours after steroids are supplemented, consider other medical problems.

Liver changes (congestion, centrolobular atrophy, and moderate to severe fatty degeneration) have been noted in dogs given mitotane. Although not commonly associated with clinical symptomatology, these effects may be more pronounced with long-term therapy or in dogs with preexisting liver disease.

In perhaps 5% of dogs treated, long-term glucocorticoid and sometimes mineralocorticoid replacement therapy may be required. All dogs receiving mitotane therapy should receive additional glucocorticoid supplementation if undergoing a stress (*e.g.,* surgery, trauma, acute illness).

Overdosage - No specific recommendations were located regarding overdoses of this medication. Because of the drug's toxicity and long half-life, emptying the stomach and administering charcoal and a cathartic should be considered after a recent ingestion. It is recommended that the patient be closely monitored and given glucocorticoids if necessary.

Drug Interactions - Mitotane may induce hepatic microsomal enzymes and, therefore, could increase the metabolism of certain drugs (*e.g.,* **barbiturates, warfarin**).

If mitotane is used concomitantly with drugs that cause **CNS depression**, additive depressant effects may be seen.

Diabetic dogs receiving **insulin**, may have their insulin requirements decreased when mitotane therapy is instituted.

In dogs, **spironolactone** has been demonstrated to block the action of mitotane. It is recommended to use an alternate diuretic if possible.

Drug/Laboratory Interactions - Mitotane will bind competitively to thyroxine-binding globulin and decreases the amount of serum protein-bound iodine. Serum thyroxine concentrations may be unchanged or slightly decreased, but free thyroxine values remain in the normal range. Mitotane does not affect the results of the resin triiodothyronine uptake test.

Mitotane can reduce the amounts measurable 17-OHCS in the urine, which may or may not reflect a decrease in serum cortisol levels or adrenal secretion.

Doses -
   Dogs:
      For medical treatment of pituitary-dependent hyperadrenocorticism (bilateral adrenal hyperplasia): **Note**: The information provided below (in "a & b") is a synopsis of the authors'

treatment protocol. It is strongly recommended to refer to the original references and read the entire discussion before instituting therapy for the first time.

a) Initiate therapy at home (preferably on a Saturday): 50 mg/kg divided twice a day PO. Do not give glucocorticoids, but owner should have a small supply of prednisolone. Give until one of the following occurs: Polydipsic dogs consume less than 60 ml/kg/day of water; dogs' with excellent appetite takes 10-30 minutes longer than before mitotane therapy to consume meals (feed two small meals twice daily); dog vomits, is listless, or has diarrhea. Beginning on 3rd day of therapy, contact owner daily to monitor the situation and encourage. If dog develops GI upset 3-4 days after starting therapy; evaluate and either temporarily halt therapy or divide dosage further.

  After 8-9 days after therapy initiated, the dog should be evaluated and history and physical repeated, ACTH response test, BUN, serum sodium and potassium redone. If the dog has responded clinically, stop mitotane until ACTH response test can be evaluated. If the response test yields normal or high cortisol values, mitotane is continued (generally for 3-7 days). Repeat ACTH response test every 7-10 days until a low post-ACTH cortisol level is obtained. Most dogs respond during the first 7-10 days and nearly all respond by the 16th day of therapy.

  Maintenance therapy: Dogs who have responded to mitotane within 10 days of initiation receive 25 mg/kg every 7 days. Recheck ACTH response every 1-3 months. Those taking longer than 10 days to respond, receive 50 mg/kg weekly. If ACTH-stimulated cortisol levels begin to increase, mitotane dosage should be increased. Dogs with recurrent signs and symptoms of PDH or post ACTH cortisol values of > 5 micrograms/dl, should undergo daily therapy as outlined above. These animals should also be evaluated for other conditions (*e.g.,* renal disease, diabetes mellitus). Should anorexia and listlessness be seen with low plasma cortisol levels, reduce dosage. (Feldman 1989)

b) 40 - 50 mg/kg/day with food until serum cortisol reaches the normal resting range (usually takes 7-10 days). Once adrenal reserve is appropriately reduced, continue at 50 mg/kg/week in 2-3 divided dosages. See full reference for more specific details regarding dosage adjustments and monitoring of therapy. (Kintzer and Peterson 1995)

For palliative medical treatment of adrenal carcinomas or medical treatment of adrenal adenomas:

a) Initially, 50 - 75 mg/kg PO in daily divided doses for 10-14 days. May supplement with predniso(lo)ne at 0.2 mg/kg/day. Stop therapy and evaluate dog if adverse effects occur. After initial therapy run ACTH-stimulation test (do not give predniso(lo)ne the morning of the test). If basal or post-ACTH serum cortisol values are decreased, but still above the therapeutic end-point (<1 micrograms/dl), repeat therapy for an additional 7-14 days and repeat testing.

  If post-ACTH serum cortisol values remain greatly elevated or unchanged, increase mitotane to 100 mg/kg/day and repeat ACTH-stimulation test at 7-14 day intervals. If continues to remain greatly elevated, increase dosage by 50 mg/kg/day every 7-14 days until response occurs or drug intolerance ensues. Adjust dosage as necessary as patient tolerates or ACTH-responsive dictates.

  Once undetectable or low-normal post-ACTH cortisol levels are attained, continue mitotane at 100 - 200 mg/kg/week in divided doses with glucocorticoid supplementation (predniso(lo)ne 0.2 mg/kg/day). Repeat ACTH-stimulation test in 1-2 months. continue at present dose if cortisols remain below 1 micrograms/dl. Should cortisols increase to 1 - 4 micrograms/dl, increase maintenance dose by 50%. If basal or post-ACTH cortisols go above 4 micrograms/dl, restart daily treatment (50 - 100 mg/kg/day) as outlined above. Once patient is stabilized, repeat ACTH-stimulation tests at 3-6 month intervals. (Kintzer and Peterson 1989)

Monitoring Parameters -
Initially and *prn* (see doses above):
1) Physical exam and history (including water and food consumption, weight)
2) BUN, CBC, Liver enzymes, Blood glucose, ACTH response test, serum electrolytes (Na$^+$/K$^+$)

Client Information - Clients must be clearly instructed in the adverse effects of the drug and the symptoms of acute hypoadrenocorticism. Because of the potential severe toxicity associated with this agent, clients should be instructed to wash their hands after administering and to keep the tablets out of reach of children or pets.

Dosage Forms/Preparations/FDA Approval Status/Withholding Times -
Veterinary-Approved Products: None
Human-Approved Products:
   Mitotane Oral Tablets (scored) 500 mg; *Lysodren*® (Bristol-Myers Oncology); (Rx)

MITOXANTRONE HCL

Chemistry - Mitoxantrone HCl is a synthetic anthracenedione antineoplastic.

Storage/Stability/Compatibility - Mitoxantrone HCl should be stored at room temperature; do not freeze. Do not mix or use the same IV line with heparin infusions (precipitate may form). At present, it is not recommended to mix with other IV drugs.

Pharmacology - By intercalation between base pairs and also a nonintercalative electrostatic interaction, mitoxantrone binds to DNA and inhibits both DNA and RNA synthesis. Mitoxantrone is not cell-cycle phase specific, but appears to be most active during the S phase.

Uses/Indications - Mitoxantrone may be useful in the treatment of several neoplastic diseases in dogs, including lymphosarcoma (Note: preliminary studies have been disappointing with using mitoxantrone in the treatment of lymphoma when compared to other drug regimens), renal adenocarcinoma, fibroid sarcoma, thyroid or transitional cell carcinomas and hemangiopericytoma.

Pharmacokinetics - Mitoxantrone is rapidly and extensively distributed after intravenous infusion. Highest concentrations of the drug are found in the liver, heart, thyroid and red blood cells. In humans, it is approximately 78% bound to plasma proteins. Mitoxantrone is metabolized in the liver, but the majority of the drug is excreted unchanged in the urine. Half life of the drug in humans averages about 5 days as a result of the drug being taken up, bound by, and then slowly released by tissues.

Contraindications/Precautions/Reproductive Safety - Mitoxantrone is relatively contraindicated (weigh risk vs. benefit) in patients with myelosuppression, concurrent infection, impaired cardiac function or those who have received prior cytotoxic drug or radiation exposure. It should be used with caution in patients with sensitivity to mitoxantrone, hyperuricemia or hyperuricuria, or impaired hepatic function.

   Mitoxantrone affected fetal birth weights in rats. In a rabbit study no teratogenic effects were noted, but there was an increased incidence of premature deliveries. Use during pregnancy only when the benefits outweigh the risks involved. While it is unknown whether mitoxantrone enters milk, it is recommended to use milk replacer for nursing puppies.

Adverse Effects/Warnings - In dogs, effects include dose-dependent GI distress (vomiting, anorexia, diarrhea) and infection secondary to bone marrow depression. White cell nadirs generally occur on day 10. Some evidence exists that by giving recombinant granulocyte-colony stimulating factor bone marrow depression severity and duration may be reduced.

   Unlike doxorubicin, cardiotoxicity has not yet been reported in dogs and only rarely occurs in humans. Other adverse effects less frequently or rarely noted in humans and potentially possible in dogs, include conjunctivitis, jaundice, renal failure, seizures, allergic reactions, thrombocytopenia, irritation or phlebitis at injection site. Tissue necrosis associated with extravasation has only been reported in a few human cases.

Overdosage/Acute Toxicity - Because of the potential serious toxicity associated with this agent, dosage determinations must be made carefully.

Drug Interactions - Use extreme caution when used concurrently with other drugs that are also myelosuppressive, including many of the **other antineoplastics and other bone marrow depressant drugs** (*e.g.*, **chloramphenicol, flucytosine, amphotericin B, or colchicine**). Bone marrow depression may be additive. In humans, enhanced bone marrow depression has occurred when used concomitantly with **trimethoprim/sulfa**. Use with other **immunosuppressant drugs** (*e.g.*, **azathioprine, cyclophosphamide, corticosteroids**) may increase the risk of infection. **Live virus vaccines** should be used with caution, if at all during therapy.

   Cardiotoxicity risks may be enhanced in patients who have previously received **doxorubicin, daunorubicin** or **radiation therapy** to the mediastinum.

Laboratory Considerations - Mitoxantrone may raise serum **uric acid** levels. Drugs such as allopurinol may be required to control hyperuricemia. **Liver function tests** may become abnormal, indicating hepatotoxicity.

Doses -
  Dogs:
     As an alternative agent for the treatment of a variety of neoplastic diseases (see Indications above):
       a) For lymphoproliferative disorders: 5 - 6 mg/m2 every 3 weeks (Gilson and Page 1994)

Cats:
> For soft-tissue sarcomas:
>> a) 6 - 6.5 mg/2 IV given every 3 - 4 weeks for 4 - 6 treatments. (Keller and Helfand 1994)

Monitoring Parameters - 1) CBC with differential and platelets (see adverse effects section); 2) Efficacy; 3) Chest radiographs, ECG or other cardiac function tests if cardiac symptomatology present; 4) Liver function tests if jaundice or other symptoms of hepatotoxicity present; 5) Serum uric acid levels for susceptible patients

Client Information - Clients should understand the potential costs and toxicities associated with therapy. A blue-green color to urine or a bluish color to sclera may be noted but is of no concern. Have clients report any symptoms associated with toxicity immediately to veterinarian.

Dosage Forms/Preparations/FDA Approval Status/Withholding Times -
  Veterinary-Approved Products: None
  Human-Approved Products:
   Mitoxantrone HCl for Injection 2 mg (of base)/ml in 10, 12.5, & 15 ml vials; *Novantrone*® (Immunex); (Rx)

MORANTEL TARTRATE

Chemistry - A tetrahydropyrimidine anthelmintic, morantel tartrate occurs as a practically odorless, off-white to pale yellow, crystalline solid that is soluble in water. It has a melting range of 167-171°C. The tartrate salt is equivalent to 59.5% of base activity.

Storage/Stability/Compatibility - Morantel tartrate products should be stored at room temperature (15-30°C) unless otherwise instructed by the manufacturer.

Pharmacology - Like pyrantel, morantel acts as depolarizing neuromuscular blocking agent in susceptible parasites, thereby paralyzing the organism. The drug possesses nicotine-like properties and acts similarly to acetylcholine. Morantel also inhibits fumarate reductase in *Haemonchus spp.*.
  Morantel is slower than pyrantel in its onset of action, but is approximately 100 times as potent.

Uses/Indications - Morantel is indicated (labeled) for the removal of the following parasites in **cattle**: Mature forms of: *Haemonchus spp., Ostertagia spp., Trichostrongylus spp., Nematodirus spp., Cooperia spp. and Oesophagostomum radiatum*. It is also used in other ruminant species.

Pharmacokinetics - After oral administration, morantel is absorbed rapidly from the upper abomasum and small intestine. Peak levels occur about 4-6 hours after dosing. The drug is promptly metabolized in the liver. Within 96 hours of administration, 17% of the drug is excreted in the urine and the remainder in the feces.

Contraindications/Precautions - There are no absolute contraindications to using this drug. The sustained-release oral cartridges (*Paratect*®) are not to be used in cattle weighing less than 90 kg. Morantel is considered to be generally safe to use during pregnancy.

Adverse Effects/Warnings - At recommended doses, adverse effects are not commonly seen. For more information, see Overdosage section below.

Overdosage/Acute Toxicity - Morantel tartrate has a large safety margin. In cattle, dosages of up to 200 mg/kg (20 times recommended dose) resulted in no toxic reactions. The LD_{50} in mice is 5 g/kg. Symptoms of toxicity that might possibly be seen include increased respiratory rates, profuse sweating (in animals able to do so), ataxia or other cholinergic effects.
  Chronic toxicity studies have been conducted in cattle and sheep. Doses of 4 times recommended were given to sheep with no detectable deleterious effects. Cattle receiving 2.5 times recommended dose for 2 weeks showed no toxic signs.

Drug Interactions - *Paratect*® cartridges should not be administered with **mineral bullets** as decreased anthelmintic efficacy can result.
  Because of similar mechanisms of action (and toxicity), morantel is recommended not to be used concurrently with **pyrantel** or **levamisole**.
  Observation for adverse effects should be intensified if used concomitantly with an **organophosphate** or **diethylcarbamazine**.
  Piperazine and morantel have antagonistic mechanisms of action; do not use together.
  Do not add to feeds containing **bentonite**.

Doses -
  Cattle:
>   For susceptible parasites:
>> a) 9.68 mg/kg PO. (Paul 1986), (Label Directions; Nematel®—Pfizer)
>> b) 8.8 mg/kg PO. (Roberson 1988b)

   c) *Paratect®* Cartridges: One cartridge PO when animal placed onto spring pasture. All cattle grazing on same pasture must be treated. Effective for 90 days. (Label Directions; *Paratect®*—Pfizer)

Sheep:
   For susceptible parasites:
     a) 10 mg/kg PO. (Roberson 1988b)

Dosage Forms/Preparations/FDA Approval Status/Withdrawal Times -
   Morantel Tartrate Oral Boluses 2.2 g (equiv. to 1.3 g base)
     Nematel® Cattle Wormer Boluses (Pfizer); (OTC) Approved for use in beef or dairy cattle. Milk withdrawal = none; Slaughter withdrawal = 14 days

   Morantel Tartrate Medicated Premix, 88 g morantel tartrate per lb.
     Rumatel® Medicated Premix-88 (Pfizer); (OTC) Approved for use in beef or dairy cattle. Milk withdrawal = none; Slaughter withdrawal = 14 days

   Morantel Tartrate Sustained-Release Oral Cartridges, 22.7 g per cartridge (13.5 g base)
     Paratect® Cartridge (Pfizer); (OTC) Approved for use in beef or dairy cattle. Milk withdrawal = none; Slaughter withdrawal = 160 days

MORPHINE SULFATE

Chemistry - The sulfate salt of a natural (derived from opium) occurring opiate analgesic, morphine sulfate occurs as white, odorless, crystals. Solubility: 1 g in 16 ml of water (62.5 mg/ml), 570 ml (1.75 mg/ml) of alcohol. Insoluble in chloroform or ether. The pH of morphine sulfate injection ranges from 2.5-6.

Storage/Stability/Compatibility - Morphine gradually darkens in color when exposed to light; protect from prolonged exposure to bright light. Does not appear to adsorb to plastic or PVC syringes, tubing or bags. Morphine sulfate has been shown to be compatible at a concentration of 16.2 mg/l with the following intravenous fluids: Dextrose 2.5%, 5%, 10% in water; Ringer's injection and Lactated Ringer's injection; Sodium Chloride 0.45% and 0.9% for injection. The following drugs have been shown to **incompatible** when mixed with morphine sulfate: aminophylline, chlorothiazide sodium, heparin sodium, meperidine, pentobarbital sodium, phenobarbital sodium, phenytoin sodium, sodium bicarbonate, and thiopental sodium. Morphine sulfate has been demonstrated to be generally **compatible** when mixed with the following agents: Atropine sulfate, benzquinamide HCl, butorphanol tartrate, chlorpromazine HCl, diphenhydramine HCl, dobutamine HCl, droperidol, fentanyl citrate, glycopyrrolate, hydroxyzine HCl, metoclopramide, pentazocine lactate, promazine HCl, scopolamine HBr, and succinylcholine chloride.

Pharmacology - Refer to the monograph: Narcotic (opiate) Analgesic Agonists, Pharmacology of, for more information. Morphine's CNS effects are irregular and are species specific. Cats, horses, sheep, goats, cattle and swine may exhibit stimulatory effects after morphine injection, while dogs, humans, and other primates exhibit CNS depression. Both dogs and cats are sensitive to the emetic effects of morphine, but significantly higher doses are required in cats before vomiting occurs. This effect is a result of a direct stimulation of the chemorecepetor trigger zone (CTZ). Other species (horses, ruminants and swine) do not respond to the emetic effects of morphine. Like meperidine, morphine can effect the release of histamine from mast cells.

   Morphine is an effective centrally acting antitussive in dogs. Following morphine administration, hypothermia may be seen in dogs and rabbits, while hyperthermia may be seen in cattle, goats, horses, and cats. Morphine can cause miosis (pinpoint pupils) in humans, rabbits and dogs.

   While morphine is considered to be a respiratory depressant, initially in dogs respirations are stimulated. Panting may ensue which may be a result of increased body temperature. Often however, body temperature may be reduced due to a resetting of the "body's thermostat". As CNS depression increases and the hyperthermia resolves, respirations can become depressed. Morphine at moderate to high doses can also cause bronchoconstriction in dogs.

   The cardiovascular effects of morphine in dogs are in direct contrast to its effects on humans. In dogs, morphine causes coronary vasoconstriction with resultant increase in coronary vascular resistance, and a transient decrease in arterial pressure. Both bradycardias and tachycardias have also been reported in dogs. While morphine has been used for years as a sedative/analgesic in the treatment of myocardial infarction and congestive heart failure in people, its effects on dogs make it a less than optimal choice in canine patients with symptoms of cardiopulmonary failure. However, its use has been recommended by several clinicians in the initial treatment for cardiogenic edema in dogs.

   The effects of morphine on the gastrointestinal (GI) tract consist primarily of a decrease in motility and secretions. The dog however, will immediately defecate following an injection of morphine and then exhibit the signs of decreased intestinal motility and ultimately constipation can reesult. Both biliary and gastric secretions are reduced following administration of morphine, but gastric secretion of HCl will later be compensated by increased (above normal) acid secretion.

Initially, morphine can induce micturation, but with higher doses (>2.4 mg/kg IV) urine secretion can be substantially reduced by an increase in anti-diuretic hormone (ADH) release. Morphine may also cause bladder hypertonia, which can lead to increased difficulty in urination.

Pharmacokinetics - Morphine is absorbed when given by IV, IM, SQ, and rectal routes. Although absorbed when given orally, bioavailability is reduced, probably as a result of a high first-pass effect. Morphine concentrates in the kidney, liver, and lungs; lower levels are found in the CNS. Although at lower levels then in the parenchymatous tissues, the majority of free morphine is found in skeletal muscle. Morphine crosses the placenta and narcotized newborns can result if mothers are given the drug before giving birth. These effects can be rapidly reversed with naloxone. Small amounts of morphine will also be distributed into the milk of nursing mothers.

The major route of elimination of morphine is by metabolism in the liver; primarily by glucuronidation. Because cats are deficient in this metabolic pathway, half-lives in cats are probably prolonged. The glucuronidated metabolite is excreted by the kidney.

In horses, the serum half-life of morphine has been reported to be 88 minutes after a dose of 0.1 mg/kg IV. At this dose the drug was detectable in the serum for 48 hours and in the urine for up to 6 days. The half-life in cats has been reported to be approximately 3 hours.

Uses/Indications - Morphine is used for the treatment of acute pain in dogs, cats, horses, swine, sheep, and goats. It may be also be used as a preanesthetic agent in dogs and swine. Additionally, it has been used as an antitussive, antidiarrheal, and as adjunctive therapy for some cardiac abnormalities (see doses) in dogs.

Contraindications/Precautions - All opiates should be used with caution in patients with hypothyroidism, severe renal insufficiency, adrenocortical insufficiency (Addison's), and in geriatric or severely debilitated patients. Morphine is contraindicated in cases where the patient is hypersensitive to narcotic analgesics, and in patients taking monamine oxidase inhibitors (MAOIs). It is also contraindicated in patients with diarrhea caused by a toxic ingestion until the toxin is eliminated from the GI tract.

Morphine should be used with extreme caution in patients with head injuries, increased intracranial pressure and acute abdominal conditions (*e.g.,* colic) as it may obscure the diagnosis or clinical course of these conditions. Morphine may also increase intracranial pressure secondary to cerebral vasodilatation as a result of increased p_aCO_2 stemming from respiratory depression. It should be used with extreme caution in patients suffering from respiratory disease or from acute respiratory dysfunction (*e.g.,* pulmonary edema secondary to smoke inhalation).

Because of its effects on vasopressin (ADH), morphine must be used cautiously in patients suffering from acute uremia. Urine flow has been reported to be decreased by as much as 90% in dogs given large doses of morphine.

Neonatal, debilitated or geriatric patients may be more susceptible to the effects of morphine and may require lower dosages. Patients with severe hepatic disease may have prolonged durations of action of the drug.

Opiate analgesics are contraindicated in patients who have been stung by the scorpion species *Centruroides sculpturatus* Ewing and *C. gertschi* Stahnke as they can potentiate these venoms.

Adverse Effects/Warnings - At usual doses, the primary concern is the effect the opioids have on respiratory function. Decreased tidal volume, depressed cough reflex and the drying of respiratory secretions may all have a detrimental effect on a susceptible patient. Bronchoconstriction (secondary to histamine release?) following IV doses has been noted in dogs.

Gastrointestinal effects may include: nausea, vomiting and decreased intestinal persitalsis. Dogs will usually defecate after an initial dose of morphine. Horses exhibiting signs of mild colic may have their symptoms masked by the administration of narcotic analgesics.

The CNS effects of morphine are dose and species specific. Animals that are stimulated by morphine, may elucidate changes in behavior, appear restless, and at very high doses, have convulsions. The CNS depressant effects seen in dogs may encumber the abilities of working animals.

Body temperature changes may be seen. Cattle, goats, horses and cats may exhibit signs of hyperthermia. while rabbits and dogs may develop hypothermia.
Chronic administration may lead to physical dependence.

Overdosage - Overdosage may produce profound respiratory and/or CNS depression in most species. Newborns may be more susceptible to these effects than adult animals. Parenteral doses greater than 100 mg/kg are thought to be fatal in dogs. Other toxic effects can include cardiovascular collapse, hypothermia, and skeletal muscle hypotonia. Some species such as horses, cats, swine, and cattle may demonstrate CNS excitability (hyperreflexia, tremors) and seizures at high doses or if given intravenously (rapidly). Naloxone is the agent of choice in treating respiratory depression. In massive overdoses, naloxone doses may need to be repeated, animals should be closely observed as naloxone's effects may diminish before sub-toxic levels of morphine are attained. Mechanical respiratory support should also be considered in cases of severe respiratory depression.

Pentobarbital has been suggested as a treatment for CNS excitement and seizures in cats. Extreme caution should be used as barbiturates and narcotics can have additive effects on respiratory depression.

Drug Interactions - Other **CNS depressants** (*e.g.,* anesthetic agents, antihistamines, phenothiazines, barbiturates, tranquilizers, alcohol, etc.) may cause increased CNS or respiratory depression when used with morphine.

Morphine is contraindicated in patients receiving **monamine oxidase (MOA) inhibitors** (rarely used in veterinary medicine) for at least 14 days after receiving MOA inhibitors in humans. Some human patients have exhibited signs of opiate overdose after receiving therapeutic doses of morphine while on these agents.

Laboratory Interactions - Plasma **amylase** and **lipase** values may be increased for up to 24 hours following administration of opiate analgesics as they may increase biliary tract pressure.

Doses -
Dogs:
As a post-operative analgesic:
    a) 0.25 - 1.0 mg/kg IM or IV prn (Reidesel)
    b) 0.25 mg/kg SQ q1-2h prn (Booth 1988a)
For analgesia:
    a) 0.5 - 1.0 mg/kg SQ, IM prn (Morgan 1988)
As a preanesthetic:
    a) 0.1 - 2 mg/kg SQ (Booth 1988a)
For adjunctive treatment of cardiogenic edema:
    a) 0.1 mg/kg IV q2-3minutes prn to effect (reduction in dyspnea and anxiety), or 0.25 mg SQ (Roudebush 1985)
For adjunctive treatment of supraventricular premature beats:
    a) 0.2 mg/kg IM or SQ (Morgan 1988)
For treatment of hypermotile diarrhea:
    a) 0.25 mg/kg (Jones 1985a)
As an antitussive:
    a) 0.1 mg/kg q6-12h SQ (Roudebush 1985)
Cats:
For analgesia:
    a) 0.05 - 0.1 mg/kg SQ, IM prn (Morgan 1988)
    b) 0.1 mg/kg q4-6h SQ or IM (Jenkins 1987), (Booth 1988a)
  Note: Use cautiously; may cause significant CNS excitement if used without a concurrent tranquilizer.
Horses:
For analgesia:
    a) 0.22 mg/kg IM or slow IV (Booth 1988a)
    b) 0.2 - 0.6 mg/kg IV (slowly); premedicate with xylazine (1 mg/kg IV) to reduce excitement (Jenkins 1987)
    c) 0.02 - 0.04 mg/kg IV (Muir 1987)
    d) 0.05 - 0.12 mg/kg IV (Thurmon and Benson 1987)
Note: Narcotics may cause CNS excitement in the horse. Some clinicians recommend pretreatment with acepromazine (0.02 - 0.04 mg/kg IV), or xylazine (0.3 - 0.5 mg/kg IV) to reduce the behavioral changes these drugs can cause.
Warning: Narcotic analgesics can mask the behavioral and cardiovascular symptoms associated with mild colic.
Swine:
As a preanesthetic/analgesic (prior to chloralose/barbiturate):
    a) 0.2 - 0.9 mg/kg IM. Note: may cause undesirable stimulation. (Booth 1988a)
As an analgesic:
    a) 0.2 mg/kg up to 20 mg total dose IM. (Jenkins 1987)
Sheep & Goats:
As an analgesic:
    a) Up to 10 mg total dose IM. (Jenkins 1987)

Monitoring Parameters -
   1) Respiratory rate/depth
   2) CNS level of depression/excitation
   3) Blood pressure if possible and indicated (especially with IV use)
   4) Analgesic activity

Client Information - When given parenterally, this agent should be used in an inpatient setting or with direct professional supervision.

Dosage Forms/Preparations/FDA Approval Status/Withholding Times -
Veterinary-Approved Products: None
Human-Approved Products:
   Morphine Sulfate for Injection: 0.5 mg/ml in 2, & 10 ml amps and 10 ml vials; 1 mg/ml in 2,
      10, 30 & 60 ml amps and 10 ml vials; 2 mg/ml in 50 ml vials and 1 & 2 ml syringes; 3
      mg/ml in 50 ml vials; 4 mg/ml in 1& 2 ml syringes; 5 mg/ml in 1 & 30 ml vials; 8 mg/ml in
      1 ml vials, amps & syringes; 10 mg/ml in 1 ml amps, vials, 10 ml vials and 20 ml amps; 15
      mg/ml in 1 & 20 ml amps, & vials; 25 mg/ml in 4, 10 , 20, & 40 ml syringes and 20 ml am-
      puls; 50 mg/ml in 10, 20 and 40 ml syringes

   Morphine Sulfate for Injection (preservative-free): 0.5 mg/ml, 10 ml amps & vials; 1 mg/ml,
      10 ml amps & vials;*Infumorph®* (Elkins-Sinn); *Astramorph PF®* (Astra)

   Morphine Sulfate Soluble Tablets: 10 mg, 15 mg, 30 mg

   Morphine Sulfate Tablets: 15 mg, 30 mg

   Morphine Sulfate Capsules: 15 mg, 30 mg

   Morphine Sulfate Oral Solution; 10 mg/5ml in 100, 120 & 500 ml btls & unit dose (2.5, 5, 10
      ml); 20 mg/5ml in 100, 120 & 500 ml btls & unit dose 5 ml; 20 mg/ml in 30 & 120 ml, in
      UD 1 ml and 1.5 ml vials; 100 mg/5 ml in 120 & 240 ml

   Morphine Sulfate Controlled-release Tablets 15 mg, 30 mg, 60 mg, 100 mg, 200 mg

   Morphine Sulfate Rectal Suppositories 5 mg, 10 mg & 20 mg, 30 mg in UD 12's and 50's

Note: All morphine products are Rx and a **Class-II controlled substance**. Very accurate record keeping is required as to use and disposition of stock. See the appendix for more information.

MOXIDECTIN

Chemistry/Storage/Stability/Compatibility - An avermectin-class antiparasitic agent, mox-idectin is a semi-synthetic methoxime derivative of nemadectin.

   The commercially available tablets for dogs should be stored at room temperature (do not store at temperatures greater than 77°F) and not be exposed to light for extended periods of time.

   The topical solution for cattle should be stored at, or below room temperature. Do not allow prolonged exposure to temperatures above 77°F. If product becomes frozen, thaw completely and shake well before using.

   The oral gel for horses should be stored at, or near room temperature (59°F-86°F); avoid freez-ing. If product becomes frozen, thaw completely before using. Partially used syringes should have the cap tightly secured.

Pharmacology - The primary mode of action of avermectins like moxidectin is to affect chloride ion channel activity in the nervous system of nematodes and arthropods. The drug binds to recep-tors that increase membrane permeability to chloride ions. This inhibits the electrical activity of nerve cells in nematodes and muscle cells in arthropods and causes paralysis and death of the parasites. Avermectins also enhance the release of gamma amino butyric acid (GABA) at presy-naptic neurons. GABA acts as an inhibitory neurotransmitter and blocks the post-synaptic stimu-lation of the adjacent neuron in nematodes or the muscle fiber in arthropods. Avermectins are generally not toxic to mammals as they do not have glutamate-gated chloride channels and these compounds do not readily cross the blood-brain barrier where mammalian GABA receptors oc-cur.

Uses/Indications - In dogs, moxidectin is indicated as a once a month oral preventative for the prevention of heartworm.

   In cattle, moxidectin is indicated for the treatment and control of the following internal [adult and fourth stage larvae (L4)] and external parasites: Gastrointestinal roundworms: *Ostertagia ostertagi* (adult and L4, including inhibited larvae), *Haemonchus placei* (adult), *Trichostrongylus axei* (adult and L4), *Trichostrongylus colubriformis* (adult), *Cooperia oncophora* (adult), *Cooperia punctata* (adult), *Bunostomum phlebotomum* (adult), *Oesophagostomum radiatum* (adult), *Nematodirus helvetianus* (adult); Lungworm: *Dictyocaulus viviparus* (adult and L4); Cattle Grubs: *Hypoderma bovis, Hypoderma lineatum.*. Mites: *Chorioptes bovis, Psoroptes ovis* (*Psoroptes communis var. bovis*); Lice: *Linognathus vituli, Haematopinus eurysternus, Solenopotes capillatus, Damalinia bovis.*; Horn flies: *Haematobia irritans.* To control infections and to protect from reinfection from *Ostertagia ostertagi* for 28 days after treatment and from *Dictyocaulus viviparus* for 42 days after treatment.

In horses and ponies, moxidectin is indicated for the treatment and control of the following stages of gastrointestinal parasites: Large strongyles: *Strongylus vulgaris* (adults and L4L5 arterial stages); *Strongylus edentatus* (adults and tissue stages); *Triodontophorus brevicauda* (adults); *Triodontophorus serratus* (adults); Small strongyles (adults and larvae): *Cyathostomum spp.* (adults); *Cylicocyclus spp.* (adults); *Cylicostephanus spp.* (adults); *Gyalocephalus capitatus* (adults); undifferentiated lumenal larvae; Encysted cyathostomes: late L3 and L4 mucosal cyathostome larvae; Ascarids: *Parascaris equorum* (adults and L4 larval stages); Pin worms: *Oxyuris equi* (adults and L4 larval stages); Hair worms: *Trichostrongylus axei* (adults); Large-mouth stomach worms: *Habronema muscae* (adults); Horse stomach bots: *Gasterophilus intestinalis* (2nd and 3rd instars).

Pharmacokinetics - Minimal information was located. In cattle, the drug apparently has a long duration of plasma residence (14-15 days). After subQ injection, approximately 5% of the dose given to the cow can be passed to the suckling calf.

Contraindications/Precautions/Reproductive Safety -
Dogs: The manufacturer warns to only use this product in dogs tested negative for heartworm infection. Adult heartworms and microfilaria should be removed prior to therapy. If more than two months pass between dosages of this, or other once a month heartworm preventative medications, the dog should be tested for heartworm infection before receiving the next dose.

Reproductive studies have demonstrated no evidence of adverse effects on fertility, reproductive performance, or offspring

Cattle: Not for use in female dairy cattle of breeding age. Thus far at labeled doses, adverse effects appear to nonexistent or minimal.

Reproductive studies performed thus far have demonstrated no evidence of adverse effects on fertility, reproductive performance, or offspring in cattle treated.

Horses: Not for horses intended for food purposes and is not labeled for use in foals younger than 4 months of age.

Reproductive studies performed thus far have demonstrated no evidence of adverse effects on fertility, reproductive performance, or offspring in horses treated.

Adverse Effects/Warnings -
Dogs: While adverse reactions to this medication apparently occur infrequently, the following adverse reactions are noted on the product label: lethargy, vomiting, ataxia, anorexia, diarrhea, nervousness, weakness, increased thirst and itching. Studies done in Collies (up to 20X) demonstrated no notable adverse effects. One Collie receiving doses of 30X demonstrated mild signs of depression, ataxia, and salivation.
Cattle: Thus far at labeled doses, adverse effects appear to nonexistent or minimal.
Horses: Thus far at labeled doses, adverse effects appear to nonexistent or minimal.

Overdosage -
Dogs: The drug apparently has a very wide margin of safety in dogs when administered orally. Dosages of up to 300X (1120 mcg/kg) demonstrated little or no effects.
Cattle: In studies done on cattle, application of the pour-on solution at 5X the recommended dose for 5 consecutive days, 10X for 2 consecutive days and 25X for one day did not produce any significant adverse clinical or pathological effects.
Horses: In one study, three of eight foals given the 3X dose became depressed or ataxic after one treatment. The author has received an anectdotal report of a miniature horse developing seizures after receiving a full tube of Quest®.

Drug Interactions - None noted.

Doses -
Dogs:
>> For heartworm prevention: 3 mcg/kg PO once monthly. (Package Insert-*ProHeart*®); Fort Dodge)

Cattle:
>> For labeled indications: 1 ml (5 mg)/10 kg (22 lb) BW applied directly to the hair and skin along the top of the back from the withers to the base of the tail. Application should be made to healthy skin avoiding mange scabs, skin lesions or extraneous foreign matter. (Label Directions—Cydectin®; Fort Dodge)

Horses:
>> For labeled indications: 0.4 mg/kg BW. Administer gel by inserting the syringe applicator into the animal's mouth through the interdental space and depositing the gel in the back of the mouth near the base of the tongue. Once the syringe is removed, the animal's head should be raised to insure proper swallowing of the gel. Horses weighing more

than 1150 lb require additional gel from a second syringe. (Label Directions—Quest®; Fort Dodge)

Dosage Forms/Preparations/FDA Approval Status -

Moxidectin Oral Tablets 30 mcg, 68 mcg, or 136 mcg; *ProHeart®* (Fort Dodge); (Rx). Approved for use in dogs 8 weeks or older.

Moxidectin 0.5% (5 mg/ml) Pour-On for Cattle in 500 ml, 1 L and 2.5 L containers. *Cydectin®* (Fort Dodge); (OTC). Approved for use in cattle; not to be used in female dairy cattle of breeding age. No meat withdrawal times required, but FDA has established tolerances of 50 ppb and 200 ppb for parent moxidectin in muscle and liver, respectively, of cattle.

Moxidectin Oral Gel containing 20 mg/ml in 11.3 g syringes (sufficient to treat one 1150 lb horse); *Quest®* (Fort Dodge) (OTC). Approved for use in horse or ponies not intended for food purposes.

NALOXONE HCL

Chemistry - An opiate antagonist, naloxone HCl is structurally related to oxymorphone. It occurs as a white to slightly off-white powder with a pK_a of 7.94. Naloxone is soluble in water and slightly soluble in alcohol. The pH range of commercially available injectable solutions are from 3-4.5. Naloxone HCl may also be known as *N*-allylnoroxymorphone HCl.

Storage/Stability/Compatibility - Naloxone HCl for injection should be stored at room temperature (15-30°C) and protected from light.

Sterile water for injection is the recommended diluent for naloxone injection. When given as an IV infusion, either D_5W or normal saline should be used. Naloxone HCl injection should not be mixed with solutions containing sulfites, bisulfites, long-chain or high molecular weight anions or any solutions at alkaline pH.

Pharmacology - Naloxone is considered to be a pure opiate antagonist and it has basically no analgesic activity. The exact mechanism for its activity is not understood, but it is believed that the drug acts as a competitive antagonist by binding to the *mu*, *kappa*, and *sigma* opioid receptor sites. The drug apparently has its highest affinity for the *mu* receptor.

Naloxone reverses the majority of effects associated with high-dose opiate administration (respiratory and CNS depression). In dogs, naloxone apparently does not reverse the emetic actions of apomorphine.

Naloxone also has other pharmacologic activity at high doses, including effects on dopaminergic mechanisms (increases dopamine levels) and GABA antagonism.

Uses/Indications - Naloxone is used in veterinary medicine almost exclusively for its opiate reversal effects, but the drug is being investigated for treating other conditions (*e.g.,* septic, hypovolemic or cardiogenic shock). Naloxone may also be employed as a test drug to see if endogenous opiate blockade will result in diminished tail-chasing or other self-mutilating behaviors.

Pharmacokinetics - Naloxone is only minimally absorbed when given orally as it is rapidly destroyed in the GI tract. Much higher doses are required if using this route of administration for any pharmacologic effect. When given IV, naloxone has a very rapid onset of action (usually 1-2 minutes). If given IM, the drug generally has an onset of action within 5 minutes of administration. The duration of action usually persists from 45-90 minutes, but may act for up to 3 hours.

Naloxone is distributed rapidly throughout the body with high levels found in the brain, kidneys, spleen, skeletal muscle, lung and heart. The drug also readily crosses the placenta.

Naloxone is metabolized in the liver, principally via glucuronidative conjugation with metabolites excreted into the urine. In humans, the serum half-life is approximately 60-100 minutes.

Contraindications/Precautions/Reproductive Safety - Naloxone is contraindicated in patients hypersensitive to it. It should be used cautiously in animals that have preexisting cardiac abnormalities or in animals that may be opioid dependent. The veterinary manufacturer states to use the drug "...cautiously in animals who have received exceedingly large doses of narcotics. ... may produce an acute withdrawal syndrome and smaller doses should be employed." (Package Insert; *P/M® Naloxone HCl Injection*—P/M; Mallinckrodt)

Naloxone is generally considered to be non-teratogenic in animals, but has precipitated withdrawal in opioid-dependent human fetuses.

Adverse Effects/Warnings - At usual doses, naloxone is relatively free of adverse effects in non-opioid dependent patients.

Because the duration of action of naloxone may be shorter than that of the narcotic being reversed, animals that are being treated for opioid intoxication or with symptoms of respiratory depression should be closely monitored as additional doses of naloxone and/or ventilatory support may be required.

Overdosage/Acute Toxicity - Naloxone is considered to be a very safe agent with a very wide margin of safety, but very high doses have initiated seizures (secondary to GABA antagonism?) in a few patients.

Drug Interactions - Naloxone also reverses the effects of opioid agonists/antagonists such as **butorphanol, pentazocine or nalbuphine**.

Doses -
Dogs & Cats:
For opioid reversal:
    a) 0.002 - 0.02 mg/kg IV or IM; duration of effect 0.5-1 hour. (Bednarski 1989)
    b) Dogs: 0.04 mg/kg IV, IM or SQ (Package Insert; *P/M® Naloxone HCl Injection —P/M*; Mallinckrodt), (Kirk 1989)
    c) Cats: 0.05 - 0.1 mg/kg IV (Muir and Swanson 1989)
    d) 0.02 - 0.04 mg/kg IV (Morgan 1988)

Rabbits/Rodents/Pocket Pets:
For opioid reversal in rodents: 0.01 -0.1 mg/kg SubQ or IP as needed (Huerkamp 1995)

Horses:
For opioid reversal:
    a) 0.01 - 0.022 mg/kg to reverse sedative and excitatory effects of narcotic agonists. (Clark and Becht 1987)
    b) 0.01 mg/kg IV to limit increases in locomotor activity secondary to narcotic agonists. (Muir 1987)
    c) 0.01 - 0.02 mg/kg IV (Robinson 1987)

Monitoring Parameters -
    1) Respiratory rate/depth
    2) CNS function
    3) Pain associated with opiate reversal

Client Information - Should be used with direct professional supervision only.

Dosage Forms/Preparations/FDA Approval Status/Withholding Times -
Veterinary-Approved Products:
Naloxone HCl Injection 0.4 mg/ml in 10 ml vials; *P/M® Naloxone HCl Injection* (Schering Plough); (Rx) Approved for use in dogs.

Human-Approved Products:
Naloxone HCl Injection 0.4 mg/ml in 1 ml amps, syringes & 1, 2, & 10 ml vials; *Narcan®* (Dupont Pharm.), Generic; (Rx)

Naloxone HCl Injection 1 mg/ml in 2 ml amps, vials & 1, 5, & 10 ml vials; *Narcan®* (Dupont Pharm.), Generic; (Rx)

Naloxone HCl Neonatal Injection 0.02 mg/ml in 2 ml amps, & vials; *Narcan®* (Dupont Pharm); Generic; (Rx)

NALTREXONE HCL

Chemistry - A synthetic opiate antagonist, naltrexone HCl occurs as white crystals having a bitter taste. 100 mg are soluble in one ml of water.

Storage/Stability/Compatibility - Naltrexone tablets should be stored at room temperature in well-closed containers.

Pharmacology - Naltrexone is an orally available narcotic antagonist. It competitively binds to opiate receptors in the CNS, thereby preventing both endogenous opiates (*e.g.*, endorphins) and exogenously administered opiate agonists or agonist/antagonists from occupying the site. Naltrexone may be more effective in blocking the euphoric aspects of the opiates and less effective at blocking the respiratory depressive or miotic effects.

Naltrexone may also increase plasma concentrations of luteinizing hormone (LH), cortisol and ACTH. In dogs with experimentally-induced hypovolemic shock, naltrexone (like naloxone) given IV in high dosages increased mean arterial pressure, cardiac output, stroke volume, and left ventricular contractility.

Uses/Indications - Naltrexone may be useful in the treatment of self-mutilating or tail-chasing behaviors in dogs or cats.

Pharmacokinetics - In humans, naltrexone is rapidly and nearly completed absorbed, but undergoes a significant first-pass effect as only 5-12% of a dose reaches the systemic circulation. Naltrexone circulates throughout the body and CSF levels are approximately 30% of those found in the plasma. Only about 20-30% is bound to plasma proteins. It is unknown whether naltrexone crosses the placenta or enters milk. Naltrexone is metabolized in the liver primarily to 6-beta-naltrexol, which has some opiate blocking activity. In humans, serum half life of naltrexone is about 4 hours; 6-beta-naltrexol, about 13 hours. Naltrexone, as metabolites are then eliminated primarily via the kidney.

Contraindications/Precautions/Reproductive Safety - Naltrexone is generally considered to be contraindicated in patients physically dependent on opiate drugs, in hepatic failure or with acute hepatitis. The benefits of the drug versus its risks should be weighed in patients with hepatic dysfunction or who have had a history of allergic reaction to naltrexone or naloxone.

Very high doses have caused increased embryotoxicity in some laboratory animals. It should be used during pregnancy only when the benefits outweigh any potential risks. It is unknown whether naltrexone enters maternal milk.

Adverse Effects/Warnings - At usual doses, naltrexone is relatively free of adverse effects in non-opioid dependent patients. Some human patients have developed abdominal cramping, nausea and vomiting, nervousness, insomnia, joint or muscle pain, skin rashes. Dose-dependent hepatotoxicity has been described in humans on occasion.

Naltrexone will block the analgesic, antidiarrheal and antitussive effects of opiate agonist or agonist/antagonist agents. Withdrawal symptoms may be precipitated in physically dependent patients.

Overdosage/Acute Toxicity - Naltrexone appears to be relatively safe even after very large doses. The LD_{50} in dogs after subcutaneous injection has been reported to be 200 mg/kg. Oral LD_{50}'s in species tested range from 1.1 g/kg in mice to 3 g/kg in monkeys (dogs or cats not tested). Death at these doses were a result of respiratory depression and/or tonic-clonic seizures. Massive overdoses should be treated using gut emptying protocols when warranted and giving supportive treatment.

Drug Interactions - In addition to blocking the effects of pure opiate agonists (*e.g.*, **morphine, meperidine, codeine, oxymorphone**, etc.) naltrexone also reverses the effects of opioid agonist/antagonists such as **butorphanol, pentazocine** or **nalbuphine**.

Laboratory Considerations - Naltrexone reportedly does not interfere with TLC, GLC, or HPLC methods of determining **urinary morphine, methadone or quinine**. Naltrexone may cause increases in hepatic function tests (*e.g.,* **AST, ALT**) (see adverse effects above).

Doses -
  Dogs:
    As adjunctive therapy in behavior disorders:
      a) For tail chasing or excessive licking: First give 0.01 mg/kg SubQ of naloxone to determine if narcotic antagonists may be effective, if so give naltrexone PO at 1 - 2 mg/kg daily. Long term therapy may be required. (Crowill-Davis 1992)
    For the adjunctive treatment of acral pruritic dermatitis:
      a) 2.2 mg/kg PO once daily for one month trial. Some dogs exhibit drowsiness and minor changes in behavior. 50-60% of patients have benefited. Expense is of concern. (Rosychuck 1991)

Monitoring Parameters - 1) Efficacy; 2) Liver enzymes if using very high dose prolonged therapy

Client Information - Stress the importance of compliance with prescribed dosing regimen. Additional behavior modification techniques may be required to alleviate symptoms.

Dosage Forms/Preparations/FDA Approval Status/Withholding Times -
  Veterinary-Approved Products: None
  Human-Approved Products:
    Naltrexone HCl Oral Tablets 50 mg; *ReVia*®(DuPont); (Rx)

NANDROLONE DECANOATE

Chemistry - An injectable anabolic steroid, nandrolone decanoate occurs as a white, to creamy white, crystalline powder. It is odorless or may have a slight odor and melts between 33-37°C. Nandrolone decanoate is soluble in alcohol and vegetable oils and is practically insoluble in water. The commercially available injectable products are generally solutions dissolved in sesame oil.

Storage/Stability/Compatibility - Nandrolone decanoate for injection should be stored at temperatures less than 40°C and preferably between 15-30°C; protect from freezing and protect from light.

Pharmacology - Nandrolone exhibits similar actions as other anabolic agents. For more information refer to the preceding monograph (Boldenone).

Many veterinary and human clinicians feel that nandrolone is clinically superior to other anabolics in its ability to stimulate erythropoiesis. It is believed that nandrolone may enhance red cell counts by directly stimulating red cell precursors in the bone marrow, increasing red cell 2,3-diphosphoglycerate and increasing erythropoietin production in the kidney.

Uses/Indications - The principle use of nandrolone in veterinary medicine has been to stimulate erythropoiesis in patients with certain anemias (*e.g.,* secondary to renal failure, aplastic anemias). It has also been suggested to be used as an appetite stimulant.

Pharmacokinetics - No specific information was located for this agent. It is generally recommended for both small animals and humans to be dosed on a weekly basis.

Contraindications/Precautions - No specific recommendations were located for this agent in veterinary species.

In humans, anabolic agents are also contraindicated in patients with hepatic dysfunction, hypercalcemia, patients with a history of myocardial infarction (can cause hypercholesterolemia), pituitary insufficiency, prostate carcinoma, in selected patients with breast carcinoma, benign prostatic hypertrophy and during the nephrotic stage of nephritis.

The anabolic agents are category X (risk of use outweighs any possible benefit) agents for use in pregnancy and are contraindicated because of possible fetal masculinization.

Adverse Effects/Warnings - Potential (from human data) adverse reactions of the anabolic agents in dogs and cats include: sodium, calcium, potassium, water, chloride and phosphate retention; hepatotoxicity, behavioral (androgenic) changes and reproductive abnormalities (oligospermia, estrus suppression).

Overdosage - No information was located for this specific agent. In humans, sodium and water retention can occur after overdosage of anabolic steroids. It is suggested to treat supportively and monitor liver function should an inadvertent overdose be administered.

Drug Interactions - Anabolic agents as a class may potentiate the effects of **anticoagulants**. Monitoring of PT's and dosage adjustment, if necessary of the anticoagulant are recommended.

Diabetic patients receiving **insulin** may need dosage adjustments if anabolic therapy is added or discontinued. Anabolics may decrease blood glucose and decrease insulin requirements.

Anabolics may enhance the edema that can be associated with **ACTH** or **adrenal steroid** therapy.

Drug/Laboratory Interactions - Concentrations of **protein bound iodine (PBI)** can be decreased in patients receiving androgen/anabolic therapy, but the clinical significance of this is probably not important. Androgen/anabolic agents can decrease amounts of **thyroxine-binding globulin** and decrease **total T4** concentrations and increase **resin uptake of T3 and T4**. Free thyroid hormones are unaltered and, clinically, there is no evidence of dysfunction.

Both **creatinine** and **creatine excretion** can be decreased by anabolic steroids. Anabolic steroids can increase the urinary excretion of **17-ketosteroids**.

Androgenic/anabolic steroids may alter **blood glucose** levels. Androgenic/-anabolic steroids may suppress **clotting factors II, V, VII, and X**. Anabolic agents can affect **liver function tests** (BSP retention, SGOT, SGPT, bilirubin, and alkaline phosphatase).

Doses -
Dogs:
    For treatment of anemia in patients with chronic renal failure:
        a) 1 - 1.5 mg/kg IM once weekly; may require 2-3 months to achieve beneficial effects. (Polzin and Osborne 1985)
        b) 5 mg/kg IM (maximum of 200 mg/week) every 2-3 weeks (Ross et al. 1988)
    For treatment of metabolic and endocrine anemias:
        a) 5 mg/kg IM once weekly (maximum of 200 mg); most resolve with correction of underlying disease process (Maggio-Price 1988)
    For aplastic anemia:
        a) 1 - 3 mg/kg IM weekly (Weiss 1986)
    As an appetite stimulant:
        a) 5 mg/kg IM (max. 200 mg/week) weekly (Macy and Ralston 1989)
Cats:
    For FELV-induced anemia or as a general bone marrow stimulant:
        a) 10 - 20 mg IM once weekly (is of questionable benefit). (Maggio-Price 1988)
    For chronic anemia secondary to feline cardiomyopathy:
        a) 50 mg IM weekly (Harpster 1986)
Monitoring Parameters -
    1) Androgenic side effects
    2) Fluid and electrolyte status, if indicated
    3) Liver function tests if indicated
    4) Red blood cell count, indices, if indicated

5) Weight, appetite

Client Information - Because of the potential for abuse of anabolic steroids by humans, many states have included, or are considering including this agent as a controlled drug. It should be kept in a secure area and out of the reach of children.

Dosage Forms/Preparations/FDA Approval Status/Withholding Times -
  Veterinary-Approved Products: None
  Human-Approved Products:
    Nandrolone Decanoate Injection (in oil) 50 mg/ml in 2 ml vials & 1 ml syringes; 100 mg/ml in 2 ml vials & 1 ml syringes; 200 mg/ml in 1 ml vials & syringes
    Available generically and under several proprietary trade names. A commonly known product is *Deca-Durabolin*® (Organon); (Rx) C-III

NAPROXEN

Chemistry - Naproxen is a propionic acid derivative, and has similar structure and pharmacologic profiles as ibuprofen and ketoprofen. It is a white to off-white crystalline powder with an apparent pK_a of 4.15. It is practically insoluble in water and freely soluble in alcohol. The sodium salt is also available commercially for human use.

Storage/Stability/Compatibility - Naproxen should be stored in well-closed, light resistant containers and stored at room temperature. Temperatures above 40° C (104°F) should be avoided.

Pharmacology - Like other NSAIDs, naproxen exhibits analgesic, anti-inflammatory, and antipyrexic activity probably through its inhibition of cyclooxygenase with resultant impediment of prostaglandin synthesis.

Pharmacokinetics - In horses, the drug is reported to have a 50% bioavailability after oral dosing and a half-life of approximately 4 hours. Absorption does not appear to be altered by the presence of food. It may take 5-7 days to see a beneficial response after starting treatment. Following a dose, the drug is metabolized in the liver. It is detectable in the urine for at least 48 hours in the horse after an oral dose.

In dogs, absorption after oral dosing is rapid and bioavailability is between 68-100%. The drug is highly bound to plasma proteins. The average half-life in dogs is very long at 74 hours.

In humans, naproxen is highly bound to plasma proteins (99%). It crosses the placenta and enters milk at levels of about 1% of those in serum.

Uses/Indications - The manufacturer lists the following indications: ".... for the relief of inflammation and associated pain and lameness exhibited with myositis and other soft tissue diseases of the musculoskeletal system of the horse." (Package Insert; *Equiproxen*®—Syntex). It has also been used as an antiinflammatory/analgesic in dogs for the treatment of osteoarthritis and other musculoskeletal inflammatory diseases (see adverse reactions below).

Contraindications/Precautions - Naproxen is relatively contraindicated in patients with a history of, or preexisting hematologic, renal or hepatic disease. It is contraindicated in patients with active GI ulcers or with a history of hypersensitivity to the drug. It should be used cautiously in patients with a history of GI ulcers, or heart failure (may cause fluid retention). Animals suffering from inflammation secondary to concomitant infection, should receive appropriate antimicrobial therapy.

In studies in rodents and in limited studies in horses, no evidence of teratogenicity or adverse effects in breeding performance have been detected following the use of naproxen. However, the potential benefits of therapy must be weighed against the potential risks of its use in pregnant animals.

Adverse Effects/Warnings - Adverse effects are apparently uncommon in horses. The possibility exists for GI (distress, diarrhea, ulcers), hematologic (hypoproteinemia, decreased hematocrit), renal (fluid retention) and CNS (neuropathies) effects.

Reports of GI ulcers and perforation associated with naproxen has occurred in dogs. Dogs may also be overly sensitive to the adverse renal effects (nephritis/nephrotic syndrome) and hepatic (increased liver enzymes) effects with naproxen. Because of the apparent very narrow therapeutic index and the seriousness of the potential adverse reactions that can be seen in dogs, many clinicians feel that the drug should not be used in this species.

Overdosage - There is very limited information regarding acute overdoses of this drug in humans and domestic animals. The reported oral LD_{50} in dogs is >1000 mg/kg. Treatment should follow standard overdose procedures (empty gut following oral ingestion, etc.). Animal studies have demonstrated that activated charcoal may bind significant amounts of naproxen. Supportive treatment should be instituted as necessary. Because naproxen may cause renal effects, monitor electrolyte and fluid balance carefully and manage renal failure using established guidelines.

One report of a dog who received 5.6 mg/kg for 7 days has been published (Gilmour and Walshaw 1987). The dog presented with symptoms of melena, vomiting, depression, regenerative anemia, and pale mucous membranes. Laboratory indices of note included, neutrophilia with a left shift, BUN of 66 mg/dl, serum creatinine of 2.1 mg/dl, serum protein:albumin of 4.0:2.1 g/dls. The dog recovered following treatment with fluids/blood, antibiotics, vitamin/iron supplementation, oral antacids and cimetidine.

Drug Interactions - Because naproxen is highly bound to plasma proteins and may displace other highly bound drugs, increased serum levels and duration of actions of **phenytoin, valproic acid, oral anticoagulants**, other **anti-inflammatory agents, salicylates, sulfonamides**, and the **sulfonylurea antidiabetic agents** can occur. If naproxen is used concurrently with **warfarin**, enhanced hypoprothrombinemic effects have not been noted, but because of the tendency of naproxen to induce GI bleeding it should be used cautiously in patients on warfarin therapy.

When **aspirin** is used concurrently with naproxen, plasma levels of naproxen may decrease as well as an increased likelihood of GI adverse effects (blood loss) developing. Concomitant administration of aspirin with naproxen is not recommended.

Probenicid may cause a significant increase in serum levels and half-life of naproxen.

Serious toxicity has occurred when NSAIDs have been used concomitantly with **methotrexate**; use together with extreme caution.

Naproxen may reduce the saluretic and diuretic effects of **furosemide**. Use with caution in patients with severe cardiac failure.

Doses -
Dogs:
a) 5 mg/kg PO initially, then 1.2 - 2.8 mg/kg PO once daily (Frey and Rieh 1981)
b) 1.1 mg/kg PO q12h (McConnell and Hughey 1987)

Horses:
a) 5 mg/kg by slow IV, then 10 mg/kg PO (top dressed in feed) twice daily for up to 14 days or 10 mg/kg PO (top dressed in feed) *bid* for up to 14 consecutive days. (Package Insert; *Equiproxen*® - Syntex Animal Health)

Monitoring Parameters -
1) Analgesic/anti-inflammatory efficacy
2) GI: appetite, feces (occult blood, diarrhea)
3) PCV (packed cell volume), hematocrit if indicated or on chronic therapy
4) WBC's if indicated or on chronic therapy

Client Information - Notify veterinarian if symptoms of GI distress (anorexia, vomiting in dogs, diarrhea, black feces or blood in stool) occur, or if animal becomes depressed.

Dosage Forms/Preparations/FDA Approval Status/Withholding Times -
Veterinary-Approved Products:
Naproxen 10% (100 mg/ml) Veterinary Solution for Injection; 2 gm vial with 19 ml vial of sterile water for injection. Use entire contents immediately after reconstituting. Makes 20 ml of 10% (100 mg/ml) solution.; *Equiproxen*® (Fort Dodge); (Rx) Approved for us in horses not intended for food.

Naproxen Veterinary Granules; Each 8 gram packet contains 4 grams of naproxen. Cartons of 14 - 8 gram packets; *Equiproxen*® (Fort Dodge); (Rx) Approved for us in horses not intended for food.

Human-Approved Products:
Naproxen Oral tablets (scored) 250 mg, 375 mg, 500 mg; *Naprosyn*® (Syntex); Generic (Rx)

Naproxen Oral Suspension 125 mg/5 ml in pints; *Naprosyn*® (Syntex); Generic (Rx)

NARCOTIC (OPIATE) AGONIST ANALGESICS, PHARMACOLOGY OF

Receptors for opiate analgesics are found in high concentrations in the limbic system, spinal cord, thalamus, hypothalamus, striatum, and midbrain. They are also found in tissues such as the gastrointestinal tract, urinary tract, and in other smooth muscle.

Opiate receptors are further broken down into five main sub-groups. *Mu* receptors are found primarily in the pain regulating areas of the brain. They are thought to contribute to the analgesia, euphoria, respiratory depression, physical dependence, miosis, and hypothermic actions of opiates. *Kappa* receptors are located primarily in the deep layers of the cerebral cortex and spinal cord. They are responsible for analgesia, sedation and miosis. *Sigma* receptors are thought to be responsible for the dysphoric effects (struggling, whining), hallucinations, respiratory and cardiac stimulation, and mydriatic effects of opiates. *Delta* receptors, located in the limbic areas of the CNS and *epsilon* receptors have also been described, but their actions have not been well explained at this time.

The morphine-like agonists (morphine, meperidine, oxymorphone) have primary activity at the *mu* receptors, with some activity possible at the *delta* receptor. The primary pharmacologic effects of these agents include: analgesia, antitussive activity, respiratory depression, sedation, emesis, physical dependence, and intestinal effects (constipation/defecation). Secondary pharmacologic effects include: CNS: euphoria, sedation, & confusion. Cardiovascular: bradycardia due to central vagal stimulation, alpha-adrenergic receptors may be depressed resulting in peripheral vasodilation, decreased peripheral resistance, and baroreceptor inhibition. Orthostatic hypotension and syncope may occur. Urinary: Increased bladder sphincter tone can induce urinary retention.

Various species may exhibit contradictory effects from these agents. For example, horses, cattle, swine, and cats may develop excitement after morphine injections and dogs may defecate after morphine. These effects are in contrast to the expected effects of sedation and constipation. Dogs and humans may develop miosis, while other species (especially cats) may develop mydriasis. For more information see the individual monographs for each agent.

Neomycin Sulfate

Chemistry - An aminoglycoside antibiotic obtained from *Streptomyces fradiae*, neomycin is actually a complex of three separate compounds, neomycin A (neamine; inactive), neomycin C and neomycin B (framycetin). The commercially available product almost entirely consists of the sulfate salt of neomycin B. It occurs as an odorless or almost odorless, white to slightly yellow, hygroscopic powder or cryodessicated solid. It is freely soluble in water and very slightly soluble in alcohol. One mg of pure neomycin sulfate is equivalent to not less than 650 Units. Oral or injectable (after reconstitution with normal saline) solutions of neomycin sulfate have a pH from 5-7.5.

Storage/Stability/Compatibility - Neomycin sulfate oral solution should be stored at room temperature (15-30°C) in tight, light-resistant containers. Unless otherwise instructed by the manufacturer, oral tablets/boluses should be stored in tight containers at room temperature. The sterile powder should be stored at room temperature and protected from light.

In the dry state, neomycin is stable for at least 2 years at room temperature.

Pharmacology - Neomycin has a mechanism of action and spectrum of activity (primarily gram negative aerobes) similar to the other aminoglycosides, but in comparison to either gentamicin or amikacin, it is significantly less effective against several species of gram negative organisms, including strains of *Klebsiella*, *E. coli* and *Pseudomonas*. However, most strains of neomycin-resistant bacteria of these species remain susceptible to amikacin. More information on the aminoglycosides mechanism of action and spectrum of activity is outlined in more detail in the amikacin monograph.

Uses/Indications - Because neomycin is more nephrotoxic and less effective against several bacterial species than either gentamicin or amikacin, its use is generally limited to the oral treatment of enteral infections, to reduce microbe numbers in the colon prior to colon surgery, and orally or in enema form to reduce ammonia-producing bacteria in the treatment of hepatic encephalopathy. Doses for parenteral administration are listed below, but should be used only with extreme caution due to the drug's toxic potential.

Pharmacokinetics - Approximately 3% of a dose of neomycin is absorbed after oral or rectal (retention enema) administration, but this can be increased if gut motility is slowed or if the bowel wall is damaged. Therapeutic levels are not attained in the systemic circulation after oral administration.

After IM administration, therapeutic levels can be attained with peak levels occurring within 1 hour of dosing. The drug apparently distributes to tissues and is eliminated like the other aminoglycosides (refer to Amikacin monograph for more details). Orally administered neomycin is nearly all excreted unchanged in the feces.

Contraindications/Precautions/Reproductive Safety - More detailed information on the contraindications, precautions and reproductive safety of the aminoglycoside antibiotics can be found in the amikacin monograph.

Oral neomycin is contraindicated in the presence of intestinal obstruction or if the patient is hypersensitive to aminoglycosides.

Chronic usage of oral aminoglycosides may result in bacterial or fungal superinfections.

Because oral neomycin is only minimally absorbed, it is unlikely significant systemic or teratogenic effects should occur. However, one group of authors (Caprile and Short 1987) recommends that the drug not be used orally in foals.

Adverse Effects/Warnings, Overdosage/Acute Toxicity - Refer to the amikacin monograph for more information regarding these topics with parenteral neomycin.

Rarely, oral neomycin may cause ototoxicity, nephrotoxicity, severe diarrhea and intestinal malabsorption.

Drug Interactions, Drug/Laboratory Interactions - Refer to the amikacin monograph for more information regarding drug interactions with parenteral neomycin. In addition: Oral neomycin should not be given concurrently with oral **penicillin VK** as malabsorption of the penicillin may occur.

Oral neomycin with orally administered **digitalis preparations** (*e.g.,* **digoxin**) may result in decreased absorption of the digitalis. Separating the doses of the two medications may not alleviate this effect. Some human patients (<10%) metabolize digoxin in the GI tract and neomycin may increase serum digoxin levels in these patients. It is recommended that if oral neomycin is added or withdrawn from the drug regimen of a patient stabilized on a digitalis glycoside, that enhanced monitoring be performed.

Oral neomycin may decrease the amount of **vitamin K** absorbed from the gut; this may have ramifications for patients receiving **oral anticoagulants**.

Methotrexate absorption may be reduced by oral neomycin but is increased by oral kanamycin (found in *Amforal*®).

Although only minimal amounts of neomycin are absorbed after oral or rectal administration, the concurrent use of **other ototoxic or nephrotoxic drugs** with neomycin should be done with caution.

Doses -
Dogs:
For treatment of hepatic encephalopathy:
   a) 22 mg/kg PO *tid-qid* (Hardy 1989)
   b) For emergency treatment of hepatic encephalopathy secondary to portosystemic shunts: Following evacuation enema instill 10 - 20 mg/kg neomycin sulfate diluted in water. Oral neomycin not recommended. (Cornelius and Bjorling 1988)
   c) 15 mg/kg as an enema every 6 hours after a cleansing enema or 10 - 20 mg/kg PO every 6 hours. May be used with lactulose. (Johnson 1986)

For GI tract bacterial overgrowth:
   a) 20 mg/kg PO *bid-tid* (Morgan 1988)

For systemic therapy (**Caution**: Very nephrotoxic):
   a) 3.5 mg/kg IV, IM or SQ q8h (Kirk 1989)

Cats:
For treatment of hepatic encephalopathy:
   a) Secondary to portosystemic shunts: 10 - 20 mg/kg PO *bid*. May be used in combination with lactulose or in cleansing enemas. (Center, Hornbuckle, and Scavelli 1986)

For systemic therapy (**Caution**: Very nephrotoxic):
   a) 3.5 mg/kg IV, IM or SQ q8h (Kirk 1989)

Cattle:
For oral administration to treat susceptible enteral infections:
   a) Cattle: 4 - 7.5 g/day PO divided 2-4 times daily at regular intervals. Calves: 2 - 3 g/day PO divided 2-4 times daily at regular intervals. Doses are not standardized; use for general guidance only. (Brander, Pugh, and Bywater 1982)
   b) 10 - 20 mg/kg q12h (general guideline only). (Jenkins 1986)
   c) 7-12 mg/kg PO q12h (Howard 1986)
   d) Feed at levels of 70-140 g/ton of feed or mix the appropriate dose in the drinking water which will be consumed by animals in 12 hours to provide 11 mg/kg or mix with reconstituted milk replacers to provide 200 - 400 mg/gallon. (Label directions; *Neomix Ag*® *325*—Upjohn)

For respiratory tract infections:
   a) 4.4 mg/kg IM q8-12h, or 22 mg/kg IM q8-12h,: may give oral form IM or SQ. At highest dose almost all *P. hemolytica* and *P. multocida* and 74% of *C. pyogenes* are inhibited. Nephrotoxicity and/or ototoxicity can occur even with low dose regimen. Monitor creatinine levels. (Beech 1987b)
   b) 6.6 - 19.8 mg/kg IM once daily. (Upson 1988)

Horses:
For oral administration to treat susceptible enteral infections:
   a) Adults: 4 - 7.5 g/day PO divided 2-4 times daily at regular intervals. Foals: 2 - 3 g/day PO divided 2-4 times daily at regular intervals. Doses are not standardized; use for general guidance only. (Brander, Pugh, and Bywater 1982)
   b) 5 - 15 mg/kg PO once daily (Robinson 1987)

For respiratory tract infections:
   a) For pleuritis and less frequently pneumonia: 4.4 mg/kg IM or IV q8-12h. Nephrotoxicity and/or ototoxicity can occur; nephrotoxicity more common in foals.

Local myositis seen with IM dosing particularly if treatment is longer than 7 days. Systemic use of oral form is not approved, but is used with penicillin to increase gram negative coverage (Beech 1987b)

Swine:
For oral administration to treat susceptible enteral infections:
  a) Young pigs: 0.75 - 1 g/day PO divided 2-4 times daily at regular intervals. Doses are not standardized; use for general guidance only. (Brander, Pugh, and Bywater 1982)
  b) 7-12 mg/kg PO q12h (Howard 1986)

Sheep & Goats:
For oral administration to treat susceptible enteral infections:
  a) Lambs: 0.75 - 1 g/day PO divided 2-4 times daily at regular intervals. Doses are not standardized; use for general guidance only. (Brander, Pugh, and Bywater 1982)
  b) Feed at levels of 70-140 g/ton of feed or mix the appropriate dose in the drinking water which will be consumed by animals in 12 hours to provide 11 mg/kg or mix with reconstituted milk replacers to provide 200 - 400 mg/gallon. (Label directions; *Neomix Ag® 325*—Upjohn)

Birds:
For bacterial enteritis:
  a) Chickens, turkeys, ducks: Feed at levels of 70-140 g/ton of feed or mix the appropriate dose in the drinking water which will be consumed by animals in 12 hours to provide 11 mg/kg. (Label directions; *Neomix Ag® 325*—Upjohn)

Snakes:
For susceptible infections:
  a) For bacterial gastritis: gentamicin 2.5 mg/kg IM every 72 hours with oral neomycin 15 mg/kg plus oral live lactobacillus. (Burke 1986)

Monitoring Parameters -
For oral use:
  1) Clinical efficacy
  2) Systemic and GI adverse effects with prolonged use

For parenteral use: Refer to Amikacin monograph

Client Information - Clients should understand that the potential exists for severe toxicity (nephrotoxicity, ototoxicity) developing from this medication when used parenterally.

Dosage Forms/Preparations/FDA Approval Status/Withholding Times -
  Veterinary-Approved Products:
  Neomycin Sulfate Oral Liquid 200 mg/ml
    Biosol® (Upjohn); (OTC) Approved for use in cattle, swine, sheep, turkeys, laying hens, and broilers. Withdrawal times: Cattle = 30 days; Sheep and swine = 20 days, Turkeys and Layers = 14 days; Broilers = 5 days.
    Also available as generically labeled products.
  Neomycin Sulfate Oral Solution 50 mg/ml in 10 ml dropper bottles
    Biosol Aquadrops® (Upjohn); (OTC) Approved for use in dogs and cats.
  Neomycin Sulfate Oral Tablets 100 mg
    Biosol® Tablets (Upjohn); (OTC) Approved for use in dogs and cats.
  Neomycin Sulfate Intrauterine or Oral Boluses 500 mg; *Biosol® Boluses* (Upjohn); (OTC) Approved for use in cattle, foals, swine, and sheep. Slaughter withdrawal times: Cattle = 30 days; Sheep and swine = 20 days. Milk withdrawal = 48 hours.
  Neomycin Sulfate Soluble Powder 3.125 g/ounce;*Biosol® Soluble Powder* (Upjohn); (OTC) Approved for use in dogs, cats, cattle, swine, sheep, and horses. Slaughter withdrawal times: Cattle = 30 days; Sheep and swine = 20 days.
  Neomycin Powder Water/Feed Additive 325 g/lb; *Biosol 325®* (Upjohn), *Neomix Ag® 325* (Upjohn); (OTC) Approved for use in chickens, turkeys, ducks, nonlactating dairy cattle, beef cattle, goats, horses, mink, sheep, and swine. Slaughter withdrawal times: Cattle = 30 days; Sheep and swine = 20 days, Turkeys & layers = 14 days; Broilers = 5 days.
  There are several combination neomycin veterinary products, the following are examples:
  Neomycin 25 mg, isopropamide 1.67 mg, prochlorperazine 3.33 mg capsules; Neomycin 75 mg, isopropamide 5 mg, prochlorperazine 10 mg capsules; *Neo-Darbazine® #1* (Pfizer); (Rx) Approved for use in dogs. *Neo-Darbazine® #3* (SKB); (Rx) Approved for use in dogs.

Human-Approved Products:

Neomycin Sulfate Oral Tablets 500 mg; *Neo-Tabs*® (Pharma-Tek) (Rx), generic (Rx)

Neomycin Sulfate Oral Solution 25 mg/ml in pints;*Mycifradin*® (Upjohn);*Neo-fradin*® (Pharma-Tek); (Rx)

NEOSTIGMINE BROMIDE
NEOSTIGMINE METHYLSULFATE

Chemistry - Synthetic quaternary ammonium parasympathomimetic agents, neostigmine bromide and neostigmine methylsulfate both occur as odorless, bitter-tasting, white, crystalline powders that are very soluble in water and soluble in alcohol. The melting point of neostigmine methylsulfate is from 144-149°. The pH of the commercially available neostigmine methylsulfate injection is from 5-6.5.

Storage/Stability/Compatibility - Neostigmine bromide tablets should be stored at room temperature in tight containers. Neostigmine methylsulfate injection should be stored at room temperature and protected from light; avoid freezing.

Neostigmine methylsulfate injection is reportedly **compatible** with the commonly used IV replacement solutions and the following drugs: glycopyrrolate, pentobarbital sodium, and thiopental sodium.

Pharmacology - Neostigmine competes with acetylcholine for acetylcholinesterase. As the neostigmine-acetylcholinesterase complex is hydrolyzed at a slower rate than that of the acetylcholine-enzyme complex, acetylcholine will accumulate with a resultant exaggeration and prolongation of its effects. These effects can include increased tone of intestinal and skeletal musculature, stimulation of salivary and sweat glands, bronchoconstriction, ureter constriction, miosis and bradycardia. Neostigmine also has a direct cholinomimetic effect on skeletal muscle.

Uses/Indications - Neostigmine is indicated for rumen atony, initiating peristalsis, emptying the bladder and stimulating skeletal muscle contractions in cattle, horses, sheep and swine (Package insert; *Stiglyn*® 1:500 - P/M; Mallinckrodt). It has also been used in the diagnosis and treatment of myasthenia gravis and in treating non-depolarizing neuromuscular blocking agents (curare-type) overdoses in dogs.

Pharmacokinetics - Information on the pharmacokinetics of neostigmine in veterinary species was not located. In humans, neostigmine bromide is poorly absorbed after oral administration with only 1-2% of the dose absorbed. Neostigmine effects on peristaltic activity in humans begin within 10-30 minutes after parenteral administration and can persist for up to 4 hours.

Neostigmine is 15-25% bound to plasma proteins. It has not been detected in human milk nor would be expected to cross the placenta when given at usual doses.

In humans, the half-life of the drug is approximately one hour. It is metabolized in the liver and also hydrolyzed by cholinesterases to 3-OH PTM which is weakly active. When administered parenterally, approximately 80% of the drug is excreted in the urine within 24 hours, with 50% excreted unchanged.

Contraindications/Precautions - Neostigmine is contraindicated in patients with peritonitis, mechanical intestinal or urinary tract obstructions, late stages of pregnancy, in animals hypersensitive to this class of compounds or treated with other cholinesterase inhibitors.

Use neostigmine with caution in patients with epilepsy, peptic ulcer disease, bronchial asthma, cardiac arrhythmias, hyperthyroidism, vagotonia or megacolon.

Adverse Effects/Warnings - Adverse effects of neostigmine are dose-related and cholinergic in nature. See overdosage section below.

Overdosage - Overdosage of neostigmine can induce a cholinergic crisis. Symptoms can include nausea, vomiting, diarrhea, excessive salivation and drooling, sweating (in animals with sweat glands), miosis, lacrimation, increased bronchial secretions, bradycardia or tachycardia, cardiospasm, bronchospasm, hypotension, muscle cramps and weakness, agitation, restlessness or paralysis. In patients with myasthenia gravis, it may be difficult to distinguish between a cholinergic crisis and myasthenic crisis. A test dose of edrophonium, should differentiate between the two.

Cholinergic crisis is treated by temporarily ceasing neostigmine therapy and instituting treatment with atropine (doses are listed in the Atropine monograph). Maintain adequate respirations using mechanical assistance if necessary.

Drug Interactions - Anticholinesterase therapy may be antagonized by administration of parenteral **magnesium** therapy, as it can have a direct depressant effect on skeletal muscle.

Drugs that possess some neuromuscular blocking activity (*e.g.*, aminoglycoside antibiotics, some antiarrhythmic and anesthetic drugs) may necessitate increased dosages of neostigmine in treating or diagnosing myasthenic patients.

Corticosteroids may decrease the anticholinesterase activity of neostigmine. After stopping corticosteroid therapy, neostigmine may cause increased anticholinesterase activity.

Neostigmine may prolong the Phase I block of **depolarizing muscle relaxants** (*e.g.,* succinyl-choline, decamethonium). Neostigmine antagonizes the actions of **non-depolarizing neuromuscular blocking agents** (pancuronium, tubocurarine, gallamine, etc.).

Atropine will antagonize the muscarinic effects of neostigmine and is often used to reduce neostigmine's side effects. Use cautiously however, as atropine can mask the early symptoms of cholinergic crisis.

Theoretically, **dexpanthenol** may have additive effects when used with neostigmine.

Doses -
Dogs:
    a) 1 - 2 mg IM as needed; 5 - 15 mg PO as needed (Kirk 1986)

For treatment of myasthenia gravis:
    a) For dogs weighing:
        less than 5 kg = 0.25 mg *qid* IM
        5 - 25 kg = 0.25 - 0.5 mg *qid* IM
        > 25 kg = 0.5 - 0.75 mg *qid* IM; Doses are initial guidelines only; titrate doses to the patient (Hurvitz and Johnessee 1985)

For diagnosis of myasthenia gravis:
    a) 0.05 mg/kg IM (Diagnostic if clinical improvement occurs in 15-30 minutes; pre-treat with atropine) (LeCouteur 1988)

For treatment of curare overdoses:
    a) 0.001 mg/kg SQ, follow with IV injection of atropine (0.04 mg/kg) (Bailey 1986)

Cattle:
    a) 1 mg/100 lbs of body weight SQ; repeat as indicated (Package Insert; *Stiglyn*® 1:500 - P/M; Mallinckrodt)

Horses:
    a) 1 mg/100 lbs of body weight SQ; repeat as indicated (Package Insert; *Stiglyn*® 1:500 - P/M; Mallinckrodt)

For treatment of paralytic ileus of large colon:
    a) 2 - 4 mg SQ q2h. Use after correction of large bowel displacement; discontinue when GI motility returns. May cause increased secretion into GI tract and therefore may be harmful in small intestinal disease. Does not produce progressive contractions of small intestine. (Stover 1987)
    b) 0.02 mg/kg SQ; duration of action may be very short (15-30 minutes); does not increase propulsive motility of jejunum and may delay gastric emptying time. (Clark and Becht 1987)

Swine:
    a) 2 - 3 mg/100 lbs of body weight IM; repeat as indicated (Package Insert; *Stiglyn*® 1:500 - P/M; Mallinckrodt)
    b) 0.03 mg/kg (Davis 1986)

Sheep:
    a) 1.0 - 1.5 mg/100 lbs of body weight SQ; repeat as indicated (Package Insert; *Stiglyn*® 1:500 - P/M; Mallinckrodt)
    b) 0.01 - 0.02 mg/kg (goats also) (Davis 1986)

Monitoring Parameters - Dependent on reason for use.
    1) Adverse reactions (see Adverse Reactions and Overdosage above)
    2) Clinical efficacy

Client Information - This product should be used by professionals in situations where the drug's effects can be monitored.

Dosage Forms/Preparations/FDA Approval Status/Withholding Times -
Veterinary-Approved Products: None

Human-Approved Products:

Neostigmine Tablets 15 mg; *Prostigmin*® (ICN); (Rx)

Neostigmine Methylsulfate Injection 1:1000 (1 mg/ml), 1:2000 (0.5 mg/ml), 1:4000 (0.25 mg/ml) in 1 ml amps and 10 ml vials; *Prostigmin*® (ICN); Generic; (Rx)

NITROFURANTOIN

Chemistry - A synthetic, nitrofuran antibacterial, nitrofurantoin occurs as a bitter tasting, lemon-yellow, crystalline powder with a pK_a of 7.2. It is very slightly soluble in water or alcohol.

Storage/Stability/Compatibility - Nitrofurantoin preparations should be stored in tight containers at room temperature and protected from light. The oral suspension should not be frozen. Nitrofurantoin will decompose if contacted with metals other than aluminum or stainless steel.

Pharmacology - Nitrofurantoin acts usually as a bacteriostatic antimicrobial, but may be bactericidal depending on the concentration of the drug and the susceptibility of the organism. The exact mechanism of action of nitrofurantoin has not been fully elucidated, but the drug apparently inhibits various bacterial enzyme systems, including acetyl coenzyme A. Nitrofurantoin has greater antibacterial activity in acidic environments.

Nitrofurantoin has activity against several gram negative and some gram positive organisms, including many strains of *E. coli, Klebsiella, Enterobacter, Enterococci, Staphylococcus aureus* and *epidermidis, Enterobacter, Citrobacter, Salmonella*, Shigella, and Corynebacterium. It has little or no activity against most strains of *Proteus, Serratia* or *Acinetobacter* and has no activity against *Pseudomonas sp.*.

Uses/Indications - Considered a urinary tract antiseptic, nitrofurantoin is used primarily in small animals, but also occasionally in horses in the treatment of lower urinary tract infections caused by susceptible bacteria. It is not effective in treating renal cortical or perinephric abscesses or other systemic infections.

Pharmacokinetics - Nitrofurantoin is rapidly absorbed from the GI tract and the presence of food may enhance the absorption of the drug. Macrocrystalline forms of the drug may be absorbed more slowly with less GI upset. Because of its slower absorption, urine levels of the drug may be prolonged.

Because of the rapid elimination of the drug after absorption, therapeutic levels in the systemic circulation are not maintained. Approximately 20-60% of the drug is bound to serum proteins. Peak urine levels occur within 30 minutes of dosing. The drug crosses the placenta and only minimal quantities of the drug are found in milk.

Approximately 40-50% of the drug is eliminated into urine unchanged via both glomerular filtration and tubular secretion. Some of the drug is metabolized, primarily in the liver. Elimination half-lives in humans with normal renal function average 20 minutes.

Contraindications/Precautions/Reproductive Safety - Nitrofurantoin is contraindicated in patients with renal impairment as the drug is much less efficacious and the development of toxicity is much more likely. The drug is also contraindicated in patients hypersensitive to it.

In humans, the drug is contraindicated in pregnant patients at term and in neonates as hemolytic anemia can occur secondary to immature enzyme systems. Safe use of the drug during earlier stages of pregnancy has not been determined. Nitrofurantoin has been implicated in causing infertility in male dogs. Use only when the benefits of therapy outweigh the potential risks.

Adverse Effects/Warnings - In dogs and cats, gastrointestinal disturbances and hepatopathy can occur with this drug. Neuropathies, chronic active hepatitis, hemolytic anemia and pneumonitis have been described in humans, but are believed to occur very rarely in animals.

Overdosage/Acute Toxicity - No specific information was located. Because the drug is rapidly absorbed and excreted. Patients with normal renal function should require little therapy when mild overdoses occur. Massive overdoses should be handled by emptying the gut using standard protocols if the ingestion was relatively recent, and then monitoring the patient for adverse effects (see above).

Drug Interactions - The uricosuric agents **sulfinpyrazone** or **probenecid** may inhibit the renal excretion of nitrofurantoin and potentially increase its toxicity and reduce its effectiveness in urinary tract infections.

Nitrofurantoin may antagonize the antimicrobial activity of the fluoroquinolones (*e.g.,* **enrofloxacin, ciprofloxacin**) and their concomitant use is not recommended.

Magnesium trisilicate containing antacids may inhibit the oral absorption of nitrofurantoin. **Food** or **anticholinergic drugs** may increase the oral bioavailability of nitrofurantoin.

Drug/Laboratory Interactions - Nitrofurantoin may cause **false-positive urine glucose** determinations if using cupric sulfate solutions (Benedict's reagent, *Clinitest*®). Tests using glucose oxidase methods (*Tes-Tape*®, *Clinistix*®) are not affected by nitrofurantoin.

Nitrofurantoin may cause decreases in **blood glucose**, and increases in serum **creatinine, bilirubin and alkaline phosphatase**.

Doses -
  Dogs:
    For susceptible bacterial urinary tract infections:
      a) 4 mg/kg PO q6h (Osborne and Lulich 1987)
      b) For recurrent UTI: Conventional dose: 4 mg/kg PO q8h; Prophylactic dose: 3-4 mg/kg PO q24h (should be given at night after micturation and immediately before bedtime). (Polzin and Osborne 1985)

c) 4 mg/kg PO *tid* (Morgan 1988)

Cats:
For susceptible bacterial urinary tract infections:
a) 4 mg/kg PO q6h (Osborne and Lulich 1987)
b) For recurrent UTI: Conventional dose: 4 mg/kg PO q8h; Prophylactic dose: 3-4 mg/kg PO q24h (should be given at night after micturation and immediately before bedtime). (Polzin and Osborne 1985)

Horses:
For susceptible urinary tract infections:
a) 2.5 - 4.5 mg/kg PO *tid* (Robinson 1987)
b) 10 mg/kg PO daily (Huber 1988a)

Monitoring Parameters -
1) Clinical efficacy
2) Adverse effects
3) Periodic liver function tests should be considered with chronic therapy

Dosage Forms/Preparations/FDA Approval Status/Withholding Times -
Veterinary-Approved Products: None

Human-Approved Products:

Nitrofurantoin Macrocrystals Capsules 25 mg, 50 mg, and 100 mg; *Macrodantin*® (Procter & Gamble Pharm); *Macrobid*® (Procter & Gamble Pharm); generic; (Rx)

Nitrofurantoin Oral Suspension 5 mg/ml in 60 ml and pint bottles; *Furadantin*® (Dura); (Rx)

NITROGLYCERIN, TOPICAL

Chemistry - Famous as an explosive, nitroglycerin (NTG) occurs undiluted as a thick, volatile, white-pale yellow flammable, explosive liquid with a sweet, burning taste. The undiluted drug is soluble in alcohol and slightly soluble in water. Because of obvious safety reasons, nitroglycerin is diluted with lactose, dextrose, propylene glycol, alcohol, etc. when used for pharmaceutical purposes. Nitroglycerin may also be called glyceryl trinitrate, or nitroglycerol.

Storage/Stability/Compatibility - For storage/stability and compatibility for dosage forms other than the topical ointment, see specialized references or the package inserts for each product. The topical ointment should be stored at room temperature and the cap firmly attached.

Pharmacology - Nitroglycerin relaxes vascular smooth muscle primarily on the venous side, but a dose related effect on arterioles may also occur. Preload (left end-diastolic pressure) is reduced from the peripheral pooling of blood and decreased venous return to the heart. Because of its arteriolar effects, afterload may also be reduced depending on the dose. Myocardial oxygen demand and workload are reduced and coronary circulation can be improved.

Uses/Indications - Topical nitroglycerin in small animal medicine is used primarily as an adjunctive vasodilator in heart failure and cardiogenic edema. It is also used as an anti-anginal agent, an antihypertensive (acute), and topically to treat Raynaud's disease in humans.

Pharmacokinetics - Nitroglycerin topical ointment is absorbed through the skin, with an onset of action usually within 1 hour and a duration of action of 2-12 hours. It is generally dosed in dogs and cats q6-8 hours (*tid-qid*). Nitroglycerine has a very short half-life (1-4 minutes in humans) and is metabolized in the liver. At least two metabolites have some vasodilator activity and have longer half-lives than NTG.

Contraindications/Precautions - Nitrates are contraindicated in patients with severe anemia or who are hypersensitive to them. They should be used with caution (if at all) in patients with cerebral hemorrhage or head trauma. Nitrates should be used with caution in patients with diuretic-induced hypovolemia or with other hypotensive conditions

Adverse Effects/Warnings - Most common side effects seen are rashes at the application sites and orthostatic hypotension. If hypotension is a problem, reduce dosage. Transient headaches are a common side effect seen in humans and may be a problem for some animals.

Overdosage - If severe hypotension results after topical administration, wash site of application to prevent any more absorption of ointment. Fluids may be administered if necessary. Epinephrine is contraindicated as it is ineffective and may complicate the animal's condition.

Drug Interactions - Use of nitroglycerin with other **antihypertensive drugs** may cause additive hypotensive effects.

Doses -
Dogs:
a) 1/4 - 1 inch cutaneously every 6-8 hours (Bonagura and Muir 1986)

b) 1/4 - 2 inches topically *tid-qid*; 1/4 - 1/2 inch topically (inside ear) for small dogs; 2 inches topically for giant breeds (Tilley and Owens 1985)

Cats:
a) 1/4 inch cutaneously every 6-8 hours (Bonagura and Muir 1986)
b) 1/8 - 1/4 inch topically *tid* (Tilley and Owens 1985)

Monitoring Parameters -
1) Clinical efficacy
2) Sites of application for rash symptoms
3) Blood pressure, if possible or if hypotensive effects are seen

Client Information - Dosage is measured in inches of ointment; use papers supplied with product to measure appropriate dose. Wear gloves (non-permeable) when applying. Do not pet animal where ointment has been applied. Rotate application sites. Recommended application sites include: groin, inside the ears, and thorax. Rub ointment into skin well. If rash develops, do not use that site again until cleared. Contact veterinarian if rash persists or animal's condition deteriorates. There is no danger of explosion or fire with the use of this product.

Dosage Forms/Preparations/FDA Approval Status/Withholding Times -
Veterinary-Approved Products: None
Human-Approved Products: Note: Many dosage forms of nitroglycerin are available for human use, including sublingual tablets, buccal tablets, lingual spray, extended-release oral capsules and tablets, transdermal patches, and parenteral solutions for IV infusion. Because the use of nitroglycerin in small animal medicine is basically limited to the use of topical ointment, those other dosage forms will not be included here.

Nitroglycerin Topical Ointment 2% in a lanolin-petrolatum base in 20, 30 and 60 gram tubes & UD 1g & 3 g; *Nitro-bid*® (Hoechst Marion Roussel); *Nitrol*® (Savage); Generic; (Rx)

NITROPRUSSIDE SODIUM

Chemistry - A vascular smooth muscle relaxant, nitroprusside sodium occurs as practically odorless, reddish-brown crystals or powder. It is freely soluble in water and slightly soluble in alcohol. After reconstitution in D5W, solutions may have a brownish, straw, or light orange color and have a pH of 3.5 - 6.

Nitroprusside sodium may also be known as sodium nitroprusside or sodium nitroferricyanide.

Storage/Stability/Compatibility - Nitroprusside sodium powder for injection should be stored protected from light and moisture and kept at room temperature (15-30°C). Nitroprusside solutions exposed to light will cause a reduction of the ferric ion to the ferrous ion with a resultant loss in potency and a change from a brownish-color to a blue color. Degradation is enhanced with nitroprusside solutions in *Viaflex*® (Baxter) plastic bags exposed to fluorescent light. After reconstitution, protect immediately by covering vial or infusion bag with aluminum foil or other opaque material. Discard solutions that turn to a blue, dark red or green color. Solutions protected from light will remain stable for 24 hours after reconstitution. IV infusion tubing need not be protected from light while the infusion is running. It is not recommended to use IV infusion solutions other than D5W or to add any other medications to the infusion solution.

Pharmacology - Nitroprusside is an immediate acting intravenous hypotensive agent that directly causes peripheral vasodilation (arterial and venous) independent of autonomic innervation. It produces a lowering of blood pressure, an increase in heart rate, mild decrease in cardiac output and significant reduction in total peripheral resistance.

Uses/Indications - In human medicine, nitroprusside is indicated for the management of hypertensive crises, acute heart failure secondary to mitral regurgitation, and severe refractory CHF (often in combination with dopamine). Its use in veterinary medicine is generally reserved for the treatment of critically ill patients with one of these conditions only when constant blood pressure monitoring can be performed.

Pharmacokinetics - After starting an IV infusion of nitroprusside, reduction in blood pressure and other pharmacologic effects begin almost immediately. Blood pressure will return to pretreatment levels within 1-10 minutes following cessation of therapy.

Nitroprusside is metabolized non-enzymatically in the blood and tissues to cyanogen (cyanide radical). Cyanogen is converted in the liver to thiocyanate where it is eliminated in the urine, feces, and exhaled air. The half-life of cyanogen is 2.7-7 days if renal function is normal, but prolonged in patients with impaired renal function or with hyponatremia.

Contraindications/Precautions - Nitroprusside is contraindicated in patients with compensatory hypertension (*e.g.*, AV shunts or coarctation of the aorta), inadequate cerebral circulation, or during emergency surgery in patients near death.

Nitroprusside must be used with caution in patients with hepatic insufficiency, severe renal impairment, hyponatremia, or hypothyroidism. When nitroprusside is used for controlled hypotension during surgery, patients may have less tolerance to hypovolemia, anemia, or blood loss. Geriatric patients may be more sensitive to the hypotensive effects of nitroprusside.

Adverse Effects/Warnings - Most adverse reactions from nitroprusside are associated with its hypotensive effects, particularly if blood pressure is reduced too rapidly. Symptoms such as nausea, retching, restlessness, apprehension, muscle twitching, dizziness, have been reported in humans. These effects disappear when the infusion rate is reduced or stopped. Nitroprusside may be irritating at the infusion site; avoid extravasation.

Overdosage - Acute overdosage is manifested by a profound hypotension. Treat by reducing or stopping the infusion and giving fluids. Monitor blood pressure constantly.

Excessive doses, prolonged therapy, a depleted hepatic thiosulfate (sulfur) supply, or severe hepatic or renal insufficiency may lead to profound hypotension, cyanogen or thiocyanate toxicity. Acid/base status should be monitored to evaluate therapy and to detect metabolic acidosis (early sign of cyanogen toxicity). Tolerance to therapy is also an early sign of nitroprusside toxicity. Hydroxocobalamin (Vitamin B_{12a}) may prevent cyanogen toxicity. Thiocyanate toxicity may be exhibited as delirium in dogs. Serum thiocyanate levels may need to be monitored in patients on prolonged therapy, especially in those patients with concurrent renal dysfunction. Serum levels >100 micrograms/ml are considered toxic. It is suggested to refer to other references for further information should cyanogen or thiocyanate toxicity be suspected.

Drug Interactions - The hypotensive effects of nitroprusside may be enhanced by concomitant administration of **ganglionic blocking agents** (*e.g.,* **trimethaphan, hexamethonium), general anesthetics** (*e.g.,* **halothane, enflurane), or other circulatory depressants.**

Patients taking other **hypotensive agents (e.g** beta-**blockers, ACE inhibitors, etc.**) may be more sensitive to the hypotensive effects of nitroprusside.

Synergistic effects (increased cardiac output and reduced wedge pressure) may result if **dobutamine** is used with nitroprusside.

Doses -
 Directions for preparation of infusion: Add 2 - 3 ml D_5W to 50 mg vial to dissolve powder. Add dissolved solution to 1000 ml of D_5W and promptly protect solution from light (using aluminum foil or other opaque covering). Resultant solution contains 50 micrograms/ml of nitroprusside. Higher concentrations may be necessary in treating large animals. The administration set need not be protected from light. Solution may have a slight brownish tint, but discard solutions that turn to a blue, dark red or green color. Solution is stable for 24 hours after reconstitution. Do not add any other medications to IV running nitroprusside.

Using a Mini-Drip IV set (for small animals) (60 drops ≈ 1 ml; 1 drop contains approximately 0.83 micrograms) and a flow control device (pump, controller, etc.). Dose to effect at a rate of **0.5 - 10 micrograms/kg/min IV constant infusion.** A dose of 3 micrograms/kg/min will control most patients. Blood pressure must be continuously monitored. Avoid extravasation at IV site. (Plumb 1988). A dosage of 1 - 10 micrograms/kg/min IV infusion is recommended for use in dogs by one author (Moses 1988).

Monitoring Parameters -
 1) Blood pressure must be constantly monitored
 2) Acid/base balance
 3) Electrolytes (especially Na^+)

Client Information - Must only be used by professionals in a setting where precise IV infusion and constant blood pressure monitoring can be performed.

Dosage Forms/Preparations/FDA Approval Status/Withholding Times -
 Veterinary-Approved Products: None
 Human-Approved Products:
  Nitroprusside Sodium Powder for Injection 50 mg/vial in 2ml & 5 ml vials; *Nitropress*® (Abbott); Generic; (Rx)

NOVOBIOCIN SODIUM

Chemistry - An antibiotic obtained from *Streptomyces niveus* or *spheroides*, novobiocin sodium occurs as white to light yellow, crystalline powder and is very soluble in water.

Storage/Stability/Compatibility - Novobiocin should be stored in tight containers and at room temperature unless otherwise directed.

Pharmacology - Novobiocin is believed to act in several ways in a bactericidal manner. It inhibits bacterial DNA gyrase, thereby interfering with protein and nucleic acid synthesis. It also interferes with bacterial cell wall synthesis. Activity of the drug is enhanced in an alkaline medium.

The spectrum of activity of novobiocin includes some gram positive cocci (Staphs, *Streptococcus pneumoni*a, and some group A streps). Activity is variable against other Streptococci and weak against the Enterococci. Most gram negative organisms are resistant to the drug, but some *Haemophilus sp., Neisseria sp.*, and *Proteus sp.* may be susceptible.

Uses/Indications - As a single agent, novobiocin is approved for use in dry dairy cattle as a mastitis tube and as a premix for chickens, turkeys, ducks, and mink. It is available in combination with procaine penicillin G to treat mastitis in lactating dairy cattle. Novobiocin is available in combination with tetracycline ± prednisolone for oral use in dogs.

Pharmacokinetics - After oral administration, novobiocin is well absorbed from the GI tract. Peak levels occur within 1-4 hours. The presence of food can decrease peak concentrations of the drug.

Novobiocin is only poorly distributed to body fluids with concentrations in synovial, pleural and ascitic fluids less than those found in the plasma. Only minimal quantities of the drug cross the blood-brain barrier, even when meninges are inflamed. Highest concentrations of novobiocin are found in the small intestine and liver. The drug is approximately 90% protein bound and is distributed into milk.

Novobiocin is primarily eliminated in the bile and feces. Approximately 3% is excreted into the urine and urine levels are usually less than those found in serum.

Contraindications/Precautions/Reproductive Safety - Novobiocin is contraindicated in patients hypersensitive to it. Additionally, the drug should be used with extreme caution in patients with preexisting hepatic or hematopoietic dysfunction.

Safety during pregnancy has not been established; use only when clearly indicated.

Adverse Effects/Warnings - Adverse effects reported with the systemic use of this drug include fever, GI disturbances (nausea, vomiting, diarrhea), rashes and blood dyscrasias. In humans, occurrances of hypersensitivity reactions, hepatotoxicity and blood dyscrasias have significantly limited the use of this drug.

Overdosage/Acute Toxicity - Little information is available regarding overdoses of this drug. It is suggested that large oral overdoses be handled by emptying the gut following standard protocols; monitor and treat adverse effects symptomatically if necessary.

Drug Interactions - Novobiocin reportedly acts similarly to probenecid by blocking the tubular transport of drugs. Although the clinical significance of this is unclear, the elimination rates of drugs excreted in this manner (*e.g.,* **penicillins, cephalosporins**) could be decreased and half-lives prolonged.

Drug/Laboratory Interactions - Novobiocin can be metabolized into a yellow-colored product that can interfere with **serum bilirubin** determinations. It may also interfere with the determination **BSP** (bromosulfophthalein, sulfobromophthaelein) uptake tests by altering BSP uptake or biliary excretion.

Doses -
  Dogs:
    For susceptible infections:
      a) 10 mg/kg q8h PO (Greene 1984)
    For susceptible infections using the combination product (with tetracycline):
      a) 22 mg/kg of each antibiotic PO q12h (Package insert; *Albaplex*®—Upjohn)
  Cattle:
    For treatment of mastitis in dry cows:
      a) Infuse contents of one syringe into each quarter at the time of drying off; not later than 30 days prior to calving. (Package directions; *Drygard*® *Suspension* —Upjohn)
    For treatment of mastitis in lactating cows:
      a) Using the penicillin/novobiocin product (Special Formula 17900-Forte®): Infuse contents of one syringe in each infected quarter. Repeat once in 24 hours. (Package Directions; *Special Formula 17900-Forte*®—Upjohn)
Client Information: Shake mastitis tubes well before using.
Monitoring Parameters -
    1) Clinical efficacy
    2) Adverse effects
    3   Periodic liver function tests and CBC's are recommended if using long-term systemically.

**Dosage Forms/Preparations/FDA Approval Status/Withholding Times -
Veterinary-Approved Products**:

Novobiocin (as the sodium) Oil Suspension 400 mg per 10 ml Mastitis tube; *Drygard®
Suspension* (Upjohn); (OTC) Approved for use in dry cows. Not to be used within 30 days
of calving. Slaughter withdrawal = 30 days.

Novobiocin Premix 17.5 g/lb, and 25 g/lb; *Albamix® Premix* (Upjohn); (OTC) Approved for
use in chickens (not layers), turkeys (not layers for human consumption), ducks, and mink.
Slaughter withdrawal = chickens and turkeys (4 days), ducks (3 days), and mink (none).

Novobiocin Combination Products:

Novobiocin (as the sodium salt) 150 mg and Penicillin G Procaine 100,000 IU per 10 ml
Mastitis Syringe; *Special Formula 17900-Forte®* (Upjohn); (OTC) Approved for use in
lactating dairy cattle. Milk withdrawal = 72 hours. Slaughter withdrawal = 15 days.

Novobiocin Sodium 60 mg and Tetracycline HCl 60 mg tablets; Novobiocin Sodium 180 mg
and Tetracycline HCl 180 mg tablets; *Albaplex®* and *Albaplex® 3X* (Upjohn); (Rx)
Approved for use in dogs.

Novobiocin Sodium 60 mg, Tetracycline HCl 60 mg & Prednisolone 1.5 mg tablets;
Novobiocin Sodium 180 mg, Tetracycline HCl 180 mg & Prednisolone 4.5 mg tablets; *Delta
Albaplex®* and *Delta Albaplex® 3X* (Upjohn); (Rx) Approved for use in dogs.

Human-Approved Products:

Novobiocin (as the sodium) 250 mg Capsules; *Albamycin®* (Upjohn); (Rx)

NYSTATIN

Chemistry - A polyene antifungal antibiotic produced by *Streptomyces noursei*, nystatin occurs
as a yellow to light tan, hygroscopic powder having a cereal-like odor. It is very slightly soluble
in water and slightly to sparingly soluble in alcohol. One mg of nystatin contains not less than
4400 Units of activity. According to the USP, nystatin used in the preparation of oral suspensions
should not contain less than 5000 Units per mg.

Storage/Stability/Compatibility - Nystatin tablets and oral suspension should be stored at room
temperature (15-30°C) in tight, light-resistant containers. Avoid freezing the oral suspension or
exposing to temperatures greater than 40°C.

Nystatin deteriorates when exposed to heat, light, air or moisture.

Pharmacology - Nystatin has a mechanism of action similar to that of amphotericin B. It binds
to sterols in the membrane of the fungal cell where it alters the permeability of the membrane allowing intracellular potassium and other cellular constituents to "leak out".

Nystatin has activity against a variety of fungal organisms, but is clinically used against topical,
oropharyngeal and gastrointestinal *Candida* infections.

Uses/Indications - Nystatin is used orally primarily for the treatment of oral or gastrointestinal
tract *Candida* infections in dogs, cats and birds. It has also been used in other species for the
same indications, but less commonly.

Nystatin is also used for the topical treatment of Candidal (Monilial) skin infections. It is a
principal ingredient in the well-known proprietary product, *Panolog®*.

Pharmacokinetics - Nystatin is not measurably absorbed after oral administration and is almost
entirely excreted unchanged in the feces. The drug is not used parenterally because it is reportedly extremely toxic to internal tissues.

Contraindications/Precautions/Reproductive Safety - Nystatin is contraindicated in patients
with known hypersensitivity to it.

Although the safety of the drug during pregnancy has not been firmly established, the lack of
appreciable absorption or case reports associating the drug with teratogenic effects appear to
make it safe to use.

Adverse Effects/Warnings - Occasionally, nystatin may cause GI upset (anorexia, vomiting, diarrhea) when administered in high dosages. Rarely, hypersensitivity reactions have been reported
in humans.

Overdosage/Acute Toxicity - Because the drug is not absorbed after oral administration, acute
toxicity after an oral overdose is extremely unlikely, but transient GI distress may result.

Drug Interactions - The veterinary-approved product for chickens and turkeys (*Myco-20®*—
Solvay) should not be administered with **tetracycline** products. It has a high calcium content in
its vehicle that may prevent oral absorption of tetracycline.

Doses -
　Dogs:
　　For oral treatment of Candidal infections:
　　　a)　100,000 Units PO q6h (Kirk 1989)
　　　b)　50,000 - 150,000 Units PO q8h (Jenkins and Boothe 1987)
　　　c)　22,000 Units/kg/day (Huber 1988b)
　Cats:
　　For oral treatment of Candidal infections:
　　　a)　100,000 Units PO q6h (Kirk 1989)
　Birds:
　　For crop mycosis and mycotic diarrhea (*Candida albicans*) in chickens and turkeys:
　　　a)　Feed at 50 grams per ton (*Mycostatin®-20*) or at 100 g/ton for 7-10 days. (Label directions; *Mycostatin®-20*—Solvay)
　　For oropharyngeal Candidal infections:
　　　a)　In caged birds: 300,000 Units/kg PO via crop tube or directly into mouth *bid* for 7-10 days. Flocks may be treated using the veterinary product (*Myco-20®*) at 5 grams of Myco-20 per pound of food. Add to either a cooked mash or other food. (Flammer 1986)
　　　b)　For treatment of candidiasis after antibiotic or in conjunction with antibiotics: One ml of the 100,000 U/ml suspension per 300 g body weight PO once, twice or 3 times daily for 7-14 days. If treating mouth lesions do not give by gavage. Hand-fed babies should receive antifungal therapy if being treated with antibiotics. (Clubb 1986)
　Reptiles:
　　For susceptible infections:
　　　a)　For turtles with enteric yeast infections: 100,000 IU/kg PO once daily for 10 days. (Gauvin 1993)
Monitoring Parameters -
　1)　Clinical efficacy
Client Information - Shake suspension well before administering.
Dosage Forms/Preparations/FDA Approval Status/Withholding Times -
　Veterinary-Approved Products: None
　Human-Approved Products:
　　Nystatin Oral Suspension 100,000 Units/ml in 5, 60, 473　and 480 ml bottles; *Nilstat®* (Lederle); *Mycostatin®* (Apothecon); *Nystex®* (Savage); generic; (Rx)

　　Nystatin Bulk Powder: 50, 150, 500 million units, 1, 2 & 5 billion units; *Nystatin®* (Paddock); *Nilstat®* (Lederle); (Rx)

　　Nystatin Oral Tablets 500,000 Units; *Nilstat®* (Lederle); *Mycostatin®* (Apothecon); generic; (Rx)

　　Also available in oral troches, vaginal tablets, topical creams, powders and ointments

o,p- DDD **- see Mitotane**

OMEPRAZOLE

Chemistry - A substituted benzimidazole proton pump inhibitor, omeprazole has a molecular weight of 345.4 and pK_a's of 4 and 8.8.

Storage/Stability/Compatibility - Omeprazole tablets should be stored at room temperature in light-resistant, tight containers. Omeprazole pellets found in the capsules are fragile and should not be crushed. If needed to administer as a slurry, it has been suggested to mix the pellets carefully with fruit juices and not water, milk or saline.

Pharmacology - A representative of a new class of agent, the substituted benzimidazoles, omeprazole is a gastric acid (proton) pump inhibitor. In an acidic environment, omeprazole is activated to a sulphenamide derivative that binds irreversibly at the secretory surface of parietal cells to the enzyme, H^+/K^+ ATPase. There it inhibits the transport of hydrogen ions into the stomach. Omeprazole inhibits acid secretion during both basal and stimulated conditions. Omeprazole also inhibits the hepatic cytochrome P-450 mixed function oxidase system (see Drug Interactions below).

Uses/Indications - Omeprazole is potentially useful in treating both gastroduodenal ulcer disease and to prevent or treat gastric erosions caused by ulcerogenic drugs (*e.g.*, aspirin). Because of the drugs recent availability and high cost, experience is limited in domestic animals.

Pharmacokinetics - Omeprazole is rapidly absorbed from the gut; the commercial product is in an enteric coated granule form as the drug is rapidly degraded by acid. Peak serum levels occur within 0.5 to 3.5 hours and onset of action within 1 hour. Omeprazole is distributed widely, but primarily in gastric parietal cells. In humans, approximately 95% is bound to albumin and alpha$_1$-acid glycoprotein. It is unknown whether omeprazole enters maternal milk.

Omeprazole is extensively metabolized in the liver to at least six different metabolites, these are excreted principally in the urine, but also via the bile into feces. Significant hepatic dysfunction will reduce the first pass effect of the drug. In humans with normal hepatic function, serum half life averages about 1 hour, but the duration of therapeutic effect may persist for 72 hours or more.

Contraindications/Precautions/Reproductive Safety - Omeprazole is contraindicated in patients hypersensitive to it. Omeprazole should be used when the benefits outweigh the risks in patients with hepatic disease or a history of hepatic disease, as the drug's half life may be prolonged and dosage adjustment may be necessary.

Omeprazole's safety during pregnancy has not been established, but a study done in rats at doses of up to 345 times those recommended did not demonstrate any teratogenic effects. Increased embryo-lethality has been noted in lab animals at very high dosages. It is unknown whether omeprazole is excreted in milk.

Adverse Effects/Warnings - While veterinary use is quite limited, the drug appears to be quite well tolerated in both dogs and cats at effective dosages. Potentially, GI distress (anorexia, colic, nausea, vomiting, flatulence, diarrhea) could occur as well as hematologic abnormalities (rare in humans), urinary tract infections, proteinuria, or CNS disturbances. Chronic very high doses in rats caused enterochromaffin-like cell hyperplasia and gastric carcinoid tumors; effects occurred in dose related manner. The clinical significance of these findings for long term low-dose clinical usage is not known. However, at the current time in humans, dosing for longer than 8 weeks is rarely recommended unless the benefits of therapy outweigh the potential risks.

Overdosage/Acute Toxicity - The LD$_{50}$ in rats after oral administration is reportedly >4 g/kg. Humans have tolerated oral dosages of 360 mg/day without significant toxicity. Should a massive overdose occur, treat symptomatically and supportively.

Drug Interactions - Because omeprazole can inhibit the cytochrome P-450 enzyme system, omeprazole may decrease the hepatic clearance of **diazepam, phenytoin or warfarin**, thereby enhancing their effects and causing potential toxicity. Additional monitoring and dosage adjustments may be required.

Because omeprazole can increase gastric pH, drugs that require low gastric pH for optimal absorption (*e.g.*, **ketoconazole, ampicillin esters or iron salts**) may have their absorption reduced. Although omeprazole causes bone marrow depression only rarely in humans, use with **other drugs that cause bone marrow depression** may lead to additive hematologic abnormalities.

Laboratory Considerations - Omeprazole may cause **increased liver enzymes.** Omeprazole will increase **serum gastrin levels** early in therapy.

Doses -
  Dogs:
    For ulcer management:
      a) 0.5 - 1 mg/kg PO once daily (Davenport 1992)
      b) 20 mg (total dose) once daily (Papich 1992)
      c) For severe ulceration unresponsive to H$_2$ blockers; severe esophagitis unresponsive to metoclopramide and H$_2$ blockers; gastrinoma (Zollinger-Ellison syndrome): 0.75 - 1 mg/kg PO once daily (q24h) - or - one 20 mg capsule for animals > 20 kg, 10 mg (1/2 capsule) for animals weighing >5 kg < 20 kg, 5 mg (1/4 capsule for animals weighing < 5 kg. When using less than a full capsule, repackage granules in a gelatin capsule to avoid gastric acid degradation. (Johnson, Sherding et al. 1994)
      d) 0.7 mg/kg (>20 kg, 20 mg/dog; <20 kg, 10 mg/dog) PO once daily (Matz 1995)
      e) For dogs less than 20 kg: 0.7 mg/kg PO once a day; for dogs > 20 kg: 20 mg PO once a day (Johnson 1996)
  Cats:
    For ulcer management:
      a) For cats: 0.7 mg/kg PO once a day (Johnson 1996)
  Horses:
    For ulcer management:
      a) 0.7 - 1.4 mg/kg PO once daily. While dosage has not been firmly established, these dosages have been shown to suppress gastric acid output for up to 24 hours. Use should probably be limited to those cases where the client prefers once a day only dosing. (Geor 1992)

Monitoring Parameters - 1) Efficacy; 2) Adverse Effects

Client Information - Brief client on drug's cost before prescribing. Give before meals, preferably in the morning.

Dosage Forms/Preparations/FDA Approval Status/Withholding Times -

Veterinary-Approved Products: None

Human-Approved Products:

Omeprazole Oral Sustained Release 10 mg & 20 mg Capsules; *Prilosec*® (*Losec*® in Canada); (Astra Merck); (Rx)

OPIATE ANTIDIARRHEALS
PAREGORIC
DIPHENOXALATE HCL/ATROPINE SULFATE
LOPERAMIDE HCL

Chemistry - Paregoric, also known as camphorated tincture of opium, contains 2 mg of anhydrous morphine (usually as powdered opium or opium tincture). Also included (per 5 ml) is 0.02 ml anise oil, 0.2 ml glycerin, 20 mg benzoic acid, 20 mg camphor and a sufficient quantity of diluted alcohol to make a total of 5 ml. Paregoric should not be confused with opium tincture (tincture of opium), which contains 50 mg or anhydrous morphine per 5 ml.

Structurally related to meperidine, diphenoxylate HCl is a synthetic phenylpiperidine-derivative opiate agonist. It occurs as an odorless, white, crystalline powder that is slightly soluble in water and sparingly soluble in alcohol. Commercially available preparations also contain a small amount of atropine sulfate to discourage the abuse of the drug for its narcotic effects. At therapeutic doses the atropine has no clinical effect.

A synthetic piperidine-derivative antidiarrheal, loperamide occurs as a white to faintly yellow, powder with a pK_a of 8.6 that is soluble in alcohol and slightly soluble in water.

Storage/Stability/Compatibility - Paregoric should be stored in tight, light-resistant containers. Avoid exposure to excessive heat or direct exposure to sunlight.

Diphenoxalate/atropine tablets should be stored at room temperature in well-closed, light-resistant containers. Diphenoxalate/atropine oral solution should be stored at room temperature in tight, light-resistant containers; avoid freezing.

Loperamide capsules or oral solution should be stored at room temperature in well-closed containers. It is recommended that the oral solution not be diluted with other solvents.

Pharmacology - Among their other actions, opiates inhibit GI motility and excessive GI propulsion. They also decrease intestinal secretion induced by cholera toxin, prostaglandin E_2 and diarrheas caused by factors in which calcium is the second messenger (non-cyclic AMP/GMP mediated). Opiates may also enhance mucosal absorption.

Uses/Indications - The opiate antidiarrheal products are generally considered to be the motility modifiers of choice in dogs with diarrhea. Their use in cats is controversial and many clinicians do not recommend their use in this species. Paregoric has also been used in large animals (see Doses below).

Pharmacokinetics - The morphine in paregoric is absorbed in a variable fashion from the GI tract. It is rapidly metabolized in the liver and serum morphine levels are considerably less than when morphine is administered parenterally.

In humans, diphenoxylate is rapidly absorbed after administration of either the tablets or oral solution. The bioavailability of the tablets is approximately 90% that of the solution, however. Generally, onset of action occurs within 45 minutes to one hour after dosing and is sustained for 3-4 hours. Diphenoxylate is found in maternal milk. Diphenoxylate is metabolized into diphenoxylic acid, an active metabolite. The serum half-lives of diphenoxylate and diphenoxylic acid, are approximately 2.5 hours and 3-14 hours respectively.

In dogs, loperamide reportedly has a faster onset of action and longer duration of action than diphenoxylate, but clinical studies confirming this appear to be lacking. In humans, loperamide's half-life is about 11 hours. It is unknown if the drug enters milk or crosses the placenta.

Contraindications/Precautions - All opiates should be used with caution in patients with hypothyroidism, severe renal insufficiency, adrenocortical insufficiency (Addison's) and in geriatric or severely debilitated patients. Opiate antidiarrheals are contraindicated in cases where the patient is hypersensitive to narcotic analgesics and in patients taking monoamine oxidase inhibitors (MAOIs). They are also contraindicated in patients with diarrhea caused by a toxic ingestion until the toxin is eliminated from the GI tract.

Opiate antidiarrheals should be used with caution in patients with head injuries or increased intracranial pressure and acute abdominal conditions (*e.g.,* colic) as it may obscure the diagnosis or clinical course of these conditions. It should be used with extreme caution in patients suffering from respiratory disease or from acute respiratory dysfunction (*e.g.,* pulmonary edema secondary to smoke inhalation). Opiate antidiarrheals should be used with extreme caution in patients with hepatic disease with CNS symptoms of hepatic encephalopathy. Hepatic coma may result.

Many clinicians recommend not using diphenoxylate or loperamide in dogs weighing less than 10 kg, but this is probably a result of the potency of the tablet or capsule forms of the drugs. Dosage titration using the liquid forms of these agents should allow their safe use in dogs when indicated.

Adverse Effects/Warnings - In dogs, constipation, bloat and sedation are the most likely adverse reactions encountered when usual doses are used. Potentially, paralytic ileus, toxic megacolon, pancreatitis and CNS effects could be seen.

Use of antidiarrheal opiates in cats is controversial; this species may react with excitatory behavior.

Opiates used in horses with acute diarrhea (or in any animal with a potentially bacterial-induced diarrhea) may have a detrimental effect. Opiates may enhance bacterial proliferation, delay the disappearance of the microbe from the feces and prolong the febrile state.

Overdosage - Acute overdosage of the opiate antidiarrheals could result in CNS, cardiovascular, GI or respiratory toxicity. Because the opiates may significantly reduce GI motility, absorption from the GI may be delayed and prolonged. For more information, refer to the meperidine and morphine monographs found in the CNS section. Naloxone may be necessary to reverse the opiate effects.

Massive overdoses of diphenoxylate/atropine sulfate may also induce atropine toxicity. Refer to the atropine monograph for more information.

Drug Interactions - Other **CNS depressants** (*e.g.,* anesthetic agents, antihistamines, phenothiazines, barbiturates, tranquilizers, alcohol, etc.) may cause increased CNS or respiratory depression when used with opiate antidiarrheal agents.

Opiate antidiarrheal agents are contraindicated in patients receiving **monoamine oxidase (MOA) inhibitors** (rarely used in veterinary medicine) for at least 14 days after receiving MOA inhibitors in humans.

Drug/Laboratory Interactions - Plasma **amylase** and **lipase** values may be increased for up to 24 hours following administration of opiates.

Doses -
  Dogs:
    Paregoric:
      a) For acute colitis: 0.06 mg/kg PO *tid* (DeNovo 1988)
      b) For maldigestion/malabsorption/antidiarrheal: 0.05 - 0.06 mg/kg PO *bid-tid* (Chiapella 1988), (Johnson 1984)
      c) As an antidiarrheal: 2 - 15 ml PO q6h (Davis 1985a)

    Diphenoxylate/Atropine:
      a) For acute colitis/irritable colon syndrome: 0.1 mg/kg PO *tid* (DeNovo 1988)
      b) As an antidiarrheal: 0.05 - 0.1 mg/kg *qid* PO; (not recommended for dogs weighing less than 10 kg) (Johnson 1984)
      c) As an antidiarrheal: 0.1 - 0.2 mg/kg PO q8h (Jergens 1995)

    Loperamide:
      a) For acute colitis: 0.08 mg/kg PO *tid* (DeNovo 1988)
      b) For maldigestion/malabsorption: 0.08 mg/kg PO *qid* (Chiapella 1988)
      c) As an antidiarrheal: 1 capsule (2 mg) per 25 kg body weight *qid* PO; (not recommended for dogs weighing less than 10 kg) (Johnson 1984)
      d) As an antidiarrheal: 0.1 - 0.2 mg/kg PO q8h (Jergens 1995)

  Cats: Note: Use of antidiarrheal opiates in cats is controversial; this species may react with excitatory behavior.
    Paregoric:
      a) For maldigestion/malabsorption/antidiarrheal: 0.05 - 0.06 mg/kg PO *bid-tid* (Chiapella 1988), (Johnson 1984)

    Diphenoxylate/Atropine:
      a) 0.063 mg/kg PO q8h (Davis 1985b)

  Cattle:
    Paregoric:
      a) Calves: 15 - 30 ml PO (Cornell 1985)

  Horses:
    Paregoric:
      a) Foals: 15 - 30 ml PO; Adults: 15 - 60 ml PO (Cornell 1985)

Monitoring Parameters -
1) Clinical efficacy
2) Fluid & electrolyte status in severe diarrhea
3) CNS effects if using high dosages

Client Information - If diarrhea persists, contact veterinarian. If animal appears listless or develops a high fever, contact veterinarian.

Dosage Forms/Preparations/FDA Approval Status/Withholding Times -
Veterinary-Approved Products: None
Human-Approved Products:

Paregoric (camphorated tincture of opium) 2 mg of morphine equiv. per 5 ml; 45% alcohol. Available in 60 ml, pints, and gallons & UD 5 ml; Generic; (Rx; Class-III controlled substance)

Diphenoxylate HCl 2.5 mg with 0.025 mg Atropine Sulfate Tablets (Class-V controlled substance; prescription only); *Logen*® (Goldline); *Lomotil*® (Searle); *Lonox*® (Geneva); Generic; (C-V)

Diphenoxylate HCl 2.5 mg with 0.025 mg Atropine Sulfate per 5 ml Oral Liquid in 60 ml dropper bottles, UD 4 & 10 ml. (Class-V controlled substance; prescription only). There are many trade names for this combination, included are: *Lomotil*® (Searle), *Lonox*® (Geneva), *Diphenatol*® (Rugby); *Lofene*® (Lannett), *Logen*® (Goldline), Generic

Loperamide HCl 1 mg/5 ml (0.2 mg/ml) & 1 mg/ml Oral Liquid; *Imodium*® A-D (McNeil-CPC); *Pepto Diarrhea Control*® (Procter & Gamble); generic (OTC)

Loperamide HCl 2 mg Capsules & Tablets; *Imodium* ® (Janssen) (OTC); *Kaopectate II Caplets*® (Upjohn) (OTC); *Maalox Anti-Diarrheal Caplets*® (R-P Rorer); *Imodium A-D Caplets*® (McNeil-CPC) (OTC); *Neo-Diaral*® (Roberts) (OTC); generic (OTC)

ORBIFLOXACIN

Chemistry/Storage/Stability/Compatibility - A 4-fluroquinolone antibiotic, orbifloxacin is slightly soluble in water at neutral pH. Solubility increases in either an acidic or basic medium. The commercially available tablets should be stored between 2-30°C (36-86°F) and protected from excessive moisture.

Pharmacology - Orbifloxacin is a concentration-dependent bactericidal agent. It acts by inhibiting bacterial DNA-gyrase (a type-II topoisomerase), thereby preventing DNA supercoiling and DNA synthesis. The net result is disruption of bacterial cell replication.

Orbifloxacin has good activity against many gram negative and gram positive bacilli and cocci, including most species and strains of *Klebsiella spp., Staphylococcus intermedius* or *aureus, E. coli, Enterobacter, Campylobacter, Shigella, Proteus, Pasturella* species. Some strains of *Pseudomonas aeruginosa* and *Pseudomonas species* are resistant and most *Enterococcus spp.* are resistant. Like other fluroquinolones, orbifloxacin has weak activity against most anaerobes and is not a good choice when treating known or suspected anaerobic infections.

Development of bacterial resistance to 4-fluroquinolones can occur.

Uses/Indications - Orbifloxacin is indicated for treatment in dogs and cats for bacterial infections susceptible to it.

Pharmacokinetics - After oral administration in dogs or cats, orbifloxacin is apparently nearly completely absorbed. The drug is well distributed (V_d=1.4 L/kg in dogs and 1.4 L/kg in cats) and only bound slight to plasma proteins (8% dogs; 15% cats). Orbifloxacin is eliminated primarily by the kidneys. Approximately 50% of the drug is excreted unchanged. Serum half lives are about 6 hours in both dogs and cats. Urine levels remain well above MIC's for susceptible organisms for at least 24 hours after dosing.

Contraindications/Precautions/Reproductive Safety - Orbifloxacin, like other fluroquinolones can cause arthropathies in immature, growing animals. Because dogs appear to be more sensitive to this effect, the manufacturer states that the drug is contraindicated in immature dogs during the rapid growth phase (between 2-8 months in small and medium-sized breeds and up to 18 months in large and giant breeds). The drug is also contraindicated in dogs and cats known to be hypersensitive to orbifloxacin or other drugs in its class (quinolones).

The manufacturer states that orbifloxacin should be used with caution in animals with known or suspected CNS disorders (e.g., seizure disorders) as rarely, drugs in this class have been associated with CNS stimulation.

Safety in breeding or pregnant dogs or cats has not been established. It is not known whether orbifloxacin enters maternal milk.

Adverse Effects/Warnings - While the manufacturer reports that no adverse effects were reported during clinical studies (at 2.5. mg/kg dosing) in adult animals, higher doses or additional experience with use of the drug may demonstrate additional adverse effects. Gastrointestinal effects (anorexia, vomiting, diarrhea) would most likely be the first adverse effects noted.

Overdosage - Dogs and cats receiving up to 5X (37.5mg/kg) for 30 days did not result in any significant adverse effects. Cats receiving the higher dosages exhibited soft feces and decreased body weight gains.

Drug Interactions - Antacids or other agents containing divalent or trivalent cations (Mg^{++}, Al^{+++}, Ca^{++}) may bind to orbifloxacin and prevent its absorption. **Sucralfate** may inhibit absorption of orbifloxacin; separate doses of these drugs by at least 2 hours.

Orbifloxacin administered with **theophylline** may increase theophylline blood levels.

Probenecid may block the tubular secretion of orbifloxacin and may increase its blood level and half-life.

Synergism may occur, but is not predictable, against some bacteria (particularly *Pseudomonas aeruginosa* or other Enterobacteriaceae) with these compounds and **aminoglycosides, 3rd generation cephalosporins agents, and extended-spectrum penicillins**. Although orbifloxacin apparently has minimal activity against anaerobes, *in vitro* synergy has been reported when other fluroquinolones have been used with **clindamycin** against strains of *Peptostreptococcus*, *Lactobacillus* and *Bacteroids fragilis*. **Nitrofurantoin** may antagonize the antimicrobial activity of the fluroquinolones and their concomitant use is not recommended. Fluroquinolones may exacerbate the nephrotoxicity of **cyclosporine** (used systemically).

Doses -

Dogs/Cats: For susceptible infections:

    a) 2.5 mg/kg - 7.5 mg/kg once daily PO. Higher end of the dosing range may be necessary in hospitalized patients, those with underlying disease (e.g., malignancy) or structural alterations (e.g. burns, complicated urinary tract infections, foreign body infections), infections associated with vascular compromise and infections caused by "problem" pathogens. (Package Insert—Orbax®)

Monitoring Parameters/Client Information - Efficacy is the most important monitoring parameter; clients should be instructed on the importance of giving the medication as instructed and not to discontinue it on their own.

Dosage Forms/Preparations/FDA Approval Status -

  Human-Approved Products: None

  Veterinary-Approved Products:

    Orbifloxacin Oral Tablets: 5.7 mg (yellow) in btls of 250; 22.7 mg (green; E-Z Break) in btls of 250; 68 mg (blue; E-Z Break) in btls of 100; *Orbax*® (Schering-Plough Animal Health); (Rx). Approved for use in dogs and cats. Federal law prohibits the use of the drug in food-producing animals.

Ormetoprim - see Sulfadimethoxine/Ormetoprim

OXACILLIN SODIUM

For general information on the penicillins, including adverse effects, contraindications, overdosage, drug interactions and monitoring parameters, refer to the monograph: Penicillins, General Information.

Chemistry - An isoxazolyl-penicillin, oxacillin sodium is a semisynthetic penicillinase-resistant penicillin. It is available commercially as the monohydrate sodium salt which occurs as a fine, white, crystalline powder that is odorless or has a slight odor. It is freely soluble in water and has a pK_a of about 2.8. One mg of oxacillin sodium contains not less than 815-950 micrograms of oxacillin. Each gram of the commercially available powder for injection contains 2.8 -3.1 mEq of sodium.

Oxacillin sodium may also be known as sodium oxacillin or methylphenyl isoxazolyl penicillin.

Storage/Stability/Compatibility - Oxacillin sodium capsules, powder for oral solution, and powder for injection should be stored at room temperature (15-30°C) in tight containers. After reconstituting with water, refrigerated and discard any remaining oral solution after 14 days. If kept at room temperature, the oral solution is stable for 3 days.

After reconstituting the sterile powder for injection with sterile water for injection or sterile sodium chloride 0.9%, the resultant solution with a concentration of 167 mg/ml is stable for 3 days at room temperature or 7 days if refrigerated. The manufacturer recommends using different quantities of diluent depending on whether the drug is to be administered IM, IV directly, or IV (piggyback). Refer to the package insert for specific instructions.

Oxacillin sodium injection is reportedly **compatible** with the following fluids/drugs: dextrose 5% & 10% in water, dextrose 5% & 10% in sodium chloride 0.9%, lactated Ringer's injection, sodium chloride 0.9% amikacin sulfate, cephapirin sodium, choramphenicol sodium succinate, dopamine HCl, potassium chloride, sodium bicarbonate and verapamil.

Oxacillin sodium injection is reportedly **incompatible** with the following fluids/drugs: oxytetracycline HCl and tetracycline HCl. Compatibility is dependent upon factors such as pH, concentration, temperature and diluents used. It is suggested to consult specialized references for more specific information (*e.g., Handbook on Injectable Drugs* by Trissel; see bibliography).

Pharmacology/Uses/Indications - Refer to the Cloxacillin monograph and the Doses section for Oxacillin for more information regarding this drug.

Pharmacokinetics (specific) - Oxacillin sodium is resistant to acid inactivation in the gut, but is only partially absorbed after oral administration. The bioavailability after oral administration in humans has been reported to range from 30-35%, and, if given with food, both the rate and extent of absorption is decreased. After IM administration, oxacillin is rapidly absorbed and peak levels generally occur within 30 minutes.

The drug is distributed to the lungs, kidneys, bone, bile, pleural fluid, synovial fluid and ascitic fluid. The volume of distribution is reportedly 0.4 L/kg in human adults and 0.3 L/kg in dogs. As with the other penicillins, only minimal amounts are distributed into the CSF, but levels are increased with meningeal inflammation. In humans, approximately 89-94% of the drug is bound to plasma proteins.

Oxacillin is partially metabolized to both active and inactive metabolites. These metabolites and the parent compound are rapidly excreted in the urine via both glomerular filtration and tubular secretion mechanisms. A small amount of the drug is also excreted in the feces via biliary elimination. The serum half-life in humans with normal renal function ranges from about 18-48 minutes. In dogs, 20-30 minutes has been reported as the elimination half-life.

Doses -
  Dogs:
    For susceptible infections:
      a) 22 - 40 mg/kg PO q8h (Vaden and Papich 1995)
      b) 5.5 - 11 mg/kg IV q8h; 27.5 - 33 mg/kg PO q8h (Aronson and Aucoin 1989)
      c) For *Staph.* infections: 10 - 20 mg/kg PO, IV, or IM *qid* (Morgan 1988)
      d) For penicillinase-producing *Staph.* endocarditis: 50 - 60 mg/kg *tid* for 4-6 weeks (route not indicated). (Sisson and Thomas 1986)
      e) For canine pyoderma: 22 mg/kg PO q8h (Ihrke 1986)
      f) For systemic therapy for *Staph.* blepharitis: 22 mg/kg PO *tid* (Laratta 1986)
      g) 7 mg/kg IM q8h; 8 -15 mg/kg PO q8h (Ford and Aronson 1985)
      h) 10 - 22 mg/kg q6-8h PO; 7 - 25 mg/kg IV or IM q4-6h (Greene 1984)
  Cats:
    For susceptible infections:
      a) 22 - 40 mg/kg PO q8h (Vaden and Papich 1995)
      b) 5.5 - 11 mg/kg IV q8h; 27.5 - 33 mg/kg PO q8h (Aronson and Aucoin 1989)
      c) For *Staph.* infections: 10 - 20 mg/kg PO, IV, or IM *qid* (Morgan 1988)
      d) 7 mg/kg IM q8h; 8 -15 mg/kg PO q8h (Ford and Aronson 1985)
      e) 10 - 22 mg/kg q6-8h PO; 7 - 25 mg/kg IV or IM q4-6h (Greene 1984)
  Horses:
    For susceptible infections:
      a) Foals: 20 - 30 mg/kg IV q6-8h (Dose extrapolated from adult horse data; use lower dose or longer interval in premature foals or those less than 7 days old.) (Caprile and Short 1987)
      b) 25 - 50 mg/kg IM, IV *bid* (Robinson 1987)

Client Information - Unless otherwise instructed by the veterinarian, this drug should be given on an empty stomach, at least 1 hour before feeding or 2 hours after. Keep oral solution in the refrigerator and discard any unused suspension after 14 days.

Dosage Forms/Preparations/FDA Approval Status -
  Veterinary-Approved Products: None
  Human-Approved Products:
    Oxacillin Sodium Capsules 250 mg, 500 mg; *Prostaphlin*® (Apothecon) (Rx), *Bactocill*® (Beecham); (Rx); generic, (Rx)

    Oxacillin Sodium Powder for Oral Solution 250 mg/5 ml in 100 ml bottles; *Prostaphlin*® (Apothecon); (Rx)

Oxacillin Sodium Powder for Injection 250 mg vials, 500 mg vials, 1 g, 2 g, & 4 g vials; 1 g & 2 g piggyback vials, 4 g and 10 g bulk vials; *Prostaphlin*® (Apothecon) (Rx); *Bactocill*® (S-K Beecham); (Rx); Oxacillin Sodium® (Apothecon) (Rx)

OXAZEPAM

Chemistry - A benzodiazepine, oxazepam occurs as a creamy white to pale yellow powder. It is practically insoluble in water.

Storage/Stability/Compatibility - Store oxazepam capsules and tablets at room temperature in well-closed containers.

Pharmacology - The subcortical levels (primarily limbic, thalamic, and hypothalamic) of the CNS are depressed by oxazepam and other benzodiazepines thus producing the anxiolytic, sedative, skeletal muscle relaxant and anticonvulsant effects seen. The exact mechanism of action is unknown, but postulated mechanisms include: antagonism of serotonin, increased release of and/or facilitation of gamma-aminobutyric acid (GABA) activity, and diminished release or turnover of acetylcholine in the CNS. Benzodiazepine specific receptors have been located in the mammalian brain, kidney, liver, lung, and heart. In all species studied, receptors are lacking in the white matter.

Uses/Indications - Oxazepam is used most frequently in small animal medicine as an appetite stimulant in cats and dogs. It may also be useful as an oral anxiolytic agent for adjunctive therapy of anxiety-related disorders.

Pharmacokinetics - Oxazepam is absorbed from the GI tract, but it is one the more slowly absorbed oral benzodiazepines. Oxazepam. like other benzodiazepines is widely distributed; it is highly bound to plasma proteins (97% in humans). While not confirmed, oxazepam may cross the placenta and enter maternal milk. Oxazepam is principally conjugated in the liver via glucuronidation to an inactive metabolite. Serum half-life in humans range from 3-21 hours.

Contraindications/Precautions/Reproductive Safety - Oxazepam is contraindicated in patients who are hypersensitive to it or other benzodiazepines or have acute narrow angle glaucoma. Benzodiazepines have been reported to exacerbate myasthenia gravis. While oxazepam is less susceptible to accumulation than many other benzodiazepines in patients with hepatic dysfunction, it should be used with caution nonetheless. Rarely, oxazepam has reportedly precipitated tonic-clonic seizures, it should be used with caution in susceptible patients.

Safe use during pregnancy has not been established; teratogenic effects of similar benzodiazepines have been noted in rabbits and rats. It is not known if the drug enters maternal milk.

Adverse Effects/Warnings - The most prevalent adverse effects seen with oxazepam in small animals is sedation and occasionally, ataxia. These may be transient and dosage adjustment may be required to alleviate. For more information on less likely occurring adverse effects with benzodiazepines, see the diazepam monograph.

Overdosage/Acute Toxicity - When used alone, oxazepam overdoses are generally limited to significant CNS depression (confusion, coma, decreased reflexes, etc.). Treatment of significant overdoses consist of standard protocols for removing and/or binding the drug in the gut if taken orally, and supportive systemic measures. The use of analeptic agents (CNS stimulants such as caffeine, amphetamines, etc) are generally not recommended.

Drug Interactions - Metabolism of oxazepam may be decreased and excessive sedation may occur if given with the following drugs: **cimetidine, erythromycin, isoniazid, ketoconazole, propranolol, & valproic acid**. This interaction is less likely to occur with oxazepam, than other benzodiazepines (*e.g.*, diazepam) because oxazepam undergoes glucuronide conjugation. **Probenecid** however, may impair the glucuronide conjugation of oxazepam.

If administered with other **CNS depressant agents (barbiturates, narcotics, anesthetics**, etc.) additive CNS depressant effects may occur.

Laboratory Considerations - Benzodiazepines may decrease the thyroidal uptake of I^{123} or I^{131}.

Doses -
  Cats:
    As an appetite stimulant:
      a) 2 mg per cat (total dose) every 12 hours. (Hartke, Rojko et al. 1992), (Hodgkins and Franks 1991)

Monitoring Parameters - Efficacy and adverse effects

Client Information - Caution clients not to discontinue medication or adjust dosage without first checking with veterinarian. Efficacy may be improved if given just prior to feeding as effects are generally seen within 30 minutes..

Dosage Forms/Preparations/FDA Approval Status/Withholding Times -
Veterinary-Approved Products: None
Human-Approved Products:

Oxazepam Oral Capsules 10 mg, 15 mg, 30 mg; *Serax*® (Wyeth-Ayerst), Generic; (Rx)

Oxazepam Oral Tablets 15 mg; *Serax*® (Wyeth-Ayerst), Generic; (Rx)

All oxazepam products are C-IV controlled substances in the USA.

OXFENDAZOLE

Chemistry - A benzimidazole anthelmintic, oxfendazole occurs as white or almost white powder possessing a characteristic odor. It is practically insoluble in water. Oxfendazole is the sulfoxide metabolite of fenbendazole.

Storage/Stability/Compatibility - Unless otherwise directed by the manufacturer, oxfendazole products should be stored at room temperature and protected from light. The manufacturer recommends discarding any unused suspension 24 hours after it has been reconstituted.

Uses/Indications - Oxfendazole is indicated (labeled) for the removal of the following parasites in **horses**: large roundworms (*Parascaris equorum*), large strongyles (*S. edentatus, S. equinus, S. vulgaris*), small strongyles and pinworms (*Oxyuris equi*).

Oxfendazole has also been used in cattle, sheep, goats, and swine; see Dosage section for more information.

Pharmacokinetics - Limited information is available regarding this compound's pharmacokinetics. Unlike most of the other benzimidazole compounds, oxfendazole is absorbed more readily from the GI tract. The elimination half-life has been reported to be about 7.5 hours in sheep and 5.25 hours in goats. Absorbed oxfendazole is metabolized (and vice-versa) to the active compound, fenbendazole (sulfoxide) and the sulfone.

Contraindications/Precautions - There are no contraindications to using this drug in horses, but it is recommended to use oxfendazole cautiously in debilitated or sick horses. Oxfendazole may be safely used in pregnant mares and foals.

Adverse Effects/Warnings - When used as labeled, it is unlikely any adverse effects will be noted. Hypersensitivity reactions secondary to antigen release by dying parasites are theoretically possible, particularly at high dosages.

Overdosage/Toxicity - Doses of 10 times those recommended elicited no adverse reactions in horses tested. It is unlikely that this compound would cause serious toxicity when given alone.

Drug Interactions - Oxfendazole or fenbendazole should not be given concurrently with the **bromsalan flukicides (Dibromsalan, Tribromsalan)**. Abortions in cattle and death in sheep have been reported after using these compounds together.

Doses -
Horses:

For susceptible parasites: 10 mg/kg PO. (Package insert; Benzelmin®—Syntex), (Roberson 1988b)

Cattle:
For susceptible parasites:
    a) 4.5 mg/kg PO. (Roberson 1988b)
    b) 5 mg/kg PO. (Brander, Pugh, and Bywater 1982)

Swine:
For susceptible parasites: 3 - 4.5 mg/kg PO. (Roberson 1988b)

Sheep:
For susceptible parasites: 5 mg/kg PO. (Roberson 1988b), (Brander, Pugh, and Bywater 1982)

Goats:
For susceptible parasites: 7.5 mg/kg PO. (Roberson 1988b)

Monitoring Parameters - Efficacy

Client Information - Not to be used in horses intended for food purposes.

Dosage Forms/Preparations/FDA Approval Status -
Veterinary-Approved Products: None

Oxfendazole Powder for Suspension 75.6 mg/gram in 30 gram packets and 300 gram bulk powder.

    Benzelmin® (Fort Dodge); (Rx) Approved for use in horses.

Oxfendazole Suspension 90.6 mg/ml in 1 liter bottles.

    Benzelmin® (Fort Dodge); (Rx) Approved for use in horses. Shake well before using.

Oxfendazole Oral Paste 375 mg/gram in 12 g and 72 g syringes. *Benzelmin®* *Paste* (Fort Dodge); (OTC) Approved for use in horses.

Oxfendazole may be known in the U.K. by the proprietary names: *Synanthic®* (Syntex) or *Systamex®* (Coopers).

Human-Approved Products: None

OXIBENDAZOLE

Chemistry - A benzimidazole anthelmintic, oxibendazole occurs as a white powder that is practically insoluble in water.

Storage/Stability/Compatibility - Unless otherwise directed by the manufacturer, oxibendazole products should be stored at room temperature; protect from freezing.

Uses/Indications - Oxibendazole is indicated (labeled) for the removal of the following parasites in horses: large roundworms (*Parascaris equorum*), large strongyles (*S. edentatus, S. equinus, S. vulgaris*), small strongyles, threadworms, and pinworms (*Oxyuris equi*).

Oxfendazole has also been used in cattle, sheep, and swine; see Dosage section for more information.

Pharmacokinetics - No information was located.

Contraindications/Precautions - Oxibendazole is stated by the manufacturer (SKB) to be contraindicated in severely debilitated horses or in horses suffering from colic, toxemia or infectious disease. Oxibendazole is considered to be safe to use in pregnant mares.

Adverse Effects/Warnings - When used in horses at recommended doses, it is unlikely any adverse effects would be seen. Hypersensitivity reactions secondary to antigen release by dying parasites are theoretically possible, particularly at high dosages.

Oxibendazole in combination with diethylcarbamazine (*Filaribits Plus®*) has been implicated in causing periportal hepatitis in dogs.

Overdosage/Toxicity - Doses of 60 times those recommended elicited no adverse reactions in horses tested. It is unlikely that this compound would cause serious toxicity when given alone to horses.

Doses -

Horses:

For susceptible parasites:
a) 10 mg/kg PO; 15 mg/kg PO for strongyloides. (Package insert; *Anthelcide EQ®*— SKB)
b) 10 mg/kg PO (Robinson 1987), (Roberson 1988b)

Cattle:

For susceptible parasites:
a) 10 - 20 mg/kg PO. (Brander, Pugh, and Bywater 1982)

Swine:

For susceptible parasites:
a) 15 mg/kg PO. (Roberson 1988b)

Sheep:

For susceptible parasites:
a) 10 - 20 mg/kg PO. (Brander, Pugh, and Bywater 1982)

Monitoring Parameters -
1) Efficacy

Client Information - Protect suspension from freezing. Shake suspension well before using. Not for use in horses intended for food.

Dosage Forms/Preparations/FDA Approval Status -

Veterinary-Approved Products:

Oxibendazole Suspension 100 mg/ml (10%) gallons. *Anthelcide EQ®* *Suspension* (Pfizer); (Rx) Approved for use in horses not used for food.

Oxibendazole Oral Paste 227 mg/gram (22.7%) in 24 gram syringes. *Anthelcide EQ®* *Paste* (Pfizer), (OTC) Approved for use in horses not used for food.

A combination product (*Filaribits Plus®*—Pfizer) containing diethylcarbamazine and oxibendazole for the prophylactic treatment of heartworm and hookworms is available for dogs. See the product's literature for more information. Oxibendazole may be known in the U.K. by the proprietary names: *Dio®* (Alan Hitchings), *Equidin®* (Univet), *Equitac®* (SKF) or *Loditac®* (SKF).

Human-Approved Products: None

OXYBUTYNIN CHLORIDE

Chemistry - A synthetic tertiary amine, oxybutynin chloride occurs as white to off-white crystals. It is freely soluble in water.

Storage/Stability/Compatibility - Tablets and oral solution should be stored at room temperature in tight containers. Protect oral solution from light. Tablets have an expiration date of 4 years after manufacture.

Pharmacology - Considered a urinary antispasmodic, oxybutynin has direct antimuscarinic (atropine-like) and spasmolytic (papaverine-like) effects on smooth muscle. Spasmolytic effects appear to be most predominant on the detrusor muscle of the bladder and small and large intestine. It does not have appreciable effects on vascular smooth muscle. Studies done in patients with neurogenic bladders showed that oxybutynin increased bladder capacity, reduced the frequency of uninhibited contractions of the detrusor muscle and delayed initial desire to void. Effects were more pronounced in patients with uninhibited neurogenic bladders than in patients with reflex neurogenic bladders. Other effects noted in lab animal studies include moderate antihistaminic, local anesthetic, mild analgesic, very low mydriatic and antisialagogue effects.

Uses/Indications - Oxybutynin may be useful for the adjunctive therapy of detrusor hyperreflexia in dogs and in cats with FeLV-associated detrusor instability.

Pharmacokinetics - Oxybutynin is apparently rapidly and well absorbed from the GI tract. Studies done in rats show the drug distributed into the brain, lungs, kidneys, and liver. While elimination characteristics have not been well documented, oxybutynin apparently is metabolized in the liver and also excreted in the urine. In humans, the duration of action is from 6-10 hours after a dose.

Contraindications/Precautions/Reproductive Safety - Because of the drug's pharmacologic actions, oxybutynin should be used when its benefits outweigh its risks when the following conditions are present: obstructive GI tract disease or intestinal atony/paralytic ileus, angle closure glaucoma, hiatal hernia, cardiac disease (particularly associated with mitral stenosis, associated arrhythmias, tachycardia, CHF, etc.), myasthenia gravis, hyperthyroidism, prostatic hypertrophy, severe ulcerative colitis, urinary retention or other obstructive uropathies.

  While safety during pregnancy has not been firmly established, studies in a variety of lab animals have demonstrated no teratogenic effect associated with the drug. While oxybutynin may inhibit lactation, no documented problems associated with its use in nursing offspring have been noted.

Adverse Effects/Warnings - While use in small animals is limited, diarrhea and sedation have been reported. Other adverse effects reported in humans, and potentially seen in animals are primarily as a result of the drug's pharmacologic effects. These can include dry mouth or eyes, urinary retention or hesitancy, constipation, tachycardia, anorexia, vomiting, weakness, or mydriasis.

Overdosage/Acute Toxicity - Overdosage may cause CNS effects (*e.g.*, restlessness, excitement, seizures), cardiovascular effects (*e.g.*, hyper or hypotension, tachycardia, circulatory failure), fever, nausea or vomiting may also be present. Massive overdoses may lead to paralysis, coma, respiratory failure and death. Treatment of overdoses should consist of general techniques to limit absorption of the drug from the GI tract and supportive care as required. Intravenous physostigmine may be useful. See the atropine monograph for more information on the use of physostigmine.

Drug Interactions - Other **drugs with anticholinergic effects** (*e.g.*, atropine, propantheline, scopolamine, isopropamide, glycopyrrolate, hyoscyamine, tricyclic antidepressants, disopyramide, procainamide, antihistamines, etc.) may intensify oxybutynin's anticholinergic effects. Other **sedating drugs** may exacerbate the sedating effects of oxybutynin.

Doses -
  Dogs/Cats:
    For detrusor hyperreflexia:
      a) 5 mg PO q8-12h (Labato 1994)
      b) Cats: 0.5 mg q12h (Lane and Barsanti 1994)

Monitoring Parameters - Efficacy and adverse effects

Dosage Forms/Preparations/FDA Approval Status/Withholding Times -
  Veterinary-Approved Products: None
  Human-Approved Products:

    Oxybutynin Chloride Oral Tablets 5 mg; *Ditropan*® (Hoechst Marion Roussel) (Rx), Generic; (Rx)

Oxybutynin Chloride Oral Solution 1 mg/ml; *Ditropan*® *Syrup* (Hoechst Marion Roussel); *Oxybutynin*® (Silarx) (Rx)

OXYMORPHONE HCL

Chemistry - A semi-synthetic phenanethrene narcotic agonist, oxymorphone HCl occurs as odorless white crystals or white to off-white powder. It will darken in color with prolonged exposure to light. One gram of oxymorphone HCl is soluble in 4 ml of water and it is sparingly soluble in alcohol and ether. The commercially available injection has a pH of 2.7 - 4.5.

Storage/Stability/Compatibility - The injection should be stored protected from light and at room temperature (15-30° C); avoid freezing. The commercially available suppositories should be stored at temperatures between 2° and 15° C. Oxymorphone has been reported to be **compatible** when mixed with acepromazine, atropine, and glycopyrrolate. It is **incompatible** when mixed with barbiturates, and diazepam.

Pharmacology - See the monograph: Narcotic (Opiate) Analgesics for more infortmation. Oxymorphone is approximately 10 times more potent an analgesic on a weight basis when compared to morphine. It has less antitussive activity than does morphine. In humans, it has more of a tendency to cause increased nausea and vomiting than does morphine, while in dogs the opposite appears to be true. At the usual doses employed, oxymorphone alone has good sedative qualities in dog. Respiratory depression can occur especially in debilitated, neonatal or geriatric patients. Bradycardia, as well as a slight decrease in cardiac contractility and blood pressure may also be seen. Like morphine, oxymorphone does initially increase the respiratory rate (panting in dogs) while actual oxygenation may be decreased and blood CO_2 levels may increase by 10 mmHg or more. Gut motility is decreased with resultant increases in stomach emptying times. Unlike either morphine or meperidine, oxymorphone does not appear to cause histamine release.

Pharmacokinetics - Oxymorphone is absorbed when given by IV, IM , SQ, and rectal routes. Although absorbed when given orally bioavailability is reduced, probably from a high first-pass effect. After IV administration, analgesic efficacy usually occurs within 3-5 minutes.

Like morphine, oxymorphone concentrates in the kidney, liver, and lungs; lower levels are found in the CNS. Oxymorphone crosses the placenta and narcotized newborns can result if mothers are given the drug before giving birth, but these effects can be rapidly reversed with naloxone.

The drug is metabolized in the liver; primarily by glucuronidation. Because cats are deficient in this metabolic pathway, half-lives in cats are probably prolonged. The glucuronidated metabolite is excreted by the kidney.

Uses/Indications - Oxymorphone is used in dogs and cats as a sedative/restraining agent, analgesic and preanesthetic and occassionally in horses as an analgesic and anesthesia induction agent. It may also be used in swine as an adjunctive analgesic with ketamine/xylazine anesthesia and in small rodents as an analgesic/anesthetic for minor surgical procedures.

Contraindications/Precautions - All opiates should be used with caution in patients with hypothyroidism, severe renal insufficiency, adrenocortical insufficiency (Addison's), and in geriatric or severely debilitated patients. Oxymorphone is contraindicated in patients hypersensitive to narcotic analgesics, and in patients taking monamine oxidase inhibitors (MAOIs). It is also contraindicated in patients with diarrhea caused by a toxic ingestion until the toxin is eliminated from the GI tract.

Oxymorphone should be used with extreme caution in patients with head injuries, increased intracranial pressure and acute abdominal conditions (*e.g.,* colic) as it may obscure the diagnosis or clinical course of these conditions. It should be used with extreme caution in patients suffering from respiratory disease or from acute respiratory dysfunction (*e.g.,* pulmonary edema secondary to smoke inhalation).

Oxymorphone can cause bradycardia and therefore should be used cautiously in patients with preexisting bradyarrhythmias.

Neonatal, debilitated or geriatric patients may be more susceptible to the effects of oxymorphone and may require lower dosages. Patients with severe hepatic disease may have prolonged durations of action of the drug. If used in cats at high dosages, the drug has been recommended to be given along with a tranquilizing agent, as oxymorphone can produce bizarre behavioral changes in this species. This also is true in cats also for the other opiate agents, such as morphine.

Opiate analgesics are also contraindicated in patients who have been stung by the scorpion species *Centruroides sculpturatus* Ewing and *C. gertschi* Stahnke as it may potentiate these venoms.

Adverse Effects/Warnings - Oxymorphone may cause respiratory depression and bradycardia (see above). When used in cats at high dosages, oxymorphone may cause ataxia, hyperesthesia and behavioral changes (without concomitant tranquilization). Decreased GI motility with resultant constipation has also been described.

Overdosage - Massive overdoses may produce profound respiratory and/or CNS depression in most species. Other effects may include cardiovascular collapse, hypothermia, and skeletal muscle hypotonia. Naloxone is the agent of choice in treating respiratory depression. In massive overdoses, naloxone doses may need to be repeated, and animals should be closely observed as naloxone's effects may diminish before sub-toxic levels of oxymorphone are attained. Mechanical respiratory support should also be considered in cases of severe respiratory depression.

Drug Interactions - Other **CNS depressants** (*e.g.*, anesthetic agents, antihistamines, phenothiazines, barbiturates, tranquilizers, alcohol, etc.) may cause increased CNS or respiratory depression when used with oxymorphone. Oxymorphone is contraindicated in patients receiving **monoamine oxidase (MOA) inhibitors** (rarely used in veterinary medicine) for at least 14 days after receiving MOA inhibitors in humans. Some human patients have exhibited signs of opiate overdose after receiving therapeutic doses of oxymorphone while on these agents.

Laboratory Interactions - Plasma **amylase** and **lipase** values may be increased for up to 24 hours following administration of opiate analgesics as they may increase biliary tract pressure.

Doses -
Dogs:
For sedation for minor procedures:
  a) up to 0.2 mg/kg IM or IV; initially a maximum of 5 mg total dose (Combine with acepromazine 0.05 - 0.1 mg/kg IM or IV) (Shaw et al. 1986)
  b) 0.05 - 0.1 mg/kg IV or 0.1 - 0.2 mg/kg IM, SQ (Morgan 1988)
For analgesia:
  a) Intraoperative: 0.025 - 0.066 mg/kg IV (Shaw et al. 1986)
  b) Postoperative: 0.05 - 0.1 mg/kg IM or IV (Shaw et al. 1986), (Reidesel)
For premedication to anesthesia in healthy dogs:
  a) 0.1 - 0.2 mg/kg IM or IV (used with acepromazine and atropine or glycopyrrolate unless contraindicated. Thiopental/thiamylal dose may be reduced to 2 - 4 mg/kg when using high end of oxymorphone dose). (Shaw et al. 1986)
Induction of anesthesia in geriatric or sick dogs:
  a) 0.1 - 0.2 mg/kg IM or IV; give incrementally to effect (administered alternately with diazepam at 0.2 - 0.5 mg/kg; use with atropine or glycopyrrolate unless contraindicated; follow with halothane, methoxyflurane or isoflurane) (Shaw et al. 1986)
Facilitation of inhalation anesthesia without thiobarbiturates or ketamine in sight hounds:
  a) up to 0.2 mg/kg IV or IM (Combine with acepromazine; use with atropine or glycopyrrolate unless contraindicated) (Shaw et al. 1986)
Cats:
For restraint/sedation for minor procedures:
  a) 0.02 mg/kg IV (Morgan 1988)
  b) 0.025 - 0.1 mg/kg IV (must be given with tranquilizer; *e.g.*, acepromazine 0.1 mg/kg) (Shaw et al. 1986)
  c) 0.02 - 0.03 mg/kg IV or IM with or without another tranquilizer (Mandsager 1988)
As a preanesthetic/analgesic:
  a) 0.1 - 0.4 mg/kg IV (Shaw et al. 1986)
As a postoperative analgesic:
  a) 0.05 - 0.15 mg/kg IM or IV (must be given with tranquilizer; *e.g.*, acepromazine 0.05 - 0.1 mg/kg IM in IV) (Shaw et al. 1986)
Horses:
As an analgesic:
  a) 0.01 - 0.02 mg/kg IV (Muir 1987)
  b) 0.01 - 0.022 mg/kg IV; up to 15mg total (divide dose into 3-4 increments and give several minutes apart (Shaw et al. 1986)
  c) 0.02 - 0.03 mg/kg IM (Robinson 1987)
  d) 0.015 - 0.03 mg/kg IV (Thurmon and Benson 1987)
Anesthetic induction in severely compromised horses:
  a) 0.01 - 0.022 mg/kg IV (after approx. 45 minutes, may be necessary to "top off" with another 1/3 of the original dose) (Shaw et al. 1986)
Note: Narcotics (oxymorphone included) may cause CNS excitement in the horse. Some clinicians recommend pretreatment with acepromazine (0.02 - 0.04 mg/kg IV), or xylazine (0.3 - 0.5 mg/kg IV) to reduce the behavioral changes these drugs can cause.

> **Warning**: Narcotic analgesics can mask the behavioral and cardiovascular symptoms associated with mild colic.

Swine:
To increase analgesia when used with ketamine (2 mg/kg)/xylazine (2 mg/kg):
a) 0.075 mg/kg IV (duration of anesthesia and recumbency: 20 - 30 minutes) (Shaw et al. 1986)

Rodents (hamsters, gerbils, rats, etc.):
Anesthetic/analgesic for minor surgical procedures:
a) 0.15 mg/kg IM (for a hamster-sized animal) (Shaw et al. 1986)

Monitoring Parameters -
1) Respiratory rate/depth
2) CNS level of depression/excitation
3) Blood pressure if possible and indicated (especially with IV use)
4) Analgesic activity
5) Cardiac rate

Client Information - When given parenterally, this agent should be used in an inpatient setting or with direct professional supervision.

Dosage Forms/Preparations/FDA Approval Status/Withholding Times -
Veterinary-Approved Products: The veterinary labeled product is reportedly discontinued.

Human-Approved Products:
Oxymorphone HCl for Injection 1 mg/ml in 1 ml amps; 1.5 mg/ml in 1 ml amps and 10 ml vials; *Numorphan*® (Du Pont); (Rx)

Oxymorphone HCl 5 mg suppositories in 6s.; *Numorphan*® (Du Pont); (Rx)

Note: Oxymorphone is a **Class-II controlled substance**. Very accurate record keeping is required as to use and disposition of stock.

OXYTETRACYCLINE
OXYTETRACYCLINE HCL

Chemistry - A tetracycline derivative obtained from *Streptomyces rimosus*, oxytetracycline base occurs as a pale yellow to tan, crystalline powder that is very slightly soluble in water and sparingly soluble in alcohol. Oxytetracycline HCl occurs as a bitter-tasting, hygroscopic, yellow, crystalline powder that is freely soluble in water and sparingly soluble in alcohol. Commercially available 50 mg/ml and 100 mg/ml oxytetracycline HCl injections are usually available in either propylene glycol or povidone based products.

Storage/Stability/Compatibility - Unless otherwise directed by the manufacturer, oxytetracycline HCl and oxytetracycline products should be stored in tight, light-resistant containers at temperatures of less than 40°C (104°) and preferably at room temperature (15-30°C); avoid freezing.

Oxytetracycline HCl is generally considered to be **compatible** with most commonly used IV infusion solutions, including D5W, sodium chloride 0.9%, and lactated Ringer's, but can become relatively unstable in solutions with a pH > 6, particularly in those containing calcium. This is apparently more of a problem with the veterinary injections that are propylene glycol based, rather than those that are povidone based. Other drugs that are reported to be **compatible** with oxytetracycline for injection include: colistimethate sodium, corticotropin, dimenhydrinate, insulin (regular), isoproterenol HCl, methyldopate HCl, norepinephrine bitartrate, polymyxin B sulfate, potassium chloride, tetracycline HCl, and vitamin B-complex with C.

Drugs that are reportedly **incompatible** with oxytetracycline, data conflicts, or compatibility is concentration/time dependent, include: amikacin sulfate, aminophylline, amphotericin B, calcium chloride/gluconate, carbenicillin disodium, cephalothin sodium, cephapirin sodium, chloramphenicol sodium succinate, erythromycin glucceptate, heparin sodium, hydrocortisone sodium succinate, iron dextran, methicillin sodium, methohexital sodium, oxacillin sodium, penicillin G potassium/sodium, pentobarbital sodium, phenobarbital sodium, and sodium bicarbonate. Compatibility is dependent upon factors such as pH, concentration, temperature and diluents used. It is suggested to consult specialized references for more specific information (*e.g., Handbook on Injectable Drugs* by Trissel; see bibliography).

Pharmacology - Tetracyclines generally act as bacteriostatic antibiotics and inhibit protein synthesis by reversibly binding to 30S ribosomal subunits of susceptible organisms, thereby preventing binding to those ribosomes of aminoacyl transfer-RNA. Tetracyclines also are believed to reversibly bind to 50S ribosomes and additionally alter cytoplasmic membrane permeability in susceptible organisms. In high concentrations, tetracyclines can also inhibit protein synthesis by mammalian cells.

As a class, the tetracyclines have activity against most *mycoplasma*, spirochetes (including the Lyme disease organism), *Chlamydia*, and *Rickettsia*. Against gram positive bacteria, the tetracyclines have activity against some strains of *staphylococcus* and *streptococci*, but resistance of these organisms is increasing. Gram positive bacteria that are usually covered by tetracyclines, include *Actinomyces sp., Bacillus anthracis, Clostridium perfringens* and *tetani, Listeria monocytogenes,* and *Nocardia*. Among gram negative bacteria that tetracyclines usually have *in vitro* and *in vivo* activity against include *Bordetella sp., Brucella, Bartonella, Haemophilus sp., Pasturella multocida, Shigella,* and *Yersinia pestis*. Many or most strains of *E. coli, Klebsiella, Bacteroides, Enterobacter, Proteus* and *Pseudomonas aeruginosa* are resistant to the tetracyclines. While most strains of *Pseudomonas aeruginosa* show *in vitro* resistance to tetracyclines, those compounds attaining high urine levels (*e.g.,* tetracycline, oxytetracycline) have been associated with clinical cures in dogs with UTI secondary to this organism.

Oxytetracycline and tetracycline share nearly identical spectrums of activity and patterns of cross-resistance and a tetracycline susceptibility disk is usually used for *in vitro* testing for oxytetracycline susceptibility.

Uses/Indications - Oxytetracycline products are approved for use in dogs and cats (no known products are being marketed, however), calves, non-lactating dairy cattle, beef cattle, swine, fish, and poultry. For more information refer to the Doses section, below.

Pharmacokinetics - Both oxytetracycline and tetracycline are readily absorbed after oral administration to fasting animals. Bioavialabilities are approximately 60-80%. The presence of food or dairy products can significantly reduce the amount of tetracycline absorbed, with reductions of 50% or more possible. After IM administration of oxytetracycline (not long-acting), peak levels may occur in 30 minutes to several hours, depending on the volume and site of injection. The long-acting product (LA-200®) has significantly slower absorption after IM injection.

Tetracyclines as a class, are widely distributed in the body, including to the heart, kidney, lungs, muscle, pleural fluid, bronchial secretions, sputum, bile, saliva, urine, synovial fluid, ascitic fluid, and aqueous and vitreous humor. Only small quantities of tetracycline and oxytetracycline are distributed to the CSF and therapeutic levels may not be attainable. While all tetracyclines distribute to the prostate and eye, doxycycline or minocycline penetrate better into these and most other tissues. Tetracyclines cross the placenta, enter fetal circulation and are distributed into milk. The volume of distribution of oxytetracycline is approximately 2.1 L/kg in small animals, 1.4 L/kg in horses, and 0.8 L/kg in cattle. The amount of plasma protein binding is about 10-40% for oxytetracycline.

Both oxytetracycline and tetracycline are eliminated unchanged primarily via glomerular filtration. Patients with impaired renal function can have prolonged elimination half-lives and may accumulate the drug with repeated dosing. These drugs apparently are not metabolized, but are excreted into the GI tract via both biliary and nonbiliary routes and may become inactive after chelation with fecal materials. The elimination half-life of oxytetracycline is approximately 4-6 hours in dogs and cats, 4.3 - 9.7 hours in cattle, 10.5 hours in horses, 6.7 hours in swine, and 3.6 hours in sheep.

Contraindications/Precautions/Reproductive Safety - Oxytetracycline is contraindicated in patients hypersensitive to it or other tetracyclines. Because tetracyclines can retard fetal skeletal development and discolor deciduous teeth, they should only be used in the last half of pregnancy when the benefits outweigh the fetal risks. Oxytetracycline and tetracycline are considered to be more likely to cause these abnormalities than either doxycycline or minocycline.

In patients with renal insufficiency or hepatic impairment, oxytetracycline and tetracycline must be used cautiously. Lower than normal dosages are recommended with enhanced monitoring of renal and hepatic function. Avoid concurrent administration of other nephrotoxic or hepatotoxic drugs if tetracyclines are administered to these patients. Monitoring of serum levels should be considered if long-term therapy is required.

Adverse Effects/Warnings - Oxytetracycline and tetracycline given to young animals can cause discoloration of bones and teeth to a yellow, brown, or gray color. High dosages or chronic administration may delay bone growth and healing.

Tetracyclines in high levels can exert an antianabolic effect which can cause an increase in BUN and/or hepatotoxicity, particularly in patients with preexisting renal dysfunction. As renal function deteriorates secondary to drug accumulation, this effect may be exacerbated.

In ruminants, high oral doses can cause ruminal microflora depression and ruminoreticular stasis. Rapid intravenous injection of undiluted propylene glycol-based products can cause intravascular hemolysis with resultant hemoglobinuria. Propylene glycol based products have also caused cardiodepressant effects when administered to calves. When administered IM, local reactions, yellow staining and necrosis may be seen at the injection site.

In small animals, tetracyclines can cause nausea, vomiting, anorexia and diarrhea. Cats do not tolerate oral tetracycline or oxytetracycline very well, and may also present with symptoms of colic, fever, hair loss and depression.

Horses who are stressed by surgery, anesthesia, trauma, etc., may break with severe diarrheas after receiving tetracyclines (especially with oral administration).

Tetracycline therapy (especially long-term) may result in overgrowth (superinfections) of non-susceptible bacteria or fungi.

Tetracyclines have also been associated with photosensitivity reactions and, rarely, hepatotoxicity or blood dyscrasias.

Overdosage/Acute Toxicity - Tetracyclines are generally well tolerated after acute overdoses. Dogs given more than 400 mg/kg/day orally or 100 mg/kg/day IM of oxytetracycline did not demonstrate any toxicity. Oral overdoses would most likely be associated with GI disturbances (vomiting, anorexia, and/or diarrhea). Should the patient develop severe emesis or diarrhea, fluids and electrolytes should be monitored and replaced if necessary. Chronic overdoses may lead to drug accumulation and nephrotoxicity.

High oral doses given to ruminants, can cause ruminal microflora depression and ruminoreticular stasis. Rapid intravenous injection of undiluted propylene glycol-based products can cause intravascular hemolysis with resultant hemoglobinuria.

Rapid intravenous injection of tetracyclines has induced transient collapse and cardiac arrhythmias in several species, presumably due to chelation with intravascular calcium ions. Overdose quantities of drug could exacerbate this effect if given too rapidly IV. If the drug must be given rapidly IV (less than 5 minutes), some clinicians recommend pre-treating the animal with intravenous calcium gluconate.

Drug Interactions - When orally administered, tetracyclines can chelate **divalent or trivalent cations** which can decrease the absorption of the tetracycline or the other drug if it contains these cations. Oral antacids, saline cathartics or other GI products containing aluminum, calcium, magnesium, zinc or bismuth cations are most commonly associated with this interaction. It is recommended that all oral tetracyclines be given at least 1-2 hours before or after the cation-containing product.

Oral iron products are also associated with decreased tetracycline absorption, and administration of iron salts should preferably be given 3 hours before or 2 hours after the tetracycline dose. **Oral sodium bicarbonate, kaolin, pectin, or bismuth subsalicylate** may impair tetracycline absorption when given together orally.

Bacteriostatic drugs like the tetracyclines, may interfere with bactericidal activity of the **penicillins, cephalosporins,** and **aminoglycosides**. There is some amount of controversy regarding the actual clinical significance of this interaction, however.

Tetracyclines may increase the bioavailability of **digoxin** in a small percentage of patients (human) and lead to digoxin toxicity. These effects may persist for months after discontinuation of the tetracycline.

Tetracyclines may depress plasma prothrombin activity and patients on **anticoagulant** (*e.g.,* **warfarin**) therapy may need dosage adjustment. Tetracyclines have been reported to increase the nephrotoxic effects of **methoxyflurane** and tetracycline HCl or oxytetracycline are not recommended to used with methoxyflurane.

GI side effects may be increased if tetracyclines are administered concurrently with **theophylline** products.

Tetracyclines have reportedly reduced **insulin** requirements in diabetic patients, but this interaction is yet to be confirmed with controlled studies.

Drug/Laboratory Interactions - Tetracyclines (not minocycline) may cause falsely elevated values of **urine catecholamines** when using fluorometric methods of determination.

Tetracyclines reportedly can cause false-positive **urine glucose** results if using the cupric sulfate method of determination (Benedict's reagent, *Clinitest®*), but this may be the result of ascorbic acid which is found in some parenteral formulations of tetracyclines. Tetracyclines have also reportedly caused false-negative results in determining urine glucose when using the glucose oxidase method (*Clinistix®, Tes-Tape®*).

Doses -
  Dogs:
      For susceptible infections:
      a)   20 mg/kg PO *tid* (Morgan 1988)
      b)   10 mg/kg IV initially, then 7.5 mg/kg IV maintenance q12h (Ford and Aronson 1985)
      c)   20 mg/kg PO q8-12h; (may give with food if GI upset occurs; avoid or reduce dose in animals with renal or severe liver failure; avoid in young, pregnant or breeding animals) (Vaden and Papich 1995)
      d)   55 - 82.5 mg/kg PO q8h (Aronson and Aucoin 1989)
      e)   20 mg/kg PO q8h or 7 mg/kg IV or IM q12h. (Kirk 1989)
      f)   For haemobartonellosis: 22 mg/kg PO *tid* for 3 weeks (Lissman 1988)

Cats:
For susceptible infections:
    a)   20 mg/kg PO *tid* (Morgan 1988)
    b)   10 mg/kg IV initially, then 7.5 mg/kg IV maintenance q12h (Ford and Aronson 1985)
    c)   20 mg/kg PO q8-12h; (may give with food if GI upset occurs; avoid or reduce dose in animals with renal or severe liver failure; avoid in young, pregnant or breeding animals) (Vaden and Papich 1995)
    d)   55 - 82.5 mg/kg PO q8h (Aronson and Aucoin 1989)
    e)   20 mg/kg PO q8h or 7 mg/kg IV or IM q12h. (Kirk 1989)
    f)   For haemobartonellosis: 16 - 20 mg/kg PO *tid* for 3 weeks (Lissman 1988)

Cattle:
For susceptible infections:
    a)   5 - 10 mg/kg IM q24h or 20 mg/kg q48-72h IM if depot form (*LA®-200*);
           2.5 - 5 mg/kg IV q24h;
           10 - 20 mg/kg PO q12h. (Jenkins 1986)
    b)   For respiratory tract infections: Using 50 mg/ml product: 11 mg/kg IM or SQ q24h or IV q12-24h.
           Using 100 mg/ml product: 20 mg/kg IM q24h
           Using 200 mg/ml product (*LA-200®*): 20 mg/kg IM q3-4 days.
           IM or SQ doses should be injected into the neck and not more than 10 ml per site. IM route may lead to myositis and abscesses. Rapid IV injection may cause collapse. Phlebitis possible with IV dosing. (Beech 1987b)
    c)   For anthrax: 4.4 mg/kg IM or IV daily; do not use in healthy animals recently vaccinated against anthrax as the protective effect of the vaccine may be negated. (Kaufmann 1986)
    d)   For bovine anaplasmosis:
           For control: At start of vector season give 6.6 - 11 mg/kg (if using 50 mg/ml or 100 mg/ml product) or 20 mg/kg (if using depot form —*LA®-200*) every 21-28 days and extending 1-2 months after vector season ends.
           To eliminate carrier state: If using 50 mg/ml or 100 mg/ml product: 22 mg/kg IM (not over 10 ml per injection site) or IV (diluted in saline) daily for 5 days; or 11 mg/kg as above for 10 days. If using depot form (*LA®-200*): Give 20 mg/kg for 4 treatments deep IM in two separate injection sites at 3 day intervals.
           For treatment of sick animals: Preferably using depot form (*LA®-200*): Give 20 mg/kg one time.
           For temporary/prolonged protection for rest of herd: If using 50 mg/ml or 100 mg/ml product: 6.6 - 11 mg/kg IM (not over 10 ml per injection site) repeat at 21-28 day intervals throughout vector season for prolonged protection. If using depot form (*LA®-200*): Give 20 mg/kg IM as above and repeat at 28 day intervals for prolonged protection. (Richey 1986)
    e)   For pneumonia: If using 50 mg/ml or 100 mg/ml product: 11 mg/kg SQ once daily. If using depot form (*LA®-200*): Give 20 mg/kg IM q48h. (Hjerpe 1986)
    f)   6 - 11 mg/kg IM or IV; 10 - 20 mg/kg PO q6h (Howard 1986)
    g)   If using 50 mg/ml or 100 mg/ml product: 10 mg/kg IM initially, then 7.5 mg/kg IM once daily. If using depot form (*LA®-200*): Give 20 mg/kg IM q48h. (Baggot 1983)
    h)   22 - 33 mg/kg once daily IM or IV.
           If using LA-200®: 39.6 mg/kg IM q48h (Upson 1988)

Horses:
For susceptible infections:
    a)   5 - 10 mg/kg IV *bid* (Robinson 1987)
    b)   For respiratory tract infections: 5 mg/kg IV q12h; do not give too rapidly. (Beech 1987b)
    c)   3 mg/kg IV q12h (Baggot and Prescott 1987)
    d)   5 - 11 mg/kg IV q12h (Upson 1988)

Swine:
For susceptible infections:
    a)   For anthrax: 4.4 mg/kg IM or IV daily; do not use in healthy animals recently vaccinated against anthrax as the protective effect of the vaccine may be negated. (Kaufmann 1986)
    b)   6 - 11 mg/kg IV or IM; 10 - 20 mg/kg PO q6h (Howard 1986)
    c)   If using 50 mg/ml or 100 mg/ml product: 10 mg/kg IM initially, then 7.5 mg/kg IM once daily. (Baggot 1983)

Sheep & Goats:

For susceptible infections:

   a) For anthrax: 4.4 mg/kg IM or IV daily; do not use in healthy animals recently vacci-
   nated against anthrax as the protective effect of the vaccine may be negated.
   (Kaufmann 1986)

   b) 6 - 11 mg/kg IV or IM; 10 - 20 mg/kg PO q6h (Howard 1986)

Birds:

For chlamydiosis (Psittacosis):

   a) Using 200 mg/ml product (*LA-200®*): 50 mg/kg IM once every 3-5 days in birds suspected or confirmed of having disease. Used in conjunction with other forms of tetracyclines. IM injections may cause severe local tissue reactions. (McDonald 1989)

   b) Using 200 mg/ml product (*LA-200®*): 200 mg/kg IM once daily for 3-5 days. Has
   worked well in treating breeding birds to control outbreak and while getting birds to
   eat oral forms doxycycline or chlortetracycline. (Clubb 1986)

Reptiles:

For susceptible infections:

   a) For turtles and tortoises: 10 mg/kg PO once daily for 7 days (useful in ulcerative
   stomatitis caused by *Vibrio*) (Gauvin 1993)

Monitoring Parameters -

   1) Adverse effects
   2) Clinical efficacy
   3) Long-term use or in susceptible patients: periodic renal, hepatic, hematologic evaluations

Client Information - Avoid giving this drug orally within 1-2 hours of feeding, giving milk or
dairy products.

Dosage Forms/Preparations/FDA Approval Status/Withholding Times -
Veterinary-Approved Products:

Oxytetracycline HCl 50 mg/ml, 100 mg/ml Injection. There are many approved oxytetracycline products marketed in these concentrations. Some are labeled for Rx (legend) use only,
while some are over-the-counter (OTC). Depending on the actual product, this drug may be
approved for use in swine, non-lactating dairy cattle, beef cattle, chickens or turkeys.
Products may also be labeled for IV, IM, or SQ use. Withdrawal times vary with regard to
individual products. Slaughter withdrawal times vary in cattle from 15-22 days, swine 20-26
days, and 5 days for chickens and turkeys. Refer to the actual labeled information for the
product used for more information. Some trade names for these products include:
Terramycin®, *Liquamycin®*, *Biomycin* (Bio-Ceutic), *Medamycin®* (TechAmerica), *Biocyl®*
(Anthony), *Oxyject®* (Fermenta), and *Oxytet®* (BI).

Oxytetracycline base 200 mg/ml Injection in 100, 250, and 500 ml bottles; *Liquamycin® LA-
200®* (Pfizer); (OTC or Rx) Approved for use in swine, non-lactating dairy cattle and beef
cattle. Slaughter withdrawal = 28 days for swine and cattle.

Oxytetracycline Oral Tablets (Boluses) 250 mg tablet; *Terramycin® Scours Tablets* (Pfizer);
(OTC) Approved for use in non-lactating dairy and beef cattle. Slaughter withdrawal = 7
days.

Oxytetracycline is also available in feed additive, premix, ophthalmic and intramammary
products.

Established residue tolerances: Uncooked edible tissues of swine, cattle, salmonids, catfish
and lobsters: 0.10 ppm. Uncooked kidneys of chickens or turkeys: 3 ppm. Uncooked muscle,
liver, fat or skin of chickens or turkeys: 1 ppm.

Human-Approved Products:

Oxytetracycline Oral Capsules 250 mg; *Terramycin®* (Pfizer); *Uri-Tet®* (American
Urologicals); generic; (Rx)

Oxytetracycline For Injection (IM only) 50 mg/ml or 125 mg/ml (both with 2% lidocaine) in 2
ml amps and 10 ml vials; *Terramycin® I.M.* (Roerig); generic, (Rx)

OXYTOCIN

Chemistry - A nonapeptide hypothalamic hormone stored in the posterior pituitary (in mammals), oxytocin occurs as a white powder that is soluble in water. The commercially available
preparations are highly purified and have virtually no antidiuretic or vasopressor activity when
administered at usual doses. Oxytocin potency is standardized according to its vasopressor activ-

ity in chickens and is expressed in USP Posterior Pituitary Units. One unit is equivalent of approximately 2.0 - 2.2 micrograms of pure hormone.

Commercial preparations of oxytocin injection have their pH adjusted with acetic acid to 2.5-4.5 and multi-dose vials generally contain chlorbutanol 0.5% as a preservative.

Storage/Stability/Compatibility - Oxytocin injection should be stored at temperatures of less than 25°C, but should not be frozen. Some manufacturers recommend storing the product under refrigeration (2-8°C), but some products have been demonstrated to be stable for up to 5 years if stored at less than 26°C.

Oxytocin is reportedly **compatible** with most commonly used intravenous fluids and the following drugs: chloramphenicol sodium succinate, metaraminol bitartrate, netilmicin sulfate, sodium bicarbonate, tetracycline HCl, thiopental sodium and verapamil HCl.

Oxytocin is reportedly **incompatible** with the following drugs: fibrinolysin, norepinephrine bitartrate, prochlorperazine edisylate and warfarin sodium. Compatibility is dependent upon factors such as pH, concentration, temperature and diluents used. It is suggested to consult specialized references for more specific information (*e.g., Handbook on Injectable Drugs* by Trissel; see bibliography).

Pharmacology - By increasing the sodium permeability of uterine myofibrils, oxytocin stimulates uterine contraction. The threshold for oxytocin-induced uterine contraction is reduced with pregnancy duration, in the presence of high estrogen levels and in patients already in labor.

Oxytocin can facilitate milk ejection, but does not have any galactopoietic properties. While oxytocin only has minimal antidiuretic properties, water intoxication can occur if it is administered at too rapid a rate and/or if excessively large volumes of electrolyte-free intravenous fluids are administered.

Uses/Indications - In veterinary medicine, oxytocin has been used for induction or enhancement of uterine contractions at parturition, treatment of postpartum retained placenta and metritis, uterine involution after manual correction of prolapsed uterus in dogs, and in treating agalactia.

Pharmacokinetics - Oxytocin is destroyed in the GI tract and, therefore, must be administered parenterally. After IV administration, uterine response occurs almost immediately. Following IM administration, the uterus responds generally within 3-5 minutes. The duration of effect in dogs after IV or IM/SQ administration has been reported to be 13 minutes and 20 minutes, respectively. While oxytocin can be administered intranasally, absorption can be erratic. Oxytocin is distributed throughout the extracellular fluid. It is believed that small quantities of the drug cross the placenta and enter the fetal circulation.

In humans, the plasma half-life of oxytocin is about 3-5 minutes. In goats, this value has been reported to be about 22 minutes. Oxytocin is metabolized rapidly in the liver and kidneys and a circulating enzyme, oxytocinase can also destroy the hormone. Very small amounts of oxytocin are excreted in the urine unchanged.

Contraindications/Precautions - Oxytocin is considered to be contraindicated in animals with dystocia due to abnormal presentation of fetus(es), unless correction is made. When used prepartum, oxytocin should be used only when the cervix is relaxed naturally or by the prior administration of estrogens (Note: Most clinicians avoid the use of estrogens, as natural relaxation is a better indicator for the proper time to induce contractions).

In humans, oxytocin is considered to be contraindicated in patients with significant cephalopelvic disproportion, unfavorable fetal positions, in obstetrical emergencies when surgical intervention is warranted, severe toxemia or when vaginal delivery is contraindicated. Oxytocin is also contraindicated in patients who are hypersensitive to it. Nasally administered oxytocin is contraindicated in pregnancy.

Before using oxytocin, treat hypoglycemia or hypocalcemia if present.

Adverse Effects/Warnings - When used appropriately at reasonable dosages, oxytocin rarely causes significant adverse reactions. Most adverse effects are as a result of using the drug in inappropriate individuals (adequate physical exam and monitoring of patient are essential) or at too high doses (see Overdosage below). Hypersensitivity reactions are a possibility in non-synthetically produced products. Repeated bolus injections of oxytocin may cause uterine cramping and discomfort.

Overdosage - Effects of overdosage on the uterus depend on the stage of the uterus and the position of the fetus(es). Hypertonic or tetanic contractions can occur leading to tumultuous labor, uterine rupture, fetal injury or death.

Water intoxication can occur if large doses are infused for a long period of time, especially if large volumes of electrolyte-free intravenous fluids are concomitantly being administered. Early symptoms can include listlessness or depression. More severe intoxication symptoms can include coma, seizures and eventually death. Treatment for mild water intoxication is stopping oxytocin therapy and restricting water access until resolved. Severe intoxication may require the use of osmotic diuretics (mannitol, urea, dextrose) with or without furosemide.

Drug Interactions - If **sympathomimetic agents** are used concurrently with oxytocin, post-partum hypertension may result. Monitor and treat if necessary. Oxytocin used concomitantly with **cyclopropane** anesthesia can result in hypotension, maternal sinus bradycardia with atrioventricular dysrhythmias. One case in humans has been reported where **thiopental** anesthesia was delayed when oxytocin was being administered. The clinical significance of this interaction has not been firmly established.

Doses -
Dogs:
To augment uterine contractions during parturition:
   a)   1 - 5 Units SQ or IM; repeat no sooner than 30 minutes if necessary (Wheaton 1989)
   b)   In bitches who fail to progress after appropriate physical exam and diagnostic tests: Oxytocin 3 - 20 Units IM and/or with calcium gluconate 10% (3 - 5 ml IV, given slowly) if low total or ionized serum Ca^{++} levels. May repeat oxytocin at 30 minute intervals. If no progress after 3 treatments, recommend cesarian section. (Johnston 1986)

To treat primary uterine inertia:
   a)   5 - 20 Units (depending on size of bitch) IM or IV infusion. If no effect, give second injection 30 minutes later. If no effect, perform cesarean section. (Barton and Wolf 1988)

To induce milk let-down in bitches with adequate milk production and who tolerate nursing:
   a)   Oxytocin nasal spray (*Syntocinon®*): 5-10 minutes prior to nursing *tid* (Loar 1988)

For adjunctive treatment of acute metritis:
   a)   To promote uterine involution and evacuation: 0.5 - 1 Unit/kg IM; may repeat in 1-2 hours. Less effective if parturition occurred several days ago. (Magne 1986)

To promote uterine involution after uterine prolapse manual reduction:
   a)   5 - 20 Units IM (Nelson 1988)

Cats:
To promote uterine involution after uterine prolapse manual reduction:
   a)   5 Units IM once (Morgan 1988)

To treat primary uterine inertia:
   a)   2.5 - 5 Units IM or by IV infusion (Morgan 1988)
   b)   5 Units IM repeated in 15 to 20 minute intervals (Lein 1989)
   c)   2 - 5 Units IM or SQ, may repeat in 45 minutes. 1 - 3 ml of 10% calcium gluconate given slowly IV, may be helpful. If no response within 45 minutes after second injection, initiate appropriate surgical intervention. (Laliberté 1986)

Cattle:
For retained placenta in patients
   a)   40 - 60 Units oxytocin q2h (often used in conjunction with intravenous calcium therapy) as necessary. Of limited value after 48 hours postpartum as uterine sensitivity is reduced. (McClary 1986)
   b)   To reduce incidence of retained placenta: 20 Units IM immediately following calving and repeated 2-4 hours later. (Hameida, Gustafsson, and Whitmore 1986)

For mild to moderate cases of acute post-partum metritis:
   a)   20 Units IM 3-4 times a day for 2-3 days (Hameida, Gustafsson, and Whitmore 1986)

To augment uterine contractions during parturition:
   a)   30 Units IM; repeat no sooner 30 minutes if necessary (Wheaton 1989)

For obstetrical use in cows:
   a)   100 Units IV, IM or SQ (Package Insert; Oxytocin Injection—Anthony Products)

For milk let-down in cows:
   a)   10 - 20 Units IV, (Package Insert; Oxytocin Injection—Anthony Products)

Horses:
To augment or initiate uterine contractions during parturition in properly evaluated mares:
   a)   20 Units IM causes slow, quiet foaling;
        40 - 60 Units IM produces, quiet, safe foaling within an hour;
        100 Units or more will result in rapid completion of a more active foaling;
        IV (bolus) doses of 2.5 - 10 Units may be used to initiate parturition. (Hillman 1987)
   b)   For induction: If cervix is dilated at least 2 cm (internal measurement): 40 - 60 Units given as IV bolus, delivery should occur within 90 minutes.
        If the cervix is closed or less than 2 cm dilated: give oxytocin in 10 unit increments IV at 15-30 minute intervals. If the cervix dilates, but no signs of labor are shown, give additional oxytocin of 40 - 60 Units. (Carleton and Threlfall 1986)

To aid in removal of retained placenta:
   a) Oxytocin Bolus: 30 - 40 Units IM at intervals of 60-90 minutes. If parturition oc-
       curred more than 24 hours prior to oxytocin, doses up to 80 - 100 Units IM may be
       used. Alternatively, IV doses of 30 - 60 Units may be used until an adequate response
       is detected via rectal palpation of the uterus.
       Oxytocin Infusion: Add 80 - 100 Units oxytocin to 500 ml normal saline and begin
       IV infusion. Adjust rate of infusion according to mare's reactions. Slow rate if mare
       exhibits symptoms of excessive abdominal pain. Retained placenta generally expelled
       within 30 minutes. Gentle traction may help speed up expulsion. If several days have
       past since parturition, doses of up to 300 Units (administered rapidly) may be neces-
       sary to activate uterine motility. (Held 1987)
For mild to moderate cases of acute post-partum metritis:
   a) 20 Units IM 3-4 times a day for 2-3 days (Hameida, Gustafsson, and Whitmore 1986)
For obstetrical use in mares:
   a) 100 Units IV, IM or SQ (Package Insert; Oxytocin Injection—Anthony Products)
Swine:
   For adjunctive treatment of agalactia syndrome (MMA) in sows:
   a) 30 - 40 Units per sow at 3-4 hours (Powe 1986)
   b) 20 - 50 Units IM or 5 - 10 Units IV (Einarsson 1986)
   For retained placenta in patients with uterine atony:
   a) 20 - 30 Units oxytocin q2-3h as necessary (with broad-spectrum antibiotics).
       (McClary 1986)
   To augment uterine contractions during parturition:
   a) 10 Units IM; repeat no sooner than 30 minutes if necessary (Wheaton 1989)
   For mild to moderate cases of acute post-partum metritis:
   a) 5 - 10 Units IM 3-4 times a day for 2-3 days (Hameida, Gustafsson, and Whitmore
       1986)
   b) 5 Units IM, may need to be repeated as effect may be as short as 30 minutes
       (Meredith 1986)
   For obstetrical use in sows:
   a) 30 - 50 Units IV, IM or SQ (Package Insert; Oxytocin Injection—Anthony Products)
   For milk let-down in sows:
   a) 5 - 20 Units IV, (Package Insert; Oxytocin Injection—Anthony Products)
Sheep & Goats:
   For retained placenta in patients with uterine atony:
   a) 10 - 20 Units oxytocin. Of limited value after 48 hours postpartum as uterine sensi-
       tivity is reduced. If signs of metritis develop, treat with antibiotics. (McClary 1986)
   For mild to moderate cases of acute post-partum metritis:
   a) 5 - 10 Units IM 3-4 times a day for 2-3 days (Hameida, Gustafsson, and Whitmore
       1986)
   To control post-extraction cervical and uterine bleeding after internal manipulations (e.g fe-
   totomy, etc.):
   a) Goats: 10 - 20 Units IV, may repeat SQ in 2 hours (Franklin 1986a)
Birds:
   For egg expulsion:
   a) 0.01 - 0.1 ml once IM. Should be administered with Vitamin A and calcium
       (injectable). (Clubb 1986)
Reptiles:
   a) For egg binding in combination with calcium (Calcium glubionate: 10 -50 mg/kg IM
       as needed until calcium levels back to normal or egg binding is resolved): oxytocin: 1
       - 10 IU/kg IM. Use care when giving multiple injections. Not as effective in lizards as
       in other species. (Gauvin 1993)
Monitoring Parameters -
   1) Uterine contractions, status of cervix
   2) Fetal monitoring if available and indicated
Client Information - Oxytocin should only be used by individuals able to adequately monitor its
effects.
Dosage Forms/Preparations/FDA Approval Status/Withholding Times -
   Veterinary-Approved Products: Oxytocin products are approved for several species, including horses, dairy cattle, beef cattle, sheep, swine, cats and dogs. There is no milk or meat withdrawal times specified for oxytocin. Oxytocin is a prescription (Rx) drug.

Oxytocin for Injection 20 USP Units/ml in 10 ml, 30 ml, & 100 ml vials; available labeled generically from several manufacturers.

Human-Approved Products:

Oxytocin for Injection (Human-labeled) 10 Units/ml in 0.5 ml & 1 ml amps, 1 & 10 ml vials; 1 ml Tubex, 1 ml Steri-Dose syringe; *Pitocin*® (Parke-Davis); *Syntocinon*® (Sandoz); Oxytocin® (Wyeth); generic, (Rx)

Oxytocin, Synthetic, Nasal Spray (Human-labeled) 40 Units/ml in 2 and 5 ml squeeze bottles; *Syntocinon*® (Sandoz) (Rx)

PANCRELIPASE

Chemistry - Pancrelipase contains pancreatic enzymes, primarily lipase but also amylase and protease and is obtained from the pancreas of hogs. Each mg of pancrelipase contains not less than 24 USP units of lipase activity, not less than 100 USP units of protease activity, and not less than 100 USP units of amylase activity. When compared on a weight basis, pancrelipase has at least 4 times the trypsin and amylase content of pancreatin, and at least 12 times the lipolytic activity of pancreatin.

Storage/Stability/Compatibility - *Viokase*® preparations should be stored at room temperature in a dry place in tight containers. When present in quantities greater than trace amounts, acids will inactivate pancrelipase.

Pharmacology - The enzymes found in pancrelipase help to digest and absorb fats, proteins and carbohydrates.

Uses/Indications - Pancrelipase is used to treat patients with exocrine pancreatic enzyme deficiency. It may also be used in the attempt to test for pancreatic insufficiency secondary to chronic pancreatitis.

Contraindications/Precautions - Pancrelipase products are contraindicated in animals who are hypersensitive to pork proteins.

Adverse Effects/Warnings - High doses may cause GI distress (diarrhea, cramping, nausea).

Overdosage - Overdosage may cause diarrhea or other intestinal upset. The effects should be temporary; treat by reducing dosage and supportively if diarrhea is severe.

Drug Interactions - **Antacids** (magnesium hydroxide, calcium carbonate) may diminish the effectiveness of pancrelipase. **Cimetidine** (or other H_2 antagonists) may increase the amount of pancrelipase that reaches the duodenum.

Doses -

Dogs:

For pancreatic exocrine insufficiency:

a) 1 - 1.5 teaspoonsful with each meal mixed with food. Mix with food thoroughly and allow to stand for 15-20 minutes before feeding. Dosage should be adjusted as necessary. Best results are usually obtained by feeding small meals frequently (at least 3 times per day). (Package Insert; *Viokase*®-*V Powder* - Fort Dodge)

b) 1 - 2 teaspoons of powder of crushed tablets with meals; adjust dose according to clinical response. Not necessary to incubate with food before administering. If enzyme supplementation is inadequate, give cimetidine (5 - 10 mg/kg PO *tid* 30 minutes before meals) to reduce gastric acid destruction of enzymes (Bunch 1988)

c) Initially, 2 tsp of powdered extract per 20 kg of body weight mixed with food immediately prior to feeding; feed twice daily. Once clinical improvement has occurred, dosage may be varied to obtain efficacy with the minimum dose required. Most animals require at least 1 tsp. Some dogs may be satisfactorily controlled with once daily feedings. (Williams 1989)

Cats:

For pancreatic exocrine insufficiency:

a) 0.5 - 0.75 teaspoonsful with each meal mixed with food. Mix with food thoroughly and allow to stand for 15-20 minutes before feeding. Dosage should be adjusted as necessary. Best results are usually obtained by feeding small meals frequently (at least 3 times per day). (Package Insert; *Viokase*®-*V Powder* - Fort Dodge)

Birds:

For pancreatic exocrine insufficiency (used in birds that are polyphagic "going light", passing whole seeds, and slow in emptying crops):

a) 1/8 tsp per kg. Mix with moistened feed or administer by gavage. Incubate with food for 15 minutes prior to gavage. (Clubb 1986)

Monitoring Parameters -
1) Animal's weight
2) Stool consistency, frequency

Client Information - Powder spilled on hands should be washed off or skin irritation may develop. Avoid inhaling powder; causes mucous membrane irritation and may trigger asthma attacks in susceptible individuals.

Dosage Forms/Preparations/FDA Approval Status/Withholding Times -Note: There are several dosage forms (both human and veterinary-label) available containing pancrelipase, including oral capsules, oral delayed-release capsules, tablets, and delayed-released tablets. Most small animal practitioners feel that the oral powder is most effective, however.

Veterinary-Approved Products:

Powder containing (approximately) per teaspoonful (2.8 grams): 57,000 U lipase; 285,000 U protease; 428,000 U amylase; 8 oz bottle; *Viokase®-V Powder* (Fort Dodge); (Rx) Approved for use in dogs and cats.

Powder containing (approximately) per teaspoonful (2.8 grams): 61,000 U lipase; 330,000 U protease; 440,000 U amylase; 8 oz bottle; *Pancrezyme® Powder* (Daniels); (Rx) Approved for use in dogs and cats.

PANCURONIUM BROMIDE

Chemistry - A synthetic, non-depolarizing neuromuscular blocker, pancuronium bromide occurs as a white, odorless, bitter-tasting, hygroscopic, fine powder. It has a melting point of 215°C and one gram is soluble in 100 ml of water; it is very soluble in alcohol. Acetic acid is used to adjust the commercially available injection to a pH of approximately 4.

Storage/Stability/Compatibility - Pancuronium injection should be stored under refrigeration (2-8°C), but, according to the manufacturer, it is stable for 6 months at room temperature.

Do not store pancuronium in plastic syringes or containers as it may be adsorbed to plastic surfaces. It may be administered in plastic syringes, however.

It is recommended that pancuronium not be mixed with barbiturates as a precipitate may form, but data are conflicting on this point. No precipitate was seen when pancuronium was mixed with either succinylcholine, meperidine, neostigmine, gallamine, tubocurarine, or promethazine.

Pharmacology - Pancuronium is a nondepolarizing neuromuscular blocking agent and acts by competitively binding at cholinergic receptor sites at the motor end-plate, thereby inhibiting the effects of acetylcholine. It is considered to be 5 times as potent as d-tubocurarine and 1/3 as potent as vecuronium (some sources say that pancuronium is equipotent with vecuronium in animals). It has little effect on the cardiovascular system other than increasing heart rate slightly and only rarely does it cause histamine release.

Uses/Indications - Pancuronium is indicated as an adjunct to general anesthesia to produce muscle relaxation during surgical procedures or mechanical ventilation and also to facilitate endotracheal intubation.

Pharmacokinetics - After intravenous administration, muscle relaxation sufficient for endotracheal intubation occurs generally within 2-3 minutes, but is dependent on the actual dose administered. Duration of action may persist 30-45 minutes, but is again dependent on the dose. Additional doses may slightly increase the magnitude of the blockade and will significantly increase the duration of action.

In humans, pancuronium is approximately 87% bound to plasma proteins, but it may be used in hypoalbuminemic patients. Activity is not affected substantially by either plasma pH or carbon dioxide levels.

The half-life in humans ranges from 90 - 161 minutes. Approximately 40% of the drug is excreted unchanged by the kidneys. The remainder is excreted in the bile (11%) or metabolized by the liver. In patients with renal failure, plasma half-lives are doubled. Atracurium may be a better choice for these patients.

Contraindications/Precautions - Pancuronium is contraindicated in patients hypersensitive to it. It should be used with caution in patients with renal dysfunction, and in patients where tachycardias may be deleterious. Lower doses may be necessary in patients with hepatic or biliary disease. Pancuronium has no analgesic or sedative/anesthetic actions. In patients with myasthenia gravis, neuromuscular blocking agents should be used with extreme caution, if at all.

Adverse Effects/Warnings - Adverse reactions seen with pancuronium include: slight elevations in cardiac rate and blood pressure, hypersalivation (if not pretreated with an anticholinergic agent), occasional rash (humans), and prolonged or profound muscular weakness and respiratory depression. Very rarely will pancuronium cause substantial histamine release with resultant hypersensitivity reactions.

Overdosage - Overdosage possibilities can be minimized by monitoring muscle twitch response to peripheral nerve stimulation. Increased risks of hypotension and histamine release occur with overdoses, as well as prolonged duration of muscle blockade.

Besides treating conservatively (mechanical ventilation, O_2, fluids, etc.), reversal of blockade may be accomplished by administering an anticholinesterase agent (edrophomium, physostigmine, or neostigmine) with an anticholinergic (atropine or glycopyrrolate). A suggested dose for neostigmine is 0.06 mg/kg IV after atropine 0.02 mg/kg IV.

Drug Interactions - The following agents may enhance the neuromuscular blocking activity of pancuronium: **quinidine, aminoglycoside antibiotics (gentamicin**, etc.**), lincomycin, clindamycin, bacitracin, magnesium sulfate, polymyxin B, enflurane, isoflurane,** and **halothane**.

Other muscle relaxant drugs may cause a synergistic or antagonistic effect. **Succinylcholine** may speed the onset of action and enhance the neuromuscular blocking actions of pancuronium. Do not give pancuronium until succinylcholine effects have subsided.

Theophylline may inhibit or reverse the neuromuscular blocking action of pancuronium and possibly induce arrhythmias.

Azathioprine may reverse pancuronium's neuromuscular blocking effects.

Doses -
  Dogs:
    a) 0.1 mg/kg IV; 0.03 mg/kg IV if using methoxyflurane; 0.06 mg/kg if using halothane. (Morgan 1988)
    b) 0.044 mg/kg IV (Muir)
    c) 0.044 - 0.11 mg/kg IV; higher dose used initially; lower doses required if repeated doses are necessary (Mandsager 1988)

  Cats:
    a) 0.044 - 0.11 mg/kg IV; higher dose used initially; lower doses required if repeated doses are necessary (Mandsager 1988)

  Swine:
    a) 0.11 mg/kg IV (Muir)

Monitoring Parameters -
  1) Level of neuromuscular blockade; cardiac rate

Client Information - This drug should only be used by professionals familiar with its use.

Dosage Forms/Preparations/FDA Approval Status/Withholding Times -
  Veterinary-Approved Products: None
  Human-Approved Products:
  Pancuronium Bromide for Injection 1 mg/ml in 10 ml vials; 2 mg/ml in 2 & 5 ml amps, vials and syringes; *Pavulon*® (Organon); generic (Rx)

Paregoric - see Opiate Antidiarrheals

PEG 3550 Products - see Saline Cathartics

PENICILLAMINE

Chemistry - A monothiol chelating agent that is a degradation product of penicillins, penicillamine occurs as a white or practically white, crystalline powder with a characteristic odor. Penicillamine is freely soluble in water and slightly soluble in alcohol and has pK_a values of 1.83, 8.03, and 10.83. Penicillamine may also be known as D-Penicillamine, beta,beta-Dimethylcysteine, or D-3-Mercaptovaline.

Storage/Stability/Compatibility - Penicillamine should be stored at room temperature (15-30°C). The capsules should be stored in tight containers and the tablets in well-closed containers.

Pharmacology - Penicillamine chelates a variety of metals, including copper, lead, iron, and mercury, forming stable water soluble complexes that are excreted by the kidneys.

Penicillamine also combines chemically with cystine to form a stable, soluble complex that can be readily excreted.

Penicillamine has antirheumatic activity. The exact mechanisms for this action are not understood, but the drug apparently improves lymphocyte function, decreases IgM rheumatoid factor and immune complexes in serum and synovial fluid.

Although penicillamine is a degradation product of penicillins, it has no antimicrobial activity.

Uses/Indications - Penicillamine is used primarily for its chelating ability in veterinary medicine. It is the drug of choice for Copper storage-associated hepatopathies in dogs, and may be used for the long-term oral treatment of lead poisoning or in cystine urolithiasis.

Although the drug may be of benefit in chronic hepatitis, doses necessary for effective treatment may be too high to be tolerated.

Pharmacokinetics - Penicillamine is well absorbed after oral administration and peak serum levels occur about one hour (in humans) after dosing. The drug apparently crosses the placenta, but otherwise little information is known about its distribution. Penicillamine that is not complexed with either a metal or cystine is thought to be metabolized in the liver and excreted in the urine and feces.

Contraindications/Precautions/Reproductive Safety - Penicillamine is contraindicated in patients who have a history of penicillamine-related blood dyscrasias.

Penicillamine has been associated with the development of birth defects in offspring of rats given 10 times the recommended dose. There are also some reports of human teratogenicity.

Adverse Effects/Warnings - In dogs, the most prevalent adverse effect associated with penicillamine is nausea and vomiting. If vomiting is a problem, attempt to alleviate by giving smaller doses of the drug on a more frequent basis. Although food probably decreases the bioavailability of the drug, many clinicians recommend mixing the drug with food or giving at mealtimes if vomiting persists. Although thought to occur infrequently or rarely, fever, lymphadenopathy, skin hypersensitivity reactions, or immune-complex glomerulonephropathy may also potentially occur.

Overdosage/Acute Toxicity - No information located.

Drug Interactions - The amount of penicillamine absorbed from the GI tract may be reduced by the concurrent administration of **food, antacids, or iron salts**.

Administration of penicillamine with **gold compounds, cytotoxic or other immunosuppressant agents** (*e.g.,* **cyclophosphamide, azathioprine, but not corticosteroids), or phenylbutazone** may increase the risk of hematologic and/or renal adverse reactions.

Concomitant administration with **4-aminoquinoline compounds** (*e.g.,* **chloroquine, quinacrine**) may increase the risks of severe dermatologic adverse effects occurring.

Penicillamine may cause **pyridoxine** deficiency in humans, but this is not believed to occur in dogs.

Drug/Laboratory Interactions - When using **technetium Tc 99m gluceptate** to visualize the kidneys, penicillamine may chelate this agent and form a compound which is excreted via the hepatobiliary system. This may result in gallbladder visualization which could confuse the results.

Doses -
  Dogs:
    For copper-associated hepatopathy:
      a) 10 - 15 mg/kg PO *bid* on an empty stomach. Only effective for long-term use, not for acute copper toxicity. (Twedt and Whitney 1989)]
      b) For Bedlington Terriers: Initially at 125 mg q12h PO. If anorexia and vomiting are significant problems, start dose at 125 mg daily and increase to 125 mg *bid* over several days. (Hardy 1989)
      c) 125 - 250 mg PO 30 minutes prior to feeding. If vomiting occurs, divide daily dosage into *bid-tid*. (Cornelius and Bjorling 1988)
    For cystine urolithiasis:
      a) 15 mg/kg PO twice daily. If nausea and vomiting occur, mix with food or give at mealtime. Some dogs may need to have the dosage slowly increased to full dose in order to tolerate the drug. (Osborne, Hoppe, and O'Brien 1989)
      b) 15 mg/kg PO *bid* with food (Lage, Polzin, and Zenoble 1988)
    For lead poisoning:
      a) After initial therapy regimen with CaEDTA and if continued therapy is desired at home, may give penicillamine at 110 mg/kg/day PO divided q6-8h for 1-2 weeks. If vomiting, depression, and anorexia occur, may reduce dose to 33 - 55 mg/kg/day divided q6-8h which should be better tolerated. (Mount 1989)
      b) As an alternate or adjunct to CaEDTA: 30 - 110 mg/kg/day divided *qid* for 7 days; may repeat after 7 days off therapy. If vomiting occurs, may give dimenhydrinate at 2 - 4 mg/kg PO 1/2 hour before penicillamine dose. (Grauer and Hjelle 1988b)
  Cats:
    For lead poisoning:
      a) After initial therapy with CaEDTA and if blood lead is greater than 0.2 ppm at 3-4 weeks post-treatment, may repeat CaEDTA or give penicillamine at 125 mg q12h PO for 5 days. (Reid and Oehme 1989)

Monitoring Parameters - Monitoring of penicillamine therapy is dependent upon the reason for its use; refer to the references in the Dose section above for further discussion on the diseases and associated monitoring of therapy.

Client Information - This drug should preferably be given on an empty stomach, at least 30 minutes before feeding. If the animal develops problems with vomiting or anorexia, three remedies have been suggested. 1) Give same total daily dose, but divide into smaller individual doses and give more frequently. 2) Temporarily reduce the daily dose and gradually increase to recommended dosage. 3) Give with meals (will probably reduce amount of drug absorbed).

Dosage Forms/Preparations/FDA Approval Status/Withholding Times -
  Veterinary-Approved Products: None
  Human-Approved Products:

    Penicillamine Oral Titratable Tablets 250 mg (scored); *Depen*® (Wallace); (Rx)

    Penicillamine Oral Capsules 125 mg, 250 mg; *Cuprimine*® (Merck) (Rx)

PENICILLINS (GENERAL INFORMATION)

Pharmacology - Penicillins are usually bactericidal against susceptible bacteria and act by inhibiting mucopeptide synthesis in the cell wall resulting in a defective barrier and an osmotically unstable spheroplast. The exact mechanism for this effect has not been definitively determined, but beta-lactam antibiotics have been shown to bind to several enzymes (carboxypeptidases, transpeptidases, endopeptidases) within the bacterial cytoplasmic membrane that are involved with cell wall synthesis. The different affinities that various beta-lactam antibiotics have for these enzymes (also known as penicillin-binding proteins; PBPs) help explain the differences in spectrums of activity the drugs have that are not explained by the influence of beta-lactamases. Like other beta-lactam antibiotics, penicillins are generally considered to be more effective against actively growing bacteria.

The clinically available penicillins encompass several distinct classes of compounds with varying spectrums of activity: The so-called natural penicillins including penicillin G and V; the penicillinase-resistant penicillins including cloxacillin, dicloxacillin, oxacillin, nafcillin and methicillin; the aminopenicillins including ampicillin, amoxicillin, cyclacillin, hetacillin and bacampicillin; extended-spectrum penicillins including carbenicillin, ticarcillin, piperacillin, azlocillin and mezlocillin; and the potentiated penicillins including amoxicillin-potassium clavulanate, ampicillin-sulbactam, and ticarcillin-potassium clavulanate.

The natural penicillins (G and K) have similar spectrums of activity, but penicillin G is slightly more active *in vitro* on a weight basis against many organisms. This class of penicillin has *in vitro* activity against most spirochetes and gram positive and gram negative aerobic cocci, but not penicillinase producing strains. They have activity against some aerobic and anaerobic gram positive bacilli such as *Bacillus anthracis, Clostridium sp.* (not *C. difficile*), *Fusobacterium* and *Actinomyces*. The natural penicillins are customarily inactive against most gram negative aerobic and anaerobic bacilli, and all *Rickettsia*, mycobacteria, fungi, *Mycoplasma* and viruses.

The penicillinase-resistant penicillins have a more narrow spectrum of activity than the natural penicillins. Their antimicrobial efficacy is aimed directly against penicillinase-producing strains of gram positive cocci, particularly *Staphylococcal* species and these drugs are sometimes called anti-staphylococcal penicillins. There are documented strains of *Staphylococcus* that are resistant to these drugs (so-called methicillin-resistant *Staph*), but these strains have not as yet been a major problem in veterinary species. While this class of penicillins do have activity against some other gram positive and gram negative aerobes and anaerobes, other antibiotics (penicillins and otherwise) are usually better choices. The penicillinase-resistant penicillins are inactive against *Rickettsia*, mycobacteria, fungi, *Mycoplasma*, and viruses.

The aminopenicillins, also called the "broad-spectrum" or ampicillin penicillins, have increased activity against many strains of gram negative aerobes not covered by either the natural penicillins or penicillinase-resistant penicillins, including some strains of *E. coli, Klebsiella,* and *Haemophilus*. Like the natural penicillins, they are susceptible to inactivation by beta-lactamase-producing bacteria (e.g *Staph aureus*). Although not as active as the natural penicillins, they do have activity against many anaerobic bacteria, including *Clostridial* organisms. Organisms that are generally not susceptible include *Pseudomonas aeruginosa, Serratia*, Indole-positive *Proteus* (*Proteus mirabilis* is susceptible), *Enterobacter, Citrobacter,* and *Acinetobacter*. The aminopenicillins also are inactive against *Rickettsia*, mycobacteria, fungi, *Mycoplasma*, and viruses.

The extended-spectrum penicillins, sometimes called anti-pseudomonal penicillins, include both alpha-carboxypenicillins (carbenicillin and ticarcillin) and acylaminopenicillins (piperacillin, azlocillin, and mezlocillin). These agents have similar spectrums of activity as the aminopenicillins but with additional activity against several gram negative organisms of the family Enterobacteriaceae, including many strains of *Pseudomonas aeruginosa*. Like the aminopenicillins, these agents are susceptible to inactivation by beta-lactamases.

In order to reduce the inactivation of penicillins by beta-lactamases, potassium clavulanate and sulbactam have been developed to inactivate these enzymes and thus extend the spectrum of those penicillins. When used with a penicillin, these combinations are often effective against many beta-lactamase-producing strains of otherwise resistant *E. coli, Pasturella spp, Staphylococcus spp, Klebsiella*, and *Proteus*. Type I beta-lactamases that are often associated with *E. coli, Enterobacter,* and *Pseudomonas* are not generally inhibited by clavulanic acid.

Uses/Indications - Penicillins have been used for a wide range of infections in various species. FDA-approved indications/species, as well as non-approved uses, are listed in the Uses/Indications and Dosage sections for each individual drug.

Pharmacokinetics (General) - The oral absorption characteristics of the penicillins are dependent upon its class. Penicillin G is the only available oral penicillin that is substantially affected by gastric pH and can be completely inactivated at pH's of less than 2. The other orally available penicillins are resistant to acid degradation but bioavailability can be decreased by the presence of food (not amoxicillin). Of the orally administered penicillins, penicillin V and amoxicillin tend to have the greatest bioavailability in their respective classes.

Penicillins are generally distributed widely throughout the body. Most drugs attain therapeutic levels in the kidneys, liver, heart, skin, lungs, intestines, bile, bone, prostate, and peritoneal, pleural and synovial fluids. Penetration into the CSF and eye only occur with inflammation and may not reach therapeutic levels. Penicillins are bound in varying degrees to plasma proteins and they cross the placenta.

Most penicillins are rapidly excreted largely unchanged by the kidneys into the urine via glomerular filtration and tubular secretion. Probenecid can prolong half-lives and increase serum levels by blocking the tubular secretion of penicillins. Eexcept for nafcillin and oxacillin, hepatic inactivation and biliary secretion is a minor route of excretion.

Contraindications/Precautions/Reproductive Safety - Penicillins are contraindicated in patients who have a history of hypersensitivity to them. Because there may be cross-reactivity, use penicillins cautiously in patients who are documented hypersensitive to other beta-lactam antibiotics (*e.g.*, cephalosporins, cefamycins, carbapenems).

Do not administer systemic antibiotics orally in patients with septicemia, shock, or other grave illnesses as absorption of the medication from the GI tract may be significantly delayed or diminished. Parenteral (preferably IV) routes should be used for these cases.

Penicillins have been shown to cross the placenta and safe use of them during pregnancy has not been firmly established, but neither have there been any documented teratogenic problems associated with these drugs. However, use only when the potential benefits outweigh the risks. Certain species (snakes, birds, turtles, Guinea pigs, and chinchillas) are reportedly sensitive to procaine penicillin G.

High doses of penicillin G sodium or potassium, particularly in small animals with a preexisting electrolyte abnormality, renal disease or congestive heart failure may cause electrolyte imbalances. Other injectable penicillins, such as ticarcillin, carbenicillin and ampicillin, have significant quantities of sodium per gram and may cause electrolyte imbalances when used in large dosages in susceptible patients.

Adverse Effects/Warnings - Adverse effects with the penicillins are usually not serious and have a relatively low frequency of occurrence.

Hypersensitivity reactions unrelated to dose can occur with these agents and can be manifested as rashes, fever, eosinophilia, neutropenia, agranulocytosis, thrombocytopenia, leukopenia, anemias, lymphadenopathy, or full blown anaphylaxis. In humans, it is estimated that up to 15% of patients hypersensitive to cephalosporins will also be hypersensitive to penicillins. The incidence of cross-reactivity in veterinary patients is unknown.

When given orally, penicillins may cause GI effects (anorexia, vomiting, diarrhea). Because the penicillins may also alter gut flora, antibiotic-associated diarrhea can occur, as well as selecting out resistant bacteria maintaining residence in the colon of the animal (superinfections).

High doses or very prolonged use has been associated with neurotoxicity (*e.g.,* ataxia in dogs). Although the penicillins are not considered to be hepatotoxic, elevated liver enzymes have been reported. Other effects reported in dogs include tachypnea, dyspnea, edema and tachycardia.

Some penicillins (ticarcillin, carbenicillin, azlocillin, mezlocillin, piperacillin and nafcillin) have been implicated in causing bleeding problems in humans. These drugs are infrequently used systemically in veterinary species at the present time and the veterinary ramifications of this effect is unclear.

Overdosage/Acute Toxicity - Acute oral penicillin overdoses are unlikely to cause significant problems other than GI distress, but other effects are possible (see Adverse effects). In humans, very high dosages of parenteral penicillins, especially in patients with renal disease, have induced CNS effects.

Drug Interactions - *In vitro* studies have demonstrated that penicillins can have synergistic or additive activity against certain bacteria when used with **aminoglycosides** or **cephalosporins**.

Use of **bacteriostatic antibiotics** (*e.g.,* **chloramphenicol, erythromycin, tetracyclines**) with penicillins is generally not recommended, particularly in acute infections where the organism is proliferating rapidly as penicillins tend to perform better on actively growing bacteria. In low concentrations, certain penicillins (*e.g.,* ampicillin, oxacillin or nafcillin) may have additive or synergistic effects against certain bacteria when used with **rifampin**, but there is apparent antagonism when the penicillin is present in high concentrations.

Probenecid competitively blocks the tubular secretion of most penicillins, thereby increasing serum levels and serum half-lives.

High dosages of certain penicillins (*e.g.,* ticarcillin, carbenicillin) have been associated with bleeding; they should be used cautiously in patients receiving **oral anticoagulants or heparin**.

Drug/Laboratory Interactions - Ampicillin may cause false-positive **urine glucose determinations** when using cupric sulfate solution (Benedict's Solution, *Clinitest*®). Tests utilizing glucose oxidase (*Tes-Tape*®, *Clinistix*®) are not affected by ampicillin.

When using the Jaffe reaction to measure **serum or urine creatinine**, cephalosporins in high dosages (not ceftazidime or cefotaxime), may falsely cause elevated values.

In humans, clavulanic acid and high dosages of piperacillin have caused a false-positive direct **Combs' test**.

As penicillins and other beta-lactams can inactivate **aminoglycosides** *in vitro* (and *in vivo* in patients in renal failure), serum concentrations of aminoglycosides may be falsely decreased if the patient is also receiving beta-lactam antibiotics and the serum is stored prior to analysis. It is recommended that if the assay is delayed, samples be frozen and, if possible, drawn at times when the beta-lactam antibiotic is at a trough.

Monitoring Parameters - Because penicillins usually have minimal toxicity associated with their use, monitoring for efficacy is usually all that is required unless toxic signs or symptoms develop. Serum levels and therapeutic drug monitoring are not routinely done with these agents.

Client Information - Owners should be instructed to give oral penicillins on an empty stomach, unless using amoxicillin or if GI effects (anorexia, vomiting) occur. Compliance with the therapeutic regimen should be stressed. Reconstituted oral suspensions should be kept refrigerated and discarded after 14 days.

PENICILLIN G

For general information on the penicillins, including adverse effects, contraindications, overdosage, drug interactions and monitoring parameters, refer to the monograph: Penicillins, General Information.

Chemistry - Penicillin G is a natural penicillin and is obtained from cultures *Penicillium chrysogenum* and is available in several different salt forms. Penicillin G potassium (also known as benzylpenicillin potassium, aqueous or crystalline penicillin) occurs as colorless or white crystals, or white crystalline powder. It is very soluble in water and sparingly soluble in alcohol. Potency of penicillin G potassium is usually expressed in terms of Units. One mg of penicillin G potassium is equivalent to 1440-1680 USP Units (1355-1595 USP Units for the powder for injection). After reconstitution, penicillin G potassium powder for injection has a pH of 6-8.5, and contains 1.7 mEq of potassium per 1 million Units.

Penicillin G sodium (also known as benzylpenicillin sodium, aqueous or crystalline penicillin) occurs as colorless or white crystals, or white to slightly yellow, crystalline powder. Approximately 25 mg is soluble in 1 ml of water. Potency of penicillin G sodium is usually expressed in terms of Units. One mg of penicillin G sodium is equivalent to 1500-1750 USP Units (1420-1667 USP Units for the powder for injection). After reconstitution, penicillin G sodium powder for injection has a pH of 6-7.5, and contains 2 mEq of sodium per 1 million Units.

Penicillin G procaine (also known as APPG, Aqueous Procaine Penicillin G, Benzylpenicillin Procaine, Procaine Penicillin G, Procaine Benzylpenicillin) is the procaine monohydrate salt of penicillin G. *In vivo* it is hydrolyzed to penicillin G and acts as a depot, or repository form of penicillin G. It occurs as white crystals or very fine, white crystalline powder. Approximately 4-4.5 mg are soluble in 1 ml of water and 3.3 mg are soluble in 1 ml of alcohol. Potency of penicillin G procaine is usually expressed in terms of Units. One mg of penicillin G procaine is equivalent to 900-1050 USP Units. The commercially available suspension for injection is buffered with sodium citrate and has a pH of 5-7.5. It is preserved with methylparaben and propylparaben.

Penicillin G Benzathine (also known as Benzathine Benzylpenicillin, Benzathine Penicillin G, Benzylpenicillin Benzathine, Dibenzylethylenediamine Benzylpenicillin) is the benzathine tetrahydrate salt of penicillin G. It is hydrolyzed *in vivo* to penicillin G and acts as a long-acting form of penicillin G. It occurs as an odorless, white, crystalline powder. Solubilities are 0.2-0.3

mg/ml of water and 15 mg/ml of alcohol. One mg of penicillin G benzathine is equivalent to 1090-1272 USP Units. The commercially available suspension for injection is buffered with sodium citrate and has a pH of 5-7.5. It is preserved with methylparaben and propylparaben.

Storage/Stability/Compatibility - Penicillin G sodium and potassium should be protected from moisture to prevent hydrolysis of the compounds. Penicillin G potassium tablets and powder for oral solution should be stored at room temperature in tight containers; avoid exposure to excessive heat. After reconstituting, the oral powder for solution should be stored from 2-8°C (refrigerated) and discarded after 14 days.

Penicillin G sodium and potassium powder for injection can be stored at room temperature (15-30°C). After reconstituting, the injectable solution is stable for 7 days when kept refrigerated (2-8°C) and for 24 hours at room temperature.

Penicillin G procaine should be stored at 2-8°C; avoid freezing. Benzathine penicillin G should be stored at 2-8°C.

All commonly used IV fluids (some Dextran products are incompatible) and the following drugs are reportedly **compatible** with **penicillin G potassium**: ascorbic acid injection, calcium chloride/gluconate, cephapirin sodium, chloramphenicol sodium succinate, cimetidine HCl, clindamycin phosphate, colistimethate sodium, corticotropin, dimenhydrinate, diphenhydramine HCl, ephedrine sulfate, erythromycin gluceptate/lactobionate, hydrocortisone sodium succinate, kanamycin sulfate, lidocaine HCl, methicillin sodium, methylprednisolone sodium succinate, metronidazole with sodium bicarbonate, nitrofurantoin sodium, polymyxin B sulfate, potassium chloride, prednisolone sodium phosphate, procaine HCl, prochlorperazine edisylate, sodium iodide, sulfisoxazole diolamine and verapamil HCl.

The following drugs/solutions are either **incompatible** or data conflicts regarding compatibility with **penicillin G potassium** injection: amikacin sulfate, aminophylline, cephalothin sodium, chlorpromazine HCl, dopamine HCl, heparin sodium, hydroxyzine HCl, lincomycin HCl, metoclopramide HCl, oxytetracycline HCl, pentobarbital sodium, prochlorperazine mesylate, promazine HCl, promethazine HCl, sodium bicarbonate, tetracycline HCl and vitamin B-complex with C.

The following drugs/solutions are reportedly **compatible** with **penicillin G sodium** injection: Dextran 40 10%, dextrose 5% (some degradation may occur if stored for 24 hours), sodium chloride 0.9% (some degradation may occur if stored for 24 hours), calcium chloride/gluconate, chloramphenicol sodium succinate, cimetidine HCl, clindamycin phosphate, colistimethate sodium, diphenhydramine HCl, erythromycin lactobionate, gentamicin sulfate, hydrocortisone sodium succinate, kanamycin sulfate, methicillin sodium, nitrofurantoin sodium, polymyxin B sulfate, prednisolone sodium phosphate, procaine HCl, verapamil HCl and vitamin B-complex with C.

The following drugs/solutions are either **incompatible** or data conflicts regarding compatibility with **penicillin G sodium** injection: amphotericin B, bleomycin sulfate, cephalothin sodium, chlorpromazine HCl, heparin sodium, hydroxyzine HCl, lincomycin HCl, methylprednisolone sodium succinate, oxytetracycline HCl, potassium chloride, prochlorperazine mesylate, promethazine HCl and tetracycline HCl. Compatibility is dependent upon factors such as pH, concentration, temperature and diluents used. It is suggested to consult specialized references for more specific information (*e.g., Handbook on Injectable Drugs* by Trissel; see bibliography).

Uses/Indications - Natural penicillins remain the drugs of choice for a variety of bacteria, including group A beta-hemolytic streptococci, many gram positive anaerobes, spirochetes, gram negative aerobic cocci, and some gram negative aerobic bacilli. Generally, if a bacteria is susceptible to a natural penicillin, either penicillin G or V is preferred for treating that infection as long as adequate penetration of the drug to the site of the infection occurs and the patient is not hypersensitive to penicillins.

Pharmacokinetics (specific) - Penicillin G potassium is poorly absorbed orally as a result of rapid acid-catalyzed hydrolysis. When administered on an empty (fasted) stomach, oral bioavailability is only about 15-30%. If given with food, absorption rate and extent will be decreased.

Penicillin G potassium and sodium salts are rapidly absorbed after IM injections and yield high peak levels usually within 20 minutes of administration. In horses, equivalent doses given either IV or IM demonstrated that IM dosing will provide serum levels above 0.5 micrograms/ml for about twice as long as IV administration [approx. 3-4 hours (IV) vs. 6-7 hours (IM)].

Procaine penicillin G is slowly hydrolyzed to penicillin G after IM injection. Peak levels are much lower than with parenterally administered aqueous penicillin G sodium or potassium, but serum levels are more prolonged.

Benzathine penicillin G is also very slowly absorbed after IM injections after being hydrolyzed to the parent compound. Serum levels can be very prolonged, but levels attained generally only exceed MIC's for the most susceptible *Streptococci*, and the use of benzathine penicillin G should be limited to these infections when other penicillin therapy is impractical.

After absorption, penicillin G is widely distributed throughout the body with the exception of the CSF, joints and milk. CSF levels are generally only 10% or less of those found in the serum when meninges are not inflamed. Levels in the CSF may be greater in patients with inflamed meninges or if probenecid is given concurrently. Binding to plasma proteins is approximately 50% in most species.

Penicillin G is principally excreted unchanged into the urine through renal mechanisms via both glomerular filtration and tubular secretion. Elimination half-lives are very rapid and are usually one hour or less in most species (if normal renal function exists).

Doses -
Dogs:
For susceptible infections:
a) Penicillin G potassium: 20,000 Units/kg IV, IM, SQ q4h or 40,000 IU/kg PO on an empty stomach q6h
Penicillin G sodium: 20,000 Units/kg IV, IM, SQ q4h
Penicillin G procaine: 20,000 Units/kg IM, SQ q12-24h
Penicillin G benzathine: 50,000 IU/kg IM q5 days (Upson 1988)
b) Penicillin G potassium/sodium: 20,000 Units/kg IV, IM, or SQ q6h
Penicillin G procaine: 22,000 Units/kg IM, SQ q12h. Doses may be increased to 80,000 IU/kg per day, *Actinomyces* infections may require 100,000 - 200,000 IU/kg IM daily. (Ford and Aronson 1985)
c) Penicillin G potassium/sodium: 20,000 Units/kg IV, IM, q4h or 40,000 IU/kg PO on an empty stomach q6h
Penicillin G procaine: 20,000 Units/kg IM, SQ q12-24h.
Penicillin G benzathine: 40,000 IU/kg q5 days IM (Kirk 1989)
d) Penicillin G sodium or potassium: 22,000 - 55,000 IU/kg IV or IM q6-8h (Aronson and Aucoin 1989)
e) For adjunctive therapy of septicemia: Penicillin G sodium/potassium: 25,000 IU/kg IV q6h. Too rapid IV infusions may cause neurologic signs; hypersensitivity may also occur. (Goodwin and Schaer 1989)

Cats:
For susceptible infections:
a) Penicillin G potassium: 20,000 Units/kg IV, IM, SQ q4h or 40,000 IU/kg PO on an empty stomach q6h
Penicillin G sodium: 20,000 Units/kg IV, IM, SQ q4h
Penicillin G procaine: 20,000 Units/kg IM, SQ q12-24h
Penicillin G benzathine: 50,000 IU/kg IM q5 days (Upson 1988)
b) Penicillin G potassium/sodium: 20,000 - 40,000 Units/kg IV, IM, q6h
Penicillin G procaine: 22,000 Units/kg IM, SQ q12h. Doses may be increased to 80,000 IU/kg per day, *Actinomyces* infections may require 100,000 - 200,000 IU/kg IM daily. (Ford and Aronson 1985)
c) Penicillin G potassium/sodium: 20,000 Units/kg IV, IM, q4h or 40,000 IU/kg PO on an empty stomach q6h
Penicillin G procaine: 20,000 Units/kg IM, SQ q12-24h.
Penicillin G benzathine: 40,000 IU/kg q5 days IM (Kirk 1989)
d) Penicillin G sodium or potassium: 22,000 - 55,000 IU/kg IV or IM q6-8h (Aronson and Aucoin 1989)

Cattle (and other ruminants unless specified):
For susceptible infections:
a) Cattle: Penicillin G procaine: 44,000 - 66,000 Units/kg IM, SQ once daily
Penicillin G benzathine: 44,000 - 66,000 Units/kg IM, or SQ q2days (Upson 1988)
b) Cattle for bovine respiratory disease complex: Procaine penicillin G 66,000 IU/kg IM or SQ once daily. Recommend 20 day slaughter withdrawal at this dosage. (Hjerpe 1986)
c) Procaine penicillin G: 40,000 IU/kg IM once daily.
Procaine penicillin G/benzathine penicillin G combination: 40,000 IU/kg IM once. (Howard 1986)
d) Procaine penicillin G: 10,000 - 20,000 IU/kg IM q12-24h.
Benzathine penicillin G: 10,000 - 20,000 IU/kg IM, SQ q48h. (Jenkins 1986)

Horses:
For susceptible infections:
a) Penicillin G potassium: 5000 - 50,000 Units/kg IV *qid*
Penicillin G sodium: 5000 - 50,000 Units/kg IV *qid*
Penicillin G procaine: 5000 - 50,000 Units/kg IM *bid* (Robinson 1987)
b) Penicillin G sodium: 25,000 - 50,000 Units/kg IV, IM q6h

Penicillin G procaine: 20,000 - 100,000 Units/kg IM q12h
Penicillin G benzathine: 50,000 Units/kg IM q2 days (Upson 1988)
c) Initially give Penicillin G (aqueous, sodium salt used in experiment) 10,000 IU/kg IM with procaine penicillin G at 15,000 IU/kg IM q12h. If infection is severe, penicillin G sodium at 10,000 IU/kg at the same time as the procaine penicillin G. (Love et al. 1983)
d) For treatment of botulism: Penicillin G sodium or potassium 22,000 - 44,000 IU/kg IV *qid* (do not use oral penicillin therapy). (Johnston and Whitlock 1987)
e) For preoperative antibiotic prophylaxis for colic: Penicillin G potassium 40,000 IU IV *qid* with gentamicin 2.2 mg/kg IV tid. (Stover 1987)
f) For respiratory infections (*Streptococci*): Initially, 20,000 - 40,000 U/kg of aqueous penicillin G (sodium/potassium) IM with 20,000 u/kg IM of procaine penicillin G which is then continued *bid*. (Beech 1987a)
g) For foals: Penicillin G Na or K: 25,000 - 50,000 U/kg IV q6-8h;
Procaine penicillin G 25,000 - 50,000 U/kg IM q12h. Use the longer dose interval or smaller dose in premature foals or those less than 7 days old. (Caprile and Short 1987)
h) Procaine penicillin G 25,000 Units/kg IM q12-24h
Penicillin G sodium: 15,000 - 20,000 U/kg IV or IM q6h (Baggot and Prescott 1987)
i) Penicillin G potassium: 12,500 - 100,000 Units/kg IV q4h
Penicillin G sodium: 12,500 - 100,000 Units/kg IV q4h
Penicillin G procaine: 20,000 - 50,000 Units/kg IM q12h (Brumbaugh 1987)

Swine:
For susceptible infections:
a) Procaine penicillin G: 40,000 IU/kg IM once daily.
Procaine penicillin G/benzathine penicillin G combination: 40,000 IU/kg IM once. (Howard 1986)
b) Procaine penicillin G: 6,600 IU/kg IM once daily for not more than 4 days.
Procaine penicillin G/benzathine penicillin G combination: 11,000 - 22,000 IU/kg IM once. (Wood 1986)

Birds:
For susceptible infections:
a) In turkeys: Procaine penicillin G/benzathine penicillin G combination: 100 mg/kg IM of each drug once a day or every 2 days. Use cautiously in small birds as it may cause procaine toxicity. (Clubb 1986)

Dosage Forms/Preparations/FDA Approval Status/Withholding Times -
Veterinary-Approved Products:
Penicillin G Procaine Injection 300,000 Units/ml in 100 ml and 250 ml bottles
Crystacillin® 300 A.S. Veterinary (Solvay); (OTC) Approved for use in cattle, sheep, horses, and swine. Do not exceed 7 days of treatment in non-lactating dairy cattle, beef cattle, swine or sheep, and 5 days in lactating dairy cattle. Milk withdrawal = 48 hours. Slaughter withdrawal: Calves (non-ruminating) 7 days; cattle 4 days; sheep 8 days; swine 6 days.
Note: These withdrawal times are for the labeled dosage of 6,600 U/kg once daily which is rarely used clinically today. Actual withdrawal times may be longer. There are other generically labeled products available that may have different withdrawal times; refer to label for more information.
Note: There are several penicillin G procaine combination products available for the veterinary market. These products may contain dihydrostreptomycin, streptomycin or novobiocin, and be available in either intramammary or injectable dosage forms.
Penicillin G Benzathine 150,000 U/ml with Penicillin G Procaine Injection 150,000 Units/ml for Injection in 100 ml and 250 ml vials
Flo-Cillin® (Fort Dodge), *Pen BP-48®* (Pfizer), *Crystiben®* (Solvay), *Dual-Pen®* (TechAmerica), generic; (OTC) Approved (most products) in dogs, horses and beef cattle. Slaughter withdrawal: cattle=30 days. Actual species approvals and withdrawal times may vary with the actual product; refer to the label of the product you are using.

Human-Approved Products:
Penicillin G (aqueous) Potassium Powder for Injection 1,000,000 units in vials, 5,000,000 units in vials, 10,000,000 units in vials, 20,000,000 units/vial (Rx) *Penicillin G Potassium®* (Apothecon); *Pfizerpen®* (Roerig) (Rx)
Penicillin G (aqueous) Potassium Premixed Frozen Injection: 1,000,000 units, 2,000,000 units & 3,000,000 units in 50 mls *Penicillin G Potassium®* (Baxter) (Rx)

Penicillin G (aqueous) Sodium Powder for Injection 5 million Units/vial; *Penicillin G Sodium*® (Apothecon) (Rx)

Penicillin G Potassium Oral Tablets 200,000 Units, 250,000 Units, 400,000 Units, 500,000 Units, 800,000 Units; *Penicillin G Potassium*® (Rugby) (Rx); *Pentids '400'*® (Apothecon) (Rx); *Pentids '800'*® (Apothecon) (Rx); generic, (Rx)

Penicillin G Potassium Oral Powder for Suspension 400,000 Units/5 ml in 100 ml and 200 ml; *Pentids '400' for Syrup*® (Apothecon) (Rx)

Penicillin G (aqueous) Procaine for Injection 300,000 Units/ml in 10 ml vials, 500,000 Units/ml (600,00 units/1.2 ml) in 12 ml vials, 600,000 Units/unit dose in 1 ml Tubex, 1.2 million Units/unit dose in 2 ml Tubex &, 2.4 million Units/unit dose in 4 ml syringes; *Crysticillin 300 A.S.*® (Apothecon); *Pfizerpen-AS*® (Roerig); *Crysticillin 600 A.S.*® (Apothecon); *Wycillin*® (Wyeth-Ayerst); (Rx)

Penicillin G Benzathine for Injection 300,000 Units/ml in 10 ml vials; 600,000 unit/dose in 1 ml Tubex; 1,200,000 units/dose in 2 ml Tubex; 2,400,000 units/dose in 4 ml syringes; *Bicillin L-A*® (Wyeth-Ayerst); *Permapen*® (Roerig) (Rx)

Penicillin G Benzathine & Procaine Combined for Injection 300,000 units/ml (150,000 units each penicillin G benzathine & penicillin G procaine) in 10 ml vials; 600,000 units/dose (300,000 units each penicillin G benzathine & penicillin G procaine) in 1 ml Tubex; 1,200,000 units/dose in 2 ml Tubex; 2,400,000 units/dose in 4 ml syringe; 900,000 units penicillin G benzathine and 300,000 units penicillin G procaine per dose in 2 ml Tubex; *Bicillin C-R*® (Wyeth-Ayerst); *Bicillin C-R 900/300*® (Wyeth-Ayerst) (Rx)

PENICILLIN V POTASSIUM

For general information on the penicillins, including adverse effects, contraindications, overdosage, drug interactions and monitoring parameters, refer to the monograph: Penicillins, General Information.

Chemistry - A natural penicillin, penicillin V is produced from *Penicillium chrysogenum* and is usually commercially available as the potassium salt. It may also be known as phenoxymethylpenicillin potassium. Penicillin V potassium occurs as an odorless, white, crystalline powder that is very soluble in water and slightly soluble in alcohol. Potency of penicillin V potassium is usually expressed in terms of weight (in mg) of penicillin V, but penicillin V units may also be used. One mg of penicillin V potassium is equivalent to 1380-1610 USP Units of penicillin V. Manufacturers, however, generally state that 125 mg of penicillin V potassium is approximately equivalent to 200,000 USP units of penicillin V.

Storage/Stability/Compatibility - Penicillin V potassium tablets and powder for oral solution should be stored in tight containers at room temperature (15-30°C). After reconstitution, the oral solution should be stored at 2-8°C (refrigerated) and any unused portion discarded after 14 days.

Pharmacology, Uses/Indications - Penicillin V may be slightly less active than penicillin G against organisms susceptible to the natural penicillins, but its superior absorptive characteristics after oral administration make it a better choice against mild to moderately severe infections when oral administration is desired in monogastric animals. For more information on the types of organisms that penicillin V generally covers, refer to the general statement on penicillins and the penicillin G monograph.

Pharmacokinetics (specific) - The pharmacokinetics of penicillin V are very similar to penicillin G with the exception of oral bioavailability and the percent of the drug that is bound to plasma proteins. Penicillin V is significantly more resistant to acid-catalyzed inactivation in the gut and bioavailability after oral administration in humans is approximately 60-73%. In veterinary species, actual bioavailability measurements have been measured in calves (30%), but studies performed in horses and dogs have demonstrated that therapeutic serum levels can be achieved with the drug after oral administration. In dogs, it has been shown that food will decrease the rate and extent of absorption of the drug from the gut.

Distribution of penicillin V follows that of penicillin G but, at least in humans, the drug is bound to a larger extent to plasma proteins (approximately 80% with penicillin VK vs. 50% with penicillin G).

Like penicillin G, penicillin V is excreted rapidly in the urine via the kidney. Elimination half-lives are generally less than 1 hour in animals with normal renal function, but an elimination half-life of 3.65 hours has been reported after oral dosing in horses (Schwark et al. 1983).

Doses -

  Dogs:

    For susceptible infections:

      a) 5.5 - 11 mg/kg PO q6-8h (Aronson and Aucoin 1989)

b) 10 mg/kg (listed as penicillin V) PO q8h (Kirk 1989)

Cats:
For susceptible infections:
a) 5.5 - 11 mg/kg PO q6-8h (Aronson and Aucoin 1989)
b) 10 mg/kg (listed as penicillin V) PO q8h (Kirk 1989)

Horses:
For susceptible infections:
a) 66,000 U/kg (41.25 mg/kg) PO gives levels greater than 0.1 micrograms/ml for greater than 325 minutes which should be effective against *Streptococci*. (Beech 1987a) (Author's (Plumb) note: Because of the post-antibiotic effect phenomenon; dosing every 6-8 hours should be sufficient)
b) 110,000 U/kg (68.75 mg/kg) PO q8h (may yield supra-optimal levels against uncomplicated infections by sensitive organisms). (Schwark et al. 1983)
c) 110,000 U/kg PO q6-12h (Brumbaugh 1987)

Client Information - Unless otherwise instructed by the veterinarian, this drug should be given on an empty stomach, at least 1 hour before feeding or 2 hours after. Keep oral suspension in the refrigerator and discard any unused suspension after 14 days.

Dosage Forms/Preparations/FDA Approval Status/Withholding Times -
Veterinary-Approved Products: None
Human-Approved Products:
Penicillin V Potassium Oral Tablets 125 mg, 250 mg, 500 mg; (Rx)

Penicillin V Potassium Oral Powder for Suspension 125 mg/5 ml in 100 ml, 150 ml and 200 ml, 250 mg/5 ml in 100 ml, 150 ml and 200 ml; (Rx)

There are a multitude of proprietary penicillin VK products, some more widely known include: *V-Cillin K®* (Lilly), *Pen-Vee K®* (Wyeth), *Veetids®* (Squibb), *Uticillin VK®* (Upjohn), *Beepen-VK®* (Beecham), *Ledercillin® VK* (Lederle)

PENTAZOCINE LACTATE
PENTAZOCINE HCL

Chemistry- A synthetic partial opiate agonist, pentazocine is commercially available as two separate salts. The hydrochloride salt, which is found in oral dosage forms, occurs as a white, crystalline powder. It is soluble in water and freely soluble in alcohol. The commercial injection is prepared from pentazocine base with the assistance of lactic acid. This allows the drug to be soluble in water. The pH of this product is adjusted to a range of 4-5. Pentazocine is a weak base with an approximate pK_a of 9.0.

Storage/Stability/Compatibility - The tablet preparations should be stored at room temperature and in tight, light-resistant containers. The injectable product should be kept at room temperature; avoid freezing.

The following agents have been reported to be **compatible** when mixed with pentazocine lactate: atropine sulfate, benzquinamide HCl, butorphanol tartrate, chlorpromazine HCl, dimenhydrinate, diphenhydramine HCl, droperidol, fentanyl citrate, hydromorphone, hydroxyzine HCl, meperidine HCl, metoclopramide, morphine sulfate, perphenazine, prochlorperazine edisylate, promazine HCl, promethazine HCl, and scopolamine HBr. The following agents have been reported to be **incompatible** when mixed with pentazocine lactate: aminophylline, amobarbital sodium, flunixin meglumine, glycopyrrolate, pentobarbital sodium, phenobarbital sodium, secobarbital sodium, and sodium bicarbonate.

Pharmacology - While considered to be a partial opiate agonist, pentazocine exhibits many of the same characteristics as the true opiate agonists. It is reported to have an analgesic potency of approximately one-half that of morphine and five times that of meperidine. It is a very weak antagonist at the *mu* opioid receptor when compared to naloxone. It will not antagonize the respiratory depression caused by drugs like morphine, but may induce symptoms of withdrawal in human patients dependent to narcotic agents.

Besides its analgesic properties, pentazocine can cause respiratory depression, decreased GI motility, sedation, and it possesses antitussive effects. Pentazocine tends to have less sedative qualities in animals than other opiates and therefore is usually not used as a pre-operative medication.

In dogs, pentazocine has been demonstrated to cause a transient decrease in blood pressure. In man, pentazocine can cause increases in cardiac output, heart rate, and blood pressure.

Pharmacokinetics - Pentazocine is well absorbed following oral, IM, or SQ administration. Because of a high first-pass effect, only about 1/5th of an oral dose will enter the systemic circulation in patients with normal hepatic function.

After absorption, the drug is distributed widely into tissues. In the equine, it has been shown to be 80% bound to plasma proteins. Pentazocine will cross the placenta and neonatal serum levels have been measured at 60-65% of maternal levels at delivery. It is not clearly known if or how much pentazocine crosses into milk.

The drug is primarily metabolized in the liver with resultant excretion by the kidneys of the metabolites. In the horse, approximately 30% of a given dose is excreted as the glucuronide. Pentazocine and its metabolites have been detected in equine urine for up to 5 days following an injection. Apparently less than 15% of the drug is excreted by the kidneys in an unchanged form.

Plasma half-lives have been reported for various species: Humans = 2-3 hrs; Ponies = 97 mins.; Dogs = 22 mins.; Cats = 84 mins.; Swine = 49 mins. Volumes of distribution range from a high of 5.09 L/kg in ponies to 2.78 L/kg in cats. In horses, the onset of action has been reported to be 2-3 minutes following IV dosing with a peak effect at 5-10 minutes.

Uses/Indications - Pentazocine is labeled for the symptomatic relief of pain of colic in horses and for the amelioration of pain accompanying postoperative recovery from fractures, trauma, and spinal disorders in dogs. It has also been used as an analgesic in cats (see adverse effects below) and in swine.

Contraindications/Precautions - All opiates should be used with caution in patients with hypothyroidism, severe renal insufficiency, adrenocortical insufficiency (Addison's), and in geriatric or severely debilitated patients.

Like other opiates, pentazocine must be used with extreme caution in patients with head trauma, increased CSF pressure or other CNS dysfunction (*e.g.,* coma). Pentazocine should not be used in place of appropriate therapy (medical &/or surgical) for equine colic, but only as adjunctive treatment for pain.

Because reproductive studies have not been done in dogs, the manufacturer does not recommend its use in pregnant bitches, or bitches intended for breeding. Studies performed in laboratory animals have not demonstrated any indications of teratogenicity.

The drug is contraindicated in patients having known hypersensitivity to it.

Adverse Effects/Warnings - In dogs, the most predominant adverse reaction following parenteral administration is salivation. Other potential side effects at usual doses include fine tremors, emesis, and swelling at the injection site. At very high doses (6 mg/kg) dogs have been noted to develop ataxia, fine tremors, convulsions, and swelling at the injection site.

Horses may develop transient ataxia, and symptoms of CNS excitement. Pulse and respiratory rates may be mildly elevated.

The use of pentazocine in cats is controversial. Some clinicians claim that the drug causes dysphoric reactions in cats which precludes its use in this species, while others disagree and state that drug may be safely used.

Overdosage - There is little information regarding acute overdose situations with pentazocine. For oral ingestions, the gut should be emptied if indicated and safe to do so. Symptoms should be managed by supportive treatment (O_2, pressor agents, IV fluids, mechanical ventilation) and respiratory depression can be treated with naloxone. Repeated doses of naloxone may be necessary.

Drug Interactions - When used with pentazocine, other **CNS depressants** (*e.g.,* anesthetic agents, antihistamines, phenothiazines, barbiturates, tranquilizers, alcohol, etc.) may cause increased CNS or respiratory depression; dosage may need to be decreased.

Doses -
Dogs:
For analgesia:
   a) Initially 1.65 mg/kg; up to 3.3 mg/kg IM. Duration of effect generally lasts 3 hours. If dose is repeated, use different injection site. (Package Insert; *Talwin®-V* - Winthrop)
   b) 0.2 - 0.5 mg/kg IM prn (Morgan 1988)
   c) 0.5 - 1.0 mg/kg IM (Kirk 1986)

Cats: Note: Pentazocine tends to cause dysphoria in cats. Alternative analgesics are recommended.
For analgesia: 2.2 - 3.3 mg/kg SQ, IM or IV (Booth 1988a)

Horses:
For analgesia:
   a) 0.33 mg/kg slowly in jugular vein. In cases of severe pain, a second dose (0.33 mg/kg) be given IM 15 minutes later (Package Insert; *Talwin®-V* - Winthrop)
   b) 0.33 - 0.66 mg/kg IV, IM or SQ (Jenkins 1987)
   c) 0.4 - 0.8 mg/kg IV (Muir 1987)
   d) 0.4 - 0.9 mg/kg IV (Thurmon and Benson 1987)
Note: Duration of analgesia may last only 10-30 minutes following an IV dose.

Swine:
Analgesia:
a) 2.0 mg/kg IM q4h prn (Jenkins 1987)

Monitoring Parameters -
1) Analgesic efficacy
2) Respiratory rate/depth
3) Appetite/bowel function
4) CNS effects

Client Information - Clients should report any significant changes in behavior, appetite, bowel or urinary function in their animals.

It is not approved for use in food producing animals (including horses to be used for food). All pentazocine products are Class-IV controlled substances.

Dosage Forms/Preparations/FDA Approval Status/Withholding Times -
Veterinary-Approved Products:

Pentazocine Lactate Injection: 30 mg/ml (as base) in 10 ml vials; *Talwin®-V* (Pharmacia & Upjohn); (Rx) Pentazocine lactate injection is approved for use in horses and dogs.

Human-Approved Products:

Pentazocine Lactate Injection: 30 mg/ml in 10 ml vials and 1, 1.5, & 2 ml amps and pre-filled 2 ml carpuject syringes; *Talwin®* (Sanofi Winthrop) (Rx)

Pentazocine HCl 50 mg & Naloxone HCl 0.5 mg Tablets (Scored); *Talwin NX®* (Sanofi Winthrop); *Pentazocine & Naloxone HCl®* (Royce) (Rx)

Pentazocine HCl 12.5 mg & Aspirin 325 mg Tablets; *Talwin Compound Caplets®* (Sanofi Winthrop) (Rx)

Pentazocine HCl 25 mg & Acetominophen 650 mg Tablets; *Talacen Caplets®* (Sanofi Winthrop) (Rx)

Note: All pentazocine products are **Class-IV controlled substances** and are prescription items only.

PENTOBARBITAL SODIUM

(Note: Combinations of pentobarbital with other agents (*e.g.,* phenytoin) for euthanasia have a separate monograph listed under Euthanasia Agents)

Chemistry - Pentobarbital sodium occurs as odorless, slightly bitter tasting, white, crystalline powder or granules. It is very soluble in water and freely soluble in alcohol. The pK_a of the drug has been reported to range from 7.85-8.03 and the pH of the injection is from 9-10.5. Alcohol or propylene glycol may be added to enhance the stability of the injectable product.

Storage/Stability/Compatibility - The injectable product should be stored at room temperature; the suppositories should be kept refrigerated. The aqueous solution is not very stable and should not be used if it contains a precipitate. Because precipitates may occur, pentobarbital sodium should not be added to acidic solutions.

The following solutions and drugs have been reported to be **compatible** with pentobarbital sodium: dextrose IV solutions, Ringer's injection, lactated Ringer's injection, Saline IV solutions, dextrose-saline combinations, dextrose-Ringer's combinations, dextrose-Ringer's lactate combinations, amikacin sulfate, aminophylline, atropine sulfate(for at least 15 minutes, not 24 hours), calcium chloride, cephapirin sodium, chloramphenicol sodium succinate, hyaluronidase, hydromorphone HCl, lidocaine HCl, neostigmine methylsulfate, scopolamine HBr, sodium bicarbonate, sodium iodide, thiopental sodium, and verapamil HCl.

The following drugs have been reported to be **incompatible** with pentobarbital sodium: benzquinamide HCl, butorphanol tartrate, chlorpromazine HCl, cimetidine HCl, chlorpheniramine maleate, codeine phosphate, diphenhydramine HCl, droperidol, fentanyl citrate, glycopyrrolate, hydrocortisone sodium succinate, hydroxyzine HCl, insulin (regular), meperidine HCl, nalbuphine HCl, norepinephrine bitartrate, oxytetracycline HCl, penicillin G potassium, pentazocine lactate, phenytoin sodium, prochlorperazine edisylate, promazine HCl, promethazine HCl, and streptomycin sulfate. Compatibility is dependent upon factors such as pH, concentration, temperature, and diluents used and it is suggested to consult specialized references for more specific information.

Pharmacology -See the monograph: Barbiturates, Pharmacology of.

Uses/Indications - Once pentobarbital was the principal agent used for general anesthesia in small animals, but has been largely superceded by the inhalant anesthetic agents. It is still commonly used as an anesthetic in laboratory situations, for rodents and occasionally as a sedative agent in dogs and cats.

Pentobarbital is considered to be a drug of choice in dogs and cats for treating intractable seizures secondary to convulsant agents (*e.g.,* strychnine) or as a result of CNS toxins (*e.g.,* tetanus). It should not be used to treat seizures caused by lidocaine intoxication.

Pentobarbital has been used as a sedative and anesthetic agent in horses, cattle, swine, sheep and goats. Often the drug is given after a preanesthetic agent to reduce pentobarbital dosages and side effects.

Pentobarbital is a major active ingredient in several euthanasia solutions. This indication is discussed later in this section in the monograph for pentobarbital euthanasia solutions.

Pharmacokinetics - Pentobarbital is absorbed quite rapidly from the gut after oral or rectal administration with peak plasma concentrations occurring between 30-60 minutes after oral dosing in humans. The onset of action usually occurs within 15-60 minutes after oral dosing and within 1 minute after IV administration.

Pentobarbital, like all barbiturates, distributes rapidly to all body tissues with highest concentrations found in the liver and brain. It is 35-45% bound to plasma proteins in humans. Although less lipophilic than the ultra-short acting barbiturates (*e.g.,* thiopental), pentobarbital is highly lipid soluble and patient fat content may alter the distributive qualities of the drug. All barbiturates cross the placenta and enter milk (at concentrations far below those of plasma).

Pentobarbital is metabolized in the liver principally by oxidation. Excretion of the drug is not appreciably enhanced by increasing urine flow or alkalinizing the urine. Ruminants (especially sheep and goats) metabolize pentobarbital at a very rapid rate. The elimination half-life in the goat has been reported to be approximately 0.9 hrs. Conversely, the half-life in dogs is approximately 8 hours and ranges from 15-50 hours in man.

Contraindications/Precautions - Use cautiously in patients who are hypovolemic, anemic, have borderline hypoadrenal function, or cardiac or respiratory disease. Large doses are contraindicated in patients with nephritis or severe respiratory dysfunction. Barbiturates are contraindicated in patients with severe liver disease or who have demonstrated previous hypersensitivity reactions to them.

When administering IV, give SLOWLY. It is not recommended to be used for cesarian section because of fetal respiratory depression. Cats tend to particularly sensitive to the respiratory depressant effects of barbiturates; use with caution in this species. Female cats are more susceptible to the effects of pentobarbital than male cats.

Adverse Effects/Warnings - Because of the respiratory depressant effects of pentobarbital, respiratory activity must be closely monitored and respiratory assistance must be readily available when using anesthetic dosages. Pentobarbital may cause excitement in dogs during recovery from anesthetic doses. Hypothermia may develop in animals receiving pentobarbital if exposed to temperatures below 27°C (80.6°F). The barbiturates can be very irritating when administered SQ or perivascularly; avoid these types of injections. Do not administer intra-arterially.

Overdosage - In dogs, the reported oral LD_{50} is 85 mg/kg and IV LD_{50} is 40 - 60 mg/kg. Fatalities from ingestion of meat from animals euthanized by pentobarbital have been reported in dogs. Treatment of pentobarbital overdose consists of removal of ingested product from the gut if appropriate and offering respiratory and cardiovascular support. Forced alkaline diuresis is of little benefit for this drug. Peritoneal or hemodialysis may be of benefit in severe intoxications.

Drug Interactions - Most clinically significant interactions have been documented in humans with phenobarbital, however, these intreactions may also be of significance in animals receiving pentobarbital, especially with chronic therapy.

The following drugs may increase the effect of pentobarbital: **Other CNS depressants (narcotics, phenothiazines, antihistamines, etc), valproic acid, and chloramphenicol.**

Pentobarbital may decrease the effect of the following drugs: **oral anticoagulants, corticosteroids, beta-Blockers (propranolol), quinidine, theophylline, metronidazole.**

Pentobarbital with **furosemide** may cause or increase postural hypotension. Barbiturates may effect the metabolism of **phenytoin**, monitoring of blood levels may be indicated.

Fatalities have been reported when dogs suffering from **lidocaine** induced seizures were treated with pentobarbital. Until this interaction is further clarified, it is suggested that lidocaine-induced seizures in dogs be treated initially with diazepam.

Drug/Lab Interactions - Barbiturates may cause increased retention of bromosulfopthalein (**BSP**; sulfobromopthalein) and give falsely elevated results. It is recommended that barbiturates not be administered within the 24 hours before BSP retention tests.

Doses - Note: In order to avoid possible confusion, doses used for euthanasia are listed separately under the monograph for pentobarbital euthanasia solutions.

Dogs:
    As a sedative:
        a) 2 - 4 mg/kg IV (Kirk 1986)
        b) 2 - 4 mg/kg PO q6h (Davis 1985a)

For anesthesia:
  a) 30 mg/kg IV to effect (Kirk 1986)
  b) 10 - 30 mg/kg IV to effect (Morgan 1988)
  c) 24 - 33 mg/kg IV (Booth 1988a)

For chemical restraint for ventilatory support:
  a) 4 mg/kg initially IV; then 2 - 4 mg/kg/hr thereafter [Given concomitantly with oxy-
      morphone: 0.2 mg/kg (up to 4.5 mg) IV; then 0.1 mg/kg every 2 hours thereafter]
      (Pascoe 1986)

For post-myelographic seizures:
  a) 2 - 4 mg/kg IV (to effect) (Walter, Feeney, and Johnston 1986)

For status epilepticus:
  a) 5 - 15 mg/kg IV to effect (Morgan 1988)
  b) 3 - 15 mg/kg IV SLOWLY to effect. Goal is heavy sedation, not surgical planes of
      anesthesia. May need to repeat in 4-8 hours. (Raffe 1986)

Cats:
  As a sedative:
  a) 2 - 4 mg/kg IV (Kirk 1986)
  b) 2 - 4 mg/kg PO q6h (Davis 1985a)

  For status epilepticus:
  a) 5 - 15 mg/kg IV to effect (Morgan 1988)
  b) 3 - 15 mg/kg IV SLOWLY to effect. Goal is heavy sedation, not surgical planes of
      anesthesia. May need to repeat in 4-8 hours. (Raffe 1986)

  For anesthesia:
  a) 25 mg/kg IV, an additional 10 mg/kg IV may be given if initial dose is inadequate
      (Booth 1988a)

Cattle:
  a) 30 mg/kg IV to effect, repeat as needed for chlorinated hydrocarbon toxicity (Smith
      1986)
  b) As an anesthetic in calves (over one month of age): 15 - 30 mg/kg IV (Thurmon and
      Benson 1986)
  c) As a sedative in cattle: 1 - 2 grams IV in an adult cow (given until animal becomes
      unsteady and rear limb weakness occurs). 3 grams will usually induce recumbency.
      (Thurmon and Benson 1986)

Horses: Note: Pentobarbital is generally not considered an ideal agent for use in the adult horse
due to possible development of excitement and injury when the animal is "knocked down".
  a) 3 - 15 mg/kg IV (Robinson 1987)
  b) 15 - 18 mg/kg IV for light anesthesia (Schultz 1986)

Swine:
  a) 30 mg/kg IV to effect (Howard 1986)
  b) As an anesthetic: 15 - 30 mg/kg IV (Thurmon and Benson 1986)

Sheep:
  As an anesthetic:
  a) 20 - 30 mg/kg IV (Thurmon and Benson 1986)
  b) Adult Sheep: 11 - 54 mg/kg IV (average dose 24 mg/kg IV). Anesthesia required for
      longer than 15-30 minutes will require additional doses.
      Lambs: 15 - 26 mg/kg IV (will induce anesthesia for 15 minutes). Additional 5.5
      mg/kg IV will give another 30 minutes of effect. (Booth 1988a)

Goats:
  As an anesthetic:
  a) 20 - 30 mg/kg IV (Thurmon and Benson 1986)
  b) 25 mg/kg IV slowly, duration of satisfactory anesthesia will last only 20 minutes or
      so. (Booth 1988a)

Monitoring Parameters -
  1) Levels of consciousness and/or seizure control
  2) Respiratory and cardiac signs
  3) Body temperature
  4) If using chronically, routine blood counts and liver function tests should be performed.

Client Information - This drug is best used in an inpatient setting or with close professional supervision. If dosage forms are dispensed to clients, they must be in instructed to keep away from
children and should be dispensed in child-resistant packaging.

Dosage Forms/Preparations/FDA Approval Status/Withholding Times -
Veterinary-Approved Products:
Pentobarbital Sodium for Injection 64.8 mg/ml (1 grain/ml) 100 ml vials
Generic; (Rx)   Approved for use in dogs and cats.

Human-Approved Products:
Pentobarbital Sodium for Injection; 50 mg/ml in 1 & 2 ml syringes, 2 ml, 20 ml and 50 ml vials; (Rx)

Pentobarbital Sodium Oral Capsules; 50 mg, 100 mg capsules; (Rx)

Pentobarbital Sodium Rectal Suppositories; 30 mg, 60 mg, 120 mg, 200 mg in 12/pkg; (Rx)

A common trade name is *Nembutal Sodium*® (Abbott). May also be known as pentobarbitone sodium. Pentobarbital is a Class-II controlled substance and detailed records must be maintained with regard to its use and disbursement.

PENTOXIFYLLINE

Chemistry/Storage/Stability/Compatibility - A synthetic xanthine derivative structurally related to caffeine and theophylline, pentoxifylline occurs as a white, odorless, bitter-tasting, crystalline powder. At room temperature, approximately 77 mg are soluble in one ml of water and 63 mg in one ml of alcohol.

The commercially available tablets should be stored in well-closed containers, protected from light and at 15-30°C. Pentoxifylline is also known as oxpentifylline or BL-191.

Pharmacology - The mechanisms for pentoxifylline's actions are not fully understood. The drug increases erythrocyte flexibility probably by inhibiting erythrocyte phosphodiesterase and decreases blood viscosity by reducing plasma fibrinogen and increasing fibrinolytic activity.

Pentoxifylline is postulated to reduce negative endotoxic effects of cytokine mediators via its phosphodiesterase inhibition.

Uses/Indications - In horses, pentoxifylline has been used as adjunctive therapy for endotoxemia and in the treatment of navicular disease. At the time of writing, the drug is still under investigation to document both safety and efficacy for these purposes.

Pentoxifylline has been used in dogs to enhance healing and reduce inflammation caused by ulcerative dermatosis in Shelties and Collies and for other conditions where improved microcirculation may be of benefit.

Pentoxifylline's major indications for humans include symptomatic treatment of peripheral vascular disease (e.g., intermittent claudication, sickle cell disease, Raynaud's, etc.) and cerebrovascular diseases where blood flow may be impaired in the microvasculature.

Pharmacokinetics - A pharmacokinetic study done in horses showed high interpatient variability in absorption of oral dosage forms with peak levels occurring 1 - 10 hours after oral dosing. No significant difference in relative bioavailability was noted between whole and crushed extended-release tablets. The drug appears to rapidly eliminated (half life of about one hour after IV dosing). Because of the wide interpatient variability, the authors were unable to make dosing recommendations for clinical use.

In humans, pentoxifylline absorption from the gastrointestinal tract is rapid and almost complete, but a significant first-pass effect occurs. Food affects the rate, but not the extent of absorption. While the distributive characteristics have not been fully described, it is known that the drug enters maternal milk. Pentoxifylline is metabolized both in the liver and in erythrocytes and all identified metabolites appear to be active.

Contraindications/Precautions/Reproductive Safety - Pentoxifylline should be considered contraindicated in patients who have been intolerant to the drug or xanthines (e.g., theophylline, caffeine, theobromine) in the past and those with cerebral hemorrhage or retinal hemorrhage. It should be used cautiously in patients with severe hepatic or renal impairment and those at risk for hemorrhage.

Although safety in pregnant, lactating or breeding animals has not been established, studies in pregnant rats and rabbits demonstrated no overt teratogenicity. As pentoxifylline and its metabolites enter maternal milk, benefits to the mother should be weighed against the risks to offspring.

Adverse Effects/Warnings - Most commonly reported adverse effects involve the GI tract (vomiting/inappetence). There are reports of dizziness and headache occurring in a small percentage of humans receiving the drug. Other adverse effects, primarily GI, CNS and cardiovascular related have been reported in people, but are considered to occur rarely. Note: Veterinary experience is limited with pentoxifylline and animal adverse effects may differ.

Overdosage - Humans overdosed with pentoxifylline have demonstrated signs of flushing, seizures, hypotension, unconsciousness, agitation, fever, somnolence, GI distress and ECG changes. One patient who ingested 80 mg/kg recovered completely. Overdoses should be treated using the usual methods of appropriate gut emptying and supportive therapies.

Drug Interactions - Use of non-steroidal antiinflammatory agents with pentoxifylline in horses is controversial. Some sources state that when used for endotoxemia in horses, pentoxyfilline's beneficial effects are negated by **NSAIDs**, but one study showed superior efficacy when flunixin and pentoxifylline were used together compared with either used alone.

Ciprofloxacin (other quinolones too?) and **cimetidine** can increase pentoxifylline serum levels. Increased adverse effects of pentoxifylline may result.

When pentoxifylline is used with **warfarin** or other anticoagulants, increased risk of bleeding may result. Use together with enhanced monitoring and caution. **Theophylline** blood levels may be increased when used concurrently with pentoxifylline.

Doses -
  Dogs:
    a) For adjunctive therapy for ulcerative dermatosis of Shelties and Collies: 400 mg (one tablet) PO once daily or every other day if vomiting is a problem. If it can be reformulated into capsules, divide daily dose and give up to 3 times daily. (Ihrke and Gross 1997)
    b) For adjunctive treatment (with corticosteroids, vitamin E, etc) of dermatomyositis: 10 mg/kg PO once a day to every other day. Give with food. May result in improvement in 2-3 months of tx. (Buerger 1997)
    c) For adjunctive treatment of ear margin seborrhea: 400 mg (one tablet) PO per day; if dog weighs less than 10 kg: use 200 mg/day. (Rosychuck and Swartout 1997)

  Horses:
    a) To reduce the cytokine effects in endotoxemia: 8.5 mg/kg PO bid (considered to be experimental therapy) (Edens and Cargile 1997)
    b) For treatment of navicular disease: 6 grams per day PO for 6 weeks (Livesay 1996)

Monitoring Parameters - Efficacy and adverse effects

Client Information - To reduce the GI effects of pentoxifylline, give with food. Clients should understand that veterinary experience with this medication is limited and that the risk versus benefit profile is not well defined.

Dosage Forms/Preparations/FDA Approval Status -
  Veterinary-Approved Products: None
  Human-Approved Products:
    Pentoxifylline 400 mg extended-release tablets (pink); *Trental*® Tablets (Hoechst Marion Roussel), Generic; (Rx)

PHENOBARBITAL SODIUM
PHENOBARBITAL

Chemistry - Phenobarbital, a barbiturate, occurs as white, glistening, odorless, small crystals or as a white, crystalline powder with a melting point of 174°-178°C and a pK_a of 7.41. One gram is soluble in approximately 1000 ml of water, and 10 ml of alcohol. Compared to other barbiturates it has a low lipid solubility.

Phenobarbital sodium occurs as bitter-tasting, white, odorless, flaky crystals or crystalline granules or powder. It is very soluble in water, soluble in alcohol, and freely soluble in propylene glycol. The injectable product has a pH of 8.5-10.5.

Storage/Stability/Compatibility - Aqueous solutions of phenobarbital are not very stable. Propylene glycol is often used in injectable products to help stabilize the solution. Solutions of phenobarbital sodium should not be added to acidic solutions nor used if they contain a precipitate or are grossly discolored.

The following solutions and drugs have been reported to be **compatible** with phenobarbital sodium: Dextrose IV solutions, Ringer's injection, lactated Ringer's injection, Saline IV solutions, dextrose-saline combinations, dextrose-Ringer's combinations, dextrose-Ringer's lactate combinations, amikacin sulfate, aminophylline, atropine sulfate (for at least 15 minutes, not 24 hours), calcium chloride and gluconate, cephapirin sodium, dimenhydrinate, polymyxin B sulfate, sodium bicarbonate, thiopental sodium, and verapamil HCl.

The following drugs have been reported to be **incompatible** with phenobarbital sodium: benzquinamide HCl, cephalothin sodium, chlorpromazine HCl, codeine phosphate, ephedrine sulfate, fentanyl citrate, glycopyrrolate, hydralazine HCl, hydrocortisone sodium succinate, hydroxyzine HCl, insulin (regular), meperidine HCl, morphine sulfate, nalbuphine HCl, norepinephrine bitartrate, oxytetracycline HCl, pentazocine lactate, procaine HCl, prochlorperazine edisylate, promazine HCl, promethazine HCl, and streptomycin sulfate. Compatibility is dependent upon factors such as pH, concentration, temperature, and diluents used and it is suggested to consult specialized references (*e.g.,* Trissel - see bibliography) for more specific information.

Pharmacology - See the monograph: Barbiturates, Pharmacology of.

Uses/Indications - Because of its favorable pharmacokinetic profile, relative safety and efficacy, low cost, and ability to treat epilepsy at sub-hypnotic doses, phenobarbital is generally considered to be the drug of first choice when treating idiopathic epilepsy in dogs and cats. It is also occasionally used as an oral sedative agent in these species. Because it has a slightly longer onset of action, it is used principally in the treatment of status epilepticus in dogs, cats and horses to prevent the recurrence of seizures after they have been halted with either a benzodiazepine or short-acting barbiturate.

In cattle, the microsomal enzyme stimulating properties of phenobarbital have been suggested for its use in speeding the detoxification of organochlorine (chlorinated hydrocarbon) insecticide poisoning. Additionally, phenobarbital has been used in the treatment and prevention of neonatal hyperbilirubinemia in human infants. It is unknown if hyperbilirubinemia is effectively treated in veterinary patients with phenobarbital.

Pharmacokinetics - The pharmacokinetics of phenobarbital have been thoroughly studied in humans and studied in a more limited fashion in dogs and horses. Phenobarbital is slowly absorbed from the GI tract. Bioavailabilities range from 70-90% in humans, approximately 90% in dogs and absorption is practically complete in adult horses. Peak levels occur in 4-8 hours after oral dosing in dogs, and in 8-12 hours in humans.

Phenobarbital is widely distributed throughout the body, but because of its lower lipid solubility it does not distribute as rapidly as most other barbiturates into the CNS. The amount of phenobarbital bound to plasma proteins has been reported to be 40-50%. The reported apparent volumes of distribution are approximately: Horse $\approx$ 0.8 L/kg; Foals $\approx$ 0.86 L/kg; Dogs $\approx$ 0.75 L/kg.

The drug is metabolized in the liver primarily by hydroxylated oxidation to *p*-hydroxyphenobarbital. Sulfate and glucuronide conjugates are also formed. The elimination half-lives reported in humans range from 2-6 days; in dogs from 37-75 hours with an average of approximately 2 days. Elimination half lives in horses are considerably shorter with values reported of approximately 13 hours in foals and 18 hours in adult horses. Phenobarbital will induce hepatic microsomal enzymes and it can be expected that elimination half-lives will decrease with time. Approximately 25% of a dose is excreted unchanged by the kidney. By alkalinizing the urine and/or substantially increasing urine flow, excretion rates can be increased. Anuric or oliguric patients may accumulate unmetabolized drug and dosage adjustments may need to be made in these patients.

Contraindications/Precautions - Use cautiously in patients who are hypovolemic, anemic, have borderline hypoadrenal function, or cardiac or respiratory disease. Large doses are contraindicated in patients with nephritis or severe respiratory dysfunction. Barbiturates are contraindicated in patients with severe liver disease or who have demonstrated previous hypersensitivity reactions to them.

When administering IV, give slowly (not more than 60 mg/minute). Too rapid IV administration may cause respiratory depression. Commercially available injectable preparations (excluding the sterile powder) must not be administered subcutaneously or perivascularly as significant tissue irritation and possible necrosis may result. Applications of moist heat and local infiltration of 0.5% procaine HCl solution have been recommended to treat these reactions.

Adverse Effects/Warnings - Dogs may exhibit increased symptoms of anxiety and agitation when initiating therapy. These effects may be transitory in nature and often will resolve with small dosage increases. Occasionally dogs will exhibit profound depression at lower dosage ranges (and plasma levels). Polydipsia, polyuria, and polyphagia are also quite commonly displayed at moderate to high serum levels; these are best controlled by limiting intake of both food and water. Sedation and/or ataxia often become significant concerns as serum levels reach the higher ends of the therapeutic range. Increases in liver enzymes and anemias are more rare, but these potentially serious adverse effects have been reported in dogs. Cats may display a similar adverse reaction picture. Although there is much less information regarding its use in horses (and in particular foals), it would be generally expected that adverse effects would mirror those seen in other species.

Overdosage - Treatment of phenobarbital overdose consists of removal of ingested product from the gut if appropriate and offering respiratory and cardiovascular support. Activated charcoal has been demonstrated to be of considerable benefit in enhancing the clearance of phenobarbital, even when the drug was administered parenterally. Charcoal acts as a "sink" for the drug to diffuse from the vasculature back into the gut. Forced alkaline diuresis can also be of substantial benefit in augmenting the elimination of phenobarbital in patients with normal renal function. Peritoneal dialysis or hemodialysis may be helpful in severe intoxications or in anuric patients.

Drug Interactions - The following drugs may increase the effect of phenobarbital: **Other CNS depressants (narcotics, phenothiazines, antihistamines, etc), valproic acid, and chloramphenicol.**

Phenobarbital may decrease the effect of the following drugs: **oral anticoagulants, chloramphenicol, corticosteroids, doxycycline,** beta-**Blockers (propranolol), quinidine, theophylline, metronidazole.** Pentobarbital with **furosemide** may cause or increase postural hypotension. Barbiturates may effect the metabolism of **phenytoin**; monitoring of blood levels may be indicated.

Rifampin may induce hepatic microsomal enzymes and reduce the half-life and effect of phenobarbital.

Phenobarbital may decrease the absorption of **griseofulvin** if given concurrently.

Drug/Lab Interactions - Barbiturates may cause increased retention of bromosulfopthalein (BSP; sulfobromopthalein) and give falsely elevated results. It is recommended that barbiturates not be administered within the 24 hours before **BSP retention tests**; or if they must, (*e.g.,* for seizure control) the results be interpreted accordingly.

Doses -

Dogs:

For treatment of idiopathic epilepsy:
  a) 1 - 2 mg/kg PO *bid* initially, then monitor and adjust dosage. Some require up to 16 mg/kg/day. (Morgan 1988)
  b) 5 - 16 mg/kg/day divided *bid* or *tid* (Bunch 1986)
  c) Initially, 2.5 mg/kg PO *bid*, then monitor (some dogs may require up to 60 mg/kg/day) (Farnbach 1985)

For treatment of status epilepticus:
  a) 3 - 30 mg/kg IV to effect (Morgan 1988)
  b) 6 mg/kg IM or IV q6-12h as needed (Kirk 1986)

For sedation:
  a) 2.2 - 6.6 mg/kg PO *bid* (Walton 1986)
  b) Treatment of irritable bowel syndrome: 2.2 mg/kg PO *bid* (Morgan 1988)
  c) 2 mg/kg PO q8-12h (Davis 1985a)

Cats:

Treatment of idiopathic epilepsy:
  a) 8 mg - 15 mg PO once to twice daily (Morgan 1988)
  b) 2.2 - 4.4 mg/kg/day divided *bid* or *tid* (Bunch 1986)

Treatment of status epilepticus:
  a) 6 mg/kg IM or IV q6-12h as needed (Kirk 1986)

Sedation:
  a) 1 mg/kg PO *bid* (Morgan 1988)
  b) 2 mg/kg PO q8-12h (Davis 1985a)

Cattle:

For enzyme induction in organochlorine toxicity:
  a) 5 grams PO for 3-4 weeks, off 3-4 weeks, the repeat for 3-4 more weeks. (Smith 1986)

Horses:
  a) 1 - 10 mg/kg IV (Robinson 1987)
  b) Loading dose of 12 mg/kg IV over 20 minutes, then 6.65 mg/kg IV over 20 minutes every 12 hours (Duran et al. 1987)
  c) 11 mg/kg PO q24 hours (Ravis et al. 1987)
  d) Foals; for seizures: 20 mg/kg diluted with normal saline to a volume of 30-35 ml infused over 25-30 minutes IV, then 9 mg/kg diluted and infused as above q8h. Recommend monitoring serum levels if possible. (Spehar et al. 1984)

Monitoring Parameters -
  1) Anticonvulsant (or sedative) efficacy
  2) Adverse effects (CNS related, PU/PD, weight gain)
  3) Serum phenobarbital levels if lack of efficacy or adverse reactions noted. Although there is some disagreement among clinicians, therapeutic serum levels in dogs are thought to mirror those in people (15 - 40 micrograms/ml).
  4) If used chronically, routine CBC's and liver enzymes at least every 6 months.

Client Information - Compliance with therapy must be stressed to clients for successful epilepsy treatment. Encourage client to give doses at the same time each day. Keep medications out of reach of children and stored in child-resistant packaging. Veterinarian should be contacted if animal develops significant adverse reactions (including symptoms of anemia and/or liver disease) or seizure control is unacceptable.

Dosage Forms/Preparations/FDA Approval Status/Withholding Times -
Veterinary-Approved Products: None
Human-Approved Products:
Phenobarbital Tablets 15 mg, 16 mg, 16.2 mg, 30 mg, 60 mg, 100 mg; Capsules 16 mg

Phenobarbital Elixir 15 mg/5ml in pt and UD 5, 10 & 20 ml, 20 mg/5ml in pt, gal, UD 5 and 7.5 ml

Phenobarbital Sodium for Injection 30 mg/ml, 60 mg/ml, 65 mg/ml, 130 mg/ml; in 1 ml amps, Tubex and vials

Also known as phenyethylmalonylurea or phenobarbitone. Other trade names may include: *Luminal*® (Winthrop-Breon), and *Barbita*® (Vortech). Phenobarbital is a **Class-IV controlled substance** and is available by prescription (Rx) only.

PHENOXYBENZAMINE HCL

Chemistry - An alpha-adrenergic blocking agent, phenoxybenzamine HCl occurs as an odorless, white crystalline powder with a melting range of 136°-141° and a pK_a of 4.4. Approximately 40 mg is soluble in 1 ml of water and 167 mg is soluble in 1 ml of alcohol.

Storage/Stability/Compatibility - Phenoxybenzamine capsules should be stored at room temperature in well-closed containers.

Pharmacology - Alpha-adrenergic response to circulating epinephrine or norepinepinephrine is noncompetitively blocked by phenoxybenzamine. The effects of phenoxybenzamine have been described as a "chemical sympathectomy". No effects on beta-adrenergic receptors or on the parasympathetic nervous system occur.

Phenoxybenzamine causes cutaneous blood flow to increase, but little effects are noted on skeletal or cerebral blood flow. Phenoxybenzamine can also block pupillary dilation, lid retraction, and nictitating membrane contraction. Both standing and supine blood pressures are decreased in humans.

Uses/Indications - Phenoxybenzamine is used in small animals primarily for its effect in reducing internal urethral sphincter tone in dogs and cats when urethral sphincter hypertonus is present. It can also be used to treat the hypertension associated with pheochromocytoma prior to surgery or as adjunctive therapy in endotoxicosis.

In horses, phenoxybenzamine has been used for preventing or treating laminitis in its early stages and to treat secretory diarrheas.

Pharmacokinetics - No information was located on the pharmacokinetics of this agent in veterinary species. In humans, phenoxybenzamine is variably absorbed from the GI, with a bioavailability of 20-30%. Onset of action of the drug is slow (several hours) and increases over several days after regular dosing. Effects persist for 3-4 days after discontinuation of the drug.

Phenoxybenzamine is highly lipid soluble and may accumulate in body fat. It is unknown if phenoxybenzamine crosses the placenta or is excreted into milk. The serum half-life of phenoxybenzamine is approximately 24 hours in humans. It is metabolized (dealkylated) and excreted in both the urine and bile.

Contraindications/Precautions - Phenoxybenzamine is contraindicated in horses with symptoms of colic and in patients when symptoms of hypotension would be undesirable (*e.g.,* shock, unless fluid replacement is adequate). One author (Labato 1988) lists glaucoma and diabetes mellitus as contraindications for the use of phenoxybenzamine in dogs.

Phenoxybenzamine should be used with caution in patients with CHF or other heart disease as drug-induced tachycardia can occur. It should be used cautiously in patients with renal damage or cerebral/coronary arteriosclerosis.

Adverse Effects/Warnings - Adverse effects associated with alpha-adrenergic blockade include: hypotension, hypertension, miosis, increased intraocular pressure, tachycardia, inhibition of ejaculation and nasal congestion. Additionally, it can cause weakness/dizziness and GI effects (*e.g.,* nausea, vomiting). Constipation may occur in horses.

Overdosage - Overdosage of phenoxybenzamine may yield signs of postural hypotension (dizziness, syncope), tachycardia, vomiting, lethargy or shock.

Treatment should consist of emptying the gut if the ingestion was recent and there are no contraindications to those procedures. Hypotension can be treated with fluid support. Epinephrine is contraindicated (see Drug Interactions) and most vasopressor drugs are ineffective in reversing the effects of alpha-blockade. Intravenous norepinephrine (levarterenol) may be beneficial, however, if symptoms are severe.

Drug Interactions - Phenoxybenzamine will antagonize the effects of alpha-adrenergic sympathomimetic agents (*e.g.,* **phenylephrine**).

If used with drugs that have both alpha– and beta–adrenergic effects (*e.g.,* **epinephrine**), increased hypotension, vasodilatation or tachycardia may result.

Doses - **Note:**Because the only dosage form available is a 10 mg capsule, doses should be rounded to the nearest 2.5 mg dose when possible.

Dogs:
Treatment of detrusor areflexia:
a) 5 mg - 15 mg PO once daily. (Chew, DiBartola, and Fenner 1986)
b) Initially, 10 mg PO once daily; if no response after 4 days, may increase dose to 10 mg PO q12h. If after 4 more days there is no response, increase dose to 10 mg PO q8h. (Polzin and Osborne 1985)
c) 2.5 - 30 mg PO *tid* (Labato 1988)

Treatment of hypertension associated with pheochromocytoma:
a) 0.2 - 1.5 mg/kg PO *bid* for 10-14 days before surgery; start at low end of dosage range and increase until blood pressure reduced to desired range. Propranolol (0.15 - 0.5 mg/kg PO *tid*) may be added to help control arrhythmias and hypertension. Beta-blockers must be used with phenoxybenzamine or severe hypertension may result. (Wheeler 1986)

For adjunctive treatment of endotoxicosis (with appropriate antimicrobial agents, steroids (if indicated), and other supportive care):
a) 0.25 - 0.5 mg/kg PO q6h. (Coppock and Mostrom 1986)

Cats:
Treatment of detrusor areflexia:
a) 0.5 mg/kg PO once daily (Usually 2.5 mg). May increase gradually by 2.5 mg to a maximum of 10 mg. Therapy should be attempted for at least 5 days before evaluation and increase in dose. (Barsanti and Finco 1986)
b) Initially 0.25 mg/kg PO q8h; may gradually increase dose to 0.5 mg/kg PO q8h, if necessary. (Polzin and Osborne 1985)

Horses:
a) 0.66 mg/kg in 500 ml saline IV (Robinson 1987)
b) 1.2 mg/kg PO, followed in 12 hours by 0.6 mg/kg PO for 2 doses (Schultz 1986)
c) 200 - 600 mg q12h for treatment of profuse, watery diarrhea. (Clark 1988)

Monitoring Parameters - 1) Clinical efficacy (adequate urination, etc.) 2) Blood pressure, if necessary/possible

Client Information - Contact veterinarian if animal has continuing problems with weakness, appears dizzy or collapses after standing, or has persistent vomiting. GI upset may be reduced if the drug is given with meals.

Dosage Forms/Preparations/FDA Approval Status/Withholding Times -
  Veterinary-Approved Products: None
  Human-Approved Products:
    Phenoxybenzamine HCl 10 mg Capsules; *Dibenzyline*® (SKF); (Rx)

PHENYLBUTAZONE

Chemistry - A synthetic pyrazolone derivative related chemically to aminopyrine, phenylbutazone occurs as a white to off-white, odorless crystalline powder that has a pK_a of 4.5. It is very slightly soluble in water and 1 gram will dissolve in 28 ml of alcohol. It is tasteless at first, but has a slightly bitter after-taste.

Storage/Stability/Compatibility - Oral products should be stored in tight, child-resistant containers if possible. The injectable product should be stored in a cool place (46 - 56° F) or kept refrigerated.

Pharmacology - Phenylbutazone has analgesic, anti-inflammatory, antipyrexic, and mild uricosuric properties. The proposed mechanism of action is by the inhibition of cyclooxygenase, thereby reducing prostaglandin synthesis. Other pharmacologic actions phenylbutazone may induce include reduced renal blood flow and decreased glomerular filtration rate, decreased platelet aggregation, and gastric mucosal damage.

Pharmacokinetics - Following oral administration, phenylbutazone is absorbed from both the stomach and small intestine. The drug is distributed throughout the body with highest levels attained in the liver, heart, lungs, kidneys, and blood. Plasma protein binding in horses exceeds 99%. Both phenylbutazone and oxyphenbutazone cross the placenta and are excreted into milk.

The serum half-life in the horse ranges from 3.5-6 hours, and like aspirin is dose-dependent. Therapeutic efficacy however, may last for more than 24 hours however, probably due to the irreversible binding of phenylbutazone to cyclooxygenase. In horses and other species, phenylbutazone is nearly completely metabolized, primarily to oxphenbutazone (active) and gamma-hydroxyphenylbutazone. Oxyphenbutazone has been detected in horse urine for up to 48 hours after a single dose. Phenylbutazone is more rapidly excreted into alkaline than into acidic urine .

Other serum half-lives reported for animals are: Cattle ≈ 40 - 55 hrs; Dogs ≈ 2.5 - 6 hrs; Swine ≈ 2 - 6 hrs.; Rabbits ≈ 3 hrs..

Uses/Indications - One manufacturer lists the following as the indications for phenylbutazone: "For the relief of inflammatory conditions associated with the musculoskeletal system in dogs and horses." (Package Insert; *Butazolidin*® — Coopers). It has been used primarily for the treatment of lameness in horses and occasionally as an analgesic/anti-inflammatory, antipyrexic in dogs, cattle, and swine.

Contraindications/Precautions - Phenylbutazone is contraindicated in patients with a history of, or preexisting hematologic or bone marrow abnormalities, preexisting GI ulcers, and in food producing animals or lactating dairy cattle. Cautious use in both foals and ponies is recommended because of increased incidences of hypoproteinemia and GI ulceration. Foals with a heavy parasite burden or that are undernourished may be more susceptible to development of adverse effects.

Phenylbutazone may cause decreased renal blood flow and sodium and water retention, and should be used cautiously in animals with preexisting renal disease or CHF.

Because phenylbutazone may mask symptoms of lameness in horses for several days following therapy, it can be used by unethical individuals to disguise lameness for "soundness" exams. States may have different standards regarding the use of phenylbutazone in track animals. Complete elimination of phenylbutazone in horses may take 2 months and it can be detected in the urine for at least 7 days following administration.

Although phenylbutazone has shown no direct teratogenic effects, rodent studies have demonstrated reduced litter sizes, increased neonatal mortality, and increased stillbirth rates. Phenylbutazone should therefore be used in pregnancy only when the potential benefits of therapy outweigh the risks associated with it.

Phenylbutazone is contraindicated in patients demonstrating previous hypersensitivity reactions to it, and should be used very cautiously in patients that have a history of allergies to other drugs.

Adverse Effects/Warnings - The primary concerns with phenylbutazone therapy in humans include its bone marrow effects (agranulocytosis, aplastic anemia), renal and cardiovascular effects (fluid retention to acute renal failure), and GI effects (dyspepsia to perforated ulcers). Other serious concerns with phenylbutazone include hypersensitivity reactions, neurologic, dermatologic, and hepatic toxicities.

While phenylbutazone is apparently a safer drug to use in horses and dogs than in people, serious adverse reactions can still occur. Toxic effects that have been reported in horses include oral and GI erosions and ulcers, hypoalbuminemia, diarrhea, anorexia, and renal effects (azotemia, renal papillary necrosis). Unlike humans, it does not appear that phenylbutazone causes much sodium and water retention in horses at usual doses, but edema has been reported. In dogs however, phenylbutazone may cause sodium and water retention, and diminished renal blood flow. Phenylbutazone-induced blood dyscrasias have also been reported in dogs.

Do not administer injectable preparation IM or SQ, as it is very irritating (swelling, to necrosis and sloughing). Intracarotid injections may cause CNS stimulation and seizures.

Therapy should be halted at first signs of any toxic reactions (*e.g.,* anorexia, oral lesions, depression, reduced plasma proteins, increased serum creatinine or BUN, leukopenia, or anemias). The use of sucralfate or the H_2 blockers (cimetidine, ranitidine) have been suggested for use in treating the GI effects. Misoprostol, a prostaglandin E analog, may also be useful in reducing the gastrointestinal effects of phenylbutazone.

Overdosage - Manifestations (human) of acute overdosage with phenylbutazone include, a prompt respiratory or metabolic acidosis with compensatory hyperventilation, seizures, coma, and acute hypotensive crisis. In an acute overdose, symptoms of renal failure (oliguric, with proteinuria and hematuria), liver injury (hepatomegaly and jaundice), bone marrow depression, and ulceration (and perforation) of the GI tract may develop. Other symptoms reported in humans include: nausea, vomiting, abdominal pain, diaphoresis, neurologic and psychiatric symptoms, edema, hypertension, respiratory depression, and cyanosis.

Standard overdose procedures should be followed (empty gut following oral ingestion, etc.). Supportive treatment should be instituted as necessary and intravenous diazepam used to help control seizures. Monitor fluid therapy carefully, as phenylbutazone may cause fluid retention.

Drug Interactions - Both phenylbutazone and the active metabolite oxyphenbutazone are highly bound to plasma proteins and may displace other highly bound drugs. This mechanism may affect serum levels and duration of actions of **phentoin, valproic acid, oral anticoagulants**, other **antiinflammatory agents, sulfonamides**, and the **sulfonylurea antidiabetic agents**.

Phenylbutazone and oxyphenbutazone can induce hepatic microsomal enzymes and increase the metabolism of drugs affected by this system (*e.g.,* **digitoxin & phenytoin**). Conversely, other microsomal enzyme inducers (*e.g.,* **barbiturates, promethazine, rifampin, corticosteroids, or chlorpheniramine, diphenhydramine**) may decrease the plasma half-life of phenylbutazone.

Phenylbutazone may increase the plasma half-life of **penicillin G or lithium**. Phenylbutazone administered concurrently with **hepatotoxic drugs** may increase the chances of hepatotoxicity developing.

Phenylbutazone may antagonize the increased renal blood flow effects caused by **furosemide**.

Concurrent use with **other NSAIDs** may increase the potential for adverse reactions developing, however many clinicians routinely use phenylbutazone concomitantly with flunixin in horses.

Laboratory Test Interference - Phenylbutazone and oxyphenbutazone may interfere with **thyroid function tests** by competing with thyroxine at protein binding sites or by inhibiting thyroid iodine uptake.

Doses -

Dogs:
- a) 14 mg/kg PO *tid* initially (maximum of 800 mg/day regardless of weight), titrate dose to lowest effective dose (Package Insert; *Butazolidin®* - Coopers)
- b) For analgesia/phlebitis: 3-5 mg/kg PO *tid*; for analgesia/spinal disorders: 8-10 mg/kg PO *tid* (max. 800 mg/day); for antiinflammation/arthritis: 13 mg/kg PO *tid* for 48 hrs, then taper dose to lowest effective dose (max. of 800 mg/day). (Morgan 1988)

Cattle:
- a) 4 mg/kg IV or orally q24h (Koritz 1986)
- b) 4 - 8 mg/kg PO or 2 - 5 mg/kg IV (Howard 1986)
- c) 10 - 20 mg/kg PO, then 2.5 - 5.0 mg/kg q24h or 10 mg/kg every 48 hours PO (Jenkins 1987)

Horses:
- a) 4.4 - 8.8 mg/kg q24hrs PO or 3-6 mg/kg q12h IV (Do not exceed 8.8 mg/kg/day (Jenkins 1987)
- b) 1 - 2 grams IV per 454 kg (1000 lb.) horse. Injection should be made slowly and with care. Limit IV administration to no more than 5 successive days of therapy. Follow with oral forms if necessary; or 2 - 4 grams PO per 454kg (1000 lb.) horse. Do not exceed 4 grams/day. Use high end of dosage range initially, then titrate to lowest effective dose. (Package Insert; *Butazolidin®* - Coopers)
- c) 4.4 mg/kg PO twice on the first day, then 2.2 mg/kg PO *bid* for 4 days, then 2.2 mg/kg PO once daily or every other day. (Taylor et al. 1983)

Swine:
- a) 4 mg/kg IV or orally q24h (Koritz 1986)
- b) 4 - 8 mg/kg PO or 2 - 5 mg/kg IV (Howard 1986)

Monitoring Parameters - 1) Analgesic/anti-inflammatory/antipyrexic effect 2) Regular complete blood counts with chronic therapy (especially in dogs). The manufacturer recommends weekly CBC's early in therapy, and biweekly with chronic therapy 3) Urinalysis &/or renal function parameters (serum creatinine/BUN) with chronic therapy 4) Plasma protein determinations, especially in ponies, foals, and debilitated animals.

Client Information/FDA Approval Status - Do not administer injectable preparation IM or SQ.

Approved for use in dogs and horses not intended for food. While phenylbutazone is not approved for use in cattle, it is used. A general guideline for meat withdrawal times are: one dose=30 days, 2 doses=35 days, and 3 doses=40 days. Phenylbutazone is a veterinary prescription drug.

Dosage Forms/Preparations (Veterinary) -

Phenylbutazone Tablets 100 mg, 400 mg, 1 gram tablets; 2 gram boluses, 4 gram boluses *; Butazolidin®* (Schering); also available generically

Phenylbutazone Paste Oral syringes containing 6 grams or 12 grams/syringe; *Butazolidin® Paste* (Schering); *Phenylzone® Paste* (Luitpold)

Phenylbutazone Oral Gel: Each 30 grams of gel contains 4 grams phenylbutazone, 30 grams (of gel) per syringe; *Butatron®* (Rhone Merieux)

Phenylbutazone Micro-encapsulated powder; *Equipalazone®* (Steri-Vet); 1 gm packets, 60's

Phenylbutazone Injection 200 mg/ml; 100 ml vials; *Butazolidin®* (Schering); generic

PHENYLEPHRINE HCL

Chemistry - An alpha-adrenergic sympathomimetic amine, phenylephrine HCl occurs as bitter-tasting, odorless, white to nearly white crystals with a melting point of 145 - 146°C. It is freely soluble in water and alcohol. The pH of the commercially available injection is 3.0 - 6.5.

Storage/Stability/Compatibility - The injectable product should be stored protected from light. Do not use solutions if they are brown or contain a precipitate. Oxidation of the drug can occur without a color change. To protect against oxidation, the air in commercially available ampules for injection is replaced with nitrogen and a sulfite added.

Phenylephrine is reported to be **compatible** with all commonly used IV solutions and the following drugs: chloramphenicol sodium succinate, dobutamine HCl, lidocaine HCl, potassium chloride, and sodium bicarbonate. While stated to be incompatible with alkalies, it is stable with sodium bicarbonate solutions. Phenylephrine is reported to be **incompatible** with ferric salts, oxidizing agents, and metals.

Pharmacology - Phenylephrine has predominantly post-synaptic alpha-adrenergic effects at therapeutic doses. At usual doses it has negligible beta effects, but beta effects can occur at high doses.

Phenylephrine's primary effects, when given intravenously, include peripheral vasoconstriction with resultant increase in diastolic and systolic blood pressures, small decreases in cardiac output and an increase in circulation time. A reflex bradycardia (blocked by atropine) can occur. Most vascular beds are constricted (renal splanchnic, pulmonary, cutaneous), but coronary blood flow is increased. Its alpha effects can cause contraction of the pregnant uterus and constriction of uterine blood vessels.

Uses/Indications - Phenylephrine has been used to treat hypotension and shock (after adequate volume replacement), but many clinicians prefer to use an agent that also has cardiostimulatory properties. It may be of benefit, however, when cardiostimulation would be undesirable, such as during general anesthesia (halothane) or if the patient is also receiving other agents that sensitize the myocardium. Phenylephrine is recommended to be used to treat hypotension secondary to drug overdoses or idiosyncratic hypotensive reactions to drugs such as phenothiazines, adrenergic blocking agents, and ganglionic blockers. Its use to treat hypotension resulting from barbiturate or other CNS depressant agents is controversial. Phenylephrine has been used to increase blood pressure to terminate attacks of paroxysmal supraventricular tachycardia, particularly when the patient is also hypotensive. Phenylephrine has been used to treat both hypotension and to prolong the effects of spinal anesthesia.

Ophthalmic uses of phenylephrine include use for some diagnostic eye examinations, to reduce posterior synchiae formation and relieve pain associated with complicated uveitis. It has been applied intranasally in an attempt to reduce nasal congestion.

Pharmacokinetics - After oral administration, phenylephrine is rapidly metabolized in the GI tract and cardiovascular effects are generally unattainable via this route of administration. Following IV administration, pressor effects begin almost immediately and will persist for up to 20 minutes. The onset of pressor action after IM administration is usually within 10-15 minutes, and will last for approximately one hour.

It is unknown if phenylephrine is excreted into milk. It is metabolized by the liver, and the effects of the drug are also terminated by uptake into tissues.

Contraindications/Precautions - Phenylephrine is contraindicated in patients with severe hypertension, ventricular tachycardia or those who are hypersensitive to it. It should be used with extreme caution in geriatric patients, patients with hyperthyroidism, bradycardia, partial heart block or with other heart disease. Phenylephrine is not a replacement for adequate volume therapy in patients with shock.

Adverse Effects/Warnings - At usual doses, a reflex bradycardia, CNS effects (excitement, restlessness, headache) and, rarely, arrhythmias are seen. Blood pressure must be monitored to prevent hypertension.

Extravasation injuries with phenylephrine can be very serious (necrosis and sloughing of surrounding tissue). Patient's IV sites should be routinely monitored. Should extravasation occur, infiltrate the site (ischemic areas) with a solution of 5-10 mg phentolamine (Regitine®) in 10-15 ml of normal saline. A syringe with a fine needle should be used to infiltrate the site with many injections.

Overdosage - Overdosage of phenylephrine can cause hypertension, seizures, vomiting, paresthesias, ventricular extrasystoles and cerebral hemorrhage. Hypertension, if severe, can be treated by the administration of phentolamine (an alpha blocking agent). Should cardiac arrhythmias require treatment, use a beta-blocking drug such as propranolol.

Drug Interactions - Higher dosages of phenylephrine may be required to attain a pressor effect, if **phenothiazines** or an alpha-blocking agent (**phentolamine**) have been used prior to therapy.

Phenylephrine may induce cardiac arrhythmias when used with **halothane** anesthesia or in **digitalized** patients.

When used concurrently with **oxytocic agents,** pressor effects may be enhanced.

Atropine will block the reflex bradycardia that phenylephrine causes. **Monoamine oxidase (MAO) inhibitors** should not be used with phenylephrine because of a pronounced pressor effect.

Doses -
Dogs:
a) As a constant rate infusion: 1 - 3 mcg/kg/minute in either 0.9% sodium chloride or D$_5$W (Dhupa and Shaffron 1995)
b) 0.1 mg IV, 1.0 mg IM (Enos and Keiser 1985)

Cats:
a) As a constant rate infusion: 1 - 3 mcg/kg/minute in either 0.9% sodium chloride or D$_5$W (Dhupa and Shaffron 1995)

Horses:
a) 5 mg IV (Enos and Keiser 1985)

Monitoring Parameters -
1) Cardiac rate/rhythm
2) Blood pressure, and blood gases if possible

Client Information - Parenteral phenylephrine should only be used by professionals in a setting where adequate monitoring is possible.

Dosage Forms/Preparations/FDA Approval Status/Withholding Times -
Veterinary-Approved Products: None
Human-Approved Products:

Phenylephrine HCl for Injection 10 mg/ml in ml amps; *Neo-Synephrine*® ((Sanofi Winthrop); generic; (Rx)

Phenylephrine is also available in ophthalmic and intranasal dosage forms and in combination with antihistamines, analgesics, decongestants, etc., for oral administration in humans.

PHENYLPROPANOLAMINE HCL

Chemistry - A sympathomimetic amine, phenylpropanolamine HCl occurs as a white, crystalline powder with a slightly aromatic odor, a melting range between 191° - 194°C, and a pK$_a$ of 9.4. One gram is soluble in approximately 1.1 ml of water or 7 ml of alcohol. Phenylpropanolamine HCl may also be known as *dl*-Norephedrine HCl.

Storage/Stability/Compatibility - Store phenylpropanolamine products at room temperature in light-resistant, tight containers.

Pharmacology - While the exact mechanism of phenylpropanolamine's actions are undetermined, it is believed that it indirectly stimulates both alpha- and beta-adrenergic receptors by causing the release of norepinephrine. Prolonged use or excessive dosing frequency can deplete norepinephrine from its storage sites, and tachyphylaxis (decreased response) may ensue. Tachyphylaxis has not been documented in dogs or cats, however, when used for urethral sphincter hypotonus.

Pharmacologic effects of phenylpropanolamine include increased vasoconstriction, heart rate, coronary blood flow, blood pressure, mild CNS stimulation, and decreased nasal congestion and appetite. Phenylpropanolamine can also increase urethral sphincter tone and produce closure of the bladder neck; its principle veterinary indications are as a result of these effects.

Uses/Indications - Phenylpropanolamine is used chiefly for the treatment of urethral sphincter hypotonus and resulting incontinence in dogs and cats. It has also been used in an attempt to treat nasal congestion in small animals.

Pharmacokinetics - No information was located on the pharmacokinetics of this agent in veterinary species. In humans, phenylpropanolamine is readily absorbed after oral administration and has an onset of action (nasal decongestion) of about 15-30 minutes and a duration of effect of approximately 3 hours (regular capsules or tablets).

Phenylpropanolamine is reportedly distributed into various tissues and fluids, including the CNS. It is unknown if it crosses the placenta or enters milk. The drug is partially metabolized to an active metabolite, but 80-90% is excreted unchanged in the urine within 24 hours of dosing. The serum half-life is approximately 3-4 hours.

Contraindications/Precautions - Phenylpropanolamine should be used with caution in patients with glaucoma, prostatic hypertrophy, hyperthyroidism, diabetes mellitus, cardiovascular disorders or hypertension. Phenylpropanolamine may cause decreased ovum implantation; uncontrolled clinical experience, however, has not demonstrated any untoward effects during pregnancy.

Adverse Effects/Warnings - Most likely side effects include restlessness, irritability and hypertension. Anorexia may be a problem in some animals.

Overdosage - Symptoms of overdosage may consist of an exacerbation of the adverse effects listed above or, if a very large overdose, severe cardiovascular (hypertension to rebound hypotension, bradycardias to tachycardias, and cardiovascular collapse) or CNS effects (stimulation to coma) can be seen.

If the overdose was recent, empty the stomach using the usual precautions and administer charcoal and a cathartic. Treat symptoms supportively as they occur.

Drug Interactions - Phenylpropanolamine should not be administered with other **sympathomimetic agents** (*e.g.,* **ephedrine**) as increased toxicity may result.

Phenylpropanolamine should not be given within two weeks of a patient receiving **monoamine oxidase inhibitors**.

An increased chance of hypertension developing can result if phenylpropanolamine is given concomitantly with **indomethicin (or other NSAIDs, including aspirin), reserpine, tricyclic antidepressants, or ganglionic blocking agents**.

An increased risk of arrhythmias developing can occur if phenylpropanolamine is administered to patients who have received **cyclopropane** or a **halogenated hydrocarbon anesthetic agent**. Propranolol may be administered should these occur.

Doses -
  Dogs:
    For urethral sphincter hypotonus:
      a) 12.5 - 50 mg PO q8h (Labato 1988), (Polzin and Osborne 1985)
      b) 1.1 mg/kg PO q8h; dosage should be rounded to the nearest 12.5 mg for practical dosing. (Plumb 1988)

  Cats:
    For urethral sphincter hypotonus:
      a) 12.5 mg PO q8h (Labato 1988), (Polzin and Osborne 1985)
      b) One 75 mg sustained-release capsule once daily PO (Cornell 1985)

Monitoring Parameters -
    1) Clinical effectiveness
    2) Adverse effects (see above)
    3) Blood pressure, if possible

Client Information - For this drug to be effective, it must be administered as directed by the veterinarian; missed doses will negate its effect. It may take several days for the full benefit of the drug to take place. Contact veterinarian if the animal demonstrates ongoing changes in behavior (restlessness, irritability) or if incontinence persists or increases.

Dosage Forms/Preparations/FDA Approval Status/Withholding Times -
  Veterinary-Approved Products: None
  Human-Approved Products: Note: Phenylpropanolamine is available in combination with many other agents, including antihistamines, analgesics, decongestants, antitussives and expectorants. Sustained release capsules and tablets are also available. Most veterinary use has been with the non-sustained release oral tablets. A listing of these products follow:

  Phenylpropanolamine 25 mg, 50 mg Tablets; *Propagest*® (Reed & Carnick); generic, (OTC)

  Phenylpropanolamine Capsules, Timed Release 75 mg; Various (OTC)

PHENYTOIN SODIUM

Chemistry - A hydantoin-derivative, phenytoin sodium occurs as a white, hygroscopic powder which is freely soluble in water and warm propylene glycol, and soluble in alcohol.

Because phenytoin sodium slowly undergoes partial hydrolysis in aqueous solutions to phenytoin (base) with the resultant solution becoming turbid, the commercial injection contains 40% propylene glycol and 10% alcohol. The pH of the injectable solution is approximately 12.

Phenytoin sodium is used in the commercially available capsules (both extended and prompt) and the injectable preparations. Phenytoin (base) is used in the oral tablets and suspensions. Each 100 mg of phenytoin sodium contains 92 mg of the base.

Storage/Stability/Compatibility - Store capsules at room temperature (below 86°F) and protect from light and moisture. Store phenytoin sodium injection at room temperature and protect from freezing. If injection is frozen or refrigerated, a precipitate may form which should resolubilize when warmed. A slight yellowish color will not affect either potency or efficacy, but do not use precipitated solutions. Injectable solutions at less than a pH of 11.5 will precipitate. No problems with adsorption to plastic have been detected thus far.

Phenytoin sodium injection is generally incompatible with most IV solutions (upon standing) and drugs. It has been successfully mixed with sodium bicarbonate and verapamil HCl.

Because an infusion of phenytoin sodium is sometimes desirable, several studies have been performed to determine whether such a procedure can be safely done. The general conclusions and recommendations of these studies are: 1) use either normal saline or lactated Ringer's; 2) a concentration of 1 mg/ml phenytoin be used; 3) start infusion immediately and complete in a relatively short time; 4) use a 0.22 μm in-line IV filter; 5) watch the admixture carefully.

Pharmacology - The anticonvulsant actions of phenytoin are thought to be caused by the promotion of sodium efflux from neurons, thereby inhibiting the spread of seizure activity in the motor cortex. It is believed that excessive stimulation or environmental changes can alter the sodium gradient which may lower the threshold for seizure spread. Hydantoins tend to stabilize this threshold and limit seizure propagation from epileptogenic foci.

The cardiac electrophysiologic effects of phenytoin are similar (not identical) to that of lidocaine (Group 1B). It depresses phase O slightly and can shorten the action potential. Its principle cardiac use is in the treatment of digitalis-induced ventricular arrhythmias.

Phenytoin can inhibit insulin and vasopressin (ADH) secretion.

Uses/Indications - Because of its undesirable pharmacokinetic profiles in dogs and cats, the use of phenytoin as an anticonvulsant for long term treatment of epilepsy has diminished over the years. It remains however, as an alternative or adjunctive therapy in dogs who have not responded to, or have developed severe adverse reactions from either phenobarbital or primidone. Prerequisites for successful therapy include: a motivated client who will be compliant with multiple daily dosing and who is willing to assume the financial burden of high dose phenytoin therapy and therapeutic drug monitoring expenses.

Although not commonly used, phenytoin has been employed as an oral or IV antiarrhythmic agent in both dogs and cats. It has been described as the drug of choice for digitalis-induced ventricular arrhythmias in dogs.

It has been suggested that phenytoin be used as adjunctive treatment of hypoglycemia secondary to hyperinsulinism, but apparently little clinical benefit has resulted from this therapy.

Pharmacokinetics - After oral administration, phenytoin is nearly completely absorbed in humans, but in dogs, bioavailabilities may only be about 40%. Phenytoin is well distributed throughout the body and is about 78% bound to plasma proteins in dogs (vs. 95% in humans). Protein binding may be reduced in uremic patients. Small amounts of phenytoin may be excreted into the milk and it readily crosses the placenta.

The drug is metabolized in the liver and with much of the drug conjugated to a glucuronide form and then excreted by the kidneys. Phenytoin will induce hepatic microsomal enzymes which may enhance the metabolism of itself and other drugs. The serum half-life (elimination) differences between various species are striking. Phenytoin has reported half-lives of 2-8 hours in dogs, 8 hours in horses, 15-24 hours in humans, and 42-108 hours in cats. Because of the pronounced induction of hepatic enzymes in dogs, phenytoin metabolism is increased with shorter half-lives within 7-9 days after starting treatment. Puppies have a smaller volumes of distribution and shorter elimination half-lives (1.6 hours) than adult dogs.

Contraindications/Precautions - Some data suggest that additive hepatotoxicity may result if phenytoin is used with either primidone or phenobarbital. Weigh the potential risks versus the benefits before adding phenytoin to either of these drugs in dogs.

Phenytoin is contraindicated in patients known to be hypersensitive to it or other hydantoins. Intravenous use of the drug is contraindicated in patients with 2nd or 3rd degree heart block, sinoatrial block, Adams-Stokes syndrome, or sinus bradycardia. Safe use of this drug has not been established during pregnancy; weigh risks versus benefits.

Adverse Effects/Warnings - Adverse effects in dogs associated with high serum levels include anorexia and vomiting, ataxia, and sedation. Liver function tests should be monitored in patients on chronic therapy as hepatotoxicity (elevated serum ALT, decreased serum albumin, hepatocellular hypertrophy and necrosis, hepatic lipidosis, and extramedullary hematopoiesis) has been reported. Gingival hyperplasia has been reported in dogs receiving chronic therapy. Oral absorption may be enhanced and GI upset decreased if given with food.

Cats exhibit ataxia, sedation, and anorexia secondary to accumulation of phenytoin and high serum levels. Cats have also been reported to develop a dermal atrophy syndrome secondary to phenytoin.

Overdosage - Symptoms of overdosage may include sedation, anorexia, and ataxia at lower levels, and coma, hypotension and respiratory depression at higher levels. Treatment of overdose symptoms in dogs is dependent on the severity of the symptoms since dogs so rapidly clear the drug. Severe intoxications should be handled supportively.

Drug Interactions - A case report of **chloramphenicol** increasing the serum half-life of phenytoin from 3 to 15 hours in a dogs has been reported.

Note: the following interactions are from the human literature, because of the significant differences in pharmacokinetics in dogs and cats their veterinary significance will be variable. This list includes only agents used commonly in small animal medicine, many more agents have been implicated in the human literature: The following agents may increase the effects of phenytoin: **allopurinol, cimetidine, chloramphenicol, diazepam, ethanol, isoniazid, phenylbutazone, sulfonamides, trimethoprim, valproic acid, salicylates, and chlorpheniramine.**

The following agents may decrease the pharmacologic activity of phenytoin: **barbiturates, diazoxide, folic acid, theophylline, antacids, antineoplastics, calcium (dietary and gluconate), enteral feedings, nitrofurantoin, and pyridoxine**.

Phenytoin may decrease the pharmacologic activity of the following agents: **corticosteroids, disopyramide, doxycycline, estrogens, quinidine, dopamine, and furosemide**.

Phenytoin may decrease the analgesic properties **meperidine**, but enhance its toxic effects.

The toxicity of **lithium** may be enhanced.

The pharmacologic effects of **primidone** may be altered. Some data suggest that additive hepatotoxicity may result if phenytoin is used with either **primidone** or **phenobarbital**. Weigh the potential risks versus the benefits before adding phenytoin to either of these drugs in dogs.

Pyridoxine (Vitamin B$_6$) may reduce the serum levels of phenytoin.

Doses -
Dogs:
  For treatment of seizures:
   a) 15 - 40 mg/kg PO *tid* (Morgan 1988)
   b) 20 - 35 mg/kg *tid* (Bunch 1986)
   c) Initially, 8.8 - 17.6 mg/kg PO in divided doses, then gradually increase or decrease dose to maintain control. May take several days for seizure control to be attained. (Package insert; *Dilantin*® Veterinary — Parke-Davis)
   Author's note: Because of the extremely fast half-life of phenytoin in dogs, it is unlikely that this dosage regimen ("c") will attain serum levels of 10 - 20 micrograms/ml which are thought to be necessary for adequate seizure control.

  For treatment of ventricular arrhythmias:
   a) Up to 10 mg/kg IV in increments of 2 - 4 mg/kg or 20 - 35 mg/kg PO *tid* (Moses 1988)
   b) 10 mg/kg IV q8h or 30 mg/kg PO q8h (Wilcke 1985)

  For treatment of hypoglycemia secondary to tumor:
   a) 6 mg/kg PO *bid-tid* (Morgan 1988)

Cats: Note: Because cats can easily accumulate this drug and develop symptoms of toxicity, the use of phenytoin is very controversial in this species. Diligent monitoring is required.

  For treatment of ventricular arrhythmias:
   a) 2 - 3 mg/kg PO q24h (Wilcke 1985)

  For treatment of seizures:
   a) 2 - 3 mg/kg daily PO; 20 mg/kg per week (Bunch 1986)

Horses:
  For seizures:
   a) 2.83 - 16.43 mg/kg PO q8h to obtain serum levels from 5 - 10 micrograms/ml. Suggest monitoring serum levels to adjust dosage. (Kowalczyk and Beech 1983)

Monitoring Parameters -
   1) Level of seizure control; sedation/ataxia
   2) Body weight (anorexia)
   3) Liver enzymes (if chronic therapy) & serum albumin
   4) Serum drug levels if signs of toxicity or lack of seizure control

Client Information - Notify veterinarian if dog becomes anorexic, lethargic, ataxic, or if seizures are not adequately controlled. The importance of regular dosing is imperative for successful therapy.

Dosage Forms/Preparations -
Veterinary-Approved Products:
  Extended Phenytoin Sodium Capsules, USP® (Fort Dodge) (Rx) 100 mg tablets. Approved for use in dogs.Note: This product may no longer be marketed.

Human-Approved Products:
  Phenytoin Sodium, Extended Oral Capsules 30 mg, 100 mg; *Dilantin*® *Kapseals*® (Parke-Davis); generic, (Rx)

Phenytoin Oral Suspension 25 mg/ml in 8 oz. bottles; *Dilantin-125*® (Parke-Davis) (Rx)

Phenytoin Oral Tablets 50 mg; *Dilantin*® *Infa-Tabs*® (Parke-Davis) (Rx)

Phenytoin Sodium for Injection 50 mg/ml (46 mg/ml phenytoin) in 2 ml and 5 ml amps, syringes and vials; 150 mg (100 mg phenytoin sodium) in 2 ml vials; 750 mg (500 mg phenytoin sodium) in 10 ml vials (Rx)

Phenytoin may also be called diphenylhydantoin or DPH.

PHOSPHATE, PARENTERAL
POTASSIUM PHOSPHATE
SODIUM PHOSPHATE

Chemistry - Potassium phosphate injection is a combination of 224 mg monobasic potassium phosphate and 236 mg dibasic potassium phosphate. The pH of the injection is 6.5 and has an osmolarity of 7357 mOsm/L.

Sodium phosphate injection is a combination of 276 mg monobasic sodium phosphate and 142 mg dibasic sodium phosphate. The pH of the injection is 5.7 and has an osmolarity of about 7000 mOsm/L.

Because commercial preparations are a combination of monobasic and dibasic forms; prescribe and dispense in terms of mMoles of phosphate.

Storage/Stability/Compatibility - Unless otherwise instructed by the manufacturer, store potassium or sodium phosphate injection at room temperature; protect from freezing.

Phosphates may be incompatible with metals such as calcium and magnesium.

Potassium phosphate injection is reportedly **compatible** with the following intravenous solutions and drugs: amino acids 4%/dextrose 25%, $D_{10}LRS$, $D_{10}Ringer's$, Dextrose 2.5%-10% injection, sodium chloride 0.45%-0.9%, magnesium sulfate, metoclopramide HCl, and verapamil HCl.

Potassium phosphate injection is reportedly **incompatible** with the following solutions or drugs: $D_{2.5}$ in half normal Ringer's or LRS, D_5 in Ringer's, D_{10}/sodium chloride 0.9%, Ringer's injection, LRS, and dobutamine HCl. Compatibility is dependent upon factors such as pH, concentration, temperature and diluents used. It is suggested to consult specialized references for more specific information (*e.g., Handbook on Injectable Drugs* by Trissel; see bibliography).

Pharmacology - Phosphate is involved in several functions in the body, including calcium metabolism, acid-base buffering, B-vitamin utilization, bone deposition, and in several enzyme systems.

Uses/Indications - Phosphate is useful in large volume parenteral fluids to correct or prevent hypophosphatemia when adequate oral phosphorous intake is not possible. Hypophosphatemia may cause hemolytic anemia, thrombocytopenia, neuromuscular and CNS disorders, bone and joint pain, and decompensation in patient's with cirrhotic liver disease.

Pharmacokinetics - Intravenously administered phosphate is eliminated via the kidneys. It is glomerularly filtered, but up to 80% is reabsorbed by the tubules.

Contraindications/Precautions - Both potassium and sodium phosphate are contraindicated in patients with hyperphosphatemia, hypocalcemia, oliguric renal failure, or if tissue necrosis is present. Potassium phosphate is contraindicated in patients with hyperkalemia. It should be used with caution in patients with cardiac or renal disease. Particular caution should be used in using this drug in patients receiving digitalis therapy.

Sodium phosphate is also contraindicated in patients with hypernatremia.

Adverse Effects/Warnings - Overuse of parenteral phosphate can result in hyperphosphatemia, resulting in hypocalcemia (refer to the Overdose section for more information). Phosphate therapy can also result in hypotension, renal failure or soft tissue mineralization. Either hyperkalemia or hypernatremia may also result in susceptible patients.

Overdosage/Acute Toxicity - Patients developing hyperphosphatemia secondary to intravenous therapy with potassium phosphate should have the infusion stopped and be given appropriate parenteral calcium therapy to restore serum calcium levels. Serum potassium should also be monitored and treated if required.

Drug Interactions - Angiotensin converting enzyme inhibitors (**ACE inhibitors**) such as **captopril**, or **potassium sparing diuretics** (*e.g.*, **spironolactone**) may cause potassium retention. When used with potassium products such as potassium phosphate, hyperkalemia can result.

Potassium salts must be used very cautiously in patients on **digitalis therapy** and should not be used in digitalized patients with heart block.

Doses - Both sodium and potassium phosphate injections must be diluted before intravenous administration.

Dogs, Cats:

For hypophosphatemia:

a) For significant hypophosphatemia (<1.5 mg/dl) in patients unable to receive oral supplementation: 0.06 - 0.18 mM/kg IV given over 6 hours (0.01 - 0.03 mM/kg/hr). Recheck serum phosphorous before continuing. Usually may stop therapy when serum phosphorous level reaches 2 mg/dl. (Hardy and Adams 1989)

b) Cats: For severe hypophosphatemia in diabetic ketoacidosis: Using potassium phosphate give 0.01 - 0.03 mM/kg/hr for 6 hours IV. Recheck serum phosphorous before continuing. In order to provide enough potassium without inducing hyperphosphatemia, supply 50-75% of patient's potassium using potassium chloride and the remainder as potassium phosphate. (Peterson and Randolph 1989)

Monitoring Parameters -

1) Serum inorganic phosphate (phosphorous)
2) Other electrolytes, including calcium

Dosage Forms/Preparations/FDA Approval Status/Withholding Times -

Veterinary-Approved Products: There are no parenteral phosphate-only products approved for veterinary medicine. There are, however, several proprietary phosphate-containing products available that may also include calcium, magnesium, potassium and/or dextrose; refer to the individual product's labeling for specific dosage information. Trade names for these products include: *Magnadex®*—Osborn, *Norcalciphos®*—SKB, *Cal-Dextro® Special, & #2,*—Fort Dodge, and *CMPK®, & Cal-Phos® #2*—(TechAmerica). They are legend (Rx) drugs.

Human-Approved Products:

Potassium Phosphate Injection; each ml provides 3 mM of phosphate (99.1 mg/dl of phosphorous) and 4.4 mEq of potassium per ml in 5, 10, 15, 30, & 50 ml vials

Generic; (Rx)

Sodium Phosphate Injection; each ml provides 3 mM of phosphate (93 mg/dl of phosphorous) and 4 mEq of sodium per ml in 10, 15, 30, and 50 ml vials; Generic; (Rx)

PHYTONADIONE
VITAMIN K₁

Chemistry - A naphthoquinone derivative identical to naturally occurring vitamin K_1, phytonadione occurs as a clear, yellow to amber, viscous liquid. It is insoluble in water, slightly soluble in alcohol and soluble in lipids. Phytonadione may also be known as Vitamin K_1, phylloquinone, or phytomenadione.

Storage/Stability/Compatibility - Phytonadione should be protected from light at all times, as it is quite sensitive to light. If used as an intravenous infusion, the container should be wrapped with an opaque material. Tablets and capsules should be stored in well-closed, light-resistant containers.

Because most veterinary clinicians state that phytonadione is contraindicated for intravenous use, and since compatibility is dependent upon factors such as pH, concentration, temperature and diluents used, it is suggested to consult specialized references (*e.g., Handbook on Injectable Drugs* by Trissel; see bibliography) for more specific information on the compatibility of phytonadione with other drugs.

Pharmacology - Vitamin K_1 is necessary for the synthesis of blood coagulation factors II, VII, IX, and X in the liver. It is believed that Vitamin K_1 is involved in the carboxylation of the inactive precursors of these factors to form active compounds.

Uses/Indications - The principal uses of exogenously administered phytonadione is in the treatment of anticoagulant rodenticide toxicity. It is also used for treating dicumarol toxicity associated with sweet clover ingestion in ruminants, sulfaquinoxaline toxicity, and in bleeding disorders associated with faulty formation of vitamin K-dependent coagulation factors.

Pharmacokinetics - Phytonadione is absorbed from the GI tract in monogastric animals via the intestinal lymphatics, but only in the presence of bile salts. Oral absorption of phytonadione may be significantly enhanced by administering with fatty foods. The relative bioavailability of the drug is increased 4-5 times in dogs given canned dog food with the dose. After oral administration, increases in clotting factors may not occur until 6-12 hours later.

Phytonadione may concentrate in the liver for a short period of time, but is not appreciably stored in the liver or other tissues. Only small amounts are distributed across the placenta in pregnant animals. Exogenously administered phytonadione enters milk. The elimination of Vitamin K_1 is not well understood.

Contraindications/Precautions/Reproductive Safety - Many veterinary clinicians state that the intravenous use of phytonadione is contraindicated because of increased risk of anaphylaxis development, but intravenous phytonadione is used in human medicine and several intravenous dosage regimens are outlined below in the Dosage section. Phytonadione is contraindicated in patients hypersensitive to it or any component of its formulation.

Vitamin K does not correct hypoprothrombinemia due to hepatocellular damage.

Phytonadione crosses the placenta only in small amounts, but its safety has not been documented in pregnant animals.

Adverse Effects/Warnings - Anaphylactoid reactions have been reported following IV administration of Vitamin K_1; use with extreme caution (See Contraindications above). Intramuscular administration may result in acute bleeding from the site of injection during the early stages of treatment. Small gauge needles are recommended for use when injecting SQ or IM. Subcutaneous injections or oral dosages may be slowly or poorly absorbed in animals that are hypovolemic.

Because 6-12 hours may be required for new clotting factors to be synthesized after phytonadione administration, emergency needs for clotting factors must be provided for by giving blood products.

Overdosage/Acute Toxicity - Phytonadione is relatively non-toxic, and it would be unlikely that toxic symptoms would result after a single overdosage. However, refer to the Adverse Effects section for more information.

Drug Interactions - As would be expected, phytonadione antagonizes the anticoagulant effects of **coumarin** (*e.g.,* **warfarin) and indandione agents**.

The following drugs may prolong or enhance the effects of anticoagulants and antagonize some of the therapeutic effects of phytonadione: **phenylbutazone, aspirin, chloramphenicol, sulfonamides (including trimethoprim-sulfa), diazoxide, allopurinol, cimetidine, metronidazole, anabolic steroids, erythromycin, ketoconazole, propranolol, and thyroid drugs.**

Concomitant administration of **Mineral Oil** may reduce the absorption of oral vitamin K. Although chronic antibiotic therapy should have no significant effect on the absorption of phytonadione, these drugs may decrease the numbers of vitamin K producing bacteria in the gut.

Doses -
Dogs & Cats:
For anticoagulant rodenticide toxicity:
a) For known warfarin or other first generation coumarin toxicity or Vitamin K_1 deficiency: Initially, 2.5 mg/kg given SQ in several sites, then 0.25 - 2.5 mg/kg PO in divided doses (*bid-tid*) for 5-7 days.

For known indandione (diphacinone) or second generation coumarin (brodifacoum) toxicity: Loading dose of 5 mg/kg SQ in several sites; then 5 mg/kg divided *bid-tid* PO for two weeks, then reevaluate coagulation status. Animal's activity should be restricted for one week after phytonadione therapy is ended. Coagulation status should then be reevaluated 3 weeks after cessation of therapy.

For unknown anticoagulant toxicity: Load with 2.5 mg/kg SQ over several sites. Then 2.5 mg/kg PO divided *bid-tid* for 7 days. Two days post cessation of therapy, reevaluate coagulation status. If one-stage prothrombin time (OSPT) is elevated continue therapy for 2 additional weeks. If not elevated, repeat OSPT in two days. If normal, the animal should be rested for one week. If abnormal, continue therapy for an additional week and recheck OSPT's as above. (Mount, Woody, and Murphy 1986)

b) For known warfarin, fumarin, pindone, or valone ingestions: 1 mg/kg PO once daily for 4-6 days.

For known bromadiolone or brodifacoum ingestions: 2.5 mg/kg PO once daily ususally for 2-3 weeks (broadiolone duration unknown).

For known diphacinone or chlorphacinone ingestions: 2.5 - 5 mg/kg PO for 3-4 weeks.

Note: ususal dosages and durations; use oral route (with one teaspoon of canned dog food) if animal not vomiting, otherwise SubQ route preferred over IV. Therapy must be continued for as long as rodenticide is inhibiting vitamin K_1 epoxide recycling. (Felice and Murphy 1995)

c) For acute cases: Handle animal gently. Avoid IM injections; give fresh, whole blood transfusion 10-20 ml/kg IV (first half rapidly, then at 20 drops/minute). Give oxygen if hypoxic; if dyspneic consider radiographs and thorocentesis for intrathoracic hemorrhage. Then give phytonadione as below.

For subacute cases: Give phytonadione at 2-3 mg/kg SQ q12h for large dogs and 5 mg/kg SQ q12h for small dogs and cats. Repeat until coagulation times are normal. Follow with oral phytonadione at 2.5 - 3 mg/kg PO divided *tid* for 4-6 days if short acting coumarin (*e.g.,* warfarin) or up to 30 days for long-acting agents. (Grauer and Hjelle 1988)

d) Cats: 15 - 25 mg total dose as a 5% solution in D5W IV slowly daily, given for 5-7 days for first generation agents and for 3-4 weeks for second generation agents. May also be given undiluted IM or orally once bleeding is controlled. Reevaluate at 3-day intervals for 9-10 days. If clotting times increase, reinstitute therapy for an additional 1-2 weeks. (Reid and Oehme 1989), (Weiser 1989a)

Cattle:

For anticoagulant rodenticide toxicity:
- a) Initially 0.5 - 2.5 mg/kg IV in D5W at a rate of 10 mg/minute. Subsequent doses may be given IM or SQ. Second generation agents may require 3-4 weeks of treatment. (Bailey 1986b)
- b) 0.5 - 2.5 mg/kg IM, if IV use is necessary (avoid if possible), dilute in saline or D5W/saline and give very slowly (not to exceed 5 mg/minute). (Upson 1988)
- c) For acute hypoprothrombinemia with hemorrhage: 0.5 - 2.5 mg/kg IV, not to exceed 10 mg/minute in mature animals and 5 mg/minute in newborn and very young animals.
  For non-acute hypoprothrombinemia: 0.5 - 2.5 mg/kg IM or SQ (Label directions; *Veda-K1*®—Vedco)

For sweet clover (dicumarol) toxicity:
- a) Give blood if necessary, then phytonadione 1 mg/kg IV or IM; repeat 2-3 times daily for 2 days. (Osweiler and Ruhr 1986)

Horses:

For warfarin (or related compounds) toxicity:
- a) 500 mg SQ q4-6h until one-stage prothrombin time (OSPT) returns to normal control values. Whole blood or fresh plasma may also be necessary early in the course of treatment. (Byars 1987)
- b) 0.5 - 2.5 mg/kg IM, if IV use is necessary (avoid if possible), dilute in saline or D5W/saline and give very slowly (not to exceed 5 mg/minute). (Upson 1988)
- c) For acute hypoprothrombinemia with hemorrhage: 0.5 - 2.5 mg/kg IV, not to exceed 10 mg/minute in mature animals and 5 mg/minute in newborn and very young animals.
  For non-acute hypoprothrombinemia: 0.5 - 2.5 mg/kg IM or SQ (Label directions; *Veda-K1*®—Vedco)

Swine:

For warfarin (or related compounds) toxicity:
- a) 0.5 - 2.5 mg/kg IM, if IV use is necessary (avoid if possible), dilute in saline or D5W/saline and give very slowly (not to exceed 5 mg/minute). (Upson 1988)
- b) For acute hypoprothrombinemia with hemorrhage: 0.5 - 2.5 mg/kg IV, not to exceed 10 mg/minute in mature animals and 5 mg/minute in newborn and very young animals.
  For non-acute hypoprothrombinemia: 0.5 - 2.5 mg/kg IM or SQ (Label directions; *Veda-K1*®—Vedco)

Sheep & Goats:

For warfarin (or related compounds) toxicity:
- a) 0.5 - 2.5 mg/kg IM, if IV use is necessary (avoid if possible), dilute in saline or D5W/saline and give very slowly (not to exceed 5 mg/minute). (Upson 1988)
- b) For acute hypoprothrombinemia with hemorrhage: 0.5 - 2.5 mg/kg IV, not to exceed 10 mg/minute in mature animals and 5 mg/minute in newborn and very young animals.
  For non-acute hypoprothrombinemia: 0.5 - 2.5 mg/kg IM or SQ (Label directions; *Veda-K1*®—Vedco)

Birds:

For hemorrhagic disorders:
- a) 0.25 - 0.5 ml/kg IM of the 10 mg/ml injectable product. Commonly used before surgery where hemorrhage is anticipated. (McDonald 1989)
- b) 0.2 - 2.5 mg/kg IM as needed; usually only 1-2 injections are required. May also be used prophylactically when amprolium and sulfas are administered. (Clubb 1986)

Monitoring Parameters -
1) Clinical efficacy (lack of hemorrhage)
2) One-stage prothrombin time (OSPT)

Client Information - Because it may take several weeks to eliminate some of the anticoagulant rodenticides from the body, clients must be counseled on the importance of continuing to administer the drug (phytonadione) for as long as instructed or renewed bleeding may occur. Unless otherwise instructed, oral phytonadione should be administered with food, preferably foods high in fat content. During therapy, animals should be kept quiet whether at home or hospitalized.

Dosage Forms/Preparations/FDA Approval Status/Withholding Times -
Veterinary-Approved Products:

Phytonadione Oral Capsules 25 mg; *Veta-K₁*® (PVL; Vedco); (Rx) Approved for use in dogs and cats.

Phytonadione Aqueous Colloidal Solution for Injection 10 mg/ml in 30 ml and 100 ml vials; *Veda-K₁*® (Vedco); (Rx) Approved for use dogs, cats, cattle, calves, horses, swine, sheep, and goats. No withdrawal times listed.

Human-Approved Products:

Phytonadione Oral Tablets 5 mg; *Mephyton*® (Merck); (Rx)

Phytonadione Injection 2 mg/ml (aqueous colloidal solution) in 0.5 ml amps and syringes and 10 mg/ml (aqueous dispersion) in 1 ml amps and 2.5 & 5 ml vials
Aqua-Mephyton (Merck); Generic (IMS); (Rx)

PIPERAZINE

Chemistry - Piperazine occurs as a white, crystalline powder that may have a slight odor. It is soluble in water and alcohol. Piperazine is available commercially in a variety of salts, including citrate, adipate, phosphate, hexahydrate and dihydrochloride. Each salt contains a variable amount of piperazine (base): adipate (37%), chloride (48%), citrate (35%), dihydrochloride (50-53%), hexahydrate (44%), phosphate (42%) and sulfate (46%).

Storage/Stability/Compatibility - Unless otherwise specified by the manufacturer, piperazine products should be stored at room temperature (15-30°C).

Pharmacology - Piperazine is thought to exert "curare-like" effects on susceptible nematodes, thereby paralyzing or narcotizing the worm and allowing it to be passed out with the feces. The neuromuscular blocking effect is believed to be caused by blocking acetylcholine at the myoneural junction. In ascarids, succinic acid production is also inhibited.

Uses/Indications - Piperazine is used for the treatment of ascarids in dogs, cats, horses, swine and poultry. Piperazine is considered to be safe to use in animals with concurrent gastroenteritis and during pregnancy.

Pharmacokinetics - Piperazine and its salts are reportedly readily absorbed from the proximal sections of the GI tract and the drug is metabolized and excreted by the kidneys. Absorptive, distribution and elimination kinetics on individual species were not located.

Contraindications/Precautions - Piperazine should be considered contraindicated in patients with chronic liver or kidney disease, and in patients with gastrointestinal hypomotility. There is some evidence in man, that piperazine may provoke seizures in patients with a seizure history or with renal disease when given in high dosages.

If used in horses with heavy infestations of *P. equorum*, rupture or blockage of intestines is possible due to the rapid death and detachment of the worm.

Adverse Effects/Warnings - Adverse effects are uncommon at recommended doses, but diarrhea, emesis and ataxia may be noted in dogs or cats. Horses and foals generally tolerate the drug quite well, even at high dosage rates, but a transient softening of the feces may be seen. Other adverse effects have been seen at toxic dosages, refer to the Overdosage section below for more information.

Overdosage - Acute massive overdosage can lead to paralysis and death, but the drug is generally considered to have a wide margin of safety. The oral LD₅₀ of piperazine adipate in mice is 11.4 g/kg.

In cats, adverse effects occur within 24 hours after a toxic dose is ingested. Emesis, weakness, dyspnea, muscular fasiculations of ears, whiskers, tail and eyes, rear limb ataxia, hypersalivation, depression, dehydration, head-pressing, positional nystagmus and slowed pupillary responses have all been described after a toxic ingestion. Many of these effects may also be seen in dogs after toxic piperazine ingestions.

Treatment is symptomatic and supportive. If ingestion was recent, use of activated charcoal and a cathartic has been suggested. Intravenous fluid therapy and keeping the animal in a quiet, dark place is also recommended. Recovery generally takes place within 3-4 days.

Drug Interactions - Although data conflicts, piperazine and **chlorpromazine** may precipitate seizures if used concomitantly.

Piperazine and **pyrantel/morantel** have antagonistic modes of action and should generally not be used together.

The use of **purgatives (laxatives)** with piperazine is not recommended as the drug may be eliminated before its full efficacy is established.

Drug/Laboratory Interactions - Piperazine can have an effect on **uric acid blood levels**, but references conflict with regard to the effect. Both falsely high and low values have been reported. Use results cautiously.

Doses - Caution: Piperazine is available in several salts that contain varying amounts of piperazine base (see Chemistry above). Many of the doses listed below do not specify what salt (if any) is used in the dosage calculations. If the dose is in question, refer to the actual product information for the product you are using.

Dogs:

For treatment of ascarids (Note: Because larval stages in the host's tissues may not be affected by the drug, many clinicians recommend retreating about 2-3 weeks after the first dose):

a) 45 - 65 mg of base/kg PO; For pups less than 2.5 kg: 150 mg maximum. (Cornelius and Roberson 1986)
b) 110 mg/kg PO (Chiapella 1988)
c) 100 mg/kg PO; repeat in 3 weeks. (Morgan 1988)
d) 20 - 30 mg/kg PO once. (Davis 1985)
e) 110 mg/kg PO; repeat in 21 days. (Kirk 1989)
f) 45 - 65 mg/kg (as base) PO. (Roberson 1988b)

Cats:

For treatment of ascarids (Note: Because larval stages in the host's tissues may not be affected by the drug, many clinicians recommend retreating about 2-3 weeks after the first dose):

a) 45 - 65 mg of base/kg PO; 150 mg maximum. (Cornelius and Roberson 1986)
b) 110 mg/kg PO (Chiapella 1988)
c) 100 mg/kg PO; repeat in 3 weeks. (Morgan 1988)
d) 20 - 30 mg/kg PO once. (Davis 1985)
e) 110 mg/kg PO; repeat in 21 days. (Kirk 1989)
f) 45 - 65 mg/kg (as base) PO. (Roberson 1988b)

Horses: There are combination products available for use in horses (see Dosage Forms/Preparations section) that contain piperazine that have increased efficacy against nematodes and other helminths. Refer to the individual products' package insert for more information.

a) 110 mg/kg (base) PO; repeat in 3-4 weeks. Retreating at 10 week intervals for *P. equorum* infections in young animals is recommended. (Roberson 1988b)
b) 200 mg/kg PO. Maximum of 80 grams in adults, 60 grams in yearlings, and 30 grams in foals. (Brander, Pugh, and Bywater 1982)

Cattle, Sheep & Goats: Because of fairly high resistance of many nematode species to piperazine, it is rarely used alone in these species.

Swine:

For *Ascaris suum* and *Oesophagostomum*:

a) 0.2 - 0.4% in the feed, or 0.1 - 0.2% in the drinking water. All medicated water or feed must be consumed within 12 hours, so fasting or withholding water overnight may be beneficial to ensure adequate dosing. Retreat in 2 months. Safe in young animals and during pregnancy. Drug withdrawal times not determined for swine. (Paul 1986)
b) 110 mg/kg (as base). Citrate salt usually used in feed as a one day treatment, and hexahydrate in drinking water. Dose must be consumed in 8-12 hours. Withholding water or feed the previous night may be beneficial. (Roberson 1988b)

Birds:

a) For ascarids in poultry (not effective in psittacines): 100 - 500 mg/kg PO once; repeat in 10-14 days. (Clubb 1986)
b) For nematodes: Piperazine citrate: 45 - 100 mg/kg single dose or 6 - 10 grams/gallon for 1-4 days. In raptors: 100 mg/kg. In parakeets and canaries: 0.5 mg/gram. (Stunkard 1984)
c) For *Ascaridia galli* in poultry: 32 mg/kg (as base) (approximately 0.3 grams for each adult) given in each of 2 successive feedings or for 2 days in drinking water. Citrate or adipate salts are usually used in feed and the hexahydrate in drinking water. (Roberson 1988b)

Monitoring Parameters -1) Clinical and/or laboratory efficacy 2) Adverse effects

Client Information - Clients should be instructed to administer only the amount prescribed and to relate any serious adverse effects to the veterinarian.

Dosage Forms/Preparations/Approval Status/Withdrawal Times -
Veterinary-Approved Products:

Piperazine Dihydrochloride tablets equivalent to 50 mg, or 250 mg base. *Pipa-Tabs*® (Vet-A-Mix); (OTC) Approved for use in dogs and cats.

Additional products and combination products may be available for a variety of species.

Human-Approved Products: None

PIRLIMYCIN HCL

Chemistry - Pirlimycin HCl is a lincosamide antibiotic. It has a molecular weight of 465.4.

Storage/Stability/Compatibility - Store syringes at or below 25°C (77°F). Protect from freezing.

Pharmacology - Like other lincosamides, pirlimycin acts by binding to the 50S ribosomal subunit of susceptible bacterial RNA, thereby interfering with bacterial protein synthesis. It is primarily active against gram positive bacteria, including a variety of species of Staphylococcus (*S. aureus, S. epidermidis, S. chromogenes, S. hyicus, S. xylosus*), Streptococcus (*S. agalactiae, S. dysgalactiae, S. Uberis, S. Bovis*) and *Enterococcus faecalis*.

Organisms with a MIC of 2 micrograms/ml or less are considered susceptible, and organisms with a MIC value of 4 micrograms/ml are considered resistant. If using a 2 micrograms disk for Kirby-Bauer plate testing, a zone diameter of less than or equal to 12 mm indicates resistance and a diameter of greater than or equal to 13 mm indicates susceptibility.

Uses/Indications - Pirlimycin mastitis tubes are indicated for the treatment of clinical and subclinical mastitis caused by susceptible organisms in lactating dairy cattle.

Pharmacokinetics - Little information is available; the manufacturer states that the drug penetrates the udder well and is absorbed systemically from the udder and then secreted into the milk of all four quarters. Tissue levels in treated quarters of pirlimycin are approximately 2-3 times those found in the extracellular fluid.

Contraindications/Precautions/Reproductive Safety - No information noted.

Adverse Effects/Warnings - No adverse affects, including udder irritation reported thus far.

Milk from untreated quarters must be disposed of during withdrawal time as residues may be detected from untreated quarters.

Overdosage/Acute Toxicity - No data located.

Drug Interactions - Because **Erythromycin** and clindamycin have shown antagonism *in vitro*, it could be expected the same may occur with pirlimycin.

Laboratory Considerations - The established tolerance of pirlimycin in milk is 0.4 ppm.

Doses -
Lactating Dairy Cattle: Infuse one syringe into each affected quarter; repeat one time in 24 hours. See label directions for more specific information on administrative techniques. (Package Insert—Pirsue®; Upjohn)

Monitoring Parameters - Efficacy and withdrawal periods

Client Information - Be sure clients understand dosage recommendations and withdrawal periods. Milk from untreated quarters must be disposed of during withdrawal time as residues may be detected from untreated quarters.

Dosage Forms/Preparations/FDA Approval Status/Withholding Times -
Veterinary-Approved Products:

Pirlimycin HCl Aqueous Gel 50 mg (equiv. to free base) in a 10 ml disposable teat syringe; Pirsue® Aqueous Gel (Upjohn); (Rx) Approved for use in lactating dairy cattle. Milk withdrawal = 36 hours after last treatment; Meat withdrawal = 28 days

Human-Approved Products: None

PIROXICAM

Chemistry - An oxicam derivative non-steroidal antiinflammatory agent, piroxicam occurs as a white, crystalline solid. It is sparingly soluble in water. Piroxicam is structurally not related to other non-steroidal antiinflammatory agents.

Storage/Stability/Compatibility - Capsules should be stored at temperatures less than 30°C in tight, light-resistant containers. When stored as recommended, capsules have an expiration date of 36 months after manufacture.

Pharmacology - Like other non-steroidal antiinflammatory agents, piroxicam has antiinflammatory, analgesic and antipyretic activity. The drug's antiinflammatory activity is thought to be primarily due to its inhibition of prostaglandin synthesis, but additional mechanisms (*e.g.*, superoxide formation inhibition) may be important. As with other NSAIDs, piroxicam can affect renal function, cause GI mucosal damage, and inhibit platelet aggregation.

Uses/Indications - In dogs, piroxicam may be beneficial in reducing the pain and inflammation associated with degenerative joint disease. It also has been used in dogs as adjunctive treatment of bladder transitional cell carcinoma.

Pharmacokinetics - After oral administration, piroxicam is well absorbed from the gut. While the presence of food will decrease the rate of absorption, it will not decrease the amount absorbed. It is not believed that antacids significantly affect absorption.

Piroxicam is highly bound to plasma proteins. In humans, synovial levels are about 40% of those found in the plasma. Maternal milk concentrations are only about 1% of plasma levels.

In humans, piroxicam has a very long plasma half-life (about 50 hours). The drug is principally excreted as metabolites in the urine after hepatic biotransformation.

Contraindications/Precautions/Reproductive Safety - Piroxicam is contraindicated in patients hypersensitive to it or who are severely allergic to aspirin or other NSAIDs. It should be used only when its potential benefits outweigh the risks in patients with active, or a history of GI ulcer disease or bleeding disorders. Because peripheral edema has been noted in some human patients, it should be used with caution in patients with severely compromised cardiac function.

Animal studies have not demonstrated any teratogenic effects associated with piroxicam. The drug is excreted into milk in very low concentrations (about 1% found in maternal plasma).

Adverse Effects/Warnings - Like other NSAIDs used in dogs, piroxicam has the potential for causing significant GI ulceration and bleeding. The therapeutic window for the drug is very narrow in dogs as doses as low as 1 mg/kg given daily have caused significant GI ulceration, renal papillary necrosis, and peritonitis. Other adverse effects reported in humans and potentially possible in dogs include CNS effects (headache, dizziness, etc.), otic effects (tinnitus), elevations in hepatic function tests, pruritus and rash, and peripheral edema.

Overdosage/Acute Toxicity - There is limited information available, but dogs may be more sensitive to the drugs ulcerative effects than are humans. Patients ingesting significant overdoses should be monitored carefully and gut removal techniques employed when warranted. Treatment is supportive.

Drug Interactions - Because piroxicam is highly bound to plasma proteins, it can displace or be displaced by other highly protein bound drugs, including **warfarin, phenylbutazone, etc**.

Because piroxicam may inhibit platelet aggregation and also cause gastrointestinal ulceration, when used with other drugs that alter hemostasis (*e.g.*, **heparin, warfarin, etc**.) and/or cause gastrointestinal erosion (*e.g.*, **aspirin, flunixin, phenylbutazone, corticosteroids, etc**.), increased likelihood of bleeding or ulceration may occur.

NSAIDs (including piroxicam) may potentially significantly reduce the excretion of **methotrexate** and cause toxicity.

Laboratory Considerations - Piroxicam may cause falsely elevated **blood glucose values** when using the glucose oxidase and peroxidase method using ABTS as a chromogen.

Doses -
  Dogs:
    As an antiinflammatory/analgesic:
      a) 0.3 mg/kg PO every other day (q48h) (Boothe 1992)
    As an adjunctive therapy of transitional cell carcinoma of the bladder:
      a) 0.3 mg/kg PO once a day (Knapp, Richardson et al. 1994)
  Cats:
    As an adjunctive therapy of transitional cell carcinoma of the bladder:
      a) The author has seen several anectdotal dosage recommendations. These generally fall into the: "0.3 mg/kg PO once a day to every other day with food" category. Use with caution as therapeutic window is very narrow. (Plumb)

Monitoring Parameters - 1) Adverse Effects (particularly GI bleeding); 2) Liver function tests should be monitored occasionally with chronic use

Client Information - Have clients monitor for GI ulceration/bleeding (anorexia, tarry stools, etc). Do not exceed dosage recommendations without veterinarian's approval. It has been suggested to give the drug with food to reduce GI upset potential.

Dosage Forms/Preparations/FDA Approval Status/Withholding Times -
  Veterinary-Approved Products: None
  Human-Approved Products:
    Piroxicam Oral Capsules 10 mg, 20 mg; *Feldene*® (Pfizer); generic, (Rx)

Plasma-Lyte - see the section on intravenous fluids in the appendix

POLYSULFATED GLYCOSAMINOGLYCAN (PSGAG)

Chemistry - Polysulfated glycosaminoglycan (PSGAG) is chemically similar to natural mucopolysaccharides found in cartilaginous tissues. PSGAG is reportedly an analog of heparin.

Storage/Stability/Compatibility - Commercial products should be stored in a cool place 8-15°C (46-59°F). The manufacturer recommends discarding the unused portion from a vial or ampule and does not recommend mixing with any other drug or chemical.

Pharmacology - In joint tissue, PSGAG inhibits proteolytic enzymes that can degrade proteoglycans (including naturally occurring glycosaminoglycans), thereby preventing or reducing decreased connective tissue flexibility, resistance to compression and resiliency. By acting as a precursor, PSGAG also increases the synthesis of proteoglycans. PSGAG also reduces inflammation by reducing concentrations of prostaglandin E_2 (released in response to joint injury) and increases hyaluronate concentrations in the joint, thereby restoring synovial fluid viscosity.

Uses/Indications - PSGAG administered either IM or IA is indicated for the treatment of non-infectious and/or traumatic joint dysfunction and associated lameness of the carpal joints in horses. Some studies have indicated that PSGAG is much less effective in joints where there has been acute trauma but without the presence of degradative enzymes.

It is also approved for the control of signs associated with non-infectious degenerative and/or traumatic arthritis in dogs..

Pharmacokinetics - PSGAG is deposited in all layers of articular cartilage and is preferentially taken up by osteoarthritic cartilage. When administered IM, articular levels will with time exceed those found in the serum. Peak joint levels are reached 48 hours after IM injection, and persist for up to 96 hours after injection.

Contraindications/Precautions/Reproductive Safety - PSGAG is contraindicated for intra-articular administration in patients hypersensitive to it. While the manufacturer states there are no contraindications for IM use of the drug, the drug should not be used in place of other therapies in cases where infection is present or suspected, or in place of surgery or joint immobilization in cases where indicated.

Some clinicians feel that PSGAG should not be used within one week of arthrotomy in the dog, because it may cause increased bleeding. This effect apparently has not been confirmed in the literature however.

Reproductive studies have apparently not been performed; use with caution during pregnancy or in breeding animals (the manufacturer does not recommend use in breeding animals).

Adverse Effects/Warnings - Adverse effects are unlikely when using the IM route. Intraarticular administration may cause a post-injection inflammation (joint pain, effusion, swelling and associated lameness) secondary to sensitivity reactions, traumatic injection technique, overdosage, number or frequency of injections. Treatment consisting of anti-inflammatory drugs, cold hydrotherapy, and rest is recommended. Although rare, joint sepsis secondary to injection is also potentially possible; strict aseptic technique should be employed to minimize its occurrence.

In dogs, a dose-related inhibition of coagulation/hemostasis has been described.

Overdosage/Acute Toxicity - Doses five times those recommended (2.5 grams) given IM to horses twice weekly for 6 weeks revealed no untoward toxic effects. Approximately 2% of horses receiving overdoses (up to 1250 mg) IA showed transient symptoms associated with joint inflammation.

Drug Interactions - While specific drug interactions have not been detailed to date, using this product in conjunction with either steroids or non-steroidal antiinflammatory agents could mask the signs and symptoms associated with septic joints.

There is some concern that since PSGAG is a heparin analog that it should not be used in conjunction with **other NSAID's** or **other anticoagulants**. Clinical significance is unclear, but use together with caution.

Doses -
Horses:
  a) For IM administration: 500 mg IM (of IM product) every 4 days for 28 days. Thoroughly cleanse injection site before injecting. Do not mix with other drugs or chemicals. (Package Insert- Adequan® I.M.)
      For intra-articular administration: 250 mg (of IA product) IA once a week for 5 weeks. Joint area should be shaved, and cleansed as if a surgical procedure, prior to injecting. Do not mix with other drugs or chemicals. (Package Insert- Adequan® I.M.)
  b) For IM injection: 500 mg IM every 3-4 days for a minimum of 4 and preferably, 7 treatments.

For intra-articular injection: As above; author recommends adding 125 mg of amikacin for injection into the IA injection to reduce potential for infection. (Nixon 1992)

Dogs:
For the treatment of traumatic, degenerative or chronic aseptic joint disease:
a) 3 - 5 mg/kg IM every 3-5 days for 3 weeks (Bloomberg 1992)
b) 1.1 - 4.8 mg/kg IM every 4 days for six doses and then as needed. (Kelly 1995)

Cats:
As a chondroprotective drug:
a) 1.1 - 4.8 mg/kg IM every 4 days for six doses and then as needed. (Kelly 1995)

Monitoring Parameters - Efficacy and joint inflammation/infection if administered IA.

Client Information - The IA product must be administered by veterinary professionals; the IM product could, with proper instruction be administered by the owner.

Dosage Forms/Preparations/FDA Approval Status/Withholding Times -
Veterinary-Approved Products:

Polysulfated glycosaminoglycan for Intra-Articular Injection 250 mg/ml in 1 ml glass ampules or 1 ml single use vials, boxes of 6; *Adequan® I.A.* (Luitpold); (Rx) Approved for use in horses (not in those intended for food).

Polysulfated glycosaminoglycan for Intra-Muscular Injection 100 mg/ml in 5 ml glass ampules or 5 ml vials, boxes of 4; *Adequan® I.M.* (Luitpold); (Rx) Approved for use in horses (not in those intended for food).

Polysulfated glycosaminoglycan for IM Injection 100 mg/ml; *Adequan® Canine* (Luitpold); (Rx) Approved for use in Dogs.

Human-Approved Products: None

Potassium Bromide - see Bromide Salts

POTASSIUM CHLORIDE
POTASSIUM GLUCONATE

Chemistry - Potassium chloride occurs as either white, granular powder or as colorless, elongated, prismatic or cubical crystals. It is odorless and has a saline taste. One gram is soluble in about 3 ml of water and is insoluble in alcohol. The pH of the injection ranges from 4-8. One gram of potassium chloride contains 13.4 mEq of potassium. A 2 mEq/ml solution has an osmolarity of 4000 mOsm/L. Potassium chloride may also be known as KCl.

Potassium gluconate occurs as white to yellowish white, crystalline powder or granules. It is odorless and has a slightly bitter taste and is freely soluble in water. One gram of potassium gluconate contains 4.3 mEq of potassium.

Storage/Stability/Compatibility - Potassium gluconate oral products should be stored in tight, light resistant containers at room temperature (15-30°C), unless otherwise instructed by the manufacturer.

Unless otherwise directed by the manufacturer, potassium chloride products should be stored in tight, containers at room temperature (15-30°C); protect from freezing.

Potassium chloride for injection is reportedly **compatible** with the following intravenous solutions and drugs (as an additive): All commonly used intravenous replacement fluids (not 10% fat emulsion), aminophylline, amiodarone HCl, bretylium tosylate, calcium gluconate, carbenicillin disodium, cephalothin sodium, cephapirin sodium, chloramphenicol sodium succinate, cimetidine HCl, clindamycin phosphate, corticotropin (ACTH), cytarabine, dimenhydrinate, dopamine HCl, erythromycin gluceptate/lactobionate, heparin sodium, hydrocortisone sodium succinate, isoproterenol HCl, lidocaine HCl, metaraminol bitartrate, methicillin sodium, methyldopate HCl, metoclopramide HCl, nafcillin sodium, norepinephrine bitartrate, oxacillin sodium, oxytetracycline HCl, penicillin G potassium, phenylephrine HCl, piperacillin sodium, sodium bicarbonate, tetracycline HCl, thiopental sodium, vancomycin HCl, verapamil HCl, and vitamin B-complex with C.

Potassium chloride for injection **compatibility information conflicts** or is dependent on diluent or concentration factors with the following drugs or solutions: fat emulsion 10%, amikacin sulfate, dobutamine HCl, methylprednisolone sodium succinate (at Y-site), penicillin G sodium, and promethazine HCl (at Y-site). Compatibility is dependent upon factors such as pH, concentration, temperature and diluents used. It is suggested to consult specialized references (*e.g., Handbook on Injectable Drugs* by Trissel; see bibliography) for more specific information.

Potassium chloride for injection is reportedly **incompatible** with the following solutions or drugs: amphotericin B, diazepam (at Y-site), and phenytoin sodium (at Y-site).

Pharmacology - Potassium is the principal intracellular cation in the body. It is essential in maintaining cellular tonicity; nerve impulse transmission; smooth, skeletal and cardiac muscle contraction; and maintenance of normal renal function. Potassium is also used in carbohydrate utilization and in protein synthesis.

Uses/Indications - Potassium supplementation is used to prevent or treat potassium deficits. When feasible and appropriate, oral or nutritional therapy is generally preferred over parenteral potassium administration, because it is generally safer.

Pharmacokinetics - Potassium is primarily (80-90%) excreted via the kidneys with the majority of the remainder excreted in the feces. Very small amounts may be excreted in perspiration (in animals with sweat glands).

Contraindications/Precautions - Potassium salts are contraindicated in patients with hyperkalemia, renal failure or severe renal impairment, severe hemolytic reactions, untreated Addison's disease, and acute dehydration. Solid oral dosage forms should not be used in patients where GI motility is impaired. Use cautiously in digitalized patients (see Drug Interactions).

Because potassium is primarily an intracellular electrolyte, serum levels may not adequately reflect the total body stores of potassium. Acid-base balance may also mask the actual potassium picture. Patients with systemic acidosis conditions may appear to have hyperkalemia when in fact they may be significantly low in total body potassium. Conversely, alkalosis may cause a falsely low serum potassium value. Assess renal and cardiac function prior to therapy and closely monitor serum potassium levels. Supplementation should generally occur over 3-5 days to allow equilibration to occur between extracellular and intracellular fluids. Some clinicians feel that if acidosis is present, use potassium acetate, citrate or bicarbonate; and if alkalosis is present, use potassium chloride.

Adverse Effects/Warnings - The major problem associated with potassium supplementation is the development of hyperkalemia. Symptoms associated with hyperkalemia can range from muscular weakness and/or GI disturbances to cardiac conduction disturbances. Clinical symptoms can be exacerbated by concomitant hypocalcemia, hyponatremia, or acidosis. Intravenous potassium salts must be diluted before administering and given slowly (see Doses).

Oral therapy can cause GI distress and IV therapy may be irritating to veins.

Overdosage/Acute Toxicity - Fatal hyperkalemia may develop if potassium salts are administered too rapidly IV or if potassium renal excretory mechanisms are impaired. Symptoms associated with hyperkalemia are noted in the Adverse Effects section above. Treatment of hyperkalemia is dependent upon the cause and/or severity of the condition and can consist of: discontinuation of the drug with ECG, acid/base and electrolyte monitoring, glucose/insulin infusions, sodium bicarbonate, calcium therapy, and polystyrene sulfonate resin. It is suggested to refer to other references appropriate for the species being treated for specific protocols for treatment of hyperkalemia.

Drug Interactions - Potassium retention may occur when potassium is given with **angiotensin converting enzyme inhibitors** (*e.g.,* **captopril, enalapril**) or with **potassium-sparing diuretics** (*e.g.,* **spironolactone**).

In patients with severe or complete heart block who are receiving **digitalis** therapy, potassium salts are not recommended to be used.

Oral potassium given with **non-steroidal antiinflammatory agents, or anticholinergic agents** may increase the risk of gastrointestinal adverse effects occurring.

Glucocorticoids, mineralocorticoids, or ACTH may cause increased renal losses of potassium.

Doses -
  Dogs & Cats:
    For hypokalemia:
      a) Intravenous replacement: If animal has normal renal function, IV KCl not to exceed 0.5 mEq/kg/hr. Use IV replacement very cautiously in animals with impaired renal function or in those receiving potassium-sparing diuretics.
        Subcutaneous replacement: If IV use is unfeasible or rapid correction is unnecessary, may add KCl to SQ fluids; do not exceed 30 mEq of potassium per liter.
        Oral replacement: Potassium gluconate PO at a rate of 2.2 mEq per 100 calories of required energy intake or potassium gluconate elixir (20 mEq/ml) for dogs at 5 ml q8-12h PO. (Bell and Osborne 1986)
      b) Oral using *Tumil-K*® (Daniels): 1/4 teaspoonful (2 mEq) per 4.5 kg body weight PO in food twice daily. Adjust dose as necessary. (Package insert; *Tumil-K*®—Daniels).

Ruminants:
For hypokalemia in "downer" cows:
a) 80 g sodium chloride and 20 g potassium chloride in 10 liters of water PO via stomach tube. Provide a bucket containing similar solution for cow to drink and another containing fresh water. (Caple 1986)

For hypokalemia:
a) 50 grams PO daily; 1 mEq/kg/hr IV drip. (Howard 1986)

Monitoring Parameters - Level and frequency of monitoring associated with potassium therapy is dependent upon the cause and/or severity of hypokalemia, acid/base abnormalities, renal function, and concomitant drugs administered or disease states and can include: 1) Serum potassium ; 2) Other electrolytes; 3) Acid/base status; 4) Glucose; 5) ECG; 6) CBC; 7) Urinalyses

Dosage Forms/Preparations/FDA Approval Status/Withholding Times -
Veterinary-Approved Products:

There are several products for parenteral use that contain potassium; refer to the tables at the end of this section or individual proprietary veterinary products (*e.g., Cal-Dextro® K*—Fort Dodge) for additional information.

Oral Products:
Potassium Gluconate Oral Powder Each 0.65 gram 4 oz (1/4 teaspoonful) contains 2 mEq of potassium; in 4 oz. containers *Tumil-K ®* (Daniels) (Rx)

   Tumil-KCaplets® (Daniels); (Rx) Approved for use in dogs and cats.

   Tumil-K Gel® (Daniels) (Rx) 5 oz/tube

Human-Approved Products: Not a complete list.
Parenteral Products:
Potassium Chloride for Injection 2 mEq/ml in 250 & 500 ml; 10 mEq in 10 & 20 ml vials, syringes, & amps; 30 mEq in 14, 20, 30 & 100 ml vials and 20 ml syringes; 40 mEq in 20, 30, 50 & 100 ml vials, 20 ml amps and syringes; 60 mEq & 90 mEq in 30 ml vials. Must be diluted before administering. (Rx)

Potassium acetate for injection and potassium phosphate for injection (see previous monograph) are also available.

There are a multitude of human-labeled potassium salts for oral use available in several dosage forms; refer to human drug references for more information on these products.

Potassium Citrate - see Citrate Salts

PRALIDOXIME CHLORIDE
2-PAM CHLORIDE

Chemistry - A quaternary ammonium oxime cholinesterase reactivator, pralidoxime chloride occurs as a white to pale yellow, crystalline powder with a pK_a of 7.8-8. It is freely soluble in water. The commercially available injection has a pH of 3.5-4.5 after reconstitution. Pralidoxime may also be known as 2-PAM Chloride, or 2-Pyridine Aldoxime Methochloride.

Storage/Stability/Compatibility - Unless otherwise instructed by the manufacturer, pralidoxime chloride powder for injection should be stored at room temperature. After reconstituting with sterile water for injection, the solution should be used within a few hours. Do not use sterile water with preservatives added.

Pharmacology - Pralidoxime reactivates cholinesterase that has been inactivated by phosphorylation secondary to certain organophosphates. Via nucleophilic attack, the drug removes and binds the offending phosphoryl group attached to the enzyme and is then excreted.

Uses/Indications - Pralidoxime is used in the treatment of organophosphate poisoning, often in conjunction with atropine and supportive therapy.

Pharmacokinetics - Pralidoxime is only marginally absorbed after oral dosing and oral dosage forms are no longer available in the United States. It is distributed primarily throughout the extracellular water. Because of its quaternary ammonium structure, it is not believed to enter the CNS in significant quantities, but recent studies and clinical responses have led some to question this.

Pralidoxime is thought to be metabolized in the liver and excreted as both metabolite(s) and unchanged drug in the urine.

Contraindications/Precautions/Reproductive Safety - Pralidoxime is contraindicated in patients hypersensitive to it. Pralidoxime is generally not recommended to be used in instances of carbamate poisoning because inhibition is rapidly reversible, but there is some controversy regarding this issue.

Pralidoxime should be used with caution in patients receiving anticholinesterase agents for the treatment of myasthenia gravis as it may precipitate a myasthenic crisis. It should also be used cautiously and at a reduced dosage rate in patients with renal impairment.

Adverse Effects/Warnings - At usual doses, pralidoxime generally is safe and free of significant adverse effects. Rapid IV injection may cause tachycardia, muscle rigidity, transient neuromuscular blockade, and laryngospasm.

Pralidoxime must generally be given within 24 hours of exposure to be effective, but some benefits may occur, particularly in large exposures, if given within 36-48 hours.

Overdosage/Acute Toxicity - The acute LD_{50} of pralidoxime in dogs is 190 mg/kg and, at high dosages, exhibits symptoms of its own anticholinesterase activity. Symptoms of toxicity in dogs may be exhibited as muscle weakness, ataxia, vomiting, hyperventilation, seizures, respiratory arrest and death.

Drug Interactions - Anticholinesterases can potentiate the action of **barbiturates**; use with caution.

Cimetidine may potentiate the action of organophosphates by slowing its metabolism.

Use of **succinylcholine, theophylline/aminophylline, reserpine, and respiratory depressant drugs** (*e.g.,* **narcotics, phenothiazines**) should be avoided in patients with organophosphate toxicity.

Doses - Note: often used in conjunction with atropine; refer to that monograph and/or the references below for more information.

Dogs & Cats:
For organophosphate poisoning:
a) Pralidoxime works best when combined with atropine. Pralidoxime at 20 mg/kg 2-3 times a day. Initial dose may be given either IM or slow IV. Subsequent doses may be given IM or SQ. (Note: Refer to reference for more specific guidelines regarding adjunctive therapy). (Fikes 1990)
b) 20 mg/kg IV *bid* (Grauer and Hjelle 1988c)
c) 10 - 15 mg/kg IM or SubQ two - three times daily and continued until recovery. Most beneficial when started within 24 hours of exposure. (Hansen 1995)
d) Dogs: 50 mg/kg; Cats 20 mg/kg. Give IV slowly or with fluids over a 30 minute period. Repeat in one hour if symptoms persist and then q8h for 24-48 hours. Author recommends using pralidoxime in animals who are severely depressed, weak, and anorectic one or more days after exposure if not previously treated with pralidoxime. In animals who have clinical signs intensified (*e.g.,* respiratory depression), reduce dose and give as repeated one hour infusions every 4-8 hours in combination with atropine (0.04 - 0.4 mg/kg) once or *prn.* (Mount 1989)
e) Cats: 20 mg/kg IM or IV within first 24 hours of exposure. May repeat q6-8h and combine with atropine or give separately. Do not use in carbamate toxicity. (Reid and Oehme 1989)

Cattle:
For organophosphate poisoning:
a) 25 - 50 mg/kg as a 20% solution IV over 6 minutes; or as a maximum of 100 mg/kg/day as an IV drip. (Smith 1986)

Horses:
For organophosphate poisoning:
a) 20 mg/kg (may require up to 35 mg/kg) IV and repeat q4-6h. (Oehme 1987c)

Monitoring Parameters - Monitoring of pralidoxime therapy is basically by monitoring the signs and symptoms associated with organophosphate poisoning. For more information, refer to one of the references outlined noted below.

Client Information - This agent should only be used with close professional supervision.

Dosage Forms/Preparations/FDA Approval Status/Withholding Times -
Veterinary-Approved Products: None
Human-Approved Products:
Pralidoxime Chloride 1 gram cake in containers of six 20 ml vials without diluent or syringes; 600 mg in one 2 ml auto-injector; *Protopam Chloride*® (Wyeth-Ayerst); (Rx); Pralidoxime Chloride® (Survival Technology) (Rx)

PRAZIQUANTEL

Chemistry - A prazinoisoquinoline derivative anthelmintic, praziquantel occurs as a white to practically white, hygroscopic, bitter tasting, crystalline powder, either odorless or having a faint odor. It is very slightly soluble in water and freely soluble in alcohol.

Storage/Stability/Compatibility - Unless otherwise instructed by the manufacturer, praziquantel tablets should be stored in tight containers at room temperature. Protect from light.

Pharmacology - Praziquantel's exact mechanism of action against cestodes has not been determined. At low concentrations *in vitro*, the drug appears to impair the function of their suckers and stimulates the worm's motility. At higher concentrations *in vitro*, praziquantel increases the contraction (irreversibly at very high concentrations) of the worm's strobilla (chain of proglottids). Also, praziquantel causes irreversible focal vacuolization with subsequent cestodal disintegration at specific sites of the cestodal integument.

In schistosomes and trematodes, praziquantel directly kills the parasite, possibly by increasing calcium ion flux into the worm. Focal vacuolization of the integument follows and the parasite is phagocytized.

Uses/Indications - Praziquantel is indicated for (approved labeling) for the treatment of *Dipylidium caninum*, *Taenia pisiformis* and *Echinococcus granulosis* in dogs, and *Dipylidium caninum* and *Taenia taeniaeformis* in cats. Fasting is not required nor is it recommended before dosing. A single dose is usually effective, but measures should be taken to prevent reinfection, particularly against *D. caninum.*

Praziquantel has been used in birds and other animals, but it is usually not economically feasible to use in large animals. In humans, praziquantel is used for schistosomiasis, other trematodes (lung, liver, intestinal flukes) and tapeworms. It is not routinely effective in treating *F. hepatica* infections in humans.

Pharmacokinetics - Praziquantel is rapidly and nearly completely absorbed after oral administration, but there is a significant first-pass effect after oral administration. Peak serum levels are achieved after 30-120 minutes in dogs.

Praziquantel is distributed throughout the body and crosses the blood-brain barrier into the CNS and across the intestinal wall.

Praziquantel is metabolized by the liver to metabolites of unknown activity. It is excreted primarily in the urine and the elimination half-life is approximately 3 hours in the dog.

Contraindications/Precautions/Reproductive Safety - The manufacturer recommends not using praziquantel in puppies less than 4 weeks old or in kittens less than 6 weeks old. However, a combination product containing praziquantel and febantel from the same manufacturer is approved for use in puppies and kittens of all ages. No other contraindications are listed for this compound by the manufacturer. In humans, praziquantel is contraindicated in patients hypersensitive to the drug. Praziquantel is considered to be safe to use in pregnant dogs or cats.

Adverse Effects/Warnings - When used orally, praziquantel can cause anorexia, vomiting, lethargy or diarrhea in dogs, but the incidence of these effects is less than 5%. In cats, adverse effects were quite rare (<2%) in field trials using oral praziquantel with salivation and diarrhea being reported.

An increased incidence of adverse effects have been reported after using the injectable product. In dogs, pain at the injection site, vomiting, drowsiness and/or a staggering gait were reported from field trials with the drug. Some cats (9.4%) showed symptoms of diarrhea, weakness, vomiting, salivation, sleepiness, transient anorexia and/or pain at the injection site.

Overdosage/Acute Toxicity - Praziquantel has a wide margin of safety. In rats and mice the oral LD_{50} is at least 2 g/kg. An oral LD_{50} could not be determined in dogs, as at doses greater than 200 mg/kg, the drug induced vomiting. Parenteral doses of 50 - 100 mg/kg in cats caused transient ataxia and depression. Injected doses at 200 mg/kg were lethal in cats.

Drug Interactions - Reportedly in humans, synergistic activity occurs with praziquantel and **oxamniquine** in the treatment of schistosomiasis. The clinical implications of this synergism in veterinary patients is not clear.

Doses -
  Dogs:
     For susceptible cestodes:
        a)   IM or SubQ using the 56.8 mg/ml injectable product:

Body weight	Dose
5 lbs or less	17 mg (0.3 ml)
6-10 lbs	28.4 mg (0.5 ml)
11-25 lbs	56.8 mg (1.0 ml)
over 25 lbs.	0.2 ml/5 lb body weight - max. of 3 ml

Oral: Using the 34 mg canine tablet:

5 lbs or less	17 mg (1/2 tab)
6-10 lbs.	34 mg (1 tab)
11-15 lbs	51 mg (1.5 tabs)
16-30 lbs	68 mg (2 tabs)
31-45 lbs	102 mg (3 tabs)
46-60 lbs	136 mg (4 tabs)
over 60 lbs.	170 mg (5 tabs - max.); (Package insert; *Droncit*® *Injectable &*

Tablets—Miles)
   b) 5 mg/kg (Chiapella 1988)
   c) For *Echinococcus granulosis*: 10 mg/kg (Sherding 1989)
   d) For *Diphyllobothrium sp*: 7.5 mg/kg PO once. (Kirkpatrick, Knochenhauer, and Jacobsen 1987)
   e) For *Spirometra mansonoides* or *Diphyllobothrium erinacei*: 7.5 mg/kg PO once daily for 2 days. (Roberson 1988a)

For treatment of Paragonimiasis:
   a) 25 mg/kg *bid* PO for 2 consecutive days. (Kirkpatrick and Shelly 1987)
   b) 23 mg/kg PO q8h for 3 days (Reinemeyer 1995)

Cats:
For susceptible cestodes:
   a) 5 mg/kg (Chiapella 1988)
   b) IM or SubQ using the 56.8 mg/ml injectable product:

Body weight	Dose
Under 5 lbs	11.4 mg (0.2 ml)
5-10 lbs	22.7 mg (0.4 ml)
10 lbs and over	34.1 mg (0.6 ml - max)

Oral: Using the 23 mg feline tab

Body weight	Dose
4 lbs and under	11.5 mg (1/2 tab)
5-11 lbs	23 mg (1 tab)
over 11 lbs	34.5 mg (1.5 tabs)

(Package insert; *Droncit*® *Injectable & Tablets*—Miles)

For treatment of Paragonimiasis:
   a) 23 mg/kg PO q8h for 3 days (Reinemeyer 1995)

Sheep & Goats:
For all species of *Moniezia, Stilesia,* or *Avitellina*:
   a) 10 - 15 mg/kg (Roberson 1988a)

Llamas:
For susceptible parasites:
   a) 5 mg/kg PO. (Fowler 1989)

Birds:
For susceptible parasites (tapeworms):
   a) 1/4 of one 23 mg tablet/kg PO; repeat in 10-14 days. Add to feed or give by gavage. Injectable form is toxic to finches. (Clubb 1986)
   b) For common tapeworms in chickens: 10 mg/kg. (Roberson 1988a)
   c) For cestodes and some trematodes: Direct dose: 5 - 10 mg/kg PO or IM as a single dose -or- 12 mg of crushed tablets baked into a 9"x9"x2" cake. Finches should have their regular food withheld and be pre-exposed to a non-medicated cake. (Marshall 1993)

Reptiles:
   a) For cestodes and some trematodes in most species: 7.5 mg/kg PO once; repeat in 2 weeks PO (Gauvin 1993)
   b) For removal of common tapeworms in snakes: 3.5 - 7 mg/kg (Roberson 1988a)

Monitoring Parameters -
   1) Clinical efficacy

Client Information - Fasting is not required nor is it recommended before dosing. A single dose is usually effective, but measures should be taken to prevent reinfection, particularly against *D. caninum*. Tablets may be crushed or mixed with food. Because tapeworms are often digested, worm fragments may not be seen in the feces after using.

Dosage Forms/Preparations/FDA Approval Status/Withholding Times -
Veterinary-Approved Products:

Praziquantel 23 mg (feline), 34 mg (canine) Tablets; *Droncit® Tablets* (Bayer); (Rx) Approved for use in cats and dogs.

Praziquantel Injection 56.8 mg/ml in 10 ml vials; *Droncit® Injection* (Bayer); (Rx) Approved for use in cats and dogs.

Praziquantel/pyrantel pamoate; *Drontal Tablets®* (Bayer) (Rx) Approved for use in cats

Praziquantel/pyrantel pamoate plus febantel; *Drontal Plus Tablets®* (Bayer) (Rx) small, medium and large dog sizes

Human-Approved Products:

Praziquantel Tablets 600 mg; *Biltricide®* (Bayer) (Rx)

PRAZOSIN HCL

Chemistry - A quinazoline-derivative postsynaptic alpha$_1$-adrenergic blocker, prazosin HCl occurs as a white to tan powder. It is slightly soluble in water and very slightly soluble in alcohol. Prazosin may also be known as Furazosin.

Storage/Stability/Compatibility - Prazosin capsules should be stored in well-closed containers at room temperature.

Pharmacology - Prazosin's effects are a result of its selective, competitive inhibition of alpha$_1$-adrenergic receptors. It reduces blood pressure and peripheral vascular resistance and unlike hydralazine, has dilatory effects on both the arterial and venous side.

Prazosin significantly reduces systemic and venous pressures, right atrial pressure and increases cardiac output in patients with CHF. Moderate reductions in blood pressure, pulmonary vascular resistance and systemic vascular resistance are seen in these patients. Heart rates can be moderately decreased or unchanged. Unlike hydralazine, prazosin does not seem to increase renin release so diuretic therapy is not mandatory with this agent (but is usually beneficial in CHF).

Uses/Indications - Prazosin is less well studied in dogs than is hydralazine, and its capsule dosage form makes it less convenient for dosing. Prazosin, however, appears to have less problems with causing tachycardia, and its venous dilation effects may be an advantage over hydralazine when preload reduction is desired. It could be considered for therapy for the adjunctive treatment of CHF, particularly when secondary to mitral or aortic valve insufficiency when hydralazine is ineffective or not tolerated. Prazosin may also be used for the treatment of systemic hypertension or pulmonary hypertension in the dog.

Pharmacokinetics - The pharmacokinetic parameters for this agent were not located for veterinary species. In humans, prazosin is variably absorbed after oral administration. Peak levels occur in 2-3 hours.

Prazosin is widely distributed throughout the body and is approximately 97% bound to plasma proteins. Prazosin is minimally distributed into milk. It is unknown if it crosses the placenta.

Prazosin is metabolized in the liver and some metabolites have activity. Metabolites and some unchanged drug (5-10%) are primarily eliminated in feces via the bile.

Contraindications/Precautions - Prazosin should be used with caution in patients with chronic renal failure or preexisting hypotensive conditions.

Adverse Effects/Warnings - Syncope secondary to orthostatic hypotension has been reported in people after the first dose of the drug. This effect may persist if the dosage is too high for the patient. CNS effects (lethargy, dizziness, etc.) may occur, but are usually transient in nature. GI effects (nausea, vomiting, diarrhea, constipation, etc) have been reported. Tachyphylaxis (drug tolerance) has been reported in man, but dosage adjustment, temporarily withdrawing the drug &/or adding an aldosterone antagonist (*e.g.,* spironolactone) usually corrects this.

Overdosage - Evacuate gastric contents and administer activated charcoal using standard precautionary measures if the ingestion was recent and if cardiovascular status has been stabilized. Treat shock using volume expanders and pressor agents if necessary. Monitor and support renal function.

Drug Interactions - As prazosin is highly bound to plasma proteins, it may displace or be displaced by other **highly protein bound drugs** (*e.g.,* sulfonamides, phenylbutazone, warfarin, etc.).

Verapamil or nifedipine may cause synergistic hypotensive effects when used concomitantly with prazosin.

Beta-blocking agents (*e.g.,* propranolol) may enhance the postural hypotensive effects seen after the first dose of prazosin. Other **antihypertensive agents** can also cause additive hypotension.

Doses -
Dogs:
  a) For treatment of heart failure, systemic hypertension, or pulmonary hypertension: 1 mg per 15 kgs of body weight PO *tid* (*bid-tid* for systemic hypertension) (Morgan 1988)
  b) For treatment of heart failure: 1 mg PO *tid* for dogs weighing less than 15 kg; 2 mg *tid* PO for dogs weighing more than 15 kg. (Kittleson 1985b)
  c) For canine dilated cardiomyopathy: 1 mg for every 15 kg of body weight PO *tid*; must use with a diuretic. (Ogburn 1988)

Monitoring Parameters -
  1) Baseline thoracic radiographs
  2) Mucous membrane color; CRT
  3) If possible, arterial blood pressure and venous pO_2

Client Information - Compliance with directions is necessary to maximize the benefits from this drug. If possible, give medication with food. Notify veterinarian if patient's condition deteriorates or if the animal becomes lethargic or depressed.

Dosage Forms/Preparations/FDA Approval Status/Withholding Times -
  Veterinary-Approved Products: None
  Human-Approved Products:
    Prazosin Capsules 1 mg, 2 mg, 5 mg; *Minipress*® (Pfizer); generic (Rx)

PREDNISOLONE
PREDNISOLONE SODIUM SUCCINATE
PREDNISOLONE ACETATE
PREDNISONE

For more information refer to the monograph: Glucocorticoids, General Information or to the manufacturer's product information for veterinary labeled products.

Note: Although separate entities, prednisone is rapidly converted by the liver *in vivo* to prednisolone. Except for patients in frank hepatic failure, the drugs can, for all intents, be considered equivalent.

Chemistry - Prednisolone and prednisone are synthetic glucocorticoids. Prednisolone and prednisolone acetate occur as odorless, white to practically white, crystalline powders. Prednisolone is very slightly soluble in water and slightly soluble in alcohol. The acetate ester is practically insoluble in water and slightly soluble in alcohol. The sodium succinate ester is highly water soluble. Prednisolone is also known as deltahydrocortisone or metacortandralone.

Prednisone occurs as an odorless, white to practically white, crystalline powder. Prednisone is very slightly soluble in water and slightly soluble in alcohol. Prednisone is also known as deltacortisone or deltadehydrocortisone.

Storage/Stability/Compatibility - Prednisolone and prednisone tablets should be stored in well-closed containers. All prednisone and prednisolone products should be stored at temperatures less than 40°, and preferably between 15-30°C; avoid freezing liquid products. Do not autoclave. Oral liquid preparations of prednisone should be stored in tight containers.

Prednisolone sodium succinate should be stored at room temperature and protected from light (store in carton). After reconstitution, the product is recommended to be used immediately and not stored.

Little data appears to be available regarding the compatibility of prednisolone sodium succinate injection (*Solu-Delta Cortef*® — Upjohn) with other products. A related compound, prednisolone sodium phosphate is reportedly **compatible** with the following drugs/solutions: ascorbic acid injection, cephalothin sodium, cytarabine, erythromycin lactobionate, fluorouracil, heparin sodium, methicillin sodium, penicillin G potassium/sodium, tetracycline HCl and vitamin B-Complex with C. It is reportedly **incompatible** with: calcium gluconate/gluceptate, dimenhydrinate, metaraminol bitartrate, methotrexate sodium, prochlorperazine edisylate, polymyxin B sulfate, promazine HCl, and promethazine HCl. Compatibility is dependent upon factors such as pH, concentration, temperature and diluents used. It is suggested to consult specialized references for more specific information (*e.g., Handbook on Injectable Drugs* by Trissel; see bibliography).

Doses -
Dogs:
  For adjunctive therapy of endotoxemic or septic shock:
    a) Prednisolone sodium succinate: 5.5 - 11 mg/kg IV; may repeat in 1, 3, 6, or 10 hours. (Jenkins 1985)

For adjunctive treatment of neoplasms:

Note: Also see the section on Chemotherapy Protocols for Treatment of Neoplastic Diseases in Small Animals found in the appendix.

a) Brain tumors (palliative therapy): Prednisone 0.5 - 1 mg/kg PO once a day to every other day. (Fenner 1988); Prednisone 0.5 - 1 mg/kg PO *bid* for several days, then decrease dosage over the next week or month, dependent on patient's needs. (LeCouteur and Turrel 1986)

b) For adjunctive therapy in canine lymphomas:

COAP (cyclophosphamide, vincristine, cytosine arabinoside, prednisone) protocol: Prednisone: 50 mg/m^2 PO every day for one week, then 25 mg/m^2 every other day.

COP (no cytosine arabinoside) protocol: Prednisone 25 mg/m^2 PO every other day.

CHOP (doxorubicin instead of cytosine arabinoside): Prednisone 25 mg/m^2 PO every other day. (Couto 1986)

c) For adjunctive therapy for multiple myeloma: Prednisone 0.5 mg/kg PO once daily. Used with melphalan: 0.1 mg/kg PO once daily for 10 days, then 0.05 mg/kg PO once daily or cyclophosphamide: 1 mg/kg PO once daily (if resistance develops to melphalan). (Jenkins 1985)

d) For macroglobulinemia: Prednisone 0.5 mg/kg PO once daily. Used with chlorambucil: 0.2 mg/kg PO once daily for 10 days, then 0.1 mg/kg PO once daily or cyclophosphamide: 1 mg/kg PO once daily (if resistance develops to chlorambucil). (Jenkins 1985)

For adjunctive treatment of respiratory disorders:

a) Chronic bronchitis: Prednisone 0.5 - 1 mg/kg PO once a day to every other day. (Bauer 1988)

b) Allergic bronchitis: Prednisolone sodium succinate: 2 - 4 mg/kg IV or IM (do not give via rapid IV infusion). In chronically symptomatic patient: prednisone 0.5 - 1.5 mg/kg/day PO. (Bauer 1988)

c) For adjunctive therapy of collapsing trachea:

Initially, prednisolone 0.25 - 0.5 mg/kg PO *bid* for 7-10 days. (Prueter 1988b)

Prednisone 0.5 mg/kg PO once or twice a day. Discontinue if no improvement in one week. Corticosteroids must be used cautiously in this condition and rarely make a difference in the long-term outcome of therapy. (Fingland 1989)

d) For allergic (eosinophilic) bronchitis or pneumonitis: Prednisone 1 - 2 mg/kg/day divided *bid-tid*. Every 7-10 days decrease total steroid dose by 1/4 - 1/2 as long as signs are controlled. After 3-4 weeks every other day or every third day therapy may be attempted. (Noone 1986)

e) For adjunctive therapy of parasitic pulmonary hypersensitivities: To suppress inflammation prior to parasite elimination: Prednisolone 1 - 2 mg/kg PO divided into 2-3 doses. (Noone 1986)

For adjunctive therapy in liver disorders:

Note: Because prednisone requires conversion to the active compound prednisolone by the liver, some clinicians believe that only prednisolone should be used in patients with liver disease.

a) For cholangitis: Prednisolone 1 - 2 mg/kg PO once daily for at least 1 month. Then give every other day for another 2-3 months and consider discontinuing and monitoring for relapse. (Cornelius and Bjorling 1988)

b) For chronic active hepatitis: Prednisolone 1 mg/kg PO *bid*; recheck in 14 days. If improved, continue at same dose for approximately 2 months, then switch to alternate day prednisolone at 2 - 4 mg/kg PO every other day for 2-3 months. If after 14 days of prednisolone therapy no improvement is noted, add azathioprine (2 - 2.5 mg/kg PO once a day. Recheck in 10-14 days. If improved, continue for 2-3 months. If not, reconsider the diagnosis. (Cornelius and Bjorling 1988)

c) Copper-induced hepatopathy: Prednisolone 0.5 - 1.0 mg/kg PO divided *bid* (used during acute stages). Used with chelation therapy and dietary copper restriction. (Cornelius and Bjorling 1988)

For adjunctive therapy of disorders of the gastrointestinal tract:

a) For eosinophilic colitis: Prednisolone 1 - 2 mg/kg PO for 7-10 days. Gradually decrease dose over following 3-4 weeks to a minimal dosage that will control clinical signs. Some cases will require additional alternate-day therapy for an another 3-4 weeks. (DeNovo 1988)

b) For eosinophilic enteritis: Prednisolone 1 - 3 mg/kg PO once daily; gradually taper to every other day dosing for maintenance. May use injectable forms if dog is vomiting

or malabsorption is severe. Therapy may be necessary for weeks to months. Do not use until intestinal biopsy sites are healed (usually 7-10 days). (Chiapella 1988);
Prednisone 0.5 mg/kg PO once daily initially; reduce gradually to alternate day therapy. (Hall and Twedt 1989);
Prednisolone 0.5 - 1 mg/kg *bid* for 5-7 days, then decrease to 0.5 mg/kg/day for 5-7 days. Taper dose to alternate-day therapy as condition dictates. Additional therapy for 3-4 weeks is often necessary. Relapses can occur. (DeNovo 1986)

c) For eosinophilic colitis when dietary and parasitic infestations have been eliminated or when other appropriate therapy has been unsuccessful: Prednisolone 0.5 - 1 mg/kg *bid*; taper dose gradually over a 3-4 week period to the lowest effective dose. (Chiapella 1986)

d) For plasmacytic/lymphocytic enteritis: Prednisolone 2.2 mg/kg PO divided twice daily for 5-10 days, then 1.1 mg/kg/day for 5-10 days. Then taper by reducing steroid dosage by 1/2 every 10-14 days until alternate-day dosage is attained or symptoms recur. (Chiapella 1988)

e) For adjunctive therapy of chronic superficial gastritis (if predominance of lymphocyte and plasma cell infiltration seen on biopsy): Prednisone 0.5 - 1.0 mg/kg PO dived *bid* initially and reduced over a 3 month period to lowest, alternate-day effective dosage. (Hall and Twedt 1989)

f) Ulcerative colitis: May cause some patients' condition to worsen. Use only after an unsuccessful trial of sulfasalazine. Use with caution. Prednisolone 1 - 2 mg/kg/day PO for 5-7 days; then 0.5 mg/kg/day for an additional 5-7 days; then 0.25 - 0.5 mg/kg PO every other day for 10-14 days. Continue sulfasalzine during steroid therapy. If significant improvement is not seen within the first 7 days of therapy, steroids are tapered and discontinued more rapidly. (DeNovo 1988)

g) For food allergy or intolerance: Prednisone 0.5 mg/kg PO once daily; taper dose weekly if clinical response dictates. Discontinue when clinical remission ensues. (Chiapella 1988)

h) For adjunctive therapy of endotoxemia secondary to GDV: Prednisolone sodium succinate: 11 mg/kg IV (Bellah 1988); Prednisolone sodium succinate 10 mg/kg (Orton 1986)

i) For eosinophilic gastritis: Prednisone 0.5 mg/kg once daily for 1-2 weeks; gradually taper to 0.12 mg/kg PO every other day. (Twedt and Magne 1986)

j) For adjunctive therapy of intestinal lymphangiectasia: prednisolone 2 - 3 mg/kg/day. Once remission is attained, may taper to a maintenance dosage. Not all cases respond. (Sherding 1986)

k) For adjunctive therapy of refractory wheat-sensitive enteropathy in Irish Setters:
Prednisolone 0.5 mg/kg every 12 hours for one month. Then begin a reducing dosage schedule. (Batt 1986)

l) For dogs who respond poorly to conventional therapy (enzyme replacement, dietary modification, vitamin supplementation, & antibiotics) for exocrine pancreatic insufficiency: Predniso(lo)ne 1 - 2 mg/kg every 12 hours for 7-14 days. May reduce over 4-6 weeks as patient tolerates. (Williams 1989)

For adrenal diseases:

a) For adjunctive treatment of hypoadrenal crisis: Prednisolone sodium succinate: 4 - 20 mg/kg IV over 2-4 minutes, preferably after ACTH response test is completed. IV normal saline is usually sufficient therapy during the first hour until ACTH response test is completed. Prednisolone sodium succinate may be repeated in 2-6 hours or dexamethasone may be added to IV infusion at 0.05 - 0.2 mg/kg q12h. Prednisolone sodium succinate possess some mineralocorticoid activity, while dexamethasone does not. (Feldman 1989)

b) For glucocorticoid supplementation in chronic or subacute adrenal insufficiency: Predniso(lo)ne 0.2 - 0.4 mg/kg PO per day. (Feldman, Schrader, and Twedt 1988)

c) For glucocorticoid supplementation if azotemia or other symptoms of glucocorticoid deficiency result: Predniso(lo)ne 0.1 - 0.3 mg/kg PO per day. (Schrader 1986)

d) For glucocorticoid coverage before and after adrenal tumor removal: Prednisolone sodium succinate 1 - 2 mg/kg IV either at 1 hour prior to surgery or at the time of anesthesia induction. May also add to IV fluids and administer IV during the procedure. Repeat dosage at end of procedure; may give IM or IV. Glucocorticoid supplementation must be maintained using an oral product (initially predniso(lo)ne 0.5 mg/kg *bid*, cortisone acetate 2.5 mg/kg *bid*, or dexamethasone 0.1 mg/kg once daily). Slowly taper to maintenance levels (predniso(lo)ne 0.2 mg/kg once a day, or cortisone acetate 0.5 mg/kg *bid*) over 7-10 days. Should complications develop during the taper, reinitiate doses at 5 times maintenance. Most dogs can stop exogenous steroid therapy in about 2 months (based on an ACTH stimulation test). (Peterson 1986)

e) For glucocorticoid "coverage" in animals who have iatrogenic secondary adrenocortical insufficiency and/or HPA suppression: Animals exhibiting mild to moderate signs of glucocorticoid deficiency: Predniso(lo)ne 0.2 mg/kg PO every other day.
For animals with HPA suppression undergoing a "stress" factor: Prednisolone sodium succinate 1 - 2 mg/kg just before and after stressful events (*e.g.,* major surgery). Continue with lower dosages until at least 3rd post-operative day. Access to a water-soluble form of glucocorticoid should be available should animal "collapse." (Kemppainen 1986)

f) For symptoms of glucocorticoid deficiency (anorexia, diarrhea, listlessness) or in well-controlled patients receiving mitotane (*Lysodren*®) therapy for hyperadrenocorticism undergoing a "stress": Prednisone 2.2 mg/kg PO for 2 days, then 1 mg/kg for 2 days, then 0.5 mg/kg for 3 days, then 0.5 mg/kg every other day for one week, then stop. Reintroduce therapy or readjust dosage should symptoms recur. (Feldman 1989)

For adjunctive or alternative medical management of hyperinsulinism:
a) Prednisone 0.5 mg/kg PO divided *bid* initially; increase dose as required to maintain euglycemia. (Kay, Kruth, and Twedt 1988)
b) Prednisolone 1 mg/kg divided twice daily PO, then decrease to a minimally effective dosage. (Lothrop 1989)

For adjunctive therapy of toxicoses:
a) For cholecalciferol toxicity: Prednisone 1 - 2 mg/kg PO *bid-tid*. (Grauer and Hjelle 1988a)
b) For adjunctive therapy of endotoxicosis secondary to garbage or carrion ingestion: Prednisolone sodium succinate 5 - 7 mg/kg IV every 4 hours. (Coppock and Mostrom 1986)

For adjunctive therapy of reproductive disorders:
a) In bitches prone to relapse after initial therapy of eclampsia (puerperal tetany): Prednisone 0.25 mg/kg PO once daily during lactation and slowly withdrawn. (Barton and Wolf 1988);
Prednisolone 0.5 mg/kg *bid* (Russo and Lees 1986)

For adjunctive therapy of heartworm disease (considered by some clinicians to be contraindicated during treatment for routine post-adulticide therapy as pulmonary thromboses may be promoted):
a) Prednisolone 1 - 2 mg/kg PO divided *bid*. Reduce dosage over next 7-14 days. (Knight 1988)
b) Dogs with severe cough, hemoptysis, or extensive parenchymal involvement: Prior to adulticide therapy, prednisolone 1 - 2 mg/kg PO divided *bid* and tapered over a 10-14 day period. (Noone 1986)
c) For pneumonitis associated with occult heartworm disease: Prednisone 1 - 2 mg/kg daily for 3 - 5 days. After steroids are stopped, give adulticide therapy immediately. (Calvert and Rawlings 1986)

For CNS disorders:
a) For granulomatous meningoencephalitis: Prednisone: 1 - 2 mg/kg PO daily for the life of the patient. (Fenner 1988); prednisone 2-3 mg/kg PO divided *bid* for 2 weeks, then slowly reduce dosage over several weeks; long-term therapy is recommended. (Schunk 1988a)
b) For reticulosis: Prednisone: 1 - 2 mg/kg/day PO until symptoms begin to subside, then begin taper. Continue low-dose once a day or every other day therapy indefinitely. (Fenner 1988); Prednisone 2-3 mg/kg PO divided *bid* for 2 weeks, then slowly reduce dosage over several weeks; long-term therapy is recommended. (Schunk 1988a); Predniso(lo)ne: 2 mg/kg PO for 1 week, then 1 mg/kg/day for 1 week, then 0.5 mg/kg/day for 1 week, then 0.5 mg/kg every other day for 1 week, then 0.25 mg/kg every other day for 1 week, then 0.25 mg/kg every 3rd day. (Riis 1986)
c) For adjunctive therapy of hydrocephalus: For long-term management, prednisone 0.5 mg/kg PO every other day may be tried. (Fenner 1988)
Prednisone 0.25 - 0.5 mg/kg PO *bid*; continue if improvement is noted within one week and decrease dosage at weekly intervals to 0.1 mg/kg PO every other day eventually. Maintain dose for at least one month. (Shores 1989)
d) For adjunctive medical therapy of intervetebral disk disease (IVD):
Cervical IVD: Prednisolone 0.5 mg/kg PO *bid* for 3 days, then 0.5 mg/kg once daily for 3-5 days.
Thoracolumbar IVD: Prednisolone 0.5 - 1.0 mg/kg SQ or PO *bid* for 2-3 days, then taper dosage over next 3-5 days. (Schunk 1988a)

e) For adjunctive therapy of spondylopathy:
Cervical: For dogs with slowly progressive course and still ambulatory, use prednisone: 1 - 2 mg/kg PO divided *bid* initially. Gradually reduce dose every 2 weeks until reach 0.5 mg/kg PO every other day.
Lumbosacral: Prednisone: 1 mg/kg PO divided *bid* initially. Gradually reduce dose to 0.5 mg/kg PO every other day. (Schunk 1988a)

f) For adjunctive therapy of White Dog Shaker Syndrome: Prednisone 0.25 mg/kg PO *bid* for 10 days, then once a day for 10 days, then every other day for 10 days. (Fenner 1988)

g) For adjunctive therapy of generalized tremor syndrome: Predniso(lo)ne 3 m/kg each AM for 5 days, then decreased to alternate mornings for 5 days, then begin a phased withdrawal of drug. May require long-term low-dose alternate day therapy. (Farrow 1986)

h) For nonbacterial suppurative meningitis: After cultures are confirmed negative, prednisone 2 mg/kg for 10 days, then taper slowly over 1 month. (Fenner 1986b)

i) For adjunctive therapy of dogs diagnosed with canine wobbler syndrome with signs of mild to moderate paraparesis, tetraparesis, or ataxia: Prednisolone 1 - 2 mg/kg twice daily initially, decrease gradually over a 5 day period to 0.5 - 1 mg/kg on alternate days. (Trotter 1986)

For hematologic disorders:

a) For autoimmune hemolytic anemia: Prednisolone 1- 4 mg/kg PO daily divided *bid*. Add immunosuppressive agent (*e.g.,* cyclophosphamide, azathioprine) if PCV does not stabilize within 48-72 hours. May take several months to wean off drugs. (Maggio-Price 1988)

b) For adjunctive therapy of pure red blood cell aplasia (PRCA): Prednisolone 2 mg/kg divided *bid*. If no increase in reticulocyte count in 2 weeks, increase to 4 mg/kg *bid*. If reticulocyte counts remain low after 4-6 weeks add cyclophosphamide (30 - 50 mg/m^2 on 4 consecutive days each week). Continue prednisolone. Discontinue cyclophosphamide if neutropenia or thrombocytopenia occur. If reticulocyte count increases, cyclophosphamide may be discontinued and prednisolone slowly tapered to alternate day therapy. (Weiss 1986)

c) For immune-mediated thrombocytopenia: Prednisolone 1 - 3 mg/kg PO divided *bid-tid*. Do not give IM injections. If platelet count increases, prednisolone dose may be tapered by 50 per cent every 1-2 weeks. Reduction ion dose should be done slowly over several months. (Johnessee and Hurvitz 1983)

For dermatologic or other immune-mediated disorders:

a) For adjunctive therapy of urticaria and angioedema: Prednisone 2 mg/kg PO or IM *bid* (Giger and Werner 1988)

b) For canine atopy: Predniso(lo)ne 0.5 mg/kg PO *bid* initially for 5-10 days, then taper to the minimum effective alternate-day dosage. (Giger and Werner 1988)

c) For adjunctive flea allergy dermatitis: Prednisolone 1 mg/kg PO once a day for 1 week, the every other day at a minimally effective dose. (Giger and Werner 1988)

d) As an immunosuppressant for auto-immune skin diseases: Predniso(lo)ne 2.2 mg/kg *bid* until remission; then taper to lowest effective every other day dosage. (Giger and Werner 1988)

e) For type II (cytotoxic) hypersensitivity: Predniso(lo)ne 2 mg/kg *bid*. Once in remission, dosage may be reduced to a maintenance level. Other immunosuppressants may be required. (Wilcke 1986)

f) For adjunctive therapy of urticaria, shock, and/or respiratory arrest secondary to contrast media hypersensitivity: Prednisolone sodium succinate 10 mg/kg IV (Walter, Feeney, and Johnston 1986)

g) For adjunctive therapy of surface pyodermas: Predniso(lo)ne 1 mg/kg/day for 5-7 days. (Ihrke 1986)

Miscellaneous Indications:

For boxer cardiomyopathy:

a) In patients not responding to antiarrhythmic agents: Prednisolone 1 mg/kg *bid* for 10 days. (Ware and Bonagura 1986)

As an appetite stimulant:

a) Prednisolone 0.25 - 0.5 mg/kg PO every day, every other day, or intermittently as needed. (Macy and Ralston 1989)

For adjunctive therapy of posterior uveitis:

a) Prednisolone 2.2 mg/kg once daily; gradually reduce dose as inflammation is controlled. (Swanson 1989)

For chronic, proliferative, pyogranulomatous laryngitis:
  a) Prednisolone 1 mg/kg *bid* PO; decrease dosage weekly. (Prueter 1988a)

For eosinophilic ulcer:
  a) Prednisolone 2 - 4.4 mg/kg PO once a day; for chronic cases use prednisolone 0.5 - 1.0 mg/kg PO every other day (DeNovo 1988)

For adjunctive or alternate therapy for hypercalcemia:
  a) Prednisolone 1 - 1.5 mg/kg PO q12h. Has a delayed onset of action and a 4-8 day duration of response. (Kruger, Osborne, and Polzin 1986)

As an anti-inflammatory in the adjunctive treatment of otitis interna:
  a) Prednisone 0.25 mg/kg/day for first 5-7 days of treatment. (Neer 1988)

For adjunctive therapy of myasthenia gravis:
  a) Prednisone 0.5 mg/kg/day PO. Increase in 0.5 mg/kg/day increments every 2-4 days until total dose of 2 mg/kg/day is attained. After remission is achieved, gradually shift to every other day therapy. Should patient worsen during period when prednisone dose is increased, reduce dose and increase the intervals between dosage increases. May take several weeks to see a positive response. After signs are controlled, reduce dosage every 4 weeks until maintenance dose is determined. Cytotoxic drugs may be indicated should symptoms not be controlled or if dosage cannot be reduced. (LeCouteur 1988)

Cats:
As an immunosuppressive agent:
  a) Predniso(lo)ne: Initially 2 - 4 mg/kg daily in divided doses. Taper to alternate day, low-dose therapy as rapidly as patient allows. (Gorman and Werner 1989)

For adjunctive treatment of respiratory disorders:
  a) Allergic bronchitis: Prednisolone sodium succinate: 1 - 3 mg/kg IV or IM (do not give via rapid IV infusion). (Bauer 1988)
  b) For adjunctive therapy of feline asthma: Predniso(lo)ne:1 - 2 mg/kg/day (Papich 1986);
  For adjunctive emergency therapy: Prednisolone sodium succinate 50 - 100 mg IV. For non-emergency cases: Prednisone 5 mg PO *tid* initially, then rapidly decrease to alternate day use (or discontinue). (Noone 1986)

For adjunctive therapy of disorders of the gastrointestinal tract:
  a) For plasmacytic/lymphocytic enteritis: Prednisolone 2.2 mg/kg PO divided twice daily for 5-10 days, then 1.1 mg/kg/day for 5-10 days, then taper by reducing steroid dosage by 1/2 every 10-14 days until alternate-day dosage is attained or symptoms recur. (Chiapella 1988)
  b) For small intestinal inflammatory bowel disease: Prednisone 1 - 2 mg/kg/day divided into 2 doses. Mild to moderate cases generally will respond to the lower dosage. If severe, use the higher dose and treat for 2-4 weeks or until symptoms resolve. In severe cases characterized by anorexia, weight loss and chronic diarrhea, use an initial dose of 4 mg/kg/day for 2 weeks. If response is good, decrease dose by 1/2 after 2 weeks and again by 1/2 at 4 weeks. Eventually, alternate day therapy can be attained and should be maintained for 3 months. Some cats may have drugs discontinued in 3 months or long-term alternate day (or every 3rd day dosing) may be required. (Tams 1986)

For adjunctive therapy of feline plasma cell gingivitis-pharyngitis:
  a) Prednisolone 1 - 2 mg/kg PO once daily. (DeNovo, Potter, and Woolfson 1988)

For eosinophilic ulcer:
  a) Prednisolone 2 - 4.4 mg/kg PO once a day; for chronic cases use prednisolone 0.5 - 1.0 mg/kg PO every other day (DeNovo, Potter, and Woolfson 1988)

For adjunctive therapy of feline heartworm disease:
  a) For crisis due to embolization; Prednisolone 4.4 mg/kg *tid* with careful IV fluid therapy. (Dillon 1986)

For dermatologic conditions:
  a) For adjunctive treatment of flea allergy: Predniso(lo)ne 1 - 2 mg/kg PO q12h for 5 days, then gradually taper to alternate-day therapy (usually 1 - 2 mg/kg every other evening). (Kwochka 1986)
  b) For idiopathic feline miliary dermatoses: Predniso(lo)ne 1 - 2 mg/kg PO q12h for 5-7 days, then reduce gradually to alternate-day therapy at 1 - 2 mg/kg. Rarely is effective for long-term use. (Kwochka 1986)
  c) For linear granulomas: Prednisolone 0.5 mg/kg *bid* initially, with taper. (Thoday 1986)

As adjunctive therapy for feline neoplasias (lymphosarcoma, acute lymphoid leukemia, mast cell neoplasms):

Note: Also see the section on Chemotherapy Protocols for Treatment of Neoplastic Diseases in Small Animals found in the appendix.

a) 20 - 50 mg/m^2 q24-48h PO, SQ or IV (Couto 1989)

Cattle:

For adjunctive therapy of cerebral edema secondary to polioencephalomalacia:

a) Prednisolone 1 - 4 mg/kg intravenously (Dill 1986)

For adjunctive therapy of aseptic laminitis:

a) Prednisolone (assuming sodium succinate salt) 100 - 200 mg IM or IV; continue therapy for 2-3 days (Berg 1986)

For glucocorticoid activity:

a) Prednisolone sodium succinate: 0.2 - 1 mg/kg IV or IM (Howard 1986)

Horses:

For adjunctive therapy of COPD:

a) Prednisolone: Initially, 600 - 800 mg IM or PO in a 450 kg horse. May be possible to decrease dose and go to alternate day dosing. Doses as low as 200 mg every other day may be effective. (Beech 1987a)

For glucocorticoid effects:

a) Prednisolone sodium succinate: 0.25 - 1 mg/kg IV, Predniso(lo)ne tablets 0.25 - 1 mg/kg PO; Prednisolone acetate: 0.25 - 1.0 mg/kg IM or 10 - 25 mg subconjunctivally. (Robinson 1987)

Llamas:

For steroid-responsive pruritic dermatoses secondary to allergic origins:

a) Prednisone: 0.5 - 1.0 mg/kg PO initially, gradually reduce dosage to lowest effective dose given every other day. (Rosychuk 1989)

Swine:

For glucocorticoid activity:

a) Prednisolone sodium succinate: 0.2 - 1 mg/kg IV or IM (Howard 1986)

Birds:

As an antiinflammatory:

a) Prednisolone: 0.2 mg/30 gram body weight, or dissolve one 5 mg tablet in 2.5 ml of water and administer 2 drops orally. Give twice daily. Decrease dosage schedule if using long-term. (Clubb 1986)

For treatment of shock:

a) Prednisolone sodium succinate (10 mg/ml): 0.1 - 0.2 ml/100 grams body weight. Repeat every 15 minutes to effect. In large birds, dosage may be decreased by 1/2. (Clubb 1986)

Reptiles:

a) For shock in most species using prednisolone sodium succinate: 5 - 10 mg/kg IV as needed. (Gauvin 1993)

Dosage Forms/Preparations/Approval Status/Withdrawal Times-
Veterinary-Approved Products:

A zero tolerance of residues in milk for these compounds have been established for dairy cattle. All these agents require a prescription (Rx). Known approved-veterinary products are indicated below.

Prednisolone Tablets 5 mg. 20 mg

Delta-Cortef® (Upjohn), *Prednis-Tab*® (Vet-A-Mix); generic (Rx). Approved for use in dogs.

Prednisolone Acetate Suspension for Injection 25 mg/ml, 50 mg/ml, 100 mg/ml

Available under several trade names and generically.

Prednisolone Sodium Succinate for Injection (Veterinary) 20 mg/ml in 50 ml vials

Solu-Delta Cortef® (Upjohn), *Sterisol-20*® (Anthony), generic; (Rx) Approved for dogs, cats, and horses. Refer to the package insert for more information on dosage and preparation of the solution before using.

Prednisolone Sodium Phosphate for Injection (Veterinary) 100 mg/vial, 500 mg/vial

Cortisate-20® (Schering). Approved for IV use in dogs. Refer to the package insert for more information on dosage, etc.

Prednisone Suspension for Injection (Veterinary) 10 mg/ml, 40 mg/ml; *Meticorten*® (Schering) Approved for dogs, cats, and horses.

Human-Approved Products:

Prednisolone Tablets: 5 mg *Delta-Cortef*® (Upjohn); generic, (Rx)
Prednisone Tablets: 1 mg, 2.5 mg, 5 mg, 10 mg, 20, mg, 50 mg (Rx)

Prednisolone Syrup: 15 mg/5 ml in 240 ml; *Prelone*® (Muro) (Rx)
Prednisone Oral Solution/Syrup: 1 mg/ml in 30 ml, 120 ml, 240 ml and 500 ml (Rx)

Prednisolone Acetate Injection: 25 mg/ml, 50 mg/ml in 10 & 30 ml vials; *Key-Pred 25*®
(Hyrex) (Rx); *Predalone 50*® (Forest) (Rx); *Predcor-50*® (Hauck) (Rx); generic

PRIMIDONE

Chemistry - An analog of phenobarbital, primidone occurs as a white, odorless, slightly bitter-tasting, crystalline powder with a melting point of 279°-284°C. One gram is soluble in approximately 2000 ml of water or 200 ml of alcohol.

Storage/Stability/Compatibility - Tablets should be stored in well-closed containers preferably at room temperature. The oral suspension should be stored in tight, light-resistant containers preferably at room temperature; avoid freezing. Commercially available suspension and tablets generally have expiration dates of 5 years after manufacture.

Pharmacology - Primidone and its active metabolites, phenylethamalonamide (PEMA) and phenobarbital have similar anticonvulsant actions. While the exact mechanisms for this activity are unknown, these agents raise seizure thresholds or alter seizure patterns.

Uses/Indications - Primidone is indicated for seizure control (idiopathic epilepsy, epileptiform convulsions) in the dog. Because it is rapidly converted into phenobarbital in this species (see pharmacokinetics below), there is some question as to whether it has any advantages over using phenobarbital alone. However, many clinicians feel that some animals not responding to phenobarbital do benefit from primidone therapy, perhaps as a result that PEMA has been demonstrated to potentiate the anticonvulsant activity of phenobarbital in animals. When compared with phenobarbital, increased incidence of hepatotoxicity associated with primidone is considered to be the major limitation to long-term therapy with this agent. Primidone is considered to be more toxic in rabbits and cats than in humans or dogs.

Pharmacokinetics - Primidone is slowly absorbed after oral administration in the dog, with peak levels occurring 2-4 hours after dosing. The bioavailability of primidone in humans has been reported as 60-80%.

Primidone is rapidly converted to PEMA and phenobarbital in the dog. Serum half-lives of primidone, PEMA, and phenobarbital have been reported to be 1.85 hrs, 7.1 hrs, and 41 hours, respectively (Yeary 1980)

Primidone, like phenobarbital (possibly due to the phenobarbital?), can induce hepatic microsomal enzymes which can increase the rate of metabolism of itself and other drugs.

For more information on the pharmacokinetics of phenobarbital, refer to its monograph earlier in this section.

Contraindications/Precautions - Many clinicians and the veterinary manufacturers of primidone feel that primidone is contraindicated in cats, other clinicians dispute this, but it is recommended that primidone be used in cats only with extreme caution. Use cautiously in patients who are hypovolemic, anemic, have borderline hypoadrenal function, or cardiac or respiratory disease. Large doses are contraindicated in patients with nephritis or severe respiratory dysfunction. Primidone is contraindicated in patients with severe liver disease or who have demonstrated previous hypersensitivity reactions to them.

Adverse Effects/Warnings - Adverse effects in dogs are similar for both primidone and phenobarbital. Dogs may exhibit increased symptoms of anxiety and agitation when initiating therapy. These effects may be transitory in nature and often will resolve with small dosage increases. Occasionally, dogs will exhibit profound depression at lower dosage ranges (and plasma levels). Polydipsia, polyuria, and polyphagia are also quite commonly displayed at moderate to high serum levels. They are best controlled by limiting intake of both food and water. Sedation and/or ataxia often become significant concerns as serum levels reach the higher ends of the therapeutic range.

Increases in liver enzymes (ALT, ALP, glutamate dehydrogenase) and decreased serum albumin with chronic therapy are common (up to 70% of dogs treated), and is more prevalent than with phenobarbital. Hepatic lipidosis, hepatocellular hypertrophy and necrosis, and extramedullary hematopoiesis can be seen after 6 months of therapy. Serious hepatic injury probably occurs in approximately 6-14% of dogs treated.

In dogs, anorexia, tachycardia, dermatitis, episodic hyperventilation, and rarely megaloblastic anemia have also been reported with primidone therapy.

Overdosage - Because primidone is rapidly metabolized to phenobarbital in dogs, similar symptoms (sedation to coma, anorexia, vomiting, nystagmus) are seen and corresponding procedures should be used for the treatment of acute primidone overdose. This includes the removal of ingested product from the gut if appropriate and offering respiratory and cardiovascular support. Activated charcoal has been demonstrated to be of considerable benefit in enhancing the clearance of phenobarbital, even when the drug was administered parenterally. Charcoal acts as a "sink" for the drug to diffuse from the vasculature back into the gut. Forced alkaline diuresis can be of considerable benefit in augmenting the elimination of phenobarbital in patients with normal renal function. Peritoneal or hemodialysis mayalso be helpful in severe intoxications or in anuric patients.

Drug Interactions - Oral **acetozolamide** may decrease the GI absorption of primidone.

Because the primary active metabolite for primidone is phenobarbital, these drug interactions may be of significance: The following drugs may increase the effect of phenobarbital: **Other CNS depressants (narcotics, phenothiazines, antihistamines, etc), valproic acid, and chloramphenicol.** The interaction with **chloramphenicol** may be of especial significance in the dog. Phenobarbital may decrease the effect of the following drugs: **oral anticoagulants, corticosteroids,** beta **blockers (propranolol), quinidine, theophylline, metronidazole.**

Phenobarbital with **furosemide** may cause or increase postural hypotension. Barbiturates may effect the metabolism of **phenytoin,** monitoring of blood levels may be indicated.

Phenobarbital may decrease the absorption of **griseofulvin;** avoid giving simultaneously.

Drug/Lab Interactions - Barbiturates may cause increased retention of bromosulfopthalein (BSP; sulfobromopthalein) and give falsely elevated results. It is recommended that barbiturates (including primidone) not be administered within the 24 hours before **BSP retention tests,** or if they must, (*e.g.,* for seizure control) the results be interpreted accordingly.

Doses -
   Dogs:
   a) 15 - 20 mg/kg per day divided *bid-tid* initially; some dogs require 50 mg/kg/day (Morgan 1988)
   b) 11 - 22 mg/kg *tid* (Kay and Aucoin 1985)
   c) Initially, 15 mg/kg divided *bid*; up to 80 mg/kg divided *bid* (Bunch 1986)
   d) 55 mg/kg PO once daily (Kirk 1986)
   e) 55 mg/kg PO daily; if seizures are frequent, divide daily dose. Reduce dosage gradually, never discontinue abruptly. (Package Insert; *Mylepsin®* - Fort Dodge)

   Cats:
   a) 11 - 22 mg/kg *tid* (Davis 1985b)
   b) 20 mg/kg PO q12h (Neff-Davis 1985)

Monitoring Parameters -
   1) Anticonvulsant efficacy
   2) Adverse effects (CNS related, PU/PD, weight gain)
   3) Serum phenobarbital levels if lack of efficacy or adverse reactions noted. Although there is some disagreement, therapeutic serum levels in dogs are thought to mirror those in people at 15-40 micrograms/ml.
   4) If used chronically, routine CBC's and liver enzymes at least every 6 months

Client Information - Compliance with therapy must be stressed to clients for successful epilepsy treatment. Encourage to give daily doses at same time each day. Veterinarian should be contacted if animal develops significant adverse reactions (including symptoms of anemia and/or liver disease) or if seizure control is unacceptable.

Dosage Forms/Preparations/FDA Approval Status/Withholding Times -
   Veterinary-Approved Products:
   Primidone 250 mg Tablets; *Neurosyn®* (Techamerica), generic; (Rx) Approved for use in dogs.

   Human-Approved Products:
   Primidone 50 mg, 250 mg Tablets; *Mysoline®* (Wyeth-Ayerst); (Rx); generic (Rx)

   Primidone Oral Suspension 50 mg/ml in 8 oz. bottles ; *Mysoline®* (Wyeth-Ayerst); (Rx)
Additional names and trade names include: *Myidone®* (Major), and Primaclone.

PROCAINAMIDE HCL

Chemistry - Structurally related to procaine, procainamide is used as an antiarrhythmic agent. Procainamide HCl differs from procaine by the substitution of an amide group for the ester group found on procaine. It occurs as an odorless, white to tan, hygroscopic, crystalline powder with a pK_a of 9.23 and a melting range from 165°-169°C. It is very soluble in water and soluble in alcohol. The pH of the injectable product ranges from 4 - 6.

Storage/Stability/Compatibility - Oxidation due to the injection of air into the vial may cause discoloration of the injectable solution. The solution may be used if the color is no darker than a light amber. Refrigeration may retard the development of oxidation, but the solution may be stored at room temperature.

The injectable product is reportedly **compatible** with sodium chloride 0.9% injection, and water for injection. Procainamide is also compatible with dobutamine HCl, lidocaine HCl, and verapamil HCl. Compatibility is dependent upon factors such as pH, concentration, temperature and diluents used. It is suggested to consult specialized references for more specific information (*e.g., Handbook on Injectable Drugs* by Trissel; see bibliography).

Pharmacology - A class 1A antiarrhythmic agent, procainamide exhibits cardiac actions similar to that of quinidine. Procainamide prolongs the refractory times in both the atria and ventricles, decreases myocardial excitability, and depresses automaticity and conduction velocity. It has anticholinergic properties which may contribute to its effects. Procainamide's effects on heart rate are unpredictable, but it usually causes only slight increases or no change in heart rate. It may exhibit negative inotropic actions on the heart, although cardiac outputs are generally not affected.

On ECG, QRS widening, and prolonged PR & QT intervals can be seen. The QRS complex and T wave may occasionally show some slight decreases in voltage.

Uses/Indications - Procainamide is indicated for the treatment of ventricular premature complexes (VPC's), ventricular tachycardia, or supraventricular tachycardia associated with Wolff-Parkinson-White (WPW) syndrome with wide QRS complexes. Higher doses may be beneficial in the treatment of supraventricular tachycardias, although procainamide cannot be considered a first-line agent for this dysrhythmia.

Pharmacokinetics - After IM or IV administration, the onset of action is practically immediate. After oral administration in humans, approximately 75-95% of a dose is absorbed in the intestine, but some patients absorb less than 50% of a dose. Food, delayed gastric emptying or decreased stomach pH may delay oral absorption. In dogs, it has been reported that the oral bioavailability is approximately 85% and the absorption half-life is 0.5 hours. However, there is an apparent large degree of variability in both bioavailability and half-life of absorption.

Distribution of procainamide is highest into the CSF, liver, spleen, kidneys, lungs, heart and muscles. The volume of distribution in dogs is approximately 1.4 - 3 L/kg. It is only approximately 20% protein bound in humans and 15% in dogs. Procainamide can cross the placenta and is excreted into milk.

The elimination half-life in dogs has been reported to be variable, most studies report values between 2-3 hours. In humans, procainamide is metabolized to *N*-acetyl-procainamide (NAPA), an active metabolite. It appears, however, that dogs do not form appreciable amounts of NAPA from procainamide. In the dog, approximately 90% (50-70% unchanged) of an intravenous dose is excreted in the urine as procainamide and metabolites within 24 hours after dosing.

Contraindications/Precautions - Procainamide may be contraindicated in patients with myasthenia gravis (see Drug Interactions). Procainamide is contraindicated in patients hypersensitive to it, procaine or other chemically related drugs. In humans, procainamide is contraindicated in patients with systemic lupus erythematosis (SLE), but it is unknown if it adversely affects dogs with this condition. Procainamide should not be used in patients with torsade de pointes, or with 2nd or 3rd degree heart block (unless artificially paced).

Procainamide should be used with extreme caution, if at all, in patients with cardiac glycoside intoxication. It should be used with caution in patients with significant hepatic or renal disease or with congestive heart failure.

Adverse Effects/Warnings - Adverse effects are generally dosage (blood level) related in the dog. Gastrointestinal effects may include anorexia, vomiting, or diarrhea. Effects related to the cardiovascular system can include weakness, hypotension, negative inotropism, widened QRS complex and QT intervals, AV block, multiform ventricular tachycardias. Fevers and leukopenias are a possibility. Profound hypotension can occur if injected too rapidly IV. In humans, an SLE syndrome can occur, but its incidence has not been established in the dog.

Dosages should usually be reduced in patients with renal failure, congestive heart failure or those who are critically ill.

Overdosage - Symptoms of overdosage can include hypotension, lethargy, confusion, nausea, vomiting, and oliguria. Cardiac signs may include widening of the QRS complex, junctional tachycardia, ventricular fibrillation, or intraventricular conduction delays.

If an oral ingestion, emptying of the gut and charcoal administration may be beneficial to remove any unabsorbed drug. IV fluids, plus dopamine, phenylephrine, or norepinephrine could be considered to treat hypotensive effects. A 1/6 molar intravenous infusion of sodium lactate may be used in an attempt to reduce the cardiotoxic effects of procainamide. Forced diuresis using fluids and diuretics along with reduction of urinary pH, can enhance the renal excretion of the drug. Temporary cardiac pacing may be necessary should severe AV block occur.

Drug Interactions - Use with caution with **other antidysrhythmic agents**, as additive cardiotoxic or other toxic effects may result.

Procainamide may antagonize the effects of **pyridostigmine, neostigmine,** or other anticholinesterases in patients with myasthenia gravis.

Procainamide may potentiate the effects of other **drugs having hypotensive effects**.

Procainamide should only be used in patients with **digitalis** intoxication when treatment with potassium, lidocaine or phenytoin is ineffective. **Cimetidine** may decrease the renal clearance of procainamide with a resultant increase in serum level of procainamide.

Procainamide may potentiate or prolong the neuromuscular blocking activity of muscle relaxants such as **succinylcholine** or other agents (*e.g.,* **aminoglycosides**) having neuromuscular blocking activity.

Doses -
Dogs:
  a) 6 - 8 mg/kg IV over 5 minutes, then a constant rate of infusion at 25 - 40 micrograms/kg/min or 6 - 20 mg/kg IM q4-6h.
  Oral dose: 8 - 20 mg/kg q6h if using regular tablets or capsules; if using *Procan*®-SR (Parke-Davis): 8 - 20 mg/kg q6-8 hours (Tilley and Miller 1986)
  b) Add 500 - 1000 mg to 500 ml of D5W and give at slow infusion at a rate of 10 - 40 micrograms/kg/min or to effect; or 10 - 20 mg/kg IM or PO *tid-qid* (Morgan 1988)
  c) Initial maintenance dose: 15 mg/kg IV slowly q4h or 17.5 mg/kg PO q4h. Predicted serum values of 8 micrograms/ml are expected with this regimen. (Papich et al. 1986)
  d) For VPC's: 6.6 - 22 mg/kg q4h PO (up to q8h if using sustained-release form—may not be absorbed).
  For V tach: 6.6 - 8.8 mg/kg IV over 5 minutes, then infuse 11 - 40 micrograms/kg/min. (Ettinger 1989)

Horses:
  a) Intravenous: 0.5 mg/kg every 10 minutes until resolution or until a total of 2 - 4 mg/kg has been given. (Muir and McGuirk 1987a)

Monitoring Parameters -
  1) ECG; continuously with IV dosing
  2) Blood pressure if possible, during IV administration
  3) Symptoms of toxicity (see Adverse Reactions/Overdosage)
  4) Serum levels
     Because of the variability in pharmacokinetics reported in the dog, it is encouraged to monitor therapy using serum drug levels. Because dogs apparently do not form the active metabolite NAPA in appreciable quantities, the therapeutic range for procainamide is controversial. Therapeutic ranges from 3 - 8 micrograms/ml to 8 - 20 micrograms/ml have been suggested. This author would suggest using the lower range as a guideline to initiate therapy, but not to hesitate increasing doses to attain the higher values if efficacy is not achieved and toxicity is not a problem. Digitalis-induced ventricular arrhythmias may require substantially higher blood levels for control. Trough levels are usually specified when monitoring oral therapy. Because NAPA is routinely monitored with procainamide in human medicine, it may be necessary to request to your laboratory that NAPA values need not be automatically run for canine patients.

Client Information - Oral products should be administered at evenly spaced intervals throughout the day/night. Unless otherwise directed, give the medication on an empty stomach at least 1/2 hour before feeding. Notify veterinarian if animal's condition deteriorates or symptoms of toxicity (*e.g.,* vomiting, diarrhea, weakness, etc.) occur.

Dosage Forms/Preparations/FDA Approval Status/Withholding Times -
Veterinary-Approved Products: None
Human-Approved Products:
Procainamide HCl for injection 100 mg/ml in 10 ml vials & 500 mg/ml in 2 ml vials and 2 & 4 ml syringes; *Pronestyl*® (Princeton Pharm.); Generic; (Rx)

Procainamide HCl Tablets or Capsules 250 mg, 375 mg, 500 mg; *Pronestyl*® (Princeton Pharm.); Generic; (Rx)

Procainamide HCl Sustained-Release Tablets 250 mg, 500 mg, 1000 mg (Extended release only) (Note: These products are not recommended for initial therapy and have not been extensively used in veterinary medicine.); *Pronestyl*® SR (Princeton Pharm.), *Procanbid*® (Parke-Davis), Generic; (Rx)

PROCHLORPERAZINE

Chemistry - Prochlorperazine, a piperazine phenothiazine derivative, is available commercially as the base in rectal formulations, the edisylate salt in injectable and oral solutions, and as the maleate salt in oral tablets and capsules. Each 8 mg of the maleate salt and 7.5 mg of the edisylate salt are approximately equivalent to 5 mg of prochlorperazine base.

The base occurs as a clear, to pale yellow, viscous liquid that is very slightly soluble in water and freely soluble in alcohol. The edisylate salt occurs as white to very light yellow, odorless, crystalline powder. 500 mg are soluble in 1 ml of water and 750 ml of alcohol. The maleate salt occurs as a white or pale yellow, practically odorless, crystalline powder. It is practically insoluble in water or alcohol.

The commercial injection is a solution of the edisylate salt in sterile water. It has a pH of 4.2-6.2.

Storage/Stability/Compatibility - Store in tight, light resistant containers at room temperature. Avoid temperatures above 40°C and below freezing. A slight yellowing of the oral or injectable solution has no effects on potency or efficacy, but do not use if a precipitate forms or the solution is substantially discolored.

The following products have been reported to be **compatible** when mixed with prochlorperazine edisylate injection: all usual IV fluids, ascorbic acid injection, atropine sulfate, butorphanol tartrate, chlorpromazine HCl, dexamethasone sodium phosphate, droperidol, fentanyl citrate, glycopyrrolate, hydroxyzine HCl, lidocaine HCl, meperidine HCl, metoclopramide, morphine sulfate, nafcillin sodium, nalbuphine HCl, pentazocine lactate, perphenazine, promazine HCl, promethazine, scopolamine HBr, sodium bicarbonate, and vitamin B complex with C.

The following drugs have been reported to be **incompatible** when mixed with prochlorperazine edisylate: aminophylline, amphotericin B, ampicillin sodium, calcium gluceptate, chorampheni-col sodium succinate, chlorothiazide sodium, dimenhydrinate, hydrocortisone sodium succinate, methohexital sodium, penicillin G sodium, phenobarbital sodium, pentobarbital sodium, and thiopental sodium. Do not mix with other drugs/diluents having parabens as preservatives. Compatibility is dependent upon factors such as pH, concentration, temperature and diluents used. It is suggested to consult specialized references for more specific information (*e.g.*, *Handbook on Injectable Drugs* by Trissel; see bibliography).

Pharmacology - The basic pharmacology of prochlorperazine is similar to that of the other phenothiazines (refer to the acepromazine monograph for more information). Prochlorperazine has weak anticholinergic effects, strong extrapyrimidal effects, and moderate sedative effects. It has strong antiemetic effects and this action is used for its primary indications in both human and veterinary medicine.

Uses/Indications - The only approved products for animals are combination products containing prochlorperazine, isopropamide, with or without neomycin (*Darbazine®, Neo-Darbazine®*, — SKB Labs). The approved indications for these products include: vomiting, non-specific gastroenteritis, drug induced diarrhea, infectious diarrhea, spastic colitis, and motion sickness in dogs and cats (injectable product only). Prochlorperazine as a single agent is used in dogs and cats as an antiemetic.

Pharmacokinetics - Little information is available regarding the pharmacokinetics of prochlorperazine in animals, although it probably follows the general patterns of other phenothiazine agents in absorption, distribution and elimination.

Contraindications/Precautions - The manufacturer lists glaucoma, pyloric obstruction or stenosis, and prostatic hypertrophy as contraindications for the combination product *Darbazine®*. For other precautions and contraindications refer to the acepromazine monograph.

Adverse Effects/Warnings - In addition to the adverse effects listed for dogs and cats in the acepromazine monograph, *Darbazine®* may cause a dry mouth, dilated pupils, constipation and urinary retention secondary to the anticholinergic ingredient. Alone, prochlorperazine is most likely to casue sedation or hypotension.

Overdosage - Refer to the information listed in the acepromazine monograph. Acute extrapyrimadal symptoms (torticollis, tremor, salivation) have been successfully treated with injectable diphenhydramine in humans.

Drug Interactions - **Drug interactions for prochlorperazine** include: Phenothiazines should not be given within one month of worming with an **organophosphate agent** as their effects may be potentiated.

Other CNS depressant agents (barbiturates, narcotics, anesthetics, etc.) may cause additive CNS depression if used with prochlorperazine.

Quinidine given with phenothiazines may cause additive cardiac depression. **Antidiarrheal mixtures** (*e.g.*, Kaolin/pectin, bismuth subsalicylate mixtures) and **antacids** may cause reduced GI absorption of oral phenothiazines. Increased blood levels of both drugs may result if **propra-**

nolol is administered with phenothiazines. Phenothiazines block alpha-adrenergic receptors, if **epinephrine** is given, unopposed beta-activity causing vasodilation and increased cardiac rate can occur.

Phenytoin metabolism may be decreased if given concurrently with phenothiazines.

Drug Interactions for Isopropamide (ingredient in *Darbazine®*): The following drugs may enhance the activity of isopropamide and its derivatives: **antihistamines, procainamide, quinidine, meperidine, benzodiazepines, phenothiazines.**

The following drugs may potentiate the adverse effects of isopropamide and its derivatives: **primidone, disopyramide, nitrates, long-term corticosteroid use** (may increase intraocular pressure).

Isopropamide and its derivatives may enhance the actions of **nitrofurantoin, thiazide diuretics, sympathomimetics.**

Isopropamide and its derivatives may antagonize the actions of **metoclopramide.**

Drug/Laboratory Interactions - Isopropamide iodide may alter thyroid function tests (due to the iodine component) and will suppress iodine[131] uptake. It is recommended that the drug be discontinued one week prior to testing or treatment.

Doses -
Dogs:
Prochlorperazine:
   As an antiemetic:
     a) 0.5 mg/kg IM or SubQ q8h (Washabau and Elie 1995)
     b) 0.5 mg/kg IM *tid-qid* or 1 mg/kg PO *bid* (Morgan 1988)
     c) 0.1 mg/kg IM q6h (DeNovo 1986)

Prochlorperazine/Isopropamide (*Darbazine®*)
     a) As an antiemetic/antidiarrheal: 0.14 - 0.22mg/kg SQ *bid* (Morgan 1988)
     b) As an antiemetic: 0.5 - 0.8mg/kg IM or SQ q12h (DeNovo 1986)
     c) Injectable: Animals weighing:
        Up to 4 pounds = 0.25 ml; 5 - 14 lb = 0.5 - 1 ml; 15 - 30 lb = 2 - 3 ml; 30 - 45 lb = 3 - 4 ml; 45 - 60 lb = 4 - 5 ml; over 60 lb = 6 ml
        Oral:
        Darbazine® #1: Weighing 2 - 7 kg: 1 capsule q12h PO; Weighing 7 - 14 kg: 2 capsules q12h PO
        Darbazine® #3: Weighing over 14 kg: 1 capsule q12h PO (Package Insert, *Darbazine®* - SKB)

Cats:
Prochlorperazine:
     a) 0.13 mg/kg q12h IM (Davis 1985b)
     b) 0.1 mg/kg IM q6h (DeNovo 1986)
     c) 0.5 mg/kg IM or SubQ q8h (Washabau and Elie 1995)

Prochlorperazine/Isopropamide (*Darbazine®*)
     a) As an antiemetic: 0.5 - 0.8 mg/kg IM or SQ q12h (DeNovo 1986)
     b) Injectable: Animals weighing:
        Up to 4 pounds = 0.25 ml;
        5 - 14 lbs = 0.5 - 1 ml (Package Insert, *Darbazine®* - SKB)

Monitoring Parameters -
   1) Cardiac rate/rhythm/blood pressure if indicated and possible to measure
   2) Anti-emetic/anti-spasmodic efficacy; hydration & electrolyte status
   3) Body temperature (especially if ambient temperature is very hot or cold)

Client Information - Observe animals for at least one hour following dosing. Dry mouth may be relieved by applying small amounts of water to animal's tongue for 10-15 minutes. May discolor the urine to a pink or red-brown color; this is not abnormal. Protracted vomiting and diarrhea can be serious; contact veterinarian if symptoms are not alleviated. Contact veterinarian if animal exhibits abnormal behavior, becomes rigid or displays other abnormal body movements.

Dosage Forms/Preparations/FDA Approval Status/Withholding Times -
  Veterinary-Approved Products:
    Prochlorperazine dimaleate/Isopropamide iodide sustained-release capsules
      Darbazine® #1 (Pfizer): 3.33 mg prochlorperazine, 1.67 mg isopropamide
      Darbazine® #3 (Pfizer): 10 mg prochlorperazine, 5 mg isopropamide
      (Rx) Approved for use in dogs.

Prochlorperazine edisylate/Isopropamide iodide Injection

Darbazine® (Pfizer): 6 mg/ml prochlorperazine, 0.38 mg/ml isopropamide iodide; (Rx) Approved for use in dogs and cats.

Human-Approved Products:

Prochlorperazine edisylate for Injection 5 mg/ml in 2 ml amps and syringes; 10 ml vials; *Compazine*® (SKF); *Prochlorperazine*® (Wyeth-Ayerst); Generic; (Rx)

Prochlorperazine edisylate oral syrup 1 mg/ml in 120 ml bottles; *Compazine*® (SKF); (Rx)

Prochlorperazine maleate 5 mg, 10 mg, 25 mg tablets and 10 mg, 15 mg, 30 mg sustained release capsules; *Compazine*® (SKF); Generic; (Rx)

Prochlorperazine (base) Suppositories 2.5 mg, 5 mg, and 25 mg; *Compazine*® (SKF); *Prochlorperazine*® (G & W Labs); (Rx)

PROMAZINE HCL

Chemistry - A propylamino phenothiazine derivative, promazine is structurally identical to chlorpromazine, but lacks the chlorine atom at the 2 position of the phenothiazine nucleus. It occurs as a bitter tasting, practically odorless, white to slight yellow crystalline powder. Promazine is freely soluble in alcohol and 333 mg are soluble in 1 ml of water at 25°C. The commercial injection has a pH from 4-4.5 and is dissolved in a solution of sterile water for injection.

Storage/Stability/Compatibility - Protect from prolonged exposure to air, protect from light, and store from 15-30°C. Avoid freezing the injectable product.

Upon prolonged exposure to air, promazine will oxidize and change to a pink or blue color. Do not use the injectable product if color changes (a slight yellowish tint is OK), or a precipitate forms.

The following products have been reported to be **compatible** when mixed with promazine injection: All usual intravenous fluids (except Ionosol B with Dextrose 5% or isotonic sodium bicarbonate), atropine sulfate, chlorpromazine HCl, chloramphenicol sodium succinate, diphenhydramine, droperidol, fentanyl citrate, glycopyrrolate, heparin sodium, hydroxyzine HCl, lidocaine HCl, meperidine, metoclopramide, metaraminol bitartrate, morphine sulfate, pentazocine lactate, promethazine, scopolamine HBr, & tetracycline HCl.

The following products have been reported as being **incompatible** when mixed with promazine: Ionosol B with dextrose 5%, aminophylline, chlorothiazide sodium, dimenhydrinate, fibrinogen, fibrinolysin (human), methohexital sodium, nafcillin sodium, penicillin g potassium, pentobarbital sodium, phenobarbital sodium, sodium bicarbonate (is reportedly compatible when 100 mg/l of promazine mixed with 2.4 mEq/l of bicarb in D$_5$W), thiopental sodium, and warfarin sodium. Compatibility is dependent upon factors such as pH, concentration, temperature and diluents used. It is suggested to consult specialized references for more specific information (*e.g., Handbook on Injectable Drugs* by Trissel; see bibliography).

Pharmacology - Promazine has pharmacologic actions similar to acepromazine; refer to that monograph for a more detailed discussion of phenothiazine actions in animals.

Uses/Indications - Used basically for the same purposes as acepromazine; refer to that monograph for more information. Promazine is approved for use in dogs, cats, and horses.

Pharmacokinetics - Promazine is absorbed when given orally to non-ruminants; the drug is also apparently absorbed to some extent in ruminants when oral granules are used as they have some efficacy. In the dog, the onset of action following an IV dose is usually within 5 minutes, and following an IM dose within 30 minutes. Onsets of action reportedly are slightly longer in large animal species after parenteral administration. In horses, the onset of action after the oral granules have been consumed average around 45 minutes. The duration of action of promazine has been described as being dose-dependent, but generally ranges between 4-6 hours.

Promazine is metabolized in the liver primarily to glucuronide conjugates and these are excreted by the kidneys. In the horse, promazine metabolites are not detectable in the urine 72 hours after the last dose.

Contraindications/Precautions - Refer to the monograph for acepromazine for more information. Additionally, there are reports of horses being unusually sensitive to noise and reacting violently to sudden stimulation.

Adverse Effects/Warnings - Refer to the monograph for acepromazine for more information.

Overdosage - Refer to the monograph for acepromazine for more information.

Drug Interactions - Refer to the monograph for acepromazine for more information.

Doses -
Dogs:
   a) 2.2 - 6.6 mg/kg IV as a preanesthetic (Barbiturate dose is then reduced by 1/3 - 1/2. (Lumb and Jones 1984)
   b) 2.2 - 4.4 mg/kg IM as a sedative (Morgan 1988)
   c) 2 - 4 mg/kg IM or IV (Davis 1985a)
   d) 2 - 6 mg/kg IM or IV repeat q4-6h *prn*; as an antiemetic reduce dose by 1/3-1/2 (Booth 1988a)

Cats:
   a) 2.2 - 4.4 mg/kg IM as a sedative (Morgan 1988)
   b) 2.2 - 4.4 mg/kg IM or IV (Kirk 1986)

Cattle:
   a) 1.1 mg/kg IV as a tranquilizer (Lumb and Jones 1984)
   b) 0.44 - 1.0 mg/kg IV or IM (Howard 1986)

Horses:
   a) 1.1 mg/kg IV as a tranquilizer (Lumb and Jones 1984)
   b) 0.4 - 1.0 mg/kg IV (Robinson 1987)
   c) 0.99 - 1.98 mg/kg PO (equivalent to 1.63 - 3.26 grams/100 lbs of body weight) One level capful of promazine granules (Fort Dodge) will treat 300 lbs of horse at a dosage of approximately 1.45 mg/kg. Onset of action generally starts in 45 minutes and lasts for 4-6 hours. (Package Insert - Promazine Granules, Fort Dodge)

Swine:
   a) 0.44 - 1.0 mg/kg IV or IM (Howard 1986)
   b) Preanesthetic: 2 mg/kg with atropine (0.07 - 0.09 mg/kg) and meperidine (1 - 2mg/kg) (Booth 1988a)

Monitoring Parameters -
   1) Cardiac rate/rhythm/blood pressure if indicated and possible to measure
   2) Degree of tranquilization
   3) Body temperature (especially if ambient temperature is very hot or cold)

Client Information - May discolor the urine to a pink or red-brown color; this is not abnormal.

Dosage Forms/Preparations/FDA Approval Status/Withholding Times -
   Veterinary-Approved Products:
   Promazine HCl Granules (Veterinary); 10.25 oz containers containing 8 grams of promazine HCl; each gram of granules contains 27.5 mg. of promazine HCl; (Fort Dodge); (Rx) Approved for use in horses.

   Human-Approved Products:
   Promazine HCl for Injection 2 mg/ml in 10 ml vials; 5 mg/ml in 2 ml, 10 ml, & 100 ml vials; *Sparine*® (Wyeth-Ayerst), generic; (Rx)

   Promazine HCl tablets 25 mg, 50 mg, 100 mg; *Sparine*® (Wyeth-Ayerst); *Prozine-50*® (Hauck); generic, (Rx)

   Promazine HCl Oral Syrup 2 mg/ml in 120 ml bottles; *Sparine*® (Wyeth); (Rx)

PROPANTHELINE BROMIDE

Chemistry - A quaternary ammonium antimuscarinic agent, propantheline bromide occurs as bitter-tasting, odorless, white or practically white crystals, with a melting range of 156-162° (with decomposition). It is very soluble in both water and alcohol.

Storage/Stability/Compatibility - Propantheline bromide tablets should be stored at room temperature in tight containers.

Pharmacology - An antimuscarinic with similar actions as atropine, propantheline is a quaternary ammonium compound, however, and does not cross appreciably into the CNS. It, therefore, should not exhibit the same extent of CNS adverse effects that atropine possesses. For further information, refer to the atropine monograph.

Uses/Indications - In small animal medicine propantheline bromide has been used for its antispasmodic/antisecretory effects in the treatment of diarrhea. It is also employed in the treatment of hyperreflexic detrusor or urge incontinence and as oral treatment in anticholinergic responsive bradycardias. In horses, propantheline has been used intravenously to reduce colonic peristalsis and to relax the rectum to allow easier rectal examination and perform surgical procedures to the rectum.

Pharmacokinetics - Quaternary anticholinergic agents are not completely absorbed after oral administration because it is completely ionized. In humans, peak levels occur about 2 hours after oral administration. Food apparently decreases the amount of drug absorbed.

The distribution of propantheline has not been extensively studied, but like other quaternary antimuscarinics, propantheline is poorly lipid soluble and does not extensively penetrate into the CNS or eye.

Propantheline is believed to be prevalently metabolized in the GI and/or liver; less than 5% of an oral dose is excreted unchanged in the urine.

Contraindications/Precautions - Use of propantheline should be considered contraindicated if the patient has a history of hypersensitivity to anticholinergic drugs, tachycardias secondary to thyrotoxicosis or cardiac insufficiency, myocardial ischemia, unstable cardiac status during acute hemorrhage, GI obstructive disease, paralytic ileus, severe ulcerative colitis, obstructive uropathy or myasthenia gravis (unless used to reverse adverse muscarinic effects secondary to therapy).

Antimuscarinic agents should be used with extreme caution in patients with known or suspected GI infections. Propantheline or other antimuscarinic agents can decrease GI motility and prolong retention of the causative agent(s) or toxin(s) resulting in prolonged symptoms. Antimuscarinic agents must also be used with extreme caution in patients with autonomic neuropathy.

Antimuscarinic agents should be used with caution in patients with hepatic disease, renal disease, hyperthyroidism, hypertension, CHF, tachyarrhythmias, prostatic hypertrophy, esophogeal reflux, and geriatric or pediatric patients.

Adverse Effects/Warnings - With the exception of fewer effects on the eye and the CNS, propantheline can be expected to have a similar adverse reaction profile as atropine (dry mouth, dry eyes, urinary hesitancy, tachycardia, constipation, etc.). High doses may lead to the development of ileus with resultant bacterial overgrowth in susceptible animals. For more information refer to the atropine monograph.

Overdosage - Because of its quaternary structure, it would be expected that minimal CNS effects would occur after an overdose of propantheline when compared to atropine. See the information listed in the atropine monograph for more information on the symptoms and signs that may be see following an overdose.

If a recent oral ingestion, emptying of gut contents and administration of activated charcoal and saline cathartics may be warranted. Treat symptoms supportively and symptomatically. Do not use phenothiazines as they may contribute to the anticholinergic effects. Fluid therapy and standard treatments for shock may be instituted.

The use of physostigmine is controversial and should probably be reserved for cases where the patient exhibits either extreme agitation and is at risk for injuring themselves or others, or for cases where supraventricular tachycardias and sinus tachycardias are severe or life-threatening. The usual dose for physostigmine (human) is 2 mg IV slowly (for average sized adult); if no response may repeat every 20 minutes until reversal of toxic antimuscarinic effects or cholinergic effects takes place. The human pediatric dose is 0.02 mg/kg slow IV (repeat q10 minutes as above) and may be a reasonable choice for treatment of small animals. Physostigmine adverse effects (bronchoconstriction, bradycardia, seizures) may be treated with small doses of IV atropine.

Drug Interactions - The following drugs may enhance the activity of propantheline and its derivatives: **antihistamines, procainamide, quinidine, meperidine, benzodiazepines, phenothiazines**.

The following drugs may potentiate the adverse effects of propantheline and its derivatives: **primidone, disopyramide, nitrates, long-term corticosteroid use** (may increase intraocular pressure).

Propantheline and its derivatives may enhance the actions of **nitrofurantoin, thiazide diuretics, sympathomimetics**.

Propantheline delays the absorption, but increases the peak serum level of **ranitidine**. The relative bioavailability of ranitidine may be increased by 23% when propantheline is administered concomitantly with ranitidine.

Propantheline may decrease the absorption of **cimetidine**.

Doses -
  Dogs:
   a) For small dogs: 7.5 mg PO q8h
     For medium dogs: 15 mg PO q8h
     For large dogs: 30 mg PO q8h (Kirk 1986)

  For detrusor hyperreflexia, urge incontinence:
   a) 0.2 mg/kg PO q6-8h; increase dose if necessary to the lowest dose which will control symptoms (Polzin and Osborne 1985)
   b) 7.5 - 30 mg PO once a day to *tid*, start low and increase until symptoms abated or side effects occur (Labato 1988)

   c) 5 - 30 mg PO *tid* (Chew, DiBartola, and Fenner 1986)

For sinus bradycardia, incomplete AV block, etc.:
   a) If injectable anticholinergic therapy is shown to be effective and desire to convert to oral therapy: 0.5 - 1.0 mg/kg PO *tid* (Moses 1988)

For colitis, irritable bowel syndrome, etc.
   a) 0.25 mg/kg PO *tid*; do not use longer than 48-72 hours (48 hours for acute colitis) (DeNovo 1988)
   b) 0.5 mg/kg *bid-tid* (Chiapella 1986)

As an antiemetic/antidiarrheal:
   a) 0.25 mg/kg PO q8h (DeNovo 1986)

Cats:
   a) 7.5 mg PO q8h (Kirk 1986)

For detrusor hyperreflexia, urge incontinence:
   a) 7.5 mg PO every 3rd day; increase dose if necessary to the lowest dose which will control symptoms (Polzin and Osborne 1985)
   b) 7.5 mg PO every 24 to 72 hours, start low and increase until symptoms are abated or side effects occur (Labato 1988)
   c) 5 - 7.5 mg PO *tid* (Chew, DiBartola, and Fenner 1986)

For sinus bradycardia, incomplete AV block, etc.:
   a) Although generally ineffective, a trial may be attempted using: 0.8 - 1.6 mg/kg *tid* (Harpster 1986)

For chronic colitis
   a) 0.5 mg/kg *bid-tid* (Chiapella 1986)

As an antiemetic/antidiarrheal:
   a) 0.25 mg/kg PO q8h (DeNovo 1986)

Horses:
   a) 0.014 mg/kg IV (Robinson 1987)
   b) 30 mg IV to inhibit peristalsis for 2 hours during rectal surgery (Merkt et al. 1979)
   Note: There is no commercially available injectable product available in the U.S.A.. Should a preparation be made from oral tablets, it should be freshly prepared and filtered through a 0.22 micron filter before administering. Use with caution.

Monitoring Parameters - Dependent of reason for use
   1) Clinical efficacy
   2) Heart rate and rhythm if indicated
   3) Adverse effects

Client Information - Dry mouth may be relieved by applying small amounts of water to animal's tongue for 10-15 minutes. Protracted vomiting and diarrhea can be serious; contact veterinarian if symptoms are not alleviated.

Dosage Forms/Preparations/FDA Approval Status/Withholding Times -
   Veterinary-Approved Products: None
   Human-Approved Products:
     Propantheline Bromide Tablets 7.5 mg, 15 mg; *Pro-Banthine*® (Schiapparelli Searle); Generic; (Rx)

PROPIONIBACTERIUM ACNES INJECTION

Chemistry - Propionibacterium acnes injection is an immunostimulant agent, containing nonviable *Propionibacterium acnes* suspended in 12.5% ethanol in saline.

Storage/Stability/Compatibility - Store refrigerated; do not freeze. Shake well before using.

Pharmacology - A non-specific immunostimulant, Propionibacterium acnes injection may induce macrophage activation, and lymphokine production, increase natural killer cell activity and enhance cell-mediated immunity.

Uses/Indications - The manufacturer's label notes the product (*Immunoregulin*®) "is indicated in the dog as adjunct to antibiotic therapy in the treatment of chronic recurring canine pyoderma to decrease the severity and extent of lesions and increase the percentage of dogs free of lesions after the appropriate therapeutic period.

  Additionally, it has been used as an immunostimulant for the adjunctive treatment of feline rhinotracheitis and feline leukemia virus-induced disease. In dogs, it may be of use in the adjunctive treatment of oral melanoma and mastocytoma. Unfortunately, controlled studies documenting its efficacy are difficult to discern for these potential indications.

Pharmacokinetics - No information noted.

Contraindications/Precautions/Reproductive Safety - Propionibacterium acnes injection is contraindicated in patients hypersensitive to it. It should be used with caution in patients with cardiac dysfunction. Safe use during pregnancy has not been established.

Adverse Effects/Warnings - Occasionally within hours after injection, lethargy, increased body temperature, chills, and anorexia may be noted. Anaphylactic reactions have also been reported. Extravasation may cause local tissue inflammation. Long term toxicity studies have demonstrated vomiting, anorexia, malaise, fever, acidosis, increased water consumption and hepatitis.

Overdosage/Acute Toxicity - No overdosage information noted; the manufacturer states that the antidote is epinephrine, presumably for the treatment of anaphylactic reactions.

Drug Interactions - The manufacturer states that the immunostimulant effects may be compromised if given concomitantly with **glucocorticoids** or other **immune suppressing drugs**; manufacturer recommends discontinuing steroids at least 7 days prior to initiating therapy.

Doses -
  Dogs:
    For labeled indications:
      a) Shake well. Give via intravenous route at the following dosages: For animals weighing up to 15 lbs. = 0.25 - 0.5 ml; 15 - 45 lbs = 0.25 - 1 ml; 45 - 75 lbs = 1 - 1.5 ml; over 75 lbs = 1.5 - 2 ml. During the first two weeks give 4 times at 3-4 day intervals, then once weekly until symptoms abate or stabilize. Maintenance doses once per month are recommended. (Package Insert - *Immunoregulin*®)

    For adjunctive therapy of chronic recurrent canine pyoderma:
      a) 0.03 - 0.07 ml/kg twice weekly for 10 weeks (combined with antibiotic therapy) (Barta 1992)

  Cats:
    For adjunctive therapy of feline retrovirus infections:
      a) 0.5 ml IV twice weekly for 2 weeks, then one injection weekly for 20 weeks or until cat is seronegative. (McCaw 1994)

Monitoring Parameters - Efficacy & adverse effects (see above)

Dosage Forms/Preparations/FDA Approval Status/Withholding Times -
  Veterinary-Approved Products:
    Propionibacterium acnes (non-viable) for Injection 0.4 mg/ml in 5 ml vials; *Immunoregulin*® (ImmunoVet); (manufacturer states that use is restricted to use by, or under the supervision of a veterinarian)

  Human-Approved Products: None

PROPOFOL

Chemistry - Propofol is an alkylphenol derivative (2,6 - diisopropylphenol). The commercially available injection is an emulsion containing 100 mg/ml of soybean oil, 22.5 mg/ml of glycerol, and 12 mg/ml of egg lecithin. The emulsion has a pH of 7-8.5. Propofol may also be known as disoprofol.

Storage/Stability/Compatibility - Store propofol injection below 22°C (72°F), but not below 4°C (40°F.); do not refrigerate or freeze. Protect from light. Shake well before using. Do not use if the emulsion has separated. The manufacturer recommends discarding any unused portion at the end of the anesthetic procedure or after 6 hours, whichever occurs sooner.

  Compatibility with other agents has not been well established. Propofol is compatible with the commonly used IV solutions (*e.g.,* LRS, D5W) when injected into a running IV line.

Pharmacology - Propofol is a short acting hypnotic unrelated to other general anesthetic agents. Its mechanism of action is not well understood.

  In dogs, propofol produces rapid, yet smooth and excitement-free anesthesia induction (in 30-60 seconds) when given slowly IV. Sub-anesthetic dosages will produce sedation, restraint and an unawareness of surroundings. Anesthetic dosages produces unconsciousness.

  Propofol's cardiovascular effects include arterial hypotension, bradycardia, (especially in combination with opiate premedicants) and negative inotropism. It causes significant respiratory depression, particularly with rapid administration or very high dosages. Propofol also decreases intraocular pressure, increases appetite and has antiemetic properties. It does not appear to precipitate malignant hyperthermia and it has little or no analgesic properties.

Uses/Indications - In appropriate patients, propofol may be useful as an induction agent (especially before endotracheal intubation or an inhalant anesthetic); as an anesthetic for outpatient diagnostic or minor procedures (*e.g.,* laceration repair, radiologic procedures, minor dentistry, minor biopsies, endoscopy, etc.). Propofol may be of particular usefulness for use in Greyhounds and in patients with preexisting cardiac dysrhythmias.

In dogs, propofol's labeled indications are: 1) for induction of anesthesia; 2) for maintenance of anesthesia for up to 20 minutes; 3) for induction of general anesthesia where maintenance is provided inhalant anesthetics.

Pharmacokinetics - After IV administration, propofol rapidly crosses the blood brain barrier and has an onset of action usually within one minute. Duration of action after a single bolus lasts about 2-5 minutes. It is highly bound to plasma proteins (95-99%), crosses the placenta, is highly lipophilic and reportedly enters maternal milk.

Propofol's short duration of action is principally due to its rapid redistribution from the CNS to other tissues. It is rapidly biotransformed in the liver via glucuronide conjugation to inactive metabolites which are then excreted primarily by the kidneys. Because cat's do not glucuronidate as well as dogs or humans, this may help explain their problems with consecutive day administration (see Adverse Effects below).

There are limited data available on propofol's pharmacokinetic parameters in dogs. The steady state volume of distribution is >3L/kg, elimination half life is about 1.4 hours and clearance is about 50 ml/kg/min.

Contraindications/Precautions/Reproductive Safety - Propofol is contraindicated in patients hypersensitive to it or any of component of the product. It should not be used in patients where general anesthesia or sedation are contraindicated. Propofol should only be used in facilities where sufficient monitoring and patient-support capabilities are available.

Because patients who are in shock, under severe stress or have undergone trauma may be overly sensitive to the cardiovascular and respiratory depressant effects of propofol, it should be used with caution in these patients. Adequate perfusion should be maintained before and during propofol anesthesia and dosage adjustments may be necessary.

Because propofol is so highly bound to plasma proteins, patients with hypoproteinemia may be susceptible to untoward effects. Other general anesthetic agents may be a safer choice in these patients.

The benefits of propofol should be weighed against its risks in patients with a history of hyperlipidemia, seizures or anaphylactic reactions. Cat's with preexisting liver disease may be susceptible to longer recovery times.

Propofol crosses the placenta and its safe use during pregnancy has not been established. High dosages (6 times those recommended) in laboratory animals caused increased maternal death and decreased offspring survival rates after birth.

Adverse Effects/Warnings - Because there is a high incidence of apnea with resultant cyanosis if propofol is given too rapidly, it should be given slowly (25% of the calculated dose every 30 seconds until desired effect).

Propofol has been documented to cause histamine release in some patients and anaphylactoid reactions (rare) have been noted in humans. Propofol has direct myocardial depressant properties and resultant arterial hypotension has been reported.

Occasionally, dogs may exhibit seizure-like symptoms (paddling, opisthotonus, myoclonic twitching) during induction, which if persist, may be treated with intravenous diazepam. Propofol may have both anticonvulsant and seizure-causing properties. It should be used with caution in patients with a history of, or active seizure disorders. However, some clinicians believe that propofol is actually better-suited to use in seizure patients or in high seizure-risk procedures (*e.g.*, myelography) than is thiopental.

While propofol is not inexpensive, it should be used in a single-use fashion as it is a good growth medium (contains no preservative) for bacteria.

When used repeatedly (once daily) in cats, increased Heinz body production, slowed recoveries, anorexia, lethargy, malaise, and diarrhea have been noted. Heinz body formation is due to oxidative injury to RBC's and has been documented in cats with other phenolic compounds as well. Consecutive use in dogs appears to be safe.

Pain upon injection has been reported in humans, but does not appear to be of major significance for dogs or cats. Extravasation of injection is not irritating nor does it cause tissue sloughing.

Overdosage/Acute Toxicity - Overdosages are likely to cause significant respiratory depression and potentially cardiovascular depression. Treatment should consist of propofol discontinuation, artificial ventilation with oxygen, and if necessary, symptomatic and supportive treatment for cardiovascular depression (*e.g.*, intravenous fluids, pressors, anticholinergics, etc.).

Drug Interactions - Propofol used in conjunction with **preanesthetic agents** (*e.g.*, **acepromazine, opiates**) may cause increased vasodilation and negative cardiac inotropy. This may be of particular concern in animals with preexisting cardiopulmonary disease, in shock, or suffering from trauma.

Propofol-induced bradycardia may be exacerbated in animals receiving **opiate premedicants**, particularly when anticholinergic agents (*e.g.*, atropine) are not given concurrently.

As would be logically expected, increased CNS depressant effects and recovery times may be noted in patients receiving other **CNS depressant medications** with propofol.

Drugs that inhibit the hepatic P-450 enzyme system (*e.g.*, chloramphenicol, cimetidine) or **other basic lipophilic drugs (*e.g.*, fentanyl, halothane)** may potentially increase the recovery times associated with propofol. Clinical significance is unclear, but in cats it may be of significance.

Doses -
  Dogs & Cats:
    a) As a single injection (25% of the calculated dose every 30 seconds until desired effect):
    For healthy, unpremedicated animal: 6 mg/kg IV
    For healthy, premedicated animal: After tranquilizer (*e.g.,* acepromazine) = 4 mg/kg IV; After sedative (*e.g.*, xylazine, opioids) = 3 mg/kg IV

    As a constant infusion:
    For sedation only: 0.1 mg/kg/minute
    For minor surgery: 0.6 mg/kg/min, or 1 ml (10 mg) per minute per 12-25 kg of body weight (Robinson, Sanderson et al. 1993)
    b) 4 - 8 mg/kg IV (Hubbell 1994)
    c) 6 mg/kg IV; in healthy animals 25% of the calculated dose is administered every 30 seconds until intubation is possible. After induction, duration of anesthesia is only 2.5 - 9.4 minutes. Maintenance anesthesia obtained using either inhalational agents or a continuous infusion of propofol at approximately 0.4 mg/kg/minute. If anesthesia appears inadequate, a small bolus of 1 mg/kg followed by an increase in the infusion rate by 25%. If infusion is too deep, discontinue infusion until suitable anesthesia level is achieved. An infusion dose of 0.1 mg/kg/min appears to be suitable dose for sedation in the dog. (Ilkiw 1992)
    d) As an induction agent for halothane or isoflurane anesthesia: 6.6 mg/kg IV given over 60 seconds to unpredmedicated dogs. Best achieved by early intubation and administration of the inhalant following propofol induction. (Bufalari, Miller et al. 1998)

Monitoring Parameters - 1) Level of anesthesia/CNS effects; 2) Respiratory depression; 3) Cardiovascular status (cardiac rate/rhythm; blood pressure)

Dosage Forms/Preparations/FDA Approval Status/Withholding Times -
  Veterinary-Approved Products:
  Propofol Injectable 10 mg/ml in 20 ml (single use) amps & vials; *Rapinovet®* (Schering); *PropoFlo®* (Abbott) (Rx). Approved for use in dogs.

  Human-Approved Products:
  Propofol Injection 10 mg/ml in 20 ml ampules and 50 & 100 ml vials for infusion; *Diprivan®* (Zeneca); (Rx)

PROPRANOLOL HCL

Chemistry - A non-specific beta-adrenergic blocking agent, propranolol HCl occurs as a bitter-tasting, odorless, white to almost white powder with a pK_a of 9.45 and a melting point of about 161°C. One gram of propranolol is soluble in about 20 ml of water or alcohol. At a pH from 4-5, solutions of propranolol will fluoresce. The commercially available injectable solutions are adjusted with citric acid to a pH 2.8 - 3.5.

Storage/Stability/Compatibility - All propranolol preparations should be stored at room temperature (15-30°C) and protected from light. Propranolol solutions will decompose rapidly at alkaline pH. Propranolol injection is reported to be compatible with D5W, 0.9% sodium chloride, or lactated Ringer's injection. It is also physically compatible with dobutamine HCl, verapamil HCl and benzquinamide HCl.

Pharmacology - Propranolol blocks both $beta_1$ and $beta_2$ adrenergic receptors in the myocardium, bronchi, and vascular smooth muscle. Propranolol does not have any intrinsic sympathomimetic activity (ISA). Additionally, propranolol possesses membrane-stabilizing effects (quinidine-like) affecting the cardiac action potential and direct myocardial depressant effects. Cardiovascular effects secondary to propranolol include: decreased sinus heart rate, depressed AV conduction, diminished cardiac output at rest and during exercise, decreased myocardial oxygen demand, decrease hepatic and renal blood flow, reduced blood pressure, and inhibition of isoproterenol-induced tachycardia. Electrophysiologic effects on the heart include decreased automaticity, increased or no effect on effective refractory period, and no effect on conduction velocity.

Additional pharmacologic effects of propranolol, include increased airway resistance (especially in patients with bronchoconstrictive disease), prevention of migraine headaches, increased uterine activity (more so in the non-pregnant uterus), decreased platelet aggregability, inhibited glycogenolysis in cardiac and skeletal muscle and increased numbers of circulating eosinophils.

Uses/Indications - While propranolol is used for hypertension, migraine headache prophylaxis and angina in human patients, it is used primarily in veterinary medicine for its antiarrhythmic effects. Dysrhythmias treated with propranolol include, atrial premature complexes, ventricular premature complexes, supraventricular premature complexes and tachyarrhythmias, ventricular or atrial tachyarrhythmias secondary to digitalis, atrial tachycardia secondary to WPW with normal QRS complexes, and atrial fibrillation (generally in combination with digoxin). Propranolol reportedly improves cardiac performance in animals with hypertrophic cardiomyopathy. It has been used to treat systemic hypertension and symptoms associated with thyrotoxicosis and pheochromocytoma.

Pharmacokinetics - Propranolol is well absorbed after oral administration, but a rapid first-pass effect through the liver reduces systemic bioavailability to approximately 2-27% in dogs, thereby explaining the significant difference between oral and intravenous dosages. These values reportedly increase with chronic dosing.

Propranolol is highly lipid soluble and readily crosses the blood-brain barrier. The apparent volume of distribution has been reported to 3.3 - 11 L/kg in the dog. Propranolol will cross the placenta and enters milk (at very low levels). In humans, propranolol is approximately 90% bound to plasma proteins.

Propranolol is principally metabolized by the liver. An active metabolite, 4-hydroxypropranolol, has been identified after oral administration in humans. Less than 1% of a dose is excreted unchanged into the urine. The half-life in dogs has been reported to range from 0.77 - 2 hours, and in horses, less than 2 hours.

Contraindications/Precautions - Propranolol is contraindicated in patients with overt heart failure, hypersensitivity to this class of agents, greater than 1st degree heart block, or sinus bradycardia. Non-specific beta-blockers are generally contraindicated in patients with CHF unless secondary to a tachyarrhythmia responsive to beta-blocker therapy. They are also relatively contraindicated in patients with bronchospastic lung disease.

Propranolol should be used cautiously in patients with significant renal or hepatic insufficiency. It should also be used cautiously in patients with sinus node dysfunction.

Propranolol can mask the symptoms associated with hypoglycemia. It can also cause hypoglycemia or hyperglycemia and, therefore, should be used cautiously in labile diabetic patients.

Propranolol can mask the symptoms associated with thyrotoxicosis, but it has been used clinically to treat the symptoms associated with this condition.

Use propranolol cautiously with digitalis or in digitalis intoxicated patients; severe bradycardias may result.

Adverse Effects/Warnings - It is reported that adverse effects most commonly occur in geriatric animals or those that have acute decompensating heart disease. Adverse effects considered to be clinically relevant include: bradycardia, lethargy and depression, impaired AV conduction, CHF or worsening of heart failure, hypotension, hypoglycemia, and bronchoconstriction. Syncope and diarrhea have also been reported in canine patients.

Exacerbation of symptoms have been reported following abrupt cessation of beta-blockers in humans. It is recommended to withdraw therapy gradually in patients who have been receiving the drug chronically.

Overdosage - The most predominant symptoms expected would be hypotension and bradycardia. Other possible effects could include: CNS (depressed consciousness to seizures), bronchospasm, hypoglycemia, hyperkalemia, respiratory depression, pulmonary edema, other arrhythmias (especially AV block), or asystole.

If overdose is secondary to a recent oral ingestion, emptying the gut and charcoal administration may be considered. Monitor ECG, blood glucose, potassium, and, if possible, blood pressure. Treatment of the cardiovascular and CNS effects are symptomatic. Use fluids, and pressor agents to treat hypotension. Bradycardia may be treated with atropine. If atropine fails, isoproterenol given cautiously has been recommended. Use of a transvenous pacemaker may be necessary. Cardiac failure can be treated with a digitalis glycosides, diuretics, oxygen and, if necessary, IV aminophylline. Glucagon (5-10 mg IV - Human dose) may increase heart rate and blood pressure and reduce the cardiodepressant effects of propranolol. Seizures generally will respond to IV diazepam.

Drug Interactions - Sympathomimetics (metaproterenol, terbutaline, beta effects of epinephrine, phenylpropanolamine, etc.) may have their actions blocked by propranolol. Additive myocardial depression may occur with the concurrent use of propranolol and myocardial depressant **anesthetic agents**. **Phenothiazines** given with propranolol may exhibit enhanced hypotensive effects. **Thyroid hormones** may decrease the effect of beta blocking agents. Propranolol doses may need to be decreased when initiating **methimazole or propylthiouracil** therapy. **Cimetidine** may decrease the metabolism of propranolol and increase blood levels. **Furosemide and hydralazine** may increase the effects of propranolol. Effects of **tubocurarine and succinylcholine** may be enhanced with propranolol therapy. Hepatic enzyme induction with **phenobarbital, rifampin or phenytoin** may increase the metabolism of propranolol. Unopposed alpha effects of **epinephrine** may lead to rapid increases in blood pressure and decrease in heart rate when given with propranolol. Propranolol may prolong the hypoglycemic effects of **insulin** therapy. **Lidocaine** clearance may be impaired by propranolol. Effects of **theophylline** (bronchodilitation) may be blocked by propranolol. Concurrent use of beta blockers with **calcium channel blockers** (or other negative inotropes should be done with caution; particularly in patients with preexisting cardiomyopathy or CHF.

Doses -
  Dogs:
- a) IV: 0.02 - 0.06 mg/kg IV slowly; PO: 0.2 - 1.0 mg/kg *tid*. (Murtaugh and Ross 1988)
- b) IV: 0.04 - 0.06 mg/kg IV slowly; PO:0.2 - 1.0 mg/kg q8h. (Miller 1985)
- c) For ventricular hypertrophy from aortic stenosis: 0.125 - 0.25 mg/kg PO *bid*
  For ventricular arrhythmias: 0.02 - 0.06 mg/kg IV over 2-3 minutes or 0.2 mg/kg PO *tid*; maximum 1 mg/kg/day.
  For hypertrophic cardiomyopathy: 0.3 - 1.0 mg/kg PO *tid*; maximum of 120 mg/day.
  For hypertension: 2.5 - 10 mg PO *bid-tid*
  For arrhythmias secondary to pheochromocytomas: 0.15 - 0.5 mg/kg PO *tid* or 0.03 - 0.10 mg/kg IV (Morgan 1988)
- d) For susceptible cardiac arrhythmias: General: 0.44 - 1.1 mg/kg q8h. Small dogs: 2.5 - 20 mg PO q8-12h *(Note: actual reference has this dose per pound, but it is believed this is an error)*; Medium and large dogs: 10 - 40 mg PO q8-12h; Large and giant breeds: 40 - 80 mg PO q8-12h.
  Intravenously: 0.25 - 0.5 mg IV no more frequently than every 1-3 minutes. (Ettinger 1989)

  Cats:
- a) 2.5 - 5.0 mg *bid* to *tid* (Murtaugh and Ross 1988)
- b) IV: 0.04 mg/kg IV slowly; PO: 2.5 - 5.0 mg PO q8-12h (Miller 1985)
- c) For hypertrophic cardiomyopathy: Cats 4.5 kg or less: 2.5 mg PO *bid- tid*; Cats 5 kg or more: 5 mg PO *bid-tid*
  For hypertension: 2.5 - 5.0 mg PO *bid- tid* (Morgan 1988)
- d) For adjunctive therapy (to control tachycardia) in feline hyperthyroidism: 2.5 mg PO q8-12h; adjust dose as necessary. (Meric 1989)
- e) For suceptible cardiac arrhythmias: 2.5 mg PO q12-24h; 0.25 - 0.5 mg IV no more frequently than every 1-3 minutes. (Ettinger 1989)

  Horses:
- a) 0.1 - 0.3 mg/kg twice a day IV administered over 1 minute (Muir and McGuirk 1987a)
- b) Oral: Days 1 & 2: 175 mg *tid*; Days 3 & 4: 275 mg *tid*; Days 5 & 6: 350 mg *tid*.
  Intravenous: Days 1 & 2: 25 mg *bid*; Days 3 & 4: 50 mg *bid*; Days 5 & 6: 75 mg *bid* (Hilwig 1987)

Monitoring Parameters -
1) ECG
2) Toxicity (see Adverse Effects/Overdosage)
3) Blood pressure if administering IV

Client Information - To be effective, the animal must receive all doses as prescribed. Notify veterinarian if animal becomes lethargic or becomes exercise intolerant, begins wheezing, has shortness of breath or cough, or develops a change in behavior or attitude.

Dosage Forms/Preparations/FDA Approval Status/Withholding Times -
  Veterinary-Approved Products: None
  Human-Approved Products:

Propranolol HCl Tablets 10 mg, 20 mg, 40 mg, 60 mg, 80 mg, 90 mg; *Inderal*® (Wyeth-Ayerst), Generic; (Rx)

Propranolol HCl Extended/Sustained-Release capsules 60 mg, 80 mg, 120 mg, 160 mg; *Inderal*® *LA* (Wyeth-Ayerst); *Betachron E-R*® (Inwood); generic, (Rx)

Propranolol for Injection 1 mg/ml in 1 ml amps or vials; *Inderal*® (Wyeth-Ayerst) (Rx), Generic; (Rx)

Propranolol Oral Solution 4 mg/ml, 8 mg/ml, 80 mg/ml concentrate in 30 ml; *Propranolol Intensol*® (Roxane); *Propranolol HCl*® (Roxane) (Rx)

Also, fixed dose combination products containing propranolol and hydrochlorothiazide are available to treat hypertension in humans.

Prostaglandin F2 alpha - see Dinoprost

PROTAMINE SULFATE

Chemistry - Simple, low molecular weight, cationic proteins, protamines occur naturally in the sperm of fish. Commercially available protamine sulfate is produced from protamine obtained from the sperm or mature testes of salmon (or related species). It occurs as a fine, white to off-white crystalline or amorphous powder that is sparingly soluble in water and very slightly soluble in alcohol. The injection is available as either a prepared solution with a pH of 6-7 or a lyophilized powder that has a pH of 6.5-7.5 after reconstituting.

Storage/Stability/Compatibility - The powder for injection should be stored at room temperature (15-30°C), and the injection (liquid) in the refrigerator (2-8°C); avoid freezing. The injection is stable at room temperature for at least 2 weeks, however. The powder for injection should be used immediately if reconstituted with Sterile Water for Injection and within 72 hours if reconstituted with Bacteriostatic Water for Injection.

Either D_5W or normal saline are recommended to be used for protamine sulfate infusions. Cimetidine HCl or Verapamil HCl are reported to be compatible with protamine sulfate for injection.

Pharmacology - Protamine is strongly basic and heparin, strongly acidic; protamine complexes with heparin to form an inactive stable salt. Protamine has intrinsic anticoagulant activity, but its effects are weak and rarely cause problems.

Uses/Indications - Protamine is used in all species for the treatment of heparin overdosage when significant bleeding occurs. It has also been suggested to be used for Bracken Fern toxicity in ruminants (see Doses).

Pharmacokinetics - After IV injection, protamine binds to heparin within 5 minutes. The exact metabolic fate of the heparin-protamine complex is not known, but there is evidence that the complex is partially metabolized and/or degraded by fibrinolysin thus freeing heparin.

Contraindications/Precautions/Reproductive Safety - Protamine is contraindicated in patients who have demonstrated hypersensitivity or intolerance to the drug in the past.

Adverse Effects/Warnings - If protamine sulfate is injected IV too rapidly, acute hypotension, bradycardia, pulmonary hypertension and dyspnea can occur. These effects are usually absent or minimized when the drug is administered slowly (over 1-3 minutes). Hypersensitivity reactions have also been reported.

A heparin "rebound" effect has also been reported; where anticoagulation and bleeding occur several hours after heparin has been apparently neutralized. This may be due to either a release of heparin from extravascular compartments or the release of heparin from the protamine-heparin complex.

Overdosage/Acute Toxicity - Because protamine has inherent anticoagulant activity, overdoses of protamine may theoretically result in hemorrhage. However, in one human study, overdoses of 600 - 800 mg resulted only in mild, transient effects on coagulation. The LD_{50} of protamine in mice is 100 mg/kg.

Drug Interactions; **Drug/Laboratory Interactions** - None located.

Doses -
  Dogs, Cats (and presumably other species):
    For heparin overdosage:
      a) Give 1 - 1.5 mg protamine sulfate to antagonize each mg (≈100 units) of heparin via slow IV injection. Reduce dose as time increases between heparin dose and start of treatment (after 30 minutes give only 0.5 mg). (Bailey 1986a)
      b) Administer 1 mg protamine for each 100 Units of heparin to be inactivated. Decrease protamine dose by 1/2 for every 30 minutes that have lapsed since heparin was administered (Author's note: This may be ineffective if heparin has been administered by deep SQ injection). Give dose slowly IV, do not give at a rate faster than 50 mg over a 10 minute period. (Adams 1988b)
  Cattle:
    For Bracken Fern (*Pteridium sp.*) poisoning:
      a) In combination with whole blood (2.25-4.5L), 1 injection of 10 ml of 1% protamine sulfate IV. (Osweiler and Ruhr 1986)

Monitoring Parameters - See the Heparin monograph.

Client Information - Should only be used in a setting where adequate monitoring facilities are available.

Dosage Forms/Preparations/FDA Approval Status/Withholding Times -
  Veterinary-Approved Products: None

  Human-Approved Products:
    Protamine Sulfate Injection 10 mg/ml in 5 & 25 ml amps, and 5 & 25 ml vials; generic; (Rx)

PSYLLIUM HYDROPHILIC MUCILLOID

Chemistry - Psyllium is obtained from the ripe seeds of varieties of *Plantago* species. The seed coating is high in content of hemicellulose mucillages which absorb and swell in the presence of water.

Storage/Stability/Compatibility - Store psyllium products in tightly closed containers; protect from excess moisture or humidity.

Pharmacology - By swelling after absorbing water, psyllium increases bulk in the intestine and is believed to induce peristalsis and decrease intestinal transit time. In the treatment of sand colic in horses, psyllium is thought to help collect sand and to help lubricate its passage through the GI tract.

Uses/Indications - Bulk forming laxatives are used in patients where constipation is a result a too little fiber in their diets or when straining to defecate may be deleterious. Psyllium is considered to be the laxative of choice in the treatment and prevention of sand colic in horses.

Psyllium has also been used to increase stool consistency in patients with chronic, watery diarrhea. The total amount of water in the stool remains unchanged.

Pharmacokinetics - Psyllium is not absorbed when administered orally. Laxative action may take up to 72 hours to occur.

Contraindications/Precautions - Bulk-forming laxatives should not be used in cases where prompt intestinal evacuation is required, or when fecal impaction (no feces being passed) or intestinal obstruction is present.

Adverse Effects/Warnings - With the exception of increased flatulence, psyllium very rarely produces any adverse reactions if adequate water is given or is available to the patient. If insufficient liquid is given, there is an increased possibility of esophogeal or bowel obstruction occurring.

Overdosage - If administered with sufficient liquid, psyllium overdose should cause only an increased amount of soft or loose stools.

Drug Interactions - Because the potential exists for bulk-forming laxatives to bind **digoxin, salicylates and nitrofurantoin**, it is recommended that bulk-forming laxatives be administered at least 3 hours apart from these drugs.

Doses -
  Dogs:
    a) 3 - 10 grams mixed with food (Davis 1985a)
    b) 2 - 10 grams q12-24h in wetted or liquid food (Schultz 1986)
    c) 1 teaspoonful - 2 tablespoonsful mixed with food every 12 hours (McConnell and Hughey 1987)
    d) 2 - 10 grams PO as needed in food (Morgan 1988)

  Cats:
    a) 3 grams mixed with food (Davis 1985a)
    b) 2 - 4 grams q12-24h in wetted or liquid food (Schultz 1986)
    c) 1 teaspoonful mixed with food every 12-24 hours (McConnell and Hughey 1987)
    d) 1 - 4 grams PO once to twice daily in food (Morgan 1988)
    e) 1 teaspoonful per day with food (Sherding 1989)

  Horses:
    For treatment of sand colic:
    a) 0.5 kg in 6-8 L (1 pound in 1.5-2 gallons) of water via stomach tube. Mix with water just before administration; simultaneously mixing water with psyllium as mixture is being pumped is ideal. May repeat as necessary as long as horse continues to pass feces and fluid does not accumulate in stomach. After initial treatment, may add up to 125 gm with each feeding; best if mixed with grain or sweet feed. Water must be available. (Calahan 1987)
    b) 0.25 kg mixed in 8 L of warm water *bid*. After obstruction is resolved may add to grain ration; may require 2-3 weeks of therapy to eliminate the majority of sand. (Clark and Becht 1987)

Monitoring Parameters -
1) Stool consistency, frequency

Client Information - Contact veterinarian if patient begins vomiting. Be sure animal has free access to water.

Dosage Forms/Preparations/FDA Approval Status/Withholding Times -
Veterinary-Approved Products:
Equi-Psyllium® (Equine Healthcare) is a product labeled for use in horses. It is available in 5 lb. jars.

Human-Approved Products: There are many human-approved products containing psyllium, most products contain approximately 3.4 grams of psyllium per rounded teaspoonful. Commonly known products include: *Metamucil*® (Procter & Gamble), *Hydrocil*® *Instant* (Reid-Rowell), *Correctol*® *Powder* (Plough), *Konsyl*® (Lafayette), *Serutan* (Beecham), *Effer-syllium*® (Stuart), *Perdiem*® *Plain* (Rorer), and *Siblin*® (Warner-Lambert). These products are all OTC.

PYRANTEL PAMOATE
PYRANTEL TARTRATE

Chemistry - A pyrimidine-derivative anthelmintic, pyrantel pamoate occurs as yellow to tan solid and is practically insoluble in water and alcohol. Pyrantel tartrate is more water soluble than is the pamoate salt. Each gram of pyrantel pamoate is approximately equivalent to 347 mg (34.7%) of the base.

Pyrantel pamoate may also be known as pyrantel embonate.

Storage/Stability/Compatibility - Pyrantel pamoate products should be stored in tight, light-resistant containers at room temperature (15-30°C) unless otherwise directed by the manufacturer.

Pharmacology - Pyrantel acts as a depolarizing neuromuscular blocking agent in susceptible parasites, thereby paralyzing the organism. The drug possesses nicotine-like properties and acts similarly to acetylcholine. It also inhibits cholinesterase.

Uses/Indications - Pyrantel has been used for the removal of the following parasites in **dogs**: ascarids *(Toxocara canis, T. leonina)*, hookworms *(Ancylostoma caninum, Uncinaria steno-cephala)* and stomach worm *(Physaloptera)*. Although not approved for use in **cats**, it is useful for similar parasites and is considered to be safe to use.

Pyrantel is indicated (labeled) for the removal of the following parasites in **horses**: *Strongylus vulgaris* and *equinus.*, *Parasacaris equorum,* and *Probstymayria vivapara.* It has variable activity against *Oxyuris equi.*, *S. edentatus* and small strongyles. Pyrantel is active against ileocecal tapeworm *(A. perfoliata)* when used at twice the recommended dose.

Although there are apparently no pyrantel products approved for use in **cattle, sheep,** or **goats,** the drug is effective (as the tartrate) for the removal of the following parasites: *Haemonchus spp., Ostertagia spp., Trichostrongylus spp., Nematodirus spp., Chabertia spp., Cooperia spp. and Oesophagostomum spp..*

Pyrantel tartrate is indicated (labeled) for the removal or prevention of the following parasites in **swine**: large roundworms *(Ascaris suum)* and *Oesophagostomum spp..* The drug also has activity against the swine stomach worm *(Hyostrongylus rubidus)*.

Although not approved, pyrantel has been used in **pet birds** and **llamas.** See the Dosage section for more information.

Pharmacokinetics - Pyrantel pamoate is poorly absorbed from the GI tract, thereby allowing it to reach the lower GI in dogs, cats and equines. Pyrantel tartrate is absorbed more readily than the pamoate salt. Pigs and dogs absorb pyrantel tartrate more so than do ruminants, with peak plasma levels occurring 2-3 hours after administration. Peak plasma levels occur at highly variable times in ruminants.

Absorbed drug is rapidly metabolized and excreted into the urine and feces.

Contraindications/Precautions/Usage in Pregnancy - Use with caution in severely debilitated animals. The manufacturers usually recommend not administering the drug to severely debilitated animals.

Pyrantel is considered to be safe to use during pregnancy and in nursing animals.

Adverse Effects/Warnings - When administered at recommended doses, adverse effects are unlikely. Emesis may occur however, in small animals receiving pyrantel pamoate.

Overdosage/Acute Toxicity - Pyrantel has a moderate margin of safety. Dosages up to approximately 7 times recommended generally result in no toxic reactions. In horses, doses of 20 times those recommended yielded no adverse effects. The LD_{50} in mice and rats for pyrantel tartrate is 170 mg/kg and is >690 mg/kg for pyrantel pamoate in dogs.

Chronic dosing of pyrantel pamoate in dogs resulted in symptoms when given at 50 mg/kg/day, but not at 20 mg/kg/day over 3 months. Symptoms of toxicity that could possibly be seen include increased respiratory rates, profuse sweating (in animals able to do so), ataxia or other cholinergic effects.

Drug Interactions - Because of similar mechanisms of action (and toxicity), pyrantel is recommended not to be used concurrently with **morantel** or **levamisole**.

Observation for adverse effects should be intensified if used concomitantly with an **organophosphate** or **diethylcarbamazine**.

Piperazine and pyrantel have antagonistic mechanisms of action; do not use together.

Doses -

All doses are for pyrantel pamoate unless otherwise noted. **Caution:** Listed dosages are often not specified as to whether using the salt or base.

Dogs:
For susceptible parasites:
a) 5 mg/kg PO, repeat in 3 weeks. (Kirk 1989)
b) 15 mg/kg PO 30 minutes after a light meal. Re-treatment recommendations: For hooks: 2 weeks; every other week for 5-6 weeks (beginning at 1 week old) if bitch previously lost pups due to hookworm anemia. For Ascarids: Every other week for 3-4 treatments beginning at 2 weeks old if pups have heavy infestation; retreatment usually not necessary for mature animals. (Cornelius and Roberson 1986)
c) 5 mg/kg PO; stir liquid before using. (Chiapella 1988)
d) For dogs weighing less than 5 lbs: 10 mg/kg (as base) PO; For dogs weighing more than 5 lbs: 5 mg/kg (as base) PO. Treat puppies at 2, 3, 4, 6, 8, and 10 weeks of age. Treat lactating bitches 2-3 weeks after whelping. Do follow-up fecal 2-4 weeks after treating to determine need for retreatment. (Label directions; *Nemex*® *Tabs*—Pfizer)

Cats:
For susceptible parasites:
a) Ascarids, Hookworms, *Physaloptera*: 5 mg/kg PO; repeat in 2 weeks (one time only for *Physaloptera*). (Dimski 1989)
b) 10 mg/kg PO, repeat in 3 weeks. (Kirk 1989)

Horses:
For susceptible parasites:
a) 6.6 mg (as base)/kg PO; 13.2 mg (as base)/kg for cestodes. (Robinson 1987), (Roberson 1988b)
b) 19 mg/kg PO (Brander, Pugh, and Bywater 1982)
c) Pyrantel tartrate: 12.5 mg/kg PO (Roberson 1988b)

Swine:
For susceptible parasites:
a) To remove *Ascaris suum* or *Oesophagostomum spp.*: Pyrantel tartrate: 22 mg/kg PO (or in feed at a rate of 800 g/ton) as a single treatment. For *Ascaris suum* only: in feed at a rate of 96 g/ton (2.6 mg/kg) for 3 days. (Paul 1986), (Label instructions from several pyrantel tartrate premix products)
b) Pyrantel tartrate: 22 mg/kg PO; maximum of 2 grams per animal (Roberson 1988b)
c) For ascarids and nodular worms in potbellied pigs: 6.6 mg/kg PO (Braun 1995)

Cattle, Sheep & Goats:
For susceptible parasites:
a) Pyrantel tartrate: 25 mg/kg PO. (Roberson 1988b)

Llamas:
For susceptible parasites:
a) 18 mg/kg PO for one day. (Cheney and Allen 1989), (Fowler 1989)

Birds:
For intestinal nematodes:
a) 4.5 mg/kg PO once. Repeat in 14 days. Suspension is non-toxic and palatable. (Clubb 1986)
b) For nematodes: 100 mg/kg PO as a single dose in psittacines and passerines. (Marshall 1993)

Client Information - Shake suspensions well before administering

Dosage Forms/Preparations/FDA Approval Status/Withholding Times -
Veterinary-Approved Products:

Pyrantel Pamoate Tablets 22.7 mg (of base), 113.5 mg (of base); *Nemex*® *Tabs* (Pfizer); (OTC) Approved for use in dogs.

Pyrantel Pamoate Oral Suspension; 2.27 mg/ml (as base)(for dogs only), 4.54 mg/ml (of base); *Nemex*®*-2* (Pfizer); RFD Liquid Wormer® (Pfizer) (OTC) Approved for use in dogs & cats.

Pyrantel Pamoate Oral Suspension 50 mg/ml (of base); *Strongid® T* (Pfizer); (OTC) Approved for use in horses not intended for food.

Pyrantel Pamoate Oral Paste 43.9% w/w pyrantel base in 23.6 g (20 ml) paste (180 mg pyrantel base/ml); *Strongid® Paste* (Pfizer); (OTC) Approved for use in horses not intended for food.

Human-Approved Products:

Pyrantel Pamoate Oral Suspension or liquid 50 mg/ml (base) in 30 & 60 ml; *Antiminth®* (Pfizer) (OTC); *Reese's Pinworm®* (Reese) (OTC); *Pin-Rid®* (Apothecary) (OTC);*Pin-X®* (Effcon) (OTC)

Pyrantel Capsules 180 mg (equivalent to 62.5 mg pyrantel base); *Pin-Rid®* (Apothecary) (OTC); Reese's Pinworm® (Reese) (OTC)

PYRIDOSTIGMINE BROMIDE

Chemistry - An anticholinesterase agent, pyridostigmine bromide is a synthetic quaternary ammonium compound that occurs as an agreeable smelling, bitter-tasting, hygroscopic, white or practically white, crystalline powder. It is freely soluble in water and in alcohol. The pH of the commercially available injection is approximately 5.

Storage/Stability/Compatibility - Unless otherwise instructed by the manufacturer, store pyridostigmine products at room temperature. The oral solution and injection should be protected from light and freezing. Pyridostigmine tablets should be kept in tight containers.

The extended-release tablets may become mottled with time, but does not affect their potency.

Pyridostigmine injection is unstable in alkaline solutions. It is reportedly compatible with glycopyrrolate, heparin sodium, hydrocortisone sodium succinate, potassium chloride, and vitamin B-complex with C. Compatibility is dependent upon factors such as pH, concentration, temperature and diluents used. It is suggested to consult specialized references (*e.g., Handbook on Injectable Drugs* by Trissel; see bibliography) for more specific information.

Pharmacology - Pyridostigmine inhibits the hydrolysis of acetylcholine by directly competing with acetylcholine for attachment to acetylcholinesterase. Because the pyridostigmine-acetylcholinesterase complex is hydrolyzed at a much slower rate than the acetylcholine-acetylcholinesterase complex, acetylcholine tends to accumulate at cholinergic synapses with resultant cholinergic activity.

At usual doses, pyridostigmine does not cross into the CNS (quaternary ammonium structure), but overdoses can cause CNS effects.

Uses/Indications - Pyridostigmine is used in the treatment of myasthenia gravis (MG) in dogs (and rarely in cats). It is considered to be much more effective in acquired MG, rather than congenital MG.

Pharmacokinetics - Pyridostigmine is only marginally absorbed from the GI tract and absorption may be more erratic from the sustained-release tablets than with the regular tablets. The onset of action after oral dosing is generally within one hour.

At usual doses, pyridostigmine is apparently distributed to most tissues, but not to the brain, intestinal wall, fat or thymus. The drug crosses the placenta.

Pyridostigmine is both metabolized by the liver and hydrolyzed by cholinesterases.

Contraindications/Precautions/Reproductive Safety - Pyridostigmine is contraindicated in patients hypersensitive to this class of compounds or bromides, or those who have mechanical or physical obstructions of the urinary or GI tract.

The drug should be used with caution in patients with bronchospastic disease, epilepsy, hyperthyroidism, bradycardia or other arrhythmias, vagotonia, or GI ulcer diseases.

Adverse Effects/Warnings - Adverse effects associated with pyridostigmine are generally dose related and cholinergic in nature. Although usually mild and easily treatable with dosage reduction, severe adverse effects are possible (see Overdosage below).

Overdosage/Acute Toxicity - Overdosage of pyridostigmine may induce a cholinergic crisis. Symptoms of cholinergic toxicity can include GI effects (nausea, vomiting, diarrhea), salivation, sweating (in animals able to do so), respiratory effects (increased bronchial secretions, bronchospasm, pulmonary edema, respiratory paralysis), ophthalmic effects (miosis, blurred vision, lacrimation), cardiovascular effects (bradycardia or tachycardia, cardiospasm, hypotension, cardiac arrest), muscle cramps and weakness.

Overdoses in myasthenic patients can be very difficult to distinguish from the effects associated with a myasthenic crisis. The time of onset of symptoms or an edrophonium challenge may help to distinguish between the two.

Treatment of pyridostigmine overdosage, consists of both respiratory and cardiac supportive therapy and atropine if necessary. Refer to the atropine monograph for more information on its use for cholinergic toxicity.

Drug Interactions - Anticholinesterase therapy may be antagonized by administration of parenteral **magnesium** therapy, as it can have a direct depressant effect on skeletal muscle. **Drugs that possess some neuromuscular blocking activity** (*e.g.,* aminoglycoside antibiotics, some antiarrhythmic and anesthetic drugs) may necessitate increased dosages of pyridostigmine in treating or diagnosing myasthenic patients.

Corticosteroids may decrease the anticholinesterase activity of pyridostigmine. After stopping corticosteroid therapy, neostigmine may cause increased anticholinesterase activity.

Pyridostigmine may prolong the Phase I block of **depolarizing muscle relaxants** (*e.g.,* succinylcholine, decamethonium). Pyridostigmine antagonizes the actions of **non-depolarizing neuromuscular blocking agents** (pancuronium, tubocurarine, gallamine, etc.).

Atropine will antagonize the muscarinic effects of pyridostigmine, but concurrent use should be used cautiously as atropine can mask the early symptoms of cholinergic crisis.

Theoretically, **dexpanthenol** may have additive effects when used with pyridostigmine.

Doses -
Dogs:
For myasthenia gravis (MG):
a) For acquired MG: After oral regurgitation is abolished with parenteral therapy (neostigmine), may begin oral therapy with pyridostigmine at 7.5 - 30 mg PO *bid*. Once patient is stable and infections have resolved, begin corticosteroid therapy (antiinflammatory doses of prednisone) and continue concurrently with anticholinesterase drugs for 2 weeks. Then pyridostigmine may be gradually reduced. (Pedroia 1989)
b) Proven efficacy for acquired MG, but of questionable value for congenital MG. Pyridostigmine: 0.2 - 2 mg/kg PO *bid-tid*. Higher dose is often too high initially. (LeCouteur 1989)
c) Initial guidelines only; titrate dose to the patient. Dogs weighing less than 5 kg: 45 mg PO *qid*; weighing 5-25 kg: 45-90 mg PO *qid*; weighing more than 25 kg: 90 - 135 mg PO *qid*. If cholinergic symptoms occur, reduce dose by 25%; atropine rarely necessary. (Hurvitz and Johnessee 1985)

Cats:
For myasthenia gravis (MG):
a) For acquired MG: Cats are sensitive to anticholinesterase agents. Do not exceed 0.25 mg/kg/day PO initially in cats. (Fenner 1989)

Monitoring Parameters - Animals should be routinely monitored for symptoms of cholinergic toxicity (see Overdose section above) and also for efficacy of the therapy.

Client Information - See Monitoring above. Clients should be instructed to report to the veterinarian symptoms of excessive salivation, GI disturbances, weakness, or difficulty breathing.

Dosage Forms/Preparations/FDA Approval Status/Withholding Times -
Veterinary-Approved Products: None
Human-Approved Products:
Pyridostigmine Br Oral Tablets 60 mg; *Mestinon*® ICN); (Rx)

Pyridostigmine Br Oral Sustained-Release Tablets 180 mg; *Mestinon*® (ICN); (Rx)

Pyridostigmine Br Oral Syrup 60 mg/5 ml (12 mg/ml) in pints; *Mestinon*® (ICN); (Rx)

Pyridostigmine Br Injection 5 mg/ml in 2 ml amps and 5 ml vials; *Mestinon*® (ICN); *Regunol*® (Organon); (Rx)

PYRILAMINE MALEATE

Chemistry - An ethylenediamine antihistamine, pyrilamine maleate occurs as a white, crystalline powder with a melting range of 99-103°. One gram is soluble in approximately 0.5 ml of water or 3 ml alcohol.

Storage/Stability/Compatibility - Avoid freezing the injectable product.

Pharmacology - Antihistamines (H_1-receptor antagonists) competitively inhibit histamine at H_1 receptor sites. They do not inactivate, nor prevent the release of histamine, but can prevent histamine's action on the cell. Besides their antihistaminic activity, these agents also have varying degrees of anticholinergic and CNS activity (sedation). Pyrilamine is considered to be less sedating and have much less anticholinergic effects when compared to most other antihistamines.

Uses/Indications - Antihistamines are used in veterinary medicine to reduce or help prevent histamine mediated adverse effects.

Pharmacokinetics - The pharmacokinetics of this agent have apparently not been extensively studied.

Contraindications/Precautions - The manufacturer indicates that the use of this product "should not supercede the use of other emergency drugs and procedures."

Adverse Effects/Warnings - Adverse effects in horses can include CNS stimulation (nervousness, insomnia, convulsions, tremors, ataxia), palpitation, GI disturbances, CNS depression (sedation), muscular weakness, anorexia, lassitude and incoordination.

Overdosage - Treatment of overdosage is basically supportive and symptomatic. The manufacturer (Schering - *Histavet-P®*) suggests using "careful titration" of barbiturates to treat convulsions, and analeptics (caffeine, ephedrine, or amphetamines) to treat CNS depression. Most toxicologists however, recommend avoiding the use of CNS stimulants in the treatment of CNS depressant overdoses. Phenytoin (IV) is recommended in the treatment of seizures caused by antihistamine overdose in humans; barbiturates and diazepam are to be avoided.

Drug Interactions - Increased sedation can occur if diphenhydramine is combined with **other CNS depressant drugs**.

Antihistamines may partially counteract the anticoagulation effects of **heparin** or **warfarin**.
Pyrilamine may enhance the effects of **epinephrine**.

Laboratory Interactions - Antihistamines can decrease the wheal and flare response to **antigen skin testing**. In humans, it is suggested that antihistamines be discontinued at least 4 days before testing.

Doses -
Dogs:
    a) 12.5 - 25 mg PO *qid*; 25 - 125 mg IM (Swinyard 1975)

Cattle:
    a) 0.5 -1.5 grams IM (Swinyard 1975)
    b) For adjunctive treatment of aseptic laminitis: 55 - 110 mg/100 kg IV or IM (Berg 1986)

Horses:
    a) 0.88 - 1.32 mg/kg (2-3 mls of 20 mg/ml solution per 100 lbs body weight) IV (slowly), IM or SQ; may repeat in 6-12 hours if necessary. Foals: 0.44 mg/kg (1 ml of 20 mg/ml solution per 100 lbs. body weight) IV (slowly), IM or SQ; may repeat in 6-12 hours if necessary. (Package Insert; *Histavet-P®* - Schering)
    b) 1 mg/kg IV, IM or SQ (Robinson 1987)
    c) 0.5 -1.5 grams IM (Swinyard 1975)

Sheep, Swine:
    a) 0.25 - 0.5 gram IM (Swinyard 1975)

Monitoring Parameters -
    1) Clinical efficacy and adverse effects

Dosage Forms/Preparations/FDA Approval Status/Withholding Times -
Veterinary-Approved Products:
    Pyrilamine Maleate Injection 20 mg/ml; 100 ml vial; *Histavet-P®* (Schering); (Rx) Approved for use in horses not intended for food only.

Human-Approved Products:
    Pyrilamine Maleate Tablets 25 mg; Generic; (Rx/OTC)

PYRIMETHAMINE

Chemistry - An aminpyrimidine agent structurally related to trimethoprim, pyrimethamine occurs as an odorless, white, or almost white, crystalline powder or crystals. It is practically insoluble in water and slightly soluble in alcohol.

Storage/Stability/Compatibility - Pyrimethamine tablets should be stored in tight, light-resistant containers.

Pyrimethamine tablets may be crushed to make oral suspensions of the drug. Although stable in an aqueous solution, sugars tend to adversely affect the stability of pyrimethamine. If cherry syrup, corn syrup, or sucrose-containing liquids are used in the preparation of the suspension, it is recommended to store the suspension at room temperature and discard after 7 days.

Pharmacology - Pyrimethamine is a folic acid antagonist similar to trimethoprim. It acts by inhibiting the enzyme, dihydrofolate reductase that catalyzes the conversion of dihydrofolic acid to tetrahydrofolic acid.

Uses/Indications - In veterinary medicine, pyrimethamine is used to treat (often in combination with sulfonamides) toxoplasmosis in small animals. In horses, it is used to treat equine protozoal myeloencephalitis, sometimes called equine toxoplasmosis.

In humans, pyrimethamine is used for the treatment of toxoplasmosis and as a prophylactic agent for malaria.

Pharmacokinetics - No pharmacokinetic data was located for veterinary species. In humans, pyrimethamine is well absorbed from the gut after oral administration. It is distributed primarily to the kidneys, liver, spleen and lungs, but does cross the blood-brain barrier. It has a volume of distribution of about 3 L/kg and is 80% bound to plasma proteins. Pyrimethamine enters milk in levels greater than those found in serum and is detected in milk for up to 48 hours after dosing.

In humans, the plasma half-life is approximately 3-5 days. It is unknown how or where the drug is metabolized, but metabolites are found in the urine.

Contraindications/Precautions/Reproductive Safety - Pyrimethamine is contraindicated in patients hypersensitive to it and should be used cautiously in patients with preexisting hematologic disorders. Pyrimethamine has been demonstrated to be teratogenic in rats. However, it has been used in treating women with toxoplasmosis during pregnancy. Clearly, the risks associated with therapy must be weighed against the potential for toxicity, the severity of the disease, and any alternative therapies available (*e.g.,* clindamycin in small animals). Concomitant administration of folinic acid has been recommended if the drug is to be used during pregnancy.

Adverse Effects/Warnings - In small animals, anorexia, malaise, vomiting, depression and bone marrow depression (anemia, thrombocytopenia, leukopenia) have been seen. Adverse effects may be more prominent in cats and may be noted 4-6 days after starting combination therapy. Hematologic effects can develop rapidly and frequent monitoring is recommended, particularly if therapy persists longer than 2 weeks. Oral administration of folinic acid at 1 mg/kg PO, folic acid 5 mg/day, or Brewer's yeast 100 mg/kg/day have been suggested to alleviate adverse effects.

The drug is unpalatable to cats when mixed with food and the 25 mg tablet dosage size makes successful dosing a challenge.

In horses, pyrimethamine when used in combination with sulfonamides has caused leukopenias, thrombocytopenia and anemias. Baker's yeast or folinic acid have been suggested to be used to antagonize these adverse effects.

Overdosage/Acute Toxicity - Reports of acute overdosage of pyrimethamine in animals was not located. In humans, vomiting, nausea, anorexia, CNS stimulation (including seizures) and hematologic effects can be seen. Recommendations for treatment include: standard procedures in emptying the gut or preventing absorption, parenteral barbiturates for seizures, folinic acid for hematologic effects and long-term monitoring (at least 1 month) of renal and hematopoietic systems.

Drug Interactions - Pyrimethamine is synergistic with **sulfonamides** in activity against toxoplasmosis (and malaria).

p-**aminobenzoic acid (PABA)** is reportedly antagonistic towards the activity of pyrimethamine; clinical significance is unclear.

Use of pyrimethamine with **trimethoprim/sulfa** is not recommended (in humans) as adverse effects may be additive, but this combination has been used clinically in horses.

Doses -
Dogs:
    For toxoplasmosis:
        a) 0.5 - 1 mg/kg PO once daily for 2 days, then 0.25 mg/kg PO once daily for 2 weeks. Given with sulfadiazine at 30 - 50 mg/kg PO divided *bid-qid* for 1-2 weeks. (Murtaugh 1988)
        b) 1 mg/kg PO once daily for 3 days, then 0.5 mg/kg PO once daily. (Kirk 1989)
        c) Pyrimethamine: 1 mg/kg PO per day with sulfadiazine at 30 mg/kg PO q12h for 7-10 days. Do not use continually for longer than 2 weeks. (Swango, Bankemper, and Kong 1989)

Cats:
    For toxoplasmosis:
        a) 0.5 - 1 mg/kg PO once daily for 2 days, then 0.25 mg/kg PO once daily for 2 weeks. Given with sulfadiazine at 30 - 50 mg/kg PO divided *bid-qid* for 1-2 weeks. (Murtaugh 1988)
        b) For enteroepithelial cycle: 2 mg/kg PO once daily. For extraintestinal cycle: 0.5 - 1 mg/kg PO divided *bid-tid* combined with sulfonamides (*e.g.,* triple sulfa, sulfadiazine) at 60 mg/kg PO or IM divided *bid-tid*. (Lappin 1989)
        c) For protozoal myocarditis: Pyrimethamine 1 mg/kg PO once daily for 3 days, then decrease dose to 0.5 mg/kg PO once a day, with sulfadimethoxine 25 mg/kg PO, IV, or IM once a day. (Ogburn 1988)

    d) Pyrimethamine: 0.5 mg/kg PO per day with sulfadiazine at 30 mg/kg PO q12h for 7-10 days. Do not use continuously for longer than 2 weeks. Supplementation with folic acid 5 mg/day or folinic acid 1 mg/kg/day may alleviate toxicity. (Swango, Bankemper, and Kong 1989) (**NOTE**: Since this reference was published, pyrimethamine dosage is now more commonly given at 1 mg/kg PO once daily—Plumb; March 1999)

Horses:
    For equine protozoal myeloencephalitis:

    a) Pyrimethamine 0.1 - 0.2 mg/kg PO once daily, with trimethoprim/sulfadiazine 15 mg/kg PO *bid*. Dosage may be continued for up to 2 months. Reinstitute therapy if animal is stressed; long-term intermittent therapy may be rational. Guarded prognosis; relapses are not uncommon. (Brewer 1987)

Monitoring Parameters -
    1) See adverse effects; CBC with platelet count; 2) Clinical efficacy

Client Information - Clients should he instructed to monitor for symptoms of abnormal bleeding, lassitude, etc. that may signal development of hematologic disorders. Accurate dosing of the tablets in cats may be very difficult as only 25 mg tablets are commercially available. Preferably, custom prepared capsules containing the accurate dosage should be prepared.

Dosage Forms/Preparations/FDA Approval Status -
  Veterinary-Approved Products: None
  Human-Approved Products:
    Pyrimethamine Tablets 25 mg; *Daraprim*® (Glaxo Wellcome); (Rx)

QUINACRINE HCL

Chemistry - A synthetic acridine derivative anthelmintic, quinacrine HCl occurs as a bright yellow, odorless, crystalline powder having a bitter taste. It is sparingly soluble in water. Quinacrine HCl may also be known as mepacrine HCl.

Storage/Stability/Compatibility - Tablets should be stored in tight, light-resistant containers at room temperature. Quinacrine is not stable in solution for any length of time; however, it may be crushed and mixed with foods to mask its very bitter taste.

Pharmacology - Quinacrine's mechanism of action for its antiprotozoal activity against Giardia is not understood, however it does bind to DNA by intercalation to adjacent base pairs, thereby inhibiting RNA transcription and translocation. Additionally, quinacrine interferes with electron transport, inhibits succinate oxidation and cholinesterase. Quinacrine binds to nucleoproteins which (in humans at least) can suppress lupus erythromatosis (LE) cell factor.

Uses/Indications - While quinacrine has activity against a variety of protozoans and helminths, its use against all but Giardia and Trichomonas has been superseded by safer or more effective agents. In humans, quinacrine may also be used for treatment of mild to moderate discoid lupus erythromatosis, transcervically as a sterilizing agent or in powder form as an intrapleural sclerosing agent.

Pharmacokinetics - Quinacrine is absorbed well from the GI tract or after intrapleural administration. It is distributed throughout the body, but CSF levels are only 1-5% of those found in the plasma. Drug is concentrated in the liver, spleen, lungs and adrenals. It is relatively highly bound to plasma proteins in humans (80-90%). Quinacrine crosses the placenta, but only small amounts enter maternal milk.

  Quinacrine is eliminated very slowly (half life in humans: 5-14 days). Quinacrine is slowly metabolized, but primarily eliminated by the kidneys. Acidifying the urine will increase renal excretion somewhat. Significant amounts may be detected in the urine up to 2 months after drug discontinuation.

Contraindications/Precautions/Reproductive Safety - In humans, quinacrine is relatively contraindicated in patients with psychotic disorders, psoriasis, or porphyria as it may exacerbate these conditions. Veterinary relevance is unknown.

  Quinacrine crosses the placenta and has been implicated in causing a case of renal agenesis and hydrocephalus in a human infant. In high doses, it also has caused increased fetal death rates in rats. Weigh the potential benefits with the risks when considering use in pregnant animals.

Adverse Effects/Warnings - In small animals, a yellowing of skin and urine color can occur, but is not of clinical importance (does not indicate jaundice). Additionally, gastrointestinal disturbances (anorexia, nausea, vomiting, diarrhea), abnormal behaviors ("fly biting", agitation), pruritus, and fever have been noted.

  Potentially hypersensitivity reactions, hepatopathy, aplastic anemia, corneal edema and retinopathy could occur (all reported rarely in humans, primarily with high dose long term use).

Overdosage/Acute Toxicity - Overdosage may be serious depending on the dose. In humans, a dose as low as 6.8 grams (administered intraduodenally) caused death. Symptoms associated with acute toxicity include CNS excitation (including seizures), GI disturbances, vascular collapse and cardiac arrhythmias. Treatment consists of gut emptying protocols, and supportive and symptomatic therapies. Urinary acidification with ammonium chloride and forced diuresis (with adequate fluid therapy) may be beneficial in enhancing urinary excretion of the drug.

Drug Interactions - Quinacrine increases the toxicity of **primaquine** (generally not used in veterinary medicine), and the two should not be used simultaneously. Quinacrine may cause a "disulfiram-reaction" if used with **alcohol**. Quinacrine concentrates in the liver and should be used with caution with **hepatotoxic drugs** (clinical significance unknown).

Laboratory Considerations - When urine is acidic, quinacrine can cause it to turn a deep yellow color. By causing an interfering fluorescence, quinacrine can cause falsely elevated values of **plasma and urine cortisol values.**

Doses - As a drug of second-choice in the treatment of Giardia or other susceptible protozoa:
Dogs:
    a) 6.6 mg/kg PO q12h for 5 days (Papich 1992), (Sherding and Johnson 1994a)

Cats:
    a) 11 mg/kg PO once daily for 5 days (Papich 1992)
    b) 6.6 mg/kg PO bid for 5 days (Barr and Bowman 1994)

Monitoring Parameters - 1) Efficacy (fecal exams, reduction in diarrhea); 2) Adverse Effects

Client Information - Quinacrine should preferably be given after meals with plenty of liquids available. Be sure clients understand the importance of compliance with directions and to watch for signs of adverse effects.

Dosage Forms/Preparations/FDA Approval Status/Withholding Times -
Veterinary-Approved Products: None
Human-Approved Products: There currently are no quinacrine products being marketed.

QUINIDINE GLUCONATE
QUINIDINE POLYGALACTURONATE
QUINIDINE SULFATE

Chemistry - Used as an antiarrhythmic agent, quinidine is an alkaloid obtained from *cinchona* or related plants, or is prepared from quinine. It is available commercially in three separate salts: gluconate, polygalacturonate, or sulfate.

Quinidine gluconate occurs as a very bitter tasting, odorless, white powder. It is freely soluble in water and slightly soluble in alcohol. The injectable form has a pH of 5.5-7.

Quinidine polygalacturonate occurs as a bitter tasting, creamy white, amorphous powder. It is sparingly soluble in water and freely soluble in hot 40% alcohol.

Quinidine sulfate occurs as very bitter tasting, odorless, fine, needle-like, white crystals that may cohere in masses. One gram is soluble in approximately 100 ml of water or 10 ml of alcohol.

Storage/Stability/Compatibility - All quinidine salts darken upon exposure to light (acquire a brownish tint) and should be stored in light-resistant, well-closed containers. Use only colorless, clear solutions of quinidine gluconate for injection.

Quinidine gluconate injection is usually administered intramuscularly, but may be given very slowly (1 ml/minute) intravenously. It may be diluted by adding 10 to 40 ml of D_5W. Quinidine gluconate is reported to be **compatible** with bretylium tosylate, cimetidine HCl, and verapamil HCl. It is reportedly **incompatible** with alkalies and iodides.

Pharmacology - A class IA antiarrhythmic, quinidine has effects similar to that of procainamide. It depresses myocardial excitability, conduction velocity and contractility. Quinidine will prolong the effective refractory period, which prevents the reentry phenomenon and increases conduction times. Quinidine also possesses anticholinergic activity which decreases vagal tone and may facilitate AV conduction.

Uses/Indications - Quinidine is indicated in small animal or equine medicine for the treatment of ventricular arrhythmias (VPC's, ventricular tachycardia), refractory supraventricular tachycardias, supraventricular arrhythmias associated with anomalous conduction in Wolff-Parkinson-White (WPW) syndrome, and acute atrial fibrillation. Oral therapy is generally not used in cats.

Pharmacokinetics - After oral administration, quinidine salts are nearly completely absorbed from the GI. However, the actual amount that reaches the systemic circulation will be reduced due to the hepatic first-pass effect. The extended-release formulations of quinidine sulfate and gluconate, as well as the polygalacturonate tablets, are more slowly absorbed than the conventional tablets or capsules.

Quinidine is distributed rapidly to all body tissues except the brain. Protein binding varies from 82-92%. The reported volumes of distribution in various species are: horses ≈ 15.1 L/kg, cattle ≈ 3.8 L/kg; dogs ≈ 2.9 L/kg; cats ≈ 2.2 L/kg. Quinidine is distributed into milk and crosses the placenta.

Quinidine is metabolized in the liver, primarily by hydroxylation. Approximately 20% of a dose may be excreted unchanged in the urine within 24 hours after dosing. Serum half-lives reported in various species are: horses ≈ 8.1 hours; cattle ≈ 2.3 hours; dogs ≈ 5.6 hours; cats ≈ 1.9 hours; swine ≈ 5.5 hours; goats ≈ 0.9 hours. Acidic urine (pH < 6) can increase renal excretion of quinidine and decrease its serum half-life.

Contraindications/Precautions - Quinidine is generally contraindicated in patients who have demonstrated previous hypersensitivity reactions to it; myasthenia gravis; complete AV block with an AV junctional or idioventricular pacemaker; intraventricular conduction defects (especially with pronounced QRS widening); digitalis intoxication with associated arrhythmias or AV conduction disorders; aberrant ectopic impulses; or abnormal rhythms secondary to escape mechanisms. It should be used with extreme caution, if at all, in any form of AV block or if any symptoms of digitalis toxicity are exhibited.

Quinidine should be used with caution in patients with uncorrected hypokalemia, hypoxia, and disorders or acid-base balance. Use cautiously in patients with hepatic or renal insufficiency as accumulation of the drug may result.

Adverse Effects/Warnings - In dogs, gastrointestinal effects may include anorexia, vomiting, or diarrhea. Effects related to the cardiovascular system can include weakness, hypotension (especially with too rapid IV administration), negative inotropism, widened QRS complex and QT intervals, AV block, and multiform ventricular tachycardias hypotension.

Horses may exhibit swelling of the nasal mucosa, laminitis, GI distress, and the development of urticarial wheals. Horses may also develop cardiac arrhythmias including AV block, circulatory collapse and sudden death.

Patients exhibiting signs of toxicity or lack of response may be candidates for therapeutic serum monitoring. The therapeutic range is thought to be 2.5 - 5.0 micrograms/ml in dogs. Toxic effects usually are not seen unless levels are >10 micrograms/ml.

Overdosage - Symptoms of overdosage can include depression, hypotension, lethargy, confusion, seizures, vomiting, diarrhea and oliguria. Cardiac signs may include depressed automaticity and conduction, or tachyarrhythmias. The CNS effects are often delayed after the onset of cardiovascular effects but may persist after the cardiovascular effects have begun to resolve.

If a recent oral ingestion, emptying of the gut and charcoal administration may be beneficial to remove any unabsorbed drug. IV fluids, plus metaraminol or norepinephrine can be considered to treat hypotensive effects. A 1/6 molar intravenous infusion of sodium lactate may be used in an attempt to reduce the cardiotoxic effects of quinidine. Forced diuresis using fluids and diuretics along with reduction of urinary pH, may enhance the renal excretion of the drug. Temporary cardiac pacing may be necessary should severe AV block occur. Hemodialysis will effectively remove quinidine, but peritoneal dialysis will not.

Drug Interactions - **Digoxin** levels may increase considerably in patients stabilized on digoxin who receive quinidine. Some cardiologists recommend decreasing the digoxin dosage by 1/2 when adding quinidine. Therapeutic drug monitoring of both quinidine and digoxin may be warranted in these cases.

Coumarin anticoagulants with quinidine may increase the likelihood of bleeding problems developing.

Quinidine may increase the neuromuscular blocking effects of drugs like **succinylcholine, tubocurarine or atracurium**.

Phenobarbital, phenytoin or rifampin may induce hepatic enzymes that metabolize quinidine thus reducing quinidine serum half-life by 50%. **Cimetidine** may increase the effects of quinidine by inhibiting hepatic microsomal enzymes.

Use with caution with **other antidysrhythmic agents**, as additive cardiotoxic or other toxic effects may result.

Quinidine may antagonize the effects of **pyridostigmine, neostigmine,** or other anticholinesterases in patients with myasthenia gravis.

Quinidine may potentiate the effects of other **drugs having hypotensive effects**.

Additive cardiac depressant effects may be seen if used with other agents that depress cardiac contractility (*e.g.,* other **antiarrhythmic drugs (procainamide, disopyramide, etc.), phenothiazines**).

Drugs that alkalinize the urine (**carbonic anhydrase inhibitors, thiazide diuretics, sodium bicarbonate, antacids**, etc.) may decrease the excretion of quinidine, prolonging its half-life. Drugs that acidify the urine (*e.g.,* **methionine, ammonium chloride**) may increase the excretion of quinidine and decrease serum levels.

Doses -
Dogs:
- a) Quinidine sulfate: 6 - 16 mg/kg PO q6h (conventional tabs/caps); q8h (Extentabs®)
  Quinidine gluconate: 6 - 20 mg/kg IM q6h; 8 - 20 mg/kg PO q6-8h (sustained-release)
  Quinidine polygalacturonate: 8 - 20 mg/kg q6-8h (Miller 1985)
- b) Quinidine gluconate (sustained-release): 8 - 20 mg/kg PO q8-12h; Injection: 8 - 20 mg/kg IM q8-12h or slow IV q8h
  Quinidine sulfate: 8 - 20 mg/kg PO q6-8h
  Quinidine polygalcturonate: 8 - 20 mg/kg PO q8-12h (Kirk 1986)
- c) For VPC's or V. tach:
  Quinidine gluconate: 6.6 - 22 mg/kg IM q2-4h or q8-12h PO (delayed dosage forms).
  Quinidine Sulfate: 6.6 - 22 mg/kg PO q6-8h; may be given initially q2h as a loading dose until arrhythmias is controlled or toxicity is induced. (Ettinger 1989)
- d) For conversion of atrial fib to sinus rhythm: Initially attempted with quinidine gluconate at 6 - 11 mg/kg IM q6h. Most dogs will convert in the first 24 hours of threapy. If rapid ventricular response occurs, may give either digoxin or a beta blocker to slow rate of conduction across AV node. (Russell and Rush 1995)

Cats:
- a) 4 - 8 mg/kg IM *tid* (Morgan 1988)
- b) 10 - 20 mg/kg q6h PO (Neff-Davis 1985)

Horses:
- a) Oral Dosing:
  Method 1: Give quinidine sulfate powder by stomach tube or in large gelatin capsules.
  Day 1: Give 5 gram test dose; if no adverse reactions (see Adverse Effects) may continue therapy
  Days 2, 3: 10 gram *bid*
  Days 4, 5: 10 gram *tid*
  Days 6, 7: 10 gram *qid*
  Days 8,9: 10 gram every 5 hours
  Day 10 and thereafter: 15 gram *qid*

  Method 2:
  Day 1: 5 gram test dose
  Day 2: 10 gram every 2 hours until a total dose of 80 grams or less has been given.
  Once the arrhythmia is halted, reduce dose total dose by 1/2 every other day until a maintenance dose is reached that prevents recurrence of arrhythmia. If treating atrial fibrillation, quinidine can usually be discontinued 1-2 days after conversion to sinus rhythm. Doses greater than 40 grams per day tend to cause undesirable effects. (Hilwig 1987)

Monitoring Parameters - 1) ECG; 2) Blood pressure if possible, during IV administration; 3) Symptoms of toxicity (see Adverse Reactions/Overdosage); 4) Serum levels. Therapeutic serum levels are believed to range from 2.5 - 5.0 micrograms/ml. Levels greater than 10 micrograms/ml are considered to be toxic.

Client Information - Oral products should be administered at evenly spaced intervals throughout the day/night. GI upset may be decreased if administered with food. Do not allow animal to chew or crush sustained-release oral dosage forms. Notify veterinarian if animal's condition deteriorates or symptoms of toxicity (*e.g.,* vomiting, diarrhea, weakness, etc.) occur.

Dosage Forms/Preparations/FDA Approval Status/Withholding Times -
Veterinary-Approved Products: None
Human-Approved Products:
Quinidine Sulfate (contains 83% anhydrous quinidine alkaloid) Tablets 200 mg, 300 mg; *Quinora*® (Key), Generic; (Rx)

Quinidine Sulfate (contains 83% anhydrous quinidine alkaloid) Sustained-Release Tablets 300 mg; *Quinidex*® *Extentabs* (Robins); (Rx)

Quinidine Gluconate (contains 62% anhydrous quinidine alkaloid); Sustained-release Tablets 324 mg; *Quinaglute*® *Dura-Tabs* (Berlex); *Quinalan*® (Lannett); Generic; (Rx)

Quinidine Gluconate Injection 80 mg/ml (50 mg/ml of quinidine), 10 ml vials; Generic (Lilly); (Rx)

Quinidine Polygalacturonate (contains 80% anhydrous quinidine alkaloid); Tablets 275 mg; *Cardioquin*® (Purdue-Frederick); (Rx)

RANITIDINE HCL

Chemistry - An H_2 receptor antagonist, ranitidine HCl occurs as a white to pale-yellow granular substance with a bitter taste and a sulfur-like odor. The drug has pK_as of 8.2 and 2.7. One gram is approximately soluble in 1.5 ml of water or 6 ml of alcohol. The commercially available injection has a pH of 6.7-7.3.

Storage/Stability/Compatibility - Ranitidine tablets should be stored in tight, light-resistant containers at room temperature. The injectable product should be stored protected from light and at a temperature less than 30°C. A slight darkening of the injectable solution does not affect the potency of the drug.

Ranitidine injection is reportedly stable for up to 48 hours when mixed with the commonly used IV solutions (including 5% sodium bicarbonate).

Pharmacology - At the H_2 receptors of the parietal cells, ranitidine competitively inhibits histamine, thereby reducing gastric acid output both during basal conditions and when stimulated by food, amino acids, pentagastrin, histamine or insulin. Ranitidine is between 3-13 times more potent (on a molar basis) as cimetidine.

Ranitidine can cause gastric emptying times to be delayed, but the clinical significance of this effect is not known. Lower esophageal sphincter pressures may be increased by ranitidine. By decreasing the amount of gastric juice produced, ranitidine also decreases the amount of pepsin secreted.

Ranitidine, unlike cimetidine, does not appear to have any appreciable effect on serum prolactin levels, although it may inhibit the release of vasopressin.

Uses/Indications - In veterinary medicine, ranitidine has been used for the treatment and/or prophylaxis of gastric, abomasal and duodenal ulcers, uremic gastritis, stress-related or drug-induced erosive gastritis, esophagitis, duodenal gastric reflux and esophageal reflux. It has also been employed to treat hypersecretory conditions associated with gastrinomas and systemic mastocytosis.

Pharmacokinetics - Pharmacokinetic data for veterinary species is limited for this product. In dogs, the oral bioavailability is approximately 81%, serum half-life is 2.2 hours and volume of distribution 2.6 L/kg.

In humans, ranitidine is absorbed rapidly after oral administration, but undergoes extensive first-pass metabolism with a net systemic bioavailability of approximately 50%. Peak levels occur at about 2-3 hours after oral dosing. Food does not appreciably alter the extent of absorption or the peak serum levels attained.

Ranitidine is distributed widely throughout the body and is only 10-19% bound to plasma proteins. Ranitidine is distributed into human milk at levels of 25-100% of those found in the plasma.

Ranitidine is both excreted in the urine by the kidneys (via glomerular filtration and tubular secretion) and metabolized in the liver to inactive metabolites; accumulation of the drug can occur in patients with renal insufficiency. The serum half-life of ranitidine in humans averages from 2-3 hours. The duration of action at usual doses is from 8-12 hours.

Contraindications/Precautions - Ranitidine is contraindicated in patients who are hypersensitive to it. It should be used cautiously and possibly at reduced dosage in patients with diminished renal function. Ranitidine has caused increased serum ALT levels in humans receiving high, IV doses for longer than 5 days. The manufacturer recommends that in high dose, chronic therapy that serum ALT values be considered for monitoring.

Adverse Effects/Warnings - Adverse effects appear to be very rare in animals at the dosages generally used. Potential adverse effects (documented in humans) that might be seen include mental confusion and headache. Rarely, agranulocytosis may develop and if given rapidly IV, transient cardiac arrhythmias may be seen. Pain at the injection site may be noted after IM administration.

Overdosage - Clinical experience with ranitidine overdosage is limited. In laboratory animals, very high dosages (225 mg/kg/day) have been associated with muscular tremors, vomiting and rapid respirations. Single doses of 1 gram/kg in rodents did not cause death.

Treatment of overdoses in animals should be handled using standard protocols for oral ingestions of drugs; symptoms may be treated symptomatically and supportively if necessary. Hemodialysis and peritoneal dialysis have been noted to remove ranitidine from the body.

Drug Interactions - Unlike cimetidine, ranitidine appears to only have minimal effects on the hepatic metabolism of drugs and is unlikely to cause clinically relevant drug interactions via this mechanism.

Propantheline Bromide delays the absorption, but increases the peak serum level of ranitidine. The relative bioavailability of ranitidine may be increased by 23% when propantheline is administered concomitantly with ranitidine.

Antacids may decrease the absorption of ranitidine; give at separate times (2 hours apart) if used concurrently.

Ranitidine may decrease the renal clearance of **procainamide**, but the clinical relevance of this interaction is unclear at this time.

The manufacturer states that ranitidine may alter the bioavailability of certain drugs through pH-dependent effects, changes in volume of distribution or an unknown effect. Further information is pending.

Drug/Laboratory Interactions - Ranitidine may cause a false-positive **urine protein** reading when using *Multistix®*. The sulfosalicylic acid reagent is recommended for determining urine protein when the patient is concomitantly receiving ranitidine.

Doses -
Dogs:
 For esophagitis:
  a) 1 - 2 mg/kg PO *bid* (Watrous 1988)
 For chronic gastritis:
  a) 0.5 mg/kg PO *bid* (Hall and Twedt 1988)
 For ulcer disease:
  a) 2 mg/kg PO q8h (Papich 1989)
  b) 2 mg/kg PO, IV q8h (Matz 1995)
  c) 0.5 mg/kg PO, IV *bid* (Chiapella 1988)
 For gastrinoma:
  a) 2 - 4 mg/kg PO *bid* (Lothrop 1989)
  b) 0.5 mg/kg PO, IV or SQ *bid* (Kay, Kruth, and Twedt 1988)
 To treat hypergastrinemia secondary to chronic renal failure:
  a) 1 - 2 mg/kg PO *bid* (Morgan 1988)
 To treat hyperhistaminemia secondary to mast cell tumors:
  a) 2 mg/kg q12h (Fox 1995b)
Cats:
 For ulcer disease:
  a) 2.5 mg/kg IV q12h or 3.5 mg/kg PO q12h (Matz 1995), (Johnson 1996)
Horses:
  a) 0.5 mg/kg *bid* PO (Robinson 1987)
  b) Foals: 150 mg PO *bid* (Clark and Becht 1987)
  c) 1 mg/kg q8h IV (Duran 1992)

Monitoring Parameters -
 1) Clinical efficacy (dependent on reason for use); monitored by decrease in symptomatology, endoscopic examination, blood in feces, etc.

Client Information - To maximize the benefit of this medication, it must be administered as prescribed by the veterinarian; symptoms may reoccur if dosages are missed.

Dosage Forms/Preparations/FDA Approval Status/Withholding Times -
Veterinary-Approved Products: None
Human-Approved Products:

Ranitidine HCl Tablets 75 mg, 150 mg, 300 mg (as base); *Zantac®* (Glaxo Wellcome); (Rx); Zantac 75® (Glaxo Wellcome) (OTC)

Rantidine HCl Effervescent Tablets & Granules: 150 mg; *Zantac EFFERdose®* (Glaxo Wellcome) (Rx)

Rantidine Capsules: 150 mg, 300 mg; *Zantac GELdose®* (Glaxo Wellcome) (Rx)

Ranitidine HCl Oral Syrup 15 mg/ml in UD 10 ml and 480 ml; *Zantac®* (Glaxo Wellcome); (Rx); Rantidine HCl (UDL) (Rx)

Ranitidine HCl Injection: 0.5 mg/ml, 25 mg/ml in 100 ml single dose containers and 2, 10, & 40 ml vials and 2 ml syringes; *Zantac®* (Glaxo Wellcome) (Rx)

Ranitidine HCl 0.5 mg/ml (preservative free in 100ml single dose containers & 25 mg/ml (as HCl) in 2 ml, 10 ml, & 40 ml vials; *Zantac®* (Glaxo); (Rx)

Rifampin

Chemistry - A semi-synthetic zwitterion derivative of rifamycin B, rifampin occurs as a red-brown, crystalline powder with a pK_a of 7.9. It is very slightly soluble in water and slightly soluble in alcohol.

Storage/Stability/Compatibility - Rifampin capsules should be stored in tight, light-resistant containers, preferably at room temperature (15-30°C).

Pharmacology - Rifampin may act as either a bactericidal or bacteriostatic antimicrobial dependent upon the susceptibility of the organism and the concentration of the drug. Rifampin acts by inhibiting DNA-dependent RNA polymerase in susceptible organisms, thereby suppressing the initiation of chain formation for RNA synthesis. It does not inhibit the mammalian enzyme.

Rifampin is active against a variety of mycobacterium species and *Staphylococcus aureus*, *Neisseria*, *Haemophilus*, and *Rhodococcus equi (C. equi)*. At very high levels, rifampin also has activity against poxviruses, adenoviruses, and *Chlamydia trachomatis*. Rifampin also has anti-fungal activity when combined with other antifungal agents.

Uses/Indications - At the present time, the principle use of rifampin in veterinary medicine is in the treatment of *Rhodococcus equi* (*Corynebacterium equi*) infections (usually with erythromycin estolate) in young horses.

In small animals, the drug is sometimes used in combination with other antifungal agents (amphotericin B and 5-FC) in the treatment of histoplasmosis or aspergillosis with CNS involvement.

Pharmacokinetics - After oral administration, rifampin is relatively well absorbed from the GI tract. Oral bioavailability is reportedly about 40-70% in horses and 37% in adult sheep. If food is given concurrently, peak plasma levels may be delayed and slightly reduced.

Rifampin is very lipophilic and penetrates most body tissues (including bone and prostate), cells and fluids (including CSF) well. It also penetrates abscesses and caseous material. Rifampin is 70-90% bound to serum proteins and is distributed into milk and crosses the placenta. Mean volume of distribution is approximately 0.9 L/kg in horses, and 1.3 L/kg in sheep.

Rifampin is metabolized in the liver to a deacetylated form which also has antibacterial activity. Both this metabolite and unchanged drug are excreted primarily in the bile, but up to 30% may be excreted in the urine. The parent drug is substantially reabsorbed in the gut, but the metabolite is not. Reported elimination half-lives for various species are: 6-8 hours (horses), 8 hours (dogs), 3-5 hours (sheep). Because rifampin can induce hepatic microsomal enzymes, elimination rates may increase with time.

Contraindications/Precautions/Reproductive Safety - Rifampin is contraindicated in patients hypersensitive to it or other rifamycins. It should be used with caution in patients with preexisting hepatic dysfunction.

Rodents given high doses of rifampin 150 - 250 mg/kg/day resulted in some congenital malformations in offspring, but the drug has been used in pregnant women with no reported increases in teratogenicity.

Adverse Effects/Warnings - Rifampin can cause red-orange colored urine, tears, sweat and saliva. There are no harmful consequences from this effect. In some species (*e.g.*, humans), rashes, GI distress, and increases in liver enzymes may occur, particularly with long-term use.

Adverse effects in horses are apparently rare when rifampin is given orally. Although not commercially available, intravenous rifampin has caused CNS depression, sweating, hemolysis and anorexia in horses.

Overdosage/Acute Toxicity - Symptoms associated with overdosage of oral rifampin generally are extensions of the adverse effects outlined above (GI, orange-red coloring of fluids, and skin), but massive overdoses may cause hepatotoxicity. Should a massive oral overdosage occur, the gut should be emptied following standard protocols. Liver enzymes should be monitored and supportive treatment initiated if necessary.

Drug Interactions - Because rifampin has been documented to induce hepatic microsomal enzymes, drugs that are metabolized by these enzymes may have their elimination half-lives shortened and serum levels decreased Drugs that may be affected by this process include **propranolol, quinidine, dapsone, chloramphenicol, corticosteroids, oral anticoagulants** (*e.g., warfarin*), **benzodiazepines** (*e.g., diazepam*), and **barbiturates** (*e.g., phenobarbital*).

Rifampin may cause decreased serum concentrations of **ketoconazole** if administered concurrently.

Drug/Laboratory Interactions - Microbiologic methods of assaying **serum folate** and **vitamin B$_{12}$** are interfered with by rifampin.

Rifampin can cause false-positive **BSP** (bromosulfophthalein, sulfobromophthalein) test results, by inhibiting the hepatic uptake of the drug.

Doses -
  Dogs:
    For CNS fungal infections (aspergillosis/histoplasmosis):
      a) Rifampin 10 - 20 mg/kg PO *tid* with amphotericin B and flucytocine. (Schunk 1988)

For actinomycosis:
    a) 10 - 20 mg/kg PO q12h PO (Hardie 1984)

Cats:
For CNS fungal infections (aspergillosis/histoplasmosis):
    a) Rifampin 10 - 20 mg/kg PO *tid* with amphotericin B and flucytocine. (Schunk 1988)

Horses:
For treatment of *C. equi* infections in foals:
    a) Rifampin 5 mg/kg PO *tid* with erythromycin estolate or ethylsuccinate 25 mg/kg PO *tid*. May cause urine to become red. Use a continuous course of rifampin as intermittent use may be associated with allergic reactions. Treat until chest radiographs and plasma fibrinogen levels return to normal. (Hillidge and Zertuche 1987)

For susceptible infections in foals:
    a) 5 mg/kg PO q12h (dose extrapolated from adult horses). Used in combination with erythromycin for *C. equi* infections (see above), but could be used with other agents (*e.g.,* penicillins) to treat other gram positive infections. Should be used with other antimicrobial agents to minimize the potential for bacterial resistance development. (Caprile and Short 1987)

Monitoring Parameters -
  1) Clinical efficacy
    a) For monitoring *C. equi* infections in foals and response to rifampin/erythromycin: Chest radiographs and plasma fibrinogen levels have been suggested as prognostic indicators when done after 1 week of therapy. (Hillidge and Zertuche 1987)
  2) Adverse effects; may consider liver function monitoring with long-term therapy

Client Information - Rifampin may cause urine and other secretions (tears, saliva, etc.) to turn red-orange in color. This is not abnormal.

Dosage Forms/Preparations/FDA Approval Status/Withholding Times -
Veterinary-Approved Products: None

Human-Approved Products:
Rifampin Capsules 150 mg, 300 mg; *Rifadin*® (Hoechst Marion Roussel); *Rimactane*® (Ciba); (Rx)

Rifampin Powder for Injection: 600 mg; *Rifadin*® (Hoechst Marion Roussel) (Rx)

SALINE/HYPEROSMOTIC LAXATIVES
MAGNESIUM SALTS
SODIUM PHOSPHATE SALTS
PEG 3350 PRODUCTS

Chemistry - Magnesium cation containing solutions of magnesium citrate, magnesium hydroxide, or magnesium sulfate act as saline laxatives. Magnesium citrate solutions contain 4.71 mEq of magnesium per 5 ml. Magnesium hydroxide contains 34.3 mEq of magnesium per gram and milk of magnesia contains 13.66 mEq per 5 ml. One gram of magnesium sulfate (epsom salt) contains approximately 8.1 mEq of magnesium.

Solutions containing phosphate anions also act as saline laxatives. These solutions generally contain monobasic and/or dibasic sodium phosphate.

Polyethylene glycol 3350 is a non-absorbable compound that acts as an osmotic agent.

Storage/Stability/Compatibility - Magnesium citrate solutions should be stored at 2-30°C. Store Milk of Magnesia at temperatures less than 35°C, but do not freeze. PEG 3350 reconstituted (from powder by the pharmacy, client, clinic, etc.) solutions should be kept refrigerated and used within 24 hours.

Pharmacology - Although unproven, it is commonly believed that the hyperosmotic effect of the poorly absorbed magnesium cation or phosphate anion causes water retention, stimulates stretch receptors and enhances peristalsis in the small intestine and colon. Recent data, however, suggests that magnesium ions may directly decrease transit times and increase cholecystokinin release.

Polyethylene glycol 3350 is a non-absorbable compound that acts as an osmotic agent. By adding sodium sulfate as the primary sodium source, sodium absorption is minimized. Other electrolytes (bicarbonate, potassium and chloride) are also added so that no net change occurs with either absorption or secretion of electrolytes or water in the gut.

Uses/Indications - The saline laxatives are used for their cathartic action to relieve constipation. They are also used to reduce intestinal transit time thereby reducing the absorption of orally ingested toxicants. Polyethylene glycol 3350 balanced electrolyte solutions are used to evacuate the colon prior to intestinal examination or surgery.

Pharmacokinetics - While it is unknown how much sodium or phosphate is absorbed after administration of sodium phosphate solutions, it is estimated that up to 20% of the phosphate dose can be absorbed. When magnesium salts are administered, up to 30% of the magnesium dose of magnesium can be absorbed.

Generally, the onset of action of saline cathartics (characterized by a loose, watery stool) occurs in 3-12 hours after dosing in monogastric animals and within 18 hours in ruminants.

Contraindications/Precautions - Saline cathartics are contraindicated for long-term or chronic use. Sodium containing laxatives are contraindicated in patients with congestive heart failure or congenital megacolon. PEG 3350 solutions are contraindicated in patients with GI obstruction, gastric retention, bowel perforation, toxic colitis or megacolon. Saline cathartics should be used with extreme caution in patients with renal insufficiency, pre-existing water-balance or electrolyte abnormalities, or cardiac disease.

Adverse Effects/Warnings - Except for possible cramping and nausea, adverse effects in otherwise healthy patients generally occur only with the saline cathartics with chronic use or overdoses. Hypermagnesemia manifested by muscle weakness, ECG changes and CNS effects can occur. Hyperphosphatemia with resultant hypocalcemia can occur with chronic overuse or overdoses of phosphate containing products. Hypernatremia can also occur when administering sodium phosphate solutions.

Cats may be particularly sensitive to the electrolyte imbalance effects of sodium phosphate enema solutions and these products are not recommended for use in this species until more data are available.

Overdosage - Symptoms of overdosage of magnesium or phosphate containing laxatives are described above. Treatment should consist of monitoring and correcting any fluid imbalances that occur with parenteral fluids.

If hypermagnesemia occurs, furosemide may be used to enhance the renal excretion of the excess magnesium. Calcium has been suggested to help antagonize the CNS effects of magnesium. Hyperphosphatemia may cause hypocalcemia and parenteral calcium therapy may be necessary.

Drug Interactions - All orally administered saline laxatives may alter the rate and extent of absorption of other drugs by decreasing intestinal transit times. The extent of these effects have not been well characterized for individual drugs, however.

Magnesium laxatives should not be administered with **tetracycline** products

Doses -
Dogs:
    Magnesium hydroxide (Milk of Magnesia) as a cathartic:
        a)   5 - 10 ml (Davis 1985a)
        b)   1 - 20 ml PO (Rossoff 1974)

    Sodium sulfate:
        a)   1 gram/kg PO (Grauer and Hjelle 1988b)
        b)   5 - 25 grams PO (Davis 1985a)

    Magnesium sulfate:
        a)   5 - 25 grams PO (Davis 1985a)
        b)   2 - 60 grams PO (Rossoff 1974)

    Polyethylene Glycol-Electrolyte Solution:
        a)   22 - 33 mls/kg PO by stomach tube before lower GI exam (Plumb 1988)

Cats:
    Magnesium hydroxide (Milk of Magnesia) as a cathartic:
        a)   2 - 6 ml (Davis 1985a)
        b)   1 - 5 ml PO (Rossoff 1974)

    Sodium sulfate:
        a)   2 - 5 grams PO (Davis 1985a)

    Magnesium sulfate:
        a)   2 - 5 grams PO (Davis 1985a), (Rossoff 1974)

Cattle:
    Magnesium sulfate (as a cathartic):
        a)   0.5 - 1 kg/500 kg orally (Whitlock 1986b)
        b)   1 - 2 gm/kg PO (Howard 1986)

    Magnesium oxide:
        a)   0.5 - 1 kg/500 kg orally (Whitlock 1986b)

    Sodium Sulfate:
        a)   1 - 3 gm/kg PO (Howard 1986)

Horses:
Magnesium sulfate (epsom salt):
a) 0.2 gm/kg diluted in 4 L of warm water administered via nasogastric tube. Administer only to well hydrated animals (ideally in conjunction with IV fluid therapy). Do not treat longer than 3 days or there is an increased risk of enteritis or magnesium toxicity occurring. (Clark and Becht 1987)
b) To reduce absorption of toxicants and GI transit time: 500 gm (as a 20% solution) PO. If mineral oil has been used initially, give saline cathartic 30-45 minutes after mineral oil. (Oehme 1987)

Swine:
Magnesium sulfate (as a cathartic):
a) 1 - 2 gm/kg PO (Howard 1986)

Birds:
Magnesium sulfate:
a) To act as a cathartic and reduce lead absorption: 0.5 -1.0 gm/kg PO as a 5% solution in drinking water (McDonald 1986)

Monitoring Parameters -
1) Fluid and electrolyte status in susceptible patients or if using high doses or chronically.
2) Clinical efficacy

Client Information - Do not give dosages greater than, or for periods of time longer than recommended by veterinarian. Contact veterinarian if patient begins vomiting.

Dosage Forms/Preparations/FDA Approval Status/Withholding Times - Saline cathartic products have apparently not been formally approved for use in domestic animals. They are available without prescription (OTC). PEG 3350 products are available only by prescription and are approved for use in humans.
Veterinary-Approved Products: None located
Human-Approved Products:
Saline Laxatives (not an inclusive list):
Magnesium Citrate (Citrate of Magnesia): powder and oral solution

Magnesium Hydroxide: powder, suspension (Milk of Magnesia)

Magnesium Sulfate (Epsom Salt): crystals, powder

Sodium Phosphate, Dibasic or Monobasic: powder

Sodium Phosphate, Dibasic 900 mg/5ml with Sodium Phosphate, Monobasic 2.4 gm/5ml oral solution
Fleet® Phospho®-Soda (Fleet)

Sodium Phosphate, Dibasic 60 mg/ml with Sodium Phosphate, Monobasic 160 mg/ml rectal solution
Fleet® Enema (Fleet), *Fleet® Pediatric Enema* (Fleet)

Hyperosmotic Laxatives (not an inclusive list):
Polyethylene Glycol-Electrolyte Solution
OCL® Solution (Abbott) per 100 ml: 146 mg Sodium Chloride, 168 mg Sodium Bicarbonate, 1.29 grams Sodium Sulfate Decahydrate, 75 mg potassium chloride, 6 grams PEG-3350 and 30 ml Polysorbate-80

CoLyte® (R&C) Packets to make 2 liters of solution: 2.92 gm Sodium Chloride, 3.36 gm Sodium Bicarbonate, 11.36 gm Sodium Sulfate, 1.49 gm potassium chloride, 120 gm PEG-3350 (Also available in 1 gallon and 6 liter sizes)

GoLYTELY® (Braintree Labs) contains per 4800 ml container: 5.86 gm Sodium Chloride, 6.74 gm Sodium Bicarbonate, 22.74 gm Sodium Sulfate, 2.97 gm potassium chloride, 236 gm PEG-3350

SELEGILINE HCL
L-DEPRENYL

Chemistry - Selegiline HCl, also commonly called l-deprenyl, occurs as a white to off-white crystalline powder that is freely soluble in water. It has a pKa of 7.5.

Storage/Stability/Compatibility - Commercially available veterinary tablets should be stored at controlled room temperature 20-25°C (68-77°F). The commercially available human-labeled tablets and capsules are recommended to be stored from 15-30°C.

Pharmacology - Selegiline's mechanism of action for treatment of Cushing's disease (pituitary dependent hyperadrenocorticism—PDH) is complex; a somewhat simplified explanation follows: In the hypothalamus, corticotropin-releasing hormone (CRH) acts to stimulate the production of ACTH in the pituitary and dopamine acts to inhibit the release of ACTH. As dogs get older, there is a tendency for a decrease in dopamine production that can contribute to the development of PDH.

As dopamine is metabolized by monamine oxidase-B (MOA-B) and selegiline inhibits MAO-B, dopamine levels can be increased at receptor sites after selegiline administration. In theory, this allows the levels of dopamine and CRH to be in balance in the hypothalamus, thereby reducing the amount of ACTH produced and ultimately, cortisol.

Two of three metabolites of selegiline are amphetamine and methamphetamine which may contribute to both the efficacy and the adverse effects of the drug.

Uses/Indications - At the time of writing, selegiline is approved for use in dogs only for the treatment of Cushing's Disease, but in Canada it is also approved for the treatment of Canine Cognitive Dysfunction (so-called "old dog dementia"). In humans, selegiline's primary indication is for the adjunctive treatment of Parkinson's disease.

Pharmacokinetics - There is only limited information on the pharmacokinetics of selegiline in dogs. A study done in 4 dogs showed that selegiline was absorbed rapidly and had an absolute bioavailability of about 10%. The volume of distribution of the central compartment was measured at approximately 7 l/kg. Terminal half life was about one hour.

In humans, selegiline pharmacokinetics have been demonstrated to have wide interpatient variability. The drug has a high first pass effect where extensive metabolism to L-desmethylselegiline, methylamphetamine and L-amphetamine occur. Each of these metabolites is active. While L-desmethylselegiline does inhibit MAO-B, the others do not, but are CNS stimulants. The drug is excreted in the urine, primarily as conjugated and unconjugated metabolites.

Contraindications/Precautions/Reproductive Safety - Selegiline is contraindicated in patients known to be hypersensitive to it. In human patients, it is contraindicated in patients receiving meperidine and possibly with other opioids as well.

The manufacturer cautions to perform appropriate diagnostic tests to confirm the diagnosis before starting therapy and not to attempt to treat hyperadrenocorticism not of pituitary origin.

Safety of selegiline in pregnant, breeding or lactating animals has not been established. Rat studies have not demonstrated overt teratogenicity.

Adverse Effects/Warnings - Adverse reports reported thus far in dogs include, vomiting and diarrhea; CNS effects manifested by restlessness, repetitive movements, or lethargy; salivation and anorexia. Diminished hearing/deafness, pruritus, licking, shivers/trembles/shakes have also been reported. Note that clinical experience with this drug is limited and the adverse effect profile may change. The manufacturer advises to observe animals carefully for atypical responses.

Adverse effects that have been reported in human patients, include nausea (10%), hallucinations, confusion, depression, loss of balance, insomnia and hypersexuality. These effects are noted because of their "subjective" nature and they could help explain untoward behavioral changes in canine patients should they also occur in that species.

Because selegiline could potentially be abused by humans, veterinarians should be alert for drug "shoppers".

Overdosage - Oral LD$_{50}$ in laboratory animals was approximately 200-445 mg/kg. In limited data, dogs receiving 3X dosages showed signs of decreased weight, salivation, decreased pupillary response, panting, stereotypic behaviors and decreased skin elasticity (dehydration). Overdoses, if severe, should be treated with appropriate gut emptying and supportive treatments.

Drug Interactions - In humans, severe agitation, hallucinations and death have occurred in some patients receiving **meperidine** and an MAO inhibitor. Until the data can be clarified, it is recommended not use selegiline and meperidine together. A separation of two weeks has been recommended. Other opioids (e.g., morphine) should be safer, but use with extreme caution, if at all.

Potentially, the so-called serotonin syndrome could occur if selegiline is used concurrently with selective serotonin reuptake inhibitors (**SSRI's**) such as **fluoxetine** (Prozac®). Concurrent use with these antidepressants or other **tricyclic/tetracyclic antidepressants** (e.g., **amitriptyline**) are not advised at this time and a 2 week separation between these compounds and selegiline is also recommended.

The manufacturer recommends not using selegiline concurrently with **amitraz** (**Mitaban**®) or **ephedrine.**

Doses -
  Dogs:
      For Cushing's Disease:
        a) 1 mg/kg PO in the AM (with food prn); Reevaluate clinically over next 2 mos.; if no improvement, may increase to 2 mg/kg once daily; if no improvement or signs in-

crease, reevaluate diagnosis or consider alternate treatment (Package Insert; *Anipryl®;—*Pfizer)

For Canine Cognitive Dysfunction:
    a) 0.5 mg/kg PO in the AM (with food prn); Reevaluate clinically over next 2 mos.; if no improvement, may increase to 1 mg/kg once daily (Canadian product label directions)

Monitoring Parameters - Clinical efficacy and adverse effects. No correlation between low dose dexamethasone suppression test results and clinical efficacy of the drug. The manufacturer recommends physical exam and history as the primary methods to measure response to therapy.

Client Information - Keep this and all medications out of reach of children. Have clients monitor closely for adverse effects. Clients should be advised on the importance of complying with the dosing recommendations so as to adequately evaluate therapeutic response to the drug.

Dosage Forms/Preparations/FDA Approval Status -
Veterinary-Approved Products:
Selegiline HCl Oral Tablets 2 mg, 5 mg, 10 mg, 15 mg, 30 mg in blister-packs of 30 tablets; *Anipryl®* (Pfizer); (Rx). Approved for use in dogs.

Human-Approved Products:
Selegiline HCl Oral Tablets and Capsules 5 mg; *Eldepryl®*; Capsules (Somerset); *Atapryl®*; Tablets(Athena); Generic Tablets; (Rx)

SODIUM BICARBONATE

Chemistry - An alkalinizing agent, sodium bicarbonate occurs as a white, crystalline powder having a slightly saline or alkaline taste. It is soluble in water and insoluble in alcohol. One gram of sodium bicarbonate contains about 12 mEq each of sodium and bicarbonate; 84 mg of sodium bicarbonate contains 1 mEq each of sodium and bicarbonate. A 1.5% solution of sodium bicarbonate is approximately isotonic. An 8.4% solution of sodium bicarbonate can be made isotonic by diluting each ml with 4.6 ml of sterile water for injection.

Sodium bicarbonate may also be known as: Baking Soda, Sodium Hydrogen Carbonate, Sodium Acid Carbonate, or by its chemical abbreviation, $NaHCO_3$.

Storage/Stability/Compatibility - Sodium bicarbonate tablets should be stored in tight containers, preferably at room temperature (15-30°C). Sodium bicarbonate injection should be stored at temperatures less than 40°C and preferably at room temperature; avoid freezing.

Sodium bicarbonate powder is stable in dry air, but will slowly decompose upon exposure to moist air.

Sodium bicarbonate is reportedly **compatible** with the following intravenous solutions and drugs: Dextrose in water, dextrose/saline combinations, dextrose-Ringer's combinations, sodium chloride injections, amikacin sulfate, aminophylline, amobarbital sodium, amphotericin B, atropine sulfate, bretylium tosylate, carbenicillin disodium, cefoxitin sodium, cephalothin sodium, cephapirin sodium, chloramphenicol sodium succinate, chlorothiazide sodium, cimetidine HCl, clindamycin phosphate, ergonavine maleate, erythromycin gluceptate/lactobionate, Innovar®, heparin sodium, hyaluronidase, hydrocortisone sodium succinate, kanamycin sulfate, lidocaine HCl, metaraminol bitartrate, methotrexate sodium, methyldopate HCl, nafcillin sodium, netilmicin sulfate, oxacillin sodium, oxytocin, phenobarbital sodium, phenylephrine HCl, phenytoin sodium, phytonadione, potassium chloride, prochlorperazine edisylate, and sodium iodide.

Sodium bicarbonate **compatibility information conflicts** or is dependent on diluent or concentration factors with the following drugs or solutions: lactated Ringer's injection, Ringer's injection, sodium lactate 1/6 M, ampicillin sodium, calcium chloride/gluconate, methicillin sodium, penicillin G potassium, pentobarbital sodium, promazine HCl, thiopental sodium, vancomycin HCl, verapamil HCl, and vitamin B-complex w/C. Compatibility is dependent upon factors such as pH, concentration, temperature and diluents used. It is suggested to consult specialized references for more specific information (*e.g., Handbook on Injectable Drugs* by Trissel; see bibliography).

Sodium bicarbonate is reportedly **incompatible** with the following solutions or drugs: alcohol 5%/dextrose 5%, D5 lactated Ringer's, amrinone lactate, ascorbic acid injection, carmustine, cisplatin, codeine phosphate, corticotropin, dobutamine HCl, epinephrine HCl, glycopyrrolate, hydromorphone HCl, imipenem-cilastatin, regular insulin, isoproterenol HCl, labetolol HCl, levorphanol bitartrate, magnesium sulfate, meperidine HCl, methadone HCl, metoclopramide HCl, norepinephrine bitartrate, oxytetracycline HCl, pentazocine lactate, procaine HCl, secobarbital sodium, streptomycin sulfate, succinylcholine chloride, tetracycline HCl,

Pharmacology - Bicarbonate ion is the conjugate base component of bicarbonate:carbonic acid buffer, the principal extracellular buffer in the body.

Uses/Indications - Sodium bicarbonate is indicated to treat metabolic acidosis and to alkalinize the urine. It is also used as adjunctive therapy in treating hypercalcemic or hyperkalemia crises.

Contraindications/Precautions/Reproductive Safety - Parenterally administered sodium bicarbonate is considered generally contraindicated in patients with metabolic or respiratory alkalosis, excessive chloride loss secondary to vomiting or GI suction, at risk for development of diuretic-induced hypochloremic alkolosis, or with hypocalcemia where alkalosis may induce tetany.

Use with extreme caution and give very slowly in patients with hypocalcemia. Because of the potential sodium load, use with caution in patients with CHF, nephrotic syndrome, hypertension, oliguria, or volume overload.

Reproductive safety studies have not been performed. Assess risk versus benefit before using.

Adverse Effects/Warnings - Sodium bicarbonate therapy (particularly high-dose parenteral use) can lead to metabolic alkalosis, hypokalemia, hypocalcemia, "overshoot" alkalosis, hypernatremia, volume overload, congestive heart failure, shifts in the oxygen dissociation curve causing decreased tissue oxygenation, and paradoxical CNS acidosis leading to respiratory arrest.

When sodium bicarbonate is used during cardiopulmonary resuscitation, hypercapnia may result if the patient is not well ventilated; patients may be predisposed to ventricular fibrillation.

Oral & parenteral bicarbonate (especially at higher doses) may contribute significant amounts of sodium and result in hypernatremia and volume overload; use with caution in patients with CHF, or acute renal failure.

Overdosage/Acute Toxicity - Sodium bicarbonate can cause severe alkalosis, with irritability or tetany if overdosed or given too rapidly. Dosages should be thoroughly checked and frequent monitoring of electrolyte and acid/base status performed.

Treatment may consist of simply discontinuing bicarbonate if alkalosis is mild, or by using a rebreathing mask. Severe alkalosis may require intravenous calcium therapy. Sodium chloride or potassium chloride may be necessary if hypokalemia is present.

Drug Interactions - Because oral sodium bicarbonate can either increase or reduce the rate and/or extent of absorption of many orally administered drugs, it is recommended to avoid giving other drugs within 1-2 hours of sodium bicarbonate. Oral sodium bicarbonate may increase the amount of **naproxen** absorbed. Oral sodium bicarbonate may reduce the amount and/or extent absorbed of the following drugs: anticholinergic agents, **Histamine2 blocking agents** (*e.g.,* **cimetidine, ranitidine**), **iron products, ketoconazole**, and **tetracyclines**. Sodium bicarbonate may reduce the efficacy of **sucralfate** if administered concurrently.

When urine is alkalinized by sodium bicarbonate, excretion of certain drugs (*e.g.,* **quinidine, amphetamines, ephedrine**) is decreased, and excretion of weakly acidic drugs (*e.g.,* **salicylates**) is increased.

The solubility of **ciprofloxacin & enrofloxacin** is decreased in an alkaline environment. Patients with alkaline urine should be monitored for signs of crystalluria.

Concurrent use of sodium bicarbonate in patients receiving potassium-wasting diuretics (*e.g.,* **thiazides, furosemide**) may cause hypochloremic alkalosis.

Patients receiving high dosages of sodium bicarbonate and **ACTH** or **glucocorticoids** may develop hypernatremia.

Doses -
Dogs, Cats:
    For severe metabolic acidosis:
      a) Main therapeutic goal should be to eliminate the underlying cause of acidosis. If causes are not readily reversible, if arterial pH is <7.2 (7.1 if diabetic ketoacidosis), and ventilatory procedures have not reduced acidemia, bicarbonate therapy should be considered. mEq of bicarbonate required = 0.5 x body weight in kgs. x (desired total CO_2 mEq/L - measured total CO_2 mEq/L). Give 1/2 of the calculated dose slowly over 3-4 hours IV. Recheck blood gases and assess the clinical status of the patient. Avoid over-alkalinization. (Schaer 1986)

    For adjunctive therapy of diabetic ketoacidosis:
      a) If plasma bicarbonate is ≤11 mEq/L give bicarbonate therapy. Dose (in mEq) = body weight in kgs. x 0.4 x (12 - patient's bicarbonate) x 0.5. Give above dose over 6 hours in IV fluids and then recheck plasma bicarbonate or total venous CO2. If still ≤11 mEq/L, recalculate dose and repeat therapy. (Nelson and Feldman 1988)

    For metabolic acidosis in acutely critical situations (cardiac arrest):
      a) 1 mEq/kg IV initially, followed by 0.5 mEq/kg at 10-15 minute intervals during CPR. (Moses 1988)
      b) Give none during the first 5-10 minutes of arrest, then 0.5 mEq/kg every 5 minutes of cardiac arrest thereafter. (Haskins 1989)

For adjunctive treatment of hypercalcemic crisis:

a) mEq of bicarbonate required = 0.3 x body weight in kgs. x (desired plasma bicarbonate mEq/L - measured plasma bicarbonate mEq/L); or 1.0 mEq/kg IV every 10-15 minutes; maximum total dose: 4 mEq/L. (Kruger, Osborne, and Polzin 1986)

For adjunctive therapy for hyperkalemic crises:

a) If serum bicarbonate or total CO_2 is unavailable: 2 - 3 mEq/kg IV over 30 minutes if patient has decreased tissue perfusion or renal failure and does not have diabetic ketoacidosis. Must be used judiciously. (Willard 1986)

Metabolic acidosis secondary to renal failure:

a) Dogs: Initial dose: 8-12 **mg**/kg PO q8h; adjust dosage to attain blood total CO_2 concentrations to 18-24 mEq/L for renal failure. Although, inferior to monitoring total CO_2, urine pH may be used as a guideline for adjusting dosage. Urine pH should be between 6.5 and 7.0. (Polzin and Osborne 1985)

b) Initial dose: 8-12 mg/kg q8h; adjust dosage to attain blood total CO_2 concentrations to 18-24 mEq/L. (Allen 1989)

To alkalinize the urine:

a) Dosage must be individualized to the patient. Initially give 10 - 90 grains (650 mg - 5.85 grams) PO per day, depending on the size of the patient and the pretreatment urine pH value. Goal of therapy is to maintain a urine pH of about 7; avoid pH > than 7.5. (Osborne et al. 1989)

b) For adjunctive therapy in dissolution and/or prevention of urate urolithiasis in dogs: 0.5 - 1 gram (1/8 - 1/4 tsp) per 5 kg of body weight *tid* PO. Goal of therapy is to attain a urine pH of from 7 - 7.5. (Senior 1989)

Horses:

For metabolic acidosis:

a) Associated with colic; if pH is <7.3 and base deficit is >10 mEq/L estimate bicarbonate requirement using the formula: bicarbonate deficit (HCO^{-3} mEq) = base deficit (mEq/L) x 0.4 x body weight (kg). May administer as a 5% sodium bicarbonate solution. Each L of solution contains 600 mEq of bicarbonate (hypertonic) and should not be administered any faster than 1 - 2 L/hr. Because acidotic horses with colic tend also to be dehydrated, may be preferable to give as isotonic sodium bicarbonate (150 mEq/L). (Stover 1987)

Ruminants:

For acidosis:

a) 2 - 5 mEq/kg IV for a 4-8 hour period. (Howard 1986)

b) For severely dehydrated (10-16 % dehydrated) acidotic calves (usually comatose): Use isotonic sodium bicarbonate (156 mEq/L). Most calves require about 2 liters of this solution given over 1-2 hours, then change to isotonic saline and sodium bicarbonate or a balanced electrolyte solution. Isotonic sodium bicarbonate may be made by dissolving 13 grams of sodium bicarbonate in 1 L of sterile water. Isotonic saline and sodium bicarbonate may be made by mixing 1 L of isotonic saline with 1 L of isotonic sodium bicarbonate. (Radostits 1986)

Birds:

For metabolic acidosis:

a) 1 mEq/kg initially IV (then SQ) for 15-30 minutes to a maximum of 4 mEq/kg. (Clubb 1986)

Monitoring Parameters -

1) Acid/base status
2) Serum electrolytes
3) Urine pH (if being used to alkalinize urine)

Dosage Forms/Preparations/FDA Approval Status/Withholding Times -

Veterinary-Approved Products:

Sodium bicarbonate 5% (0.6 mEq/ml) in 500 ml vials (297.5 mEq/500 ml)

Sodium bicarbonate 8.4% (1 mEq/ml) in 50 ml (50 mEq/vial), 100 ml (100 mEq/vial) and 500 ml (500 mEq/vial) vials

Available generically labeled; (Rx). Approval status unknown.

Human-Approved Products:

Injectable Products:

Sodium bicarbonate 4% (0.48 mEq/ml) in 5 & 10 ml vials

Sodium bicarbonate 4.2% (0.5 mEq/ml) in 5 & 10 ml syringes

Sodium bicarbonate 5% (0.6 mEq/ml) in 500 ml vials (297.5 mEq/500 ml)

Sodium bicarbonate 7.5% (0.9 mEq/ml) in 50 ml amps, syringes and vials (44.6 mEq/50 ml)

Sodium bicarbonate 8.4% (1 mEq/ml) in 10 ml syringes (10 mEq) & 50 ml vials (50 mEq/vial)

Available generically labeled; (Rx).

Oral Products:

Oral Tablets 325 mg (5 grain), 650 mg (10 grain)

May be labeled generically or as Soda Mint; (OTC)

Sodium Bromide - see Bromide Salts

Sodium Chloride Injections - see the Intravenous Fluids section in the appendix

Sodium Citrate - see Citrate Salts

Sodium Hyaluronate - see Hyaluronate Sodium

SODIUM IODIDE

Chemistry - Sodium iodide occurs as colorless, odorless crystals or white crystalline powder. It will develop a brown tint upon degradation. Approximately 1 gram is soluble in 0.6 ml of water and 2 ml of alcohol.

Storage/Stability/Compatibility - Commercially available veterinary injectable products should generally be stored at room temperature (15- 30° C). Sodium iodide injection is reportedly incompatible with vitamins B & C injection.

Pharmacology - While the exact mode of action for its efficacy in treating actinobacillosis is unknown, iodides probably have some effect on the granulomatous inflammatory process. Iodides have little, if any *in vitro* antibiotic activity.

Uses/Indications - The primary use for sodium iodide is in the treatment of actinobacillosis and actinomycosis in cattle. It has been used as an expectorant with little success in a variety of species and occasionally as a supplement for iodine deficiency disorders. In horses, oral sodium iodide has been the classical treatment for sporotrichosis.

Pharmacokinetics - Little published information appears to be available. Therapeutic efficacy of intravenous sodium iodide for actinobacillosis is rapid, with beneficial effects usually seen within 48 hours of therapy.

Contraindications/Precautions/Reproductive Safety - Sodium iodide injection labels state that it should not be given to lactating animals or to animals with hyperthyroidism. Do not inject intramuscularly (IM).

Iodides should be given slowly intravenously and with caution to horses as severe generalized reactions have been reported.

Anecdotal reports that iodides can cause abortion in cattle persist and label information of some veterinary products state not to use in pregnant animals. Clearly, potential risks versus benefits of therapy must be weighed.

Adverse Effects/Warnings - In ruminants, the adverse effect profile is related to excessive iodine (see Overdosage below). Young animals may be more susceptible to iodism than adults. Foals have developed goiter when mares have been excessively supplemented.

Overdosage - Excessive iodine in animals can cause excessive tearing, nasal discharge, scaly haircoats/dandruff, hyperthermia, decreased milk production and weight gain, coughing, inappetence and diarrhea.

Drug Interactions - Iodides may enhance the efficacy of **thyroid medications** and may decrease the efficacy of **antithyroid** medications.

Doses -

Cattle, Sheep & Goats:

For treatment of actinobacillosis (woody tongue):

a) 70 mg/kg IV given as a 10% or 20% solution; repeat at least one more time at a 7-10 day interval. Refractory cases may require more frequent (2-3 day intervals) treatment. Severe, generalized, or refractory cases may require adjunctive tx with antibiotics (sulfas, aminoglycoside or tetracyclines). (Smith 1996a)

For treatment of actinomycosis (lumpy jaw):

a) 70 mg/kg IV given as a 10% or 20% solution at 7-10 day intervals or more frequently until signs of iodism occur (see Overdose above). Also requires adjunctive tx with antibiotics: isoniazid (10 mg/kg/day PO for one month), penicillin (10, 000 U/kg bid) and an aminoglycoside where treating a valuable animal or twice daily dosing for 7-14 days is possible. (Smith 1996b)

For treatment of actinobacillosis or actinomycosis in sheep:
a) 20 ml of a 10% solution subQ; repeated weekly for 4-5 weeks (Howard 1986)

Horses:
For treatment of sporotrichosis:
a) Sodium iodide 20 - 40 mg/kg orally daily for several weeks (Fadok 1992)

Monitoring Parameters/Client Information - Ruminants: 1) Clinical efficacy 2) Signs of iodism (excessive tearing, nasal discharge, scaly haircoats/dandruff, hyperthermia, decreased milk production and weight gain, coughing, inappetence, and diarrhea). Although formal withholding times were not located, there is concern about using this product in animals about to be slaughtered. In the interest of public health, author recommends not using within 30 days of slaughter.

Dosage Forms/Preparations/FDA Approval Status -
Veterinary-Approved Products:
Sodium Iodide Injection 20 g/100 ml (20%; 200 mg/ml) in 250 ml vials—available as multi- or single use vials; Generic; (Rx)

Human-Approved Products: NOTE: The following are listed for information purposes. The above monograph pertains to the veterinary injectable product only.
Sodium Iodide[123] Oral Capsules 3.7 mBq and 7.4 mBq (Note: Radioactive isotope used for thyroid diagnostic procedures) (Mallinckrodt); (Rx)
Sodium Iodide[131] Capsules and Oral solution (Note: Radioactive isotope used for treatment of hyperthyroidism and thyroid carcinoma; requires NRC approval for use); (Bracco, Mallinckrodt); (Rx)

Sodium Phosphate - see Phosphate, Sodium

SODIUM POLYSTYRENE SULFONATE

Chemistry - A sulfonated cation exchange resin, sodium polystyrene sulfonate (SPS) occurs as a golden brown, fine powder. It is odorless and tasteless. Each gram contains 4.1 mEq of sodium and has an *in vitro* exchange capacity of about 3.1 mEq of potassium (in actuality a maximum of 1 mEq is usually exchanged)..

Storage/Stability/Compatibility - Store products in well-closed containers at room temperature; do not heat. Suspensions should be freshly prepared and used within 24 hours.

Pharmacology - SPS is a resin that exchanges sodium for other cations. After being given orally, hydrogen ions will be exchanged for sodium (in an acidic environment). As the resin travels through the intestinal tract, the hydrogen ions will be exchanged with other more concentrated cations. Primary exchange with potassium occurs predominantly in the large intestine. When given as a retention enema, SPS generally exchanges sodium for potassium directly in the colorectum. While theoretically, up to 3.1 mEq of potassium could be exchanged per gram of SPS, it is unlikely that more than one mEq will be exchanged per gram of resin administered.

Uses/Indications - SPS is indicated as adjunctive treatment of hyperkalemia. The cause of the hyperkalemia should be elucidated and corrected if possible.

Pharmacokinetics - SPS is not absorbed from the GI tract. Its onset of action may be from hours to days, so severe hyperkalemia may require other treatments (*e.g.,* dialysis) in the interim.

Contraindications/Precautions/Reproductive Safety - Because large quantities of sodium may be released and absorbed, patients on severely restricted sodium diets (severe CHF, hypertension, oliguria) may benefit from alternative methods of treatment. Overdosage/overuse may lead to hypokalemia, hypocalcemia and hypomagnesemia.

While reproductive studies have apparently not been performed, it is unlikely the drug carries much teratogenic potential.

Adverse Effects/Warnings - Large doses may cause constipation (fecal impactions have been reported rarely), anorexia, vomiting or nausea. Dose related hypocalcemia, hypokalemia and sodium retention have also been noted. To hasten the drug's action and to prevent constipation, SPS is generally mixed with 70% sorbitol (3-4 ml per one gram of resin).

Overdosage/Acute Toxicity - Overdosage may cause the adverse effects noted above. Treat symptomatically.

Drug Interactions - SPS may bind with magnesium or calcium found in **laxatives** (milk of magnesia, magnesium sulfate, etc.) or **antacids** which can prevent bicarbonate ion neutralization and lead to metabolic alkalosis. Concurrent use is not recommended during SPS therapy.

Doses - To hasten the drug's action and to prevent constipation, SPS is generally mixed with 70% sorbitol (3-4 ml per one gram of resin); shake well before using.

Dogs:
    For hyperkalemia:
        a) 2 grams of resin/kg of body weight (each gram should be suspended in 3-4 ml of water; or use commercially prepared suspension products) divided into 3 daily doses. If given orally, give with a cathartic. Do not use a cathartic if using as a retention enema as it must be in the colon for at least 30 minutes. To prepare a retention enema from the powder: add 15 grams per 100 ml of a 1% methylcellulose solution or 10% dextrose. If hyperkalemia is severe: 3-4 times the normal amount of resin may be given. (Willard 1986)

Monitoring Parameters - 1) Serum electrolytes (sodium, potassium (at least once a day), calcium, magnesium; 2) acid/base status, ECG, if warranted

Dosage Forms/Preparations/FDA Approval Status/Withholding Times -
  Veterinary-Approved Products: None
  Human-Approved Products:
    Sodium Polystyrene Sulfonate Powder for Suspension (for rectal or oral use) in 1 lb. jars; *Kayexalate®* (Sanofi Winthrop), (Rx)

    Sodium Polystyrene Sulfonate Suspension: 15 g/60 ml (sodium 1.5 g, 65 mEq) in 120, 480 ml and UD 60 ml; 15 g/60 ml in 50, 120, 200, & 500 ml; *SPS®* (Carolina Medical Products Co); *Sodium Polystyrene Sulfonate* (Roxane) (Rx)

SODIUM SULFATE
GLAUBER'S SALT

Chemistry - Sodium sulfate (hexahydrate form) occurs as large, colorless, odorless, crystals or white crystalline powder. It will effloresce in dry air and partially dissolve in its own water of crystallization at about 33°C. 1 gram is soluble in about 2.5 ml of water.

Storage/Stability/Compatibility - Store in tight containers at temperatures not exceeding 30°C.

Pharmacology - When given orally, sodium sulfate acts as a saline cathartic (draws water into small intestine). Sodium sulfate is considered to be the most effective saline cathartic on a molar basis. Sulfates also react with a variety of cations to form non-absorbable compounds, which may explain its efficacy in reducing copper loads and to reduce gut calcium.

Uses/Indications - Sodium sulfate is used as a saline cathartic, primarily in food animals.

Pharmacokinetics - Sodium sulfate is not appreciably absorbed from the GI tract and thereby acts a saline cathartic. Sodium may be absorbed however, after exchanging with other cations.

Contraindications/Precautions - Saline cathartics should not be used in dehydrated animals. Because of the drug's high sodium content, it should be used with caution in patients with severe CHF or in patients otherwise susceptible to sodium retention.

Adverse Effects/Warnings - Diarrhea, cramping and flatulence may result. Electrolyte abnormalities may occur with chronic use.

Doses -
Cattle:
    As a cathartic:
        a) 500 - 750 g PO as a 6% solution via stomach tube (Davis 1993)

Sheep & Goats:
    As a cathartic: 60 g PO as a 6% solution via stomach tube (Davis 1993)

Swine:
    As a cathartic: 30 - 60 g PO as a 6% solution via stomach tube (Davis 1993)

Dosage Forms/Preparations/FDA Approval Status/Withholding Times -
  Veterinary-Approved Products: None
  Human-Approved Products: None
    Sodium sulfate (hexahydrate) is available from chemical supply houses.

SODIUM THIOSULFATE

Chemistry - Used systemically for cyanide or arsenic poisoning and topically as an antifungal, sodium thiosulfate occurs as large, colorless crystals or coarse, crystalline powder. It is very soluble in water, deliquescent in moist air and effloresces in dry air at temperatures >33°C.

Storage/Stability/Compatibility - Unless otherwise stated by the manufacturer, store at room temperature. Crystals should be stored in tight containers.

Pharmacology - By administering thiosulfate, an exogenous source of sulfur is available to the body, thereby allowing it hasten the detoxification of cyanide using the enzyme rhodanese. Rhodanese (thiosulfate cyanide sulfurtransferase) converts cyanide to the relatively nontoxic thiocyanate ion. Thiocyanate is then excreted in the urine.

Sodium thiosulfate's topical antifungal activity is probably due to its slow release of colloidal sulfur.

While sodium thiosulfate has been recommended for treating arsenic (and some other heavy metal) poisoning, it's proposed mechanism of action is not known. Presumably the sulfate moiety may react with and chelate the metal, allowing its removal.

Uses/Indications - Sodium thiosulfate (alone or in combination with sodium nitrite) is useful in the treatment of cyanide toxicity. It has been touted for use in treating arsenic or other heavy metal poisonings, but its efficacy is in question for these purposes. However, because sodium thiosulfate is relatively non-toxic and inexpensive, it may be tried to treat arsenic poisoning. When used in combination with sodium molybdate sodium thiosulfate may be useful for the treatment of copper poisoning.

Sodium thiosulfate may also be useful for the topical treatment for some fungal infections (Tinea). In humans, sodium thiosulfate has been used to reduce the nephrotoxicity of cisplatin therapy.

Pharmacokinetics - Sodium thiosulfate is relatively poorly absorbed from the GI tract. When substantial doses are given PO, it acts a saline cathartic. When administered intravenously, it is distributed in the extracellular fluid and then rapidly excreted via the urine.

Contraindications/Precautions/Reproductive Safety - There are no absolute contraindications to the use of the drug. Safe use during pregnancy has not been established; use when benefits outweigh the potential risks.

Adverse Effects/Warnings - The drug is relatively non-toxic. Large doses by mouth may cause profuse diarrhea. Injectable forms should be given slowly IV.

Doses -
Horses:

> For cyanide toxicity: First give sodium nitrite at a dose of 16 mg/kg IV followed with a 20% solution of sodium thiosulfate given at a dose of 30 - 40 mg/kg IV. If repeating treatment, use sodium thiosulfate only. (Bailey and Garland 1992a)

Ruminants:

> In combination with sodium molybdate for the treatment of copper poisoning: In conjunction with fluid replacement therapy, 500 mg sodium thiosulfate in combination with 200 mg ammonium or sodium molybdate PO daily for up to 3 weeks will help decrease total body burden of copper. (Thompson and Buck 1993b)

> For treatment of cyanide toxicity secondary to cyanogenic plants: 660 mg/kg IV sodium thiosulfate in a 30% solution given rapidly using a 12 or 14 gauge needle. (Nicholson 1993)

> For treatment of arsenic poisoning: 30 - 60 grams PO every 6 hours for 3-4 days and 30 - 60 grams as a 10-20% solution IV may be potentially useful in binding arsenic. Adjunctive fluid and electrolyte replacement is necessary. (Galey 1993)

Dosage Forms/Preparations/FDA Approval Status/Withholding Times -
Veterinary-Approved Products:

> Sodium Thiosulfate for Injection 500 mg multidose vials, 300 mg/mL.*Cya-dote Injection*® (Anthony) (Rx). Approved for use in animal not to be used for food or lactating dairy animals.

Human-Approved Products:

> Sodium Thiosulfate for Injection 25% (250 mg/ml) in 50 ml vials; Generic; (Rx)

SPECTINOMYCIN HCL

Chemistry - An aminocyclitol antibiotic obtained from *Streptomyces spectabilis*, spectinomycin is available as the dihydrochloride pentahydrate. It occurs as a white to pale buff, crystalline powder with pK_as of 7 and 8.7. It is freely soluble in water and practically insoluble in alcohol.

Storage/Stability/Compatibility - Unless otherwise instructed by the manufacturer, spectinomycin products should be stored at room temperature (15-30°C).

Pharmacology - Spectinomycin is primarily a bacteriostatic antibiotic that inhibits protein synthesis in susceptible bacteria by binding to the 30S ribosomal subunit.

Spectinomycin has activity against a wide variety of gram positive and gram negative bacteria, including *E. coli, Klebsiella, Proteus, Enterobacter, Salmonella, Streptococci, Staphylococcus* and *Mycoplasma*. It has minimal activity against anaerobes, most strains of *Pseudomonas, Chlamydia*, or *Treponema*.

In human medicine, spectinomycin is used principally for its activity against *Neissiera gonorrhoeae*.

Uses/Indications - Although occasionally used in dogs, cats, horses and cattle for susceptible infections, spectinomycin is only approved for use in chickens, turkeys and swine. Refer to the Dosage section below for more information on approved uses.

Pharmacokinetics - After oral administration only about 7% of the dose is absorbed, but the drug that remains in the GI tract is active. When injected SQ or IM, the drug is reportedly well absorbed with peak levels occurring in about 1 hour.

Tissue levels of absorbed drug are lower than those found in the serum. Spectinomycin does not appreciably enter the CSF or the eye and is not bound significantly to plasma proteins. It is unknown whether spectinomycin crosses the placenta or enters milk.

Absorbed drug is excreted via glomerular filtration into the urine mostly unchanged. No specific pharmacokinetic parameters were located for veterinary species.

Contraindications/Precautions/Reproductive Safety - Spectinomycin is contraindicated in patients hypersensitive to it. The reproductive safety of the drug is not known.

Adverse Effects/Warnings - When used as labeled, adverse effects are unlikely with this drug. It is reported that parenteral use of this drug is much safer than with other aminocyclitol antibiotics, but little is known regarding prolonged use of the drug. It is probably safe to say that spectinomycin is significantly less ototoxic and nephrotoxic than other commonly used aminocyclitol antibiotics, but can cause neuromuscular blockade. Parenteral calcium administration will generally reverse the blockade.

Adverse effects that have been reported in human patients receiving the drug in single or multi-dose studies include soreness at injection site, increases in BUN, alkaline phosphatase and SGPT, and decreases in hemoglobin, hematocrit and creatinine clearance. Although increases in BUN and decreases in creatinine clearance and urine output have been noted, overt renal toxicity has not been demonstrated with this drug.

Overdosage/Acute Toxicity - No specific information was located on oral overdoses, but because the drug is negligibly absorbed after oral administration, significant toxicity is unlikely via this route.

Injected doses of 90 mg produced transient ataxia in turkey poults.

Drug Interactions - Antagonism has been reported when spectinomycin is used with **chloramphenicol** or **tetracycline**.

Doses -
  Dogs:
    For susceptible infections:
      a) 5.5 - 11 mg/kg q12h IM or 22 mg/kg PO q12h (for enteric infections; not absorbed). (Kirk 1989)
      b) 5 - 10 mg/kg IM q12h. (Davis 1985)
      c) For acute infectious gastroenteritis: 5 - 12 mg/kg IM q12h (DeNovo 1986)
  Cats:
    For susceptible infections:
      a) For acute infectious gastroenteritis: 5 - 12 mg/kg IM q12h (DeNovo 1986)
  Cattle:
    For susceptible infections:
      a) For bronchopneumonia and fibrinous pneumonia: 33 mg/kg SQ q8h. Suggested withdrawal time is 60 days. (Hjerpe 1986)
      b) 22 - 39.6 mg/kg/day IM divided *tid* (Upson 1988)
  Horses:
    For susceptible infections:
      a) 20 mg/kg IM *tid* (Robinson 1987)
      b) For pneumonia: 20 mg/kg IM q8h; may cause local myositis. Insufficient data to comment on use. (Beech 1987b)
  Swine:
    For susceptible enteric infections:
      a) 10 mg/kg PO q12h (Howard 1986)
      b) For bacterial enteritis (white scours) in baby pigs associated with *E.coli* susceptible to spectinomycin: 50 mg/10 lbs of body weight PO *bid* for 3-5 days. (Label directions; *Spectam Scour-Halt*®—Ceva)

    c) 10 mg/kg IM q12h (Baggot 1983)

Birds:
    a) For airsacculitis associated with *M. meleagridis* or chronic respiratory disease associated with *E.coli* in turkey poults (1-3 day old): Inject 0.1 ml (10 mg) SQ in the base of the neck.

        For control and to lessen mortality due to infections from *M. synoviae, S. typhimurium, S. infantis*, and *E. coli* in newly hatched chicks: Dilute injection with normal saline to a concentration of 2.5 - 5 mg/0.2 ml and inject SQ. (Label directions; *Spectam® Injectable*—Ceva)

    b) For prevention and control of chronic respiratory disease associated with *mycoplasma gallisepticum* in broilers: Add sufficient amount to drinking water to attain a final concentration of 2 g/gallon.

        For infectious synovitis associated with *Mycoplasma synoviae* in broilers: Add sufficient amount to drinking water to attain a final concentration of 1 g/gallon.

        For improved weight gain/feed efficiency in floor-raised broilers: Add sufficient amount to drinking water to attain a final concentration of 0.5 g/gallon. (Label directions; *Spectam® Water-Soluble*—Ceva)

Monitoring Parameters -
    1) Clinical efficacy

Dosage Forms/Preparations/FDA Approval Status/Withholding Times -
Veterinary-Approved Products:

Spectinomycin Injection 100 mg/ml 500 ml vials; *Spectam® Injectable* (Rhone Merieux); (OTC) Approved for use in turkey poults and newly hatched chicks.

Spectinomycin Water Soluble Concentrate 50% Powder in 128 g (64 g spectinomycin), 200 g (100 g spectinomycin), 1000 g (500 g spectinomycin) packets; *Spectam® Water Soluble Concentrate* (Rhone Merieux); (OTC) Approved for use in chickens (not layers). Slaughter withdrawal = 5 days.

Spectinomycin Oral Solution 50 mg/ml in 240 ml pump bottle and 500 and 1000 ml refill bottles; *Spectam Scour-Halt®* (Rhone Merieux); (OTC) Approved for use in swine (Not older than 4 weeks of age or greater than 15 lbs of b.w.). Slaughter w'drawal = 21 days.

Spectinomycin Oral Solution 50 mg/ml in 240 ml pump bottle and 500 and 1000 ml refill bottles; *Spectinomycin Oral Liquid* (Syntex); (OTC) Approved for use in swine (Not older than 4 weeks of age or greater than 15 lbs of b.w.). Slaughter w'drawal = 21 days.

Spectinomycin combination products:
    Spectinomycin/Lincomycin in a 2:1 ratio Soluble Powder
        LS 50 Water Soluble Powder (Upjohn); (OTC) Approved for use in chickens. No withdrawal time required.

Human-Approved Products:
Spectinomycin Powder for Injection 400 mg (as the HCl) per ml after reconstitution. 2 g vial with 3.2 ml diluent and 4 g vial with 6.2 ml diluent.; *Trobicin®* (Upjohn); (Rx)

SPIRONOLACTONE

Chemistry - A synthetically produced aldosterone antagonist, spironolactone occurs as a cream-colored to light tan, crystalline powder with a faint mercaptan-like odor. It has a melting range of 198°-207°, with decomposition. Spironolactone is practically insoluble in water and soluble in alcohol.

Storage/Stability/Compatibility - Spironolactone tablets should be stored at room-temperature in tight, light-resistant containers. An extemporaneously prepared oral suspension can be prepared by pulverizing commercially available tablets and adding cherry syrup. This preparation is reportedly stable for at least one month when refrigerated.

Pharmacology - Aldosterone is competitively inhibited by spironolactone in the distal renal tubules with resultant increased excretion of sodium, chloride and water, and decreased excretion of potassium, ammonium, phosphate and titratable acid. Spironolactone has no effect on carbonic anhydrase or renal transport mechanisms and has its greatest effect in patients with hyperaldosteronism.

  Spironolactone is not commonly used alone as most sodium is reabsorbed at the proximal tubules. Combining it with a thiazide or loop diuretic will yield maximum diuretic effect.

Uses/Indications - The use of spironolactone in veterinary medicine is rather limited. It may be used in patients who develop hypokalemia on other diuretics and are unwilling or unable to supplement with exogenous potassium sources. It may also be effective in treating ascites as it has less potential to increase ammonia levels than other diuretics.

Pharmacokinetics - No information was found regarding the pharmacokinetics of spironolactone in veterinary species. In humans, spironolactone is >90% bioavailable and peak levels are reached within 1-2 hours. The diuretic action of spironolactone (when used alone) is gradually attained and generally reaches its maximal effect on the third day of therapy.

Spironolactone and its active metabolite canrenone, are both about 98% bound to plasma proteins. Both spironolactone and its metabolites may cross the placenta. Canrenone has been detected in breast milk. Spironolactone is rapidly metabolized (half-life of 1-2 hours) to several metabolites, including canrenone, which has diuretic activity. Canrenone is more slowly eliminated, with an average half-life of around 20 hours.

Contraindications/Precautions - Spironolactone is contraindicated in patients with hyperkalemia, anuria, acute renal failure or significant renal impairment. It should be used cautiously in patients with any renal impairment or hepatic disease.

Adverse Effects/Warnings - Adverse effects are usually considered mild and reversible upon discontinuation of the drug. Electrolyte (hyperkalemia, hyponatremia) and water balance (dehydration) abnormalities are the most likely effects with spironolactone therapy. Transient increases in BUN and mild acidosis may occur in patients with renal impairment. GI distress (vomiting, anorexia, etc.), CNS effects (lethargy, ataxia, headache, etc.) and endocrine changes (gynecomastia in human males) are all possible.

Use of spironolactone in patients with renal impairment may lead to hyperkalemia. Spironolactone reportedly inhibits the synthesis of testosterone and may increase the peripheral conversion of testosterone to estradiol. Long-term toxicity studies in rats have demonstrated that spironolactone is tumorigenic in that species. Safe use of this drug has not been established during pregnancy and, as canrenone is distributed into milk, nursing should be discontinued if therapy with the drug is required.

Overdosage - Information on overdosage of spironolactone is apparently unavailable. Should an acute overdose occur, it is suggested to follow the guidelines outlined in the chlorothiazide and furosemide monographs (preceeding this one).

Drug Interactions - Do not use spironolactone concurrently with **other potassium-sparing diuretics** (*e.g.,* amiloride, triamterene) as hyperkalemia may result. Other drugs that may increase the risk of hyperkalemia if used concomitantly with spironolactone include **indomethacin** and **ACE inhibitors** (*e.g.,* **captopril, enalapril,** etc.)

Spironolactone may increase the half-life of **digoxin** and may either decrease or increase the half-life of **digitoxin**. Enhanced monitoring of digitalis serum levels and effects are warranted when spironolactone is used with these agents. Spironolactone may mute the effects of **mitotane** if given concurrently, but very limited information is available on this potential interaction; monitor carefully.

Spironolactone's diuretic effects may be decreased if **aspirin** (or other salicylates) are administered concomitantly.

Vascular responses to **norepinephrine** and regional or general **anesthesia** may be diminished in patients also receiving spironolactone.

Additive or potentiated effects may occur if spironolactone is added to other **diuretics** or **antihypertensive agents**; dosage adjustments and increased monitoring may be necessary.

Food may enhance the absorption of spironolactone.

Drug/Lab Interactions - Spironolactone may give falsely elevated **digoxin** values, if using a radioimmune assay (RIA) method. Fluorometric methods of determining plasma and urinary 17-hydroxycorticosteroids (**cortisol**) may be interfered with by spironolactone.

Doses -
  Dogs:
    As a diuretic in CHF:
      a) 2 - 4 mg/kg/day PO (Kittleson 1985)

    For treating ascites:
      a) 1 - 2 mg/kg PO *bid*; if no response in 4-5 days, double dose for an additional 4-5 days; if no response, may double again (4 - 8 mg/kg *bid*). Monitor (weigh) patients daily and do not allow patient to become dehydrated or to lose more than 0.25 - 0.5 kg/day. (Hardy 1985)

  Cats:
    As a diuretic in CHF:
      a) 2 - 4 mg/kg/day PO (Kittleson 1985)
      b) 1 mg/kg q12h PO when serum potassium is low (Bonagura 1989)

Monitoring Parameters -
  1) Serum electrolytes, BUN, creatinine
  2) Hydration status
  3) Blood pressure, if indicated
  4) Symptoms of edema/ascites; patient weight, if indicated

Client Information - Notify veterinarian if GI symptoms (*e.g.,* vomiting, diarrhea, anorexia), lethargy or other CNS effects are severe or persist.

Dosage Forms/Preparations/FDA Approval Status/Withholding Times -
  Veterinary-Approved Products: None
  Human-Approved Products:
    Spironolactone Tablets 25 mg, 50 mg, 100 mg; *Aldactone*® (Searle), Generic; (Rx)

    Also available in combination with hydrochlorothiazide.

STANOZOLOL

Chemistry - An anabolic steroid, stanozolol occurs as an odorless, nearly colorless, crystalline powder that can exist in two forms: prisms, melting at approximately 235°C, and needles that melt at about 155°C. It is sparingly soluble in alcohol and insoluble in water.

Storage/Stability/Compatibility - Stanozolol tablets should be stored in tight, light-resistant packaging, preferably at room temperature.

Pharmacology - Stanozolol possess the actions of other anabolic agents. It may be less androgenic than other anabolics that are routinely used in veterinary medicine, however. Refer to the discussion in the Boldenone monograph for more information.

Uses/Indications - Labeled indications for the stanozolol product *Winstrol*®-*V* (Winthrop/Upjohn) include "... to improve appetite, promote weight gain, and increase strength and vitality..." in dogs, cats and horses. The manufacturer also states that "Anabolic therapy is intended primarily as an adjunct to other specific and supportive therapy, including nutritional therapy."

  Like nandrolone, stanozolol has been used to treat anemia of chronic disease. Because stanozolol has been demonstrated to enhance fibrinolysis after parenteral injection, it may be efficacious in the treatment of feline aortic thromboembolism or in the treatment of thrombosis in nephrotic syndrome. However, at present, clinical studies and/or experience are apparently lacking for this indication.

Pharmacokinetics - No specific information was located for this agent. It is generally recommended that the injectable suspension be dosed on a weekly basis in both small animals and horses.

Contraindications/Precautions - Stanozolol is contraindicated in pregnant animals and in breeding stallions and should not be administered to horses intended for food purposes.

  The manufacturer recommends using stanozolol cautiously in patients with cardiac and renal function and with enhanced fluid and electrolyte monitoring.

  In humans, anabolic agents are also contraindicated in patients with hepatic dysfunction, hypercalcemia, patients with a history of myocardial infarction (can cause hypercholesterolemia), pituitary insufficiency, prostate carcinoma, in selected patients with breast carcinoma, benign prostatic hypertrophy and during the nephrotic stage of nephritis.

  The anabolic agents are category X (risk of use outweighs any possible benefit) agents for use in pregnancy and are contraindicated because of possible fetal masculinization.

Adverse Effects/Warnings - The manufacturer (Winthrop/Upjohn) lists as adverse effects in dogs, cats and horses only "mild androgenic effects" and then only when used with excessively high doses for a prolonged period of time.

  Potentially (from human data), adverse reactions of the anabolic agents in dogs and cats could include: sodium, calcium, potassium, water, chloride, and phosphate retention; hepatotoxicity, behavioral (androgenic) changes and reproductive abnormalities (oligospermia, estrus suppression).

Overdosage - No information was located for this specific agent. In humans, sodium and water retention can occur after overdosage of anabolic steroids. It is suggested to treat supportively and monitor liver function should an inadvertent overdose be administered.

Drug Interactions - Anabolic agents as a class may potentiate the effects of **anticoagulants**. Monitoring of PT's and dosage adjustment, if necessary of the anticoagulant are recommended.

  Diabetic patients receiving **insulin** may need dosage adjustments if anabolic therapy is added or discontinued. Anabolics may decrease blood glucose and decrease insulin requirements.

  Anabolics may enhance the edema that can be associated with **ACTH** or **adrenal steroid** therapy.

Drug/Laboratory Interactions - Concentrations of **protein bound iodine (PBI)** can be decreased in patients receiving androgen/anabolic therapy, but the clinical significance of this is probably not important. Androgen/anabolic agents can decrease amounts of **thyroxine-binding globulin** and decrease **total T4** concentrations and increase **resin uptake of T3 and T4**. Free thyroid hormones are unaltered and, clinically, there is no evidence of dysfunction.

Both **creatinine** and **creatine excretion** can be decreased by anabolic steroids. Anabolic steroids can increase the urinary excretion of **17-ketosteroids**.

Androgenic/anabolic steroids may alter **blood glucose** levels. Androgenic/anabolic steroids may suppress **clotting factors II, V, VII, and X**. Anabolic agents can affect **liver function tests** (BSP retention, SGOT, SGPT, bilirubin, and alkaline phosphatase).

Doses -
Dogs:
   As an anabolic agent per labeled indications:
      a) Small Breeds: 1 - 2 mg PO *bid*; or 25 mg deep IM, may repeat weekly.
          Large Breeds: 2 - 4 mg PO *bid*; or 50 mg deep IM, may repeat weekly.
          Treatment should continue for several weeks, depending on response and condition of animal. (Package Insert; *Winstrol®-V* —Winthrop/Upjohn)
   For anemia secondary to chronic renal failure:
      a) 1 - 4 mg PO once daily (Ross et al. 1988)
      b) For anemias secondary to uremia: 2 - 10 mg PO *bid* (Maggio-Price 1988)
   As an anabolic/appetite stimulant:
      a) 1 - 4 mg PO *bid* (Weller 1988)
      b) 1 - 2 mg PO *bid* or 25 - 50 mg IM weekly (Macy and Ralston 1989)

Cats:
   As an anabolic agent per labeled indications:
      a) 1 - 2 mg PO *bid*; or 25 mg deep IM, may repeat weekly.
          Treatment should continue for several weeks, depending on response and condition of animal. (Package Insert; *Winstrol®-V* —Winthrop/Upjohn)
   For chronic anemia secondary to feline cardiomyopathy:
      a) 2 mg PO once daily (Harpster 1986)
   For anemia secondary to chronic renal failure:
      a) 1 - 4 mg PO once daily (Ross et al. 1988)
      b) For anemias secondary to uremia: 1 - 2 mg PO *bid* (Maggio-Price 1988)

Horses:
   As an anabolic agent per labeled indications:
      a) 0.55 mg/kg (25 mg per 100 pounds of body weight) IM deeply. May repeat weekly for up to and including 4 weeks. (Package Insert; *Winstrol®-V* —Winthrop/Upjohn)

Sheep & Goats:
   For acute or subacute aflatoxicosis in ruminants:
      a) Stanozolol 2 mg/kg IM (plus activated charcoal 6.7 mg/kg as a 30% w/v slurry in M/15, pH 7 phosphate buffer). Do not combine with oxytetracycline therapy. (Hatch 1988)

Birds:
   As an anabolic agent to promote weight gain and recovery from disease:
      a) 0.5 - 1 ml/kg (25 - 50 mg/kg) IM once or twice weekly. Use with caution in birds with renal disease. (Clubb 1986)

Reptiles:
      a) For most species post-surgically and in very debilitated animals: 5 mg/kg IM once a week as needed. (Gauvin 1993)

Monitoring Parameters - 1) Androgenic side effects; 2) Fluid and electrolyte status, if indicated; 3) Liver function tests if indicated; 4) RBC count, indices, if indicated; 5) Weight, appetite

Client Information - Tablets may be crushed and administered with food. Because of the potential for abuse of anabolic steroids by humans, many states have included, or are considering including this agent as a controlled drug. It should be kept in a secure area and out of the reach of children.

Dosage Forms/Preparations/FDA Approval Status/Withholding Times -
Veterinary-Approved Products:

   Stanozolol Suspension for Injection 50 mg/ml in 10 ml and 30 ml vials; *Winstrol®-V* (Upjohn); (Rx) Approved for cats, dogs and horses.

Stanozolol Oral Tablets 2 mg; Oral Chewable Tablets 2 mg (dogs only); *Winstrol®-V* (Upjohn); (Rx) Approved for cats, dogs and horses. In horses, the manufacturer recommends using the injectable product only.

Human-Approved Products:

Stanozolol Oral Tablets 2 mg; *Winstrol®* (Winthrop); (Rx)

Note: All stanozolol products are now controlled drugs (C-IV) in the USA.

SUCCINYLCHOLINE CHLORIDE

Chemistry - A depolarizing neuromuscular blocking agent, succinylcholine chloride occurs as an odorless, white, crystalline powder. The dihydrate form melts at 190°C and the anhydrous form at 160°C. Aqueous solutions are acidic with a pH of approximately 4. One gram is soluble in about 1 ml of water and about 350 ml of alcohol. Commercially available injections have a pH from 3-4.5. Succinylcholine may also be known as suxemethonium chloride.

Storage/Stability/Compatibility - Commercial injectable solutions should be stored refrigerated (2°-8°C). One manufacturer (Glaxo Wellcome - *Anectine®*) states that multiple dose vials are stable for up to 2 weeks at room temperature with no significant loss of potency.

The powder forms of the drug are stable indefinitely when stored unopened at room temperature. After reconstitution with either D_5W or normal saline, they are stable for 4 weeks at 5°C or 1 week at room temperature, but because they contain no preservative, it is recommended they be used within 24 hours.

Succinylcholine chloride is **compatible** with all commonly used IV solutions, amikacin sulfate, cephapirin sodium, isoproterenol HCl, meperidine HCl, norepinephrine bitartrate, scopolamine HBr. It may not be compatible with pentobarbital sodium and is **incompatible** with sodium bicarbonate and thiopental sodium.

Pharmacology - An ultrashort-acting depolarizing skeletal muscle relaxant, succinylcholine bonds with motor endplate cholinergic receptors to produce depolarization (perceived as fasiculations). The neuromuscular block remains as long as sufficient quantities of succinylcholine remain, and is characterized by a flaccid paralysis. Other pharmacologic effects are discussed in the precautions and adverse effects sections.

Uses/Indications - Succinylcholine chloride is indicated for short-term muscle relaxation needed for surgical or diagnostic procedures, to facilitate endotracheal intubation in some species, and to reduce the intensity of muscle contractions associated with electro- or pharmacological- induced convulsions. Dogs, cats, and horses are the primary veterinary species where succinylcholine chloride has been used.

Pharmacokinetics - The onset of action, with complete muscle relaxation, after IV administration is usually within 30 seconds to 1 minute. In humans this effect lasts for 2-3 minutes and then gradually diminishes within 10 minutes. The very short duration of action after a single IV dose is thought to occur because the drug diffuses away from the motor end-plate. If multiple injections or a continuous infusion is performed, the brief activity is a result of rapid hydrolysis by pseudocholinesterases at the site of action. After IM injection, the onset of action is generally within 2-3 minutes and may persist for 10-30 minutes. Dogs exhibit a prolonged duration of action (≈ 20 minutes); this species appears unique in this idiosyncratic response.

Succinylcholine is metabolized by plasma pseudocholinesterases to succinylmonocholine and choline and 10% of it is excreted unchanged in the urine. Succinylmonocholine is partially excreted in the urine and may accumulate in patients with impaired renal function. Succinylmonocholine has approximately 1/20th the neuromuscular blocking activity of succinylcholine, but if it accumulates, prolonged periods of apnea may result.

Contraindications/Precautions - Succinylcholine is contraindicated in patients with severe liver disease, chronic anemias, malnourishment (chronic), glaucoma or penetrating eye injuries, predisposition to malignant hyperthermia, and increased CPK values with resultant myopathies. As succinylcholine can exacerbate the effects of hyperkalemia, it should be used with extreme caution in patients who have suffered traumatic wounds or burns, are receiving quinidine or digitalis therapy, have preexisting hyperkalemia or electrolyte imbalances, as arrhythmias or cardiac arrest may occur. It should also be used with caution in patients with pulmonary, renal, cardiovascular, metabolic or hepatic dysfunction.

It is unknown if succinylcholine can cause fetal harm. The drug does cross the placenta in low concentrations and a newly delivered neonate may show signs of neuromuscular blockade if the mother received high doses or prolonged administration of the drug prior to delivery.

Succinylcholine should not be used if organophosphate agents have been given or applied recently.

Succinylcholine chloride does not have analgesic effects; and should be used with appropriate analgesic/sedative/anesthetic agents.

In horses, the following additional recommendations have been made by the American Association of Equine Practitioners:
1) Inform the owner that succinylcholine chloride is to be used as a restraining agent, not as an anesthetic.
2) Obtain history before use; do not use in horses if within 30 days they have received, an antibiotic ending in "mycin", organophosphate insecticides or anthelmintics, any other cholinesterase inhibitor, or procaine.
3) Do not use in debilitated, excited, or exhausted horses.
4) If possible, withhold food for 4-6 hours before use.
5) Dosage of 0.088mg/kg IV may be used to paralyze skeletal muscles without causing respiratory depression. Higher doses may cause apnea and death without respiratory support. Lower doses may be possible if animal is used with a preanesthetic agent.
6) After administration, have someone hold the horse that is familiar with the actions of succinylcholine chloride so that the animal does not fall forward on its nose. Be prepared to administer oxygen and artificial respiration.
7) If death occurs, a necropsy should be performed.

Adverse Effects/Warnings - Succinylcholine chloride can cause muscle soreness, histamine release, malignant hyperthermia, excessive salivation, hyperkalemia, rash, and myoglobinemia/myoglobinuria. Cardiovascular effects can include bradycardia, tachycardia, hypertension, hypotension, or arrhythmias.

Overdosage - Inadvertent overdoses, or patients deficient in pseudocholinesterase may result in prolonged apnea. Mechanical ventilation with O_2 should be used until recovery.

Repeated or prolonged high dosages may cause patients to convert from a phase I to a phase II block.

Drug Interactions - **Furosemide, phenothiazines, oxytocin, quinidine, procainamide,** beta-adrenergic blockers (propranolol), lidocaine, magnesium salts, and isoflurane** may enhance the actions of succinylcholine.

Diazepam may reduce the duration of action of succinylcholine.

Succinylcholine may cause a sudden outflux of potassium from muscle cells, thus causing arrhythmias in **digitilized** patients.

Drugs such as **neostigmine or organophosphates,** which can inhibit pseudocholinesterases, should not be used with succinylcholine.

Intravenous **procaine** (competes for the pseudocholinesterase enzyme) and **cyclophosphamide** (decreases plasma pseudocholinesterase) may prolong succinylcholine's effects.

Thiazide diuretics and **Amphotericin B** may increase succinylcholine's effects by causing electrolyte imbalances.

Increased incidences of bradycardia and sinus arrest may occur if used concurrently with **narcotic analgesics.**

Concomitant administration with **inhalation anesthetics (halothane, cyclopropane, nitrous oxide, diethyl ether)** may induce increased incidences of cardiac effects (bradycardia, arrhythmias, sinus arrest and apnea) and in susceptible patients, malignant hyperthermia.

Doses -
Dogs:
      a) 0.07 mg/kg IV (Morgan 1988)
      b) 0.22 mg/kg IV (Mandsager 1988)

Cats:
      a) 0.06 mg/kg IV (Morgan 1988)
      b) 0.11 mg/kg IV (Mandsager 1988)

Horses: See Precautions above.
      a) 0.088 mg/kg (Muir)
      b) 0.088 - 0.11 mg/kg IV, IM (Mandsager 1988)

Monitoring Parameters -
1) Level of muscle relaxation
2) Cardiac rate/rhythm
3) Respiratory depressant effect

Client Information - This drug should only be used by professionals familiar with its use.

Dosage Forms/Preparations/FDA Approval Status/Withholding Times -
Veterinary-Approved Products: None
Human-Approved Products:
Succinylcholine Chloride for Injection 20 mg/ml, 50 mg/ml, 100 mg/ml in 10 ml vials and amps and 5 ml syringes; *Anectine*® (Glaxo Wellcome); *Quelicin*® (Abbott): Succinylcholine Chloride (Organon) (Rx)

Succinylcholine Chloride Powder for Infusion 500 mg or 1 gram vials; *Anectine Flo-Pak*® (Glaxo Wellcome); (Rx)

SUCRALFATE

Chemistry - A basic, aluminum complex of sucrose sulfate, sucralfate occurs as a white, amorphous powder. It is practically insoluble in alcohol or water.

Sucralfate is structurally related to heparin, but does not posses any appreciable anticoagulant activity. It is also structurally related to sucrose, but is not utilized as a sugar by the body. Sucralfate is also known as aluminum sucrose sulfate, basic.

Storage/Stability/Compatibility - Store sucralfate tablets in tight containers at room temperature.

Pharmacology - While the exact mechanism of action of sucralfate as an antiulcer agent is not known, the drug has a local effect rather than a systemic one. After oral administration, sucralfate reacts with hydrochloric acid in the stomach to form a paste-like complex that will bind to the proteinaceous exudates that generally are found at ulcer sites. This insoluble complex forms a barrier at the site and protects the ulcer from further damage caused by pepsin, acid or bile.

Sucralfate may have some cytoprotective effects, possibly by stimulation of prostaglandin E_2 and I_2. Sucralfate also has some antacid activity, but it is believed that this is not of clinical importance.

Sucralfate does not significantly affect gastric acid output, or trypsin or pancreatic amylase activity. It may decrease the rate of gastric emptying.

Uses/Indications - Sucralfate has been used in the treatment of oral, esophageal, gastric and duodenal ulcers. It has also been employed to prevent drug-induced (*e.g.,* aspirin) gastric erosions.

Pharmacokinetics - Animal studies have indicated that only 3-5% of an oral dose is absorbed which is excreted in the urine unchanged within 48 hours. The remainder of the drug is converted to sucrose sulfate in the gut by reacting with hydrochloric acid and is excreted in the feces within 48 hours. The duration of action (binding to ulcer site) may persist up to 6 hours after oral dosing.

Contraindications/Precautions - There are no known contraindications to the use of sucralfate. Because it may cause constipation, it should be used with caution in animals where decreased intestinal transit times may be deleterious.

It is unknown if sucralfate crosses the placenta and whether it may be used safely during pregnancy. In rats, dosages up to 38 times those used in humans caused no impaired fertility and doses up to 5O times normal caused no symptoms of teratogenicity.

Adverse Effects/Warnings - Adverse effects are uncommon with sucralfate therapy. Constipation is the most prominent adverse effect reported in humans (2%) and dogs taking the drug.

Overdosage - Overdosage is unlikely to cause any significant problems. Laboratory animals receiving up to 12 grams/kg orally demonstrated no incidence of mortality.

Drug Interactions - **Cimetidine, tetracycline, phenytoin and digoxin** bioavailability may be reduced if administered with sucralfate. To avoid this problem, give sucralfate at least 2 hours apart from these other drugs. Because sucralfate requires an acidic environment to be effective, give sucralfate doses before (at least 1/2 hour) **cimetidine (or other H$_2$ antagonist) or antacids**.

Doses -
Dogs:
a) Large dogs: 1 gram (1 tablet) PO q8h
    Small dogs: 0.5 gram (1/2 tablet) PO q8h (Papich 1989)
b) 0.5 - 1 gram PO q8-12h (Matz 1995)
c) Dogs weighing < 20 kg: 0.5 gram PO *tid-qid*
    Dogs weighing > 20 kg: 1 gram PO *tid-qid* (Morgan 1988)

Cats:
a) 1/4 - 1/2 tablet q8-12h (Papich 1989)
b) 0.25 gram PO q8-12h (Matz 1995)

Horses:
a) Foals: 1 - 2 grams PO *qid* (Clark and Becht 1987)
b) 2 mg/kg PO *tid* (Robinson 1987)

Reptiles:
a) For GI irritation in most species: 500 - 1,000 mg/kg PO q6-8h (Gauvin 1993)

Monitoring Parameters -
1) Clinical efficacy (dependent on reason for use); monitored by decrease in symptomatology, endoscopic examination, blood in feces, etc.

Client Information - To maximize the benefit of this medication, it must be administered as prescribed by the veterinarian; symptoms may reoccur if dosages are missed. Unless otherwise instructed, give this medication on an empty stomach (1 hour before feeding or 2 hours after) and at bedtime.

Dosage Forms/Preparations/FDA Approval Status/Withholding Times -
Veterinary-Approved Products: None
Human-Approved Products:
Sucralfate 1 gram tablets (scored); *Carafate*® (Hoechst Marion Roussel); Generic. (Rx)
Sucralfate Suspension: 1 g/10 ml in 420 ml; *Carafate*® (Hoechst Marion Roussel) (Rx)

SULFACHLORPYRIDAZINE SODIUM

Chemistry - Sulfachlorpyridazine sodium is listed as a short to intermediate-acting, low lipid soluble sulfonamide antibacterial. It is reportedly very soluble in urine at usual pH's.

Storage/Stability/Compatibility -The injection should be stored at room temperature and protected from light; avoid freezing. The oral suspension should be stored at room temperature; avoid freezing. The oral boluses and powder should be stored at room temperature; avoid excessive heat (above 40°C/104°F).

No information was located regarding the compatibility of sulfachlorpyridazine with other fluids or agents.

Pharmacology - Sulfonamides are usually bacteriostatic agents when used alone. They are thought to prevent bacterial replication by competing with para-aminobenzoic acid (PABA) in the biosynthesis of tetrahydrofolic acid in the pathway to form folic acid. Only microorganisms that synthesize their own folic acid are affected by sulfas.

Microorganisms that are usually affected by sulfonamides include some gram positive bacteria, including some strains of streptococci, staphylococcus, *Bacillus anthracis, Clostridium tetani, C. perfringens* and many strains of Nocardia. Sulfas also have *in vitro* activity against some gram negative species, including some strains of *Shigella, Salmonella, E. coli, Klebsiella, Enterobacter, Pasturella* and *Proteus*. Sulfas also have activity against some rickettsia, and protozoa (Toxoplasma, Coccidia). Unfortunately, resistance to sulfas is a progressing phenomenon and many strains of bacteria that were once susceptible to this class of antibacterial are now resistant. The sulfas are less efficacious in pus, necrotic tissue or in areas with extensive cellular debris.

Uses/Indications - Sulfachlorpyridazine is indicated for the treatment of diarrhea caused or complicated by *E. coli* in calves less than one month of age or for the treatment of colibacillosis in swine. It is also used parenterally as a general purpose sulfonamide in adult cattle and other species.

Pharmacokinetics - Very limited information is available on the specific pharmacokinetics for this agent. In general, sulfonamides are readily absorbed from the GI tract of non-ruminants, but absorption can vary depending on the drug, species, disease process, etc.. Food delays the rate, but usually not the extent of absorption. Peak levels occur within 1-2 hours in non-ruminant (and young pre-ruminant) animals. Adult ruminants may have significant delays before the drug is absorbed orally.

Sulfas are well distributed throughout the body and some reach significant levels in the CSF. Levels of the drugs tends to be highest in liver, kidney and lung, and lower in muscle and bone. The sulfas can be highly bound to serum proteins, but the extent of binding is species and drug dependent. When bound to proteins the sulfa is not active.

Sulfas cross the placenta and may reach fetal levels of 50% or greater of those found in maternal serum. Sulfonamides also are distributed into milk.

Sulfonamides are both renally excreted and metabolized. Renal excretion of unchanged drug occurs via both tubular secretion and glomerular filtration. Protein bound drug is not filtered by the glomeruli. Metabolism is performed principally by the liver, but extra-hepatic metabolism is also involved. Mechanisms of metabolism are usually acetylation and glucuronidation. The acetylated metabolites may be less soluble and crystallization in the urine can occur with some sulfonamides, particularly at lower pH. The serum half-life of sulfachlorpyridazine is approximately 1.2 hours in cattle.

Contraindications/Precautions/Reproductive Safety - Sulfonamides are contraindicated in patients hypersensitive to them, thiazides, or sulfonylurea agents. They are also considered contraindicated in patients with severe renal or hepatic impairment and should be used with caution in patients with diminished renal or hepatic function, or urinary obstruction.

Oral sulfonamides can depress the normal cellulytic function of the ruminoreticulum, but this effect is generally temporary and the animal adapts.

Sulfas cross the placenta and teratogenicity has been reported in some laboratory animals when given at very high doses. They should be used in pregnant animals only when the benefits clearly outweigh the risks of therapy.

Adverse Effects/Warnings - Sulfonamides (or their metabolites) can precipitate in the urine, particularly in an acidic environment resulting in crystalluria, hematouria and renal tubule obstruction. Different sulfonamides have different solubilities at various pH's. Alkalinization of the urine using sodium bicarbonate may prevent crystalluria, but it also decreases the amount available for tubular reabsorption. Crystalluria can usually be avoided with most of the commercially available sulfonamides by maintaining an adequate urine flow. Normal urine pH in herbivores is usually 8 or more so crystalluria is not frequently a problem in those species. Sulfonamides can also cause various hypersensitivity reactions or diarrhea by altering the normal gut flora.

Too rapid intravenous injection of the sulfas can cause muscle weakness, blindness, ataxia and collapse.

In dogs, keratoconjunctivitis sicca has been reported with sulfonamide therapy. Also, in dogs, bone marrow depression, hypersensitivity reactions (rashes, dermatitis), focal retinitis, fever, vomiting and nonseptic polyarthritis have been reported.

Oral sulfonamides can depress the normal cellulytic function of the ruminoreticulum, but this effect is generally temporary and the animal adapts.

Because solutions of sulfonamides are usually alkaline, they can cause tissue irritation and necrosis if injected intramuscularly or subcutaneously.

Overdosage/Acute Toxicity - Acute toxicity secondary to overdoses apparently occurs only rarely in veterinary species. In addition to the adverse effects listed above, CNS stimulation and myelin degeneration have been noted after very high dosages.

Drug Interactions - Sulfachlorpyridazine or other sulfonamides may displace highly protein bound drugs, such as **methotrexate, warfarin, phenylbutazone, thiazide diuretics, salicylates, probenicid and phenytoin.** Although the clinical significance of these interactions is not entirely clear, patients should be monitored for enhanced effects of the displaced agents. **Antacids** may decrease the oral bioavailability of sulfonamides if administered concurrently.

Drug/Laboratory Interactions - Sulfonamides may give false-positive results for **urine glucose** determinations when using the Benedict's method.

Doses -
Cattle:
a) 88 - 110 mg/kg IV once to twice daily. (Upson 1988)
b) 30 mg/kg PO q8h (Burrows 1980)
c) For bronchopneumonia and fibrinous pneumonia: 33 - 50 mg/kg q12h (method of administration not specified) (Hjerpe 1986)
d) In calves for labeled indications: 33 - 49.5 mg/kg PO, or IV *bid* for 1-5 days; suggest initiating therapy with intravenous preparation and then changing to oral if possible. (Package insert; *Vetisulid®*—Solvay)

Swine:
a) In swine for labeled indications: 44 - 77 mg/kg PO per day (divide dose and give twice daily if treating individual animals) for 1-5 days (Package insert; *Vetisulid®*—Solvay)

Birds:
For enteric bacterial infections:
a) Using the oral powder: Mix 1/4 teaspoonful per liter of water and use as only supply of drinking water for 5-10 days. May be effective for many E. coli enteric infections. (Clubb 1986)
b) Using the oral powder: Mix 3/4 teaspoonful per 2 quarts of water. Fairly effective for enteric infections, particularly E.coli. Reserved for clients who are unable to give other medications by mouth or parenterally. (McDonald 1989)

Monitoring Parameters -
1) Clinical efficacy
2) Adverse effects

Client Information - To help reduce the possibility of crystalluria occurring, animals should have free access to water; avoid dehydration.

Dosage Forms/Preparations/FDA Approval Status/Withholding Times -
Veterinary-Approved Products:

Sulfachlorpyridazine Sodium Injection 215 mg/ml in 250 ml bottles; *Vetisulid® Injection* (Fort Dodge); (OTC) Approved for use in nonlactating dairy cattle and beef cattle. Slaughter withdrawal = 5 days for cattle.

Sulfachlorpyridazine Sodium Oral Boluses 2 g bottles of 50 or 100; *Vetisulid® Bolus* (Fort Dodge); (OTC) Indicated for use in calves under one month of age. Slaughter withdrawal = 7 days.

Sulfachlorpyridazine Sodium Oral Powder 54 grams per bottle; *Vetisulid® Powder* (Fort Dodge); (OTC) Indicated for use in calves under one month of age and swine. Slaughter withdrawal = 7 days for cattle and 4 days for swine.

Sulfachlorpyridazine Sodium Oral Suspension 50 mg/ml in 180 ml bottles; *Vetisulid® Oral Suspension* (Fort Dodge); (OTC) Approved for use in swine. Slaughter withdrawal = 4 days for swine.

Human-Approved Products: None

SULFADIAZINE/TRIMETHOPRIM
SULFAMETHOXAZOLE/TRIMETHOPRIM

Note: In the practice of veterinary medicine in the United States, two separate combinations with trimethoprim are used clinically. There are trimethoprim/sulfadiazine products approved for use in dogs, cats and horses in both parenteral and oral dosage forms. Many veterinarians also will use the human approved, trimethoprim/sulfamethoxazole oral products because of economic considerations. In Canada, sulfadoxine is available in combination with trimethoprim for veterinary use.

Chemistry - Trimethoprim occurs as odorless, bitter-tasting, white to cream-colored crystals or crystalline powder. It is very slightly soluble in water and slightly soluble in alcohol.

Sulfadiazine occurs as an odorless or nearly odorless, white to slightly yellow powder. It is practically insoluble in water and sparingly soluble in alcohol.

Sulfamethoxazole occurs as a practically odorless, white to off-white, crystalline powder. Approximately 0.29 mg is soluble in 1 ml of water and 20 mg are soluble in 1 ml of alcohol.

In combination, these products may be known as: Co-trimoxazole, SMX-TMP, TMP-SMX, trimethoprim-sulfamethoxazole, sulfamethoxazole-trimethoprim, sulfadiazine-trimethoprim, trimethoprim-sulfadiazine, TMP-SDZ, SDZ-TMP, Co-trimazine or by their various trade names.

Storage/Stability/Compatibility - Unless otherwise instructed by the manufacturer, trimethoprim/sulfadiazine and co-trimoxazole products should be stored at room temperature (15-30°C) in tight containers.

Pharmacology - Alone, sulfonamides are bacteriostatic agents and trimethoprim is bactericidal, but in combination, the potentiated sulfas are bactericidal. Potentiated sulfas sequentially inhibit enzymes in the folic acid pathway, thereby inhibiting bacterial thymidine synthesis. The sulfonamide blocks the conversion of para-aminobenzoic acid (PABA) to dihydrofolic acid (DFA), and trimethoprim blocks the conversion of DFA to tetrahydrofolic acid by inhibiting dihydrofolate reductase.

The *in vitro* optimal ratio for most susceptible bacteria is approximately 1:20 (trimethoprim:sulfa), but synergistic activity can reportedly occur with ratios of 1:1 - 1:40. The serum concentration of the trimethoprim component is considered to be more important than the sulfa concentration. For most susceptible bacteria, the MIC's for TMP are generally above 0.5 micrograms/ml.

The potentiated sulfas have a fairly broad spectrum of activity. Gram positive bacteria that are generally susceptible include most streptococci, many strains of staphylococcus and *Nocardia*. Many gram negative organisms of the family Enterobacteriaceae are susceptible to the potentiated sulfas, but not *Pseudomonas aeruginosa*. Some protozoa (*Pneumocystis carinii*, Coccidia and Toxoplasma) are also inhibited by the combination. Potentiated sulfas reportedly have little activity against most anaerobes, but opinions on this vary.

Resistance will develop slower to the combination of drugs than to either one alone. In gram negative organisms, resistance is usually plasmid-mediated.

Uses/Indications - Although only approved for use in dogs and horses, trimethoprim/sulfadiazine *et al* is used in many species to treat infections caused by susceptible organisms. See Dosage section for more information.

Pharmacokinetics - Trimethoprim/sulfa is well absorbed after oral administration, with peak levels occurring about 1-4 hours after dosing. The drug is more slowly absorbed after subcutaneous absorption, however. In ruminants, the trimethoprim is apparently trapped in the ruminoreticulum after oral administration and undergoes some degradation.

Trimethoprim/sulfa is well distributed in the body. When meninges are inflamed, the drugs enter the CSF in levels of about 50% of those found in the serum. Both drugs cross the placenta and are distributed into milk. The volume of distribution for trimethoprim in various species are: 1.49 L/kg (dogs), and 0.59-1.51 L/kg (horses). The volume of distribution for sulfadiazine in dogs is 1.02 L/kg.

Trimethoprim/sulfa is both renally excreted unchanged via glomerular filtration and tubular secretion and metabolized by the liver. The sulfas are primarily acetylated and conjugated with glucuronic acid and trimethoprim is metabolized to oxide and hydroxylated metabolites. Trimethoprim may be more extensively metabolized by the liver in adult ruminants than in other species. The serum elimination half-lives for trimethoprim in various species are: 2.5 hours (dogs), 1.91-3 hours (horses), 1.5 hours (cattle). The serum elimination half-lives for sulfadiazine in various species are: 9.84 hours (dogs), 2.71 hours (horses), 2.5 hours (cattle). While trimethoprim is quite rapidly eliminated from the serum, the drug may persist for a longer period of time in tissues.

Because of the number of variables involved it is extremely difficult to apply pharmacokinetic values in making dosage recommendations with these combinations. Each drug (trimethoprim and the sulfa) has different pharmacokinetic parameters (absorption, distribution, elimination) in each species. Since different organisms have different MIC values and the optimal ratio of trimethoprim to sulfa also differs from organism to organism, this problem is exacerbated.

There is considerable controversy regarding the frequency of administration of these combinations. The veterinary product, trimethoprim/sulfadiazine is labeled for once daily administration in dogs and horses, but many clinicians believe that the drug is more efficacious if given twice daily, regardless of which sulfa is used.

Contraindications/Precautions/Reproductive Safety - The manufacturer states that trimethoprim/sulfadiazine should not be used in dogs or horses showing marked liver parenchymal damage, blood dyscrasias, or in those with a history of sulfonamide sensitivity. It is not for use in horses (or approved for other animals) intended for food.

This combination should be used with caution in patients with pre-existing hepatic disease.

Safety of trimethoprim/sulfa has not been clearly established in pregnant animals. Reports of teratogenicity (cleft palate) have been reported in some rat studies. Fetal mortality was also increased in rabbits receiving high doses of trimethoprim. Dog studies have not demonstrated any teratogenic effects. However, this combination should be used in pregnant females only when the benefits clearly outweigh the risks of use. Studies thus far in male animals have not demonstrated any decreases in reproductive performance.

Adverse Effects/Warnings - Adverse effects noted in dogs: keratoconjunctivitis sicca (which may be irreversible), acute neutrophilic hepatitis with icterus, vomiting, anorexia, diarrhea, fever, hemolytic anemia, urticaria, polyarthritis, facial swelling, polydipsia, polyuria and cholestasis. Potentiated sulfonamides may cause hypothyroidism in the dog, particularly with extended therapy. Acute hypersensitivity reactions manifesting as Type I (anaphylaxis) or Type III reaction (serum sickness) can also be seen. Hypersensitivity reactions appear to be more common in large breed dogs; Doberman Pinschers may possibly be more susceptible to this effect than other breeds. Other hematologic effects (anemias, agranulocytosis) are possible, but are fairly rare in dogs.

Adverse effects noted in cats may include anorexia, leukopenias and anemias.

In horses, transient pruritis has been noted after intravenous injection. Oral therapy has resulted in diarrhea development in some horses. If the 48% injectable product is injected IM, SQ, or extravasates after IV administration, swelling, pain and minor tissue damage may result. Hypersensitivity reactions and hematologic effects (anemias, thrombocytopenia, or leukopenias) may also be seen; long term therapy should include periodic hematologic monitoring.

Overdosage/Acute Toxicity - Manifestations of an acute overdosage can include symptoms of GI distress (nausea, vomiting, diarrhea), CNS toxicity (depression, headache, and confusion), facial swelling, bone marrow depression and increases in serum aminotransferases. Oral overdoses can be treated by emptying the stomach (following usual protocols) and initiating symptomatic and supportive therapy. Acidification of the urine may increase the renal elimination of trimethoprim, but could also cause sulfonamide crystalluria, particularly with sulfadiazine containing products. Complete blood counts (and other laboratory parameters) should be monitored as necessary. Bone marrow suppression associated with chronic overdoses may be treated with folinic acid (leucovorin) if severe. Peritoneal dialysis is not effective in removing TMP or sulfas from the circulation.

Drug Interactions - Trimethoprim/sulfa may prolong the clotting times in patients receiving **coumarin (warfarin)** anticoagulants. Sulfonamides may displace other highly bound drugs, such as **methotrexate, phenylbutazone, thiazide diuretics, salicylates, probenicid and phenytoin.**

Although the clinical significance of these interactions is not entirely clear, patients should be monitored for enhanced effects of the displaced agents. **Antacids** may decrease the bioavailability of sulfonamides if administered concurrently. Trimethoprim may decrease the therapeutic effect of **cyclosporine (systemic)** and increase the risk of nephrotoxicity developing.

Drug/Laboratory Interactions - When using the Jaffe alkaline picrate reaction assay for **creatinine** determination, trimethoprim/sulfa may cause an overestimation of approximately 10%. Sulfonamides may give false-positive results for **urine glucose** determinations when using the Benedict's method.

Doses -

Note: There is significant controversy regarding the frequency of dosing these drugs. See the pharmacokinetic section above for more information. Unless otherwise noted, doses are for combined amounts of trimethoprim/sulfa.

Dogs:

For susceptible infections:
a) 30 mg/kg PO or IV q12h (avoid or reduce dose in patients with renal failure; avoid in pregnant or breeding animals (Vaden and Papich 1995)
b) 30 mg/kg q12h (if treating Nocardia, double dose) (Ford and Aronson 1985)
c) 15 mg/kg PO or SQ q12h or 30 mg/kg PO, SQ q24h (Kirk 1989)
d) 30 mg/kg PO or 26.4 mg/kg SQ once daily (Package insert; *Tribrissen®*—Coopers)
e) For routine infections: 15 mg/kg PO, SQ *bid*
   For meningitis: 15 mg/kg PO, IV *bid-tid*
   For pneumocystis carinii: 15 mg/kg PO *tid* for 14 days
   For mastitis: 30 mg/kg PO *bid* for 7 days
   For toxoplasmosis: 15 mg/kg PO *bid-tid* (Morgan 1988)
f) For coccidiosis: 30 mg/kg PO once daily for 10 days (Matz 1995)

Cats:

For susceptible infections:
a) 30 mg/kg PO or SQ q12-24h (Papich 1988)
b) 30 mg/kg q12h (if treating Nocardia, double dose) (Ford and Aronson 1985)
c) For toxoplasmosis: 15 mg/kg PO bid has resulted in resolution of CNS disease in some cats. (Lappin 1995)

Pocket Pets/Rodents:

For empiric antibiotic therapy:
a) 15 - 30 mg/kg PO q12h (Oglesbee 1995)

Cattle:

For susceptible infections:
a) 44 mg/kg once daily IM or IV using 48% suspension. (Upson 1988)
b) 25 mg/kg IV or IM q24h (Burrows 1980)
c) Calves: 48 mg/kg IV or IM q24h (Baggot 1983)

Horses:

For susceptible infections:
a) 15 mg/kg IV q8-12h (Brumbaugh 1987)
b) Foals: 15 mg/kg IV q12h (dose extrapolated from adult horses) (Caprile and Short 1987)
c) 22 mg/kg IV q24h or 30 mg/kg PO q24h (Upson 1988)
d) 30 mg/kg PO once daily or 21.3 mg/kg IV once daily (Package inserts; *Tribrissen®*—Coopers)
e) 24 mg/kg PO, IV or IM q12h (Baggot and Prescott 1987)

Swine:

For susceptible infections:
a) 48 mg/kg IM q24h (Baggot 1983)

Birds:

For susceptible infections:
a) Using TMP/SMX oral suspension (240 mg/5 ml): 2 ml/kg PO *bid*. Good for many gram positive and negative enteric and respiratory infections, particularly in hand-fed babies. May cause emesis in macaws. (McDonald 1989)
b) For respiratory and enteric infections in psittacines using the 24% injectable suspension: 0.22 ml/kg IM once to twice daily.
   For coccidiosis in toucans and mynahs using TMP/SMX oral suspension (240 mg/5 ml): 2.2 ml/kg once daily for 5 days. May be added to feed.

For respiratory and enteric infections in hand-fed baby psittacines using TMP/SMX oral suspension (240 mg/5 ml): 0.22 ml/30 grams *bid* to *tid* for 5-7 days. (Clubb 1986)

   c) Using oral suspension: 50 -100 mg/kg (of combined product) PO q12h (Hoeffer 1995)

Reptiles:

For susceptible infections:

   a) For most species: 30 mg/kg IM (upper part of body) once daily for 2 treatments, then every othe day for 5-12 treatments. May be useful for enteric infections. (Gauvin 1993)

Monitoring Parameters -

   1) Clinical efficacy

   2) Adverse effects; with chronic therapy, periodic complete blood counts should be considered.

   3) Thyroid function tests should be considered (baseline and ongoing) particularly in dogs recieving long term treatment

Client Information - If using suspension, shake well before using. Does not need to be refrigerated. Animals must be allowed free access to water and must not become dehydrated while on therapy.

Dosage Forms/Preparations/FDA Approval Status/Withholding Times -

Veterinary-Approved Products:

Trimethoprim (TMP)/Sulfadiazine (SDZ) Oral Tablets:

   30's: 5 mg TMP/25 mg SDZ (coated tablets)

   120's: 20 mg TMP/100 mg SDZ (coated tablets)

   480's: 80 mg TMP/400 mg SDZ (uncoated, scored tablets)

   960's: 160 mg TMP/800 mg SDZ (uncoated, unscored tablets)

Tribrissen® (Schering), (Rx) Approved for use in dogs.

Trimethoprim (TMP)/Sulfadiazine (SDZ) Oral Paste. Each gram contains 67 mg trimethoprim and 333 mg sulfadiazine. Available in 37.5 gram (total weight) syringes.; *Tribrissen*® *400 Oral Paste* (Schering) (Rx) Approved for use in horses.

In Canada, trimethoprim and sulfadoxine are available for use in cattle and swine (*Trivetrin*®—Wellcome; *Borgal*®—Hoechst). They have a slaughter withdrawal of 10 days and milk withdrawal of 96 hours.

Human-Approved Products:

Trimethoprim (alone) Tablets: 100 mg and 200 mg; *Proloprim*® (Glaxo Wellcome); *Trimpex*® (Roche); generic, (Rx)

Trimethoprim 80 mg and Sulfamethoxazole 400 mg Tablets; Trimethoprim 160 mg and Sulfamethoxazole 800 mg Tablets; *Bactrim*®, *Bactrim-DS*® (Roche); *Septra*®, *Septra*® DS, (Glaxo Wellcome); *Cotrim*®, *Cotrim-DS*® (Lemmon), generic; (Rx)

Trimethoprim 8 mg/ml and Sulfamethoxazole 40 mg/ml oral suspension in pint bottles; *Bactrim Pediatric*® (Roche); *Septra*® (Glaxo Wellcome); *Cotrim Pediatric*® (Lemmon) (Rx), Sulfatrim, generic (Rx); generic; (Rx)

Trimethoprim 16 mg/ml and Sulfamethoxazole 80 mg/ml for IV infusion in 5, 10, 20 and 30 ml vials ; *Bactrim*® *IV*(Roche); *Septra*® *IV*(Glaxo Wellcome); generic (Rx)

Because of the unavailability of veterinary trimethoprim/sulfadiazine injection in the USA, the human injectable product has been used. Before giving IV, the product must be diluted, generally at a rate of 1 ml of TMP/SMZ injection per 25 mls of dextrose 5% injection. Once diluted the injection should be used within 6 hours. Some reports of administering the drug SubQ to ruminants have also been received. To minimize potential local reactions, the injection should be diluted at a rate of about 1 ml TMP/SMZ injection to 5 ml dextrose 5%.

SULFADIMETHOXINE

Chemistry - A long-acting sulfonamide, sulfadimethoxine occurs as an odorless or almost odorless, creamy white powder. It is very slightly soluble in water and slightly soluble in alcohol.

Storage/Stability/Compatibility - Unless otherwise instructed by the manufacturer, store sulfadimethoxine products at room temperature and protect from light. Sulfadimethoxine injection should be stored at room temperature (15-30°C). If crystals form due to exposure to cold temperatures, either warm the vial or store at room temperature for several days to resolubolize the drug. Efficacy is not impaired by this process.

Information on the Pharmacology, Contraindications, Precautions, Reproductive Safety, Adverse Effects, Warnings, Overdosage, Acute Toxicity, Drug Interactions, Drug/Laboratory Interactions, Monitoring Parameters & Client Information for the sulfon-amide agents can be found in the Sulfachlorpyridazine and the TMP/Sulfa monographs.

Uses/Indications - Sulfadimethoxine injection and tablets are approved for use in dogs and cats for respiratory, genitourinary, enteric and soft tissue infections caused by susceptible organisms. Sulfadimethoxine is also used in the treatment of coccidiosis in dogs although not approved for this indication.

In horses, sulfadimethoxine injection is approved for the treatment of respiratory infections caused by *Streptococcus equi*.

In cattle, the drug is approved for treating shipping fever complex, calf diphtheria, bacterial pneumonia and foot rot caused by susceptible organisms.

In poultry, sulfadimethoxine is added to drinking water to treat coccidiosis, fowl cholera and infectious coryza.

Pharmacokinetics - In dogs, cats, swine and sheep, sulfadimethoxine is reportedly readily absorbed and well distributed. Relative volumes of distribution range from 0.17 L/kg in sheep to 0.35 L/kg in cattle and horses. The drug is also highly protein bound.

In most species, sulfadimethoxine is acetylated in the liver to acetylsulfadimethoxine and excreted unchanged in the liver. In dogs, the drug is not appreciably hepatically metabolized and renal excretion is the basis for the majority of elimination of the drug. Sulfadimethoxine's long elimination half-lives are a result of its appreciable reabsorption in the renal tubules. Serum half-lives reported in various species are: swine (14 hours), sheep (15 hours) and horses (11.3 hours).

Doses -

Dogs:
For susceptible infections:
a) 25 mg/kg PO, IV, or IM once daily (Davis 1985), (Kirk 1989)
b) 100 mg/kg PO, IV or IM once daily (Upson 1988)
c) 55 mg/kg PO, or IV, or SQ initially, then 27.5 mg/kg once daily thereafter. (Package insert; *Albon*®—Roche)

For coccidiosis:
a) 55 mg/kg PO initially on the first day of therapy, then 27.5 mg/kg PO once daily for 9 days (Matz 1995)
b) 50 mg/kg once daily for the first day, then 25 mg/kg once daily for 14-20 days. Sulfas are coccidiostatic. It is important that supportive care, including fluids and good nutrition be maintained during therapy. (Cornelius and Roberson 1986)

Cats:
For susceptible infections:
a) 25 mg/kg PO, IV, or IM once daily (Davis 1985), (Kirk 1989)
b) 100 mg/kg PO, IV or IM once daily (Upson 1988)
c) 55 mg/kg PO, or IV, or SQ initially, then 27.5 mg/kg once daily thereafter. (Package insert; *Albon*®—Roche)

For coccidiosis:
a) 50 mg/kg once daily for the first day, then 25 mg/kg once daily for 14-20 days. Sulfas are coccidiostatic. It is important that supportive care, including fluids and good nutrition be maintained during therapy. (Cornelius and Roberson 1986)

Cattle:
For susceptible infections:
a) 110 mg/kg PO or IV once daily (Upson 1988)
b) 55 mg/kg IV initially, then 27.5 mg/kg IV once daily. (Baggot 1983)
c) 110 mg/kg PO q24h (Burrows 1980)
d) 55 mg/kg PO or IV initially, then 27.5 mg/kg q24h. (Jenkins 1986)
e) 55 mg/kg IV or PO initially, then 27.5 mg/kg q24h IV or PO for up to 5 days. If using sustained release boluses: 137.5 mg/kg PO every 4 days. (Package insert; *Albon*®—Roche)

Horses:
For susceptible infections:
a) 55 mg/kg PO or IV q12h (Upson 1988)
b) 55 mg/kg IV or PO initially, then 27.5 mg/kg q24h IV (Package insert; *Albon*®—Roche)

Dosage Forms/Preparations/FDA Approval Status/Withholding Times -
Veterinary-Approved Products:

Sulfadimethoxine Injection 400 mg/ml (40%) in 100 ml and 250 ml vials

Albon® (Pfizer); (Rx) Approved for use in dogs, cats, horses and cattle. Not to be used in horses intended for food or calves to be processed for veal. Slaughter withdrawal = 5 days (cattle); milk withdrawal = 60 hours.

Sulfadimethoxine Oral Tablets 125 mg, 250 mg, 500 mg

Albon® (Pfizer), (Rx) Approved for use in dogs and cats.

Sulfadimethoxine Oral Suspension 50 mg/ml in 1 oz. and 16 oz. bottles

Albon® (Pfizer); (Rx) Approved for use in dogs and cats.

Sulfadimethoxine Oral Suspension 125 mg/ml 5% in 2 and 16 oz. bottles

Albon® (Pfizer) (Rx) Approved for use in dogs and cats.

Sulfadimethoxine Oral Boluses 5 g, & 15 g

Albon® (Pfizer); (OTC) Approved for use in cattle. Slaughter withdrawal = 7 days (cattle); milk withdrawal = 60 hours.

Sulfadimethoxine Oral Boluses Sustained-Release 12.5 g

Albon® (Pfizer); (Rx) Approved for use in non-lactating cattle. Slaughter withdrawal = 21 days (cattle)

Sulfadimethoxine Soluble Powder 94.6 g/packet (for addition to drinking water)

Albon® (Pfizer); (OTC) Approved for use in dairy calves, dairy heifers, beef cattle, broiler and replacement chickens only, and meat-producing turkeys. Slaughter withdrawal = 7 days (cattle); 5 days (poultry—do not use in chickens over 16 weeks old or in turkeys over 24 weeks old).

Sulfadimethoxine 12.5% Concentrated Solution (for addition to drinking water); *Albon*® (Pfizer); Generic (OTC) Approved for use in chickens, turkeys and cattle. Slaughter withdrawal = 7 days (cattle); 5 days (poultry—do not use in chickens over 16 weeks old or in turkeys over 24 weeks old).

Human-Approved Products: None

SULFADIMETHOXINE/ORMETOPRIM

Chemistry - A diaminopyrimidine structurally related to trimethoprim, ormetoprim occurs as a white, almost tasteless powder. The chemistry of sulfadimethoxine is described in the previous monograph.

Storage/Stability/Compatibility - Unless otherwise instructed by the manufacturer, store tablets in tight, light resistant containers at room temperature.

Pharmacology - Sulfadimethoxine/ormetoprim shares mechanisms of action and probably the bacterial spectrum of activity with trimethoprim/sulfa. Alone, sulfonamides are bacteriostatic agents, but in combination with either ormetoprim or trimethoprim, the potentiated sulfas are bactericidal. Potentiated sulfas sequentially inhibit enzymes in the folic acid pathway, thereby inhibiting bacterial thymidine synthesis. The sulfonamide blocks the conversion of para-aminobenzoic acid (PABA) to dihydrofolic acid (DFA) and ormetoprim blocks the conversion of DFA to tetrahydrofolic acid by inhibiting dihydrofolate reductase.

The potentiated sulfas have a fairly broad spectrum of activity. Gram positive bacteria that are generally susceptible include, most streptococci, many strains of staphylococcus, and *Nocardia*. Many gram negative organisms of the family Enterobacteriaceae are susceptible to the potentiated sulfas, but not *Pseudomonas aeruginosa*. Some protozoa (*Pneumocystis carinii*, Coccidia and Toxoplasma) are also inhibited by the combination. Potentiated sulfas reportedly have little activity against most anaerobes, but opinions on this vary.

Resistance will develop slower to the combination of drugs, than to either one alone. In gram negative organisms, resistance is usually plasmid-mediated.

Uses/Indications - The present approved indications for this combination are for the treatment of skin and soft tissue infections in dogs caused by susceptible strains of *Staphylococcus aureus* and *E. coli*. Because clinical experience with this drug is extremely limited at the time of this writing, further uses and indications may be forthcoming.

Pharmacokinetics - The pharmacokinetics of sulfadimethoxine are outlined in the previous monograph. Pharmacokinetic data for ormetoprim is not available at the time of this writing, but the manufacturer claims that therapeutic levels are maintained over 24 hours at recommended doses.

Contraindications/Precautions/Reproductive Safety - The manufacturer states that ormetoprim/sulfadimethoxine should not be used in dogs or horses showing marked liver parenchymal damage, blood dyscrasias, or in those with a history of sulfonamide sensitivity.

This combination should be used with caution in patients with pre-existing hepatic or thyroid disease.

Safety of ormetoprim/sulfadimethoxine has not been established in pregnant animals. Reports of teratogenicity (cleft palate) have been reported in some lab animals with trimethoprim/sulfa.

Adverse Effects/Warnings - Adverse effects with this combination have not been reported at recommended doses, but the number of evaluated patients is very small at the time of this writing. This combination would be expected to exhibit an adverse reaction profile in dogs similar to that seen with trimethoprim/sulfa, including: keratoconjunctivitis sicca (which may be irreversible), acute neutrophilic hepatitis with icterus, vomiting, anorexia, diarrhea, fever, hemolytic anemia, urticaria, polyarthritis, facial swelling, polydipsia, polyuria and cholestasis. Acute hypersensitivity reactions manifesting as Type I (anaphylaxis) or Type III reaction (serum sickness) can also be seen. Hypersensitivity reactions appear to be more common in large breed dogs; Doberman Pinschers may possibly be more susceptible to this effect than other breeds. Other hematologic effects (anemias, agranulocytosis) are possible, but fairly rare in dogs.

Long-term (8 weeks) therapy at recommended doses with ormetoprim/sulfadimethoxine (27.5 mg/kg once daily) resulted in elevated serum cholesterol, thyroid and liver weights, mild follicular thyroid hyperplasia and enlarged basophilic cells in the pituitary. The manufacturer states that the principal treatment-related effect of extended or excessive usage is hypothyroidism.

Overdosage/Acute Toxicity - In experimental studies in dogs, doses greater than 80 mg/kg resulted in slight tremors and increased motor activity in some dogs. Higher doses may result in depression, anorexia or seizures.

It is suggested that very high oral overdoses be handled by emptying the gut using standard precautions and protocols and by treating symptoms supportively and symptomatically.

Drug Interactions; Drug/Laboratory Interactions - None have been noted for this combination, but it would be expected that the potential interactions outlined for the trimethoprim/sulfa monograph would also apply to this combination; refer to that monograph for more information.

Doses -
  Dogs:
    For susceptible infections:
      a) Initially 55 mg/kg (combined drug) PO on the first day of therapy, then 27.5 mg/kg PO once daily for at least 2 days after remission of clinical signs. Not approved for treatment longer than 21 days. (Package insert; *Primor*®—SKB)

Monitoring Parameters -
  1) Clinical efficacy
  2) Adverse effects

Client Information - Animals must be allowed free access to water and must not become dehydrated while on therapy.

Dosage Forms/Preparations/FDA Approval Status/Withholding Times -
Veterinary-Approved Products:
Sulfadimethoxine/Ormetoprim Tablets (scored)
  120's: 100 mg Sulfadimethoxine, 20 mg Ormetoprim
  240's: 200 mg Sulfadimethoxine, 40 mg Ormetoprim
  600's: 500 mg Sulfadimethoxine, 100 mg Ormetoprim
  1200's: 1000 mg Sulfadimethoxine, 200 mg Ormetoprim
    Primor® (Pfizer); (Rx) Approved for use in dogs.

  Human-Approved Products: None

SULFASALAZINE

Chemistry - Sulfasalazine is basically a molecule of sulfapyridine linked by a diazo bond to the diazonium salt of salicylic acid. It occurs as an odorless, bright yellow to brownish-yellow fine powder. Less than 0.1 mg is soluble in 1 ml of water and about 0.34 mg is soluble in 1 ml of alcohol. It is also known as salazosulfapyridine or salicylazosulfapyridine.

Storage/Stability/Compatibility - Sulfasalazine tablets (either plain or enteric-coated) should be stored at temperatures less than 40°C and preferably at room temperature (15-30°C) in well-closed containers. The oral suspension should be stored at room temperature (15-30°C); avoid freezing.

Pharmacology - While the exact mechanism of action for its therapeutic effects in treating colitis in small animals has not been determined, it is believed that after sulfasalazine is cleaved into sulfapyridine and 5-aminosalicylic acid (5-ASA, mesalamine) by bacteria in the gut the antibacterial (sulfapyridine) and/or anti-inflammatory (5-ASA) activity alters the symptoms/course of the disease. Levels of both drugs in the colon are higher then by giving them orally as separate agents.

Uses/Indications - Sulfasalazine is used for the treatment of inflammatory bowel disease in dogs and cats.

Pharmacokinetics - Only about 10-33% of an orally administered dose of sulfasalazine is absorbed. Apparently, some of this absorbed drug is then excreted unchanged in the bile. Unabsorbed and biliary excreted drug is cleaved into 5-ASA and sulfapyridine in the colon by bacterial flora. The sulfapyridine component is rapidly absorbed, but only a small percentage of the 5-ASA is absorbed.

Absorbed sulfapyridine and 5-ASA are hepatically metabolized and then renally excreted.

Contraindications/Precautions/Reproductive Safety - Sulfasalazine is contraindicated in animals hypersensitive to it, sulfonamides or salicylates. It is also contraindicated in patients with intestinal or urinary obstructions. It should be used with caution in animals with preexisting liver, renal or hematologic diseases. Because cats can be sensitive to salicylates (see the aspirin monograph), use caution when using this drug in that species.

Although sulfasalazine has not been proven to be harmful to use during pregnancy and incidences of neonatal kernicterus in infants born to women taking sulfasalazine are low, it should only be used when clearly indicated. In laboratory animal studies (rats, rabbits), doses of 6 times normal (human) caused impairment of fertility in male animals This effect is thought to be caused by the sulfapyridine component and was reversible upon discontinuation of the drug.

Adverse Effects/Warnings - Although adverse effects do occur in dogs, with keratoconjunctivitis sicca (KCS) reported most frequently, they are considered to occur relatively uncommonly. Other potential adverse effects include cholestatic jaundice, hemolytic anemia, leukopenia, vomiting, decreased sperm counts and an allergic dermatitis.

Cats can occasionally develop anorexia and vomiting which may be alleviated through the use of the enteric-coated tablets. Anemias secondary to sulfasalazine are also potentially possible in cats.

Overdosage/Acute Toxicity - Little specific information is available regarding overdoses with this agent, but because massive overdoses could cause significant salicylate and/or sulfonamide toxicity, standard protocols (empty stomach, cathartics, etc.) should be considered. Urine alkalinization and forced diuresis may also be beneficial in selected cases.

Drug Interactions - Sulfasalazine shares the interactive potential with other sulfonamides and may displace highly protein bound drugs, such as **methotrexate, warfarin, phenylbutazone, thiazide diuretics, salicylates, probenicid and phenytoin.** Although the clinical significance of these interactions is not entirely clear, patients should be monitored for enhanced effects of the displaced agents.

Antacids may decrease the oral bioavailability of sulfonamides if administered concurrently.

Sulfasalazine may decrease the bioavailability of **folic acid** or **digoxin**; enhanced digoxin monitoring is warranted if both drugs are necessary and folic acid supplementation may be required with chronic therapy.

Ferrous sulfate or other iron salts may decrease the blood levels of sulfasalazine if administered concurrently; clinical significance is unknown.

Doses -
  Dogs:
    For inflammatory bowel disease:
      a) Initially, 20 - 30 mg/kg q8h PO. If lesions are mild (histologically), the drug can be usually stopped in 3 weeks. Severe cases may require therapy for 6 weeks or more. (Richter 1989)
      b) Chronic (Ulcerative) colitis: 10 - 15 mg/kg PO *tid-qid*; maximum of 3 grams per day. Although response is variable, most dogs respond in 4-5 weeks. Then decrease dose to 10 - 15 mg/kg once to twice daily for another 2-3 weeks. Some cases require treatment for several months; use trial and error to find dose that maintains remission (2 weeks of therapy before assessing efficacy). (DeNovo 1988)
      c) For chronic enterocolitis: 10 - 15 mg/kg q6h PO. (DeNovo 1986)
      d) For chronic colitis: 35 - 50 mg/kg/day divided into 3-4 equal doses. Reevaluate at 2-4 weeks of therapy; only animals with severe forms of colitis (*e.g.*, ulcerative colitis) require long-term sulfasalazine therapy. (Chiapella 1986)
  Cats:
    For inflammatory bowel disease:
      a) 20 - 25 mg/kg q12h- q24h PO. (Richter 1989)

    b) Lymphocytic-plasmacytic enteritis where colon is involved: 10 - 20 mg/kg q12h PO. For idiopathic colitis: 10 - 20 mg/kg q12h PO or 250 mg total dose (1/2 - 500 mg tablet) once daily. (Sherding 1989)

    c) 10 - 20 mg/kg PO q8-12h (maximum of 10 days) (Dimski 1995)

Monitoring Parameters -
1) Efficacy
2) Adverse effects, particularly KCS
3) Occasional CBC, liver function tests are warranted with chronic therapy

Client Information - Clients should monitor for symptoms of KCS (dry cornea, blepharospasm, bilateral mucopurulent discharge) and be instructed to report such to the veterinarian immediately.

Dosage Forms/Preparations/FDA Approval Status/Withholding Times -
  Veterinary-Approved Products: None
  Human-Approved Products:

    Sulfasalazine Oral Tablets 500 mg; *Azulfidine®* (Pharmacia), generic; (Rx)

    Sulfasalazine 500 mg Enteric-coated Tablets; *Azulfidine® EN-tabs®* (Pharmacia), generic; (Rx)

Syrup of Ipecac - see Ipecac

TERBUTALINE SULFATE

Chemistry - A synthetic sympathomimetic amine, terbutaline sulfate occurs as a slightly bitter-tasting, white to gray-white, crystalline powder that may have a faint odor of acetic acid. One gram is soluble in 1.5 ml of water or 250 ml of alcohol. The commercially available injection has its pH adjusted to 3-5 with hydrochloric acid.

Storage/Stability/Compatibility - Terbutaline tablets should be stored in tight containers at room temperature (15-30°C). Tablets have an expiration date of 3 years beyond the date of manufacture. Terbutaline injection should be stored at room temperature (15-30°C), and protected from light. The injection has an expiration date of 2 years after the date of manufacture.

Terbutaline injection is stable over a pH range of 1-7. Discolored solutions should not be used. It is compatible with D_5W and aminophylline.

Pharmacology - Terbutaline stimulates beta-adrenergic receptors found principally in bronchial, vascular, and uterine smooth muscles ($beta_2$) and bronchial and vascular smooth muscle relaxation occurs with resultant reduced airway resistance. At usual doses it has little effect on cardiac ($beta_1$) receptors and usually does not cause direct cardiostimulatory effects. Occasionally, a tachycardia develops which may be a result of either direct beta stimulation or a reflex response secondary to peripheral vasodilation. Terbutaline has virtually no alpha-adrenergic activity.

Uses/Indications - Terbutaline is used as a bronchodilating agent in the adjunctive treatment of cardiopulmonary diseases (including tracheobronchitis, collapsing trachea, pulmonary edema, and allergic bronchitis) in small animals.

It has been used occasionally in horses for its bronchodilating effects, but adverse effects have limited its use in this species. A related compound, clenbuterol, has been used to a much greater extent for treating bronchoconstriction in the horse, but it is not available commercially in the United States.

Oral and intravenous terbutaline has been used successfully (in humans) in the inhibition of premature labor symptoms.

Pharmacokinetics - The pharmacokinetics of this agent have apparently not been thoroughly studied in domestic animals. In humans, only about 33-50% of an oral dose is absorbed; peak bronchial effects occur within 2-3 hours and activity persists for up to 8 hours. Terbutaline is well absorbed following SQ administration with an onset of action occurring within 15 minutes, peak effects at 30-60 minutes, and a duration of activity for up to 4 hours.

Terbutaline is distributed into milk, but at levels of approximately 1% of the oral dose given to the mother. Terbutaline is principally excreted unchanged in the urine (60%), but is also metabolized in the liver to an inactive sulfate conjugate.

Contraindications/Precautions - Terbutaline is contraindicated in patients hypersensitive to it. One veterinary school formulary (Schultz 1986) states that terbutaline is contraindicated in dogs and cats with heart disease, especially with CHF or cardiomyopathy. It should be used with caution in patients with diabetes, hyperthyroidism, hypertension, seizure disorders, or cardiac disease (especially with concurrent arrhythmias).

Adverse Effects/Warnings - Most adverse effects are dose-related and are those that would be expected with sympathomimetic agents, including increased heart rate, tremors, CNS excitement (nervousness) and dizziness. These effects are generally transient and mild and do not require discontinuation of therapy. After parenteral injection in horses, sweating and CNS excitation have been reported.

Transient hypokalemia has been reported in humans receiving beta-adrenergic agents. If an animal is susceptible to developing hypokalemia, it is suggested that additional serum potassium monitoring be done early in therapy.

Overdosage - Symptoms of significant overdose after systemic administration may include arrhythmias (bradycardia, tachycardia, heart block, extrasystoles), hypertension, fever, vomiting, mydriasis, and CNS stimulation. If a recent oral ingestion, it should be handled like other overdoses (empty gut, give activated charcoal and a cathartic) if the animal does not have significant cardiac or CNS effects. If cardiac arrhythmias require treatment, a beta blocking agent (*e.g.,* propranolol) can be used, but may precipitate bronchoconstriction.

Drug Interactions - Use of terbutaline with **other sympathomimetic amines** may increase the risk of developing adverse cardiovascular effects. **Beta-adrenergic blocking agents** (*e.g.,* propranolol) may antagonize the actions of terbutaline. **Tricyclic antidepressants or monoamine oxidase inhibitors** may potentiate the vascular effects of terbutaline. Use with inhalation anesthetics (*e.g.,* **halothane, isoflurane, methoxyflurane**), may predispose the patient to ventricular arrhythmias, particularly in patients with preexisting cardiac disease—use cautiously. Use with **digitalis** glycosides may increase the risk of cardiac arrhythmias.

Doses -
Dogs:
- a) 0.01 mg/kg SQ q4h; 0.03 mg/kg PO q8h (Davis 1985)
- b) 2.5 mg PO q8h (Papich 1986)
- c) 2.5 - 5 mg PO q8h; 0.625 mg/10 lbs body weight PO q8h (McConnell and Hughey 1987)

Cats:
- a) 0.01 mg/kg SQ q4h; 0.03 mg/kg PO q8h (Davis 1985)
- b) 1.25 mg PO q12h (Papich 1986)

Horses:
- a) 0.0033 mg/kg IV (Robinson 1987)
- b) 0.025 mg/kg once daily PO; 0.0033 mg/kg IV (Schultz 1986)
- c) 0.13 mg/kg PO q8h (McConnell and Hughey 1987)
- d) 30 mg PO *tid* (in a 450 kg horse); usually used in combination with aminphylline and prednisone. (Duran 1992)

Monitoring Parameters -
1) Clinical symptom improvement; auscultation
2) Cardiac rate, rhythm (if indicated)
3) Serum potassium, early in therapy if animal susceptible to hypokalemia

Client Information - Contact veterinarian if animal's condition deteriorates or becomes acutely ill.

Dosage Forms/Preparations/FDA Approval Status/Withholding Times -
Veterinary-Approved Products: None
Human-Approved Products:

Terbutaline Sulfate Oral Tablets 2.5 mg, 5 mg; *Brethine*® (Geigy); *Bricanyl*® (Hoechst Marion Roussel); (Rx)

Terbutaline Injection 1 mg/ml in 2 ml amps with 1 ml fill; *Brethine*® (Geigy), *Bricanyl*®S (Hoechst Marion Roussel); (Rx)

Also available in a metered-dose inhaler.

TESTOSTERONE CYPIONATE
TESTOSTERONE ENANTHATE
TESTOSTERONE PROPRIONATE

Chemistry - The esterified compounds, testosterone cypionate, enanthate, and propionate are available commercially as injectable products. Testosterone cypionate occurs as an odorless to having a faint odor, creamy white to white, crystalline powder. It is insoluble in water, soluble in vegetable oils, and freely soluble in alcohol. Testosterone cypionate has a melting range of 98°-104°C. It may also be known as testosterone cyclopentylpropionate.

Testosterone enanthate occurs as an odorless to having a faint odor, creamy white to white, crystalline powder. It is soluble in vegetable oils, insoluble in water and melts between 34-39°C.

Testosterone propionate occurs as odorless, creamy white to white, crystals or crystalline powder. It is insoluble in water, freely soluble in alcohol and soluble in vegetable oils. Testosterone propionate melts between 118-123°C.

Storage/Stability/Compatibility - The commercially available injectable preparations of testosterone cypionate, enanthate and propionate should be stored at room temperature; avoid freezing or exposing to temperatures greater than 40°C. If exposed to low temperature a precipitate may form, but should redissolve with shaking and rewarming. If a wet needle or syringe is used to draw up the parenteral solutions, cloudy solutions may result, but will not affect the drugs' potency.

Pharmacology - The principle endogenous androgenic steroid, testosterone is responsible for many secondary sex characteristic of the male as well as the maturation and growth of the male reproductive organs and increasing libido.

Testosterone has anabolic activity with resultant increased protein anabolism and decreased protein catabolism. Testosterone causes nitrogen, sodium, potassium and phosphorus retention and decreases the urinary excretion of calcium. Nitrogen balance is improved only when an adequate intake of both calories and protein occurs.

By stimulating erythropoeitic stimulating factor, testosterone can stimulate the production of red blood cells. Large doses of exogenous testosterone can inhibit spermatogenesis through a negative feedback mechanism inhibiting lutenizing hormone (LH).

Testosterone may help maintain the normal urethral muscle tone and the integrity of the urethral mucosa in male dogs. It may also be necessary to prevent some types of dermatoses.

Uses/Indications - The use of injectable esters of testosterone in veterinary medicine is limited primarily to its use in dogs (and perhaps cats) for the treatment of testosterone-responsive urinary incontinence in neutered males. Testosterone has been used to treat a rare form of dermatitis (exhibited by bilateral alopeci) in neutered male dogs. These drugs are also used in bovine medicine to produce an estrus-detector (teaser) animal in cull cows, heifers, steers.

The use of testosterone to increase libido, treat hypogonadism, aspermia and infertility in domestic animals has been disappointing.

Pharmacokinetics - Orally administered testosterone is rapidly metabolized by the GI mucosa and the liver (first-pass effect) and very little reaches the systemic circulation. The esterified compounds, testosterone enanthate and cypionate are less polar than testosterone and more slowly absorbed from lipid tissue after IM injection. The duration of action of these compounds may persist for 2-4 weeks after IM injection. Testosterone propionate reportedly has a much shorter duration of action than either the enanthate or cypionate ester. Because absorption is dependent upon several factors (volume injected, perfusion, etc.), durations of action may be variable.

Testosterone is highly bound to a specific testosterone-estradiol globulin (98% in humans). The quantity of this globulin determines the amount of drug that is in the free or bound form. The free form concentration determines the plasma half-life of the hormone.

Testosterone is metabolized in the liver and is, with its metabolites, excreted in the urine (≈90%) and the feces (≈6%). The plasma half-life of testosterone has been reported to be between 10-100 minutes in humans. The plasma half-life of testosterone cypionate has been reported to be 8 days.

Contraindications/Precautions - Testosterone therapy is contraindicated in patients with known hypersensitivity to the drug or prostate carcinoma. It should be used with caution in patients with renal, cardiac or hepatic dysfunction.

Adverse Effects/Warnings - Adverse effects are reportedly uncommon when injectable testosterone products are used in male dogs to treat hormone-responsive incontinence. Perianal adenomas, perineal hernias, prostatic disorders and behavior changes are all possible, however. Polycythemia has been reported in humans receiving high dosages of testosterone. High dosages or chronic usage may result in oligospermia or infertility in intact males.

Overdosage - No specific information was located; refer to the Adverse effects section for further information.

Drug Interactions - Testosterone administered with **oral anticoagulants** may cause increased bleeding in some patients. Diligent monitoring is necessary if patients are receiving androgens and oral anticoagulants. Anticoagulant dosage adjustments may be necessary when adding or discontinuing androgen therapy.

Diabetic patients receiving **insulin** may need dosage adjustments if androgen therapy is added or discontinued. Androgens may decrease blood glucose and decrease insulin requirements.

Androgens may enhance the edema that can be associated with **ACTH** or **adrenal steroid** therapy.

Drug/Laboratory Interactions - Concentrations of **protein bound iodine** (PBI) can be decreased in patients receiving testosterone therapy, but the clinical significance of this is probably not important. Androgen agents can decrease amounts of **thyroxine-binding globulin** and decrease total **T4** concentrations and increase **resin uptake of T3 and T4.** Free thyroid hormones are unaltered and clinically, there is no evidence of dysfunction.

Both **creatinine** and **creatine excretion** can be decreased by testosterone. Testosterone can increase the urinary excretion of **17-ketosteroids.**

Androgenic/anabolic steroids may alter **blood glucose** levels.

Androgenic/anabolic steroids may suppress **clotting factors II, V, VII, and X**.

Doses -
  Dogs:
      For testosterone-responsive urinary incontinence (may be used with phenylpropanolamine):
          a) Testosterone propionate: approximately 2 mg/kg IM or SQ 3 times per week.
              Testosterone cypionate: 200 mg IM once per month. (LaBato 1988), (Polzin and Osborne 1985)
          b) Testosterone propionate: 2.2 mg/kg IM q2-3 days.
              Testosterone cypionate: 2.2 mg/kg IM once per month. (Moreau and Lappin 1989), (Chew, DiBartola, and Fenner 1986)

  Cats:
      For testosterone-responsive urinary incontinence (may be used with phenylpropanolamine):
          a) Testosterone propionate 5 - 10 mg IM (Barsanti and Finco 1986)

  Cattle:
      To produce an estrus-detector (teaser) animal (cull cows, heifers, steers):
          a) Testosterone propionate 200 mg IM on day 1 and on days 4-9. On day 10, give 1 gram IM and attach a chinball marker and put with the breeding herd. To maintain the teaser give 1 gram booster every 10-14 days.
              Alternatively, initially give testosterone enanthate 0.5 gram IM and 1.5 gram SQ (divided in two separate locations). After 4 days attach chinball marker and put in with breeding herd. To maintain, give 0.5 - 0.75 gram SQ every 10-14 days. (Wolfe 1986)

Monitoring Parameters -
    1) Efficacy
    2) Adverse effects

Dosage Forms/Preparations/FDA Approval Status/Withholding Times -
  Veterinary-Approved Products: No known testosterone products (with the exception of combinations with estradiol as growth promotant implants) approved for use in veterinary species were located. Testosterone propionate (200 mg) is also available in combination with estradiol benzoate (20 mg) as a growth promotant in beef cattle. Trade names include *HEIFER-oid*® (Bio-Ceutic) and *Synovex-H*® (Syntex); (Rx)

  Human-Approved Products:
      Testosterone Cypionate (in oil) for injection 50 mg/ml, 100 mg/ml, & 200 mg/ml in 1 & 10 ml vials. Available generically and in many proprietary labeled products. A commonly known trade name is *Depo-Testosterone*® (Upjohn); (Rx).

      Testosterone Enanthate (in oil) for injection 100 mg/ml and 200 mg/ml in 5 and 10 ml vials & 1 ml syringes; Available generically and in many proprietary labeled products; (Rx)

      Testosterone Propionate Injection (in oil): 100 mg/ml in 10 ml vials 25 mg/ml, 50 mg/ml, & 100 mg/ml in 10 ml and 30 ml vials; Available generically; (Rx)

      Testosterone products are now controlled substances (C-III).

TETRACYCLINE HCL

Chemistry - An antibiotic obtained from *Streptomyces aureofaciens*, or derived semisynthetically from oxytetracycline, tetracycline HCl occurs as a moderately hygroscopic, yellow, crystalline powder. About 100 mg/ml is soluble in water and 10 mg/ml soluble in alcohol. Tetracycline base has a solubility of about 0.4 mg per ml of water and 20 mg per ml of alcohol. Commercially available tetracycline HCl for IM injection also contains magnesium chloride, procaine HCl and ascorbic acid.

Storage/Stability/Compatibility - Unless otherwise instructed by the manufacturer, tetracycline oral tablets and capsules should be stored in tight, light resistant containers at room temperature (15-30°C). The oral suspension and powder for injection should be stored at room temperature. Avoid freezing the oral suspension.

After reconstituting the IM product, it may be stored at room temperature but should be used within 24 hours of reconstitution. After reconstituting the intravenous product with sterile water to a concentration of 50 mg/ml, the preparation is stable for 12 hours at room temperature. If further diluted in an appropriate IV fluid, use immediately.

Tetracycline HCl for intravenous injection is reportedly **compatible** with the following IV fluids and drugs: 0.9% sodium chloride, D5W, D5W in normal saline, Ringer's injection, lactated Ringer's injection, 10% invert sugar, dextrose-Ringer's and lactated Ringer's combinations, ascorbic acid, cimetidine HCl, colistimethate sodium, corticotropin, ephedrine sulfate, isoproterenol HCl, kanamycin sulfate, lidocaine HCl, metaraminol bitartrate, norepinephrine bitartrate, oxytetracycline HCl, oxytocin, potassium chloride, prednisolone sodium phosphate, procaine HCl, promazine HCl, and vitamin B complex with C.

Drugs that are reportedly **incompatible** with tetracycline, data conflicts, or compatibility is concentration/time dependent, include: amikacin sulfate, aminophylline, ampicillin sodium, amobarbital sodium, amphotericin B, calcium chloride/gluconate, carbenicillin disodium, cephalothin sodium, cephapirin sodium, chloramphenicol sodium succinate, dimenhydrinate, erythromycin glucceptate/lactobionate, heparin sodium, hydrocortisone sodium succinate, meperidine HCl, morphine sulfate, methicillin sodium, methohexital sodium, methyldopate HCl, oxacillin sodium, penicillin G potassium/sodium, phenobarbital sodium, sodium bicarbonate, thiopental sodium, and warfarin sodium. Compatibility is dependent upon factors such as pH, concentration, temperature and diluents used. It is suggested to consult specialized references for more specific information (*e.g., Handbook on Injectable Drugs* by Trissel; see bibliography).

Pharmacology/Uses/Indications - Refer to the oxytetracycline monograph just preceding this one for information for tetracycline.

Pharmacokinetics - Both oxytetracycline and tetracycline are readily absorbed after oral administration to fasting animals. Bioavailabilities are approximately 60-80%. The presence of food or dairy products can significantly reduce the amount of tetracycline absorbed, with reductions of 50% or more possible. After IM administration, tetracycline is erratically and poorly absorbed with serum levels usually lower than those attainable with oral therapy.

Tetracyclines as a class, are widely distributed to heart, kidney, lungs, muscle, pleural fluid, bronchial secretions, sputum, bile, saliva, urine, synovial fluid, ascitic fluid, and aqueous and vitreous humor. Only small quantities of tetracycline and oxytetracycline are distributed to the CSF, and therapeutic levels may not be achievable. While all tetracyclines distribute to the prostate and eye, doxycycline or minocycline penetrate better into these and most other tissues. Tetracyclines cross the placenta, enter fetal circulation and are distributed into milk. The volume of distribution of tetracycline is approximately 1.2 - 1.3 L/kg in small animals. The amount of plasma protein binding is about 20 - 67% for tetracycline.

Both oxytetracycline and tetracycline are eliminated unchanged primarily via glomerular filtration. Patients with impaired renal function can have prolonged elimination half-lives and may accumulate the drug with repeated dosing. These drugs apparently are not metabolized, but are excreted into the GI tract via both biliary and nonbiliary routes and may become inactive after chelation with fecal materials. The elimination half-life of tetracycline is approximately 5-6 hours in dogs and cats.

Contraindications/Precautions/Reproductive Safety/
Adverse Effects/Warnings/ Overdosage/Acute Toxicity/Drug Interactions/-Drug-Laboratory Interactions - Refer to the oxytetracycline monograph preceding this one for information for tetracycline.

Doses -
  Dogs:
    For susceptible infections:
      a) For UTI: 55 mg/kg/day divided into 3 daily dosages PO (Rogers and Lees 1989)
      b) 20 mg/kg PO q8h; 7 mg/kg IV or IM q12h (Kirk 1989)
      c) 20 mg/kg PO q8-12h; (may give with food if GI upset occurs; avoid or reduce dose in animals with renal or severe liver failure; avoid in young, pregnant or breeding animals) (Vaden and Papich 1995)
      d) 22 - 33 mg/kg PO q8h (Aronson and Aucoin 1989)
      e) For Lyme Disease: 22 mg/kg PO *tid* (Lissman 1986)
      d) For acute colitis: 22 mg/kg PO *tid* (Morgan 1988)
      e) For brucellosis: 10 - 20 mg/kg PO *tid* for 28 days (Morgan 1988)
      f) For *Yersinia pestis* infections: 15 mg/kg PO *tid* (Morgan 1988)
      g) For mastitis: 10 mg/kg PO *tid* for 21 days (Morgan 1988)
      h) For Rocky Mountain Spotted Fever/ehrlichiosis: 22 mg/kg PO *tid* for 2 weeks. (Greene 1986)
      i) For rickettsial diseases:
        Ehrlichiosis: 22 mg/kg PO *tid* for at least 14 days
        Salmon Poisoning: 22 mg/kg PO *tid* for 10-14 days or 7 mg/kg IV *tid*
        Rocky Mountain Spotted Fever: 22 mg/kg PO *tid* for 10-14 days (Lissman 1988)

> j) For canine ehrlichiosis: 22 mg/kg every 8 hours for 2-3 months (duration of treatment based upon preliminary data). For prophylaxis in endemic areas: 6 mg/kg once daily. (Greene 1995)
>
> k) For Rocky Mountain Spotted Fever: 22 mg/kg q8h for 14-21 days (Sellon and Breitschwerdt 1995)

For facial tear staining:
  a) 5 - 10 mg/kg/day or 50 mg per dog per day. Results are variable. (Kern 1986)

For pleurodesis:
  a) Using capsules or aqueous solution; mix 20 mg/kg in 4 ml per kg of saline and infuse into pleural space. (Morgan 1988)

Cats:
For susceptible infections:
  a) 20 mg/kg PO q8h; 7 mg/kg IV or IM q12h (Kirk 1989)
  b) For rickettsial diseases: 16 mg/kg PO *tid* for 21 days (Morgan 1988)
  c) 20 mg/kg PO q8-12h; (may give with food if GI upset occurs; avoid or reduce dose in animals with renal or severe liver failure; avoid in young, pregnant or breeding animals) (Vaden and Papich 1995)
  d) 22 - 33 mg/kg PO q8h (Aronson and Aucoin 1989)

Cattle:
For susceptible infections in calves:
  a) 11 mg/kg orally (Howard 1986)
  b) 11 mg/kg PO *bid* for up to 5 days (Label directions; *Polyotic*®—American Cyanamid)

Sheep:
For susceptible infections:
  a) 11 mg/kg PO *bid* for up to 5 days (Label directions; *Polyotic*®—American Cyanamid)

Horses:
For susceptible infections:
  a) 5 - 7.5 mg/kg IV q12h (Brumbaugh 1987)

Swine:
For susceptible infections:
  a) 22 mg/kg PO for 3 to 5 days in drinking water (Label directions; *Polyotic*®—American Cyanamid)

Birds:
For susceptible infections:
  a) For treatment of psittacossis in conjunction with LA-200® (see oxytetracycline doses) and/or medicated pellets and/or Keet Life: Using 25 mg/ml oral suspension, mix 2 teaspoonsful to 1 cup of soft food.
     For mild respiratory disease (especially flock treatment): Mix 1 teaspoonful of 10 g/6.4 oz. soluble powder per gallon of drinking water. Used as an adjunct for psittacossis with other tetracycline forms. Will not reach therapeutic levels by itself. Prepare fresh solution twice daily as potency is rapidly lost. (McDonald 1989)
  b) Mix 1 teaspoonful of 10 g/6.4 oz. soluble powder per gallon of drinking water and administer for 5-10 days. Prepare fresh solution 2-3 times daily as potency is rapidly lost.
     For converting regimen to pelleted feeds administer oral suspension by gavage at 200 - 250 mg/kg once or twice daily until feeds are accepted. Is not adequate therapy for long-term chlamydiosis (psittacosis) treatment. (Clubb 1986)

Monitoring Parameters -
  1) Adverse effects
  2) Clinical efficacy
  3) Long-term use or in susceptible patients: periodic renal, hepatic, hematologic evaluations

Client Information - Avoid giving this drug orally within 1-2 hours of feeding, giving milk or dairy products. If gastrointestinal upset occurs, giving with a small amount of food may help, but this will also reduce the amount drug absorbed.

Dosage Forms/Preparations/FDA Approval Status/Withholding Times -
Veterinary -Approved Products:
Tetracycline Oral Suspension 100 mg/ml (approximately 5 mg/drop) in 15 ml and 30 ml bottles
>   *Panmycin Aquadrops*® (Upjohn); (Rx) Approved for use in dogs and cats.

Tetracycline HCl Oral Boluses 500 mg
>   *Polyotic*® *Oblets*® (American Cyanimid) (Rx) Approved for use in calves and sheep. Slaughter withdrawal = 12 days calves; = 5 days sheep.
>   *Panmycin*® *Oral Boluses* (Upjohn); (OTC) Approved for use in calves. Slaughter withdrawal = 12 days.

Tetracycline HCl Soluble Powder as a water additive
>   *Polyotic Soluble Powder*® (10 g or 25 g tetracycline HCl/lb); (OTC)
>   *Polyotic Soluble Powder Concentrate*® (102.4 g tetracycline HCl/lb); (OTC) Both are approved for use in calves, and swine. Slaughter withdrawal = 4 days calves; = 7 days swine
>   *Tetracycline HCl Soluble Powder-324*® (324 g tetracycline HCl/lb); (OTC) Approved for use in calves, swine, chickens, and turkeys. Slaughter withdrawal = 4 days swine, chickens, and turkeys; = 5 days calves

Human-Approved Products:
Tetracycline HCl Oral Capsules: 100 mg (capsules only from Richlyn Labs), 250 mg, 500 mg; Many trade names, including: *Achromycin-V*® (Lederle), *Sumycin '250'*® & 500 (Apothecon); *Panmycin*® (Upjohn), generic; (Rx)

Tetracycline HCl Tablets: 500 mg; *Tetracycline*® (Dr's Pharm); *Sumycin 500*® (Apothecon) (Rx)

Tetracycline HCl Oral Suspension 25 mg/ml in 60, 473, & 480 ml; *Achromycin-V*® (Lederle) (Rx), *Sumycin Syrup*® (Apothecon);*Tetralan Syrup*® (Lannett); generic; (Rx)

Tetracycline HCl Fiber: 12.7 mg/23 cm *Actisite*® (Alza) (Rx)

Tetracycline HCl Topical solution: 2.2 mg/ml *Topicycline*® (Roberts) (Rx)

Theophylline - see Aminophylline

THIABENDAZOLE

Chemistry - The prototypic benzimidazole, thiabendazole occurs as an odorless or nearly odorless, tasteless, white to practically white powder. It has a melting range of 296°-303°C and a pK_a of 4.7. Thiabendazole is practically insoluble in water and slightly soluble in alcohol.

Storage/Stability/Compatibility - Thiabendazole tablets, boluses and oral suspension should be stored in tight containers.

Uses/Indications - Thiabendazole has been used for the removal of the following parasites in **dogs**: ascarids (*Toxocara canis, T. leonina*), *Strongyloides stercoralis*, and *Filaroides*. It has also been used systemically as an anti-fungal agent in the treatment of nasal aspergillosis and penicillinosis. Topical and otic use of thiabendazole for the treatment of various fungi is also commonly employed.

Thiabendazole is indicated (labeled) for the removal of the following parasites in **cattle**: *Haemonchus spp., Ostertagia spp., Trichostrongylus spp., Nematodirus spp., Cooperia spp. and Oesophagostomum radiatum*.

Thiabendazole is indicated (labeled) for the removal of the following parasites in **sheep** and **goats**: *Haemonchus spp., Ostertagia spp., Trichostrongylus spp., Nematodirus spp., Cooperia spp., Chabertia spp., Bunostomum spp. and Oesophagostomum spp.*.

Thiabendazole is indicated (labeled) for the removal of the following parasites in **horses**: *Strongylus spp., craterstomum spp., Oesphagodontus spp., Posteriostomum spp., Cyathostomum spp., Cylicocylus spp., Cylicostephanus spp., Oxyuris spp.*, and *Parasacaris spp.*.

Thiabendazole is indicated (labeled) for the removal or prevention of the following parasites in **swine**: large roundworms (*Ascaris suum*) (prevention), and in baby pigs infested with *Strongyloides ransomi*.

Although not approved, thiabendazole has been used in pet birds and llamas. See the Dosage section for more information.

In many geographic areas, significant thiabendazole resistance problems have developed and for many parasites other anthelmintics would be a better choice for treatment.

Pharmacokinetics - Thiabendazole is relatively well absorbed (for a benzimidazole) and is distributed throughout body tissues. Peak levels occur in approximately 2-7 hours after dosing. Absorbed drug is rapidly metabolized in the liver by hydroxylation, glucuronidation and sulfate formation. Within 48 hours of dosing, 90% of the drug is excreted in the urine (as metabolites) and 5% in the feces. Less than 1% of the drug is excreted in the urine unchanged. Five days after a dose, the drug is virtually eliminated from the body.

Contraindications/Precautions - Thiabendazole has not been demonstrated to be a teratogen and is considered to be generally safe to use during pregnancy. However, in high doses it has been implicated in causing toxemia in ewes.

Adverse Effects/Warnings - At recommended doses, thiabendazole is usually well tolerated by approved species. In dogs, vomiting, diarrhea, hair loss and lethargy are possible side effects, notably with high dose or long-term therapy. Dachshunds have been reported to be particularly sensitive to thiabendazole. Toxic epidermal necrolysis (TEN) has been reported in dogs receiving thiabendazole, but the incidence appears to be very rare.

Overdosage/Toxicity - Thiabendazole has a safety margin of at least 20 times the recommended dose in horses. Doses of 800 - 1000 mg/kg are necessary to cause anorexia and depression in sheep. The minimum lethal dose is 700 mg/kg in cattle and 1200 mg/kg in sheep.

It is unlikely that a modest overdose would cause significant problems. If a massive overdose occurs, treat supportively and symptomatically. See the Adverse effects section for more information.

Drug Interactions - Thiabendazole may compete with **xanthines** (*e.g.,* **theophylline, aminophylline**) for metabolizing sites in the liver, thereby increasing xanthine blood levels.

Doses -
  Dogs:
    As an antiparasitic agent:
    a) For treatment of *Strongyloides stercoralis*: 50 - 60 mg/kg PO. (Todd, Paul, and DiPietro 1985)
    b) For treatment of *Filaroides* infections: 30 - 70 mg/kg divided q12h PO in food for 20-45 days. (Roudebush 1985)
    c) For treatment of *Filaroides* infections: 70 mg/kg PO *bid* for 2 days; then 35 mg/kg PO *bid* for 20 days. (Morgan 1988)
    d) 50 mg/kg PO once daily for 3 days; repeat in one month. (Kirk 1989)

    As an antifungal agent:
    a) For treatment of nasal aspergillosis/penicillinosis infections: 30 - 70 mg/kg divided q12h PO in food for 20-45 days. (Roudebush 1985)
    b) For the treatment of aspergillosis: 20 mg/kg PO, once a day or divided *bid*; (with or without ketoconazole: 20 mg/kg PO, once a day or divided *bid*). Maintenance therapy: 10 - 20 mg/kg PO once a day. (Greene, O'Neal, and Barsanti 1984)
    c) For penicillinosis: With appropriate adjunctive surgical curettage and topical therapy, thiabendazole: 20 mg/kg/day PO for 4-6 weeks. (Barsanti 1984)
    d) For aspergillosis: Administer 10 mg/kg as nasal flush. Dilute in 10-20 ml of water. Flush twice daily for 10 days.
      Orally: 20 mg/kg/day divided *bid* for 6 weeks. (Morgan 1988)
    e) For treatment of nasal aspergillosis: 20 mg/kg divided q12h PO for 6-8 weeks. If anorexia or nausea develop, may withdraw drug and then gradually reintroduce gradually to the full dosage. Administer with food to enhance absorption and reduce anorexia. May be effective in 40-50% of dogs treated. (Sharp 1989)

  Cattle:
    For susceptible parasites:
    a) 66 mg/kg PO; 110 mg/kg PO for *Cooperia* and severe infections of other susceptible nematodes. Retreat in 2-3 weeks if indicated. (Paul 1986), (Roberson 1988b)
    b) 50 - 100 mg/kg PO. (Brander, Pugh, and Bywater 1982)

  Horses:
    For susceptible parasites:
    a) 44 mg/kg PO. (Robinson 1987)
    b) 44 mg/kg; 88 mg/kg for ascarids. (Roberson 1988b)
    c) 50 - 100 mg/kg PO (Brander, Pugh, and Bywater 1982)

  Swine:
    For susceptible parasites:
    a) For baby pigs with *Strongyloides ransomi*: 62 - 83 mg/kg PO, retreat in 5-7 days if necessary. To prevent *Ascaris suum*: Feed at 0.05 - 0.1% per ton of feed for 2 weeks, then 0.005 - 0.02% per ton for 8-14 weeks. (Paul 1986)
    b) 75 mg/kg PO (Roberson 1988b)

    c) 50 mg/kg PO. (Brander, Pugh, and Bywater 1982)

Sheep & Goats:
    For susceptible parasites:
        a) 44 mg/kg PO; 66 mg/kg PO for severe infections in goats. (Paul 1986), (Roberson 1988b)
        b) 50 - 100 mg/kg PO (sheep). (Brander, Pugh, and Bywater 1982)

Llamas:
    For susceptible parasites:
        a) 50 - 100 mg/kg PO for 1-3 days. Use higher dosage rate over several days when animal is severely parasitized. (Cheney and Allen 1989)
        b) 66 mg/kg PO. (Fowler 1989)

Birds:
    For susceptible parasites:
        a) For ascarids: 250 - 500 mg/kg PO once. Repeat in 10-14 days.
            For *Syngamus trachea*: 100 mg/kg PO once a day for 7-10 days. (Clubb 1986)
        b) For ascarids, Capillaria, gapeworms:
            Chickens, pheasants, turkeys, and pigeons: Mix 0.5% in feed for 10 days or administer orally at 44 mg/kg as a single dose.
            Psittacines: 44 mg/kg PO; do not exceed this dose.
            Falcons: 100 mg/kg PO as a single dose. (Stunkard 1984)
        c) For thorny headed worms in water fowl and raptors: 250 mg/lb. (Stunkard 1984)

Client Information - Shake suspension well before using. Follow veterinarian's or label directions carefully.

Dosage Forms/Preparations/FDA Approval Status/Withdrawal Times- Food residue tolerances: 0.1 ppm in uncooked meat of cattle, pheasants, swine, sheep and goats. 0.05 ppm in milk.

  Veterinary-Approved Products:
    Thiabendazole Oral Suspension 4 g/fl. oz. (135 mg/ml)
      Equizole® Suspension (MSD); (OTC) Approved for use in dairy and beef cattle, sheep, goats, and horses. Milk withdrawal = 96 hours. Slaughter withdrawal = 3 days (cattle); 30 days (sheep & goats)
    Thiabendazole Oral Suspension 6 g/fl. oz. (203 mg/ml)
      Omnizole®-Six Wormer Suspension (MSD); (OTC) Approved for use in dairy and beef cattle, sheep, goats, and horses. Milk withdrawal = 96 hours. Slaughter withdrawal = 3 days (cattle); 30 days (sheep & goats)
    Thiabendazole Oral Suspension (Drench) 25 g/fl. oz. (845 mg/ml)
      TBZ® Cattle Wormer (Drench) (MSD); (OTC) Approved for use in dairy and beef cattle. Milk withdrawal = 96 hours. Slaughter withdrawal = 3 days
    Thiabendazole Oral Suspension 17.5 g/fl. oz. (592 mg/ml)
      Thibenzole® Sheep and Goat Wormer (MSD); (OTC) Approved for use in sheep and goats. Milk withdrawal = 96 hours. Slaughter withdrawal = 30 days
    Thiabendazole Oral Paste 50% (500 mg/g), 43% (430 mg/g), 20% (200 mg/g)
      TBZ® Cattle Wormer Paste 50%, TBZ® Wormer Paste 43% (MSD); (OTC) Approved for use in dairy and beef cattle. Milk withdrawal=96 hours. Slaughter withdrawal = 3 days
    Thiabendazole Oral Boluses (Tablets) 15 g (cattle), 2 g (calf, sheep, goat)
      TBZ® Calf, Sheep, and Goat Wormer (MSD); (OTC) Approved for use in non-lactating dairy and beef cattle, goats, and sheep. Slaughter withdrawal = 3 days (calves); 30 days (goats, sheep)
    Thiabendazole Medicated Premixes are available in: 22%, 44.1%, 66.1%, 88.2% concentrations. A thiabendazole medicated block (15 g/lb) is also available. An oral suspension of thiabendazole (2 g/oz) in combination with piperazine (2.5 g/oz) is available for use in horses.
    It is a prescription only medication (Rx) with the proprietary name: *Equizole® A* (MSD).

  Human-Approved Products:
    Thiabendazole Oral Chewable Scored Tablets 500 mg; *Mintezol®* (Merck); (Rx)
    Thiabendazole Oral Suspension 100 500 mg/5 ml, 120 ml bottle; *Mintezol®* (Merck); (Rx)

THIACETARSEMIDE SODIUM

Chemistry - A phenylarsenoxide, thiacetarsemide sodium is an organic arsenical compound. The commercially available injection is actually a combination of thiacetarsemide and *p*-arsenosobenzamide. It is available commercially in a 10 mg/ml (1%) solution and may also be known as sodium thiacetarsemide.

Storage/Stability/Compatibility - Thiacetarsemide should be stored in the refrigerator (2°-8°C) and protected from light or freezing. The manufacturer recommends discarding opened containers from the refrigerator after 3 months. If the solution develops a yellow or orange color or if precipitates are seen, the solution should be discarded.

Pharmacology - The exact mechanism of action of thiacetarsemide is not known. It is believed the adulticidal activity of the compound is due to an arsenical moiety that reacts with sulfhydryl groups in essential enzyme systems and is not due directly to the elemental arsenic. There is evidence that worm mortality is increased the greater the length of time it is exposed at effective concentrations to the compound and is not increased by obtaining higher thiacetarsemide blood levels. Thiacetarsemide is effective against adult heartworms only and has no clinical efficacy against microfilaria.

Uses/Indications - Thiacetarsemide is indicated for the removal of adult heartworms (*D. Immitis*) in dogs. The drug is also labeled to be given every 6 months to dogs when other larvacidal drugs are impractical to be administered. Use of thiacetarsamide is largely being supplanted by melarsomine, as the latter drug has increased efficacy and a significantly lower incidence of serious adverse effects.

Although not approved, thiacetarsemide has also been used to treat adult heartworms or hemobartenella in cats.

Pharmacokinetics - After IV injection in dogs, thiacetarsemide has an elimination half-life of about 43 minutes and a clearance of approximately 200 ml/kg/min, but significant interpatient variation exists. Thiacetarsemide is metabolized and excreted via the bile into the feces and also in the urine. Approximately 85% of the dose is recovered within 48 hours, primarily in the feces (66%). The drug is widely distributed in the body, but concentrates in the liver and to a lesser extent, the kidneys. Adult heartworms concentrate the drug in quantities greater than the liver.

Contraindications/Precautions/Reproductive Safety - Because of the serious consequences that may occur as a result of thiacetarsemide treatment, animals with significantantly impaired hepatic, renal (azotemia, protein-losing nephropathy), cardiopulmonary (*e.g.,* right heart failure, vena caval syndrome, pulmonary thromboembolism, allergic pneumonitis) systems or in DIC should generally not be given (at least temporarily) thiacetarsemide. The manufacturer recommends surgically removing worms from the vena cava if they are blocking this vessel before starting therapy.

Animals with concurrent diabetes mellitus, gastrointestinal disease, renal disease (moderate) or hypoadrenocorticism should receive thiacetarsemide only with intensified monitoring.

Extreme care must be taken to avoid perivascular leakage (extravasation) when injecting this agent. Fortunately most minor extravasation injuries are minor and result only in swelling and pain at the site, but skin sloughing can occur. Topical treatment with hot packs and topical DMSO (or DMSO/steroid product—*Synotic®* q4-6h), and/or dexamethasone/saline infiltration has been suggested should extravasation occur.

Microfilaricide therapy should not be started for approximately 4 weeks after thiacetarsemide or until the clinical complications of thiacetarsemide-related therapy have subsided.

No specific information was located regarding this drug's effects on developing fetuses. If possible, treatment with thiacetarsemide should be postponed until after parturition.

Adverse Effects/Warnings - Adverse effects that can develop with thiacetarsemide therapy can be severe and life-threatening. With the exception of azotemic patients, there is apparently no correlation between any patient factors (age, sex, breed) and the incidence of adverse effects. Because heartworm disease can cause significant heart, pulmonary, kidney and liver damage, treatment should be started as soon as possible to both reduce the long-term sequelae associated with the disease and to maximize the animal's health status to improve toleration of the therapy.

Vomiting after dosing is the most common adverse reaction seen with thiacetarsemide and usually occurs after the first or second injection. Emesis alone is not an indication to halt therapy, unless other signs or symptoms (*e.g.,* anorexia, depression, etc.) develop.

Nephrotoxicity may occur after thiacetarsemide therapy, with tubular casts seen in the urine sediment most commonly noted. Casts alone are generally not an indication that therapy must be halted, but in conjunction with other symptoms may be an indicator to stop therapy. Azotemia is uncommon during thiacetarsemide therapy and treatment may usually be continued if BUN remains below 100 mg/dl as long as the patient receives adequate fluid and electrolyte replacement during and after treatment.

Hepatotoxicity can occur during thiacetarsemide therapy, but the mechanism of its hepatotoxic effects are unknown. Approximately 20% of patients receiving thiacetarsemide acquire increased serum ALT's and Alkaline Phosphatase, but there are no factors that have been determined to be predictive for hepatotoxicity development. Signs and symptoms can occur within 1-3 days after dosing and can be acute in onset. These can include: anorexia, vomiting, depression, bilirubin-uria, hyperbilirubinemia/icterus, melena, stupor, coma or death. Bilirubinuria is often the first sign of impending hepatoxicity. Gross bilirubinuria seen after the first or second injection is usually an indication to stop therapy. Should bilirubinuria be seen after the third injection, therapy may usually be continued unless other signs/symptoms are seen. Should liver toxicity occur, thiacetarsemide should be discontinued and supportive/symptomatic treatment for liver disease be instituted as necessary.

Patients whose therapy is aborted because of the onset of acute adverse effects should not be retreated for 4 weeks. At that time, therapy may be reconsidered, often without a recurrence of adversity.

After thiacetarsemide treatment, adult worms begin to die within days and continue to die over a 3 week period with resultant degrees of pulmonary artery emboli developing. The caudal lung lobes are routinely affected. Dogs with pre-existing pulmonary emboli, periarterial granulomas or severe pulmonary artery enlargement are at greatest risk to develop severe complications. Signs/symptoms of embolic disease generally begin 5-7 days after treatment is completed and usually peak at 10-14 days. Early symptoms noted include coughing, fevers, anorexia and lethargy. Dyspnea, high fevers or hemoptysis are signs of severe pulmonary emboli and/or preex-isting pulmonary disease. To minimize the morbidity/mortality associated with pulmonary em-bolic disease, animals should be kept on strict cage rest, usually for a month following therapy. Aspirin at doses of 5 - 10 mg/kg PO once daily (see Aspirin monograph for more information) has been recommended in animals with severe pulmonary artery disease to reduce thiac-etarsemide-induced pulmonary effects, but aspirin may exacerbate pulmonary parenchymal dis-ease in some animals and cause additional clotting problems should thrombocytopenia develop (see below).

Glucocorticoids (Predniso(lo)ne 0.5 - 1 mg/kg PO *bid* in decreasing doses over 7-14 days) have also been recommended to treat symptoms associated with pulmonary thromboembolism after thiacetarsemide therapy, but its use is controversial (see Drug Interactions section below).

Thrombocytopenia is common and is seen from 5-21 days after therapy is completed. Platelet counts usually reach their nadir at 10-14 days. Aspirin therapy should be cut back or stopped if platelet counts decrease below 50,000/mm^3 or if hemoptysis develops. Vincristine (0.4 mg/m^2 IV once) has been suggested to be given if platelet counts approach 50,000/ mm^3 to stimulate platelet production. Disseminated Intravascular Coagulation (DIC) is possible and often precedes death.

Overdosage/Acute Toxicity - Thiacetarsemide has a very narrow therapeutic index and margin for safety. An accidental overdose of 7.3 mg/kg in a dog resulted in respiratory depression and pulmonary edema and the animal died despite aggressive supportive therapy. Clearly, dosages must be accurately determined (using appropriate syringes and weighing the animal accurately) to avoid these disasters. It is not known if chelating therapies used for arsenic toxicity (*e.g.,* dimercaprol/BAL, Dimercaptosuccinic acid/DMSA) are of any value in these cases, but dimer-caprol at 8.8 mg/kg/day in 4 divided doses has been recommended to treat acute toxicity by one clinician (Roberson 1988b).

Drug Interactions - One clinician (Noone 1986), notes that **glucocorticoids** have a protective effect on adult heartworms, and therefore thiacetarsemide and glucocorticoids should not be used together. Also, glucocorticoids cause increased intimal proliferation and can lead to greater vas-cular obstruction and should therefore, be reserved for use in patients who develop severe acute emboli and fever after aldulticide therapy.

Doses -
  Dogs:
    For elimination of adult heartworms:
      a) 2.2 mg/kg (0.22 ml/kg of a 1% solution) given twice a day for 2 days. Use an in-dwelling intravenous catheter or winged infusion set to avoid extravasation injuries. (Kittleson 1985)
      b) 2.2 mg/kg for 4 doses; may space doses from 6-12 hours apart, but entire dose should be given within 36 hours. (Hoskins 1989)
      c) 2.2 mg/kg IV *bid* for two days. Daily doses should be administered 4-8 hours apart and the interval between the 2nd and 3rd dose should not be longer than 16 hours. (Knight 1987)
  Cats:
    For elimination of adult heartworms:
      a) 2.2 mg/kg IV *bid* for 2 days. (Dillon 1986)
      b) 2.2 mg/kg IV q12h for 2 days. (Calvert 1989)

For *Hemobartonella felis*:
  a) 1 mg/kg IV once; repeat in 2 days. Contraindicated in icteric patients; side effects are common. Oxytetracycline usually drug of first choice. (Maggio-Price 1988)
  b) 0.25 mg/kg IV once and repeated 2 days later; potentially toxic. Oxytetracycline usually drug of first choice. (Lissman 1988)

Monitoring Parameters - Prior to therapy and after treatment *prn* (see Adverse effects section): Thorough physical exam, CBC with platelets, UA, blood chemistry profile, thoracic radiographs, ECG, vital signs, appetite, weight.

Client Information - Clients must understand the potential risks associated with therapy before treating (see Adverse Effects section) and be able to monitor at home for adverse effects (temperature, appetite, breathing (rate/effort, coughing), attitude and state of hydration). Clients should be given guidelines as to when to contact the veterinarian should adverse reactions occur. The importance of keeping the dog quiet during the month after treatment must be emphasized.

Dosage Forms/Preparations/FDA Approval Status/Withholding Times -
  Veterinary-Approved Products:

  Thiacetarsemide Sodium 10 mg/ml (1%) in 50 ml multi-dose vials; *Caparsolate*® (Rhone Merieux); (Rx) Approved for use in dogs.

  Human-Approved Products: None

THIAMINE HCL
VITAMIN B₁

Chemistry - A water-soluble B-complex vitamin, thiamine HCl occurs as bitter-tasting, white, small hygroscopic crystals, or crystalline powder that has a characteristic yeast-like odor. Thiamine HCl is freely soluble in water and slightly soluble in alcohol and has pK_as of 4.8 & 9.0. The commercially available injection has a pH of 2.5-4.5. Thiamine HCl may also be known as Aneurine HCl, Thiamin HCl, Thiamine Chloride, Thiaminium Chloride Hydrochloride, or Vitamin B₁.

Storage/Stability/Compatibility - Thiamine HCl for injection should be protected from light and stored at temperatures less than 40°C and preferably between 15-30°C; avoid freezing.

Thiamine HCl is unstable in alkaline or neutral solutions or with oxidizing or reducing agents. It is most stable at a pH of 2.

Thiamine HCl is reportedly **compatible** with all commonly used intravenous replacement fluids. Compatibility is dependent upon factors such as pH, concentration, temperature and diluents used. It is suggested to consult specialized references for more specific information (*e.g.*, *Handbook on Injectable Drugs* by Trissel; see bibliography).

Pharmacology - Thiamine combines with adenosine triphosphate (ATP) to form a compound (thiamine diphosphate/thiamine pyrophosphate) that is employed for carbohydrate metabolism, but does not effect blood glucose concentrations.

Absence of thiamine results in decreased transketolase activity in red blood cells and increased pyruvic acid blood concentrations. Without thiamine triphosphate, pyruvic acid is not converted into acetyl-CoA, diminished NADH results with anaerobic glycolysis producing lactic acid. Lactic acid production is further increased secondary to pyruvic acid conversion. Lactic acidosis may occur.

Uses/Indications - Thiamine is indicated in the treatment or prevention of thiamine deficiency states. Symptoms of thiamine deficiency may be manifested as gastrointestinal (anorexia, salivation), neuromuscular/CNS signs (ataxia, seizures, loss of reflexes), or cardiac effects (brady- or tachyarrhythmias). Deficiency states may be secondary to either a lack of thiamine in the diet or the presence of thiamine destroying compounds in the diet (*e.g.,* bracken fern, raw fish, amprolium, thiaminase-producing bacteria in ruminants).

Thiamine has also been used in the adjunctive treatment of lead poisoning and ethylene glycol toxicity (to facilitate the conversion of glyoxylate to nontoxic metabolites).

Pharmacokinetics - Thiamine is absorbed from the GI tract and is metabolized by the liver. Elimination is renal, the majority being metabolites.

Contraindications/Precautions/Reproductive Safety - Thiamine injection is contraindicated in animals hypersensitive to it or any component of it.

Adverse Effects/Warnings - Hypersensitivity reactions have occurred after injecting this agent. Some tenderness or muscle soreness may result after IM injection.

Overdosage/Acute Toxicity - Very large doses of thiamine in laboratory animals have been associated with neuromuscular or ganglionic blockade, but the clinical significance is unknown. Hypotension and respiratory depression may also occur with massive doses. A lethal dose of 350 mg/kg has been reported. Generally, no treatment should be required with most overdoses.

Drug Interactions - Thiamine may enhance the activity of **neuromuscular blocking agents**; clinical significance is unknown.

Drug/Laboratory Interactions - Thiamine may cause false-positive serum **uric acid** results when using the phosphotungstate method of determination or **urobilinogen** urine spot tests using Ehrlich's reagent. The Schack and Wexler method of determining **theophylline** concentrations may be interfered with by large doses of thiamine.

Doses -
Dogs:
For thiamine deficiency:
   a)   5 - 50 mg IM, SQ, or IV (depending on formulation) (Phillips 1988b)
   b)   1 - 2 mg IM (Greene and Braund 1989)
   c)   2 mg/kg PO once daily (Davis 1985)
   d)   100 - 250 mg SQ *bid* for several days until regression of symptoms with complete recovery. (Hoskins 1988)

For ethylene glycol toxicity:
   a)   100 mg/day PO (Morgan 1988)

Cats:
For thiamine deficiency:
   a)   100 - 250 mg parenterally twice a day (experimentally, as little as 1 mg is effective). (Armstrong and Hand 1989)
   b)   1 - 2 mg IM (Greene and Braund 1989)
   c)   4 mg/kg PO once daily (Davis 1985)
   d)   100 - 250 mg SQ *bid* for several days until regression of symptoms with complete recovery. (Hoskins 1988)
   e)   10 - 20 mg/kg IM or SQ *bid-tid* until signs abate, then 10 mg/kg PO once daily for 21 days. (Morgan 1988)

Cattle:
For thiamine deficiency:
   a)   For polioencephalomalacia: Initially, 10 mg/kg IV, then 10 mg/kg IM *bid* for 2-3 days. If no improvement within 4 days, may be advisable to recommend slaughter. (Dill 1986)
   b)   Calves: 5 - 50 mg; Ox: 200 - 1000 mg IM, SQ, or IV (depending on formulation). (Phillips 1988b)

For adjunctive therapy of lead poisoning:
   a)   2 mg/kg IM (at same time as CaEDTA therapy); total daily dose 8 mg/kg. (Brattan and Kowalczyk 1989)

Horses:
For thiamine deficiency:
   a)   0.5 - 5 mg/kg IV, IM or PO (Robinson 1987)
   b)   100 - 1000 mg IM, SQ, or IV (depending on formulation). (Phillips 1988b)

Swine:
For thiamine deficiency:
   a)   5 - 100 mg IM, SQ, or IV (depending on formulation). (Phillips 1988b)

Sheep, Goats:
For thiamine deficiency:
   a)   For polioencephalomalacia: Initially, 10 mg/kg IV, then 10 mg/kg IM *bid* for 2-3 days. If no improvement within 4 days, may be advisable to recommend slaughter. (Dill 1986)
   b)   Sheep: 20 - 200 mg IM, SQ, or IV (depending on formulation). (Phillips 1988b)

Monitoring Parameters -
   1)   Efficacy

Client Information - Epidemiologic investigation as to the cause of thiamine deficiency (diet, plants, raw fish, etc.) should be performed with necessary changes made to prevent recurrence.

Dosage Forms/Preparations/FDA Approval Status/Withholding Times -
Veterinary-Approved Products:
   Thiamine HCl for Injection 200 mg/ml and 500 mg/ml in 30 and 100 ml vials
      Available generically labeled; (Rx) Labeled for use in small and large animals. Approval status is uncertain.

   There are several B-complex vitamin preparations available that may also have thiamine included.

Human-Approved Products:

Thiamine Oral Tablets 50 mg, 100 mg, 250 mg, & 500 mg; Available generically labeled; (OTC)

Thiamine Enteric Coated Tablets 20 mg; *Thiamilate®* (Tyson) (OTC)

Thiamine HCl for Injection 100 mg/ml in 1, 2, 10 and 30 ml vials & 1 ml amps; Available generically labeled; (Rx)

THIAMYLAL SODIUM

Note: Thiamylal is not available commercially at the time of this update but is still listed in the FDA's "Green Book". Most veterinary anestheisologists are recommending using thiopental as an alternative. The monograph remains in the VDH with the hope that the product may find its way back to the market in the near future.

Chemistry - A thiobarbiturate, thiamylal sodium occurs as a pale yellow, hygroscopic powder with an unpleasant odor. It is soluble in water and a 5% solution in water has a pH of 10.5-11.5.

Storage/Stability/Compatibility - Thiamylal is stable in the dry form when stored in airtight vials. Thiamylal should be diluted with only sterile water for injection, sodium chloride injection, or D5W (Note: A veterinary manufacturer (Bio-Ceutic) recommends using only sterile water or sodium chloride for injection). After reconstitution, solutions are stable for 2 days when refrigerated (6 days according to some sources), but should generally be used within 24 hours. Do not administer any solution that has a visible precipitate. Little specific compatibility information is available other than not mixing with atropine, succinylcholine or tubocararine. Because of their chemical similarities, the compatibility listings in the thiopental monograph may be used as general guidelines with regard to thiamylal.

Pharmacology - The thiobarbiturates, because of their high lipid solubility, rapidly enter the CNS and produce profound hypnosis and anesthesia. See the monograph: Barbiturates, Pharmacology of, for more information.

Uses/Indications - Because of their rapid action and short duration, the thiobarbiturates are excellent induction agents for general anesthesia when used with other anesthetics or as the sole anesthetic agent for very short procedures.

Pharmacokinetics - Following IV injection of therapeutic doses, hypnosis and anesthesia occur within one minute. The drug rapidly enters the CNS and then redistributes to muscle and adipose tissue in the body. The short duration of action of these agents is due less to rapid metabolism than to this redistribution out of the CNS and into muscle and fat stores. Greyhounds and other sight hounds may exhibit longer recovery times than other breeds, which may be due to these breed's low body fat levels or differences in the metabolic handling of these agents.

Thiamylal is metabolized by the hepatic microsomal system. There was no information found regarding specific pharmacokinetic parameters in humans, dogs or horses. A paper on the pharmacokinetics of thiamylal in cats (Wertz et al. 1988) found a rapid first distribution phase ($t_{1/2}$ = 1.91 minutes) followed by a second slower distributory phase ($t_{1/2}$ = 26.5 minutes). The elimination half-life in cats was found to average 14.3 hours with a short period of anesthesia induced (dosage of 13.2 mg/kg IV) followed by a prolonged state of sedation. The authors concluded that based on the pharmacokinetic profile in cats, thiamylal should be used as an induction agent only followed by other anesthetic agents (*e.g.,* halothane).

Contraindications/Precautions - The following are considered to be absolute contraindications to the use of thiobarbiturates: abscence of suitable veins for IV administration, history of hypersensitivity reactions to the barbiturates, and status asthmaticus. Relative contraindications include: metabolic acidosis, severe cardiovascular disease or preexisting ventricular arrhythmias, shock, increased intracranial pressure, myasthenia gravis, asthma, and conditions where hypnotic effects may be prolonged (*e.g.,* severe hepatic disease, myxedema, severe anemia, excessive premedication, etc). These relative contraindications do not preclude the use of thiamylal, but dosage adjustments must be considered and the drug must be given slowly and cautiously.

Because greyhounds (and other sight hounds) metabolize thiobarbiturates much more slowly than methohexital, many clinicians recommend using methohexital instead. Siamese cats may develop more CNS depression than other feline breeds.

Thiobarbiturates readily crosses the placental barrier and should be used with caution during pregnancy.

Extravasation and intra-arterial injections should be avoided because of the high alkalinity of the solution. Severe CNS toxicity and tissue damage has resulted in horses receiving intra-carotid injections of thiobarbiturates. Do not administer intrapleurally or intraperitoneally.

Adverse Effects/Warnings - The manufacturer (Bio-Ceutic) lists the following possible adverse reactions: circulatory depression, thrombophlebitis, pain at injection site, respiratory depression including apnea, laryngospasm, bronchospasm, salivation, emergence delirium, injury to nerves adjacent to injection site, skin rashes, urticaria, nausea, and emesis.

In dogs, thiamylal has an approximate arrhythmogenic incidence of 60-85%. Ventricular bigeminy is the most common arrhythmia seen, is usually transient (over within 2 minutes) and generally responds to additional oxygen. Incidence may be reduced to approximately 25% by using a phenothiazine tranquilizer pre-operatively. Although the incidence of arrhythmias is higher with thiamylal than thiopental, thiamylal is considered to be less cardiotoxic. Administration of catecholamines may augment the arrhythmogenic effects of the thiobarbiturates, while lidocaine may inhibit it. Systemic arterial pressure may be increased, but this is probably only clinically significant in patients with preexisting small vessel disease.

Repeated administration of thiamylal is not advised as recovery times can be become significantly prolonged. Should parasympathetic side effects (*e.g.,* salivation, bradycardia) occur, they may be managed with the use of anticholinergic agents (atropine, glycopyrrolate).

Overdosage - Treatment of thiobarbiturate overdosage consists of supporting respirations (O_2, mechanical ventilation) and giving cardiovascular support (do not use catecholamines, *e.g.,* epinephrine, etc).

Drug Interactions - A fatal interaction has been reported in a dog receiving the proprietary product, *Diathal®* (procaine penicillin G, dihydrostreptomycin sulfate, diphemanil methylsulfate, and chlorpheniramine maleate) and thiamylal. Avoid using thiamylal with this combination.

The ventricular fibrillatory effects of **epinephrine** and **norepinephrine** are potentiated when used with thiobarbiturates and halothane.

CNS and respiratory depressant effects of **CNS depressants (narcotics, phenothiazines, antihistamines, etc.)** may be enhanced by thiobarbiturate administration.

Thiamylal with **furosemide** may cause or increase postural hypotension. **Sulfisoxasole** IV has been shown to compete with thiopental at plasma protein binding sites. This may also occur with thiamylal and other sulfonamides.

Doses -

Note: Atropine sulfate or glycopyrrolate are often administered prior to thiobarbiturate anesthesia to prevent parasympathetic side effects. Some clinicians question, however, whether routine administration of the anticholinergic agents are necessary.

Thiobarbiturates are administered strictly to effect; doses are guidelines only.

The manufacturer (Bio-Ceutic) recommends rapid injection 1/3 - 1/2 of the calculated dosage to carry the patient through the excitatory phase, then, if no apnea or severe respiratory depressant effects are seen, administer to the level of anesthesia desired.

Dogs:
   a) 17.6 mg/kg IV; if narcotic premedication is used: 8.8 mg/kg IV. Use lower dosages for larger, older, brachiocephalic breeds, and animals in poor condition. Younger and smaller animals may require higher dosages. (Package Insert; *Bio-Tal®* — Bio-Ceutic)
   b) Average dose of 17.6 mg/kg IV; will produce surgical anesthesia for about 15 minutes. (Booth 1988a)
   c) 17.6 mg/kg IV (unpremedicated); 8.8 - 13.3 mg/kg after tranquilization; 4.4 - 6.6 mg/kg after narcotic premedication. (Mandsager 1988)

Cats:
   a) 17.6 mg/kg IV; if narcotic premedication is used: 8.8 mg/kg IV. Use lower dosages for larger, older, brachiocephalic breeds, and animals in poor condition. Younger and smaller animals may require higher dosages. (Package Insert; *Bio-Tal®* — Bio-Ceutic)
   b) 17.6 mg/kg IV (unpremedicated); 8.8 - 13.3 mg/kg after tranquilization; 4.4 - 6.6 mg/kg after narcotic premedication. (Mandsager 1988)

Cattle:
   a) 8.8 mg/kg IV (jugular) for short duration; 12.5 mg/kg IV (jugular) for longer duration (Package Insert; *Bio-Tal®* — Bio-Ceutic)
   b) 4.4 mg/kg IV after sedation and guaifenesin; or 6.6 - 8.8 mg/kg IV after tranquilization. (Mandsager 1988)

Horses:
   a) For light anesthesia: One gram IV (jugular) for an animal weighing from 500 - 1100 lbs.;   Deeper anesthesia: 7.3 mg/kg IV (Package Insert; *Bio-Tal®* — Bio-Ceutic)
   b) 4.4 - 6.6 mg/kg IV after sedation and guaifenesin; or 6.6 - 8.8 mg/kg IV after tranquilization. (Mandsager 1988)

Swine:
   a) 17.6 mg/kg IV to effect (Package Insert; *Bio-Tal®* — Bio-Ceutic)

   b) 6.6 - 11.0 mg/kg IV (Mandsager 1988)

Sheep:
   a) 13.2 mg/kg IV (will produce anesthesia for approximately 8 ± 4 minutes); anesthesia may be prolonged for 35 minutes or so by giving 14.3 mg/kg pentobarbital IV 7 minutes after thiamylal. (Booth 1988a)
   b) 8.8 - 13.2 mg/kg IV (Mandsager 1988)

Goats:
   a) 8.8 - 13.2 mg/kg IV (Mandsager 1988)

Monitoring Parameters -
   1) Level of hypnosis/anesthesia
   2) Respiratory status; cardiac status (rate/rhythm/blood pressure)

Client Information - This drug should only be used by professionals familiar with its effects in a setting where adequate respiratory support can be performed.

Dosage Forms/Preparations/FDA Approval Status/Withholding Times -
Note: Thiamylal is not currently available, it was (and perhaps again?) available as:

   Thiamylal Sodium for Injection; available in 1 gram, 5 gram, & 10 gram vials for reconstitution and 5 gram ampules (Note: Veterinary products are available in 1 & 5 gram vials only)
   Bio-Tal® (Bio-Ceutic), *Surital*® (Parke-Davis); (Rx) Approved for use in dogs, cats, cattle, horses, and swine. No milk or meat withdrawal times are required.

Preparation of Solution for Administration-
The following table may be used to determine amount of diluent necessary to obtain desired concentrations:

% Solution	mg/ml (calc.)	1 GRAM VIAL mls to add	5 GRAM VIAL mls to add
0.5%	5	200 ml	1000 ml
2.0%	20	50 ml	250 ml
2.5%	25	40 ml	200 ml
4.0%	40	25 ml	125 ml

Sterile water for injection is the preferred diluent. If preparing solutions for a maintenance continuous drip, use D_5W or sterile isotonic saline to avoid hypotonic solutions. Some dextrose solutions may be acidic enough to cause precipitation. Do not use cloudy or precipitated solutions.

THIOGUANINE

Chemistry - A purine analog antineoplastic agent, thioguanine occurs as a pale yellow, odorless or practically odorless, crystalline powder. It is insoluble in water or alcohol. Thioguanine may also be known as 6- thioguanine, TG, 6-TG, or 2-Amino-6-mercaptopurine.

Storage/Stability/Compatibility - Store tablets in tight containers at room temperature.

Pharmacology - Intracellularly, thioguanine is converted to ribonucleotides that cause the synthesis and utilization of purine nucleotides to be blocked. The drug's cytotoxic effects are believed to occur when these substituted nucleotides are inserted into RNA and DNA. Thioguanine also has limited immunosuppressive activity. Extensive cross-resistance usually occurs between thioguanine and mercaptopurine.

Uses/Indications - Thioguanine may be useful as adjunctive therapy for acute lymphocytic or granulocytic leukemia in dogs or cats.

Pharmacokinetics - Thioguanine is administered orally, but absorption is variable. In humans, only about 30% of a dose is absorbed. Thioguanine is distributed into the DNA and RNA of bone marrow, but several doses may be necessary for this to occur. It does not apparently enter the CNS, but does cross the placenta. It is unknown whether it enters maternal milk.

Thioguanine is rapidly metabolized primarily in the liver to methylate derivative that is less active (and toxic) than the parent compound. This and other metabolites are then eliminated in the urine.

Contraindications/Precautions/Reproductive Safety - Thioguanine is contraindicated in patients hypersensitive to it. The drug should be used cautiously (risk versus benefit) in patients with hepatic dysfunction, bone marrow depression, infection, renal function impairment (adjust dosage) or have a history of urate urinary stones. Thioguanine has a very low therapeutic index and should only be used by clinicians with experience in the use of cytotoxic agents and able to monitor therapy appropriately.

Thioguanine is potentially mutagenic and teratogenic and is not recommended for use during pregnancy. Although it is unknown whether thioguanine enters milk, use of milk replacer is recommended for nursing bitches or queens.

Adverse Effects/Warnings - At usual doses, GI effects (nausea, anorexia, vomiting, diarrhea) may occur in small animals. However, bone marrow suppression, hepatotoxicity, pancreatitis, GI (including oral) ulceration, and dermatologic reactions are potentially possible. Cats may be particularly susceptible to the hematologic effects of thioguanine.

Overdosage/Acute Toxicity - Toxicity may present acutely (GI effects) or be delayed (bone marrow depression, hepatotoxicity, gastroenteritis). It is suggested to use standard protocols to empty the GI tract if ingestion was recent and to treat supportively.

Drug Interactions - Use extreme caution when used concurrently with other drugs that are also myelosuppressive, including many of the **other antineoplastics and other bone marrow depressant drugs** (*e.g.*, **chloramphenicol, flucytosine, amphotericin B, or colchicine**). Bone marrow depression may be additive. Use with other **immunosuppressant drugs** (*e.g.*, **azathioprine, cyclophosphamide, corticosteroids**) may increase the risk of infection. **Live virus vaccines** should be used with caution, if at all during therapy.

Thioguanine should be used cautiously with **other drugs that can cause hepatotoxicity** (*e.g.*, halothane, ketoconazole, valproic acid, phenobarbital, primidone, etc.).

Laboratory Considerations - Thioguanine may increase serum uric acid levels in some patients.

Doses - For acute lymphocytic and granulocytic leukemia:

Dogs:
   a) 40 mg/m^2 PO once daily (q24 hours) for 4-5 days, then every 3rd day thereafter. (Jacobs, Lumsden et al. 1992)

Cats:
   a) 25 mg/m^2 PO once daily (q24 hours) for 1-5 days, then every 30 days thereafter as necessary. (Jacobs, Lumsden et al. 1992)

Monitoring Parameters - 1) Hemograms (including platelets) should be monitored closely; initially every 1-2 weeks and every 1-2 months once on maintenance therapy. It is recommended by some clinicians that if the WBC count drops to between 5,000-7,000 cells/mm^3 the dose be reduced by 25%. If WBC count drops below 5,000 cells/mm^3 treatment should be discontinued until leukopenia resolves; 2) Liver function tests; serum amylase, if indicated; 3) Efficacy

Client Information - Clients must be briefed on the possibilities of severe toxicity developing from this drug, including drug-related neoplasms or mortality. Clients should contact veterinarian should the animal exhibit symptoms of abnormal bleeding, bruising, anorexia, vomiting, jaundice or infection.

Although, no special precautions are necessary with handling intact tablets, it is recommended to wash hands after administering the drug.

Dosage Forms/Preparations/FDA Approval Status/Withholding Times -
   Veterinary-Approved Products: None
   Human-Approved Products:
   Thioguanine Oral Tablets 40 mg; *Thioguanine* (Glaxo Wellcome); (Rx)

THIOPENTAL SODIUM

Chemistry - A thiobarbiturate, thiopental occurs as a bitter-tasting, white to off-white, crystalline powder or a yellow-white hygroscopic powder. It is soluble in water (1 gram in 1.5 ml) and alcohol. Thiopental has a pK$_a$ of 7.6 and is a weak organic acid.

Storage/Stability/Compatibility - When stored in the dry form, thiopental sodium is stable indefinitely. Thiopental should be diluted with only sterile water for injection, sodium chloride injection, or D$_5$W. Concentrations of less than 2% in sterile water should not be used as they may cause hemolysis. After reconstitution, solutions are stable for 3 days at room temperature and for 7 days if refrigerated. However, as no preservative is present, it is recommended it be used within 24 hours after reconstitution. After 48 hours, the solution has been reported to attack the glass bottles it is stored in. Thiopental may also adsorb to plastic IV tubing and bags. Do not administer any solution that has a visible precipitate.

The following agents have been reported to be **compatible** when mixed with thiopental: aminophylline, chloramphenicol sodium succinate, hyaluronidase, hydrocortisone sodium succinate, neostigmine methylsulfate, oxytocin, pentobarbital sodium, phenobarbital sodium, potassium chloride, scopolamine HBr, sodium iodide, and tubocurarine chloride (recommendations conflict with regard to tubocurarine; some clinicians recommend not mixing with thiopental).

The following agents have been reported to be **incompatible** when mixed with thiopental: Ringer's injection, Ringer's injection lactate, amikacin sulfate, atropine sulfate, benzquinamide, cephapirin sodium, chlorpromazine, codeine phosphate, dimenhydrinate, diphenhydramine, ephedrine sulfate, glycopyrrolate, hydromorphone, insulin (regular), levorphanol bitartrate, meperidine, metaraminol, morphine sulfate, norepinephrine bitartrate, penicillin G potassium, prochlorperazine edisylate, promazine HCl, promethazine HCl, succinylcholine chloride, and tetracycline HCl. Compatibility is dependent upon factors such as pH, concentration, temperature and diluents used. It is suggested to consult specialized references for more specific information (*e.g., Handbook on Injectable Drugs* by Trissel; see bibliography).

Pharmacology - Because of their high lipid solubility, thiobarbiturates rapidly enter the CNS and produce profound hypnosis and anesthesia. They are also known as ultrashort-acting barbiturates. See the monograph: Barbiturates, Pharmacology of, for additional information.

Uses/Indications - Because of their rapid action and short duration, the thiobarbiturates are excellent induction agents for general anesthesia with other anesthetics or as the sole anesthetic agent for very short procedures.

Pharmacokinetics - Following IV injection of therapeutic doses, hypnosis and anesthesia occur within one minute. The drug rapidly enters the CNS and then redistributes to muscle and adipose tissue in the body. The short duration of action of these agents is due less to rapid metabolism than to this redistribution out of the CNS and into muscle and fat stores. Greyhounds and other sight hounds may exhibit longer recovery times than other breeds. This may be due to these breeds low body fat levels or differences in the metabolic handling of the thiobarbiturates.

Thiopental is metabolized by the hepatic microsomal system and several metabolites have been isolated. The elimination half-life in dogs has been reported as being approximately 7 hours and in sheep, 3-4 hours. Very little of the drug is excreted unchanged in the urine (0.3% in humans), so dosage adjustments are not necessary in patients with chronic renal failure.

Contraindications/Precautions - The following are considered to be absolute contraindications to the use of thiopental: absence of suitable veins for IV administration, history of hypersensitivity reactions to the barbiturates, and status asthmaticus. Relative contraindications include: severe cardiovascular disease or preexisting ventricular arrhythmias, shock, increased intracranial pressure, myasthenia gravis, asthma, and conditions where hypnotic effects may be prolonged (*e.g.,* severe hepatic disease, myxedema, severe anemia, excessive premedication, etc). These relative contraindications do not preclude the use of thiopental, but dosage adjustments must be considered and the drug must be given slowly and cautiously.

Because greyhounds (and other sight hounds) metabolize thiobarbiturates much more slowly than methohexital, many clinicians recommend using methohexital instead.

Thiopental readily crosses the placental barrier and should be used with caution during pregnancy.

In horses, thiopental should not be used if the patient has preexisting leukopenia. Some clinicians feel that thiopental should not be used alone in the horse as it may cause excessive ataxia and excitement.

Concentrations of less than 2% in sterile water should not be used as they may cause hemolysis. Extravasation and intra-arterial injections should be avoided because of the high alkalinity of the solution. Severe CNS toxicity and tissue damage has resulted in horses receiving intra-carotid injections of thiobarbiturates.

Adverse Effects/Warnings - In dogs, thiopental has an approximate arrhythmogenic incidence of 40%. Ventricular bigeminy is the most common arrhythmia seen and is usually transient and generally responds to additional oxygen. Administration of catecholamines may augment the arrhythmogenic effects of the thiobarbiturates, while lidocaine may inhibit it. Cardiac output may also be reduced, but is probably only clinically significant in patients experiencing heart failure.

Cats are susceptible to developing apnea after injection and may also develop a mild arterial hypotension.

Horses can exhibit symptoms of excitement and severe ataxia during the recovery period if the drug is used alone. Horses also can develop transient leukopenias and hyperglycemia after administration. A period of apnea and moderate tachycardia and a mild respiratory acidosis may also develop after dosing.

Too rapid IV administration can cause significant vascular dilatation and hypoglycemia. Repeated administration of thiopental is not advised as recovery times can become significantly prolonged. Parasympathetic side effects (*e.g.,* salivation, bradycardia) may be managed with the use of anticholinergic agents (atropine, glycopyrrolate).

Overdosage - Treatment of thiobarbiturate overdosage consists of supporting respirations (O_2, mechanical ventilation) and giving cardiovascular support (do not use catecholamines, *e.g.,* epinephrine, etc).

Drug Interactions - A fatal interaction has been reported in a dog receiving the proprietary product, ***Diathal***® (procaine penicillin G, dihydrostreptomycin sulfate, diphemanil methylsulfate, and chlorpheniramine maleate) and the related compound thiamylal. Avoid using thiopental with this product.

The ventricular fibrillatory effects of **epinephrine** and **norepinephrine** are potentiated when used with thiobarbiturates and halothane.

CNS and respiratory depressant effects of **CNS depressants (narcotics, phenothiazines, antihistamines, etc.)** may be enhanced by thiobarbiturate administration.

Thiopental with **furosemide** may cause or increase postural hypotension. **Sulfisoxasole** IV has been shown to compete with thiopental at plasma protein binding sites. This may also occur with other sulfonamides.

Doses - Note: Atropine sulfate or glycopyrrolate are often administered prior to thiobarbiturate anesthesia to prevent parasympathetic side effects. Some clinicians question, however, whether routine administration of the anticholinergic agents are necessary.

Thiobarbiturates are administered strictly to effect; doses are guidelines only.

Dogs:
a) 13.2 - 26.4 mg/kg IV depending on duration of anesthesia required. (*Pentothal*® package insert— Ceva Laboratories)
b) 15 - 17 mg/kg IV for brief (7-10 minutes) anesthesia; 18 - 22 mg/kg IV for moderate (10-15 minutes) duration; 22 - 29 mg/kg IV for longer (15-25 minutes) duration (Booth 1988a)
c) 22 mg/kg IV; or 15.4 mg/kg IV after tranquilization; or 11 mg/kg IV after narcotic premedication. (Mandsager 1988)

Cats:
a) 13.2 - 26.4 mg/kg IV depending on duration of anesthesia required. (*Pentothal*® package insert, Ceva Laboratories)
b) 22 mg/kg IV; or 15.4 mg/kg IV after tranquilization; or 11 mg/kg IV after narcotic premedication. (Mandsager 1988)

Cattle:
a) Cattle: 8.14 - 15.4 mg/kg IV;
For unweaned calves from which food has been withheld for 6-12 hours: no more than 6.6 mg/kg IV for deep surgical anesthesia. (*Pentothal*® package insert; Ceva Laboratories)
b) For calves under 2 weeks of age: 15 - 22 mg/kg IV slowly until complete muscular relaxation takes place, duration of anesthesia usually lasts 10-12 minutes. (Booth 1988a)
c) 5.5 mg/kg IV after sedation and administration with guaifenesin; or 8.8-11 mg/kg IV after tranquilization. (Mandsager 1988)

Horses:
a) With preanesthetic tranquilization: 6 - 12 mg/kg IV (an average of 8.25 mg/kg is recommended); Without preanesthetic tranquilization: 8.8-15.4 mg/kg IV (an average horse: 9.9 - 11 mg/kg IV) (*Pentothal*® package insert; Ceva Laboratories)
b) One gram of thiopental per 90 kg body weight as a 10% solution given evenly over 20 seconds 15 minutes after premedication with either 0.22 mg/kg IV xylazine or 0.05 mg/kg IV acepromazine. (Booth 1988a)
c) 5.5 mg/kg IV after sedation and administration with guaifenesin; or 8.8 - 11 mg/kg IV after tranquilization. (Mandsager 1988)

Swine:
a) 5.5 - 11 mg/kg IV (*Pentothal*® package insert, Ceva Laboratories)
b) For swine weighing 5 - 50 kg: 10 - 11 mg/kg IV (Booth 1988a)

Sheep:
a) 9.9 - 15 mg/kg IV depending on depth of anesthesia required (*Pentothal*® package insert, Ceva Laboratories)

Goats:
a) 20 - 22 mg/kg IV after atropine (0.7 mg/kg) IM (Booth 1988a)

Monitoring Parameters -
1) Level of hypnosis/anesthesia
2) Respiratory status; cardiac status (rate/rhythm/blood pressure)

Client Information - This drug should only be used by professionals familiar with its effects in a setting where adequate respiratory support can be performed.

Dosage Forms/Preparations -
Veterinary-Approved Products: None
Human-Approved Products:
Thiopental Sodium Powder for Injection: 2% (20 mg/ml) in 1, 2.5 & 5 g kits, 400 mg syringes; 2.5% (25 mg/ml) in 250 & 500 mg vials and 500 mg, 1, 2.5, 5 and 10 g kits, 250 & 500 mg syringes; *Pentothal*® (Abbott/Ceva); Generic; (Rx) (C-III)

Preparation of Solution for Administration: The veterinary labeled product comes in a 5 gram kit for dilution to 2.5% or 5%. If using other products without diluent, use only sterile water for injection, normal saline, or D5W to dilute. A 5 gram vial diluted with 100 mls will yield a 5% solution and diluted with 200 ml will yield a 2.5% solution. Discard reconstituted solutions after 24 hours.

Also known as thiopentone sodium, thiopental is a Class-III controlled substance and is a legend (Rx) drug.

THIOTEPA

Chemistry - An ethylene derivative alkylating agent antineoplastic, thiotepa occurs as fine, white crystalline flakes. The drug has a faint odor and is freely soluble in water or alcohol. Thiotepa may also be known as triethylenethiophosphoramide, TESPA, or TSPA.

Storage/Stability/Compatibility - Store both the powder and the reconstituted solution refrigerated (2-8°C) and protected from light. Do not use solution that is grossly opaque (slightly opaque is OK) or if a precipitate is present. If refrigerated, reconstituted solutions are stable for up to 5 days.

Pharmacology - Thiotepa is an alkylating agent, thereby interfering with DNA replication and RNA transcription. It is cell-cycle non-specific. Thiotepa also has some immunosuppressive activity. When given via the intracavitary route, thiotepa is thought to control malignant effusions by a direct antineoplastic effect.

Uses/Indications - Veterinary indications for thiotepa include: systemic use for adjunctive therapy against carcinomas, intravesical administration for transitional cell tumors, and intracavitary use for neoplastic effusions.

Pharmacokinetics - Thiotepa is poorly absorbed from the GI tract. Systemic absorption is variable from the pleural cavity, bladder and after IM injection. Some studies in humans have shown that absorption from bladder mucosa ranges from 10-100% of an administered dose. Distribution characteristics are not well described; it is unknown if the drug enters maternal milk. Thiotepa is extensively metabolized and then excreted in the urine.

Contraindications/Precautions/Reproductive Safety - Thiotepa is contraindicated in patients hypersensitive to it. The drug should be used cautiously (weigh risk versus benefit) in patients with hepatic dysfunction, bone marrow depression, infection, tumor cell infiltration of bone marrow, renal function impairment (adjust dosage) or have a history of urate urinary stones. Thiotepa has a very low therapeutic index and should only be used by clinicians with experience in the use of cytotoxic agents and able to monitor therapy appropriately.

Thiotepa is potentially mutagenic and teratogenic and is not recommended for use during pregnancy. Although it is unknown whether thiotepa enters milk, use of milk replacer is recommended for nursing bitches or queens.

Adverse Effects/Warnings - When used systemically, leukopenia is the most likely adverse effect seen in small animals. Other hematopoietic toxicity (thrombocytopenia, anemia, pancytopenia) may also be noted. Intracavitary or intravesical instillation of thiotepa may also cause hematologic toxicity. GI toxicity (vomiting, diarrhea, stomatitis, intestinal ulceration) may be noted and human patients have reported dizziness and headache as well.

Overdosage/Acute Toxicity - There is no specific antidote for thiotepa overdose. Supportive therapy, including transfusions of appropriate blood products may be beneficial for treatment of hematologic toxicity.

Drug Interactions - Use extreme caution when used concurrently with other drugs that are also myelosuppressive, including many of the **other antineoplastics and other bone marrow depressant drugs (*e.g.*, chloramphenicol, flucytosine, amphotericin B, or colchicine)**. Bone marrow depression may be additive. Use with other **immunosuppressant drugs (*e.g.*, azathioprine, cyclophosphamide, corticosteroids)** may increase the risk of infection. **Live virus vaccines** should be used with caution, if at all during therapy.

By activating plasminogen and increasing the amount of drug in tumor tissue, **urokinase** may enhance the anti-tumor activity of thiotepa in the bladder.

Laboratory Considerations - Thiotepa may increase **serum uric acid** levels in some patients.

Doses -
  Dogs:
    For intracavitary use neoplastic effusions or systemically for adjunctive therapy of carcinomas:
      a) 0.2 - 0.5 mg/m2 intracavitary; IV. (Jacobs, Lumsden et al. 1992)

Monitoring Parameters - 1) Efficacy; 2) CBC w/platelets

Client Information - Clients must be briefed on the possibilities of severe toxicity developing from this drug, including drug-related neoplasms or mortality. Clients should contact veterinarian should the animal exhibit symptoms of abnormal bleeding, bruising, anorexia, vomiting, jaundice or infection.

Dosage Forms/Preparations/FDA Approval Status/Withholding Times -
  Veterinary-Approved Products: None
  Human-Approved Products:
    Thiotepa Powder for Injection 15 mg in vials; *Thiotepa*® (Immunex); (Rx)

THYROTROPIN (THYROID-STIMULATING HORMONE; TSH)

Chemistry - Obtained from bovine anterior pituitary glands, thyrotropin is a highly purified preparation of thyroid-stimulating hormone (TSH). Thyrotropin is a glycoprotein and has a molecular weight of approximately 28,000 - 30,000. Thyrotropin is measured in International Units (IU), with 7.5 micrograms of thyrotropin approximately equivalent to 0.037 units. Commercially available thyrotropin is available as a lyophilized powder for reconstitution and is practically free of any adrenocorticotropic, somatotropic, gonadotropic and posterior pituitary hormones.

Thyrotropin may also be known as TSH, thyrotrophin, thyroid-stimulating hormone or thyrotropic hormone.

Storage/Stability/Compatibility - Thyrotropin lyophilized powder for injection is reportedly stable in the dry state. However, the veterinary manufacturer recommends storing the powder below 59°F, and after reconstituting, storing in the refrigerator and discarding any unused drug after 48 hours. However, recent information has suggested that reconstituted TSH is stable for at least 3 weeks when refrigerated. The human-approved product may be kept refrigerated (2-8°C) for up to 2 weeks after reconstituting.

Pharmacology - Thyrotropin increases iodine uptake by the thyroid gland and increases the production and secretion of thyroid hormones. With prolonged use, hyperplasia of thyroid cells may occur.

Uses/Indications - The labeled indications for *Dermathycin*® (Coopers/P/M; Mallinckrodt) is for "the treatment of acanthosis nigricans and for temporary supportive therapy in hypothyroidism in dogs." In actuality however, TSH is used in veterinary medicine principally as a diagnostic agent in the TSH stimulation test to diagnose primary hypothyroidism.

Pharmacokinetics - No specific information was located; exogenously administered TSH apparently exerts maximal increases in circulating T4 approximately 4-8 hours after IM or IV administration.

Contraindications/Precautions - The veterinary manufacturer (Coopers) lists adrenocortical insufficiency and hyperthyroidism as contraindications to TSH use for treatment purposes in dogs. In humans, TSH is contraindicated in patients with coronary thrombosis, hypersensitive to bovine thyrotropin, or with untreated Addison's disease.

Adverse Effects/Warnings - Because the product is derived from bovine sources, anaphylaxis may occur in patients sensitive to bovine proteins, particularly with repeated use.

Overdosage - Chronic administration at high dosages can produce symptoms of hyperthyroidism. Massive overdoses can cause symptoms resembling thyroid storm. Refer to the levothyroxine monograph for more information on treatment.

Drug Interactions; **Drug/Laboratory Interactions -** For reference, refer to the information listed in the Levothyroxine monograph for more information.

Doses -
  Dogs:
    For TSH stimulation test:
      a) Draw pre-dose baseline sample. Administer 0.1 IU/kg IV (maximum of 5 IU). Collect sample for T4 6 hours after dose. (Peterson and Ferguson 1989)
      b) 5 IU IV or 0.1 IU/kg IV. Measure serum T4 at 0 hours (pre-sample) and 4 or 6 hours after dose. (Morgan 1988)

    For treatment of acanthosis nigricans or temporary supportive therapy in hypothyroidism (labeled indications):
      a) 1 - 2 IU SQ once daily for 5 days. (Package Insert; *Dermathycin*®—Coopers)
  Cats:
    For TSH stimulation test:
      a) Draw pre-dose baseline sample. Administer 1 IU/kg IV or 2.5 IU IM. Collect sample for T4 6 hours after dose. (Peterson and Ferguson 1989)

b) 2.5 IU IV. Measure serum T4 at 0 hours (pre-sample) and 4 or 6 hours after dose. (Morgan 1988)

Horses:

For TSH stimulation test:

a) Draw pre-dose sample, then 5 - 10 IU of bovine TSH IV. Draw follow-up samples 4-8 hours after dosing. Normal thyroid gland should produce a 2-4 times increase in serum T3 and T4 levels. (Chen and Li 1987)

Client Information - Usually TSH will be used by professional staff. If the drug is to be used at home, the owner should follow directions carefully, shake the vial well after reconstituting, and store in the refrigerator.

Dosage Forms/Preparations/FDA Approval Status -

Veterinary-Approved Products:

Thyroid Stimulating Hormone (Veterinary) 5 IU per vial (with 5 ml of Water for Injection as diluent); *Dermathycin*® (Schering Plough); (Rx) Approved for use in dogs. This product may not be currently on the market.

Human-Approved Products:

Thyrotropin (Thyroid Stimulating Hormone) Powder for Injection 10 IU per vial (with diluent); *Thyrotropar*® (Armour); (Rx)

Thyroxine Sodium - See Levothyroxine

TIAMULIN

Chemistry - A semisynthetic diterpene-class antibiotic derived from pleuromulin, tiamulin is available commercially for oral use as the hydrogen fumurate salt. It occurs as white to yellow, crystalline powder with a faint but characteristic odor. Approximately 60 mg of the drug are soluble in 1 ml of water.

Storage/Stability/Compatibility - Protect from moisture; store in a dry place. In unopened packets, the powder is stable for up to 5 years. Fresh solutions should be prepared daily when using clinically.

Pharmacology - Tiamulin is usually a bacteriostatic antibiotic, but can be bactericidal in very high concentrations against susceptible organisms. The drug acts by binding to the 50S ribosomal subunit, thereby inhibiting bacterial protein synthesis.

Tiamulin has good activity against many gram positive cocci, including most Staphylococci and Streptococci (not group D streps). It also has good activity against Mycoplasma and spirochetes. With the exception of *Haemophilus sp.* and some *E. coli* and *Klebsiella* strains, the drug's activity is quite poor against gram negative organisms.

Uses/Indications - Tiamulin is approved for use in swine to treat pneumonia caused by susceptible strains of *Haemophilus pleuropneumoniae* and swine dysentery caused by *Treponema hyodysenteriae*. As a feed additive it also used to cause increased weight gain in swine.

Pharmacokinetics - Tiamulin is well absorbed orally by swine. Approximately 85% of a dose is absorbed and peak levels occur between 2-4 hours after a single oral dose. Tiamulin is apparently well distributed, with highest levels found in the lungs.

Tiamulin is extensively metabolized to over 20 metabolites, some having antibacterial activity. Approximately 30% of these metabolites are excreted in the urine with the remainder excreted in the feces.

Contraindications/Precautions/Reproductive Safety - Tiamulin should not be administered to animals having access to feeds containing polyether ionophores (*e.g.,* monensin, lasalocid, narasin, or salinomycin) as adverse reactions may occur. Not for use in swine over 250 pounds.

Teratogenicity studies done in rodents demonstrated no teratogenic effects at doses up to 300 mg/kg. The manufacturer has concluded that the drug is not tumorigenic, carcinogenic, teratogenic or mutagenic.

Adverse Effects/Warnings - Adverse effects occurring with this drug at usual doses are considered unlikely. Rarely, redness of the skin, primarily over the ham and underline, has been observed. It is recommended to discontinue the medication, provide clean drinking water and hose down the area or move affected animals to clean pens.

Overdosage/Acute Toxicity - Oral overdoses in pigs may cause transient salivation, vomiting and CNS depression (calming effect). Discontinue drug and treat symptomatically and supportively if necessary.

Drug Interactions - Tiamulin should not be administered to animals having access to feeds containing polyether ionophores (*e.g.,* **monensin, lasalocid, narasin,** or **salinomycin**) as adverse reactions may occur. Although not confirmed with this drug, concomitant use with other antibiotics that bind to the 50S ribosome (*e.g.,* **clindamycin, lincomycin, erythromycin, tylosin**) could lead to decreased efficacy due to competition at the site of action.

Doses -
  Swine:
    For swine dysentery:
      a) 7.7 mg/kg PO daily in drinking water for 5 days. See package directions for dilution instructions. (Package insert; *Denagard*® *Soluble Antibiotic*)
    For *Haemophilus* pneumonia:
      a) 23.1 mg/kg PO daily in drinking water for 5 days. See package directions for dilution instructions. (Package insert; *Denagard*® *Soluble Antibiotic*)

Monitoring Parameters -
  1) Clinical efficacy

Client Information - Prepare fresh medicated water daily. Avoid contact with skin or mucous membranes as irritation may occur.

Dosage Forms/Preparations/FDA Approval Status/Withholding Times -
  Tiamulin Soluble Powder 25.3 g packets (each containing 11.4 g tiamulin) or 64.6 g packets (each containing 29.1 g tiamulin); *Denagard*® *Soluble Antibiotic* (Boehringer Ingelheim); (OTC) Approved for use in swine less than 250 pounds in weight. Slaughter withdrawal= 3 days at swine dysentery rate (7.7 mg/kg PO daily) and 7 days at Haemophilus pneumonia rate (23.1 mg/kg PO daily).

  Also available in an oral Premix form (*Denagard*® *10*—Boehringer Ingelheim).

TICARCILLIN DISODIUM

For general information on the penicillins, including adverse effects, contraindications, overdosage, drug interactions and monitoring parameters, refer to the monograph: Penicillins, General Information.

Chemistry - An alpha-carboxypenicillin, ticarcillin disodium occurs as a white to pale yellow, hygroscopic powder or lyophilized cake with pK_as of 2.55 and 3.42. More than 600 mg is soluble in 1 ml of water. Potency of ticarcillin disodium is expressed in terms of ticarcillin and one gram of the disodium contains not less than 800 mg of ticarcillin anhydrous. One gram of the commercially available injection contains 5.2-6.5 mEq of sodium and after reconstituting the injection has a pH of 6-8.

Storage/Stability/Compatibility - Ticarcillin injectable powder for injection should be stored at temperatures of less than 30°C (room temperature or colder).

  If stored at room temperature after reconstitution, polymer conjugates can form that may increase the likelihood of hypersensitivity reactions occurring. Therefore, many clinicians recommend either refrigerating the solution or administering within 30 minutes of reconstitution. From a potency standpoint, the drug should be used generally within 24 hours if stored at room temperature and 72 hours if refrigerated, but the manufacturer has specific recommendations depending on the concentration of the drug and the solution. Refer to the package insert for more specific recommendations. Frozen solutions are reportedly stable for at least 30 days when stored at -20°C.

Ticarcillin disodium solutions are reportedly physically **compatible** with the following solutions and drugs: D5W, Ringer's Injection, Lactated Ringer's Injection, Sodium chloride 0.9%, Sterile water for injection, acyclovir sodium, hydromorphone HCl, meperidine HCl, methylprednisolone sodium succinate, morphine Sulfate, ranitidine HCl, perphenazine and verapamil HCl.

Ticarcillin disodium solutions are reportedly physically **incompatible** with the aminoglycoside antibiotics; refer to the drug interaction information in the Penicillins, General Information monograph for more information. Compatibility is dependent upon factors such as pH, concentration, temperature and diluents used. It is suggested to consult specialized references for more specific information (*e.g., Handbook on Injectable Drugs* by Trissel; see bibliography).

Pharmacology/Uses/Indications - A ticarcillin disodium product is approved for intrauterine use in horses in the treatment of endometritis in horses caused by *beta hemolytic streptococci*.

Ticarcillin disodium injection is used in veterinary species in the treatment of systemic *Pseudomonas aeruginosa* infections, often in combination with an appropriate aminoglycoside agent. When compared with carbenicillin, ticarcillin is about twice as potent (on a weight basis) in the treatment against susceptible *Pseudomonas*. Synergy may occur against some *Pseudomonas* strains when used in combination with aminoglycosides, but *in vitro* inactivation of the aminoglycoside may also occur (see Drug Interactions) if the drugs are physically mixed together or in patients with severe renal failure.

Pharmacokinetics (specific) - Ticarcillin is not appreciably absorbed after oral administration and must be given parenterally to achieve therapeutic serum levels. When given IM to humans, the drug is readily absorbed with peak levels occurring about 30-60 minutes after dosing. The reported bioavailability in the horse after IM administration is about 65%.

After parenteral injection, ticarcillin is distributed into pleural fluid, interstitial fluid, bile, sputum and bone. Like other penicillins, CSF levels are low in patients with normal meninges (about 6% of serum levels), but increased (39% of serum levels) if meninges are inflamed. The volume of distribution is reportedly 0.34 L/kg in dogs and 0.22-0.25 L/kg in the horse. The drug is 45-65% bound to serum proteins (human). Ticarcillin is thought to cross the placenta and is found in small quantities in milk. In cattle, mastitic milk levels of ticarcillin are approximately twice those found in normal milk, but are too low to treat most causal organisms.

Ticarcillin is eliminated primarily by the kidneys, via both tubular secretion and glomerular filtration. Concurrent probenecid administration can slow elimination and increase blood levels. In humans, about 10-15% of the drug is metabolized by hydrolysis to inactive compounds. The half-life in dogs and cats is reportedly 45-80 minutes and about 54 minutes in the horse. Clearance is 4.3 ml/kg/min in the dog and 2.8-3.2 ml/kg/min in the horse.

Doses -
 Dogs:
  For susceptible infections:
   a) 15 - 25 mg/kg IV, or IM q8h (Davis 1985)
   b) 55 - 110 mg/kg IV, IM or SQ q8h (Aronson and Aucoin 1989)
   c) Using the ticarcillin/clavulanate product (usually for *Pseudomonas spp.* infections): 40 - 110 mg/kg IV or IM q6h (Vaden and Papich 1995)

 Cats:
  For susceptible infections:
   a) 15 - 25 mg/kg IV, or IM q8h (Davis 1985)
   b) 55 - 110 mg/kg IV, IM or SQ q8h (Aronson and Aucoin 1989)

 Horses:
  For susceptible systemic infections:
   a) 44 mg/kg q5h IV or *tid* IM. (Robinson 1987)
   b) Foals: 50 mg/kg IV q6-8h (Dose extrapolated from data obtained from adult horses; use lower dose or longer interval in premature foals or those less than 7 days old.) (Caprile and Short 1987)

  For treatment of endometritis secondary to susceptible bacteria:
   a) 6 grams intrauterine per day for 3 days during estrus. Reconstitute vial with 25 ml of Sterile Water for Injection, USP or Sodium Chloride Injection, USP. After dissolved, further dilute to a total volume of 100-500 ml with sterile water or sterile normal saline and aseptically instill into uterus. (Package insert; *Ticillin®*—Beecham)

 Birds:
  For susceptible infections:
   a) 200 mg/kg IV or IM *bid, tid* or *qid* (Clubb 1986)
   b) 200 mg/kg IM or IV q8h (Hoeffer 1995)

Dosage Forms/Preparations/FDA Approval Status/Withholding Times -
Veterinary-Approved Products:
  Ticarcillin Disodium Sterile Powder for Intrauterine Infusion 6 g vial; *Ticillin®* (Pfizer); (Rx) Approved for use in horses.

 Human-Approved Products:
  Ticarcillin Disodium Powder for Injection (contains 5.2 mEq sodium./g) 1 g, 3 g, 6 g, 20 g, & 30 g in vials; *Ticar®* (SK-Beecham); (Rx)

Also available with human approval is a ticarcillin/clavulanic acid injectable preparation (*Timentin®*—Beecham) that would be effective against many penicillinase-producing strains of bacteria, such as most *Staphylococcus* species.

TILETAMINE HCL/ZOLAZEPAM HCL
 (*Telazol®*)

Chemistry - Tiletamine is an injectable anesthetic agent chemically related to ketamine. Zolazepam is a diazepinone minor tranquilizer. The pH of the injectable product after reconstitution is 2.2 - 2.8.

Storage/Stability/Compatibility - After reconstitution, solutions may be stored for 4 days at room temperature and 14 days if refrigerated. Do not use solutions that contain a precipitate or are discolored.

Pharmacology - In cats, tiletamine decreases cardiac rate and blood pressure after IM injections. Its effect on respiratory activity is controversial, and until these effects have been clarified respiratory function should be closely monitored. The pharmacology of this drug combination is similar to that of ketamine and diazepam. For more information refer to the monographs for those agents.

Uses/Indications - *Telazol®* is indicated for restraint or anesthesia combined with muscle relaxation in cats, and for restraint and minor procedures of short duration (≈30 minutes) which require mild to moderate analgesia in dogs. Although not officially approved, it has been used also in horses and many exotic and wild species.

Pharmacokinetics - Little pharmacokinetic information is available for these agents. The onset of action may be variable and be very rapid; animals should be observed carefully after injection.

In cats, the onset of action is reported to be within 1-7 minutes after IM injection. Duration of anesthesia is dependent on dosage, but is usually about 0.33-1 hour at peak effect. This is reported to be approximately 3 times the duration of ketamine anesthesia. The duration of effect of the zolazepam component is longer than that of the tiletamine, so there is a greater degree of tranquilization than anesthesia during the recovery period. The recovery times vary in length from approximately 1-5.5 hours.

In dogs, the onset of action following IM injection averages 7.5 minutes. The mean duration of surgical anesthesia is about 27 minutes, with recovery times averaging approximately 4 hours. The duration of the tiletamine effect is longer than that of zolazepam, so there is a shorter duration of tranquilization than there is anesthesia. Less than 4% of the drugs are reported to be excreted unchanged in the urine in the dog.

Contraindications/Precautions - *Telazol®* is contraindicated in animals with pancreatic disease, severe cardiac or pulmonary disease. Animals with renal disease may have prolonged durations of anesthetic action or recovery times.

Telazol® crosses the placenta and may cause respiratory depression in newborns; the manufacturer lists its use in cesarian section as being contraindicated. The teratogenic potential of the drug is unknown, and it is not recommended to be used during any stage of pregnancy.

Because *Telazol®* may cause hypothermia, susceptible animals (small body surface area, low ambient temperatures) should be monitored carefully and supplemental heat applied if needed. Like ketamine, *Telazol®* does not abolish pinnal, palpebral, pedal, laryngeal, and pharyngeal reflexes and its use (alone) may not be adequate if surgery is to be performed on these areas.

This drug has been reported to be contraindicated in rabbits.

Cat's eyes remain open after receiving *Telazol®* , and they should be protected from injury and an ophthalmic lubricant (*e.g., Lacrilube®*) should be applied to prevent excessive drying of the cornea. Cats reportedly do not tolerate endotracheal tubes well with this agent.

Dosages may need to be reduced in geriatric, debilitated, or animals with renal dysfunction.

Adverse Effects/Warnings - Respiratory depression is a definite possibility, especially with higher dosages of this product. Apnea may occur; observe animal carefully. Pain after IM injection (especially in cats) has been noted which may be a result of the low pH of the solution. Athetoid movements (constant succession of slow, writhing, involuntary movements of flexion, extension, pronation, etc) may occur; do not give additional *Telazol®* in the attempt to diminish these actions.

In dogs, tachycardia may be a common effect and may last for 30 minutes. Insufficient anesthesia after recommended doses has been reported in dogs.

Other adverse effects listed by the manufacturer include: emesis during emergence, excessive salivation and bronchial/tracheal secretions (if atropine not administered beforehand), transient apnea, vocalization, erratic and/or prolonged recovery, involuntary muscular twitching, hypertonia, cyanosis, cardiac arrest, pulmonary edema, muscle rigidity, and either hypertension or hypotension.

Overdosage - The manufacturer claims a 2X margin of safety in dogs, and a 4.5 times margin of safety in cats. A preliminary study in dogs (Hatch et al. 1988) suggests that doxapram at 5.5 mg/kg will enhance respirations and arousal after *Telazol®*. In massive overdoses, it is suggested that mechanically assisted ventilation be performed if necessary and other symptoms be treated symptomatically and supportively.

Drug Interactions - Little specific information is available presently on drug interactions with this product. In dogs, **chloramphenicol** apparently has no effect on recovery times with *Telazol®*, but in cats, anesthesia is prolonged on average of 30 minutes by chloramphenicol. Cats wearing flea collars have not been demonstrated to have prolonged anesthesia times.

Phenothiazines can cause increased respiratory and cardiac depression when used with this product.

The dosage of **barbiturate** or **volatile anesthetics** may need to be reduced when used concomitantly with *Telazol®*. For general guidelines with regard to drug interactions with this product, please refer to the ketamine and diazepam monographs.

Doses -
Dogs:
- a) For diagnostic purposes: 6.6 - 9.9 mg/kg IM
   For minor procedures of short duration: 9.9 - 13.2 mg/kg IM
   If supplemental doses are necessary, give doses less than the initial dose and total dosage should not exceed 26.4 mg/kg. Atropine 0.04 mg/kg should be used concurrently to control hypersalivation. (Package Insert; *Telazol®* - Robins)
- b) For surgical interventions of 30-60 minutes: 6 - 13 mg/kg IM (Booth 1988a)

Cats:
- a) 9.7 - 11.9 mg/kg IM for procedures such as dentistry, abscess treatment, foreign body removal, etc. For procedures that require mild to moderate levels of analgesia (lacerations, castration, etc.) use 10.6 - 12.5 mg/kg IM.
   For ovariohysterectomy and onychectomy use 14.3 - 15.8 mg/kg IM.
   If supplemental doses are necessary, give doses less than the initial dose and the total dosage should not exceed 72 mg/kg. Atropine 0.04 mg/kg should be used concurrently to control hypersalivation. (Package Insert; *Telazol®* - Robins)
- b) For surgical interventions of 30-60 minutes: 6 - 13 mg/kg IM (Booth 1988a)

Pocket Pets:
   Gerbils: 20 mg/kg IP (in combination with xylazine 10 mg/kg) (Huerkamp 1995)

Horses:
- a) Xylazine 1.1 mg/kg IV, 5 minutes prior to *Telazol®* at 1.65 - 2.2 mg/kg IV (Hubbell, Bednarski, and Muir 1989)

Exotic Species:
- a) An extensive list of suggested *Telazol®* dosages may be found in the article by E. Schobert entitled, "*Telazol®* Use in Wild and Exotic Animals" in the October 1987 issue of *Veterinary Medicine*.

Monitoring Parameters -
1) Level of anesthesia/analgesia
2) Respiratory function; cardiovascular status (rate, rhythm, BP if possible)
3) Monitor eyes to prevent drying or injury
4) Body temperature

Client Information - Should only be administered by individuals familiar with its use.

Dosage Forms/Preparations/FDA Approval Status/Withholding Times -
Veterinary-Approved Products:
   Tiletamine HCl (equivalent to 250 mg free base) & Zolazepam HCl (equivalent to 250 mg free base) as lyophilized powder/vial in 5 ml vials. When 5 ml of sterile diluent (sterile water) is added a concentration of 50 mg/ml of each drug (100 mg/ml combined) is produced.; *Telazol®* (Fort Dodge); (Rx) Approved for use in cats and dogs. *Telazol®* is a Class III controlled substance.

Human-Approved Products: None

TILMICOSIN

Chemistry - A semi-synthetic macrolide antibiotic, tilmicosin phosphate is commercially available in a 300 mg/ml (of tilmicosin base) injection with 25% propylene glycol.

Storage/Stability/Compatibility - Store the injection at or below room temperature. Avoid exposure to direct sunlight.

Pharmacology - Like other macrolides, tilmicosin has activity primarily against gram positive bacteria, although some gram negative bacteria are affected and the drug reportedly has some activity against mycoplasma. Preliminary studies have shown that 95% of studied isolates of *Pasturella haemolytica* are sensitive.

Uses/Indications - Tilmicosin is indicated fort the treatment of bovine respiratory diseases (BRD) caused by *Pasturella haemolytica*.

Pharmacokinetics - Tilmicosin apparently concentrates in lung tissue. At 3 days post injection, the lung:serum ratio is about 60:1. MIC_{95} concentrations (3.12 micrograms/ml) for *P. Haemolytica* persist for a minimum of 3 days after a single injection.

Contraindications/Precautions/Reproductive Safety - Not to be used in automatically powered syringes or to be given intravenously as fatalities may result. Tilmicosin has been shown to be fatal in swine, non-human primates and potentially fatal in horses.

Safe use in pregnant animals or in animals to be used for breeding purposes has not been demonstrated.

Adverse Effects/Warnings - If administered IM, a local tissue reaction may occur resulting in trim loss. Edema may be noted at the site of subcutaneous injection.

Avoid contact with eyes.

Overdosage/Acute Toxicity - The cardiovascular system is apparently the target of toxicity in animals. In cattle, doses up to 50 mg/kg did not cause death, but SQ doses of 150 mg/kg did cause fatalities. Doses as low as 10 mg/kg in swine caused increased respiration, emesis and seizures; 20 mg/kg caused deaths in most animals tested. In monkeys, 10 mg/kg administered once caused no signs of toxicity, but 20 mg/kg caused vomiting and 30 mg/kg caused death.

In cases of human injection, contact physician immediately. The manufacturer has emergency telephone numbers to assist in dealing with exposure: 1-800-722-0987 or 1-317-276-2000.

Drug Interactions - In swine, **epinephrine** increased the mortality associated with tilmicosin. No other specific information noted; refer to the erythromycin monograph for potential interactions.

Doses -
  Cattle:
    For susceptible infections (subcutaneous injection behind the shoulders and over the ribs is suggested).
      a) For treatment of pneumonic pasteurellosis in cattle: 10 mg/kg SQ every 72 hours. (Shewen and Bateman 1993)
      b) Package insert (*Micotil*® 300; Elanco): 10 mg/kg SubQ (not more than 15 ml per injection site)

Monitoring Parameters - 1) Efficacy; 2) Withdrawal times

Client Information - If clients are administering the drug, they should be warned about the potential toxicity to humans, swine and horses if accidentally injected. They should also be carefully instructed in proper injection techniques. Avoid contact with eyes.

Dosage Forms/Preparations/FDA Approval Status/Withholding Times -
  Veterinary-Approved Products:
    Tilmicosin for Subcutaneous Injection 300 mg/ml in 100 ml and 250 ml multi-dose vials; *Micotil*® *300 Injection* (Elanco); (Rx) Approved for use in cattle. Not approved for use in female dairy cattle 20 months or older. Do not use in veal calves. Slaughter withdrawal = 28 days.

  Human-Approved Products: None

TIOPRONIN

Chemistry - A sulfhydryl compound related to penicillamine, tiopronin has a molecular weight of 163.2. It is also known as thiopronine or *N*-(2-Mercaptopropionyl)-glycine (MPG).

Storage/Stability/Compatibility - Store tablets at room temperature in tight containers.

Pharmacology - Tiopronin is considered to be an antiurolithic agent. It undergoes thiol-disulfide exchange with cystine (cysteine-cysteine disulfide) to form tiopronin-cystine disulfide. This complex is more water soluble and is readily excreted thereby preventing cystine calculi from forming.

Uses/Indications - Tiopronin is indicated for the prevention of cystine urolithiasis in patients where dietary therapy combined with urinary alkalinization is not completely effective. It may also be useful in combination with urine alkalinization to dissolve stones.

Pharmacokinetics - Tiopronin has a rapid onset of action and in humans, up to 48% of a dose is found in the urine within 4 hours of dosing. Tiopronin has a relatively short duration of action and its effect in humans disappears in about 10 hours. Elimination is primarily via renal routes.

Contraindications/Precautions/Reproductive Safety - Tiopronin's risks versus its benefits should be considered before using in patients with agranulocytosis, aplastic anemia, thrombocytopenia or other significant hematologic abnormality, impaired renal or hepatic function, or sensitivity to either tiopronin or penicillamine.

There is limited information on the reproductive safety of tiopronin. Skeletal defects, cleft palates and increased resorptions were noted when rats were given 10 times the human dose of penicillamine and, therefore, may also be of concern with tiopronin. Other animals studies have suggested that tiopronin may affect fetus viability at high doses. Because tiopronin may be excreted in milk, at present it is not recommended for use in nursing animals.

Adverse Effects/Warnings - There is limited information available on the adverse effect profile of tiopronin in dogs. While tiopronin is thought to have fewer adverse effects than penicillamine in humans, it has been associated with Coombs'-positive regenerative spherocyte anemia in dogs. Should this effect occur, the drug should be discontinued and appropriate treatment started (corticosteroids, blood component therapy *prn*). Adverse effects noted in humans that occur more frequently include dermatologic effects (ecchymosis, itching, rashes, mouth ulcers, jaundice) and GI distress. Less frequently allergic reactions (specifically adenopathy), arthralgias, dyspnea, fever, hematologic abnormalities, edema, and nephrotic syndrome have been noted in humans.

Overdosage/Acute Toxicity - There is little information available. It is suggested to contact an animal poison center for further information in the event of an overdose situation.

Drug Interactions - Potentially use of tiopronin with **other drugs causing nephrotoxicity, hepatotoxicity, or bone marrow depression** could cause additive toxic effects. Clinical significance is not clear.

Doses -
  Dogs:
    For treatment or prevention of recurrence of cystine urinary calculi:
      a) In conjunction with an alkalinizing, protein & sodium restricted diet (*e.g.*, U/D®), 30 - 40 mg/kg PO divided into two daily doses. (Cowan 1994)

Monitoring Parameters - 1) Efficacy (stone size); 2) CBC w/ platelets; 3) Urinalyses including urine pH; 4) In humans, serum albumin and liver function tests have been recommended

Client Information - Clients should be counseled on the importance of adequate compliance with this drug to maximize efficacy and detailed on the symptoms to watch for regarding adverse effects.

Dosage Forms/Preparations/FDA Approval Status/Withholding Times -
  Veterinary-Approved Products: None
  Human-Approved Products:
    Tiopronin Tablets 100 mg; *Thiola*® (Mission); (Rx)

TOBRAMYCIN SULFATE

Chemistry - An aminoglycoside derived from *Streptomyces tenebrarius*, tobramycin occurs as a white to off-white, hygroscopic powder that is freely soluble in water and very slightly soluble in alcohol. The sulfate salt is formed during the manufacturing process. The commercial injection is a clear, colorless solution and the pH is adjusted to 6-8 with sulfuric acid and/or sodium hydroxide.

Storage/Stability/Compatibility - Tobramycin sulfate for injection should be stored at room temperature (15-30°C); avoid freezing and temperatures above 40°C. Do not use the product if discolored.

While the manufacturers state that tobramycin should not be mixed with other drugs, it is reportedly **compatible** and stable in most commonly used intravenous solutions (not compatible with dextrose and alcohol solutions, Polysal, Polysal M, or Isolyte E, M or P) and compatible with the following drugs: aztreonam, bleomycin sulfate, calcium gluconate, cefoxitin sodium, ciprofloxacin lactate, clindamycin phosphate (not in syringes), floxacillin sodium, metronidazole (with or without sodium bicarbonate), ranitidine HCl, and verapamil HCl. Several other drugs have been demonstrated to be compatible at Y-sites (see Trissell for more info).

The following drugs or solutions are reportedly **incompatible** or only compatible in specific situations with tobramycin: cefamandole naftate, furosemide and heparin sodium. Compatibility is dependent upon factors such as pH, concentration, temperature and diluents used. It is suggested to consult specialized references for more specific information (*e.g., Handbook on Injectable Drugs* by Trissel; see bibliography).

In vitro inactivation of aminoglycoside antibiotics by beta-lactam antibiotics is well documented. See also the information in the Drug Interaction and Drug/Lab Interaction sections.

Pharmacology - Tobramycin, like the other aminoglycoside antibiotics, act on susceptible bacteria presumably by irreversibly binding to the 30S ribosomal subunit thereby inhibiting protein synthesis. It is considered to be a bactericidal antibiotic.

Tobramycin's spectrum of activity include coverage against many aerobic gram negative and some aerobic gram positive bacteria, including most species of *E. coli, Klebsiella, Proteus, Pseudomonas, Salmonella, Enterobacter, Serratia, Shigella, Mycoplasma*, and *Staphylococcus*.

Antimicrobial activity of the aminoglycosides are enhanced in an alkaline environment.

The aminoglycoside antibiotics are inactive against fungi, viruses and most anaerobic bacteria.

Uses/Indications - While there are no approved veterinary tobramycin products in the U.S., tobramycin may be useful clinically to treat serious gram negative infections in most species. It is often used in settings where gentamicin-resistant bacteria are a clinical problem. The inherent toxicity of the aminoglycosides limit their systemic use to serious infections when there is either a documented lack of susceptibility to other less toxic antibiotics or when the clinical situation dictates immediate treatment of a presumed gram negative infection before culture and susceptibility results are reported.

Whether tobramycin is less nephrotoxic than either gentamicin or amikacin when used clinically is controversial. Laboratory studies indicate that in a controlled setting in laboratory animals, it may indeed be so.

Pharmacokinetics - Tobramycin, like the other aminoglycosides is not appreciably absorbed after oral or intrauterine administration, but it is absorbed from topical administration (not skin or urinary bladder) when used in irrigations during surgical procedures. Patients receiving oral aminoglycosides with hemorrhagic or necrotic enteritises may absorb appreciable quantities of the drug. Subcutaneous injection results in slightly delayed peak levels and with more variability than after IM injection. Bioavailability from extravascular injection (IM or SQ) is greater than 90%.

After absorption, aminoglycosides are distributed primarily in the extracellular fluid. They are found in ascitic, pleural, pericardial, peritoneal, synovial and abscess fluids, and high levels are found in sputum, bronchial secretions and bile. Aminoglycosides (other than streptomycin) are minimally protein bound (<20%) to plasma proteins. Aminoglycosides do not readily cross the blood-brain barrier nor penetrate ocular tissue. CSF levels are unpredictable and range from 0-50% of those found in the serum. Therapeutic levels are found in bone, heart, gallbladder and lung tissues after parenteral dosing. Aminoglycosides tend to accumulate in certain tissues such as the inner ear and kidneys, that may help explain their toxicity. Aminoglycosides cross the placenta and fetal concentrations range from 15-50% of those found in maternal serum.

Elimination of aminoglycosides after parenteral administration occurs almost entirely by glomerular filtration. Patients with decreased renal function can have significantly prolonged half-lives. In humans with normal renal function, elimination rates can be highly variable with the aminoglycoside antibiotics.

Contraindications/Precautions/Reproductive Safety - Aminoglycosides are contraindicated in patients who are hypersensitive to them. Because these drugs are often the only effective agents in severe gram-negative infections, there are no other absolute contraindications to their use. However, they should be used with extreme caution in patients with preexisting renal disease with concomitant monitoring and dosage interval adjustments made. Other risk factors for the development of toxicity include age (both neonatal and geriatric patients), fever, sepsis and dehydration.

Because aminoglycosides can cause irreversible ototoxicity, they should be used with caution in "working" dogs (*e.g.*, "seeing-eye", herding, dogs for the hearing impaired, etc.).

Aminoglycosides should be used with caution in patients with neuromuscular disorders (*e.g.*, myasthenia gravis) due to their neuromuscular blocking activity.

Because aminoglycosides are eliminated primarily through renal mechanisms, they should be used cautiously, preferably with serum monitoring and dosage adjustment in neonatal or geriatric animals.

Aminoglycosides are generally considered contraindicated in rabbits/hares as they adversely affect the GI flora balance in these animals.

Tobramycin can cross the placenta. It has been demonstrated to concentrate in fetal kidneys and while rare, may cause 8th cranial nerve toxicity or nephrotoxicity in fetuses. Total irreversible deafness has been reported in some human babies whose mothers received tobramycin during pregnancy. Because the drug should only be used in serious infections, the benefits of therapy may exceed the potential risks.

Adverse Effects/Warnings - The aminoglycosides are infamous for their nephrotoxic and ototoxic effects. The nephrotoxic (tubular necrosis) mechanisms of these drugs are not completely understood, but are probably related to interference with phospholipid metabolism in the lysosomes of proximal renal tubular cells, resulting in leakage of proteolytic enzymes into the cytoplasm. Nephrotoxicity is usually manifested by increases in BUN, creatinine, nonprotein nitrogen in the serum and decreases in urine specific gravity and creatinine clearance. Proteinuria and cells or casts may also be seen in the urine. Nephrotoxicity is usually reversible once the drug is discontinued. While gentamicin may be more nephrotoxic than the other aminoglycosides, the incidences of nephrotoxicity with all of these agents require equal caution and monitoring.

Ototoxicity (8th cranial nerve toxicity) of the aminoglycosides can be manifested by either auditory and/or vestibular symptoms and may be irreversible. Vestibular symptoms are more frequent with streptomycin, gentamicin, or tobramycin. Auditory symptoms are more frequent with amikacin, neomycin, or kanamycin, but either forms can occur with any of the drugs. Cats are apparently very sensitive to the vestibular effects of the aminoglycosides.

The aminoglycosides can also cause neuromuscular blockade, facial edema, pain/inflammation at injection site, peripheral neuropathy and hypersensitivity reactions. Rarely, GI symptoms, hematologic and hepatic effects have been reported.

Overdosage/Acute Toxicity - Should an inadvertent overdosage be administered, three treatments have been recommended. Hemodialysis is very effective in reducing serum levels of the drug, but is not a viable option for most veterinary patients. Peritoneal dialysis also will reduce serum levels, but is much less efficacious. Complexation of drug with either carbenicillin or ticarcillin (12-20 g/day in humans) is reportedly nearly as effective as hemodialysis.

Drug Interactions - Aminoglycosides should be used with caution with other nephrotoxic, ototoxic, and neurotoxic drugs. These include **amphotericin B**, **other aminoglycosides**, **acyclovir**, **bacitracin** (parenteral use), **cisplatin**, **methoxyflurane**, **polymyxin B**, or **vancomycin**.

The concurrent use of aminoglycosides with **cephalosporins** is controversial. Potentially, cephalosporins could cause additive nephrotoxicity when used with aminoglycosides, but this interaction has only been well documented with cephaloridine (no longer marketed) and cephalothin.

Concurrent use with loop (**furosemide, ethacrynic acid**) or osmotic diuretics (**mannitol, urea**) may increase the nephrotoxic or ototoxic potential of the aminoglycosides.

Concomitant use with **general anesthetics** or **neuromuscular blocking agents** could potentiate neuromuscular blockade.

Synergism against *Pseudomonas aeruginosa* and *enterococci* may occur with beta-**lactam antibiotics** and the aminoglycosides. This effect is apparently not predictable and its clinical usefulness is in question.

Drug/Laboratory Interactions - Tobramycin **serum concentrations** may be falsely decreased if the patient is also receiving beta-lactam antibiotics and the serum is stored prior analysis. It is recommended that if assay is delayed, samples be frozen and if possible, drawn at times when the beta-lactam antibiotic is at a trough level.

Doses - Note: There is significant inter-patient variability with regards to aminoglycoside pharmacokinetic parameters. To insure therapeutic levels and to minimize the risks for toxicity development, it is recommended to consider monitoring serum levels for this drug.

For small animals, one pair of authors (Aronson and Aucoin 1989) make the following recommendations with regard to minimizing risks of toxicity, yet maximizing efficacy:

1) Dose according to animal size. The larger the animal, the smaller the dose (on a mg/kg basis).
2) The more risk factors (age, fever, sepsis, renal disease, dehydration) the smaller the dose.
3) In old patients or those suspected of renal disease, increase dosing interval from q8h to q16-24h.
4) Determine serum creatinine prior to therapy and adjust by changes in level even if it remains in "normal range".
5) Monitor urine for changes in sediment (*e.g.,* casts) or concentrating ability. Not very useful in patients with UTI.
6) Therapeutic drug monitoring is recommended when possible.

Dogs/Cats:
    a) 2 mg/kg IV, IM, or SubQ q8h (avoid use or reduce dosage in patients with renal failure; recommend therapeutic drug monitoring, particularly in young animals) (Vaden and Papich 1995)

Horses:
    For susceptible infections: 1 - 1.7 mg/kg q8h IV (slowly) or IM (Note: This is a human dose and should be used as a general guideline only) (Walker 1992)

Birds:
    For susceptible infections:
    a) 5 mg/kg IM every 12 hours (Bauck and Hoefer 1993)

Reptiles:
    For susceptible infections:
    a) 2.5 mg/kg once daily IM (Gauvin 1993)

Monitoring Parameters - 1) Efficacy (cultures, clinical signs and symptoms associated with infection); 2) Renal toxicity; baseline urinalysis, serum creatinine/BUN. Casts in the urine are often the initial sign of impending nephrotoxicity. Frequency of monitoring during therapy is controversial. It can be said that monitoring daily urinalyses early in the course of treatment or daily creatinines once casts are seen or increases are noted in serum creatinine levels are not too frequent; 3) Gross monitoring of vestibular or auditory toxicity is recommended; 4) Serum levels if possible; see the reference by Aronson and Aucoin in Ettinger (Aronson and Aucoin 1989) for more information.

Client Information - With appropriate training, owners may give subcutaneous injections at home, but routine monitoring of therapy for efficacy and toxicity must still be done. Clients should also understand that the potential exists for severe toxicity (nephrotoxicity, ototoxicity) developing from this medication.

Dosage Forms/Preparations/FDA Approval Status -
Veterinary-Approved Products: None
Human-Approved Products:

Tobramycin Sulfate Injection 10 mg/ml in 6 & 7 ml vials and 40 mg/ml in 1.5 & 2 ml syringes and 2 & 30 ml vials ; *Nebcin*® (Lilly); Generic; (Rx)

Tobramycin Sulfate Powder for Injection: 30 mg/ml in 1.2 g vials *Nebcin*® (Lilly); Generic (Rx)

Also available in ophthalmic preparations.

TOCAINIDE HCL

Chemistry - An amide-type local anesthetic, tocainide HCl occurs as a bitter-tasting, white, crystalline powder with a pK_a of 7.8. It is freely soluble in both water and alcohol. Tocainide is structurally related to lidocaine, but it is a primary amine where lidocaine is a tertiary amine. This modification allows tocainide to be resistant to extensive first-pass metabolism after oral administration.

Storage/Stability/Compatibility - Protect tablets from light and store in well-closed containers. An expiration date of 4 years after manufacture is assigned to the commercially available tablets when packaged in high-density polyethylene bottles.

Pharmacology - Tocainide is considered to be a class IB (membrane-stabilizing) antidysrhythmic agent which demonstrates rapid rates of attachment and dissociation to sodium channels. Like lidocaine, tocainide produces a dose-dependent decrease in potassium and sodium conductance which results in decreased excitability of myocardial cells. Automaticity, conduction velocity and effective refractory periods are decreased at therapeutic levels. Little or no increases in PR interval, QRS complex, or QT interval is seen at therapeutic levels. Like lidocaine, tocainide has little, if any effect, on autonomic tone.

Uses/Indications - Tocainide is a relatively recent addition to the armamentarium, and veterinary experience with it is quite limited. At this time, dogs are the only veterinary species where enough clinical experience has been garnered to recommend its use. It is indicated for the oral therapy of ventricular arrhythmias, principally ventricular tachycardia and ventricular premature complexes. In humans, response to lidocaine can usually predict whether tocainide might be effective.

Pharmacokinetics - Following oral administration, tocainide is rapidly and almost completely absorbed. The presence of food in the stomach may alter the rate, but not the extent of absorption. Unlike lidocaine, the hepatic first-pass effect is minimal with tocainide. In humans, peak plasma levels occur between 0.5-2 hours when administered on an empty stomach.

The distribution aspects of tocainide have not been fully described. In humans, the volume of distribution ranges from 1.5 - 4 L/kg and has been reported to be 1.7 L/kg in dogs. Tocainide is minimally bound to plasma proteins. It is unknown if it crosses the placenta or enters into the milk.

Tocainide is metabolized by the liver, but up to 50% of a dose is excreted unchanged by the kidneys into the urine. Alkalinization of the urine may result in a substantial decrease in the amount of tocainide that is excreted unchanged into the urine, but acidification of the urine reportedly does not enhance the excretion rate.

Contraindications/Precautions - Tocainide is contraindicated in patients who have demonstrated previous hypersensitivity reactions to it or amide-type local anesthetics, or who have 2nd or 3rd degree AV block and are not being artificially paced.

Use tocainide cautiously in patients with heart failure as it has the potential to aggravate the condition. Use with caution in patients with hematologic abnormalities or preexisting bone marrow failure.

Adverse Effects/Warnings - It is expected that tocainide would exhibit a similar adverse reaction profile as lidocaine. Although side effects are common in human patients, they are usually dose related, mild, and reversible upon discontinuation of the drug. CNS effects can include drowsiness, depression, ataxia, muscle tremors, etc. Nausea and vomiting may occur, but are usually transient. Cardiovascular effects reported include hypotension, bradycardia, tachycardia, other arrhythmias, and exacerbation of CHF. Rarely (<1% incidence), symptoms of bone marrow depression or pulmonary effects (pulmonary fibrosis, pneumonia, respiratory arrest, pulmonary edema, etc.) have been reported in humans.

Overdosage - Dogs tend to be rather resistant to the acute toxic effects of the drug. In one study, dogs were administered 750 mg/kg over 6 hours and emesis was the only frequent effect seen, but ECG changes were also seen in some animals.

There is no specific antidote for tocainide overdose and treatment tends to be supportive and symptomatic. For more information, see the Lidocaine monograph. Tocainide can be removed with hemodialysis.

Drug Interactions - Toxicities may be additive, with little or no therapeutic gain, if tocainide is used concurrently with other Class IB antidysrhythmics (*e.g.,* **lidocaine, phenytoin, mexiletine**). Use caution, when converting from one Class IB agent to another.

Tocainide used concomitantly with **metoprolol** (a beta-adrenergic antagonist) can have additive effects on cardiac index and wedge pressure. This may clinically significant, particularly in patients with sick sinus syndrome and impaired AV conduction. Because experience with tocainide is still limited, use caution when administering to patients on multiple-drug therapy.

Doses - From the wide variation of suggested dosages listed below, it is obvious that more clinical work is necessary before a "consensus" dosage range is available. Until that time it is recommended to use this drug cautiously and consider monitoring serum levels to guide therapy.

Dogs:
- a) 5 mg/kg 2 - 3 times a day PO (Murtaugh and Ross 1988)
- b) For large dogs (60-80 pounds): 17 - 20 mg/kg PO q8h;
  For small dogs: 30 mg/kg PO q8h (McConnell and Hughey 1987)
- c) 50 - 100 mg/kg PO q12h (Wilcke 1985)
- d) For suppression of symptomatic ventricular arrhythmias: 15.4 - 110 mg/kg q8-12h PO. May need to use other Class I drugs to improve effect. (Ettinger 1989)

Monitoring Parameters -
1) ECG
2) Symptoms of toxicity (see Adverse Reactions); may wish to monitor CBC's if treating chronically (Note: For human patients, the manufacturer recommends weekly CBC's with differential and platelets, be run at weekly intervals for the first 3 months of therapy and periodically thereafter.)
3) Serum levels (therapeutic levels in humans are usually 3 - 10 micrograms/ml), especially if symptoms of toxicity or lack of efficacy are noted.

Client Information - To be effective, the animal must receive all doses as prescribed. Notify veterinarian if the animal exhibits any abnormal bleeding or bruising, develops wheezing, shortness of breath, or a cough. If dog vomits or becomes anorexic after dosing, give with food. If vomiting persists or animal develops a change in behavior or attitude, notify veterinarian.

Dosage Forms/Preparations/FDA Approval Status/Withholding Times -
Veterinary-Approved Products: None
Human-Approved Products:
Tocainide HCl Oral Tablets 400 mg, 600 mg; *Tonocard*® (Astra Merck); (Rx)

TOLAZOLINE HCL

Chemistry - An alpha adrenergic blocking agent, tolazoline HCl is structurally related to phentolamine. It occurs as a white to off-white, crystalline powder possessing a bitter taste and a slight aromatic odor. Tolazoline is freely soluble in ethanol or water. The commercially available (human) injection has pH between 3 and 4.

Storage/Stability/Compatibility - Commercially available injection products should be stored between 15-30°C and protected from light. The drug is reportedly physically compatible with the commonly used IV solutions.

Pharmacology - By directly relaxing vascular smooth muscle, tolazoline has peripheral vasodilating effects and decreases total peripheral resistance. Tolazoline also is a competitive alpha$_1$ and alpha$_2$ adrenergic blocking agent, explaining its mechanism for reversing the effects of xylazine. Tolazoline is rapid acting (usually within 5 minutes of IV administration), but has a short duration of action and repeat doses may be required.

Uses/Indications - Tolazoline is approved and indicated for the reversal of effects associated with xylazine in horses. It has also been used for this purpose in a variety of other species as well, but less safety and efficacy data is available.

In humans, the primary uses for tolazoline are: treatment of persistent pulmonary hypertension in newborns, adjunctive treatment and diagnosis of peripheral vasospastic disorders and as a provocative test for glaucoma after subconjunctival injection.

Pharmacokinetics - After IV injection in horses, tolazoline is widely distributed. Animal studies have demonstrated that tolazoline is concentrated in the liver and kidneys. Half life in horses at recommended doses is approximately 1 hour.

Contraindications/Precautions/Reproductive Safety - The manufacturer does not recommend use in horses exhibiting signs of stress, debilitation, cardiac disease, sympathetic blockage, hypovolemia or shock. Safe use for foals has not been established.

Tolazoline should be considered contraindicated in patients known to be hypersensitive to it, or who have coronary artery or cerebrovascular disease. Humans having any of the above contraindicative conditions, should use extra caution when handling the agent.

Safety during pregnancy, in breeding or lactating animals has not been established. It is unknown if the drug enters maternal milk.

Adverse Effects/Warnings - In horses adverse effects that may occur include: transient tachycardia; peripheral vasodilatation presenting as sweating and injected mucous membranes of the gingiva and conjunctiva; hyperalgesia of the lips (licking, flipping of lips); piloerection; clear lacrimal and nasal discharge; muscle fasciculations; apprehensiveness. Adverse effects should diminish with time and generally disappear within 2 hours of dosing. Potential for adverse effects increase if tolazoline is given at higher than recommended dosages or if xylazine has not be previously administered.

Overdosage - In horses given tolazoline alone (no previous xylazine), doses of 5X recommended resulted in gastrointestinal hypermotility with resultant flatulence and defecation or attempt to defecate. Some horses exhibited mild colic and transient diarrhea. Intraventricular conduction may be slowed when horses are overdosed, with a prolongation of the QRS-complex noted. Ventricular arrhythmias may occur resulting in death with higher overdoses (5X). In humans, ephedrine (NOT epinephrine or norepinephrine) has been recommended to treat serious tolazoline-induced hypotension.

Drug Interactions - If large doses of tolazoline are given with either **norepinephrine** or **epinephrine**, a paradoxical drop in blood pressure can occur followed by a precipitous increase in blood pressure. Accumulation of acetaldehyde can occur if tolazoline and **alcohol** are given simultaneously.

Doses -

  Horses:

    For reversal of xylazine effects:

      a) 4 mg/kg slow IV (4 ml/220 lb. of body weight); administration rate should approximate 1 ml/second. (Package Insert; Tolazine®—Lloyd Laboratories)

  Dogs/Cats:

    For reversal of xylazine effects:

      a) 4 mg/kg slow IV (4 ml/220 lb. of body weight); administration rate should approximate 1 ml/second. (Package Insert; Tolazine®—Lloyd Laboratories-New Zealand)

      NOTE: If reversal is warranted, the high concentration (100 mg/ml) of the veterinary drug may make accurate dosing difficult; yohimbine or the human-labeled tolazoline product (25 mg/ml) may be safer alternatives than Tolazine® (100 mg/ml). Note: Tolazoline is not approved for use in dogs and cats in the USA and the US manufacturer does not recommend its use

Warning: Although dosages are listed for food-producing animals below, the drug is not approved in the USA for use in these species.

  Deer:

    For reversal of xylazine effects:

      a) 2 - 4 mg/kg slow IV; titrate to effect; Slaughter withdrawal: 30 days (Label Directions; Tolazine®—Lloyd Laboratories-New Zealand)

  Cattle:

    For reversal of xylazine effects:

      a) 2 - 4 mg/kg slow IV; titrate to effect; Slaughter withdrawal: 30 days (Label Directions; Tolazine®—Lloyd Laboratories-New Zealand)

  Sheep & Goats:

    For reversal of xylazine effects:

      a) 2 - 4 mg/kg slow IV; titrate to effect; Slaughter withdrawal: 30 days (Label Directions; Tolazine®—Lloyd Laboratories-New Zealand)

Monitoring Parameters/Client Information- 1) Reversal effects (efficacy) 2) Adverse effects (see above). Because of the risks associated with the use of xylazine and reversal by tolazoline, these drugs should be administered and monitored by veterinary professionals only.

Dosage Forms/Preparations/FDA Approval Status -

Veterinary-Approved Products:

Tolazoline HCl Injection 100 mg/ml in 100 ml multi-dose vials; *Tolazine®* (Lloyd); (Rx). Approved for use in horses; not to be used in food-producing animals.

Human-Approved Products:

Tolazoline HCl Injection 25 mg/ml; *Priscoline®; HCl* (Novartis); (Rx)

TRIAMCINOLONE ACETONIDE

Note: For more information refer to the monograph: Glucocorticoids, General Information or to the manufacturer's product information.

Chemistry - Triamcinolone acetonide, a synthetic glucocorticoid, occurs as slightly odorous, white to cream-colored, crystalline powder with a melting point between 290 - 294°C. It is practically insoluble in water, very soluble in dehydrated alcohol and slightly soluble in alcohol. The commercially available sterile suspensions have a pH range of 5-7.5.

Storage/Stability/Compatibility - Triamcinolone acetonide products should be stored at room temperature (15-30°C); the injection should be protected from light.

Doses -

Dogs:

For glucocorticoid effects:

   a) 0.25 - 2 mg PO once daily for 7 days; 0.11 - 0.22 mg/kg IM or SQ. (Kirk 1989)

   b) 0.11 - 0.22 mg/kg PO, IM or SQ once daily. (Jenkins 1985)

   c) For tablets: 0.11 mg/kg PO initially once a day, may increase to 0.22 mg/kg PO once daily if initial response is unsatisfactory. As soon as possible, but not later than 2 weeks, reduce dose gradually to 0.028 - 0.055 mg/kg/day. (Booth 1988), (Package insert; *Vetalog® Tablets*—Solvay)

   d) For injectable product: 0.11 - 0.22 mg/kg for inflammatory or allergic disorders, and 0.22 mg/kg for dermatological disorders. Effects generally persist for 7-15 days; if symptoms recur, may repeat or institute oral therapy.

     For intralesional injection: Usual dose is 1.2 - 1.8 mg; inject around lesion at 0.5 - 2.5 cm intervals. Do not exceed 0.6 mg at any one site or 6 mg total dose. May repeat as necessary. (Package insert; *Vetalog® Injection*—Solvay)

   e) As an antiinflammatory agent: 0.05 mg/kg PO *bid-tid* (Morgan 1988)

Cats:

For glucocorticoid effects:

   a) 0.25 - 0.5 mg PO once daily for 7 days. (Kirk 1989)

   b) 0.11 - 0.22 mg/kg PO, IM or SQ once daily. Maximum of 0.5 mg. (Jenkins 1985)

   c) For tablets: 0.11 mg/kg PO initially once a day, may increase to 0.22 mg/kg PO once daily if initial response is unsatisfactory. As soon as possible, but not later than 2 weeks, reduce dose gradually to 0.028 - 0.055 mg/kg/day. (Booth 1988), (Package insert; *Vetalog® Tablets*—Solvay)

   d) For injectable product: 0.11 - 0.22 mg/kg for inflammatory or allergic disorders, and 0.22 mg/kg for dermatological disorders. Effects generally persist for 7-15 days; if symptoms recur, may repeat or institute oral therapy.

     For intralesional injection: Usual dose is 1.2 - 1.8 mg; inject around lesion at 0.5 - 2.5 cm intervals. Do not exceed 0.6 mg at any one site or 6 mg total dose. May repeat as necessary. (Package insert; *Vetalog® Injection*—Solvay)

For feline plasma cell gingivitis-pharyngitis:

   a) 2 - 4 mg PO once a day to every other day. (DeNovo, Potter, and Woolfson 1988)

For feline polymyopathy:

   a) 0.5 - 1.0 mg/kg PO once a day. (Knaack 1988)

Cattle:

For glucocorticoid effects:

   a) 0.02 - 0.04 mg/kg IM; 6 - 18 mg intra-articularly. (Howard 1986)

Horses:

For glucocorticoid effects:

   a) 0.1 - 0.2 mg/kg IM or SQ; 3 - 6 mg subconjunctivally. (Robinson 1987)

   b) 0.011 - 0.022 mg/kg PO *bid*;

     0.011 - 0.022 mg/kg IM or SQ;

     6 - 18 mg intra-articularly or intrasynovially, may repeat after 3-4 days; (Package inserts; *Vetalog® Powder and Injection*—Solvay)

Dosage Forms/Preparations/Approval Status/Withdrawal Times - All require a prescription (Rx).

Veterinary-Approved Products: Note: marketing status of oral preparations is in question.

Triamcinolone Tablets 0.5 mg, 1.5 mg; *Vetalog® Tablets* (Fort Dodge), generic. Approved for use in dogs and cats

Triamcinolone Acetonide Oral Powder 15 gram packets containing 10 grams of triamcinolone acetonide.; *Vetalog® Oral Powder* (Fort Dodge). Approved for use in horses.

Triamcinolone acetonide suspension for injection 2 mg/ml; 6 mg/ml ; *Vetalog® Parenteral Veterinary* (Fort Dodge); Generic. (Rx). Approved for use in dogs, cats, and horses.

Human-Approved Products include:

Triamcinolone Tablets 1 mg, 2 mg, 4 mg, 8 mg; *Aristocort®* (Fujisawa); Generic (Rx)

Triamcinolone Oral Syrup 4 mg/5ml *Kenacort®* (Apothecon); (Rx)

Triamcinolone Acetonide Sterile Suspension for injection 3 mg/ml, 10 mg/ml, 40 mg/ml; many tradenames; Generic, (Rx)

Many topical preparations are available, alone and in combination with other agents and inhaled products are also approved.

TRIMEPRAZINE TARTRATE
TRIMEPRAZINE TARTRATE WITH PREDNISOLONE

Chemistry - A phenothiazine antihistamine related to promethazine, trimeprazine tartrate occurs as an odorless, white, to off-white crystalline powder with a melting range of 160-164°C. Approximately 0.5 gm is soluble in 1 ml water, and 0.05 gm is soluble in 1 ml of alcohol. Trimeprazine may also be known as alimenazine tartrate.

Storage/Stability/Compatibility - Store trimeprazine products at room temperature (15-30°C); avoid freezing the oral solution. Tablets and capsules should be kept in well-closed containers and the oral solution should be kept in tight containers. Protect the oral solution and tablets from light.

Pharmacology - Trimeprazine has antihistaminic, sedative, antitussive and antipruritic qualities. The veterinary-approved product also has prednisolone in its formulation which provides additional anti-inflammatory effects.

Uses/Indications - Trimeprazine is used alone for the treatment of pruritic conditions, especially if induced by allergic conditions. The veterinary combination product is suggested (by the manufacturer) to be used in dogs for either pruritic conditions or as an antitussive.

Pharmacokinetics - The pharmacokinetics of trimeprazine have apparently not been studied.

Contraindications/Precautions - The contraindications and precautions of this product follow those of the other phenothiazines and antihistaminic agents. For more information it is suggested to review the acepromazine, and chlorpheniramine monographs. The manufacturer of the veterinary combination product *(Temaril®-P)* warns that corticosteroids can induce the first stages of parturition if administered during the last trimester of pregnancy.

Adverse Effects/Warnings - For trimeprazine, possible adverse reactions include: sedation, depression, hypotension and extrapyrimidal reactions (rigidity, tremors, weakness, restlessness, etc.).

Additional adverse effects, if using the product containing steroids include: elevated liver enzymes, weight loss, polyuria/polydypsia, vomiting and diarrhea. If used chronically, therapy must be withdrawn gradually and Cushing's Syndrome may develop.

The manufacturer of the veterinary combination product *(Temaril®-P)* includes the following adverse effects in its package insert: sodium retention and potassium loss, negative nitrogen balance, suppressed adrenocortical function, delayed wound healing, osteoporosis, possible increased susceptibility to and/or exacerbation of bacterial infections, sedation, protruding nictitating membrane, blood dyscrasias. Also, intensification and prolongation of the action of sedatives, analgesics or anesthetics can be noted and potentiation of organophosphate toxicity and of procaine HCl activity.

Overdosage - Acute overdosage should be handled as per the acepromazine monograph found at the beginning of the book..

Drug Interactions - **Other CNS depressant agents (barbiturates, narcotics, anesthetics**, etc.) may cause additive CNS depression if used with phenothiazines.

Quinidine when given with phenothiazines may cause additive cardiac depression.

Antidiarrheal mixtures (*e.g.,* Kaolin/pectin, bismuth subsalicylate mixtures) and **antacids** may cause reduced GI absorption of oral·phenothiazines. Increased blood levels of both drugs may result if **propranolol** is administered with phenothiazines.

Phenothiazines block alpha-adrenergic receptors; if **epinephrine** is also given, unopposed beta activity causing vasodilation and increased cardiac rate can occur. **Phenytoin** metabolism may be decreased if given concurrently with phenothiazines.

If using the product containing prednisolone, the following interactions may also occur: **Amphotericin B** or potassium-depleting diuretics (**furosemide, thiazides**) when administered concomitantly with steroids may lead to hypokalemia. Steroids may reduce **salicylate** blood levels. **Insulin** requirements may increase in patients taking glucocorticoids. **Phenytoin or phenobarbital** may increase the metabolism of glucocorticoids.

Laboratory Interactions - Antihistamines can decrease the wheal and flare response to **antigen skin testing**. In humans, it is suggested that antihistamines be discontinued at least 4 days before testing. Glucocorticoids may increase **urine glucose levels** and decrease T_3 & T_4 values.

Doses -
Trimeprazine:
a) In general, for all species, all routes: 1.1 - 4.4 mg/kg *qid* (Swinyard 1975)
Dogs:
a) 2.5 mg/10 lbs up to 40 pounds; for patients over 40 lb.: 15 mg *bid*, after 4 days, reduce the dose to 1/2 of the initial dose (Swinyard 1975)

Trimeprazine/Prednisolone (*Temaril®-P*):
Dogs:

Wt. of patient:	≤10 lb.	11-20 lb.	21-40 lb.	>40 lb.
# of #1 caps:	1	2	4	6
# of #2 caps:	-	1	2	3
# of tabs	1/2	1	2	3

Give capsules once daily PO, and tablets *bid* PO; after 4 days reduce dose to 1/2 of initial dose; adjust as necessary. (Package Insert; *Temaril®-P* - SKB)

Monitoring Parameters -
1) Efficacy
2) Degree of sedation, and anticholinergic effects
3) Adverse effects associated with corticosteroids if using combination product

Client Information - Trimeprazine is approved for use in humans and is a prescription drug. Trimeprazine in combination with prednisolone is approved for use in dogs only and is a veterinary prescription drug.

Dosage Forms/Preparations/FDA Approval Status/Withholding Times -
Veterinary-Approved Products:
No single agent trimeprazine products are approved for veterinary medicine.
Trimeprazine Tartrate 5 mg; Prednisolone 2 mg Tablets; *Temaril-P®* *Tablets* (Pfizer); (Rx) Approved for use in dogs.
Human-Approved Products: None

Trimethoprim/Sulfa - See Sulfa/Trimethoprim

TRIPELENNAMINE HCL

Chemistry - An ethylenediamine-derivative antihistamine, tripelennamine HCl occurs as a white, crystalline powder which will slowly darken upon exposure to light. It has a melting range of 188-192°C and pK_as of 3.9 and 9.0. One gram is soluble in 1 ml of water or 6 ml of alcohol.

Storage/Stability/Compatibility - Store the injection at room temperature and protect from light; avoid freezing or excessive heat. Tablets should also be stored at room temperature in tight containers.

Pharmacology - Antihistamines (H_1-receptor antagonists) competitively inhibit histamine at H_1 receptor sites. They do not inactivate or prevent the release of histamine, but can prevent histamine's action on the cell. Besides their antihistaminic activity, these agents also have varying degrees of anticholinergic and CNS activity (sedation). Tripelennamine is considered to have moderate sedative activity and minimal anticholinergic activity when compared to other antihistamines.

Uses/Indications - Antihistamines are used in veterinary medicine to reduce or help prevent histamine mediated adverse effects. Tripelennamine has been used as a CNS stimulant in "Downer cows" when administered slow IV.

Pharmacokinetics - The pharmacokinetics of tripelennamine have apparently not been thoroughly studied in domestic animals or humans.

Pharmacokinetics - The pharmacokinetics of tripelennamine have apparently not been thoroughly studied in domestic animals or humans.

Contraindications/Precautions - Tripelennamine is not recommended to be given IV in horses (see Adverse Effects).

Adverse Effects/Warnings - CNS stimulation (hyperexcitability, nervousness, & muscle tremors) lasting up to 20 minutes, has been noted in horses after receiving tripelennamine intravenously. Other effects seen (in all species), include CNS depression, incoordination, and GI disturbances.

Tripelennamine has been mixed with pentazocine and injected by human opiate addicts and drug abusers. Be alert for clients suggesting that this drug be dispensed for their animals.

Overdosage - Overdosage of tripelennamine reportedly can cause CNS excitation, seizures and ataxia. Treat symptomatically and supportively if symptoms are severe. Phenytoin (IV) is recommended in the treatment of seizures caused by antihistamine overdose in humans; barbiturates and diazepam are generally avoided.

Drug Interactions - Increased sedation can occur if chlorpheniramine is combined with **other CNS depressant drugs**. Antihistamines may partially counteract the anti-coagulation effects of **heparin** or **warfarin**.

Laboratory Interactions - Antihistamines can decrease the wheal and flare response to antigen skin testing. In humans, it is suggested that antihistamines be discontinued at least 4 days prior to testing.

Doses - It is recommended to warm the solution to near body temperature before injecting; give IM injections into large muscle areas.

Dogs:
> a) 1.1 mg/kg IM q6-12h *prn* (Package Insert; *Re-Covr®* - Solvay)
> b) 1 mg/kg PO q12h; 1 mg/kg IM (Kirk 1986)

Cats:
> a) 1.1 mg/kg IM q6-12h *prn* (Package Insert; *Re-Covr®* - Solvay)
> b) 1 mg/kg PO q12h; 1 mg/kg IM (Kirk 1986)

Cattle:
> a) 1.1 mg/kg (2.5 ml per 100 lbs body weight) IV (for more immediate effect) or IM q6-12h *prn* (Package Insert; *Re-Covr®* - Solvay)
> b) As adjunctive treatment in "Downer Cow Syndrome" as a CNS stimulant: 0.5 mg/kg slow IV in conjunction with parenteral mineral treatment (Caple 1986)
> c) 1 mg/kg IV or IM (Howard 1986)

Horses:
> a) 1.1 mg/kg (2.5 ml per 100 lbs body weight) IM q6-12h *prn* (Package Insert; *Re-Covr®* - Solvay)
> b) 1 mg/kg IM (Robinson 1987)

Swine:
> a) 1 mg/kg IV or IM (Howard 1986)

Monitoring Parameters -
> 1) Clinical efficacy and adverse effects

Dosage Forms/Preparations/FDA Approval Status/Withholding Times -
Veterinary-Approved Products:
> Tripelennamine HCl for Injection (Veterinary) 20 mg/ml in 20 ml, 100 ml, and 250 ml vials; Generic (Phoenix) (Rx) Tripelennamine HCl injection is approved for use in cattle, horses, dogs, and cats. Treated cattle must not be slaughtered for food purposes for four days following the last treatment. Milk must not be used for food for 24 hours (2 milkings) after treatment. No specific tolerance for residues have been published

Human-Approved Products:
> Tripelennamine HCl Oral Tablets 25 mg, 50 mg; *PBZ®* (Geigy);*Pelamine®* (Major); Generic; (Rx)

> Tripelennamine HCl Extended-release tablets 100 mg; *PBZ-SR®* (Geigy); (Rx)

> Tripelennamine HCl Elixir: 37.5 mg (equivalent to 25 mg HCl) per 5 ml in 473 mls; *PBZ®* (Geigy) (Rx)

TSH - See Thyrotropin

TYLOSIN

Chemistry - A macrolide antibiotic related structurally to erythromycin, tylosin is produced from *Streptomyces fradiae*. It occurs as an almost white to buff-colored powder with a pK$_a$ of 7.1. It is slightly soluble in water and soluble in alcohol. Tylosin is considered to be highly lipid soluble. The tartrate salt is soluble in water. The injectable form of the drug (as the base) is in a 50% propylene glycol solution.

Storage/Stability/Compatibility - Unless otherwise instructed by the manufacturer, injectable tylosin should be stored in well-closed containers at room temperature. Tylosin, like erythromycin, is unstable in acidic (pH <4) media. It is not recommended to mix the parenteral injection with other drugs.

Pharmacology - Tylosin is thought to have the same mechanism of action as erythromycin (binds to 50S ribosome and inhibits protein synthesis) and exhibits a similar spectrum of activity. It is a bacteriostatic antibiotic. For more specific information on organisms that tylosin is usually active against, refer to the erythromycin monograph just prior to this one. Cross resistance with erythromycin occurs.

Uses/Indications - Although the injectable form of tylosin is approved for use in dogs and cats, it is rarely used parenterally in those species. Oral tylosin is sometimes recommended for the treatment of chronic colitis in small animals (see Doses), but controlled studies documenting its efficacy have not been performed.

Tylosin is also used in clinically in cattle and swine for infections caused by susceptible organisms.

Pharmacokinetics - Tylosin tartrate is well absorbed from the GI tract, primarily from the intestine. The phosphate salt is less well absorbed after oral administration. Tylosin base injected SQ or IM is reportedly rapidly absorbed.

Like erythromycin, tylosin is well distributed in the body after systemic absorption, with the exception of penetration into the CSF. The volume of distribution of tylosin is reportedly 1.7 L/kg in small animals. Tylosin enters milk in concentrations of approximately 20% of those found in serum.

Tylosin is eliminated in the urine and bile apparently as unchanged drug. The elimination half life of tylosin is reportedly 54 minutes in small animals, 139 minutes in newborn calves and 64 minutes in calves 2 months of age or older.

Contraindications/Precautions/Reproductive Safety - Tylosin is contraindicated in patients hypersensitive to it or other macrolide antibiotics (*e.g.,* erythromycin). Most clinicians feel that tylosin is contraindicated in horses, as severe and sometimes fatal diarrheas may result from its use in that species.

No information was located with regards to the reproductive safety of tylosin, but it is unlikely to have serious teratogenic potential.

Adverse Effects/Warnings - Most likely adverse effects with tylosin are pain and local reactions at intramuscular injection sites, and mild GI upset (anorexia, and diarrhea). Tylosin may induce severe diarrheas if administered orally to ruminants or by any route to horses. In swine, adverse effects reported include edema of rectal mucosa and mild anal protrusion with pruritis, erythema, and diarrhea.

Overdosage/Acute Toxicity - Tylosin is relatively safe in most overdose situations. The LD$_{50}$ in pigs is greater than 5 g/kg orally, and approximately 1 g/kg IM. Dogs are reported to tolerate oral doses of 800 mg/kg. Long-term (2 year) oral administration of up to 400 mg/kg produced no organ toxicity in dogs. Shock and death have been reported in baby pigs overdosed with tylosin, however.

Drug Interactions - Drug interactions with tylosin have not been well documented. It has been suggested that it may increase **digitalis glycoside** blood levels with resultant toxicity. It is suggested to refer to the erythromycin monograph for more information on potential interactions.

Drug/Laboratory Interactions - Macrolide antibiotics may cause falsely elevated values of **AST** (SGOT), and **ALT** (SGPT) when using colorimetric assays.

Fluorometric determinations of **urinary catecholamines** can be altered by concomitant macrolide administration.

Doses -

Dogs:

For susceptible infections:
   a) 6.6 - 11 mg/kg IM q12-24h (Ford and Aronson 1985)
   b) For chronic colitis: *Tylan*® *Plus Vitamins*: 40 - 80 mg/kg/day in 2-3 divided doses; either mixed with food (tastes bitter) or as a bolus mixed with water. Use at recommended dose for 2 weeks and then gradually taper as animal's diet is adjusted. Some animals may require long-term therapy. (Chiapella 1986)

c) For chronic colitis: *Tylan® Plus Vitamins*: 20 - 40 mg/kg *bid*; mixed with food (tastes bitter). May alternate with sulfasalazine for long-term maintenance therapy. (DeNovo 1988)

Note: *Tylan® plus Vitamins* has recently been discontinued by the manufacturer. *Tylan® Soluble Powder* ≈ 4,000 mg/teaspoonsful may be substituted, but this product is much more concentrated and may require dilution for accurate dosing.

Cats:
For susceptible infections:
  a) 6.6 - 11 mg/kg IM q12-24h (Ford and Aronson 1985)
  b) 10 mg/kg IM q12h (Jenkins 1987b)
  c) For chronic colitis: *Tylan® Plus Vitamins* (approximately 470 mg/teaspoonful): 10 - 20 mg/kg/day in 2 divided doses; either mixed with food (tastes bitter) or as a bolus mixed with water. Use at recommended dose for 2 weeks and then gradually taper as animal's diet is adjusted. Some animals may require long-term therapy. (Chiapella 1986)
  d) For chronic colitis: *Tylan® Plus Vitamins* (approximately 400 mg/teaspoonful): 5 - 10 mg/kg *bid*; mixed with food (tastes bitter). May alternate with sulfasalazine for long-term maintenance therapy. (DeNovo 1988)

Note: *Tylan® plus Vitamins* has recently been discontinued by the manufacturer. *Tylan® Soluble Powder* ≈ 4,000 mg/teaspoonsful may be substituted, but this product is much more concentrated and may require dilution for accurate dosing.

Cattle:
For susceptible infections:
  a) 17.6 mg/kg IM once daily. Continue treatment for 24 hours after symptoms have stopped, not to exceed 5 days. Do not inject more than 10 ml per site. Use the 50 mg/ml formulation in calves weighing less than 200 pounds. (Package insert; Tylosin Injection—TechAmerica)
  b) For bronchopneumonia and fibrinous pneumonia in cattle associated with penicillin G-refractory C. pyogenes infections or other bacteria sensitive to tylosin and resistant to sulfas, penicillin G and tetracyclines: using Tylosin 200 mg/ml : 44 mg/kg IM q24h. Recommend a 21 day slaughter withdrawal at this dosage. (Hjerpe 1986)
  c) 5 - 10 mg/kg IM or slow IV once daily; not to exceed 5 days. (Huber 1988a)
  d) Tylosin base injectable: 10 mg/kg IM initially, then 6 mg/kg IM q8h (q8-12h in calves). (Baggot 1983)

Swine:
For susceptible infections:
  a) 8.8 mg/kg IM twice daily. Continue treatment for 24 hours after symptoms have stopped, not to exceed 3 days. Do not inject more than 5 ml per site. (Package insert; Tylosin Injection—TechAmerica)
  b) 5 - 10 mg/kg until 24 hours after remission of disease signs; not to exceed 3 days therapy. (Huber 1988a)
  c) Tylosin base injectable: 12.5 mg/kg IM q12h. (Baggot 1983)

Sheep & Goats:
For susceptible infections:
  a) 10 mg/kg, treatment not to exceed 5 days. (Huber 1988a)

Birds:
For susceptible infections:
  a) For initial therapy in caged birds for upper respiratory infections (especially if mycoplasma suspected).
  Using 200 mg/ml injectable: 40 mg/kg IM. Used in combination with aminoglycosides.
  Using *Tylan® Plus Vitamins*: 1/4 teaspoonful per 8 oz of drinking water. (McDonald 1989)
  b) For initial therapy of upper respiratory infections and air sacculitis. Using 50 mg/ml or 200 mg/ml injectable: 10 - 40 mg/kg IM *bid* or *tid*.
  For chronic respiratory disease using *Tylan® Plus Vitamins*: 2 teaspoonsful per gallon of drinking water. 10 days on, 5 days off, and 10 days on. Tastes bitter. May divide dosage between food and water. (Clubb 1986)
  c) 30 mg/kg IM q12h (Hoeffer 1995)

Reptiles:
For susceptible infections:
a) For tortoises: 5 mg/kg IM once daily for at least 10 days. Used primarily for chronic respiratory infections or when Mycoplasma is suspected (Gauvin 1993)

Monitoring Parameters -
1) Clinical efficacy
2) Adverse effects

Dosage Forms/Preparations/FDA Approval Status/Withholding Times -
Veterinary-Approved Products:
Tylosin Injection 50 mg/ml, 200 mg/ml; *Tylan*® (Elanco), generic; (OTC) Approved for use in nonlactating dairy cattle, beef cattle, swine, dogs, and cats. Slaughter withdrawal = cattle 21 days; swine 14 days.
(Note: Although this author was unable to locate parenteral products approved for use in lactating dairy animals, one source (Huber 1988a) states that tylosin has a 72 hour milk withdrawal for dairy cattle, and 48 hour milk withdrawal in dairy goats and sheep.)

Tylosin tartrate (approximately 4000 mg/teaspoonsful) in 100 g bottles; *Tylan*® *Soluble* (Elanco); (OTC) Approved for use in turkeys (not layers), chickens (not layers) and swine. Slaughter withdrawal swine = 2 days; chickens = 1 day; turkeys = 5 days.

There are many approved tylosin products for addition to feed or water for use in beef cattle, swine, and poultry. Many of these products also have other active ingredients included in their formulations.

Human-Approved Products: None.

URSODIOL

Chemistry - A naturally occurring bile acid, ursodiol, also known as ursodeoxycholic acid has a molecular weight of 392.6.

Storage/Stability/Compatibility - Unless otherwise specified by the manufacturer, ursodiol capsules should be stored at room temperature (15-30°C) in tight containers.

Pharmacology - After oral administration, ursodiol suppresses hepatic synthesis and secretion of cholesterol. Ursodiol also decreases intestinal absorption of cholesterol. By reducing cholesterol saturation in the bile it is thought that ursodiol allows solubilization of cholesterol-containing gallstones. Ursodiol also increases bile flow and in patients with chronic liver disease it apparently reduces the hepatocyte toxic effects of bile salts by decreasing their detergent action, and may protect hepatic cells from toxic bile acids (*e.g.*, lithocholate, deoxycholate and chenodeoxycholate).

Uses/Indications - In small animals, ursodiol may be useful as adjunctive therapy for the medical management of cholesterol-containing gallstones and/or in patients with chronic liver disease, particularly where cholestasis (bile toxicity) plays an important role.

Pharmacokinetics - Ursodiol is well absorbed from the small intestine after oral administration. In humans, up to 90% of dose is absorbed. After absorption, it enters the portal circulation. In the liver it is extracted and combined (conjugated) with either taurine or glycine and secreted into the bile. Only very small quantities enter the systemic circulation and very little is detected in the urine. After each entero-hepatic cycle, some quantities of conjugated and free drug undergoes bacterial degradation and eventually most of the drug is eliminated in the feces after being oxidized or reduced to less soluble compounds. Ursodiol detected in the systemic circulation is highly bound to plasma proteins.

Contraindications/Precautions/Reproductive Safety - Patients sensitive to other bile acid products may also be sensitive to ursodiol. The benefits of using ursodiol should be weighed against its risks in patients with complications associated with gallstones (*e.g.*, biliary obstruction, biliary fistulas, cholecystitis, pancreatitis, cholangitis). While ursodiol may be useful in treating patients with chronic liver disease, some patients may experience further impairment of bile acid metabolism.

Ursodiol's safety during pregnancy has not been unequivocally established, but studies in rats at doses up to 100 times those given therapeutically in humans demonstrated no adversity to fetuses. It is unknown whether the drug enters breast milk, but no problems have thus far been reported and it would unlikely be of concern (due to the very low systemic levels of the drug present).

Adverse Effects/Warnings - While hepatotoxicity has not been associated with ursodiol therapy, some human patients have an inability to sulfate lithocholic acid (a naturally occurring bile acid and also a metabolite of ursodiol). Lithocholic acid is a known hepatotoxin; veterinary significance is unclear. Diarrhea and other GI effects have rarely been noted in humans taking ursodiol. Ursodiol will not dissolve calcified, radiopaque stones or radiolucent bile pigment stones.

Overdosage/Acute Toxicity - Overdosage of ursodiol would most likely cause diarrhea. Treatment, if required, could include supportive therapy; oral administration of an aluminum-containing antacid (*e.g.*, aluminum hydroxide suspension); gastric emptying (if large overdose) with concurrent administration of activated charcoal or cholestyramine suspension.

Drug Interactions - **Aluminum-containing antacids** or **cholestyramine-resin** may bind to ursodiol, thereby reducing its efficacy.

Doses -
  Dogs:
    For adjunctive treatment of chronic hepatitis:
      a) 5 - 15 mg/kg PO divided q12h, with immunosuppressive therapy. (Note: Use of this drug at this dose is preliminary, but promising) (Johnson and Sherding 1994)
      b) 10 - 15 mg/kg PO once daily (Leveille-Webster and Center 1995)

  Cats:
    For adjunctive treatment of chronic hepatitis:
      a) 10 - 15 mg/kg PO once daily (Leveille-Webster and Center 1995)

Monitoring Parameters - 1) Efficacy (ultrasonography for gallstones; improved liver function tests for chronic hepatic disease); 2) Monitoring of SGPT/SGOT (AST/ALT) on a routine basis (in humans these tests are recommended to be performed at the initiation of therapy and at 1 and 3 months after starting therapy; then every 6 months).

Client Information - Because ursodiol dissolves more rapidly in the presence of bile or pancreatic juice, it should be given with food.

Dosage Forms/Preparations/FDA Approval Status/Withholding Times -
  Veterinary-Approved Products: None
  Human-Approved Products:
    Ursodiol Capsules 300 mg; *Actigall*® (Ciba)(Rx)

VALPROIC ACID
VALPROATE SODIUM
DIVALPROEX SODIUM

Chemistry - Structurally unrelated to other anticonvulsant agents, valproic acid, valproate sodium, divalproex sodium are derivatives of carboxylic acid. Valproic acid occurs as a colorless to pale yellow clear liquid. It is slightly viscous, has a characteristic odor, a pK_a of 4.8, is slightly soluble in water and freely soluble in alcohol. It is also known as Dipropylacetic acid, DPA, 2-propylpentanoic acid, and 2-propylvaleric acid.

Valproate sodium occurs as a white, crystalline, saline tasting, very hygroscopic powder. It is very soluble in water and in alcohol. The commercially available oral solution has a pH of 7-8.

Divalproex sodium is a stable compound in a 1:1 molar ratio of valproic acid and valproate sodium. It occurs as a white powder with a characteristic odor. It is insoluble in water and very soluble in alcohol.

Storage/Stability/Compatibility - Valproic acid capsules should be stored at room temperature (15-30°C) and in tight containers; avoid freezing. Valproate sodium oral solution should be stored at room temperature and in tight containers; avoid freezing. Divalproex sodium enteric-coated tablets should be stored at room temperature in tight, light resistant containers.

Pharmacology - The mechanism of the anticonvulsant activity of valproic acid is not understood. Animal studies have demonstrated that valproic acid inhibits GABA transferase and succinic aldehyde dehydrogenase causing increased CNS levels of GABA. Additionally, one study has demonstrated that valproic acid inhibits neuronal activity by increasing potassium conductance.

Uses/Indications - Because of its cost, apparent unfavorable pharmacokinetic profile, and potential hepatotoxicity, valproic acid must be considered at this time to be a third-line drug in the treatment of seizures in the dog. Some clinicians feel it is of benefit when added to phenobarbital in patients not adequately controlled with that drug alone. Additionally, it is less protein bound in dogs than in man, so the human serum therapeutic range of the drug (40 - 100 micrograms/ml) may be too high in dogs. The drug (free form) actually may concentrate in the CSF, and anticonvulsant effects may persist even after valproate levels are non-detectable in CSF, leading to the prospect that serum levels do not accurately reflect clinical efficacy. Clearly, additional studies are needed to determine the clinical efficacy of this drug.

Pharmacokinetics - Sodium valproate is rapidly converted to valproic acid in the acidic environment of the stomach where it is rapidly absorbed from the GI tract. The bioavailability reported in dogs following oral administration is approximately 80% and peak levels occur in approximately one hour. Food may delay absorption, but does not alter the extent of it. Divalproex in its enteric-coated form has an approximately 1 hour delay in its oral absorption. Patients who exhibit GI (nausea, vomiting) adverse effects may benefit from this dosage form.

Valproic acid is rapidly distributed throughout the extracellular water spaces and plasma. It is approximately 80-95% plasma protein bound in humans, and 78-80% plasma protein bound in dogs. CSF levels are approximately 10% of those found in the plasma. Milk levels are 1-10% of those found in the plasma and it readily crosses the placenta.

Valproic acid is metabolized in the liver and is conjugated with glucuronide. These metabolic conjugates are excreted in the urine; only very small amounts of unchanged drug are excreted in the urine. The elimination half-life in humans ranges from 5-20 hours, and in dogs from 1.5-2.8 hours.

Contraindications/Precautions - Valproic acid is contraindicated in patients with significant hepatic disease or dysfunction, or exhibiting previous hypersensitivity to the drug. It should be used with caution in patients with thrombocytopenia or altered platelet aggregation function.

A 1-2% incidence of neural tube defects in children born of mothers taking valproic acid during the first trimester of pregnancy has been reported. Use in pregnant dogs only when the benefits outweigh the risks of therapy.

Adverse Effects/Warnings - Because of the limited experience with this agent, the following adverse effects may not be complete nor totally valid for dogs: Gastrointestinal effects consisting of nausea, vomiting, anorexia, diarrhea are the most common adverse effects seen in people and also apparently in dogs. Hepatotoxicity is the most serious potential adverse (human) reaction reported and must be also considered for canine patients. Dose related increases in liver enzymes may be seen and, rarely, hepatic failure and death may occur. In humans, incidences of hepatotoxicty are greater in very young (<2 yrs old) patients, those on other anticonvulsants, or with multiple congenital abnormalities.

Other potential adverse effects include: CNS (sedation, ataxia, behavioral changes, etc), dermatologic (alopecia, rash, etc), hematologic (thrombocytopenia, reduced platelet aggregation, leukopenias, anemias, etc.), pancreatitis, and edema.

Overdosage - Severe overdoses can cause profound CNS depression, asterixis, motor restlessness, hallucinations, and death. One human patient recovered after a serum level of 2000 micrograms/ml (20 times over therapeutic) was measured. Treatment consists of supportive measures and maintenance of adequate urine output is considered to be mandatory. Because the drug is rapidly absorbed, emesis or gastric lavage may be of limited value. Because of its delayed absorptive characteristics, the divalproex form may be removed by lavage or emesis if ingestion occurred recently. Naloxone is reported to be of benefit in reversing some of the CNS effects of valproic acid, but may also reverse the anticonvulsant properties of the drug.

Drug Interactions - VPA may enhance the CNS depressant effects of other **CNS active drugs**.

Valproic acid may increase serum levels of **phenobarbital and primidone**. Valproic acid may have effects on platelet aggregation; use with caution with other drugs that affect coagulation status (*e.g.,* **warfarin, ASA**).

Salicylates may displace valproic acid from plasma protein sites, thus increasing valproic acid levels.

The sedative effects of **clonazepam** may be enhanced by valproic acid and the anticonvulsant efficacy of both may be diminished.

Drug/Lab Interactions - A keto-metabolite of valproic acid is excreted into the urine and may yield false positive **urine ketone** tests. Altered **thyroid function tests** have been reported in humans with unknown clinical significance.

Doses -
Dogs:
   a) 75 - 200 mg/kg PO *tid* (Bunch 1986)
   b) 30 - 180 mg/kg/day PO divided *tid* (Schunk 1988)
   c) 170 - 185 mg/kg/day divided *bid-tid* (Kay and Aucoin 1985)

Monitoring Parameters -
   1) Anticonvulsant efficacy
   2) If used chronically, routine CBC's and liver enzymes at least every 6 months

Client Information - Compliance with therapy must be stressed to clients for successful epilepsy treatment. Encourage to give daily doses at same time each day. Veterinarian should be contacted if animal develops significant adverse reactions (including symptoms of anemia and/or liver disease) or if seizure control is unacceptable.

Dosage Forms/Preparations/FDA Approval Status/Withholding Times -
Veterinary-Approved Products: None
Human-Approved Products:

Valproic Acid Capsules 250 mg; *Depakene*® (Abbott); generic; (Rx)

Valproate Sodium Oral Syrup 50 mg/ml in 480 ml bottles; *Depakene*® (Abbott); generic (Rx)

Divalproex Sodium Delayed Release Tablets: 125 mg, 250 mg, 500 mg; *Depakote*® (Abbott) (Rx)

Divalproex Sodium Capsules (Sprinkle) 125 mg; *Depakote*® (Abbott) (Rx)

Valproate Sodium Injection 100 mg/ml in 5 ml in single dose vials; *Depacon*® (Abbott) (Rx)

VASOPRESSIN

Note: Vasopressin tannate is no longer commercially available in the USA.

Chemistry - A hypothalamic hormone stored in the posterior pituitary, vasopressin is a 9-amino acid polypeptide with a disulfide bond. In most mammals (including dogs and humans), the natural hormone is arginine vasopressin, while in swine the arginine is replaced with lysine. Lysine vasopressin has only about 1/2 the antidiuretic activity of arginine vasopressin. The commercially available vasopressin products may be a combination of arginine or lysine vasopressin derived from natural sources or synthetically prepared. The products are standardized by their pressor activity in rats [USP Posterior Pituitary (pressor) Units]; their antidiuretic activity can be variable. Commercially available vasopressin has little, if any, oxytocic activity at usual doses.

Vasopressin injection occurs as a clear, colorless or practically colorless liquid with a faint, characteristic odor. Vasopressin is soluble in water.

Vasopressin may also be known as antidiuretic hormone, ADH, 8-arginine-vasopressin or beta-hypophamine.

Storage/Stability/Compatibility - Vasopressin (aqueous) injection should be stored at room temperature; avoid freezing.

If the aqueous injection is to be administered as an intravenous or intra-arterial infusion, it may be diluted in either D5W or normal saline. For infusion use in humans, it is usually diluted to a concentration of 0.1 - 1 Unit/ml.

Pharmacology - Vasopressin or antidiuretic hormone (ADH) promotes the renal reabsorption of solute-free water in the distal convoluted tubules and collecting duct. ADH increases cyclic adenosine monophosphate (cAMP) at the tubule which increases water permeability at the luminal surface resulting in increased urine osmolality and decreased urine flow. Without vasopressin, urine flow can be increased up to 90% greater than normal.

At doses above those necessary for antidiuretic activity, vasopressin can cause smooth muscle contraction. Capillaries and small arterioles are most affected, with resultant decreased blood flow to several systems. Hepatic flow may actually be increased, however.

Vasopressin can cause contraction of smooth muscle of the bladder and gall bladder and can increase intestinal peristalsis, particularly of the colon. Vasopressin may also decrease gastric secretions and increase GI sphincter pressure. Gastric acid concentration remains unchanged.

Vasopressin possess minimal oxytocic effects, but at large doses may stimulate uterine contraction. Vasopressin also causes the release of corticotropin, growth hormone and follicle-stimulating hormone (FSH).

Uses/Indications - Vasopressin is used in veterinary medicine as a diagnostic agent and in the treatment of diabetes insipidus in small animals.

In human medicine, vasopressin has also been used to treat acute GI hemorrhage, stimulate GI peristalsis. Prior to radiographic procedures it has been used to dispel interfering gas shadows or to help concentrate contrast media.

Pharmacokinetics - Vasopressin is destroyed in the GI prior to being absorbed and therefore must be administered either intranasally or parenterally. After IM or SQ administration in dogs, aqueous vasopressin has antidiuretic activity for 2-8 hours.

Vasopressin is distributed throughout the extracellular fluid. The hormone apparently is not bound to plasma proteins.

Vasopressin is rapidly destroyed by the liver and kidneys. The plasma half-life has been reported to be only 10-20 minutes in humans.

Contraindications/Precautions - In humans, vasopressin is contraindicated in patients with chronic nephritis until nitrogen retention is resolved to reasonable levels. It is also contraindicated in patients who are hypersensitive to it.

Because of its effects on other systems, particularly at high doses, vasopressin should be used with caution in patients with vascular disease, seizure disorders, heart failure or asthma.

Although the drug has minimal effects on uterine contractions at usual doses, it should be used with caution in pregnant animals.

Adverse Effects/Warnings - Adverse effects that can be seen include local irritation at the injection site (including sterile abscesses), skin reactions, abdominal pain, hematuria and, rarely, a hypersensitivity (urticarial) reaction. Overdosage can lead to water intoxication (see below).

Overdosage - Overdosage can lead to water intoxication. Early symptoms can include listlessness or depression. More severe intoxication symptoms can include coma, seizures and eventually death. Treatment for mild intoxication is stopping vasopressin therapy and restricting water access until resolved. Severe intoxication may require the use of osmotic diuretics (mannitol, urea or dextrose) with or without furosemide.

Drug Interactions - The following drugs may inhibit the activity of vasopressin: **lithium,** large doses of **epinephrine, demeclocycline, heparin,** and **alcohol.**

The following drugs may potentiate the effects of vasopressin: **chlorpropamide, urea, carbamazepine,** and **fludrocortisone.**

Doses -
Dogs:
As a diagnostic agent after the water deprivation test (WDT); monitor carefully. The WDT is considered to be contraindicated in animals that are dehydrated or have known renal disease and is used to characterize whether DI is central or nephrogenic in origin. It is suggested to refer to either *Current Veterinary Therapy X: Small Animal Practice*, Kirk, R.W., Ed., 1989 pp. 973-978 or *Handbook of Small Animal Practice*, Morgan R.V., Ed. 1988, pp. 504-506, for more information:

    a) Exogenous vasopressin test: After WDT, empty bladder and start IV catheter and slowly reintroduce water. Give aqueous vasopressin in D5W IV at a dose of 2.5 mU/kg over one hour. To make one liter of a 5 mU/ml solution add 5 Units of vasopressin to one liter of D5W. Empty bladder and collect urine at 30 minutes, 60 minutes, and 90 minutes. If urine specific gravity >1.1015 = ADH-responsive DI; if <1.015 = either nephrogenic DI or medullary washout effect. (Nichols and Miller 1988)

For treatment of central (ADH-responsive) diabetes insipidus: For treatment of central diabetes insipidus: (Note: Because vasopressin tannate in oil is no longer commercially available; most clinicians are using desmopressin (DDAVP) for treating central DI. Refer to that monograph for more information.

Cats:
As a diagnostic agent after the water deprivation test (WDT). The WDT is generally considered to be contraindicated in animals that are dehydrated or have known renal disease and is used to characterize whether DI is central or nephrogenic in origin.:

    a) Immediately after the end-point of the WDT, give aqueous vasopressin 0.5 U/kg IM; continue to withhold food and water. At 30, 60, and 120 minutes after vasopressin, empty bladder and determine specific gravity (osmolality). Upon completion, the cat is gradually allowed access to water. Inability to concentrate urine during the water deprivation test followed by a rise in urine specific gravity above 1.025 following the vasopressin is indicative of central DI. (Peterson and Randolph 1989)

For treatment of central diabetes insipidus: (Note: Because vasopressin tannate in oil is no longer commercially available; most clinicians are using desmopressin (DDAVP) for treating central DI. Refer to that monograph for more information.

Monitoring Parameters -
    1) Urine output/frequency
    2) Water consumption
    3) Urine specific gravity &/or osmolality

Client Information - When instructing owners in injecting the medication, stress the importance of proper mixing of the tannate suspension (see below).

Dosage Forms/Preparations/FDA Approval Status/Withholding Times -
Veterinary-Approved Products: None
Human-Approved Products:
Vasopressin Injection, 20 Units/ml in 0.5, 1 ml & 10 ml vials; 0.5 and 1 ml ampules; *Pitressin*® *Synthetic* (Parke-Davis); Generic; (Rx)

Vasopressin Tannate Sterile Suspension in oil is no longer commercially available.

VECURONIUM BROMIDE

Chemistry - Structurally similar to pancuronium, vecuronium bromide is a synthetic, nondepolarizing neuromuscular blocking agent. It contains the steroid (androstane) nucleus, but is devoid of steroid activity. It occurs as white to off-white, or slightly pink crystals or crystalline powder. In aqueous solution it has a pK_a of 8.97, and the commercial injection has a pH of 4 after reconstitution. 9 mg are soluble in 1 ml of water; 23 mg are soluble in 1 ml of alcohol. Vecuronium may also be called:Org NC 45.

Storage/Stability/Compatibility - The commercially available powder for injection should be stored at room temperature and protected from light. After reconstitution with sterile water for injection, vecuronium bromide is stable for 24 hours at either 2-8°C or at room temperature (less than 30°C) if stored in the original container. As it contains no preservative, unused portions should be discarded after reconstitution. It has been demonstrated that the drug is stable for 48 hours when refrigerated or kept at room temperature when stored in plastic or glass syringes, but the manufacturer recommends that it be used within 24 hours.

Vecuronium bromide has been shown to be physically compatible with D5W, normal saline, D5 in normal saline, and lactated Ringer's. It should not be mixed with alkaline solutions (*e.g.,* thiobarbiturates).

Pharmacology - Vecuronium is a nondepolarizing neuromuscular blocking agent and acts by competitively binding at cholinergic receptor sites at the motor end-plate, thereby inhibiting the effects of acetylcholine. The potency of vecuronium when compared to pancuronium has been described as being from 3 times as potent to equipotent on a weight basis.

Uses/Indications - Vecuronium is indicated as an adjunct to general anesthesia to produce muscle relaxation during surgical procedures or mechanical ventilation and also to facilitate endotracheal intubation. It has very minimal cardiac effects and generally does not cause the release of histamine.

Pharmacokinetics - The onset of neuromuscular blockade after IV injection is dependent upon the dose administered. In dogs administered 0.1 mg/kg IV, full neuromuscular block occurs within 2 minutes and the duration of action at this dose is approximately 25 minutes (also receiving halothane anesthesia). Vecuronium has a shorter duration of action than pancuronium (approx. 1/3 - 1/2 as long), but is very similar to that of atracurium.

Vecuronium is partially metabolized; it and its metabolites are excreted into the bile and urine. Prolonged recovery times may result in patients with significant renal or hepatic disease.

Contraindications/Precautions - Vecuronium is contraindicated in patients hypersensitive to it. It should be used with caution in patients with severe renal dysfunction. Lower doses may be necessary in patients with hepatic or biliary disease. Vecuronium has no analgesic or sedative/anesthetic actions. In patients with myasthenia gravis, neuromuscular blocking agents should be used with extreme caution, if at all. One case of successful use in a dog with myasthenia gravis has been reported.

Adverse Effects/Warnings - In human studies and in one limited dog study, adverse effects other than what would be seen pharmacologically (skeletal muscle weakness to profound, prolonged musculoskeletal paralysis) have not been reported.

Overdosage - No cases of vecuronium overdosage have yet been reported (human or veterinary). Should an inadvertent overdose occur, treat conservatively (mechanical ventilation, O_2, fluids, etc.). Reversal of blockade might be accomplished by administering an anticholinesterase agent (edrophomium, physostigmine, or neostigmine) with an anticholinergic (atropine or glycopyrrolate). A suggested dose for neostigmine is 0.06 mg/kg IV after atropine 0.02 mg/kg IV.

Drug Interactions - The following agents may enhance or prolong the neuromuscular blocking activity of vecuronium: **quinidine, aminoglycoside antibiotics (gentamicin**, etc), **lincomycin, clindamycin, bacitracin, magnesium sulfate, polymyxin B, enflurane, isoflurane,** and **halothane. Other non-depolarizing muscle relaxant drugs** may have a synergistic effect if used with vecuronium. **Succinylcholine** may speed the onset of action and enhance the neuromuscular blocking actions of vecuronium. Do not give vecuronium until succinylcholine effects have subsided.

Doses -
  Dogs:
        a) 0.1 mg/kg IV initially (after meperidine and/or acepromazine preop 30 minutes before); may give subsequent incremental doses of 0.04 mg/kg IV. Duration of action after initial dose averages 25 minutes. (Jones and Seymour 1985)

Monitoring Parameters -
    1) Level of neuromuscular relaxation

Client Information - This drug should only be used by professionals familiar with its use.

Dosage Forms/Preparations/FDA Approval Status/Withholding Times -
Veterinary-Approved Products: None
Human-Approved Products:

Vecuronium Bromide powder for injection 10 mg & 20 mg; in 10 ml & 20 ml vials with and without diluent; *Norcuron*® (Organon); (Rx)

VERAPAMIL HCL

Chemistry - A calcium channel blocking agent, verapamil HCl occurs as a bitter-tasting, nearly white, crystalline powder. It is soluble in water and the injectable product has a pH of 4 - 6.5.

Storage/Stability/Compatibility - Verapamil HCl tablets should be stored at room temperature (15-30°C); the injectable product should be stored at room temperature (15-30°C) and be protected from light and freezing.

Verapamil HCl for injection is compatible when mixed with all commonly used intravenous solutions. However a crystalline precipitate may form if verapamil is added to an infusion line with 0.45% sodium chloride with sodium bicarbonate running. Verapamil is reported to be **compatible** with the following drugs: amikacin sulfate, aminophylline, ampicillin sodium, ascorbic acid, atropine sulfate, bretylium tosylate, calcium chloride/gluconate, carbenicillin disodium, cefamandole naftate, cefazolin sodium, cefotaxime sodium, cefoxitin sodium, cephapirin sodium, chloramphenicol sodium succinate, cimetidine HCl, clindamycin phosphate, dexamethasone sodium phosphate, diazepam, digoxin, dobutamine HCl (slight discoloration due to dobutamine oxidation), dopamine HCl, epinephrine HCl, furosemide, gentamicin sulfate, heparin sodium, hydrocortisone sodium phosphate, hydromorphone HCl, insulin, isoproterenol, lidocaine HCl, magnesium sulfate, mannitol, meperidine HCl, metaraminol bitartrate, methicillin sodium, methylprednisolone sodium succinate, metoclopramide HCl, morphine sulfate, multivitamin infusion, nitroglycerin, norepinephrine bitartrate, oxytocin, pancuronium Br, penicillin G potassium/sodium, pentobarbital sodium, phenobarbital sodium, phentolamine mesylate, phenytoin sodium, potassium chloride/phosphate, procainamide HCl, propranolol HCl, protamine sulfate, quinidine gluconate, sodium bicarbonate, sodium nitroprusside, ticarcillin disodium, tobramycin sulfate, vasopressin, and vitamin B complex w/C.

The following drugs have been reported to be physically **incompatible** with verapamil: albumin injection, amphotericin B, hydralazine HCl, nafcillin sodium, and trimethoprim/sulfamethoxazole. Compatibility is dependent upon factors such as pH, concentration, temperature, and diluents used and it is suggested to consult specialized references for more specific information.

Pharmacology - A slow-channel calcium blocking agent, verapamil is classified as a class IV antiarrhythmic drug. Verapamil exerts its actions by blocking the transmembrane influx of extracellular calcium ions across membranes of vascular smooth muscle cells and myocardial cells. The results of this blocking is to inhibit the contractile mechanisms of vascular and cardiac smooth muscle. Verapamil also has inhibitory effects on the cardiac conduction system and these effects produce its antiarrhythmic properties. Electrophysiologic effects include increased effective refractory period of the AV node, decreased automaticity and substantially decreased AV node conduction. On ECG, heart rate and RR intervals can be increased or decreased, PR and A-H intervals are increased. Verapamil has negative effects on myocardial contractility and decreases peripheral vascular resistance.

Uses/Indications - Veterinary experience with this agent is still rather limited, but in dogs verapamil is indicated for supraventricular tachycardias and possibly for the treatment of atrial flutter or fibrillation.

Pharmacokinetics - In humans, about 90% of a dose of verapamil is rapidly absorbed after oral administration, but because of a high first-pass effect, only about 20-30% is available to the systemic circulation. Patients with significant hepatic dysfunction, may have considerably higher percentages of the drug bioavailable. Food will decrease the rate and extent of absorption of the sustained-release tablets, but less so with the conventional tablets.

Verapamil's volume of distribution is between 4.5-7 L/kg in humans and has been reported to be approximately 4.5 L/kg in dogs. In humans, approximately 90% of the drug in the serum is bound to plasma proteins. Verapamil crosses the placenta and milk levels may approach those in the plasma.

Verapamil is metabolized in the liver to at least 12 separate metabolites, with norverapamil being the most predominant. The majority of the amount of these metabolites are excreted into the urine. Only 3-4% is excreted unchanged in the urine. In humans, the half-life of the drug is 2-8 hours after a single IV dose, but it can increase after 1-2 days of oral therapy (presumably due to a saturable process of the hepatic enzymes). Serum half-lives of 0.8 hours and 2.5 hours have been reported in the dog.

Contraindications/Precautions - Verapamil is contraindicated in patients with cardiogenic shock or severe CHF (unless secondary to a supraventricular tachycardia amenable to verapamil therapy), hypotension (<90 mmHg systolic), sick sinus syndrome, 2nd or 3rd degree AV block, digitalis-intoxicated, or if patient is hypersensitive to verapamil.

IV verapamil is contraindicated within a few hours of IV beta-adrenergic blocking agents (*e.g.,* propranolol) as they both can depress myocardial contractility and AV node conduction. Use of this combination in patients with wide complex ventricular tachycardia (QRS > 0.11 seconds) can cause rapid hemodynamic deterioration and ventricular fibrillation.

Verapamil should be used with caution in patients with heart failure, hypertrophic cardiomyopathy, and hepatic or renal impairment. Toxicity may be potentiated in patients with hepatic dysfunction. It should be used very cautiously in patients with atrial fibrillation and Wolf-Parkinson-White (WPW) syndrome as fatal arrhythmias may result.

Adverse Effects/Warnings - While clinical experience with verapamil is limited, the following adverse reactions may occur: hypotension, bradycardia, tachycardia, exacerbation of CHF, peripheral edema, AV block, pulmonary edema, nausea, constipation, dizziness, headache or fatigue.

Overdosage - Symptoms of overdosage may include bradycardia, hypotension, junctional rhythms, and 2nd or 3rd degree AV block.

If overdose is secondary to a recent oral ingestion, emptying the gut and charcoal administration may be considered. Treatment is generally supportive in nature; vigorously monitor cardiac and respiratory function. Intravenous calcium salts (1 ml of 10% solution per 10 kgs of body weight) have been suggested to treat the negative inotropic symptoms, but may not adequately treat symptoms of heart block. Use of fluids, and pressor agents (e.g dopamine, norepinephrine, etc) may be utilized to treat hypotensive symptoms. The AV block and/or bradycardia can be treated with isoproterenol, norepinephrine, atropine, or cardiac pacing. Patients who develop a rapid ventricular rate after verapamil due to antegrade conduction in flutter/fibrillation with WPW syndrome, have been treated with D.C. cardioversion, lidocaine, or procainamide.

Drug Interactions - beta-**adrenergic blockers** (*e.g.,* **propranolol**) and verapamil both are negative cardiac inotropes and chronotropes. If given concurrently, these effects may be additive and significantly affect cardiac function.

Verapamil activity may be adversely affected by **Vitamin D or calcium salts**.

Cimetidine may increase the effects of verapamil.

Verapamil may increase the blood levels of **digoxin or digitoxin**. Monitoring of "dig" serum levels recommended if using concurrently.

The neuromuscular blocking effects of **nondepolarizing muscle relaxants** may be enhanced by verapamil.

Quinidine effects may be altered and hypotension may occur in patients also receiving verapamil.

Rifampin may significantly reduce the effects of oral verapamil; these effects may persist for several days after rifampin is discontinued.

Verapamil may increase serum levels of **theophylline** and lead to toxicity. Verapamil may displace highly protein bound agents (*e.g.,* **warfarin**) from plasma proteins.

Calcium channel blockers may increase intracellular **vincristine** by inhibiting the drug's outflow from the cell.

Doses -
  Dogs:
  a) Intravenous: If normal myocardial function: 1 mg/kg IV; If myocardial function impaired: 0.05 - 0.1 mg/kg IV to effect; maximum of 0.3 mg/kg within 20 minutes.
     Oral: If normal myocardial function: up to 5 - 10 mg/kg 3 times daily; If myocardial function diminished: 0.1 - 0.2 mg/kg 3 times daily to start, titrate to effect (Murtaugh and Ross 1988)
  b) 0.05 - 0.15 mg/kg IV slowly over 5 minutes, followed by IV infusion of 2 - 10 micrograms/kg/min or by repeated slow injections in 30 minutes (Novotney and Adams 1986)
  c) Intravenous: 0.05 - 0.15 mg/kg IV bolus, followed by IV infusion of 2 - 10 micrograms/kg/minute.
     Oral: 10 - 15 mg/kg divided *bid* - *tid* PO (Moses 1988)
  d) For conversion of rapid supraventricular tachycardia (especially pre-excitation type): 1.1 - 4.4 mg/kg PO q8-12h; 0.11 - 0.33 mg/kg IV slowly. (Ettinger 1989)

Monitoring Parameters -
  1) ECG
  2) Symptoms of toxicity (see Adverse Reactions)
  3) Blood pressure if possible, during acute IV therapy

Client Information - To be effective, the animal must receive all doses as prescribed. If animal becomes lethargic or becomes exercise intolerant, begins wheezing, has shortness of breath or cough, or develops a change in behavior or attitude, notify veterinarian.

Dosage Forms/Preparations/FDA Approval Status/Withholding Times -
  Veterinary-Approved Products: None
  Human-Approved Products:
    Verapamil HCl Tablets 40 mg, 80 mg, 120 mg; *Calan®* (Searle), *Isoptin®* (Knoll), Generic. (Rx)

    Verapamil HCl Tablets Sustained-Release Tablets and Capsules: 120 mg, 180 mg, 240 mg & 360 mg; *Calan® SR Caplets* (Searle; *Isoptin® SR* (Knoll); *Covera-HS®* (Searle); *Verelan®* (Lederle); generic; (Rx)

    Verapamil HCl for Injection 5 mg/2 ml in 2, 4, & 5 ml vials; 2 & 4 ml amps & disposable syringes; *Isoptin®* (Knoll), Generic (Rx)

VINBLASTINE SULFATE

Chemistry - Commonly referred to as a vinca alklaoid, vinblastine sulfate is isolated from the plant *Cantharanthus roseus* (*Vinca rosea* Linn) and occurs as a white or slightly yellow, hygroscopic, amorphous or crystalline powder that is freely soluble in water. The commercially available injection has a pH of 3-5.5. Vinblastine sulfate may also be known as vincaleukoblastine sulfate or by the initials VLB.

Storage/Stability/Compatibility - The sterile powder for injection, solution for injection and reconstituted powder for injection should all be protected from light. The powder for injection and injection should be stored in the refrigerator (2-8°C). The intact powder for injection is stable at room temperature for at least one month. After reconstituting with bacteriostatic saline, the powder for injection is stable for 30 days if refrigerated.

Vinblastine sulfate is reportedly **compatible** with the following intravenous solutions and drugs: D5W and bleomycin sulfate. In syringes or at Y-sites with: bleomycin sulfate, cisplatin, cyclophosphamide, droperidol, fluorouracil, leucovorin calcium, methotrexate sodium, metoclopramide HCl, mitomycin, and vincristine sulfate.

Vinblastine sulfate **compatibility information conflicts** or is dependent on diluent or concentration factors with the following drugs or solutions: doxorubicin HCl, and heparin sodium (in syringes). Compatibility is dependent upon factors such as pH, concentration, temperature and diluents used. It is suggested to consult specialized references for more specific information (*e.g., Handbook on Injectable Drugs* by Trissel; see bibliography).

Vinblastine sulfate is reportedly **incompatible** with the following solutions or drugs: furosemide.

Pharmacology - Vinblastine apparently binds to microtubular proteins (tubulin) in the mitotic spindle, thereby preventing cell division during metaphase. It also interferes with amino acid metabolism by inhibiting glutamic acid utilization and preventing purine synthesis, citric acid cycle and urea formation.

Uses/Indications - Vinblastine may be employed in the treatment of lymphomas, carcinomas, mastocytomas and splenic tumors in small animals.

Pharmacokinetics - Vinblastine is administered IV. After injection it is rapidly distributed to tissues. In humans, approximately 75% is bound to tissue proteins and the drug does not appreciably enter the CNS.

Vinblastine is extensively metabolized by the liver and is primarily excreted in the bile/feces. Lesser amounts are eliminated in the urine.

Contraindications/Precautions/Reproductive Safety - Vinblastine is contraindicated in patients with preexisting leukopenia or granulocytopenia (unless a result of the disease being treated), or active bacterial infection.

As vinblastine may be a skin irritant, gloves and protective clothing should be worn when preparing or administering the medication. If skin/mucous membrane exposure occurs, thoroughly wash area with soap and water.

Little is known about the effects of vinblastine on developing fetuses, but it is believed that the drug possesses some teratogenic and embryotoxic properties. It may also cause aspermia in males.

Adverse Effects/Warnings - Vinblastine can cause gastroenterocolitis (nausea/vomiting) and can be myelosuppressive at usual dosages (nadir at 4-9 days after treatment; recovery at 7-14 days). Vinblastine may not possess the degree of peripheral neurotoxic effects seen with vincristine, but at high doses these effects may also be seen. Additionally, vinblastine may cause constipation, alopecia, stomatitis, ileus, inappropriate ADH secretion, jaw and muscle pain, and loss of deep tendon reflexes.

Extravasation of vinblastine may cause significant tissue irritation and cellulitis. Because of the vessicant action of this drug, it is recommended to use a different needle for injecting the drug than the one used to withdraw the drug from the vial. Should symptoms of extravasation be noted, discontinue infusion immediately at that site and apply moderate heat to the area to help disperse the drug. Injections of hyaluronidase have also been suggested to diffuse the drug.

Overdosage/Acute Toxicity - In dogs, the lethal dose for vinblastine has been reported as 0.2 mg/kg. Effects of an overdosage of vinblastine are basically exacerbations of the adverse effects outlined above. Additionally, neurotoxic effects similar to those associated with vincristine may also be noted.

In humans, treatment of overdoses of vinblastine include supportive care and the attempt to prevent the effects associated with the syndrome of inappropriate antidiuretic hormone (fluid restriction and loop diuretics to maintain serum osmolality), anticonvulsants, prevention of ileus, and cardiovascular and hematologic monitoring.

Drug Interactions - In humans who have previously or simultaneously received **mitomycin-C** with vinca alkaloids, severe bronchospasm has occurred.

Drug/Laboratory Interactions - Vinblastine may significantly increase both blood and urine concentrations of **uric acid**.

Doses - For more information, refer to the Protocols found in the appendix, including: *Handbook of Small Animal Practice* (Stann 1988b).

Dogs:
For susceptible neoplastic diseases:
- a) 2 mg/m^2 IV every 7-14 days. (O'Keefe and Harris 1990), (Thompson 1989a)
- b) 3 mg/m^2 weekly, or 0.1 - 0.4 mg/kg weekly. (Macy 1986)
  Note: According to reference by O'Keefe and Harris (above), 0.2 mg/kg can be a lethal dose in the dog. Until the safety of doses above 0.2 mg/kg can be verified, it is suggested to use the mg/m^2 method of figuring the dose.
- c) For lymphoma and mastocytoma: 2 mg/m^2 weekly.
- d) For lymphosarcoma and various carcinomas: 2.5 mg/m^2 IV weekly. (MacEwen and Rosenthal 1989), (Rosenthal 1985)
- e) 2 mg/m^2 slow IV every 7-14 days. (Golden and Langston 1988)

Cats:
For susceptible neoplastic diseases:
- a) For lymphosarcoma and mast cell neoplasms: 2 mg/m^2 IV every 7-14 days. (Couto 1989b)
- b) 2 mg/m^2 slow IV every 7-14 days. (Golden and Langston 1988)

Monitoring Parameters -
1. Efficacy
2. Toxicity
   - a) Complete blood counts with platelets
   - b) Liver function tests prior to therapy and repeated *prn*
   - c) Serum uric acid

Client Information - Clients must be briefed on the possibilities of severe toxicity developing from this drug, including drug-related mortality. Clients should contact the veterinarian should the patient exhibit any symptoms of profound depression, abnormal bleeding (including bloody diarrhea) and/or bruising.

Dosage Forms/Preparations/FDA Approval Status/Withholding Times -
Veterinary-Approved Products: None
Human-Approved Products:
Vinblastine Sulfate for Injection 1 mg/ml in 10 ml & 25 ml vials; *Velban*® (Lilly) (Rx); generic; (Rx)

Vinblastine Powder for Injection 10 mg/vial. Generic (LyphoMed), (Quad) (Rx)

VINCRISTINE SULFATE

Chemistry - Commonly referred to as a vinca alkaloid, vincristine sulfate is isolated from the plant *Cantharanthus roseus* (*Vinca rosea* Linn) and occurs as a white or slightly yellow, hygroscopic, amorphous or crystalline powder that is freely soluble in water and slightly soluble in alcohol. The commercially available injection has a pH of 3-5.5. Vincristine sulfate has pK$_{as}$ of 5 and 7.4 and may also be known as leurocristine sulfate or by the initials VCR, or LCR.

Storage/Stability/Compatibility - Vincristine sulfate injection should be protected from light and stored in the refrigerator (2-8°C).

Vincristine sulfate is reportedly **compatible** with the following intravenous solutions and drugs: D5W, bleomycin sulfate, cytarabine, fluorouracil, and methotrexate sodium. In syringes or at Y-sites with: bleomycin sulfate, cisplatin, cyclophosphamide, doxorubicin HCl, droperidol, fluorouracil, heparin sodium, leucovorin calcium, methotrexate sodium, metoclopramide HCl, mitomycin, and vinblastine sulfate.

Vincristine sulfate is reportedly **incompatible** with the following solutions or drugs: furosemide. Compatibility is dependent upon factors such as pH, concentration, temperature and diluents used. It is suggested to consult specialized references for more specific information (*e.g., Handbook on Injectable Drugs* by Trissel; see bibliography).

Pharmacology - Vincristine apparently binds to microtubular proteins (tubulin) in the mitotic spindle, thereby preventing cell division during metaphase. It also interferes with amino acid metabolism by inhibiting glutamic acid utilization and preventing purine synthesis, citric acid cycle and urea formation. Tumor resistance to one vinca alkaloid does not imply resistance to another.

Vincristine also can induce thrombocytosis (mechanism unknown) and has some immunosuppressant activity.

Uses/Indications - Vincristine is used as an antineoplastic primarily in combination drug protocols in dogs and cats in the treatment of lymphoid and hematopoietic neoplasms. In dogs, it may be used alone in the therapy of transmissible venereal neoplasms.

Because vincristine can induce thrombocytosis (at low doses) and has some immunosuppressant activity, it may also be employed in the treatment of immune-mediated thrombocytopenia.

Pharmacokinetics - Vincristine is administered IV as it is unpredictably absorbed from the GI tract. After injection it is rapidly distributed to tissues. In humans, approximately 75% is bound to tissue proteins and the drug does not appreciably enter the CNS.

Vincristine is extensively metabolized, presumably by the liver and is primarily excreted in the bile/feces. Lesser amounts are eliminated in the urine. The elimination half-life in dogs is reportedly biphasic, with an alpha half-life of 13 minutes and a beta half life of 75 minutes.

Contraindications/Precautions/Reproductive Safety - Vincristine should be used with caution in patients with hepatic disease, leukopenia, infection, or preexisiting neuromuscular disease.

Doses of vincristine are recommended to be reduced in patients with hepatic disease, but no clear guidelines have been established as to when, or how much to reduce the dose.

As vincristine may be a skin irritant, gloves and protective clothing should be worn when preparing or administering the medication. If skin/mucous membrane exposure occurs, thoroughly wash area with soap and water.

Little is known about the effects of vincristine on developing fetuses, but it is believed that the drug possesses some teratogenic and embryotoxic properties. It may also cause aspermia in males.

Adverse Effects/Warnings - Although structurally related to, and having a similar mechanism of action as vinblastine, vincristine has a different adverse reaction profile. Vincristine is much less myelosuppressive (mild leukopenia) at usual doses than is vinblastine, but may cause more peripheral neurotoxic effects. Neuropathic symptoms may include proprioceptive deficits, spinal hyporeflexia, or paralytic ileus with resulting constipation. In humans, vincristine commonly causes mild sensory impairment and peripheral paresthesias. These may also occur in animals, but are not usually noted due to difficulty in detection. Additionally, in small animals, vincristine may cause increased liver enzymes, inappropriate ADH secretion, jaw pain, alopecia, stomatitis or seizures.

Extravasation injuries associated with perivascular injection of vincristine can range from irritation to necrosis and tissue sloughing. Because of the vessicant action of this drug, it is recommended to use a different needle for injecting the drug than the one used to withdraw it from the vial. Recommendations of therapy for extravasation include discontinuing the infusion immediately at that site and applying moderate heat to the area to help disperse the drug. Injections of hyaluronidase have also been suggested to diffuse the drug. Others have suggested to apply ice to the area to limit the drug's diffusion and minimize the area affected. Topical dimethyl sulfoxide (DMSO) has also been recommended by some to treat the area involved.

Overdosage/Acute Toxicity - In dogs, it is reported that the maximally tolerated dose of vincristine is 0.06 mg/kg every 7 days for 6 weeks. Animals receiving this dose showed signs of slight anemia, leukopenia, increased liver enzymes, and neuronal shrinkage in the peripheral and central nervous systems.

In cats, the lethal dose of vincristine is reportedly 0.1 mg/kg. Cats receiving toxic doses showed symptoms of weight loss, seizures, leukopenia, and general debilitation.

In humans, treatment of overdoses of vincristine include supportive care and attempting to prevent the effects associated with the syndrome of inappropriate antidiuretic hormone (fluid restriction and loop diuretics to maintain serum osmolality), anticonvulsants, prevention of ileus, cardiovascular and hematologic monitoring. There have been some reports of leucovorin calcium being used to treat vincristine overdoses in humans, but efficacy of this treatment has not yet been confirmed.

Drug Interactions - In humans who have previously or simultaneously received **mitomycin-C** with vinca alkaloids, severe bronchospasm has occurred.

When used with **asparaginase**, additive neurotoxicity may occur. This is apparently less common when asparaginase is administered after vincristine.

Drug/Laboratory Interactions - Vincristine may significantly increase both blood and urine concentrations of **uric acid**.

Doses - For more information, refer to the protocol references found in the appendix or other protocols found in numerous references, including: *Handbook of Small Animal Practice* (Ogilvie 1988), (Cotter 1988), (Stann 1988a); *Handbook of Small Animal Therapeutics* (Rosenthal 1985); *Current Veterinary Therapy X: Small Animal Practice* (Helfand 1989), (Matus 1989); and *Textbook of Veterinary Internal Medicine, 3rd Edition* (Couto 1989a).

Dogs:
   For neoplastic diseases (usually used in combination protocols with other drugs):
   a) 0.5 - 0.75 mg/m^2 IV every 7-14 days (O'Keefe and Harris 1990)
   b) 0.5 mg/m^2 every 7-14 days. (Coppoc 1988)
   c) 0.5 mg/m^2 IV weekly. (MacEwen and Rosenthal 1989)
   d) For transmissible venereal tumor: 0.025 mg/kg (maximum dose 1 mg) IV once weekly. Generally requires 3-6 weeks of therapy. Usually tumor regression noted within 2 weeks of initial treatment. (Herron 1988)
   e) For transmissible venereal tumor: 0.5 mg/m^2 (maximum dose 1 mg) IV every 7 days until there is no evidence of disease. Generally requires 4-6 weeks of therapy. (Rosenthal 1985)

   For immune-mediated thrombocytopenia:
   a) If corticosteroids alone are ineffective, may use instead or add: vincristine 0.010 - 0.025 mg/kg IV at minimum of 7-10 day intervals. Alternatively, may use azathioprine, or cyclophosphamide. (Young 1988)
   b) Used only when other therapies are ineffective and bone marrow aspirate demonstrates adequate megakaryocytopoiesis: 0.02 mg/kg IV once weekly. (Feldman 1989)
   c) 0.010 - 0.025 mg/kg IV (maximum dose 1.5 mg) once every 4-7 days. (Hurvitz and Johnessee 1985)

Cats:
   For neoplastic diseases (usually used in combination protocols with other drugs):
   a) 0.5 - 0.75 mg/m^2 IV once a week. (Couto 1989b)

Monitoring Parameters -
   1. Efficacy (tumor burden reduction or platelet count); 2. Toxicity: a) Peripheral neuropathic clinical symptoms; b) Complete blood counts with platelets; c) Liver function tests prior to therapy and repeated if necessary; d) Serum uric acid

Client Information - Clients must be briefed on the possibilities of severe toxicity developing from this drug, including drug-related mortality. Clients should contact the veterinarian should the patient exhibit any symptoms of profound depression, abnormal bleeding (including bloody diarrhea) and/or bruising, severe constipation, or severe peripheral neuropathic symptoms.

Dosage Forms/Preparations/FDA Approval Status/Withholding Times -
   Veterinary-Approved Products: None
   Human-Approved Products:
   Vincristine Sulfate Injection 1 mg/ml in 1 ml, 2 ml and 5 ml vials & 1 & 2 ml Hyporets; *Oncovin*® (Lilly), *Vincasar PFS*® (Adria), generic; (Rx)

VITAMIN E/SELENIUM
VITAMIN E

Chemistry - Vitamin E is a lipid soluble vitamin that can be found in either liquid or solid forms. The liquid forms occur as clear, yellow to brownish red, viscous oils that are insoluble in water, soluble in alcohol and miscible with vegetable oils. Solid forms occur as white to tan-white granular powders that disperse in water to form cloudy suspensions. Vitamin E may also be known as alpha tocopherol.

Selenium in commercially available veterinary injections is found as sodium selenite. Each mg of sodium selenite contains approximately 460 micrograms (46%) of selenium.

Storage/Stability/Compatibility - Vitamin E/Selenium for injection should be stored at temperatures less than 25°C (77°F).

Pharmacology - Both vitamin E and selenium are involved with cellular metabolism of sulfur. Vitamin E has antioxidant properties and, with selenium, it protects against red blood cell hemolysis and prevents the action of peroxidase on unsaturated bonds in cell membranes.

Uses/Indications - Depending on the actual product and species, vitamin E/selenium is indicated for the treatment or prophylaxis of selenium-tocopheral deficiency (STD) syndromes in ewes and lambs (white muscle disease), sows, weanling and baby pigs (hepatic necrosis, mulberry heart disease, white muscle disease), calves and breeding cows (white muscle disease), and horses (myositis associated with STD).

A vitamin E/selenium product (*Seletoc®*—Schering) is also indicated for the adjunctive treatment of acute symptoms of arthritic conditions in dogs, but its efficacy for this indication has been questioned.

Pharmacokinetics - After absorption, vitamin E is transported in the circulatory system via beta-lipoproteins. It is distributed to all tissues and is stored in adipose tissue. Vitamin E is only marginally transported across the placenta. Vitamin E is metabolized in the liver and excreted primarily into the bile.

Pharmacokinetic parameters for selenium were not located.

Contraindications/Precautions/Reproductive Safety - Vitamin E/selenium products should only be used in the species in which they are approved. Because selenium can be extremely toxic, the use of these products promiscuously cannot be condoned.

When administering intravenously to horses, give slowly.

Adverse Effects/Warnings - Anaphylactoid reactions have been reported. Intramuscular injections may be associated with transient muscle soreness. Other adverse effects are generally associated with overdoses of selenium (see below).

Overdosage/Acute Toxicity - Selenium is quite toxic in overdose quantities, but has a fairly wide safety margin. Cattle have tolerated chronic doses of 0.6 mg/kg/day with no adverse effects (approximate therapeutic dose is 0.06 mg/kg). Symptoms of selenium toxicity include depression, ataxia, dyspnea, blindness, diarrhea, muscle weakness, and a "garlic" odor on the breath. Horses suffering from selenium toxicity may become blind, paralyzed, slough their hooves, and lose hair from the tail and mane. Dogs may exhibit symptoms of anorexia, vomiting, and diarrhea at high dosages.

Drug Interactions - **Vitamin A** absorption, utilization and storage may be enhanced by vitamin E.

Large doses of vitamin E may delay the hematologic response to **iron** therapy in patients with iron deficiency anemia.

Mineral oil may reduce the absorption of orally administered vitamin E.

Monitoring Parameters -
1) Clinical efficacy
2) Blood selenium levels. Normal values for selenium have been reported as: >1.14 micromol/L in calves, >0.63 micromol/L in cattle, >1.26 micromol/L in sheep, and >0.6 micromol/L in pigs. Values indicating deficiency are: <0.40 micromol/L in cattle, <0.60 micromol/L in sheep, and <0.20 micromol/L in pigs. Intermediate values may result in suboptimal production.
3) Optionally, glutathione peroxidase activity may be monitored

Dosage Forms/Preparations/FDA Approval Status/Withholding Times/Doses (per manufacturer) -

Veterinary-Approved Products: **Vitamin E/Selenium Oral:**

Equ-SeE (one teaspoonful contains 1 mg selenium and 228 IU vitamin E) & *Equ-Se5E®* (one teaspoonful contains 1 mg selenium and approximately 1100 IU vitamin E); (Vet-a-Mix) (OTC) Approved for oral use in horses.

Veterinary-Approved Products: **Vitamin E/Selenium Injection:**

Mu-Se® (Schering); (Rx): Each ml contains: selenium 5 mg (as sodium selenite); Vitamin E 68 IU; 100 ml vial for injection. Approved for use in non-lactating dairy cattle and beef cattle. Slaughter withdrawal = 30 days.

    Dose: For weanling calves: 1 ml per 200 lbs. body weight IM or SQ.

    For breeding beef cows: 1 ml per 200 lbs. body weight during middle third of pregnancy and 30 days before calving IM or SQ.

Bo-Se® (Schering); (Rx): Each ml contains selenium 1 mg (as sodium selenite) & Vitamin E 68 IU; 100 ml vial for injection. Approved for use in calves, swine and sheep. Slaughter withdrawal = 30 days (calves); 14 days (lambs, ewes, sows, and pigs).

> **Dose**: Calves: 2.5 - 3.75 mls/100 lbs body weight (depending on severity of condition and geographical area) IM or SQ.
> Lambs (2 weeks of age or older): 1 ml per 40 lbs. body weight IM or SQ (1 ml minimum).
> Ewes: 2.5 mls/100 lbs. body weight IM or SQ.
> Sows and weanling pigs: 1 ml/40 lbs. body weight IM or SQ (1 ml minimum). Do not use on newborn pigs.

L-Se® (Schering); (Rx): Each ml contains: selenium 0.25 mg (as sodium selenite) and Vitamin E 68 IU in 30 ml vials. Approved for use in lambs and baby pigs. Slaughter withdrawal = 14 days.

> **Dose**:Lambs: 1 ml SQ or IM in newborns and 4 ml SQ or IM in lambs 2 weeks of age or older
> Baby Pigs: 1 ml SQ or IM.

E-Se® (Schering); (Rx): Each ml contains selenium 2.5 mg (as sodium selenite) and Vitamin E 68 IU in 100 ml vials. Approved for use in horses.

> **Dose**: Equine: 1 ml/100 lbs. body weight slow IV or deep IM (in 2 or more sites; gluteal or cervical muscles). May be repeated at 5-10 day intervals.

Seletoc® (Schering); (Rx): Each ml contains selenium 1 mg (as sodium selenite) and Vitamin E 68 IU in 10 ml vials. Approved for use in dogs.

> **Dose**: Dogs: Initially, 1 ml per 20 pounds of body weight (minimum 0.25 ml; maximum 5 ml) SQ, or IM in divided doses in 2 or more sites. Repeat dose at 3 day intervals until satisfactory results then switch to maintenance dose. If no response in 14 days reevaluate. Maintenance dose: 1 ml per 40 lbs body weight (minimum 0.25 ml) repeat at 3-7 day intervals (or longer) to maintain.

Also available is a sustained-release selenium oral bolus (*Dura Se*®-*120*—Schering) that provides 3 mg of selenium per day for up to 4 months.

> **Human-Approved Products**: There are no approved vitamin E/selenium products, but there are many products that contain either vitamin E (alone, or in combination with other vitamins ±minerals) or selenium (as an injection alone or in combination with other trace elements) available.

WARFARIN SODIUM

Chemistry - A coumarin derivative, warfarin sodium occurs as a slightly bitter tasting, white, amorphous or crystalline powder. It is very soluble in water and freely soluble in alcohol. The commercially available products contain a racemic mixture of the two optical isomers.

Storage/Stability/Compatibility - Warfarin sodium tablets should be stored in tight, light-resistant containers at temperatures less than 40°C and, preferably, at room temperature. Warfarin sodium powder for injection should be protected from light and used immediately after reconstituting.

Pharmacology - Warfarin acts indirectly as an anticoagulant (it has no direct anticoagulant effect) by interfering with the action of vitamin K_1 in the synthesis of the coagulation factors II, VII, IX, and X. Sufficient amounts of vitamin K_1 can override this effect.

Uses/Indications - In veterinary medicine, warfarin is used primarily for the oral, long-term treatment (or prevention of recurrence) of thrombotic conditions, usually in cats, dogs or horses.

Pharmacokinetics - Warfarin is rapidly and completely absorbed in humans after oral administration; absorption data for veterinary species were not located.

After absorption, warfarin is highly bound to plasma proteins in humans, with approximately 99% of the drug bound. It is reported that there are wide species variations with regard to protein binding; horses have a higher free (unbound) fraction of the drug than do rats, sheep or swine. Only free (unbound) warfarin is active. While other coumarin and indandione anticoagulants are distributed in milk, in humans at least, warfarin does not enter milk.

Warfarin is principally metabolized in the liver to inactive metabolites which are excreted in the urine and in the bile (and then reabsorbed and excreted in the urine). The plasma half-life of warfarin may be several hours to several days, depending on the patient (and species?).

Contraindications/Precautions/Reproductive Safety - Warfarin is contraindicated in patients with preexistent hemorrhagic tendencies or diseases, those undergoing or contemplating eye or CNS surgery, major regional lumbar block anesthesia, or surgery of large, open surfaces. It should not be used in patients with active bleeding from the GI, respiratory or GU tract. Contraindications also include aneurysm, acute nephritis, cerebrovascular hemorrhage, blood dyscrasias, uncontrolled or malignant hypertension, hepatic insufficiency, pericardial effusion and visceral carcinomas.

Warfarin is embryotoxic, can cause congenital malformations and is considered contraindicated during pregnancy. If anticoagulant therapy is required during pregnancy, most clinicians recommend using low-dose heparin.

Adverse Effects/Warnings - The principal adverse effect of warfarin use is dose-related hemorrhage, which may be manifested by signs or symptoms of anemia, thrombocytopenia, weakness, hematomas and ecchymoses, epistaxis, hematemesis, hematuria, melena, hematochezia, hemathrosis, hemothorax, intracranial and/or pericardial hemorrhage, and death.

Overdosage/Acute Toxicity - Acute overdosages of warfarin may result in life-threatening hemorrhage. In dogs and cats, single doses of 5 - 50 mg/kg have been associated with toxicity. It must be remembered that a lag time of 2-5 days may occur before signs and symptoms of toxicity occur and animals must be monitored and treated accordingly.

Cumulative toxic doses of warfarin have been reported as 1 - 5 mg/kg for 5-15 days in dogs and 1 mg/kg for 7 days in cats.

If overdosage is detected early, prevent absorption from the gut using standard protocols. If symptoms are noted, they should be treated with blood products and vitamin K_1 (phytonadione). Refer to the phytonadione monograph for more information.

Drug Interactions - A multitude of drugs have been documented or theorized to interact with warfarin. The following drugs may increase the anticoagulant response of warfarin: **allopurinol, amiodarone, anabolic steroids, chloral hydrate, chloramphenicol, cimetidine, clofibrate, co-trimoxazole (trimethoprim/sulfa), danazol, dextrothyroxine sodium, diazoxide, diflunisal, disulfiram, erythromycin, ethacrynic acid, fenoprofen, glucagon, ibuprofen, indomethicin, isoniazid, ketoprofen, meclofenamic acid (meclofenamate), metronidazole, miconazole, nalidixic acid, oral neomycin, pentoxyfilline, phenylbutazone, propoxyphene, propylthiouracil, quinidine, and salicylates**.

The following drugs may decrease the anticoagulant response of warfarin: **barbiturates (phenobarbital, etc.), carbamazepine, corticosteroids, corticotropin, griseofulvin, mercaptopurine, estrogen-containing products, rifampin, spironolactone, sucralfate, and vitamin K**.

Should concurrent use of any of the above drugs with warfarin be necessary, enhanced monitoring is required. It is also recommended to refer to other references on drug interactions for more specific information.

Drug/Laboratory Interactions - Warfarin may cause falsely decreased **theophylline** values if using the Schack and Waxler ultraviolet method of assay.

Doses -
Dogs:
For adjunctive therapy of thromboemboli:
a) For pulmonary thromboemboli: 0.1 mg/kg PO once daily. Monitor PT (begin 3-4 days after starting therapy) and aim for an increase to 1.5 - 2 times baseline value. (Bauer 1988)
b) For pulmonary thromboembolism: 0.2 mg/kg PO once daily then 0.05 - 0.1 mg/kg PO once daily. Adjust dosage to increase PT to 1.5 - 2.5 times baseline. Heparin may be stopped once appropriate warfarin dosage is established. If PT exceeds 2.5 times baseline, reduce dose. If bleeding develops, stop dose and institute blood or phytonadione therapy as appropriate. (Roudebush 1985)

Cats:
For adjunctive therapy of thromboembolism:
a) For feline aortic thromboembolism: 0.06 - 0.1 mg/kg once daily PO. Evaluate using PT, APTT, or preferably PIVKA (proteins induced by vitamin K antagonists) daily during initial titration (3 days), then every other day (2 times) and weekly thereafter until stable. New steady state may require one week after dosage adjustments. Long-term therapy should be monitored at least one monthly. (Pion and Kittleson 1989)
b) For chronic management/prevention of recurrence: 0.1 - 0.2 mg/kg PO once daily. Adjust dosage to prolong PT to 2 - 2.5 times normal. Collect blood sample 8 hours after dosing. Requires 48-72 hours to achieve effective anticoagulation. Monitor PT weekly for 1 month, then at monthly intervals. Also determine hematocrit with each PT. (Harpster 1988)
c) For pulmonary thromboembolism: 0.2 mg/kg PO once daily then 0.05 - 0.1 mg/kg PO once daily. Adjust dosage to increase PT to 1.5 - 2.5 times baseline. Heparin may be stopped once appropriate warfarin dosage is established. If PT exceeds 2.5 times baseline, reduce dose. If bleeding develops, stop dose and institute blood or phytonadione therapy as appropriate. (Roudebush 1985)

Horses:

As an anticoagulant:

a) 30 - 75 mg/450 kg body weight PO. (Robinson 1987)

b) Initially, 0.018 mg/kg PO once daily and increase dose by 20% every day until baseline PT is doubled. Final dose rates may be from 0.012 mg/kg to 0.57 mg/kg daily. (Vrins, Carlson, and Feldman 1983)

Monitoring Parameters - Note: The frequency of monitoring is controversial, and is dependent on several factors including dose, patient's condition, concomitant problems, etc. See the *Dosage* section above for more information.

1) While Prothrombin Times (PT) are most commonly used to monitor warfarin, PIVKA (proteins induced by vitamin K antagonists) has been suggested as being more sensitive.

2) Platelet counts and hematocrit (PCV) should be done periodically

3) Occult blood in stool and urine; other observations for bleeding

4) Clinical efficacy

Client Information - Clients must be counseled on both the importance of administering the drug as directed and also to immediately report any signs or symptoms of hemorrhage.

Dosage Forms/Preparations/FDA Approval Status/Withholding Times -

Veterinary-Approved Products: None.

Human-Approved Products:

Warfarin Sodium Tablets (scored) 1 mg, 2 mg, 2.5 mg, 3 mg, 4 mg, 5 mg, 6 mg, 7.5 mg, 10 mg; *Coumadin®* (DuPont), (Rx)

Warfarin Sodium Powder for Injection lyophilized 2 mg in 5 mg vials; *Coumadin®* (DuPont); (Rx)

A method of suspending warfarin tablets in an oral suspension has been described (Enos 1989). To make 30 ml of a 0.25 mg/ml suspension: Crush three 2.5 mg tablets in a mortar and pestle. Add 10 ml glycerin to form a paste. Then 10 ml of water; and q.s. to 30 ml with dark corn syrup (*Karo®*). Warm gently. Shake well and use within 30 days.

XYLAZINE HCL

Chemistry - Xylazine HCl is a alpha$_2$-adrenergic agonist structurally related to clonidine. The pH of the commercially prepared injections is approximately 5.5. Dosages and bottle concentrations are expressed in terms of the base.

Storage/Stability/Compatibility - Do not store above 30°C (86°F). Xylazine is reportedly compatible in the same syringe with several compounds, including: acepromazine, buprenorphine, butorphanol, chloral hydrate, and meperidine.

Pharmacology - A potent alpha$_2$-adrenergic agonist, xylazine is classified as a sedative/analgesic with muscle relaxant properties. Although xylazine possesses several of the same pharmacologic actions as morphine, it does not cause CNS excitation in cats, horses or cattle, but causes sedation and CNS depression. In horses, the visceral analgesia produced has been demonstrated to be superior to that produced by meperidine, butorphanol or pentazocine.

Xylazine causes skeletal muscle relaxation through central mediated pathways. Emesis is often seen in cats, and is also seen occasionally in dogs receiving xylazine. While thought to be centrally mediated, neither dopaminergic blockers (*e.g.,* phenothiazines) or alpha-blockers (yohimbine, tolazoline) block the emetic effect. Xylazine does not cause emesis in horses, cattle, sheep or goats. Xylazine depresses thermoregulatory mechanisms and either hypothermia or hyperthermia is a possibility depending on ambient air temperatures.

Effects on the cardiovascular system include an initial increase in total peripheral resistance with increased blood pressure followed by a longer period of lowered blood pressures (below baseline). A bradycardic effect can be seen with some animals developing a second degree heart block or other arrhythmias. An overall decrease in cardiac output of up to 30% may be seen. Xylazine has been demonstrated to enhance the arryhthmogenic effects of epinephrine in dogs with or without concurrent halothane.

Xylazine's effects on respiratory function are usually clinically insignificant, but at high dosages, it can cause respiratory depression with decreased tidal volumes and respiratory rates and an overall decreased minute volume. Brachycephalic dogs and horses with upper airway disease may develop dyspnea.

Xylazine can induce increases in blood glucose secondary to decreased serum levels of insulin. In non-diabetic animals, there appears to be little clinical significance associated with this effect.

In horses, sedatory signs include a lowering of the head with relaxed facial muscles and drooping of the lower lip. The retractor muscle is relaxed in male horses, but unlike acepromazine, no reports of permanent penile paralysis has been reported. Although, the animal may appear to be thoroughly sedated, auditory stimuli may provoke arousal with kicking and avoidance responses.

With regard to the sensitivity of species to xylazine definite differences are seen. Ruminants are extremely sensitive to xylazine when compared with horses, dogs, or cats. Ruminants generally require approximately 1/10th the dosage that is required for horses to exhibit the same effect. In cattle (and occasionally cats and horses), polyuria is seen following xylazine administration, probably as a result of decreased production of vasopressin (anti-diuretic hormone, ADH). Bradycardia and hypersalivation are also seen in cattle and are diminished by pretreating with atropine. Swine, require 20-30 times the ruminant dose and therefore, xylazine is not routinely used in this species.

Uses/Indications - Xylazine is approved for use in dogs, cats, horses, deer, and elk. It is indicated in dogs, cats and horses to produce a state of sedation with a shorter period of analgesia, and as a preanesthetic before local or general anesthesia. Because of the emetic action of xylazine in cats, it is occasionally used to induce vomiting after ingesting toxins.

Pharmacokinetics - Absorption is rapid following IM injection, but bioavailabilities are incomplete and variable. Bioavailabilities of 40-48% in the horse, 17-73% in the sheep, and 52-90% in the dog have been reported after IM administration.

In horses, the onset of action following IV dosage occurs within 1-2 minutes with a maximum effect 3-10 minutes after injection. The duration of effect is dose dependent but may last for approximately 1.5 hours. The serum half-life after a single dose of xylazine is approximately 50 minutes in the horse and recovery times generally take from 2-3 hours.

In dogs and cats, the onset of action following an IM or SQ dose is approximately 10-15 minutes, and 3-5 minutes following an IV dose. The analgesic effects may persist for only 15-30 minutes, but the sedative actions may last for 1-2 hours depending on the dose given. The serum half-live of xylazine in dogs has been reported as averaging 30 minutes. Complete recovery after dosing may take from 2-4 hours in dogs and cats.

Xylazine is not detected in milk of lactating dairy cattle at 5 & 21 hours post-dose, but the FDA has not approved the use of this agent in dairy cattle and no meat or milk withdrawal times have been specified.

Contraindications/Precautions - Xylazine is contraindicated in animals receiving epinephrine or having active ventricular arrhythmias. It should be used with extreme caution in animals with preexisting cardiac dysfunction, hypotension or shock, respiratory dysfunction, severe hepatic or renal insufficiency, preexisting seizure disorders, or if severely debilitated. Because it may induce premature parturition, it should generally not be used in the last trimester of pregnancy, particularly in cattle.

Be certain of product concentration when drawing up into syringe, especially if treating ruminants. Do not give to ruminants that are dehydrated, have urinary tract obstruction, or are debilitated. It is not approved for any species to be consumed for food purposes.

Horses have been known to kick after a stimulatory event (usually auditory); use caution. Avoid intra-arterial injection; may cause severe seizures and collapse. The manufacturers warn against using in conjunction with other tranquilizers.

Adverse Effects/Warnings - Emesis is generally seen within 3-5 minutes after xylazine administration in cats and occasionally in dogs. To prevent aspiration, do not induce further anesthesia until this time period has lapsed. Other adverse effects listed in the package insert (*Gemini*®, Butler) for dogs and cats include: muscle tremors, bradycardia with partial A-V block, reduced respiratory rate, movement in response to sharp auditory stimuli, and increased urination in cats.

Dogs may develop bloat from aerophagia which may require decompression. Because of gaseous distention of the stomach, xylazine's use before radiography can make test interpretation difficult.

Adverse effects listed in the package insert (*AnaSed*®, Lloyd) for horses include: muscle tremors, bradycardia with partial A-V block, reduced respiratory rate, movement in response to sharp auditory stimuli, and sweating (rarely profuse). Additionally, large animals may become ataxic following dosing and caution should be observed.

Adverse reactions reported in cattle include salivation, ruminal atony, bloating and regurgitation, hypothermia, diarrhea, and bradycardia. The hypersalivation and bradycardia may be alleviated by pretreating with atropine. Xylazine may induce premature parturition in cattle.

Overdosage - In the event of an accidental overdosage, cardiac arrhythmias, hypotension, and profound CNS and respiratory depression may occur. Seizures have also been reported after overdoses. There has been much interest in using alpha-blocking agents as antidotes or reversal agents to xylazine. Yohimbine or tolazoline have been suggested to be used alone and in combination to reverse the effects of xylazine or speed recovery times. A separate monograph for yohimbine is available which discusses suggested doses, etc.

To treat the respiratory depressant effects of xylazine toxicity, mechanical respiratory support with respiratory stimulants (*e.g.,* doxapram) have been recommended for use.

Drug Interactions - The use of **epinephrine** with & without the concurrent use of halothane concomitantly with xylazine may induce the development of ventricular arrhythmias.

The combination use of **acepromazine** with xylazine is generally considered to be safe, but there is potential for additive hypotensive effects and this combination should be used cautiously in animals susceptible to hemodynamic complications.

Other CNS depressant agents (barbiturates, narcotics, anesthetics, phenothiazines, etc.) may cause additive CNS depression if used with xylazine. Dosages of these agents may need to be reduced.

A case report of a horse developing colic-like symptoms after **reserpine** and xylazine has been reported. Until more is known about this potential interaction, use together of these two agents together should be avoided.

The manufacturers warn against using xylazine in conjunction with other tranquilizers.

Doses -
Dogs:
      a) 1.1 mg/kg IV, 1.1 - 2.2 mg/kg IM or SQ (Package Insert; *Rompun*® - Miles)
      b) 0.6 mg/kg IV IM as a sedative (Morgan 1988)
      c) To treat a hypoglycemic crises (with IV dextrose): 1.1 mg/kg IM (Schall 1985)
      d) 0.5 - 1.0 mg/kg IV or 1 - 2 mg/kg IM (Davis 1985b)
      e) 0.55 mg/kg IM (Mandsager 1988)

Cats:
      a) 1.1 mg/kg IV, 1.1 - 2.2 mg/kg IM or SQ (Package Insert; *Rompun*®—Miles)
      b) As an emetic: 0.44 mg/kg IM (Morgan 1988), (Riviere 1985)
      c) 0.5 - 1.0 mg/kg IV or 1 - 2 mg/kg IM (Davis 1985b)
      d) 0.55 mg/kg IM (Mandsager 1988)

Rabbits/Rodents/Pocket Pets:
    Rabbits: For minimally invasive procedures lasting less than 30-45 minutes: 5 mg/kg once SubQ or IM in combination with ketamine (35 mg/kg)
    Mice/Rats: General anesthesia 13 mg/kg once IP in combination with ketamine (87 mg/kg)
    Hamsters/Guinea pigs: General anesthesia 8 - 10 mg/kg once IP in combination with ketamine (200 mg/kg for hamsters & 60 mg/kg for Guinea pigs) (Huerkamp 1995)

Cattle:
    Caution: Cattle are extremely sensitive to xylazine's effects; be certain of dose and dosage form. Pretreatment with atropine can decrease the bradycardia and hypersalivation seen.
      a) 0.05 - 0.15 mg/kg IV; 0.10 - 0.33 mg/kg IM. If administering IM use an 18 or 20 gauge needle at least 1.5 inches long. Intravenous route may stress cardiovascular function. (Thurmon and Benson 1986)
      b) 0.044 - 0.11 mg/kg IV; 0.22 mg/kg IM (Mandsager 1988)

Horses:
      a) 1.1 mg/kg IV; 2.2 mg/kg IM. Allow animal to rest quietly until full effect is reached. (Package Insert; *Rompun*® - Miles)
      b) Sedative/analgesic for colic: 0.3 - 0.5 mg/kg IV; repeat as necessary (Muir 1987)
      c) Prior to guaifenesin/thiobarbiturate anesthesia: 0.55 mg/kg IV; Prior to ketamine induction: 1.1 mg/kg IV; In combination with opioid/tranquilizers (all IV doses):
         1) xylazine 0.66 mg/kg; meperidine 1.1 mg/kg
         2) xylazine 1.1 mg/kg; butorphanol 0.01 - 0.02 mg/kg
         3) xylazine 0.6 mg/kg; acepromazine 0.02 mg/kg
    Note: the manufacturers state that xylazine should not be used in conjunction with tranquilizers (Thurmon and Benson 1987)

Sheep & Goats: Note: Use xyalazine with extreme caution in these species.
      a) 0.05 - 0.10 mg/kg IV; 0.10 - 0. 22 IM (Thurmon and Benson 1986)
      b) 0.044 - 0.11 mg/kg IV; 0.22 mg/kg IM (Mandsager 1988)

Exotics:
      a) An excellent list of suggested dosages can be found on page 359 of Veterinary Pharmacology and Therapeutics, 6th Ed., Booth, NH & McDonald, LE, Eds.; 1988; Iowa State University Press; Ames, Iowa

Monitoring Parameters - 1) Level of anesthesia/analgesia; 2) Respiratory function; cardiovascular status (rate, rhythm, BP if possible); 3) Hydration status if polyuria present

Client Information - Xylazine should only be used by individuals familiar with its use.

Dosage Forms/Preparations/FDA Approval Status/Withholding Times -
Veterinary-Approved Products:
   Rompun® (Bayer) *Gemini*® (Butler); *AnaSed*® (Lloyd);*Sedazine*® (Fort Dodge) (Rx)
Approved for use (depending on strength) in dogs, cats, horses, deer, and elk.

While xyalzine is not approved for use in cattle in the USA, at labeled doses in Canada it reportedly has been assigned withdrawal times of 3 days for meat and 48 hours for milk. FARAD has reportedly suggested a withdrawal of 7 days for meat and 72 hours for milk for extra-label use in the USA.

Human-Approved Products: None

YOHIMBINE HCL

Chemistry - A Rauwolfia or indolealkylamine alkaloid, yohimbine HCl has a molecular weight of 390.9. It is chemically related to reserpine.

Storage/Stability/Compatibility - Yohimbine injection should be stored at room temperature (15-30°C); (*Antagonil*®-store in refrigerator), and protected from light and heat.

Pharmacology - Yohimbine is an alpha$_2$-adrenergic antagonist that can antagonize the effects of xylazine. Alone, yohimbine increases heart rate, blood pressure, causes CNS stimulation and antidiuresis, and has hyperinsulinemic effects.

By blocking central alpha$_2$-receptors, yohimbine causes sympathetic outflow (norepinephrine) to be enhanced. Peripheral alpha$_2$-receptors are also found in the cardiovascular system, genitourinary system, GI tract, in platelets, and adipose tissue.

Uses/Indications - Yohimbine is indicated to reverse the effects of xyalzine in dogs, but it is being used clinically in several other species as well.

Yohimbine may be efficacious in reversing some of the toxic effects associated with other agents as well (*e.g.,* amitraz), but additional research must be performed before additional recommendations for its use can be made.

Pharmacokinetics - The pharmacokinetics of this drug have been reported in steers, dogs, and horses (Jernigan et al. 1988). The apparent volume of distribution (steady-state) is approximately 5 L/kg in steers, 2 - 5 L/kg in horses, and 4.5 L/kg in dogs. The total body clearance is approximately 70 ml/min/kg in steers, 35 ml/min/kg in horses, and 30 ml/min/kg in dogs. The half-life of the drug is approximately 0.5 - 1 hours in steers, 0.5 - 1.5 hours in horses, and 1.5 - 2 hours in dogs.

Yohimbine is believed to penetrate the CNS quite readily and when used to reverse the effects of xylazine, onset of action generally occurs within 3 minutes. The metabolic fate of the drug is not known.

Contraindications/Precautions/Reproductive Safety - Yohimbine is contraindicated in patients hypersensitive to it. In humans, yohimbine is contraindicated in patients with renal disease.

Yohimbine should be used cautiously in patients with seizure disorders. When used to reverse the effects xyalzine, normal pain perception may result.

Safe use of yohimbine in pregnant animals has not been established.

Adverse Effects/Warnings - Yohimbine may cause transient apprehension or CNS excitement, muscle tremors, salivation, increased respiratory rates, and hyperemic mucous membranes. Adverse effects appear to be more probable in small animals than in large animals.

Overdosage/Acute Toxicity - Dogs receiving 0.55 mg/kg (5 times recommended dose) exhibited symptoms of transient seizures and muscle tremors.

Drug Interactions - Little information is available, use with caution with other alpha$_2$-adrenergic antagonists or other drugs that can cause CNS stimulation. In humans, yohimbine is recommended not to be used with antidepressants or other mood-altering agents.

Doses -
  Dogs:
    For xylazine reversal:
      a) 0.11 mg/kg IV slowly (Package insert; *Yobine*®—Lloyd)
      b) 0.1 mg/kg IV (Gross and Tranquilli 1989)
      c) As an antiemetic: 0.25 - 0.5 mg/kg q12h subQ or IM (Washabau and Elie 1995)
  Cats:
    For xylazine reversal:
      a) As an antiemetic: 0.25 - 0.5 mg/kg q12h subQ or IM (Washabau and Elie 1995)

Rabbits/Rodents/Pocket Pets:
To reverse the effects of xylazine and to partially antagonize the effects of ketamine and acepromazine: Rabbits: 0.2 mg/kg IV as needed; Mice/Rats: 0.2 mg/kg IP as needed (Huerkamp 1995)

Cattle:
For xylazine reversal:
a) 0.125 mg/kg IV (Gross and Tranquilli 1989)

Horses:
For xylazine reversal:
a) 0.075 mg/kg IV (Gross and Tranquilli 1989)

Llamas:
For xylazine reversal:
a) 0.25 mg/kg IV or IM (Fowler 1989)

Deer:
For xylazine reversal:
a) In wild, exotic and ranched deer: 0.2 - 0.3 mg/kg IV (Package Insert—*Antagonil*®-Wildlife Labs)
Note: Yohimbine has also been used as a reversal agent in several exotic species. Several dosages are listed in the chapter on Stimulants by Booth in Veterinary Pharmacology and Therapeutics, 6th Edition. Booth, NH & McDonald, LE Eds., Iowa State University Press. Ames. 1988

Monitoring Parameters -
1) CNS status (arousal level, etc.)
2) Cardiac rate; rhythm (if indicated), blood pressure (if indicated and practical)
3) Respiratory rate

Client Information - This agent should be used with direct professional supervision only.

Dosage Forms/Preparations/FDA Approval Status/Withholding Times -
Veterinary-Approved Products:
Yohimbine Sterile Solution for Injection 2 mg/ml in 20 ml vials *Yobine*® (Lloyd); (Rx) Approved for use in dogs.

Yohimbine HCl Sterile Solution for Injection 5 mg/ml in 20 ml vials; *Antagonil*® (Wildlife Labs); (Rx) Approved for use in deer.

Human-Approved Products: Oral 5.4 mg tablets are available, but would unlikely to be of veterinary benefit.

Zolazepam - see Tiletamine/Zolazepam

ZINC ACETATE
ZINC SULFATE

Chemistry - Zinc acetate occurs as white crystals or granules. It has a faint acetous odor and effloresces slightly. One gram is soluble in 2.5 ml of water and in 30 ml of alcohol.

Zinc sulfate occurs as a colorless granular powder, small needles, or transparent prisms. It is odorless but has an astringent metallic taste. 1.67 grams are soluble in one ml of water. Zinc sulfate is insoluble in alcohol and contains 23% zinc by weight.

Storage/Stability/Compatibility - Store zinc acetate crystals in tight containers. Unless otherwise recommended by the manufacturer, store zinc sulfate products in tight containers at room temperature.

Pharmacology - Zinc is a necessary nutritional supplement; it is required by over 200 metalloenzymes for proper function. Enzyme systems that require zinc include alkaline phosphatase, alcohol dehydrogenase, carbonic anhydrase and RNA polymerase. Zinc is also necessary to maintain structural integrity of cell membranes and nucleic acids. Zinc dependent physiological processes include sexual maturation and reproduction, cell growth and division, vision, night vision, wound healing, immune response, and taste acuity.

When administered orally, large doses of zinc can inhibit the absorption of copper.

Uses/Indications - Zinc sulfate is used systemically as a nutritional supplement in a variety of species. Oral zinc acetate has been shown to reduce copper toxicity in susceptible dog breeds (Bedlington Terriers, West Highland White Terriers) with hepatic copper toxicosis. Zinc sulfate is also used topically as an astringent and as weak antiseptic both for dermatologic and ophthalmic conditions.

Pharmacokinetics - About 20-30% of dietary zinc is absorbed, principally from the duodenum and ileum. Bioavailability is dependent upon the food in which it is present. Phytates can chelate zinc and form insoluble complexes in an alkaline pH. Zinc is stored mostly in red and white blood cells, but is also found in the muscle, skin, bone, retina, pancreas, liver, kidney and prostate. Elimination is primarily via the feces, but some is also excreted by the kidneys and in sweat. Zinc found in feces may be reabsorbed in the colon.

Contraindications/Precautions/Reproductive Safety - Zinc supplementation should be carefully considered before administering to patients with copper deficiency.

No documented adverse effects associated with zinc therapy during pregnancy apparently exist, but neither have adequate, well-controlled studies been performed.

Adverse Effects/Warnings - Large doses may cause GI disturbances. Hematologic abnormalities may occur with large doses, particularly if a coexistent copper deficiency exists.

Overdosage/Acute Toxicity - Signs associated with overdoses of zinc, include hemolytic anemia, hypotension, jaundice, vomiting and pulmonary edema. Suggestions for treatment of overdoses of oral zinc, include removing the source, dilution with milk or water and chelation therapy using edetate calcium disodium (Calcium EDTA). Refer to that monograph for possible doses and usage information.

Drug Interactions - Large doses of zinc can inhibit **copper** absorption in the intestine. If this interaction is desirable, separate copper and zinc supplements by at least two hours. **Penicillamine** and **ursodiol** may potentially inhibit zinc absorption; clinical significance is not clear. Zinc salts may chelate oral **tetracycline** and reduce its absorption; separate doses by at least two hours. Zinc salts may reduce the absorption of some fluroquinolones (*e.g.,* **enrofloxacin**).

Doses -
Dogs:
For treatment and prophylaxis of hepatic copper toxicosis in Bedlington and West Highland White Terriers:
a) Initially, give a loading dose of 100 mg <u>elemental</u> zinc (zinc acetate used in this study) twice daily (separate doses by at least 8 hours) for about 3 months; then reduce dose to 50 mg (elemental zinc) twice daily. If animal vomits, give with doses with a small piece of meat. Do not give within one hour of a meal. Monitoring of zinc levels every 2-3 months initially is recommended. Target zinc levels are 200 - 500 micrograms/dl. DO not allow levels to raise higher than 1000 micrograms/dl. May require 3-6 months of therapy before significant efficacy is noted. (Brewer, Dick et al. 1992)
b) 5 - 10 mg/kg elemental zinc q12h; use high end of dosage range initially, then the reduce dose for maintenance; separate dosage from meals by 1-2 hours. Zinc gluconate may be less irritating to the GI than other salts. If vomiting occurs, capsule may be opened and mixed with a small amount of hamburger or tuna. In dogs with active copper-induced hepatitis do not use zinc alone, but in combination with a chelator (*e.g.,* D-Penicillamine, trientine). Target zinc plasma levels >200 micrograms/dl but <1000 micrograms/dl. Monitor levels every 3-4 months and adjust dosage as necessary. (Johnson and Sherding 1994)
For cases of idiopathic hepatitis where liver copper levels are elevated:
a) 1 mg/kg PO of zinc gluconate *tid* (Mack 1993)
For zinc-related dermatoses:
a) Rapidly growing dogs: 10 mg/kg day PO of zinc sulfate. (Willemse 1992)
b) For zinc-responsive dermatoses found in Siberian huskies, Alaskan malamutes, Great Danes, and Doberman pinschers: Zinc sulfate: 10 mg/kg PO with food either once daily or divided q12h. Alternatively, zinc methionine: 2 mg/kg PO once daily. Correct any dietary imbalances (high calcium and phytate). Lifetime therapy usually required. If vomiting occurs, lower dose or give with food.
For syndrome seen in puppies: Dietary corrections alone usually resolve the syndrome, but zinc supplementation as above, can expedite process. Some puppies require supplementation until maturity. (Kwochka 1994)

Cats:
For adjunctive therapy of severe hepatic lipidosis:
a) 7 -10 mg/kg PO once daily, in B-Complex mixture if possible. (Center 1994)
Monitoring Parameters/Client Information - See above

Dosage Forms/Preparations/FDA Approval Status/Withholding Times -
Veterinary-Approved Products: None (for systemic use).
Several vitamin/mineral supplements contain zinc, however.

Human-Approved Products:

Zinc Acetate is available from chemical supply houses.

Zine Sulfate Injection: 1 mg/ml (as sulfate) in 10 & 30 ml vials; 5 mg/ml in 5 & 10 ml vials; 1 mg/ml (as 2.09 mg chloride) in 10 ml vials; *Zinca-Pak*® (Smith & Nephew SoloPak); generic, (Rx)

Zinc Sulfate Oral Tablets 66 mg (15 mg zinc); 110 mg (25 mg zinc); 200 mg (45 mg zinc); *Zinc 15*® (Mericon);*Orazinc*® (Mericon); Generic; (OTC)

Zinc Sulfate Oral Capsules 220 mg (50 mg zinc); *Orazinc*® (Mericon), *Verazinc*® (Forest), *Zinc-220*® (Alto), *Zincate*® (Paddock), generic; (Rx or OTC depending on product)

Zinc sulfate is also available in topical ophthalmic preparations.

Appendix
Ophthalmic Products, Topical

The following section lists the majority of veterinary-labeled ophthalmic topical products and some of the more commonly used human-labeled products in veterinary medicine. It was written in cooperation with Dennis K. Olivero, DVM, DACVO to whom I would like to express my gratitude. Drugs are listed by therapeutic class. All doses (in italics) are from Dr. Olivero, unless otherwise noted.

For additional information, an excellent review on veterinary ophthalmic pharmacology and therapeutics can be found in the chapter by A. Regnier and P.L. Toutain in: *Veterinary Ophthalmology*, 2nd Edition; Kirk N. Gelatt, Editor; Lea & Febiger, Philadelphia, 1991. 765 pp.

Glaucoma, Topical Agents

Note: Generally, once acute congestive primary glaucoma is noted in one eye it is treated as an emergency using mannitol/glycerin systemically, a systemic carbonic anhydrase inhibitor, a miotic and then surgery is considered for lasting control of intraocular pressure. The following topical drugs are used "in general" as a preventative measure to prevent the occurrence of primary glaucoma in the unaffected eye. Topical ocular antihypertensive medications are sometimes employed for pressure control with secondary glaucomas also.

TIMOLOL MALEATE (OPHTHALMIC)

Indications/Pharmacology - Timolol maleate is used primarily to prevent the development of primary glaucoma in the contralateral eye of a dog which has developed primary glaucoma in one eye. It only reduces intraocular pressure 3-10 mmHg and, therefore is of minimal usefulness in patients requiring treatment of primary acute congestive glaucoma. Timolol's mechanism of action: decreases cyclic-AMP synthesis in non-pigmented ciliary epithelium resulting in decreased aqueous humor production. It may also cause slight miosis in dogs and cats.

Suggested Dosage/Precautions/Adverse Effects - One drop twice daily of the 0.5% solution. The 0.25% concentration has minimal efficacy in animals and is not worth using. While problems have rarely been noted in veterinary medicine, ophthalmic beta blockers should be used with caution in patients with bronchoconstrictive disease or congestive heart failure.

Dosage Forms/Preparations/FDA Approval Status -
   Veterinary-Approved Products: None
   Human-Approved Products: Timolol Maleate 0.25% (see dosage above) or 0.5% solution in 2.5, 5, 10, and 15 ml Ocumeter® bottles; *Timoptic®* (MSD); (Rx)

METIPRANOLOL (OPHTHALMIC)

Indications/Pharmacology - Metipranolol HCl can be used as a substitute for timolol maleate (see above). Metipranolol is a nonselective beta blocking agent and reduces intraocular pressure minimally in animals by decreasing cyclic-AMP synthesis in the ciliary body. Pilot studies have suggested that metipranolol is as effective as timolol maleate, but is significantly less expensive. Metipranolol has been useful in the author's (DKO) clinic for the management of primary open angle glaucoma in cats.

Suggested Dosage/Precautions/Adverse Effects - One drop twice daily of the 0.3% solution. While problems have rarely been noted in veterinary medicine, ophthalmic beta blockers should be used with caution in patients with bronchoconstrictive disease or congestive heart failure.

Dosage Forms/Preparations/FDA Approval Status -
   Veterinary Labeled Products: None
   Human-Approved Products: 0.3% Metipranolol Solution in 2, 5, & 10 ml *OptiPranolol®* (Bausch & Lomb); (Rx)

LEVOBUNOLOL HCL (OPHTHALMIC)

Indications/Pharmacology - Levobunolol HCl is a beta1 and beta2 blocking agent similar to timolol and metipranolol above but without the potential for myocardial depression or airway constriction noted rarely in veterinary medicine and occasionally in human patients. Levobunolol is used in humans with glaucoma responsive to beta adrenergic blocking agents but who suffer cardiac and respiratory side effects associated with timolol.

Suggested Dosage/Precautions/Adverse Effects - One drop twice daily of the 0.5% concentration. Miosis may develop in veterinary patients after application of topical beta blocking antiglaucoma medications.

Dosage Forms/Preparations/FDA Approval Status-
   Veterinary Labeled Products: None
   Human-Approved Products: Levobunolol HCl 0.25% or 0.5% solution in 5, 10, & 15ml. *Betagan®* (Allergan); (Rx)

PILOCARPINE HCL (OPHTHALMIC)

Indications/Pharmacology - Pilocarpine is a miotic agent that is used in the treatment of primary glaucoma only. Pilocarpine causes the ciliary body muscle to constrict placing posteriorly directed tension on the base of the iris to mechanically pull open the iridocorneal angle structures. By causing miosis, it may prevent closure of the iridocorneal angle by preventing excess iris tissue from peripherally compromising the outflow of aqueous humor.

   The lacrimal glands of dogs and cats are predominately under parasympathetic stimulation. Pilocarpine was used in the 1970's and early 1980's as a stimulant of tear production, delivered either topically or by applying it (the eyedrop preparation) on the food of dogs with keratoconjunctivitis sicca. Toxicity problems with excessive salivation, vomiting and diarrhea complicated its use. It does not directly address the issue of autoimmunity thought to be the etiopathogenesis behind most cases of keratoconjunctivitis sicca in the dog. The popularity of treatment of KCS with ophthalmic cyclosporine ointment has been associated with a decline in the use of pilocarpine for this disease.

Suggested Dosage/Precautions/Adverse Effects - One drop in affected eye(s) 3 times daily. Usually 1% or 2% is most commonly used in veterinary medicine. Pilocarpine can cause local irritation initially. In humans, this irritation reportedly diminishes after 3 days of therapy. It may also cause inflammation of the uveal tract, especially with repeated applications and can cause hyphema. Pilocarpine should not be used in secondary glaucoma cases. With repeated use, pilocarpine may cause systemic effects (vomiting, diarrhea, and increased salivation).

Dosage Forms/Preparations/FDA Approval Status -
   Veterinary-Approved Products: None
   Human-Approved Products:
      Pilocarpine HCl Ophthalmic Solution 0.25%, 0.5%, 1%, 2%, 3%, 4%, and 6% (in addition there are 8% and 10% solutions and a 4% gel is available from Alcon) in 15 ml and 30 ml containers. There are many products and trade names associated with pilocarpine, including I*sopto Carpine®* (Alcon), *Ocu-Carpine®* (Iomed), *Piloptic®* (Optopics), *Pilostat®* (Bausch and Lomb) and many generically labeled products. All are Rx.
      See also the epinephrine monograph for information on epinephrine/pilocarpine fixed dose combination products.

DEMECARIUM (OPHTHALMIC)

Indications/Pharmacology - Demecarium is a potent carbamate inhibitor that may reduce intraocular pressures for up to 48 hours in canines. Demecarium reversibly inhibits anticholinesterase thereby causing miosis. Demecarium is generally used in preventive management of the contralateral eye in patients after the diagnosis of an acute congestive crisis of primary glaucoma in the other eye. It is not used in secondary glaucoma. Demecarium has the advantage of once or twice daily dosing.

Suggested Dosage/Precautions/Adverse Effects - One drop once or twice daily. Demecarium is contraindicated during pregnancy. Because of additive effects, demecarium should be used with caution with other cholinesterase inhibitors (e.g., carbamate/organophosphate antiparasiticides), or succinylcholine. Demecarium may cause local inflammation and systemic adverse effects (vomiting, diarrhea, increased salivation, cardiac effects) are possible, particularly with high dosages or in very small dogs.

Dosage Forms/Preparations/FDA Approval Status -
   Veterinary-Approved Products: None
   Human-Approved Products:
      Demecarium 0.125% or 0.25% in 5 ml dropper bottles, *Humorsol®* (Merck); (Rx). Do not freeze and protect from heat.

EPINEPHRINE, TOPICAL (OPHTHALMIC)

Indications/Pharmacology - Epinephrine (usually in combination with pilocarpine due to epinephrine's mydriatic effects) is usually used as a preventative measure to prevent glaucoma in the unaffected eye. Epinephrine acts on both alpha and beta adrenergic receptors, thereby causing conjunctival decongestion, transient mydriasis (less so in cats) and decreased IOP (intraocular pressure). Decreased IOP is probably due primarily to increased aqueous humor outflow, but decreased aqueous humor production may occur secondary to vasoconstriction.

Suggested Dosage/Precautions/Adverse Effects - One drop 2-3 times daily in the unaffected eye. Epinephrine may cause ocular discomfort upon instillation.

Dosage Forms/Preparations/FDA Approval Status -
    Veterinary-Approved Products: None
    Human-Approved Products:
        Epinephrine (HCl) 0.25%, 0.5%, 1% & 2% in 10 or 15 ml btls.; *Epifrin®* (Allergan), *Glaucon®* (Alcon); (Rx)
        Epinephrine (Borate) 0.5%, 1% & 2% in 7.5 ml btls; *Eppy/N®* (Pilkington/Barnes-Hind), *Epinal®* (Alcon); (Rx)
        Epinephrine Bitartrate 1% in combination with Pilocarpine HCl (either 1%, 2%, 3%, 4% or 6%) *E-Pilo-1®* (2, 3, etc.) (Iolab); *P1*(2, 3, etc.)*E1* (Alcon); (Rx)

DORZOLAMIDE HCL (OPHTHALMIC)

Indications/Pharmacology - Dorzolamide is often used in the contralateral eye of a dog with primary glaucoma to prevent development of bilateral disease. It is also an excellent agent to consider for most secondary glaucomas in dogs and cats because it has no effect on pupil size. Like the related oral carbonic anhydrase inhibitors (dichlorphenamide or *Daranide®*, methazolamide or *Neptazane®*), dorzolamide decreases aqueous humor production by the ciliary body epithelium by altering pH and affecting the H^+/Na^+ active transport exchange mechanism. Oral carbonic anhydrase inhibitors cause numerous systemic side effects such as metabolic acidosis and panting, diarrhea, vomiting, anorexia and others, all of which can be avoided with topical carbonic anhydrase inhibitors.

Suggested Dosage/Precautions/Adverse Effects - One drop three times daily is the standard treatment frequency, adjusted based on clinical response. Dorzolamide may cause stinging upon topical application.

Dosage Forms/Preparations/FDA Approval Status -
    Veterinary-Approved Products: None
    Human-Approved Products: Dorzolamide HCl 2% 5, 10, 15ml; *Trusopt®* (Merck); (Rx)

LATANOPROST (OPHTHALMIC)

Indications/Pharmacology - Latanoprost is a prostaglandin F_2alpha analogue which reduces intraocular pressure by increasing aqueous humor outflow via the uveoscleral outflow mechanism. The major outflow mechanism in animals and people is through the iridocorneal angle termed the conventional outflow mechanism. A species variable alternative pathway directly across the surface of the iris into the iridal venous supply accounts for some outflow in people and animals. The horse apparently has the highest uveoscleral outflow of the domestic species studied. Latanoprost dramatically increases uveoscleral outflow and is an exciting agent for glaucoma patients because this medication directly increases alternative drainage of aqueous humor, which logically would seem superior to reducing production or attempting to increase outflow through a failing conventional outflow system. Latanoprost is marketed for once daily usage in people and clinical studies show reduced effectiveness when once daily treatment is exceeded. In the author's clinic (DKO) with limited cases, the intraocular pressure reduction associated with the use of this agent has been impressive and can exceed even that possible with oral or topical carbonic anhydrase inhibitors. Latanoprost has been used in veterinary ophthalmology to treat primary and secondary glaucomas although clinicians should assess the possibility of profound miosis associated with the use of this medication in their secondary glaucoma cases.

Suggested Dosage/Precautions/Adverse Effects - One drop is applied in the PM. Latanoprost may cause topical irritation. Conjunctival hyperemia is commonly noted in patients using this medication. A direct stimulation of iris melanocytes results in excess melanin production in the iris of people using this medication, causing a dark brown color change to the iris. Profound miosis is noted with the use of latanoprost in dogs and cats.

Dosage Forms/Preparations/FDA Approval Status -
   Veterinary-Approved Products: None
   Human-Approved Products: Latanoprost 0.005% 2.5 ml; *Xalantan®* (Pharmacia & Upjohn) (Rx).
    Store under refrigeration until use; at room temp for 6 weeks after opened.

Vasoconstrictors/Mydriatics
PHENYLEPHRINE HCL (OPHTHALMIC)

Indications/Pharmacology - Phenylephrine is used to differentiate conjunctival vascular injection (blanches with phenylephrine application) versus deep episcleral injection (blanches incompletely) associated with uveitis, glaucoma, or scleritis. It is also used prior to conjunctival surgery to reduce hemorrhage and in combination with atropine prior to cataract or other intraocular surgeries which require maximal pupillary dilation. Phenylephrine can be used to confirm the diagnosis of Horner's syndrome. Dilution of 2.5% phenylephrine solution with saline (1:10) produces a 0.25% solution. Normal eyes will not demonstrate mydriasis in response to this low concentration of phenylephrine. Third order Horner's syndrome of greater than two weeks duration is associated with receptor up regulation and therefore a response to 0.25% phenylephrine is noted. In this way, the diagnosis of Horner's is confirmed and a suggestion as to whether or not the condition is 2nd or 3rd order in nature.

In dogs, maximum mydriasis persists for about 2 hours and effects may last for up to 18 hours. Phenylephrine has significant alpha adrenergic effects (vasoconstriction and pupillary dilation) and minimal effects on beta receptors. When used alone, phenylephrine is reportedly not efficacious in the cat unless used with other mydriatics.

Suggested Dosage/Precautions/Adverse Effects - For diagnosis and characterization of Horner's syndrome: Apply 0.25% solution (see above) in both eyes. If there is a response in the miotic eye; 3rd order. If no response, apply 2.5% solution; if there is a response in both eyes it confirms Horner's and probably is 2nd order.

For treatment of Horner's Syndrome: Treatment is indicated only if patient experiences visual difficulty because third eyelid is elevated over pupil; then given on an as needed basis with an average duration of effect of 3-6 hours.

Prior to cataract or intraocular surgery: 2.5% or 10% given every 15 minutes for two hours. Monitor for hypertension and/or cardiac arrhythmia in small patients especially when using the 10% solution.

Local discomfort may occur after instillation and chronic use may lead to inflammation. In some species (cat, rabbit, humans) transient stromal clouding may occur if used when corneal epithelium is damaged.

Dosage Forms/Preparations/FDA Approval Status -
   Veterinary-Approved Products: None
   Human-Approved Products:
    Phenylephrine HCl 0.12% in 15 ml or 20 ml bottles (OTC)
    Phenylephrine HCl 2.5% in 2, 5 or 15 ml bottles (Rx)
    Phenylephrine HCl 10% available in 1, 2, 5 or 15 ml bottles (Rx). Available generically and under several proprietary names. A well known trade name is *Neo-Synephrine®* (Sanofi Winthrop). A viscous form of the 10% is also available.

Cycloplegic Mydriatics
ATROPINE SULFATE (OPHTHALMIC)

Indications/Pharmacology - Atropine, when used topically on the eye, acts by blocking the cholinergic responses of the sphincter muscle of the iris and the ciliary body to cause mydriasis (pupillary dilation) and accommodation paralysis (cycloplegia). Atropine may be useful in the control of pain secondary to corneal and uveal disease; to maximally dilate the pupil prior to intraocular surgery; to dilate the pupil and prevent pupillary block in glaucoma and uveitis. In the dog, atropine causes maximal mydriasis in about 1 hour and it may persist for up to 120 hours. Cats also show a delayed onset of action and mydriasis may persist for up to 144 hours (dose dependent). Atropine is particularly long acting in horses.

Atropine may be used in combination with 10% phenylephrine to achieve mydriasis and cycloplegia in cases of anterior uveitis.

Suggested Dosages/Precautions/Adverse Effects - Ointments or drops are routinely used in dogs. One percent is commonly used, but 2% solutions may be required in severe cases of uveitis. Ointments are generally used in cats to prevent hypersalivation associated with the bitter taste of this medication. Dosage frequencies are variable depending on the condition and its severity. Commonly, atropine is given as one drop 2-3 times a day until pupillary dilation is achieved and once daily thereafter to maintain this response.

Atropine may precipitate acute, congestive primary glaucoma in dogs predisposed to primary glaucoma; do not use in primary glaucoma. Repeated topical application prior to surgery can result in systemic atropine toxicosis (mania, hyperthermia, etc.). Salivation may result in dogs as well as cats (see above) secondary to the bitter taste.

Reportedly, very frequent treatment with atropine may induce colic in horses secondary to systemic absorption and atropine's vagal parasympathetic effects. However, clinically this effect is only rarely noted.

Dosage Forms/Preparations/FDA Approval Status -
  Veterinary-Approved Products:
    Atropine Sulfate Ophthalmic Ointment 10 mg/gm (1%) in 3.5 gm tubes; *Atrophate*® (Schering-Plough); (Rx)
  Human-Approved Products:
    Atropine Sulfate Ophthalmic Ointment 5 mg/gm (0.5%), 10 mg/gm (1%) in 3.5 gm tubes; Generic and various trade names; (Rx)
    Atropine Sulfate Ophthalmic Solution 0.5%, 1%, and 2% in unit dose droppers; 2, 5, & 15 ml bottles; Generic and various trade names; (Rx)

TROPICAMIDE (OPHTHALMIC)

Indications/Pharmacology - Tropicamide, like atropine, causes mydriasis and cycloplegia, but has more mydriatic than cycloplegic activity. Tropicamide has a more rapid onset (maximum mydriasis in 15-30 minutes) of action and a shorter duration of action (pupil returns to normal in 6-12 hours in most animals) than does atropine, thereby making it more useful for funduscopic examinations. In dogs, intraocular pressure is apparently not affected by tropicamide.

Suggested Dosages/Precautions/Adverse Effects - Once or twice application to eye, prior to exam. Following cataract surgery: apply 2-3 times daily to keep pupil constantly changing in size and reduce formation of synechiae associated with prolonged pupillary dilation (atropine). Note: a current trend away from the use of mydriatics after intraocular surgery has developed in recognition of immediate postoperative pressure elevations in some animals following surgery.

Tropicamide is less effective in pain control (cycloplegia) than atropine.

Tropicamide may cause salivation, particularly in cats and may also sting when applied. Tropicamide may precipitate acute congestive glaucoma in predisposed patients.

Dosage Forms/Preparations/FDA Approval Status -
  Veterinary Approved Products: None
  Human-Approved Products: Tropicamide Solution 0.5% and 1% in 2 ml & 15 ml bottles; *Mydriacyl*® (Alcon), *Opticyl*® (Optopics), *Tropicacyl*® (Akorn), Generic; (Rx)

Topical Anesthetics

PROPARACAINE HCL (OPHTHALMIC)

Indications/Pharmacology - Proparacaine is a rapid acting topical anesthetic useful for a variety of ophthalmic procedures including tonometry (intraocular pressure measurement), relief of corneal pain to facilitate examination, biopsy/sample collection, and to distinguish between corneal and uveal pain. Proparacaine primarily anesthetizes the cornea; with limited penetration into conjunctiva. Anesthesia is of short duration (5-10 minutes).

Suggested Dosages/Precautions/Adverse Effects- Usual dose is 1 - 2 drops prior to examination or procedure. For prolonged procedures only requiring local anesthesia; may repeat 1 drop doses every 5-10 minutes for 5-7 doses.

Topical anesthetics should not be used to treat painful eye disease. Prolonged use may retard wound healing and cause corneal epithelial ulcers. Because the blink reflex may be suppressed, the eye should be protected from external injury during use. Repeated use may lead to rapid development of tolerance. Local allergic-type reactions have been rarely reported in humans.

Dosage Forms/Preparations/FDA Approval Status -
  Veterinary-Approved Products:
    Proparacaine HCl Solution 0.5% in 15 ml bottles; *Ophthaine*® (Solvay); (Rx)
    Protect from light. Refrigerate.

Human-Approved Products:
Proparacaine HCl Solution 0.5% in 2 & 15 ml bottles; *Ophthetic®* (Allergan), *Alcaine®* (Alcon), *Ophthaine®* (Squibb), *AK-Taine®* (Akorn), Generic; (Rx)
Protect from light. Some products should be refrigerated; check label.

Non-Steroidal Antiinflammatory Agents

FLURBIPROFEN SODIUM (OPHTHALMIC)

Indications/Pharmacology - Flurbiprofen is a non-steroidal anti-inflammatory agent that probably acts by inhibiting the cyclo-oxygenase enzyme system, thereby reducing the biosynthesis of prostaglandins. Prostaglandins may mediate certain kinds of ocular inflammation. They may disrupt the blood-aqueous humor barrier, cause vasodilation, increase intraocular pressure and leukocytosis, and increase vascular permeability. Prostaglandins may also cause iris sphincter constriction (miosis) independent of cholinergic mechanisms. Flurbiprofen can inhibit this intraocular miosis and may also be useful in the management of uveal inflammation (usually in addition to topical steroids).

Suggested Dosages/Precautions/Adverse Effects - Prior to surgery: One drop 4 times at 20 minute intervals.
Because flurbiprofen may be as immunosuppressive as topical corticosteroids, it should not be used in patients with infected corneal ulcers. By blocking prostaglandin synthesis, arachidonic acid metabolites may be shunted into leukotriene pathways and this effect may result in a transient increase in intraocular pressure commonly noted after intraocular surgery. Postoperative pressure spikes following cataract surgery have been the subject of much study in recent years and a general trend away from the use of flurbiprofen prior to cataract surgery has resulted from these studies.

Dosage Forms/Preparations/FDA Approval Status -
  Veterinary-Approved Products: None
  Human-Approved Products:
    Flurbiprofen Sodium 0.03% Solution in 2.5, 5 & 10 ml btls; *Ocufen®* (Allergan); (Rx)

KETOROLAC TROMETHAMINE (OPHTHALMIC)

Indications/Pharmacology - Ketorolac tromethamine is a pyrrolol-pyrrole nonsteroidal anti-inflammatory agent that inhibits prostaglandin formation. Prostaglandins mediate inflammation within the eye by disrupting the blood-aqueous barrier, inducing vasodilation and increasing intraocular pressure. Prostaglandins may also cause iris sphincter constriction (miosis) independent of cholinergic mechanisms. Ketorolac tromethamine is marketed for use before cataract extraction in human patients (to prevent miosis during surgery) and for control of post surgical inflammation, especially following cataract surgery. It is also approved for management of conjunctivitis associated with seasonal allergy in people. In veterinary medicine, ketorolac tromethamine is primarily used to control surgical or nonsurgical uveitis particularly in cases with concurrent corneal infection when topical corticosteroids are contraindicated or in diabetic patients, especially smaller patients, adversely affected by systemic uptake of topically applied corticosteroids. Nonsteroidal agents like ketorolac tromethamine can be combined with topical steroids in patients with severe uveal inflammation.

Suggested Dosages/Precautions/Adverse Effects - Prior to surgery: One drop 4 times at 20 minute intervals. One drop four times daily following cataract surgery or for treatment of uveitis or for management of allergic conjunctivitis.
The manufacturer indicates that ketorolac tromethamine does not enhance the spread of preexisting corneal fungal, viral or bacterial infections in animals models. Ketorolac tromethamine does not in and of itself induce postoperative pressure elevation other then that which frequently follows cataract extraction in people and animals.

Dosage Forms/Preparations/FDA Approval Status -
  Veterinary-Approved Products: None
  Human-Approved Products:
    Ketorolac Tromethamine Solution 0.5% 3, 5, 10 ml; *Acular®* (Allergan); (Rx)

DICLOFENAC SODIUM (OPHTHALMIC)

Indications/Pharmacology - Diclofenac sodium is a phenylacetic acid that inhibits cyclooxygenase, inhibiting prostaglandin synthesis. Diclofenac sodium topical solution reduces inflammation following cataract extraction in people and counteracts photophobia in humans having refractive corneal surgery. In veterinary medicine, diclofenac sodium is used for treatment of uveitis following surgery on the eye or other causes of uveitis especially when corneal infection is suspected or in diabetic patients whose insulin regulation could be altered by the systemic uptake of topical corticosteroids. Diclofenac can be combined with topical corticosteroids for better control of uveitis in animals when the condition is severe.

Suggested Dosages/Precautions/Adverse Effects - Prior to surgery: One drop 4 times at 20 minute intervals. One drop four times daily following cataract surgery or for the treatment of uveitis. Caution should be used when applying any anti-inflammatory agent on the cornea in the face of corneal stromal infection because of the positive role inflammation plays in the immune response to microbial invasion of tissue. A stinging sensation is noted in 15% of people using this medication.

Dosage Forms/Preparations/FDA Approval Status -
   Veterinary-Approved Products: None
   Human-Approved Products: Diclofenac Sodium 0.1% in 2.5, 5 ml; *Voltaren*® (Ciba Vision); (Rx)

Antiinflammatory Mast Cell Stabilizers
LODOXAMINE TROMETHAMINE (OPHTHALMIC)

Indications/Pharmacology - Lodoxamine tromethamine is a mast cell stabilizer that inhibits Type I hypersensitivity responses by preventing antigen mediated histamine release. Lodoxamine stabilizes mast cells by blocking calcium influx into the cell upon antigen recognition, thereby blocking histamine release. Lodoxamine has no intrinsic vasoconstrictor, antihistaminic, cyclooxygenase inhibition or other anti-inflammatory properties. Lodoxamine is used in people for management of conjunctivitis associated with seasonal allergy and other histamine mediated disorders. In veterinary medicine, lodoxamine tromethamine has been used in horses and small animal patients with presumed allergic conjunctivitis.

Suggested Dosages/Precautions/Adverse Effects - Prior to surgery: One drop 2-4 times daily. A stinging sensation is noted in a low percentage of people using this medication.

Dosage Forms/Preparations/FDA Approval Status -
   Veterinary-Approved Products: None
   Human-Approved Products: Lodoxamine Tromethamine 0.1% 10ml; *Alomide*® (Alcon); (Rx)

CROMOLYN SODIUM (OPHTHALMIC)

Indications/Pharmacology - Cromolyn sodium is a mast cell stabilizing agent that blocks release of histamine and slow-reacting substance of anaphylaxis from mast cells following antigen recognition. Similar to lodoxamine tromethamine, cromolyn sodium has no intrinsic vasoconstrictor, antihistaminic, cyclooxygenase inhibition or other anti-inflammatory properties. Mast cell stabilizing agents are most useful in animal patients suffering from allergic conjunctivitis.

Suggested Dosages/Precautions/Adverse Effects - Prior to surgery: One drop 2-6 times daily. A stinging sensation is noted in a low percentage of people using this medication.

Dosage Forms/Preparations/FDA Approval Status -
   Veterinary-Approved Products: None
   Human-Approved Products: Cromolyn Sodium 4% in 2.5, 10ml; *Crolom*® (Bausch & Lomb); (Rx)

CORTICOSTEROIDS, TOPICAL (OPHTHALMIC)
   (see also Antibiotic & Corticosteroid Combinations)

Indications/Dosages/Precautions - Topical corticosteroids are used to treat diseases of the eye involving the conjunctiva, sclera, cornea, and anterior chamber. Penetration of topically applied corticosteroids into the eyelids is poor as is penetration to the posterior segment of the eye. Corticosteroid-responsive conditions affecting these areas are usually managed with systemically administered agents (with or without adjunctive topically applied medications).

Conjunctivitis in animals is often treated symptomatically, particularly during the first occurrence of the condition for any particular patient. Antibiotic agents with hydrocortisone or dexamethasone, or antibiotic agents alone initially, are used for conjunctivitis in the dog and the horse. Allergic and eosinophilic conjunctivitis are rare diagnoses in the cat. Topically applied corticosteroids should not be used to treat conjunctivitis in cats. Herpes virus is the most common feline conjunctival pathogen and topically applied steroids can induce prolonged disease, steroid dependency and corneal complications including ulcerative keratitis and/or corneal sequestrum formation.

Inflammatory conditions of the canine sclera and episclera include episcleritis, scleritis, nodular granulomatous episclerokeratitis, Collie granuloma and others. Potency and penetration of corticosteroid agents is important in the management of these conditions. Dexamethasone sodium phosphate ointment is often employed and the relatively reduced penetration of the fibrous ocular tunics of this medication compared with that of 1% prednisolone acetate ophthalmic suspension is made up for by increased contact time of the ointment form of this drug and by the increased potency of dexamethasone (30X cortisone) relative to prednisolone (4-5X cortisone). Dexamethasone products alone (without antibiotics) are becoming increasingly scarce in the marketplace and because of this, dexamethasone is often used in combination with an antibiotic for availability reasons only. Four times daily treatment is often the initial frequency with tapering paralleled to clinical response. Topical treatment is often used following subconjunctival injection of corticosteroid agents into or adjacent to the lesion (if focal). Systemic steroid treatment is usually not necessary.

Nonulcerative inflammatory conditions of the cornea of animals include chronic superficial keratitis (pannus) of the German Shepherd and other breeds, eosinophilic keratitis of the cat and certain, often poorly understood, keratopathies of the equine, including Onchocerca related keratitis. German Shepherd pannus may be better managed using cyclosporine ophthalmic solution or ointment with or without concurrent topical steroids initially followed by long term management with cyclosporine ophthalmic alone (see cyclosporine ophthalmic). Eosinophilic keratitis is often treated with subconjunctival corticosteroids in addition to topical 0.1% dexamethasone ophthalmic ointment or solution or 1% prednisolone acetate ophthalmic suspension 4 times daily, tapering the dosage frequency based on clinical response. Recent research reveals that eosinophilic keratitis may be an unusual immune response to latent feline herpes virus in the corneal stroma, calling into question the value of topical steroids in the management of a disease with an infectious etiology. Equine keratopathies are treated with 0.1% dexamethasone ointment 4 times daily with tapering of the treatment frequency based on the clinical response.

Corticosteroids are also used to manage anterior uveal inflammatory disease of companion animals. In small animals, 1% prednisolone acetate ophthalmic suspension is generally used for this purpose because of superior penetration into the anterior segment of the eye in comparison with dexamethasone products. The frequency of treatment depends on the severity of the condition. Severe anterior uveitis can be treated with subconjunctival corticosteroids given in combination with hourly topical corticosteroids with reevaluation performed again 24 hours after beginning treatment. Moderate to mild uveitis and that found following surgery of the anterior segment is often treated initially at the QID level with tapering based on clinical response. Anterior uveitis in animals can often be associated with an underlying systemic infectious or neoplastic condition in animals. Clinicians are advised to evaluate the patient for generalized infectious or neoplastic conditions prior to or concurrent with a course of corticosteroid antiinflammatory therapy, particularly if the condition dictates systemic treatment with these agents in combination with subconjunctival and topical treatment. Uveitis in the equine species is often treated with either 1% prednisolone acetate ophthalmic suspension or with 0.1% dexamethasone ointment. Many clinicians prefer to use the ointment because of increased contact time and potency and the logistics of frequent treatment of this species. 1% prednisolone acetate can be passed through a subpalpebral lavage catheter very frequently to treat equine patients with anterior uveitis when necessary.

Pred Forte®, Econopred Plus® or generic 1% prednisolone acetate ophthalmic suspension are the prednisolone products most used by veterinary ophthalmologists. There are few indications for *Econopred®* or *Pred Mild®* in veterinary ophthalmology.

Inflammatory condition of the posterior segment require systemic treatment because of poor penetration of topically applied agents.

Dosage Forms/Preparations/FDA Approval Status -
  Veterinary-Approved Products: None
  Human-Approved Products:
    Prednisolone Acetate Drops: 0.12% Suspension *Pred Mild®* (Allergan); 0.125% Suspension *Econopred®* (Alcon); 1% Suspension; *Econopred Plus®* (Alcon); *Pred Forte®* (Allerga_n; Generic; (Rx)

    Prednisolone Sodium Phosphate Drops: 0.125% Solution (various manufacturers); 1% Solution (various); (Rx)

Combination of Prednisolone (0.25%) and Atropine (1%) Drops: *Mydrapred®* (Alcon) in 5 ml bottles; (Rx)

Also available: Fluorometholone or Medrysone drops.

Other routes of administration: Systemically administered corticosteroids (usually orally) may be indicated for non-infectious inflammatory ocular conditions and following intraocular surgery. Subconjunctival steroids are useful in anterior segment inflammatory disease and following cataract surgery and intraocular glaucoma surgery. Subconjunctival steroids may be absorbed systemically and should be used with caution in patients with endocrinopathies (e.g., diabetes mellitus) or infectious diseases.

Antibiotics, Single and Combination Agents

Indications/Pharmacology/General Use Considerations - Topical antibiotic agents are commonly used to treat conjunctivitis and ulcerative keratitis complicated by bacterial infection of the corneal stroma. These agents are also used to prevent infection following surgery of the eyelids, conjunctiva, cornea, and the anterior segment. Conjunctivitis in animals is a common clinical entity. Because in most instances the condition does not threaten vision, it is often treated symptomatically with antibiotic agents or antibiotic agents in combination with topical steroids (see antibiotic/corticosteroid combination agents). Conjunctivitis is an exclusion diagnosis in animals, ruling out other causes for ocular discomfort and discharge, including anterior uveitis, glaucoma and inflammatory disease of the sclera, episclera and cornea. Triple antibiotic products (neomycin, bacitracin and polymyxin B) are often employed for this purpose, with or without hydrocortisone, because these drugs are not used systemically and because the combination of antibiotics is broad spectrum. Triple antibiotic or triple antibiotic HC is often used in dogs 4 times daily for 1 to 2 weeks for conjunctivitis. Chronic or recurrent cases of conjunctivitis would indicate further diagnostic evaluation to determine an underlying cause. Tetracycline ophthalmic ointment is often used QID in cats for nonspecific or undiagnosed conjunctivitis. The rationale for this treatment is the efficacy of tetracycline for Chlamydia spp. and Mycoplasma spp., two infectious agents reported to cause conjunctivitis in the cat. Antibiotic agents with corticosteroids should not be used for the treatment of conjunctivitis in the cat. The majority of cases are related to primary or recurring infection with feline herpes virus and recent evidence indicates that topical or systemic steroid therapy can potentially prolong the duration of the viral infection and result in corneal complications in cases which otherwise may have remained a conjunctival infection. Triple antibiotic with or without hydrocortisone is often used to treat conjunctivitis in the equine species. Sensitivity to triple antibiotic in dogs and cats has been noted and is reportedly the result of neomycin allergy, as is noted in people.

Antibiotic therapy for corneal disease varies from prophylactic therapy to prevent infection to treatment of established corneal infections. Following an acute superficial injury to the cornea in the dog, cat or horse, treatment with triple antibiotic ointment or drops 4 times daily is usually sufficient to prevent bacterial infection of the corneal stroma. Reevaluation of the patient 24-48 hours after the injury is indicated. Progressive edema, pain, and white opacification of the cornea (cellular infiltrate) would suggest that the antibiotic protocol (agent and frequency) has failed to prevent bacterial infection.

Established bacterial infection of the corneal stroma is managed medically or surgically depending on the depth of infection. Ulcerative keratitis with bacterial infection causing deterioration of 50-75% of the stromal thickness is usually treated with conjunctival or corneal grafting in addition to antibiotic therapy. This is done to introduce immune system components and a blood supply to the cornea (conjunctival graft) in addition to replacing lost stromal tissue. Conjunctival grafting will usually stabilize stromal deterioration secondary to bacterial infection but carries the disadvantage of permanent opacification of the cornea in the site of previous ulcerative keratitis (unless other surgeries are performed). Aggressive medical management with topical antibiotic agents is often successful in controlling corneal infection which involves 75% or less of the depth of the cornea. The slit lamp biomicroscope is used by ophthalmologists at referral centers and specialty clinics to determine the depth of corneal involvement.

Clinical signs of bacterial infection of the corneal stroma includes increasing pain, progressive corneal opacity, hypopyon, and the development of a progressively expanding indentation or crater in the surface of the cornea. Cytology is indicated in the management of such patients. Gram staining is usually not necessary. Cocci noted with Dif-Quick® or related stains are considered to be gram positive cocci. Those cocci forming chains are considered to be Streptococcus organisms. Those cocci of variable size and shape and forming grape clusters are considered to be Staphylococcal organisms. Rods are considered to be gram negative organisms and Pseudomonas spp. is suspected. A degree of suspicion for fungal keratitis should be maintained while evaluating cytologic material collected from the cornea of the horse. Fungal hyphae stain dark blue with Dif-Quick® type stains. Culture and sensitivity tests are informative but the information is available at a time when the efficacy of the antibiotic therapy chosen has already been established. In 24-48 hours the case will show signs of improvement, indicating efficacy of the therapeutic protocol or the condition will have advanced and surgery will be under consideration. Sensitivities are relatively meaningless because aggressive medical treatment can result in corneal drug concentrations several times the MIC and sometimes beyond that considered toxic on a systemic basis. The use of eyedrops rather than ointments is recommended for aggressive medical management protocols.

Cytologic evaluation of material from the cornea will dictate antibiotic selection for aggressive medical management of corneal ulcers. Cocci are often treated with frequent application of triple antibiotic drops. Gentamicin has limited spectrum for Streptococci spp. and would not be a first choice agent when cocci forming chains are noted on cytologic evaluation of material from an infected corneal ulcer. Gentamicin has efficacy for some Staphylococcal spp. Chloramphenicol is also an antibiotic available for treatment of gram positive infections of the cornea. Gram negative infections of the cornea are often treated with gentamicin, tobramycin or the quinolones. Several studies indicate that a bacterial infection of the corneal stroma that responds to tobramycin is usually as responsive to gentamicin applied frequently making the newer aminoglycoside and quinolone antibiotics rarely necessary. These agents are reserved for very specific instances of stromal infection with highly resistant organisms and should not be considered for prophylactic treatment. Applied very frequently, bactericidal concentrations of either triple antibiotic or gentamicin ophthalmic solutions can be achieved in the corneal stroma making these two agents effective for the vast majority of corneal infections in companion animals. Relative penetration of antibiotic agents into the cornea is irrelevant during the treatment of ulcerative keratitis. All agents are water soluble (eye drops) and would penetrate the corneal stroma similarly. Penetration of various antibiotic agents into the cornea is a consideration when the corneal epithelium is intact as is often noted with the development of stromal abscessation in equines.

Aggressive medical management protocols involve hourly or q30 minute application of topical antibiotics. Sometimes two agents are used with synergistic properties (for example an aminoglycoside and a cephalosporin). One agent is applied on the hour and the other on the half hour. Single agents are usually applied hourly. The case is reevaluated 18-24 hours after initiation of the treatment regimen. Increased patient comfort, reduced corneal edema and no increase in the depth or width of the corneal ulcer are signs of efficacy of the selected treatment plan. In some cases at 24 hours and most cases by 30 hours, the peripheral "rim" of the corneal ulcer will fail to take on fluorescein stain, indicating early epithelialization of the corneal ulcer. It is the author's (DKO) impression that epithelialization of the ulcer will not occur until the stromal infection has been arrested. Cytologic evaluation of material collected from the cornea can be repeated to evaluate efficacy of the drug(s) selected. Clinical improvement signals the clinician to begin reducing treatment frequency slowly over the next two days, working towards the QID level. Long term aggressive medical management is not recommended because several agents, especially the aminoglycosides, are epitheliotoxic and prolonged once per hour treatment likely would delay healing rather than improve the case.

Aggressive medical management usually requires hospitalization in an intensive care unit for careful treatment and monitoring of the case. The advantage of aggressive medical management is reduced opacity in the cornea in comparison with conjunctival grafting. This is associated with an improved visual result, particularly if the injury is central. Medical management is usually less expensive than surgical treatment. General anesthesia is not necessary for aggressive medical management. Although aggressive medical management may result in halting further bacterial deterioration of stromal tissue in very deep corneal ulcers, reepithelialization of Descemet's membrane or a thin layer of corneal stroma interposed between Descemet's membrane and the corneal epithelium leaves the cornea dangerously thin. Minor trauma to the eye could result in rupture of the cornea across this area and loss of the anterior chamber.

Post surgical prophylactic medical treatment usually involves triple antibiotic agents because of their broad spectrum and because they are not agents used systemically. Four times daily treatment is recommended. Ointments are commonly used after surgery of the eyelids, conjunctiva or cornea. Eyedrops are usually used following surgery of the cornea or anterior segment. Bacterial infection of the anterior chamber alone is uncommon. Bacterial endophthalmitis carries a poor prognosis for saving vision or the globe in animals and is usually managed surgically in people. Gentamicin is sometimes used for prophylactic therapy of the equine species because of a greater number of gram negative organisms in the environment of this species, although the aminoglycosides would not be a first choice agent for prophylactic medical treatment of small animals. Tobramycin and the quinolones would not be considered for prophylactic treatment following surgery performed under sterile conditions.

CHLORAMPHENICOL (OPHTHALMIC)

Indications/Pharmacology - A broad spectrum antibiotic, chloramphenicol has the ability to cross the corneal barrier and enter the anterior chamber. However, there are very few infections that occur in the anterior chamber and if bacteria are actually present there, the blood ocular barrier is lost and systemically administered antibiotics can achieve therapeutic levels.

Because of the potential toxicity associated with chloramphenicol to humans, chloramphenicol's use in veterinary ophthalmology is becoming less widespread. It may be useful, however, in treating cats with suspected Mycoplasma or chlamydia conjunctivitis.

Suggested Dosages/Precautions/Adverse Effects - For prophylaxis following surgery or for cats with Mycoplasma or chlamydial conjunctivitis: One drop (or 1/4 inch strip if using ointment) four times daily. For established corneal infection: Application may be very frequent (up to hourly).

Chloramphenicol exposure in humans has resulted in fatal aplastic anemia. For this reason, this drug should be used with caution in veterinary patients and some ophthalmologists avoid its use entirely. Clients should be cautioned to use appropriate safeguards when applying the drug and avoiding contact with drops or solutions after application.

Labels state to not use longer than 7 days in cats, but *tid* application of ointment for 21 days to cats did not cause toxicity. Must not be used in any food producing animal.

Dosage Forms/Preparations/FDA Approval Status -
   Veterinary-Approved Products:
      Chloramphenicol 1% Ophthalmic Ointment in 3.5 gm; *Bemacol®*-(Pfizer); *Chlorbiotic®*-(Schering); *Chloricol®* (Evsco); Generic; (Rx)
      Chloramphenicol 0.5% Ophthalmic Drops in 7.5 ml btls tubes; *Chlorasol®*-(Evsco); (Rx). Refrigerate until dispensed.
      Approved for use in dogs and cats.

   Human-Approved Products:
      Chloramphenicol 1% Ophthalmic Ointment in 3.5 gm tubes; *Chloromycetin®* (Parke Davis); *Chloroptic®* (Allergan); Generic (Rx)
      Chloramphenicol 0.5% Ophthalmic Drops in 7.5 ml btls tubes; *Chloroptic®* (Allergan); Generic; (Rx). Refrigerate until dispensed.

CIPROFLOXACIN (OPHTHALMIC)
NORFLOXACIN (OPHTHALMIC)
OFLOXACIN (OPHTHALMIC)

Indications/Pharmacology - These fluroquinolone ophthalmic antibiotics are primarily useful for established gram negative corneal infections. They are not recommended for prophylactic use prior to or after surgery. See the main enrofloxacin/ciprofloxacin monograph for additional pharmacologic information.

Precautions/Adverse Effects - Ciprofloxacin may cause crusting or crystalline precipitates in the superficial portion of corneal defects. Other potential adverse effects with quinolones include: conjunctival hyperemia, bad taste in mouth, itching foreign body sensation, photophobia, lid edema, tearing keratitis and nausea. Allergic reactions have been reported with quinolone eye preps.

Dosage Forms/Preparations/FDA Approval Status -
   Veterinary-Approved Products: None
   Human-Approved Products:
      Ciprofloxacin 3 mg/ml drops in 2.5 & 5 ml btls; *Ciloxan®* (Alcon); Rx
      Norfloxacin 3 mg/ml drops in 5 ml btls; *Chibroxin®* (Merck); Rx
      Ofloxacin 3 mg/ml drops in 5 ml btls; *Ocuflox®* (Allergan); Rx

GENTAMICIN (OPHTHALMIC)
TOBRAMYCIN (OPHTHALMIC)

Indications/Pharmacology - The aminoglycosides are excellent drugs for gram negative or staphylococcal corneal infections. With frequent application, clinicians can establish corneal drug levels far in excess of MIC for most organisms without exceeding toxic systemic levels. Therefore, MIC reports may not be meaningful. Because of the high levels attainable, gentamicin usually exhibits similar efficacy to tobramycin, except in certain resistant gram-negative infections (e.g., Pseudomonas aeruginosa).

For serious gram negative or staphylococcal corneal ulcer infections, some ophthalmologists use cefazolin eye drops (compounded preparation) in combination with gentamicin or tobramycin. Synergism may result.

Precautions/Adverse Effects - Hypersensitivity, and localized ocular toxicity (lid itching, swelling and conjunctival erythema) have been reported rarely. Mydriasis and conjunctival paresthesias may also occur.

Dosage Forms/Preparations/FDA Approval Status -
  Veterinary-Approved Products:
      Gentamicin Ophthalmic Ointment 3 mg/g in 3.5 gm tubes; *Gentocin®* (Schering); (Rx). Approved for use in dogs and cats.
      Gentamicin Ophthalmic Drops 3 mg/ml in 5 ml btls *Gentocin®* (Schering); (Rx). Approved for use in dogs and cats.

  Human-Approved Products:
      Gentamicin Ophthalmic Ointment 3 mg/g in 3.5 gm tubes; *Garamycin®* (Schering); *Genoptic®* (Allergan); various; (Rx)
      Gentamicin Ophthalmic Drops 3 mg/ml in 5 ml btls *Garamycin®* (Schering); *Genoptic®* (Allergan); various; (Rx)

      Tobramycin Ophthalmic Ointment 3 mg/g in 3.5 gm tubes; *Tobrex®* (Alcon); (Rx)
      Tobramycin Ophthalmic Drops 3 mg/ml in 5 ml btls *Tobrex®* (Alcon); (Rx)

TETRACYCLINE (OPHTHALMIC)

Indications/Pharmacology - The tetracyclines are most useful in cats for the treatment Chlamydial and Mycoplasma conjunctivitis as well as nonspecific or symptomatic therapy for undiagnosed (causative organism not determined) conjunctivitis in cats. While its use in dogs and horses is questionable, it may be useful in goats for Chlamydial/Mycoplasma keratoconjunctivitis.

Tetracycline is often used to "back into" the diagnosis of herpes virus conjunctivitis in cats. Since the majority of conjunctivitis cases in cats are caused by herpes virus (approx. 90%) and the bulk of the remainder are caused either by Chlamydia or Mycoplasma, if the cat fails to respond to tetracycline, the cause is most likely due to herpes virus.

Suggested Dosages/Precautions/Adverse Effects - For Chlamydial/Mycoplasma keratoconjunctivitis: Apply 4 times daily. Dramatic improvement should be noted in 3-4 days, but treatment should continue for 3-4 weeks for Chlamydia to break the reproductive cycle of this organism.

Dosage Forms/Preparations/FDA Approval Status -
  Veterinary-Approved Products: None
  Human-Approved Products:
      Tetracycline HCl Ointment 10 mg/g in 3.75 g tubes *Achromycin®* (Storz/Lederle); (Rx)
      Tetracycline HCl Suspension 10 mg/ml in 4 ml btls *Achromycin®* (Storz/Lederle); (Rx)

      Other available ophthalmic antibiotics: Chlortetracycline: *Aureomycin®* (Storz Lederle); Bacitracin (alone); Erythromycin Ointment; Polymyxin B powder for solution; Sodium Sulfacetamide.

ANTIBIOTIC COMBINATIONS (OPHTHALMIC)

Indications/Pharmacology - These combination products exhibit a broad-spectrum of activity and are considered the first choice for symptomatic treatment of conjunctivitis in dogs and for prophylactic treatment of small animals prior to or after eye surgery. These agents are also used prophylactically for corneal injuries/wounds.

Suggested Dosages/Precautions/Adverse Effects - Usually applied 4 times daily to prevent infection and up to every 30 minutes in established corneal infections. See individual product label information and the information noted previously.

Neomycin has been reported to cause allergic reactions in dogs and cats, particularly after prolonged usage.

Dosage Forms/Preparations/FDA Approval Status -
Veterinary-Approved Products:
      Ointments:

Bacitracin zinc 400 units/Neomycin 3.5 mg/Polymyxin B Sulfate 10,000 Units per gram in 3.5 gm tubes *Mycitracin®* (Upjohn) (Note: contains 500 mg bacitracin/gm); *Neobacimyx®* (Schering); *Trioptic-P®* (Pfizer); *Vetropolycin®* (Pitman-Moore); Generic. All are Rx and approved for dogs and cats.

Oxytetracycline HCl 5 mg/Polymyxin B Sulfate 10,000 U/gm in 3.5 gm tubes *Terramycin® Ophthalmic Ointment* (Pfizer); OTC. Approved for use in dogs, cats, sheep, cattle, and horses.

Drops:

Neomycin 3.5 mg/Polymyxin B Sulfate 10,000 Units per ml: *Optiprime®*-(Syntex); Rx. Approved for use in dogs.

Human-Approved Products:

There are a wide variety of human-labeled ophthalmic combination products available. Most are a combination of bacitracin/neomycin/polymyxin B. However, there are variations of this theme (e.g., gramicidin in place of bacitracin in topical solutions-Neosporin® Ophthalmic Solution). All these products require a prescription.

ANTIBIOTIC & CORTICOSTEROID COMBINATIONS (OPHTHALMIC)

Indications/Pharmacology - There are three basic categories of these products that are routinely used in veterinary medicine; antibiotic combinations with hydrocortisone, antibiotic combinations with dexamethasone, and individual antibiotics (e.g., gentamicin or chloramphenicol) with a steroid.

Antibiotic combinations with hydrocortisone (ointment or solution) are used in dogs and horses for conjunctivitis as nonspecific therapy after ruling out other causes for red painful eyes, including glaucoma and anterior uveitis. They generally are applied 4 times daily and then on a tapering schedule based on the response to therapy. The hydrocortisone is relatively weak as an antiinflammatory agent and is not effective for intraocular inflammatory disease such as anterior uveitis. The relative penetration and potency of hydrocortisone in these preparations makes them relatively ineffective for immune mediated extraocular disease including scleritis, episcleritis and or nodular granulomatous episclerokeratitis. Anterior uveitis is statistically more common in horses than simple conjunctivitis and the steroid in these agents would not be helpful in improving the clinical signs of immune mediated uveitis.

Antibiotic combinations with dexamethasone are valuable for use in cases of more severe canine or equine conjunctivitis, nonulcerative keratitis and for immune-mediated scleral or corneal conditions such as chronic superficial keratitis (German Shepherd pannus), feline eosinophilic keratitis, scleritis, episcleritis and nodular granulomatous episclerokeratitis. For these conditions the antibiotic agent is not necessary but dexamethasone-only products are not always available. These medications are also used in the equine species with equine uveitis because the ointment forms persist on the cornea longer than drops and because they are less expensive than prednisolone acetate ophthalmic suspensions.

Single agent antibiotic (gentamicin) and potent steroid (betamethasone) combination products (e.g., *Gentocin Durafilm®*) are commonly used in veterinary medicine. However, there are few instances in veterinary ophthalmology in which a very potent corticosteroid agent and an aminoglycoside antibiotic are necessary in combination. Simple conjunctivitis in dogs and horses is adequately treated with antibiotic combinations with hydrocortisone. Avoid use of this agent in cats with conjunctivitis for the reasons noted below.

Suggested Dosages/Precautions/Adverse Effects - See individual product label information and the information noted above.

Avoid use of antibiotic/steroid combination agents in cats with conjunctivitis as the most common cause of conjunctivitis in the cat is primary or recurring infection with exposure to, or reactivation of, latent feline herpes virus. Recent research indicates that topical steroids increase the length of the typical course of feline herpes virus related conjunctivitis and/or keratitis and can induce corneal involvement in cases which might otherwise have remained confined to conjunctiva. Corneal sequestration has been noted to occur in cats with herpes virus conjunctivitis after treatment with topical steroids. Recommended treatment for feline herpes virus conjunctivitis is tetracycline ointment *QID* during active disease, as this drug is effective against Mycoplasma and chlamydia (other causes of infectious conjunctivitis in the cat).

Dosage Forms/Preparations/FDA Approval Status -
  Veterinary-Approved Products:
    Triple Antibiotic Ointments with Hydrocortisone:

Bacitracin zinc 400 units/Neomycin 3.5 mg/Polymyxin B Sulfate 10,000 Units & Hydrocortisone acetate 1% per gram in 3.5 gm tubes *Neobacimyx H®* (Schering); *Trioptic-S®* (Pfizer); *Vetropolycin HC®-* (Pitman-Moore); Generic. All are Rx and approved for dogs and cats.

Other Antibiotic/Steroid Ointments:

Neomycin Sulfate 5 mg & Prednisolone 2 mg (0.2%) per gram in 3.5 gram tubes *(Optisone®-*Evsco); (Rx). Approved for use in dogs and cats.

Neomycin Sulfate 5 mg & Isoflupredone acetate 1 mg (0.1%) per gram in 3.5 & 5 gram tubes *Neo-Predef® Sterile Ointment®* (Upjohn); (Rx). Approved for use in horses, cattle, dogs and cats.

Chloramphenicol 1% and Prednisolone acetate 2.5 mg (0.25%) in 3.5 gm tubes; *Chlorasone®* (Evsco) (Rx). Approved for use dogs and cats.

Drops:

Gentamicin Ophthalmic Drops 3 mg/ml & Betamethasone acetate 1 m/ml in 5 ml btls *Gentocin Durafilm®* (Schering); (Rx). Approved for use in dogs.

Human-Approved Products:

There are a wide variety of human-labeled ophthalmic antibiotic/steroid combination products available. Some of the more commonly used combinations include:

Ointments:

Bacitracin/Neomycin/Polymyxin B and Hydrocortisone *Cortisporin®* (BW)

Neomycin/Polymyxin B & Dexamethasone *Maxitrol®* (Alcon); (Rx)

Neomycin and Dexamethasone *NeoDecadron®* (Merck); (Rx)

Drops:

Neomycin/Polymyxin B and Hydrocortisone *Cortisporin®* (BW, etc.); (Rx)

Neomycin/Polymyxin B & Dexamethasone *Maxitrol®* (Alcon); (Rx)

Neomycin and Dexamethasone *NeoDecadron®* (Merck); (Rx)

Antifungals (Ophthalmic)

Fungal keratitis is a serious corneal disease, most commonly reported in the horse. The species selectivity of this disease is related to the environment of this animal, which is often contaminated with fungal elements. An increased incidence of fungal keratitis in people was directly related to the development of multiple topical steroid agents for treatment of eye diseases. In the horse, many cases of fungal keratitis are noted in association with prior treatment of conjunctival and/or corneal diseases with topical steroid agents. Aspergillus is the most common cause of fungal keratitis in the horse, although there is a great deal of variation in fungal isolates from the cornea depending upon geographical location. Studies in people and anecdotal reports from veterinarians suggest that fungal keratitises due to Fusarium organisms are more resistant to therapy than are those caused by aspergillus. Most studies in the equine suggest that about 50% of cases of fungal keratitis in the horse result in perforation of the corneal and enucleation of the eye. Medical and surgical therapy (keratectomy, corneal debridement, and conjunctival grafting) are used to treat such cases with the goals of therapy including arresting infection, mechanical removal of organisms from the cornea, and support of the cornea. All antifungal agents available for use in the equine suffer from poor penetration into the corneal stroma. Conjunctival grafting may further hinder drug penetration as a trade off to improving vascular availability to the cornea and mechanical support. Pathologic specimens from horses with fungal keratitis indicate that fungal organisms, unlike bacterial organisms, have a propensity to multiply deep in the stroma, directly adjacent to Descemet's membrane, making corneal penetration an important issue. Because the prognosis for return of vision and saving the globe in cases of fungal keratitis cases is guarded and because treatment is labor intensive, referral to teaching or other hospitals for 24 hour care and observation is recommended.

NATAMYCIN (OPHTHALMIC)

Indications/Pharmacology - Natamycin is a semisynthetic polyene antibiotic. Natamycin is poorly water soluble and will not penetrate the intact corneal epithelium. Natamycin is the only antifungal agent approved for use on the eye and the only commercially available eye drug for treatment of fungal keratitis.

Suggested Dosages/Precautions/Adverse Effects - The product comes as a thick white suspension which complicates the use of subpalpebral lavage apparatus for frequent treatment of the cornea of the horse. The drug tends to plug up the tubing systems used for medication. It will cause dramatic swelling and pain in the upper eyelid if it leaks out of the tubing into the subcutaneous tissues of the eyelid. Corneal penetration is poor and the medication is very expensive. Fungal keratitis cases are treated aggressively with hourly or bi-hourly treatment the first 1 to 3 days and gradual reduction in treatment frequency with signs of clinical improvement. Cytology and repeated cultures of the cornea are used to indicate treatment effectiveness. Worsening of the corneal edema and cellular infiltration can be a sign of treatment response. This is thought to be due to antigenic release associated with killing of fungal organisms (like the pulmonary response noted in dogs with institution of antifungal therapy for blastomycosis, etc.). Four to six weeks of treatment is not uncommon for fungal keratitis cases.

Dosage Forms/Preparations/FDA Approval Status -
   Veterinary-Approved Products: None
   Human-Approved Products:
     Natamycin Ophthalmic Suspension 5% in 15 ml btls *Natacyn®* (Alcon); (Rx)

MICONAZOLE (OPHTHALMIC)

Indications/Pharmacology - Miconazole is a broad spectrum imidazole antifungal agent with some antibacterial activity. Miconazole will penetrate the intact corneal epithelium. Topical miconazole therapy has been a favorite first choice agent for treatment of fungal keratitis in the horse by veterinary ophthalmologists for several years. Miconazole may be delivered by subconjunctival route, but with some local irritation, and topical use is the most commonly employed treatment method.

Suggested Dosages/Precautions/Adverse Effects - Miconazole is formulated at 10 mg/ml for IV use in humans. It can be directly taken from the glass ampule for IV use and applied to the cornea of horses. It is a clear solution readily delivered through subpalpebral lavage apparatus systems. The medication is significantly less expensive compared with natamycin and its corneal penetration is more favorable, although still less than optimal. Treatment is generally delivered hourly or bi-hourly during the first several days of treatment. Once clinical improvement is noted and cytology specimens and repeated cultures indicate eradication of fungal organisms, the treatment frequency is gradually reduced. Most fungal keratitis cases are treated 4 to 6 weeks.

Dosage Forms/Preparations/FDA Approval Status -
   Veterinary-Approved Products: None
   Human-Approved Products:
     Miconazole Injection 10 mg/ml in 20 ml glass ampules *Monistat-i.v.®* (Janssen); Rx

SILVER SULFADIAZINE (OPHTHALMIC)

Indications/Pharmacology - Silver Sulfadiazine Cream is a broad spectrum agent which covers bacteria (gram positive and negative) and fungal agents. It has been used extensively in people suffering from skin burns. It is nontoxic to the skin, conjunctiva and cornea and has been used in the last several years for cases of fungal keratitis. Particularly good results have been noted in cases of superficial keratitis prior to development of advanced disease. Clinical response is better when used early in the course of the disease. Treatment with silver sulfadiazine is considered non-conventional in people. It is gaining in popularity in the treatment of equine fungal keratitis by veterinary ophthalmologists. For medico-legal reasons, in very expensive horses in which litigation may be an issue, treatment with more conventional therapy (Natamycin) may be indicated first, or consideration can be given to signed consent regarding treatment with Silver Sulfadiazine. The initial response to this drug has been promising, however.

Suggested Dosages/Precautions/Adverse Effects - The commercially available product is a cream, but can be delivered into the conjunctival sac using a tuberculin syringe, without the needle. A typical treatment dose is 0.2 ml drawn into a syringe. It will not pass through standard sized subpalpebral lavage catheters, although it may be administered through large medication administration systems using red rubber feeding tubes passed through the lid, with variable results getting the medication to pass through the tube. It is probably best applied manually. The cream sticks well to the cornea which probably improves effectiveness, similar to natamycin, as compared to miconazole. Treatment regimes are similar to the other antifungal agents with very frequent applications necessary during the early phases of the treatment and reduction in therapy based upon clinical response. Daily debridement of the necrotic corneal stroma and epithelium will improve penetration of the drug and the clinical response.

  The medication is inexpensive and is available from any pharmacy, but it is not labeled for use in eyes. The label (package insert) specifically states "not to be used in eyes" so liability for use in eyes rests solely with the prescribing veterinarian and some pharmacists may be unwilling to dispense this medication for ophthalmic use.

Dosage Forms/Preparations/FDA Approval Status -
 Veterinary-Approved Products: None
 Human-Approved Products:
  Silver Sulfadiazine Topical (not an ophthalmic product) 10 mg per gram in a water miscible cream base. Available in 20, 50, 400, and 1000 g containers; *Silvadene®*-(Marion); *Flint SSD®* (Flint); Rx

Antivirals (Ophthalmic)

Antiviral drugs are used most commonly in clinical practice for the treatment of feline ocular herpes virus infections. Simple acute conjunctivitis is best managed with symptomatic antibiotic therapy alone (i.e., tetracycline treatment). The development of concurrent corneal disease, however, indicates that consideration should be given to the use of antiviral drugs. Persistent cases of conjunctivitis in the cat due to feline herpes virus infection may also benefit from treatment with topical antiviral drugs.

TRIFLURIDINE (TRIFLUOROTHYMIDINE)

Indications/Pharmacology - Trifluridine (trifluorothymidine; *Viroptic®*) is a pyrimidine nucleoside analog. It is structurally related to 2-deoxythymidine, the natural precursor of DNA synthesis. Trifluridine is poorly absorbed by the cornea and is virostatic. *Viroptic®* interrupts viral replication by substituting in "nonsense" pyrimidine analogues. For this reason, a competent surface immunity is necessary to resolve ocular disease, with or without antiviral therapy. A recent in vitro study in which several strains of feline herpes virus were collected from the United States and were used to infect kidney epithelial cells showed that trifluridine was more effective at lower concentrations compared with several other agents. For this reason, trifluridine is often the first choice drug employed in the treatment of feline herpes virus ocular disease. Antiviral agents have also been used in the treatment of superficial punctate keratitis in the horse, thought to be associated with equine herpes virus-2 (EHV-2) infection of the cornea.

Suggested Dosages/Precautions/Adverse Effects - Trifluridine must be applied very frequently. The author (DKO) recommends treatment every 2 hours (waking hours) during the first 2 days of therapy to establish effective corneal drug levels. After this time, treatment 4-6 times daily is indicated. Because trifluridine is virostatic and not viricidal, treatment 1 week beyond the resolution of clinical signs is recommended, to prevent a rebound effect associated with poor surface immunity in combination with residual active viral agents.

Anecdotally, improvement with antiviral agents is noted in about 50% of cats in which the treatment is employed. In some cats the ocular disease persists despite treatment with antiviral agents. It is not certain if these are truly cases of feline herpes virus infection or other disease as the confirmation of feline herpes virus infection is exceedingly difficult in practice, (except in the acute disease with respiratory and ocular involvement, because of the logistics of viral isolation tests for doctors in clinical practice (usually only available at major institutions or referral centers) and because of the high degree of false negatives with herpes virus FA tests and with available polymerase chain reaction (DNA amplification) technology). Chronic conjunctivitis in the cat seems to be the most resistant to treatment with antiviral agents.

Dosage Forms/Preparations/FDA Approval Status -
 Veterinary-Approved Products: None
 Human-Approved Products:
  Trifluridine Ophthalmic Solution 1% in 7.5 ml btls *Viroptic®* (B-W); (Rx)

Agents for Keratoconjunctivitis Sicca

Keratoconjunctivitis sicca (KCS) is a common ocular disorder in dogs. Recent research efforts indicate that KCS in dogs is an immune mediated disease. It is similar to Sjogren's Syndrome in humans except we do not recognize a connective tissue disorder in the dog compared to this disease in people (man-dry eye, dry mouth, and connective tissue disorder like rheumatoid arthritis; dogs just dry eye). Immune mediated lacrimal adenitis can result in complete destruction of tear producing glands in dogs. Glandular fibrosis produces absolute sicca and these cases may be better managed with a parotid duct transposition surgery because there may be little remaining gland tissue to treat.

CYCLOSPORINE (OPHTHALMIC)

Indications/Pharmacology - Cyclosporine is a polypeptide agent first isolated from a fungus. The agent interferes with interleukin synthesis by T lymphocytes and in so doing has been employed extensively in people following major organ transplantation to prevent immune rejection. Cyclosporine is extremely hydrophobic and was originally compounded by pharmacists in virgin olive oil or purified corn oil for the topical application to dogs with keratoconjunctivitis sicca. Topical cyclosporine is now commercially available as a 0.2% ointment (*Optimmune®*-Schering). The mechanism of action of cyclosporine in the treatment of keratoconjunctivitis sicca is still not fully understood, although it has been employed in the treatment of KCS in dogs for several years. It stimulates increased tear production in normal dogs and for this reason it is thought to have a direct stimulatory effect on the tear gland. It may do this acting as a prolactin analog, fitting onto lacrimal prolactin receptors. Its interleukin blocking effects likely are the major mechanism of action. Halting local inflammatory mediator production appears to arrest self perpetuating lacrimal adenitis resulting in resumption of normal or improved tear production after several weeks of therapy. Cyclosporine in the cornea, appears to have the ability to lessen granulation and pigment development. This property appears to be unrelated to its tear producing ability.

The reported success rate of alleviating the signs of KCS in dogs with treatment with cyclosporine is 75-85%. Some studies indicate that the higher the Schirmer value prior to starting therapy, the more likely that the dog will be well managed with cyclosporine drops alone. Absolute sicca may be associated with extensive fibrosis of the tear glands, leaving little tissue for stimulation or repair.

Cyclosporine is effective in the management of German Shepherd Pannus or chronic superficial keratitis in the dog. This condition is an immune disease of the cornea and likely is interleukin mediated. Cyclosporine may be preferred for the treatment of pannus because of the lack of systemic side effects noted in dogs with chronic topical administration of cyclosporine. Chronic topical corticosteroid treatment is associated with biochemical changes in the blood of large and small dogs.

Cyclosporine has been tried in the management of the rare case of keratoconjunctivitis sicca in the cat. Dry eye in cats is usually associated with herpes virus destruction of lacrimal epithelial cells and or stenosis of the ductules or openings of the ductules due to chronic viral conjunctivitis. Preliminary results have not been promising. Topical cyclosporine often aggravates ophthalmic herpes virus infections in people. Cyclosporine has not shown promising effects in the management of feline eosinophilic keratitis, a condition now thought to be related to chronic stromal herpes virus infection in cats.

Suggested Dosages/Precautions/Adverse Effects - Cyclosporine is initiated generally as the first course of therapy for confirmed dry eye cases in the dog. The topical half life of cyclosporine is about 8 hours and most canine cases of KCS are managed with twice daily therapy with 0.2% ointment (*Optimmune®*). Three times a day therapy has been employed during the initial phases of treatment in more difficult or slow responding cases. For some uncertain reason (reversal of lacrimal adenitis→ reorganization of lacrimal epithelial cell function→ formation of secretory granules→ tear production) 3-8 weeks of therapy are necessary before a dramatic increase in the Schirmer tear test becomes evident. Patients are generally maintained for life on cyclosporine ophthalmic once or twice daily depending on the response. Discontinuation of therapy is usually associated with the return of clinical signs of KCS within a few days. Reinstitution of therapy at this time, is usually associated with an almost immediate return of tear production (versus the initial lag phase noted). This likely is related to the degree of inflammatory disease noted with short discontinuation of therapy versus that present initially, prior to the diagnosis of KCS.

If tear production is very low, cyclosporine is often used in combination with artificial tears during the initial phases of therapy. Once tear production is improved, artificial tears can generally be removed completely or their frequency reduced in the treatment plan. After treatment is initiated, reevaluation of tear production in one month is recommended. If ulcerative keratitis complicates keratoconjunctivitis sicca in the dog, more frequent evaluation is necessary. Cyclosporine, although an immunomodulating agent, is considered safe in the face of ulcerative keratitis, with concurrent antibiotic therapy. Caution is advised, however.

When cyclosporin is delivered topically, no systemic toxicity has been noted in dogs given this drug chronically. This is probably associated with the poor absorption of this drug across the GI tract and because it is delivered to the eye at very low concentrations which even if 100% absorbed, when divided over the body weight of the dog is well below even the therapeutic dose. Advanced detection methods have made it possible to measure trace levels of cyclosporine in the blood of dogs being topically treated for dry eye. The clinical implications of this finding is uncertain at this time.

Dosage Forms/Preparations/FDA Approval Status - *Optimmune®* ointment is the approved formulation of topical cyclosporine for the management of dry eye in dogs. Compounding of topical cyclosporine drops was popular before the introduction, approval, and marketing of *Optimmune®* ointment. Clinicians persistently using compounded formulations of cyclosporine eye drops may be outside of expected ethical and legal standards of practice except under very specific situations. The use of commercially available ophthalmic products instead of compounded medications is highly recommended. Optimmune® is first applied 2 or 3 times daily and frequency of daily application is adjusted based on clinical response.

Veterinary-Approved Products:
Cyclosporine Ophthalmic Ointment 0.2%; *Optimmune*® (Schering-Plough); (Rx)
Human-Approved Products:
Orphan products are available for human uses.

ARTIFICIAL TEAR PRODUCTS; OCULAR LUBRICANTS

Indications/Pharmacology - Artificial tear solutions are aqueous isotonic, pH buffered viscous solutions that serve as a lubricant for dry eyes and associated eye irritation due to dry eye syndromes. They are often useful adjuncts in keratoconjunctivitis sicca in dogs early in cyclosporine therapy.

Ocular lubricants are white petrolatum-based products that serve to lubricate and protect eyes. They are particularly useful during anesthetic procedures where animals' eyes may remain open and during which time tear production is dramatically reduced.

Dosage Forms/Preparations/FDA Approval Status -
Veterinary-Approved Products: None
Human-Approved Products:

There are a plethora of products available with a variety of formulations and trade names. All are OTC. Some commonly known products include:Artificial Tear Products (Methylcellulose-based): *Adsorbotear*® (Alcon); *Comfort Tears*® (Pilkington Barnes Hind); *Isopto-Tears*® (Alcon); *Tears Naturale*® (Alcon); *Lacril*® (Allergan)

Artificial Tear Products (Polyvinyl Alcohol-based): *Hypotears*® (Iolab); *Liquifilm Tears* (Allergan); *Tears Plus*® (Allergan)

Artificial Tear Products (Glycerin-based): *Dry Eye Therapy*® (Bausch & Lomb); *Eye Lube A* (Optopics)

Ocular Lubricants (Petrolatum-based): *Lacri-Lube*® *S.O.P.* (Allergan); *Akwa Tears*® (Akorn)

OPHTHALMIC IRRIGANTS

Indications/Pharmacology - Sterile isotonic solutions are used for flushing the nasolacrimal system and for removing debris from the eye. They are also used to remove excess stain after diagnostic staining of the cornea. Sterile lactated Ringer's solution (LRS) is well tolerated by the surface of the eye as is a balanced salt solution (BSS). Extraocular irrigating solutions may contain preservatives. Intraocular irrigating solutions (used during surgical procedures) do not contain preservatives and also contain electrolytes that are required for normal cell function.

Suggested Dosages/Precautions/Adverse Effects - Extraocular: Use to flush eye as necessary; control rate of flow by exerting pressure on bottle. Intraocular: Refer to both established practices for each surgical procedure as well as the specific manufacturers' recommendations.

Dosage Forms/Preparations/FDA Approval Status -
Veterinary-Approved Products:
Eye Rinse® (Butler); (OTC): Contains: water, boric acid, zinc sulfate, glycerin, camphor. Note: This product is not labeled to be used as an irrigant per se, but as an aid in cleaning the eye and removing eye stains.

Human-Approved Products:
Common trade name products for extraocular irrigation: *AK-Rinse*® (Akorn), *Blinx*® (Pilkington Barnes Hind), *Collyrium for Fresh Eyes Eye Wash*® (Wyeth-Ayerst), *Dacriose*® (Iolab), *Eye Irrigating Solution*® (Rugby), *Eye-Stream*® (Alcon), *Eye Wash*® (several manufacturers), *Eye Irrigating Wash*® (Roberts Hauck), *Irrigate Eye Wash*® (Optopics), *Optigene*® (Pfeiffer), *Star-Optic Eye Wash*® (Stellar), *Visual-Eyes* ® (Optopics). All are OTC.

Common trade name products for intraocular irrigation: Note: Most of these products contain Balanced Salt Solution (BSS) = NaCl 0.64%, KCl 0.075%, CaCl2•2H20 0.048%, MgCl2•6H20 0.03%, Na acetate trihydrate 0.39%, sodium citrate dihydrate 0.17%, sodium hydroxide and/or hydrochloric acid to adjust pH, and water: Balanced Salt Solution (various manufacturers), *BSS*® (Alcon), *Iocare Balanced Salt Solution*® (Iolab); All are Rx.

BSS + solutions that also contain dextrose, glutathione, bicarbonate, phosphate are also available as: *BSS Plus®* (Alcon) and *AMO Endosol Extra®* (Allergan); All are Rx.

Diagnostics

FLUORESCEIN SODIUM (OPHTHALMIC)

Indications/Pharmacology - Fluorescein sodium is a yellow water soluble dye. It is used most commonly to delineate full thickness loss of corneal epithelium. In this instance it will stain the corneal stroma. The epithelium is not stained because its outer lipid cell membrane repels the stain. Descemet's membrane will not stain with fluorescein stain and this is used to indicate descemetocele formation, an ocular emergency.

Fluorescein stain is applied to the precorneal tear film in dogs and cats and the break-up of this stain with time, as observed through a slit lamp biomicroscope using a cobalt blue light source, is used to determine the tear film break-up time (normal 19s), an indicator of tear film quality.

Fluorescein stain is applied to the tear film of dogs to determine patency of the nasolacrimal outflow system. The normal wait time is 2-5 minutes in dogs and up to 10 minutes in cats. A positive test indicates patency of the system. A negative test is not indicative of disease as the test is negative in a large percentage of normal animals. Fluorescein stain, then, can be added to irrigating solution to flush the nasolacrimal system, making detecting the irrigation solution at the nose more obvious during flushing of the system.

Suggested Dosages/Precautions/Adverse Effects - Fluorescein stain is applied by dropping a drop of irrigating solution onto the sterile strip and then allowing the drop to fall on the eye. The strip should not contact the cornea or it will cause false positive stain retention at the site of contact with the epithelial cells. After a few seconds, the excess fluorescein is irrigated from the eye, staining areas of full thickness epithelial loss.

Conjunctival or corneal epithelial cells for fluorescent antibody testing should be collected prior to application of fluorescein stain, which can cause a false positive test for several days after application of the stain.

Fluorescein may rarely cause hypersensitivity reactions. Temporary staining of fur and skin may result. Do not use during intraocular surgery.

Dosage Forms/Preparations/FDA Approval Status -
Veterinary-Approved Products: None
Human-Approved Products: Sterile strips of paper impregnated with fluorescein sodium are the most commonly used form in veterinary medicine. Solutions (2%) of fluorescein are available, however they are not popular following one study indicating that Pseudomonas is readily grown in such solutions. Injectable products are also available (for ophthalmic angiography), but are not routinely used in veterinary medicine.

Fluorescein Sodium Strips 0.6 mg *Ful-Glo®* (Barnes Hind); 1 mg *Fluorets®* (Akorn), *Fluor-I-Strip®-A.T.* (W-A); 9 mg *Fluor-I-Strip®* (W-A); All Rx.

ROSE BENGAL (OPHTHALMIC)

Indications/Pharmacology - Rose Bengal is a vital stain and stains dead epithelial cells and mucus. Full thickness loss of the corneal epithelium is not necessary (only dead cells need be present) to obtain Rose Bengal stain uptake. It does not stain epithelial defects and does not pass into intercellular spaces.

Rose Bengal stain is most commonly employed in the detection of the presence of viral keratitis in the cat. Because feline herpes virus tends to infect one cell, moving then to an adjacent cell (causing the so called dendritic tracts in the cornea) without full thickness loss of corneal epithelium initially, Rose Bengal is an ideal diagnostic agent for this infection. Rose Bengal can also be used to detect damaged corneal epithelium on the dorsal cornea in early cases of keratitis sicca. Rose Bengal stain is virucidal although no information is available relative to its use as a therapeutic agent.

Suggested Dosages/Precautions/Adverse Effects - Rose Bengal is applied as a solution (1-2 drops in conjunctival sac before examination) or from an impregnated strip (saturate tip of strip with sterile irrigating solution; touch bulbar conjunctiva or lower fornix with moistened strip; cause patient to blink several times to distribute the stain).

Rose Bengal is apparently toxic to the cornea and conjunctiva and should be thoroughly flushed from the eye after use to prevent irritation. Hypersensitivity reactions are possible. May stain clothing.

Dosage Forms/Preparations/FDA Approval Status -
  Veterinary-Approved Products: None
  Human-Approved Products:
      Rose Bengal Solution 1% in 5 ml dropper bottles (Akorn); Rx
      Rose Bengal Strips 1.3 mg per strip; *Rosets*® (Akorn), Generic (Barnes-Hind); Rx

Small Animal Therapeutic Diets

Editor's Note: The following information is reprinted with permission from the Nutrition Support Service at the College of Veterinary Medicine at The Ohio State University and was authored by C.A. Tony Buffington, DVM, PhD, DACVN, Professor of Veterinary Clinical Sciences and Cheryl Holloway, RVT, Nutrition Support Specialist. For the latest updates on the ever changing aspect of veterinary nutrition, the reader is referred to the service's web site: **http://nss.vet.ohio-state.edu/**

Veterinary Food Tables
Introduction:
The following tables contain some nutrient parameters of the veterinary foods available in our hospital. The diets are classified as veterinary foods because they are to be used only under veterinary supervision. Commercially available foods also may be appropriate for some of the conditions listed (as described where appropriate in the tables). The tables are based on the most commonly recognized nutrient modifications for a particular disease. This format was chosen because veterinarians commonly make the diagnosis, decide on necessary nutrient modifications, then choose the most appropriate diet for their particular patient. Some foods are used for more conditions than are mentioned in the tables.

All tables contain a title, brief introduction if necessary, a table of indications, contraindications, major nutrient modifications, and commercial substitutions if available. The nutrient tables are ordered by dog, canned and dry followed by cat, canned and dry. Table columns include:

1. **Diet** - the type, canned or dry, and the name of the diet.
2. **Mfg.** - the manufacturer of the diet.
3. **Unit** - the unit of feeding, can for canned foods, cup for dry foods.
4. **Weight** - the net weight, in ounces (oz.), of the unit.
5. **Energy** - the number of kilocalories (kcal) contained in each unit.
6. **Nutrient amount per 100 kcal** - the grams of Protein, Fat, Carbohydrate (CHO). Fiber and Water, and milligrams (mg) of Calcium (Ca), Phosphorus (P), Sodium (Na), Potassium (K), and Magnesium (Mg) contained in 100 kcal of each diet as fed.

To estimate the % of kcal as protein, or carbohydrate, multiply the grams by 4; for fat multiply by 9.

All data was obtained from manufacturer's advertising literature available in the Fall of 1998.

The data in the tables can be used to compare the nutrient content of different diets and, to compare nutrient content of a diet with the nutrient needs of a patient:

To compare diets:
    a. **of similar moisture content and energy density, one can use the amount of nutrient per unit as fed** - AAFCO regulations require that minimum percentages of protein and fat, and maximums for moisture and fiber, be reported on all pet foods.
    b. **of differing moisture content (e.g., dry vs. canned) and similar energy density, one can use the amount of nutrient per unit dry matter**. For example, a dry diet containing 20% protein and 9% water (=91% dry matter) on an as fed basis contains 20/91 * 100 = 22% protein on a dry matter basis, whereas a canned diet containing 5% protein and 77% water (=23% dry matter) on an as fed basis contains 5/23 * 100 = 22% protein on a dry matter basis.
    c. **of differing energy density (e.g., high vs. low fat), one can use the amount of nutrient per 100 kcal** - For example, a diet containing 25% protein and 7% fat on a dry matter basis contains 8 grams of protein per 100 kcal, whereas a diet containing 25% protein and 21% fat on a dry matter basis contains only 5 grams of protein per 100 kcal.

To compare nutrient content of a diet with the nutrient needs of a patient, use the amount per unit body weight per day - because many veterinary foods contain restricted amounts of some nutrients, one must compare the number of grams of nutrient in the amount of food consumed with the needs of the animal to ensure that deficiencies are avoided. This is of practical concern for protein and sodium. For example, the minimum protein intake to sustain protein reserves in dogs is approximately 1 gram per pound per day. If a dog with advanced renal failure consumes 20 kcal per pound body weight per day, the diet would need to contain at least 5 grams per 100 kcal to provide enough protein to meet the dog's needs. If the dog consumed 30 kcal per pound body weight per day, only 3.3 grams protein per 100 kcal diet would be necessary.

Because diet therapy for a number of diseases consists of restriction of nutrient intake, and because many (most?) patients with nutrient-sensitive diseases are older and don't eat much, the risk of nutrient deficiencies must be considered. This is particularly true when the therapy is anticipated to continue for months or years. For these reasons, estimates of daily minimum intakes of some essential nutrients (amount per pound body weight) for adult, average-sized pets are presented below:

Nutrient	Dog	Cat
Energy	10 kcal	
Water	10 ml	
Protein	1 gm	2 gm
Sodium	10 mg	
Phosphorus	20 mg	

Veterinary foods often are sold as containing "high" or "low" levels of some nutrients. Currently, no generally accepted definition of these terms exists. My own definitions, many extrapolated from humans, follow:

Definition of "high" and "low" nutrient densities

Nutrient	Dog	Cat
Low calorie	< 3 kcal/gm dry matter	< 3 kcal/gm dry matter
High calorie	>4.5 kcal/gm dry matter	>4.5 kcal/gm dry matter
Low protein	<5 gm/100 kcal	<7 gm/100 kcal
High protein	>8 gm/100 kcal	>10 gm/100 kcal
Low fat	<2 gm/100 kcal	<2 gm/100 kcal
High fat	>5 gm/100 kcal	>5 gm/100 kcal
Low fiber	<0.25 gm/100 kcal	<0.25 gm/100 kcal
High fiber	>1.5 gm/100 kcal	>1.5 gm/100 kcal
Low sodium	<100 mg/100 kcal	<100 mg/100 kcal

General feeding suggestions: <u>Remember, It is always better for a patient to eat some of the "wrong" diet than none of the "right" diet</u>!

1. Introduce diet gradually, once the patient's condition is improving, to avoid creating a learned aversion, which is the association of an adverse stimulus with a novel diet. If one intends to feed a particular diet long-term, it should be introduced when the patient is feeling better so it is associated with feelings of improving health.
2. Amount- use the "Energy needs of sedentary dogs and cats" graph for initial guidelines, or offer ~20 kcal per pound body weight per day to cats and most dogs (~10 kcal/pound if > ~100 pounds), adjusting intake as necessary to maintain a moderate body condition.
3. Follow instructions in the section entitled "treating inappetence" when patient food intake falls below the above intake estimates.

Diet Table for Dogs (Diet tables for cats begin on page 686)

Disease	Diets
Colitis (idiopathic)	Modified Fiber, p.677 Novel Protein, p.678 and Reduced Fat, p.681
Congestive heart failure-advanced	Modified Fiber, p.677 and Reduced Sodium, p.682
Constipation	Modified Fiber, p.677
Critical Care	Nutrient Dense, p.680
Dermatitis due to food allergy	Novel Protein, p.678
Diabetes	Modified Fiber, p.677
Exocrine pancreatic insufficiency	Reduced Fat, p.681
Fluid Overload	Reduced Sodium, p.682
Hyperlipidemia	Reduced Fat, p.681
Hypertension	Reduced Protein, Phosphorus, p.683
Kidney failure-advanced	Reduced Protein, Phosphorus, p.683
Inflammatory bowel disease	Novel Protein, p.678 and Reduced Fat?, p.681
Liver Failure	Reduced Protein, Phosphorus, p.683
Obesity	Modified Fiber, p.677 and Reduced Energy ,p.684
Maldigestion, Malabsorption	Reduced Fat, p.681
	Reduced Fat, p.681
Small bowel diarrhea	Modified Fiber, p.677 and Reduced Fat, p.681
Urolithiasis	Restricted Mineral ,p.685
Volume Restriction	Nutrient Dense, p.680

Modified Fiber Diets for Dogs

The term "dietary fiber" describes a class of chemical compounds derived from plants. The effects of fiber consumption on physiological function depends on the type(s) of fiber ingested, effects of processing on fiber properties, and the amount consumed. Potentially desirable functions of fiber in small animal patients include bulking (insoluble or nonfermentable), and fermenting and gelling (soluble or fermentable). Increasing fiber intake has been suggested as part of treatment of the following problems:

Disease	Fiber Type	Fiber Type
	Bulking	Fermenting and Gelling
Constipation	-	+
Diabetes	+	+
Idiopathic colitis	+	+
Small bowel diarrhea	-	+
Obesity	?	?

We currently cannot predict fiber function inpatients very accurately. Rational use of dietary fiber will depend on results of clinical trials of commercial products, and assurance of consistency in formulation (dietary fiber is like wine in that the soil, weather, harvest and post-harvest practices all affect the quality and consistency of the final product).

Marketed for use in patients with:	Avoid feeding to patients with:	Nutrient Modifications	Commercial Substitutions
Colitis	Increased nutrient needs	increased fiber	increased fiber products
Constipation	Increased nutrient needs	increased fiber	increased fiber products
Diabetes mellitus	Increased nutrient needs	increased fiber	increased fiber products
Hyperlipidemia	increased nutrient needs	reduced fat	low fat foods
Obesity	Increased nutrient needs	reduced energy density	reduced calorie foods; sold as "lite" or "lean"

Diets - Listed in decreasing order of fiber gm/100 kcal

		Dog				Amount per 100 kcal							
Mfg. Diet	Unit	weight	energy	Protein (% of kcal)	Fat	CHO	Fiber	H2O	Ca	P	Na	K	Mg
Canned		oz.	Kcal/ unit	gm	gm	gm	gm	gm	mg	mg	mg	mg	mg
Hills r/d	Can	14.75	234	10.6	2.9	15.2	11.0	129	190	170	120	360	59
Purina OM	Can	12	182	17.8	3.4	8.8	7.7	146	470	430	110	430	NA
Hills w/d	Can	14.75	359	5.1	3.7	16.6	4.2	84	160	160	90	180	23
DRY		oz.	Kcal/ unit	gm	gm	gm	gm	gm	mg	mg	mg	mg	mg
Hill r/d	Cup	2.7	205	8.3	2.9	12.8	8	3	230	180	100	260	53
Purina OM	Cup	3.8	276	8.2	2.2	17.4	5.5	.07	490	380	90	340	NA
Hill w/d	Cup	2.7	223	5.1	2.1	16.8	5.1	3	170	150	60	240	37
PURINA DCO	Cup	3.6	338	6.9	3.4	13	2.1	2.7	330	250	60	160	30
Waltham High Fiber	Cup	2.5	223	6.3	2.4	NA	1.4	3.8	350	410	90	320	50

FEEDING DIRECTIONS

Fiber also can be purchased separately and added (gradually, to effect) to the patient's current diet; some examples are given in the table below. Recommended dosages range widely; I recommend starting with 1 tablespoon per cup or can of food, and increasing to achieve the desired clinical effect. Clients should be told that the increase in feces volume and frequency that results from increased bulking fiber consumption is the intended effect.

Food	Amount per Tablespoon	Total fiber	insoluble	soluble
	gm	gm	gm	gm
Wheat bran	5.3	2.7	2.3	0.3
100% Bran cereal	6.4	1.8	1.6	0.2
Oat Bran	6.7	1	0.5	0.5
Metamucil	5.8	3.4	0.7	2.7

Novel Protein Diets for Dogs

These diets are among the many foods available that contain proteins to which an allergic patient has not been exposed. They have been recommended for use in patients with skin or gastrointestinal signs of disease caused by food allergies. Providing a novel protein source, and decreasing the amount of protein ingested (see, e.g., d/d) both may be beneficial. Because of the many proteins included in commercial pet foods, finding a only one, novel protein may not be easy. Home-made diets also have been recommended, especially for diagnosis of food allergy, and are presented in that section.

Marketed for use in patients with:	Avoid feeding to patients with:	Nutrient Modifications	Commercial Substitutions
Dermatitis caused by food allergy	Increased nutrient needs	Protein to which the patient has not been exposed	Any containing a protein novel to the patient
Inflammatory bowel disease			

Dog				Amount per 100 kcal									
Mfg. Diet	unit	wt.	energy	Protein (% of kcal)	Fat	CHO	Fiber	H20	Ca	P	Na	K	Mg
CANNED	oz.		Kcal/unit	gm	gm	gm	gm	gm	mg	mg	mg	mg	mg
Hills d/d - lamb & rice	Can	14.75	578	3.3	4.7	10.6	0.9	51	100	60	70	120	8
Hills d/d - white fish & rice	Can	14.75	459	3.9	4.4	13.7	1.1	NA	160	90	90	170	12
Iams Response	Can	14	518	8	6.7	5.8	0.3	60	293	206	158	491	24
Waltham Selected Protein	Can	13.2	440	7.3	7.6	NA	0.4	66	260	240	200	140	20
DRY	oz.		Kcal/unit	gm	gm	gm	gm	gm	mg	mg	mg	mg	mg
Hills d/d - egg & rice	Cup	3.5	399	3.7	2.8	15.1	0.4	2	140	80	90	100	11
Iams Response	Cup	2.6	301	5.5	3.1	11.6	0.5	2	238	216	127	370	34
Purina HA	Cup	NA	363	5.3	2.6	14.9	0.4	NA	350	260	60	170	30
Purina LA	Cup	NA	414	7.1	4.2	11.4	0.5	NA	450	270	60	180	40
Waltham Select Protein Rice & Catfish	Cup	2.8	295	7.3	2.4	NA	1.4	2.9	540	340	120	370	30

IVD Innovative Diets				Amount per 100 kcal									
Diet	unit	Wt.	Energy	Protein (% of kcal)	Fat	CHO	Fiber	H20	Ca	P	Na	K	Mg
CANNED		oz.	Kcal/unit	gm	gm	gm	gm	gm	mg	mg	mg	mg	mg
Venison & Potato	Can	15	423	7.1	6.4	6.1	0.2	NA	377	377	40	109	6
White Fish & Potato	Can	15	409	7.9	6.0	2.3	0.3	NA	622	564	82	62	82
Rabbit & Potato	Can	15	407	6.5	6.1	7.3	0.2	NA	557	454	62	144	62
Lamb & Potato	Can	45	459	5.9	7.6	4.3	0.4	NA	467	320	82	137	64
Duck & Potato	Can	15	423	7.1	6.4	6.1	0.2	NA	377	377	40	109	60
DRY		oz.	Kcal/unit	gm	gm	gm	gm	gm	mg	mg	mg	mg	mg
Venison & Potato	Cup	3.5	330	5.8	3.1	15.2	1.0	NA	312	365	42	24	24
Rabbit & Potato	Cup	3.5	330	5.8	3.1	15.2	1.0	NA	342	279	50	350	27
Lamb & Potato	Cup	3.5	336	5.8	3.2	14.9	0.7	NA	409	277	35	321	26
Duck & Potato	Cup	3.5	330	5.8	3.1	15.2	1.0	NA	312	279	42	356	24

Feeding directions

Once a diagnosis of food allergy is made and a diet found that the patient does not react to, it will be important that the owner understand the importance of not permitting the patient to consume any foods that may contain provocative antigens.

NUTRIENT DENSE DIETS FOR DOGS

Marketed for use in patients with:	Avoid feeding to patients with:	Nutrient Modifications	Commercial substitutions
Increased nutrient needs	Decreased nutrient needs	Increased nutrient density	High protein, high fat canned dog or cat foods, meat baby foods
Volume restriction	"	"	"

Diets - listed in order of decreasing energy density

Mfg. Diet	unit	Wt.	Energy	Protein (% kcal)	Fat	CHO	Fiber	H2O	Ca	P	Na	K	Mg
								Amount per 100 kcal					
Canned	oz.		Kcal/unit (per gm)	Gm	gm	gm	gm	gm	mg	mg	mg	mg	mg
Iams Recovery	Can	6	340 (2.1)	7.5 (26)	7.1	1.3	0.3	33	190	150	55	180	13
Hills p/d	Can	14.75	587 (1.4)	6.4 (30)	5.9	7.1	0.2	49	273	200	100	130	28
Chicken baby food	Heinz	2.5	100 (1.4)	9.8	7.2	0	0	33	64	120	40	135	
Purina CNM-CV	Can	5.5	223 (1.4)	8.7	5.5	4.7	0.2	50	250	190	50	270	20
Hills a/d	Can	5.5	197 (1.2)	11 (46)	7.1	2.5	0.1	61	250	200	110	180	20
Abbott Clinicare	Can	8	237 (1)	5.7	6.5	7.1	NA	NA	177	135	58	177	13
Kal-Kan Sheba	Tin	3.5	78 (0.78)	13.8	5.3	NA	3.4	NA	470	310	281	320	17
DRY	oz.		Kcal/unit	gm	gm	gm	gm	gm	mg	mg	mg	mg	mg
Iams Recovery	cup	4.8	633 (4.6)	7.7	5.6	4.4	0.5	2.0	258	204	84	295	18

Specific Feeding Directions
1. Consider usual diet when choosing dry or canned form.
2. Feed favorite foods if risk of learned aversion is present.
3. Fed small frequent meals if appetite is poor.
4. Monitor food intake. If less than recommended in "energy needs of sedentary dogs and cats" see the section entitled "treating inappetance."

REDUCED FAT DIETS FOR DOGS

Marketed for use in patients with:	Enteritis, Exocrine Pancreatic Insufficiency, Pancreatitis (Convalescence phase), or Maldigestion, Malabsorption
Avoid feeding to patients with:	Increased nutrient needs
Nutrient Modifications:	moderate to reduced fat, fiber AND increased digestibility
Commercial substitutions:	restricted fat and fiber diets

Diets - Listed in decreasing order of fat gm/100 kcal

	Dog			Amount per 100 kcal									
Mfg. Diet	unit	Wt.	Energy	Protein (% of kcal)	Fat	CHO	Fiber	H2O	Ca	P	Na	K	Mg
CANNED		oz.	Kcal/unit	gm	gm	gm	gm	gm	mg	mg	mg	mg	mg
Purina EN	Can	12.5	424	7.6	3.4	12.1	0.2	58	220	130	90	150	NA
Hills i/d	Can	14.75	544	5.8	3.2	11.7	0.2	55	230	180	100	210	19
Waltham Canine low fat	Can	14.1	420	8.5	2.1	NA	0.6	7.3	370	330	190	240	40
DRY		oz.	Kcal/unit	gm	gm	gm	gm	gm	mg	mg	mg	mg	mg
Purina EN	Cup	3.7	397	6.1	2.8	13.1	0.3	2.4	330	210	90	140	NA
Hills i/d	Cup	3.5	379	6.3	3.3	12.4	0.3	2	270	190	110	220	22
Waltham Canine low fat	Cup	3.1	280	6.8	1.5	NA	0.1	10.6	220	250	130	250	30
Iams Adult Low Residue	Cup	2.9	328	5.9	2.5	129	0.5	NA	226	181	106	206	NA
Iams Puppy Low Residue	Cup	3.3	435	6.7	4.5	0.4	7.2	NA	241	188	157	88	NA

Feeding Directions
Small, frequent (>TID) feedings may enhance utilization and decrease signs

REDUCED SODIUM DIETS FOR DOGS

These diets may be used in conjunction with diuretics to treat fluid retention. In patients with congestive heart failure, one must consider that consumption of less that 10 mg sodium per pound (by normal dogs) has been reported to activate the renin-angiotensin-aldosterone system. Such activation may antagonize the effects of angiotensin-converting enzyme inhibitors.

Marketed for use in patients with:	Avoid feeding to patients with:	Nutrient Modifications	Commercial substitutions
Congestive heart failure with fluid retention, hypertension, ascites, edema	Increased nutrient needs, dehydration, diarrhea	Reduced sodium	Some geriatric diets and baby foods

Diets - listed in decreasing order of sodium mg/100 kcal

Dog				Amount per 100 kcal									
Mfg. Diet	unit	wt.	Energy	Protein (% of kcal)	Fat	CHO	Fiber	H2O	Ca	P	Na	K	Mg
CANNED		oz.	Kcal/ unit	gm	gm	gm	gm	gm	mg	mg	mg	mg	mg
Hills h/d	Can	14.75	538	3.7	6.2	10.4	0.2	55	150	120	20	180	27
Purina CV	Can	12.5	638	3.6	6.5	10.1	0.3	37	150	80	20	250	10
DRY		oz.	Kcal/ unit	gm	gm	gm	gm	gm	mg	mg	mg	mg	mg
Hills h/d	Cup	3.5	429	3.7	4.3	12.1	0.2	2	180	130	10	160	25

Feeding direction:
Dry diets may be preferable to decrease obligatory water intake. Canned canine diets should be used with caution for the reasons mentioned above. Dogs consuming 20 kcal per pound per day would receive only approximately 4 mg sodium per pound per day.

REDUCED PROTEIN, PHOSPHORUS DIETS FOR DOGS

Marketed for use in patients with:	Avoid feeding to patients with:	Nutrient modifications	Commercial Substitutions
Advanced kidney failure	Increased nutrient needs	Decreased phosphorus protein	Some geriatric diets
Advanced liver failure	Increased nutrient needs	Decreased protein	Some geriatric diets
Hypertension	Increased nutrient needs	Decreased sodium	Some geriatric diets

Diets - Listed in decreasing order of protein gm/100 kcal

Amount per 100 kcal

Mfg. Diet	unit	wt.	Energy	Protein (% kcal)	Fat	CHO	Fiber	H2O	Ca	P	Na	K	Mg
CANNED	oz.	Kcal/can	gm	gm	gm	gm	gm	mg	mg	mg	mg	mg
Waltham Med. Protein	Can	13.6	420	5.2 (21)	7	8.5	0.3	68	264	114	143	186	21
Waltham Low protein	Can	13.6	650	4.0	5.5	16	0.2	59	260	110	130	190	20
Modif. formula	Heinz	14	525	3.6 (13)	4.8	12.3	0.3	66	181	76	45	174	15
Purina NF	Can	12.5	500	3.5	5.9	10.8	0.4	NA	110	60	50	160	10
Hills k/d	Can	14.75	14.75	3.2	5.9	10.8	0.6	71	170	40	50	70	6
Hills u/d	Can	14.75	593	2.2	5.3	11.2	0.3	50	60	30	50	80	5
DRY	wt.	Energy Kcal/cup	Protein (% kcal)	Fat	CHO	Fiber	H2O	Ca	P	Na	K	Mg
Iams Early stage	Cup	2.4	264	4.7	3.1	8.1	1.0	2.6	200	101	122	162	NA
Waltham Med. Protein	Cup	3.2	280	4.6	3.6	NA	0.5	3.8	170	100	40	150	20
Purina NF	Cup	3.5	416	3.6	3.6	14.3	0.2	2.5	170	70	50	190	20
Waltham Low protein	Cup	3.2	310	3.5	2.7	NA	0.1	3.0	160	90	60	170	15
Iams Adv. Stage	Cup	2.4	292	3.0	2.8	6.7	0.9	2.3	145	54	108	126	NA
Hills k/d	Cup	3.5	414	3.3	4.3	13.7	0.2	2	190	70	40	70	14
Modif. formula	Heinz	2.9	362	3.1	4.2	12.6	0.4	15	183	76	60	189	20
Hills u/d	Hill's	2.7	346	1.9	4.2	13.1	0.5	2	80	40	50	120	7

Feeding Directions:
- Canned diets may be preferable to increase obligatory water intake in patients with chronic renal disease.
- Physical signs of protein depletion should be monitored in patients fed diets containing less than 5 (dogs) or 10 (cats) gm protein per 100 kcal if food intake is less than 20 kcal per pound per day.

REDUCED ENERGY DIETS FOR DOGS

Long term obesity therapy includes portion control and psychological support of the client. Diets with restricted fat, added fiber and/or water to "dilute" the calories may help ease the problem of acceptance of portion control. Unfortunately, no studies describing successful obesity therapy, which is maintenance of the lost weight for the life of the patient, are available. The following diets also may be used to maintain moderate body condition of patients with low energy needs (<approx. 15 kcal/pound/day).

Marketed for use in patients with:	Avoid feeding to patients with:	Nutrient Modifications	Commercial Substitutions
Obesity	Increased nutrient needs	Decreased fat, increased fiber, increased moisture	Reduced calorie diets

Diets - Listed in increasing order of kcal per gram

				Amount per 100 kcal									
Diet	Mfg	wt.	Energy	Protein (% kcal)	Fat	CHO	Fiber	H2O	Ca	P	Na	K	Mg
CANNED		oz.	Kcal/ unit (per gm)	gm	gm	gm	gm	gm	mg	mg	mg	mg	mg
Purina OM-Formula	Can	12	182 (0.53)	17.8	3.4	8.8	7.7	146	470	430	110	430	NA
Waltham Calorie control	Can	12.7	200 (0.55)	11.7	6.4	0.5	0.7	49	441	525	180	475	71
Hills r/d	Can	14.75	234 (0.58)	10.6	2.9	15.2	11	129	190	170	120	360	59
Hills w/d	Can	14.75	359 (0.87)	5.1	3.7	16.6	4.2	84	160	160	90	180	23
DRY		oz.	Kcal/ unit (per gm)	gm	gm	gm	gm	gm	mg	mg	mg	mg	mg
Purina OM-Formula	Cup	3.8	276 (2.6)	8.2	2.2	17.4	15.5	2.5	490	380	90	340	NA
Hills r/d	Cup	2.7	205 (2.7)	8.3	2.9	12.8	8	3	230	180	100	260	53
Hills w/d	Cup	2.7	223 (2.9)	5.1	2.1	16.8	5.1	3	170	150	60	240	37
Waltham Calorie Control	Cup	2.9	255 (3.4)	8.4	3.2	0.3	0.5	3.2	580	550	110	370	50
Iams Restricted-Calorie	Can	2.3	238 (3.6)	4.7	1.6	17.2	0.5	2.7	200	181	101	181	NA

Feeding directions: Please see <u>Guidelines for Obesity Therapy</u>

RESTRICTED MINERAL DIETS FOR DOGS

Restricted mineral diets are used to treat and/or reduce the risk of recurrence of urinary stones. The two most common stone types in dogs and cats are magnesium ammonium phosphate (struvite) and calcium oxalate. Two general cornerstones of therapy for stone disease are reduction of urine specific gravity to approximately 1.020, and elimination of urinary tract infection when present. For struvite, reduction of urine pH to 6-6.5, and reduction of solute excretion are desirable. For patients, a urine pH of approximately 7 should increase endogenous citrate excretion, and reduce urine calcium excretion. Diets containing less than 5 grams protein per 100 kcal should be used with appropriate caution to prevent protein depletion in patients consuming them.

Dogs

Marketed for use in canine patients with:	Avoid feeding to patients with:	Nutrient Modifications	Commercial Substitutions
Urolithiasis	Increased nutrient needs	Reduced minerals	Depends on stone type
Struvite	Oxalate urolithiasis	less protein (?), P, Mg, urine pH	Most dry cat foods
Oxalate		less protein (?), Ca; more Mg, citrate, urine pH	
Urate		less protein; more urine pH	

Diets - Listed in alphabetical order of manufacturer

		Dog		Amount per 100 kcal										
Mfg. Diet	unit	weight	Energy	Protein (% of kcal)	Fat	CHO	Fiber	H2O	Ca	P	Na	K	Mg
CANNED	oz.	Kcal/ unit	gm	gm	gm	gm	gm	mg	mg	mg	mg	mg		
Hills c/d	Can	14.75	436	5.9	6.2	12.5	0.2	69	160	120	80	130	70
Hills k/d	Can	I4.75	527	3.2	5.9	10.8	0.6	71	170	40	50	70	6
Hills s/d	Can	14.75	573	1.6	5.5	12.3	0.6	51	60	20	270	100	4
Hills u/d	Can	14.75	593	2.2	5.3	11.2	0.3	50	60	30	50	80	5
DRY	oz.	Kcal/ unit	gm	gm	gm	gm	gm	mg	mg	mg	mg	mg		
Hills c/d	Cup	3.5	413	4.8	4.6	11.1	0.5	2	140	110	60	130	24
Hills k/d	Cup	3.5	414	3.3	4.3	13.7	0.2	2	190	70	40	70	14
Hills u/d	Cup	2.7	346	1.9	4.2	13.1	0.5	2	80	40	50	120	7

Specific feeding directions:

Canned diets, or 1 cup water per cup dry diet, may be preferable to increase obligatory water intake. Addition of KCl, provided in gelatin capsules twice daily with meals, also has been recommended to increase water intake. Sodium chloride (NaCl) should not be used to increase water intake, because increasing urine sodium excretion may increase urine calcium excretion, and decrease urine citrate excretion. Addition of water or KCl should continue gradually until the urine specific gravity is in the range of 1.020.

Diet Table for Cats

Disease	Diets
Colitis (idiopathic)	Modified Fiber, p.686 Novel Protein, p.688
Congestive heart failure-advanced	Modified Fiber, p.686 and Reduced Sodium, p.691
Constipation	Modified Fiber, p.686
Critical Care	Nutrient Dense, p.689
Dermatitis due to food allergy	Novel Protein, p.688
Diabetes	Modified Fiber, p.686
Exocrine pancreatic insufficiency	Reduced Fat, p.690
Fluid Overload	Reduced Sodium, p.691
Hyperlipidemia	Reduced Fat, p.690
Hypertension	Reduced Protein, Phosphorus, p.690
Kidney failure-advanced	Reduced Protein, Phosphorus, p.690
Inflammatory bowel disease	Novel Protein, p.688
Liver Failure	Reduced Protein, Phosphorus, p.690
Obesity	Modified Fiber, p.686 and Reduced Energy ,p.692
Maldigestion, Malabsorption	Reduced Fat, p.690
Pancreatitis	Reduced Fat, p.690
Small bowel diarrhea	Nutrient Dense, p.689
Urolithiasis	Restricted Mineral ,p.693
Volume Restriction	Nutrient Dense, p.689

MODIFIED FIBER DIETS FOR CATS

The term "dietary fiber" describes a class of chemical compounds derived from plants. The effects of fiber consumption on physiological function depends on the type(s) of fiber ingested, effects of processing on fiber properties, and the amount consumed. Potentially desirable functions of fiber in small animal patients include bulking (insoluble or nonfermentable), and fermenting and gelling (soluble or fermentable). Increasing fiber intake has been suggested as part of treatment of the following problems:

Disease	Fiber Type	
	bulking	fermenting and gelling
Constipation	-	+
Diabetes	+	+
Idiopathic colitis	+	+
Small bowel diarrhea	-	+
Obesity	?	?

We currently cannot predict fiber function in patients very accurately. Rational use of dietary fiber will depend on results of clinical trials of commercial products, and assurance of consistency in formulation (dietary fiber is like wine in that the soil, weather, harvest and post-harvest practices all affect the quality and consistency of the final product).

Marketed for use in patients with:	Avoid feeding to patients with:	Nutrient Modifications	Commercial substitutions
Colitis	Increased nutrient needs	increased fiber	increased fiber products
Constipation	Increased nutrient needs	increased fiber	increased fiber products
Diabetes mellitus	Increased nutrient needs	increased fiber	increased fiber products
Hyperlipidemia	Increased nutrient needs	reduced fat	low fat foods
Obesity	Increased nutrient needs	reduced energy density	reduced calorie foods; sold as "lite" or "lean"

Diets - Listed in decreasing order of fiber gm/100kcal

	Cat			Amount per 100 kcal									
Mfg. Diet	unit	wt.	Energy	Protein (% of kcal)	Fat	CHO	Fiber	H2O	Ca	P	Na	K	Mg
CANNED		oz.	Kcal /unit	gm	gm	gm	gm	gm	mg	mg	mg	mg	mg
Hills r/d	Can	14.25 (5.5)	251 (98)	13.5	2.9	7.8	11.1	157	240	210	110	270	15.9
Hills w/d	Can	14.25 (5.5)	364 (142)	11.4	4.6	6.6	3.4	82	180	150	120	240	14
DRY		oz.	Kcal/ unit	gm	gm	gm	gm	gm	mg	mg	mg	mg	mg
Hills r/d	Cup	2.7	224	11.6	2.6	9.7	5.2	3	310	250	90	220	23
Purina OM	Cup	3.6	283	12.2	2.5	12	3.8	2.8	420	320	100	270	30
Hills w/d	Cup	2.7	246	11	2.7	10.2	2.5	3	290	240	70	200	21

Feeding directions:

Fiber also can be purchased separately and added (gradually, to effect) to the patient's current diet; some examples are given in the table below. Recommended dosages range widely; I recommend starting with 1 tablespoon per cup or can of food, and increasing to achieve the desired clinical effect. Clients should be told that the increase in feces volume and frequency that results from increased bulking fiber consumption is the intended effect.

Food	Amount per Tablespoon	Total fiber	Insoluble	Soluble
	gm	gm	gm	gm
Wheat bran	5.3	2.7	2.3	0.3
100% Bran cereal	6.4	1.8	1.6	0.2
Oat Bran	6.7	1	0.5	0.5
Metamucil	5.8	3.4	0.7	2.7

NOVEL PROTEIN DIETS FOR CATS

These diets are among the many foods available that contain proteins to which an allergic patient has not been exposed. They have been recommended for use in patients with skin or gastrointestinal signs of disease caused b y food allergies. Providing a novel protein source, and decreasing the amount of protein ingested (see, e.g., d/d) both may be beneficial. Because of the many proteins included in commercial pet foods, finding a only one, novel protein may not be easy. Home-made diets also have been recommended, especially for diagnosis of food allergy, and are presented in that section.

Marketed for use in patients with:	Avoid feeding to patients with:	Nutrient Modifications	Commercial substitutions
Dermatitis caused by food allergy	Increased nutrient needs	Protein to which the patient has not been exposed	Any containing a protein novel to the patient
Inflammatory bowel disease			

Diets - Listed in alphabetical order by manufacturer

	Cat				Amount per 100 kcal									
Mfg. Diet	unit	wt.	Energy	Protein (% of Kcal)	Fat	CHO	Fiber	H2O	Ca	P	Na	K	Mg
CANNED	oz.		Kcal/ unit	gm	gm	gm	gm	gm	mg	mg	mg	mg	mg
Hills d/d Lamb & Rice	Can	14.25 (5.5)	578 (224)	3.3	4.7	10.6	0.9	51	100	60	70	120	8
Iams Lamb & Barley	Can	6	222	7.9	4.9	9.6	0.3	159	251	206	76	130	12
Waltham Select Protein Venison	Can	6	165	9.8	5.8	7.5	0.7	101	330	270	230	290	20
DRY	oz.		Kcal/ unit	gm	gm	gm	gm	gm	mg	mg	mg	mg	mg
Iams Lamb & Rice	Cup	3.6	461	7.3	5.0	6.5	0.3	1.6	231	204	98	200	20
Iams Ocean fish & Rice	Cup	3.6	460	7.6	5.8	6.2	0.3	2.2	220	167	71	163	182
Waltham Select Protein Duck & Rice	Cup	NA	280	10	3.3	NA	1.2	630	370	200	250	25	NA

IVD INNOVATIVE DIETS

Diet								Amount per 100 kcal						
Cats	unit	wt.	Energy	Protein (% of kcal)	Fat	CHO	Fiber	H2O	Ca	P	Na	K	Mg
CANNED		oz.	Kcal/ unit	gm	gm	gm	gm	gm	mg	mg	mg	mg	mg
Venison & Potato	Ca n	5.5	183	9.2	7.5	1.2	0.1	NA	177	169	76	135	8
Rabbit & Potato	Ca n	5.5	176	7.9	7.0	3.5	0.2	NA	201	201	61	114	9
DRY		oz.	Kcal/ unit	gm	gm	gm	gm	gm	mg	mg	mg	mg	mg
Venison & Potato	Cu p	3.5	340	7.3	3.0	14.0	0.6	NA	248	202	61	231	17

Feeding directions:
Once a diagnosis of food allergy is made and a diet found that the patient does not react to, it will be important that the owner understand the importance of not permitting the patient to consume any foods that may contain provocative antigens.

NUTRIENT DENSE DIETS FOR CATS

Marketed for use in patients with:	Avoid feeding to patients with:	Nutrient Modifications (varies with diet)	Commercial substitutions
Increased nutrient needs	Decreased nutrient needs	Increased nutrient density	High protein high fat canned cat foods, meat baby foods
Volume restriction	"	"	"
Cats with diarrhea	"	"	"

Diets - listed in order of decreasing energy density

Diet	Mfg.	wt.	Energy					Amount per 100 kcal						
				Protein (% Kcal)	Fat	CHO	Fiber	H2O	Ca	P	Na	K	Mg
CANNED		oz/ca n	Kcal/ can (/gm)	gm	gm	gm	gm	gm	mg	mg	mg	mg	mg
Iams Recovery	Can	6	340 (2.1)	7.5 (26)	7.1	1.3	0.3	33	190	150	55	180	13
Hills p/d	Can	14.25	561 (1.4)	11	7.1	2.5	0.1	47	250	200	110	180	20
Chicken baby food	Heinz	2.5	100 (1.4)	9.8	7.2	0	0	33	64	120	40	135	NA
Hills a/d	Can	5.5	203 (1.3)	8.3	5.2	3.2	0.2	64	190	190	140	170	20
Abbott Clinicare	Can	8	237 (1)	8.6	5.3	7.1	NA	NA	152	126	63	157	11
Kal-Kan Sheba	Tin	3.5	78 (0.78)	13.8	5.3	NA	3.4	NA	470	310	281	320	17
DRY		oz./cu p	Kcal/ cup (/gm)	gm	gm	gm	gm	gm	mg	mg	mg	mg	mg
Iams Recovery	Cup	4.4	603 (4.8)	8.2 (29)	5.5	3.5	0.3	2.0	248	199	101	168	17

Specific Feeding Suggestions:
- Consider usual diet when choosing dry or canned form.
- Feed favorite foods if risk of learned aversion is present.
- Feed small frequent meals if appetite is poor.
- Monitor food intake. If less than recommended in "energy needs of sedentary dogs and cats", see the section entitled "treating inappetance".

REDUCED FAT DIETS FOR CATS

Marketed for use in patients with:	Enteritis, Exocrine Pancreatic Insufficiency, Pancreatitis (convalescence phase), or Maldigestion, Malabsorption
Avoid feeding to patients with:	Increased nutrient needs
Commercial substitutions:	Low fat, fiber diets

Diets - Listed in decreasing order of fat gm/100 kcal

		Cat			Amount per 100 kcal									
Mfg. Diet	unit	weight	Energy	Protein (% of kcal)	Fat	CHO	Fiber	H2O	Ca	P	Na	K	Mg
CANNED		oz.	Kcal/ unit	gm	gm	gm	gm	gm	mg	mg	mg	mg	mg
Hills i/d	Can	5.5	165	9.5	4.8	7.2	0.4	NA	280	190	90	250	22
DRY		oz.	Kcal/ unit	gm	gm	gm	gm	gm	mg	mg	mg	mg	mg
Hills i/d	Cup	4.3	473	9.5	4.8	7.6	0.3	NA	260	200	90	230	17
Purina EN	Pouch	1.5	117	9.5	3.8	7.3	0.2	14	380	450	70	180	30

Feeding directions:
Small, frequent (>TID) feedings may enhance utilization and decrease signs.

REDUCED PROTEIN, PHOSPHORUS DIETS FOR CATS

Marketed for use in patients with:	Avoid feeding to patients with:	Nutrient Modifications	Commercial Substitutions
Advanced kidney failure	Increased nutrient needs	Decreased phosphorus protein	Some geriatric diets
Advanced liver failure	Increased nutrient needs	Decreased protein	Some geriatric diets
Hypertension	Increased nutrient needs	Decreased sodium	Some geriatric diets

Diets - Listed in decreasing order of protein gm/100 kcal

Cat				Amount per 100 kcal									
Mfg./Diet	unit	wt.	Energy	Protein (% of kcal)	Fat	CHO	Fiber	H2O	Ca	P	Na	K	Mg
CANNED		oz.	Kcal/ can	gm	gm	gm	gm	gm	mg	mg	mg	mg	mg
Abbott Clinicare RF	Can	8	237	8.6	5.3	7.1	NA	NA	152	126	63	157	11.4
Waltham Low Protein	Can	6	250	6.1 (24)	9	4	0.1	51	210	95	100	190	20
Purina NF	Can	5.5	234	6.0	5.7	5.9	0.5	NA	200	100	30	190	20
Hills k/d	Can	14.25 (5.5)	584 (228)	5.6	7.8	4.7	0.5	49	110	100	30	190	8
Modif. formula	Heinz	14	618	6 (24)	9	1.3	0.3	47	122	83	39	116	10

DRY		oz.	Kcal/ cup	Protein	Fat	CHO	Fiber	H2O	Ca	P	Na	K	Mg
Purina NF	Cup	3.6	398	7.2 (29)	3	11.9	0.3	1.8	160	100	50	210	20
Modif. formula	Heinz	3.8	440	6.5 (23)	5	10.0	0.3	1	175	122	63	205	16
Hills k/d	Cup	4.3	519	6.1	6	8.4	0.1	2	170	130	60	140	11
Waltham Low Protein	Cup	3.4	385	5.4	5	NA	1.2	3	150	100	40	180	20

Feeding Directions:
- Canned diets may be preferable to increase obligatory water intake in patients with chronic renal disease.
- Physical signs of protein depletion should be monitored in patients fed diets containing less than 10 gm protein per 100 kcal if food intake is less than 20 kcal per pound per day.

REDUCED SODIUM DIETS FOR CATS

These diets may be used in conjunction with diuretics to treat fluid retention. In patients with congestive heart failure, one must consider that consumption of less than 10 mg sodium per pound (by normal dogs) has been reported to activate the renin-angiotensin-aldosterone system. Such activation may antagonize the effects of angiotensin-converting enzyme inhibitors.

Marketed for use in patients with:	Avoid feeding to patients with:	Nutrient Modifications	Commercial Substitutions
Congestive heart failure with fluid retention, hypertension, ascites, edema	Increased nutrient needs, dehydration, diarrhea	Reduced sodium	Some geriatric diets and baby foods

Diets - listed in decreasing order of sodium mg/100 kcal

Mfg. Diet	unit	wt.	Energy	Amount per 100 kcal									
				Protein (% of kcal)	Fat	CH O	Fibe r	H2 O	Ca	P	Na	K	Mg
CANNED		oz.	Kcal/ unit	gm	gm	gm	gm	gm	mg	mg	mg	mg	mg
Hills h/d	Can	14.25 (5.5)	538 (199)	10	6.2	5.3	0.1	56	180	160	70	210	16
Purina CV	Can	5.5	223	8.7	5.5	4.7	0.2	50	250	190	50	270	20

Feeding directions:
Dry diets may be preferable to decrease obligatory water intake. Canned canine diets should be used with caution for the reasons mentioned above.

REDUCED ENERGY DIETS FOR CATS

One aspect of obesity therapy, along with portion control and psychological support of the client, is provision of a diet with fewer calories than the one currently consumed, or a diet with added fiber or water to "dilute" the calories contained in the food. Unfortunately, no studies describing successful obesity therapy, defined as maintenance of the lost weight for the life of the patient, are available. The following diets also may be (better?) used to maintain moderate body condition of patients with low energy needs (<approximately 15 kcal/pound/day).

Marketed for use in patients with:	Avoid feeding to patients with:	Nutrient Modifications (varies with diet)	Commercial substitutions
Obesity	Increased nutrient needs	Decreased fat, increased fiber, moisture	Reduced calorie diets

Diets - Listed in increasing order of kcal per gram

Diet	Mfg.	wt.	Energy	Protein (% kcal)	Amount per 100 kcal									
					Fat	CHO	Fiber	H2O	Ca	P	Na	K	Mg
CANNED		oz.	Kcal/U (/gm)	gm	gm	gm	gm	gm	mg	mg	mg	mg	mg
Waltham Calorie Control	Can	6	100 (0.59)	12.5	4.8	NA	0.5	148	520	400	330	370	20
Hills r/d	Can	14.25	251 (0.63)	13.5	2.9	7.8	11	121	240	210	110	270	15.9
Hills w/d	Can	14.25	364 (0.91)	11.4	4.6	6.6	3.4	82	180	150	120	240	14
DRY		oz.	Kcal/U (/gm)	gm	gm	gm	gm	gm	mg	mg	mg	mg	mg
Purina OM	Cup	3.6	283 (2.7)	12.2 (43)	2.5	12	3.8	3	420	320	100	270	30
Hills r/d	Cup	2.7	224 (3.0)	11.6	2.6	9.7	5.2	3	310	280	90	220	23
Hills w/d	Cup	2.7	246 (3.2)	11.1 (39)	2.7	10.2	2.5	3	290	240	70	200	21
Waltham Calorie Control	Cup	2.4	228 (3.3)	13.0	2.3	NA	1.4	3.6	640	410	210	320	20

Feeding directions   Please see <u>Guidelines for Obesity Therapy</u>

RESTRICTED MINERAL DIETS FOR CATS

Restricted mineral diets are used to treat and/or reduce the risk of recurrence of urinary stones. The two most common stone types in dogs and cats are magnesium ammonium phosphate (struvite) and calcium oxalate. Two general cornerstones of therapy for stone disease are reduction of urine specific gravity to approximately 1.020, and elimination of urinary tract infection when present. For struvite, reduction of urine pH to 6-6.5, and reduction of solute excretion are desirable. For patients, a urine pH of -7 should increase endogenous citrate excretion, and reduce urine calcium excretion. Diets containing less than 5 grams protein per 100 kcal should be used with appropriate caution to prevent protein depletion in patients consuming them.

Marketed for use in feline patients with:	Avoid feeding to patients with:	Nutrient Modifications	Commercial substitutions
Urolithiasis	Increased nutrient needs	Reduced minerals	Depends on stone type
Struvite		less Mg, urine pH	Many commercial diets
Oxalate		less Ca; more Mg, citrate, urine pH	Canned diets not modified to reduce struvite risk

Mfg. Diet	unit	wt.	Energy	Protein	Fat	CHO	Fiber	H20	Ca	P	Na	K	Mg
								Amount per 100 kcal					
CANNED	oz.		Kcal/unit	gm	gm	gm	gm		mg	mg	mg	mg	mg
Struvite													
Hills c/d-S	Can	14.25 (5.5)	423 (164)	9.9	5	5.7	0.74		140	120	140	190	13.4
Hills s/d	Can	14.25 (5.5)	552 (245)	8.8	7.1	3.4	0.3		130	110	180	200	9
Iams pH/S	Can	6	197	9.5	6.2	3.5	0.2		242	190	95	181	21
Purina UR	Can	12.5 (5.5)	493 (217)	8.6	7.6	3.4	0.02		190	170	90	200	10
Waltham Control pH	Can	6	175	7.2	8.4	1.0	0.1		250	210	220	250	20
Oxalate		oz.	Energy	Protein	Fat	CHO	Fiber		Ca	P	Na	K	Mg
Iams pH/O	Can	6	197	9.2	5.9	3.2	0.2		233	173	99	267	23
Hills c/d-O	Can	5.5	162	9.6	4.5	7.1	0.43		150	130	70	200	20.2
DRY			Add 1 cup water/cup food and soak for at least 5 minutes before feeding										
Struvite		oz.	Energy	Protein	Fat	CHO	Fiber		Ca	P	Na	K	Mg
Hills c/d-S	Cup	2.7	285	8.5	4	10.5	0.2		210	160	90	200	13.3
Hills s/d	Cup	4.3	521	7.5	5.6	7.1	0.1		150	180	150	160	12
Iams pH/S	Cup	3.6	437	7.8	3.9	8	0.4		236	203	112	198	18
Purina UR	Cup	3.3	366	8.3	2.7	10.7	0.3		260	200	60	200	20
Waltham Control pH	Cup	3.2	410	9.4	4.6	32	0.5		190	200	210	270	20
Oxalate		oz.	Energy	Protein	Fat	CHO	Fiber		Ca	P	Na	K	Mg
Iams pH/O	Cup	3.7	450	7.7	3.9	8	0.4		238	205	104	305	19
Hills c/d-O	Cup	2.7	286	8.4	4.1	10.3	0.3		200	160	100	200	19.6

Specific feeding directions:
Canned diets, or 1 cup water per cup dry diet, may be preferable to increase obligatory water intake. ADDITION OF KCl, provided in gelatin capsules twice daily with meals, also has been recommended to increase water intake. Sodium chloride (NaCl) should not be used to increase water intake, because increasing urine sodium excretion may increase urine calcium excretion, and decrease urine citrate excretion. Addition of water or KCl should continue gradually until the urine specific gravity is in the range of 1.020.

Chemotherapy Protocols for Treatment of Neoplastic Diseases In Small Animals

Carrie A. Wood, DVM, Jeffrey S. Klausner, DVM, MS,
Chand Khanna, DVM, PhD, & Ford Watson Bell, DVM, MS

Editor's Note: The following protocols are presently being used by the Veterinary Comparative Oncology group at the University of Minnesota Veterinary Teaching Hospitals. Other protocols for chemotherapeutic agents to treat neoplastic diseases may be found in numerous references. Because there is considerable ongoing clinical research in veterinary oncology, the reader is urged to follow the current literature, as therapeutic protocols for animals with neoplastic diseases will be continuously modified.

Canine Lymphoma Treatment Protocol

Week 1
    A. Prednisone 40 mg/m^2 PO; continue once daily throughout 12 weeks
    B. L-Asparaginase injection 20,000U/m^2 SQ

Week 2
    A. Vincristine injection 0.65 mg/m^2 IV
    B. Cyclophosphamide tablets 50 mg/m^2 on days 3, 4, 5, and 6 of week 2

Week 3
    A. Perform CBC; must have results before treating
    B. Doxorubicin 30 mg/m^2 IV

Week 4
    A. Perform CBC; must have results before treating
    B. Vincristine injection 0.65 mg/m^2 IV

Week 5
    A. Vincristine injection 0.65 mg/m^2 IV
    B. Cyclophosphamide tablets 50 mg/m^2 PO on days 3, 4, 5, and 6 of week 5

Week 6
    A. Perform CBC; must have results before treating
    B. Doxorubicin 30 mg/m^2 IV

Week 7
    A. Off; No chemotherapy

Week 8
    A. Vincristine injection 0.65 mg/m^2 IV
    B. Cyclophosphamide tablets 50 mg/m^2 PO on days 3, 4, 5, and 6 of week 8

Week 9
    A. Perform CBC; must have results before treating
    B. Doxorubicin 30 mg/m^2 IV

Week 10
    A. Perform CBC; must have results before treating
    B. Vincristine injection 0.65 mg/m^2 IV

Week 11
    A. Vincristine injection 0.65 mg/m^2 IV
    B. Cyclophosphamide tablets 50 mg/m^2 on days 3, 4, 5, and 6 of week 11

Week 12
    A. Vincristine injection 0.65 mg/m^2 IV
    B. Chlorambucil 4 mg/m^2 PO every other day
    C. Prednisone 40 mg/m^2 PO every other day

Maintenance
    A. Vincristine injection 0.65 mg/m^2 IV every 3 weeks
    B. Chlorambucil 4 mg/m^2 PO every other day
    C. Prednisone 40 mg/m^2 PO every other day

Doxorubicin Protocol for Canine Lymphosarcoma

1. Induction Phase

    A. Doxorubicin (*Adriamycin*®): 30 mg/M^2 given intravenously once ever 14 days for 5 cycles.

2. Maintenance Phase

There is no maintenance therapy on this protocol. Animals completing the induction phase should be evaluated every 2-3 months.

B. Special Precautions

1. Avoid extravasation of the drug. Use an indwelling catheter.
2. Reconstituted drug should be administered over a period of about 20 minutes into the side port of a freely running intravenous infusion of 0.9% NaCl.
3. Allergic reactions to the drug during administration may occur. Premedication with diphenhydramine (Benadryl) is recommended at a rate of 10 mg for dogs less that 20 pounds; 20 mg for dogs 20-60 pounds; and 30 mg for dogs over 60 pounds.
4. Doxorubicin can cause dose-dependent cardiotoxicity. Dogs should not receive more than 150 mg/M^2 cumulative total dose. Preexisting cardiac disease should be ruled out with a ECG and echocardiogram. Generally, dogs with severe arrhythmias or a decreased ventricular shortening fraction should not receive doxorubicin.
5. Anorexia, vomiting and/or diarrhea may be observed 2-5 days post therapy. Clinical signs vary from mild to severe.
6. Doxorubicin may cause severe neutropenia. A CBC should be evaluated 7 days following the first doxorubicin injection and prior to subsequent injections. If neutrophil count decreased to <1000/µl, the drug should not be administered and the dose reduced 25% at the next administration.
7. Special precautions for handling doxorubicin:
    a. Doxorubicin should be reconstituted in a biologic safety hood, if possible.
    b. Skin contact with the drug should be avoided.
    c. Care should be taken to avoid inhalation of the powder.
    d. Double gloves should be worn when handling the drug.
    e. Pregnant females should avoid handling or administering the drug.

Canine Lymphosarcoma Reinduction of Remission Protocol

INDICATIONS: For use in patients that have come out of remission on other protocols.

1. DRUGS:

    A. L-Asparginase: 20,000 units/m^2 SQ on week one
    B. Doxorubicin: 30 mg/M^2 intravenously on days 8, 22, 36, & 50

    CBC's: 7 days post doxorubicin

Canine Sarcoma and Carcinoma Treatment Protocol "AC"

I. INDICATIONS

This protocol is indicated for the treatment of thyroid and mamary carcinomas in the dog, either as primary therapy for non-resectable tumors or as adjuvant therapy following surgery.

II. DRUGS

    A. Doxorubicin (*Adriamycin*®): 30 mg/M^2 IV on day 1
    B. Cyclophosphamide (*Cytoxan*®): 50 mg/M^2 PO on days 3-6
    C. Repeat every 21 days for a total of 3 cycles.

III. TOXICITIES

Doxorubicin may be associated with a variety of toxicities in the dog. Acute toxicities include anaphylaxis and cardiac arrhythmias. Short-term toxicities may include gastrointestinal toxicity and myelosuppression. The principal chronic toxicity is a cummulative, dose dependant, cardiac toxicity leading to myocardial degeneration and irreversible congestive heart failure. Total doxorubicin dose should not exceed 250 mg/M^2. A CBC, including a platelet count should be monitored 10 days following initial therapy and subsequently prior to each new cycle. If the neutrophil count falls below 1,000/µl or platelet counts fall below 50,000/µl, treatment should be suspended until these counts return to normal.

IV. ANAPHALAXIS PREVENTION

10-30 mg diphenhydramine should be given intravenously prior to administration of doxorubicin (or IM 1/2 hour prior to administration of doxorubicin).

V. MISCELLANEOUS

A. If *Cytoxan*® tablets need to be split, have this done by the pharmacy. Also advise clients to wear gloves during administration.

B. Doxorubicin and its metabollites are excreted in the urine. Clients who are pregnant should not come in contact with urine from treated animals for at least 72 hours following therapy.

C. Doxorubicin should be reconstituted under a laminar-flow hood. Delivery of the drug should be done with extreme care, including double-gloving of the administrator and holder.

Canine Osteogenic Sarcoma Adjuvant Protocol

I. INDICATIONS: use following limb amputation in dogs with osteogenic sarcoma

II. DRUGS

A. Carboplatin: 300 mg/m2 IV every 3weeks for 3 courses; CBC at 21 days

B. Alternatively: May use the **Doxorubicin Protocol for Canine Lymphosarcoma** outlined previosuly .

Canine Multiple Myeloma Chemotherapy Protocol

I. DRUGS

A. Melphalan: 0.1 mg/kg PO daily for 10 days; then 0.05 mg/kg daily, **continuously**

B. Prednisone: 0.5 mg/kg PO daily for 10 days; then 0.5 mg/kg on alternate days, **continuously.**

II. ADMINISTRATION AND USES

A. Melphalan is an alkylating agent which tends to be less toxic than cyclophosphamide. However, bone marrow suppression may occur. Monthly re-checks are advisable during chronic therapy with melphalan. Long term administration commonly results in thrombocytopenia.

B. Myeloma patients are extremely susceptible to infection. Care should be taken with invasive procedures. On-going infections should be treated following results of culture and sensitivity testing.

C. Cyclophosphamide may be substituted for melphalan when resistance develops, but beware of hemorraghic cystitis secondary to cyclophosphamide and discontinue at first sign.

D. Careful staging work-up is important and should include: serum and urine electropheresis and a bone marrow biopsy and aspirate.

Treatment Protocol For Canine Mast Cell Sarcoma

First occurrence of a single tumor w/o metastasis and well differentiated: (Grade I)

1. Wide Surgical Excision (No follow-up therapy if surgical margins are clean)

First occurrence of a single tumor w/o metastasis and intermediate or poorly differentiated

1. Wide Surgical Excision*
2. Radiation Therapy Following Excision--Probably Best Alternative (94% disease free interval at 1 year, n=342 in recent AMC study)
3. Prednisone and Lomustine Therapy Following Excision--Alternative Therapy

Single Tumor with LN Metastasis: Any Histologic Stage

1. Wide Surgical Excision of Tumor and Lymph Node
2. Radiation Therapy to Excision Site(s)--Best Alternative
3. Prednisone and Lomustine Following Excision (in addition to radiation or alone if radiation is not selected)

Prednisone Dose: 40-50 mg/M^2 PO for a week, then 20-25 mg/M^2 PO every other day
Lomustine (CCNU) Dose: 90 mg/M^2 PO every 4 weeks for 6 months (Note: Neutorpenia at 7 days post tx and thrombocytopenia at 21 days post tx and with long term administration)

* Local injection of a glucocorticoid is an alternative to surgery and radiation therapy although ability to achieve local control is significantly reduced. Triamcinolone acetonide, 1 mg intralesionally per cm of tumor every 2-3 weeks can be used.

Feline Lymphoma Treatment Protocol "COPA"

Week 1
    A. Prednisone 40 mg/m^2 PO; continue once daily to week 7s
    B. Vincristine injection 0.65 mg/m^2 IV
    C. Cyclophosphamide tablets 300 mg/m^2 PO (given at clinic)

Week 2
    A. Perform CBC; must have results before treating
    B. Vincristine injection 0.65 mg/m^2 IV

Week 3
    A. Vincristine injection 0.65 mg/m^2 IV

Week 4
    A. Vincristine injection 0.65 mg/m^2 IV
    B. Cyclophosphamide tablets 300 mg/m^2 PO (given at clinic)

Week 5
    A. Perform CBC and serum creatinine

Week 7
    A. Doxorubicin 25 mg/m^2 IV
    B. Begin taper of prednisone dosage

Week 8
    A. Perform CBC and serum creatinine

Week 10
    A. Doxorubicin 25 mg/m^2 IV

Week 11
    A. Perform CBC and serum creatinine

Week 13
    A. Doxorubicin 25 mg/m^2 IV

Week 16
    A. Doxorubicin 25 mg/m^2 IV

Week 19
    A. Doxorubicin 25 mg/m^2 IV

Week 20
    A. Perform CBC and serum creatinine

Week 22
    A. Doxorubicin 25 mg/m^2 IV

Week 25
    A. Doxorubicin 25 mg/m^2 IV

Week 26
    A. Perform CBC and serum creatinine

Chemotherapy agents should be administered on the same day of each week; if not possble, give the following day. After 26 week protocol completed, once monthly rechecks are recommended to ensure that cat is maintaining remission.

Conversion Tables for Weight in Kilograms to Body Surface Area (m^2)

The following tables are derived from the equation:

Approximate Surface area in m^2 = $\dfrac{10.1\ (\textit{10.0 for cats})\ \times\ (\text{weight in grams})^{2/3}}{10000}$

DOGS

Kg	m^2		Kg	m^2
0.5	0.06		33	1.03
1	0.10		34	1.05
2	0.15		35	1.07
3	0.20		36	1.09
4	0.25		37	1.11
5	0.29		38	1.13
6	0.33		39	1.15
7	0.36		40	1.17
8	0.40		41	1.19
9	0.43		42	1.21
10	0.46		43	1.23
11	0.49		44	1.25
12	0.52		45	1.26
13	0.55		46	1.28
14	0.58		47	1.30
15	0.60		48	1.32
16	0.63		49	1.34
17	0.66		50	1.36
18	0.69		52	1.41
19	0.71		54	1.44
20	0.74		56	1.48
21	0.76		58	1.51
22	0.78		60	1.55
23	0.81		62	1.58
24	0.83		64	1.62
25	0.85		66	1.65
26	0.88		68	1.68
27	0.90		70	1.72
28	0.92		72	1.75
29	0.94		74	1.78
30	0.96		76	1.81
31	0.99		78	1.84
32	1.01		80	1.88

CATS

Kg	m^2
2.0	0.159
2.5	0.184
3.0	0.208
3.5	0.231
4.0	0.252
4.5	0.273
5.0	0.292
5.5	0.311
6.0	0.330
6.5	0.348
7.0	0.366
7.5	0.383
8.0	0.400
8.5	0.416
9.0	0.432
9.5	0.449
10	0.464

Tables of Parenteral Fluids

(Not a complete listing; includes both human- and veterinary-approved products.)

SODIUM CHLORIDE INJECTIONS

Solution	Sodium (mEq/L)	Chloride (mEq/L)	Osmolality (mOsm/L)	Available as:
Sodium Chloride 0.2%	34	34	69	3 ml
Sodium Chloride 0.45% (Half-Normal Saline)	77	77	155	3, 5, 500, and 1000 ml
Sodium Chloride 0.9% (Normal Saline)	154	154	310	1, 2, 2.5. 3, 4, 5, 10, 20, 25, 30, 50, 100, 130, 150, 250, 500, & 1000 ml
Sodium Chloride 3%	513	513	1030	500 ml
Sodium Chloride 5%	855	855	1710	500 ml

DEXTROSE SOLUTIONS

Solution	Dextrose (g/L)	Calories (kCal/L)	Osmolality (mOsm/L)	Available as:
Dextrose 2.5%	25	85	126	250, 500, & 1000 ml
Dextrose 5%	50	170	253	10, 25, 50, 100, 130, 150, 250, 400, 500, 1000 ml
Dextrose 10%	100	340	505	250, 500, & 1000 ml
Dextrose 20%	200	680	1010	500 & 1000 ml
Dextrose 25%	250	850	1330	in 10 ml syringes
Dextrose 30%	300	1020	1515	500 & 1000 ml
Dextrose 38.5%	385	1310	1945	1000 ml
Dextrose 40%	400	1360	2020	500 & 1000 ml
Dextrose 50%	500	1700	2525	50, 250, 500, & 1000 ml
Dextrose 60%	600	2040	3030	500 & 1000 ml
Dextrose 70%	700	2380	3535	250, 500, & 1000 ml

DEXTROSE/ELECTROLYTE COMBINATIONS

Solution	D$_5$ in Ringer's	D$_{2.5}$ in half-strength Lactated Ringers	D$_5$ in Lactated Ringers	Normosol® -M w/D$_5$; Plasma-Lyte 56 w/D$_5$	Plasma-Lyte® 148 and D$_5$	Normosol® -R and D$_5$
Dextrose (g/L)	50	25	50	50	50	50
Calories (kCal/L)	170	89	179	170	190	185
Na$^+$ (mEq/L)	147	65.5	130	40	140	140
K$^+$ (mEq/L)	4	2	4	13	5	5
Ca^{++} (mEq/L)	4.5	1.4	2.7			
Mg^{++} (mEq/L)				3	3	3
Cl$^-$ (mEq/L)	156	54	109	40	98	98
Gluconate (mEq/L)					23	23
Lactate (mEq/L)		14	28			
Acetate (mEq/L)				16	27	27
Osmolarity (mOsm/L)	562	263	527	368 (363)	547	552
Available as:	500 & 1000 ml	250, 500 & 1000 ml	250, 500 & 1000 ml	500 & 1000 ml	500 & 1000 ml	500 & 1000 ml

ELECTROLYTE COMBINATION INJECTIONS

Solution	Ringer's Injection	Lactated Ringer's Injection (LRS)	Plasma-Lyte® 56	Plasma-Lyte® R	Plasma-Lyte A; Normosol® -R pH 7.4	Isolyte® S pH 7.4
Na$^+$ (mEq/L)	147	130	40	140	140	141
K$^+$ (mEq/L)	4	4	13	10	5	5
Ca^{++} (mEq/L)	4	3		5		
Mg^{++} (mEq/L)			3	3	3	3
Cl$^-$ (mEq/L)	156	109	40	103	98	98
Gluconate (mEq/L)					23	23
Lactate (mEq/L)		28		8		
Acetate (mEq/L)			16	47	27	29
Osmolarity (mOsm/L)	310	272	111	312	294 (295)	295
Available as:	250, 500, 1000 ml	250, 500, 1000, 5000 ml	500 & 1000 ml	1000 ml	500, 1000, & 5000 ml	500 & 1000 ml

DEXTROSE/SALINE COMBINATIONS

Solution	Na$^+$ (mEq/L)	Cl$^-$ (mEq/L)	Dextrose (g/L)	Calories (kCal/L)	Osmolality (mOsm/L)	Available as:
D$_{2.5}$ & 0.45% NaCl	77	77	25	85	280	250, 500, & 1000 ml
D$_5$ & 0.11% NaCl	19	19	50	170	290	500 & 1000 ml
D$_5$ & 0.2% NaCl	34	34	50	170	320	250, 500, & 1000 ml
D$_5$ & 0.33% NaCl	56	56	50	170	365	250, 500, & 1000 ml
D$_5$ & 0.45% NaCl	77	77	50	170	405	250, 500, & 1000 ml
D$_5$ & 0.9% NaCl	154	154	100	170	560	250, 500, & 1000 ml
D$_{10}$ & 0.45% NaCl	77	77	100	340	660	1000 ml
D$_{10}$ & 0.9% NaCl	154	154	100	340	815	500 & 1000 ml

ABBREVIATIONS USED IN PRESCRIPTION WRITING

A warning; and the strange case of S.I.D.: Although prescription abbreviations are used throughout this reference and they are fairly well recognized, they do increase the potential for mistakes to occur. When writing a prescription, this author recommends writing out the directions in plain English and avoiding the use of abbreviations entirely. If abbreviations are to be used, definitely avoid q.d., q.o.d., and s.i.d. because they can be easily confused with other abbreviations.

S.I.D. is virtually unknown to health professionals outside of veterinary medicine and the vast majority of pharmacists have never seen it used. S.I.D. should be eliminated from all veterinary usage.

a.c.	before meals		o.s.	left eye
a.d.	right ear		o.u.	both eyes
a.s.	left ear		p.c.	after meals
a.u.	both ears		p.o.	by mouth
amp.	ampule		p.r.n.	as needed
b.i.d.	twice a day		q.	every
c.	with		q4h, etc	every 4 hours
cap.	capsule		q.i.d.	four times a day
cc	cubic centimeter		q.o.d.	every other day
disp.	dispense		q.s.	a sufficient quantity
g or gm	gram		q4h	every 4 hours, etc.
gtt(s).	drop(s)		s.i.d.	once a day
h.	hour		Sig:	directions to pt.
h.s.	at bedtime		stat	immediately
IM	intramuscular		SubQ, SQ, SC, Subcut	
IP	intraperitoneal			subcutaneous
IV	intravenous		susp.	suspension
lb.	pound		t.i.d.	three times a day
m^2	meter squared		tab	tablet
mg.	milligram		Tbsp.	tablespoon (15 ml)
ml.	milliliter		tsp.	teaspoon (5 ml)
o.d.	right eye		Ut dict.	as directed

Solubility Definitions

The following definitions are used throughout the book in the chemistry section for each agent:

Descriptive Term	Parts of Solvent for 1 part of solute
Very Soluble...........................	Less than 1
Freely Soluble..........................	From 1 to 10
Soluble..................................	From 10 to 30
Sparingly Soluble.....................	From 30 to 100
Slightly Soluble........................	From 100 to 1000
Very Slightly Soluble..................	From 1000 to 10,000
Practically Insoluble, or Insoluble	More than 10,000

CONVERSION TABLES

WEIGHTS:

1 Pound (lb.) = 0.454 kg = 454 grams = 16 ounces

1 kilogram (kg) = 2.2 pounds = 1000 grams

1 grain (gr.) = 64.8 mg (often rounded to 60 or 65 mg)

1 gram = 15.43 grains = 1000 mg

1 ounce = 28.4 grams

1 gram = 1000 mg

1 milligram (mg) = 1000 mcg (μg)

1 microgram (mcg or μg) = 1000 nanograms (ng)

LIQUID MEASURE:

1 gallon (gal.) = 4 qts. = 8 pts. = 128 fl. oz. = 3.785 liters = 3785 ml

1 quart (qt) = 2 pints = 32 fl. oz. = 946 ml

1 pint = 2 cups = 16 fl. oz. = 473 ml

1 cup = 8 fl. oz = 237 ml = 16 tablespoons

1 tablespoon = 15 ml = 3 teaspoons

1 teaspoon = 5 ml

4 liters = 1.057 gals.

1 liter = 1000 ml = 10 deciliters

1 deciliter (dl) = 100 ml

1 milliliter (ml) = 1 cubic centimeter (cc) = 1000 microliters (μl)

TEMPERATURE CONVERSION:

9 x (°C) = (5 x °F) - 160;   °C to °F = (°C x 1.8) + 32 = °F;   °F to °C = (°F - 32) x .555 = °C

MILLEQUIVALENTS & MOLECULAR WEIGHTS

Milliequivalents: The term milliequivalents (mEq) is usually used to express the quantities of electrolytes administered to patients. A mEq is 1/1000 of an equivalent (Eq). For pharmaceutical purposes an equivalent may be thought of as equal to the equivalent weight of a given substance. This, in practical terms, is the molecular weight of the substance divided by the valence or the radical. For example:

How many milligrams are equivalent to 1 mEq of potassium chloride (KCl)?
1. Determine the equivalent weight = gram atomic weight ÷ valence
   Molecular weight of KCl = 74.5
   Valence = 1 (K^+; Cl^-)
   Equivalent weight = 74.5 ÷ 1 = 74.5 grams

2. Determine the mEq weight
   Equivalent weight ÷ 1000
   74.5 ÷ 1000 = 74.5 mg = 1 mEq of KCl = 1 mEq of K^+ & 1 mEq of Cl^-

If the substance would have been $CaCl_2$, the process would be identical using the gram molecular weight of $CaCl_2$ (MW 111 if anhydrous; 147 if dihydrate) and a valence of 2.

Listed below are several commonly used electrolytes with their molecular weights and valences in parentheses:

Sodium Chloride	58.44 (1)	Calcium Chloride	
Sodium Bicarbonate	84 (1)	anhydrous	111 (2)
Sodium Acetate		dihydrate	147 (2)
anhydrous	82 (1)	Magnesium Sulfate	
trihydrate	136 (1)	heptahydrate	246.5 (2)
Sodium Lactate	112 (1)	anhydrous	120.4 (2)
Potassium Chloride	74.55 (1)	Magnesium Chloride	
Potassium Gluconate	234.25 (1)	anhydrous	95.21 (2)
Calcium Gluconate	430.4 (2)	hexahydrate	203.3 (2)
Calcium Lactate (anhydrous) 218.22 (2)			

"Normal" Vital Signs

Temperature (Rectal) : Temperatures will normally fluctuate over the course of the day. The following may increase body temperature: Time of day (evening), food intake, muscular activity, approaching estrus, during gestation, high external temperatures. The following may decrease body temperature: intake of large quantities of cool fluids, time of day (morning), and low atmospheric temperature.

	Celsius (°C)	Fahrenheit (°F)
Cattle		
up to 1 year old	38.6 - 39.4	101.5 - 103.5
over 1 year	37.8 - 39.2	100 - 102.5
Cat	37.8 - 39.5	100 - 103.1
Dog	37.5 - 39.2	99.5 - 102.5

(Small breeds tend to have higher normal temps than large breeds)

	Celsius (°C)	Fahrenheit (°F)
Ferret	37.8 - 39.2	100 - 102.5
Goat	38.5 - 40.2	101.3 - 104.5
Horse		
adult	37.2 - 38.5	99 - 101.3
foal	37.5 - 39.3	99.5 - 102.7
Rabbit	38.5 - 40.5	100.4 - 105
Sheep	38.5 - 40	101.3 - 104
Swine		
piglet	38.9 - 40	102 - 104
adult	37.8 - 38.9	100 - 102

Pulse Rates (resting and healthy) in beats per minute (BPM)
Pulse rates for very young animals are usually in the higher ranges and older animals in the lower ranges of those values listed.

Cattle	
calves	100 - 120
adults	55 - 80
Cat	
Young	130 - 140
Old	100 - 120
Dog	
Young	110 - 120
Adult, large breed	80 - 120
Ferret	300
Goat	70 - 120
Horse	
adult	28 - 40
3 mos - 2 yr.	40 - 80
foals to 3 mos.	64 - 128
Rabbit	120 - 150
Sheep	55 - 115
Swine	
young	100 - 130
adult	60 - 90

Respiratory Rates (resting & healthy) respirations per minute

Cat	20 - 30
Cattle	
Young	15 - 40
Adult	10 - 30
Dog	15 - 30
Ferret	33 - 36
Horse	10 - 14
Pigs	8 - 18
Rabbit	50 - 60
Sheep, Goat	10 - 30

Estrus and Gestation Periods for Dogs & Cats

	DOG	**CAT**
Appearance of first estrus at the age of:	7 - 9 months	4 - 12 months
Estrous cycle in animals not served:	Mean = 7 mos. Range = q5 - 8 mos.	every 4 - 30 days (14-19 day model) if constant photoperiod
Duration of estrus period:	7 - 42 days (proestrus + estrus)	2 - 19 days
First occurrence after parturition:	see estrous cycle; pregnancy does not alter interval	7 - 9 days
Gestation period :	Mean = 63 days Range = 58-71 days Probably not related to size	Mean = 63 days Range = 58-70 days
Number of Young:	8 - 12 Large Breeds 6 - 10 Med. Breeds 2 - 4 Small Breeds	4 - 6
Suckling Period:	3 - 6 weeks	3 - 6 weeks

Conversion of Conventional Chemistry Units to SI Units

The Système Internationale d'Unites (SI), or the International System of Units was recommended for use in the health professions by the World Health Assembly in 1977. It is slowly being adopted in the United States and many journals now require its use. The following is an abbreviated table of conversion values for some of the more commonly encountered tests that may now be reported in SI Units.

Albumin	g/dl x 10 = g/L
Ammonia	μg/dl x 0.5872 = μmol/L
Bilirubin	mg/dl x 17.10 = μmol/L
Calcium	mg/dl x 0.2495 = mmol/L
Cholesterol	mg/dl x 0.02586 = mmol/L
CO_2 pressure, pCO_2	mmHg x 0.1333 = kPa
Creatinine	mg/dl x 88.4 = μmol/L
Glucose	mg/dl x 0.05551 = mmol/L
Lactate	mg/dl x 0.111 = mmol/L
Magnesium	mg/dl x 0.4114 = mmol/L
O_2 pressure, pO_2	mmHg x 0.1333 = kPa
Phosphorus	mg/dl x 0.3229 = mmol/L
Protein	g/dl x 10 = g/L
Urea Nitrogen	mg/dl x 0.7140 = mmol/L
Amylase	IU/L = U/L
AST (SGOT)	IU/L = U/L
ALT (SGPT)	IU/L = U/L
Lipase	IU/L = U/L
ALP	IU/L = U/L
SDH (Sorbitol)	IU/L = U/L

Bicarbonate, Chloride, CO_2 (total), Potassium, & Sodium do not require conversion from conventional to SI units.

Reference Laboratory Values: Dogs & Cats

The following reference values are those presently being used at the University of Minnesota, Veterinary Teaching Hospital. They should be used as a general reference only; refer to the laboratory normals from the lab you are using for specific reference values applicable to your practice situation.

HEMATOLOGY

	DOG	CAT
PCV (%)	37.0 - 55.0	24.0 - 45.0
Hct	29.8 - 57.5	25.8 - 41.8
Hb (g/dl)	12.4 - 19.1	8.5 - 14.4
RBC ($\times 10^6/\mu l$)	5.2 - 8.06	4.95 - 10.53
WBC ($\times 10^3$)	5.4 - 15.3	3.8 - 19
Total Protein (TPP) (g/dl)	5.8 - 7.2	5.7 - 7.5
MCV (fl)	62.7 - 72	36 - 50
MCH (pg)	22.2 - 25.4	12.2 - 16.8
MCHC (g/dl)	34 - 36.6	32.4 - 35.2
Reticulocytes (%)	0 - 1.5	0.2 - 1.6
RBC diameter (microns)	6.7 - 7.2	5.5 - 6.3
RBC life (days)	100 - 120	66 - 78
M:E ratio	0.75 - 2.5 : 10	0.6 - 3.9 : 10
Platelets ($\times 10^3/\mu l$)	160 - 525	160 - 660
Icterus Index	2 - 5	2 - 5
Fibrinogen (mg/dl)	200 - 400	150 - 300
RDW	12.2 - 14.9	14.1 - 18.4
PCT	.182 - .416	.179 - .916
MPV	6.6 - 10.9	10.0 - 15.5
PDW	14.5 - 16.0	14.4.- 17

WBC Diff. - Absolute count/μl (% of total)

	DOG	CAT
stabs	0 - 150 (0 - 1)	0 - 190 (0 - 1)
segs	2750 - 12850 (51 - 84)	1290 - 15950 (34 - 84)
lymphs	430 - 5800 (8 - 38)	260 - 11400 (7 - 60)
monos	50 - 1400 (1 - 9)	0 - 950 (0 - 5)
eos	0 - 1400 (0 - 9)	0 - 2300 (0 - 12)
basos	rare (0 - 1)	0 - 400 (0 - 2)

Coagulation (secs)

	DOG	CAT
PT	6. - 8.4	8.7 - 10.5
PTT	11.0 - 17.4	12.3 - 16.7
TT	4.3 - 7.1	5.6 - 9.0

CHEMISTRY - SERUM

Small Animal Profile

	DOG	**CAT**
Albumin (ALB) (g/dl)	2.6 - 4.0	2.6 - 4.3
Alk. Phosphatase (ALP) (U/l)	3 - 60	3 - 61
Alanine Transaminase (ALT) (U/l)	4 - 91	13 - 75
Amylase (AMYL) (U/l)	220 - 1070	400 - 1590
Bilirubin Total (T Bili) (mg/dl)	0 - 0.7	0 - 0.6
Blood Urea Nitrogen (BUN) (mg/dl)	7 - 26	10 - 30
Calcium, Total (mg/dl)	9.6 - 11.6	9.3 - 11.7
Creatinine (mg/dl)	0.6 - 1.4	0.8 - 2.0
Creatine Kinase (CK) (IU/l)	36 - 155	21 - 275
Glucose (g/dl)	79 - 126	63 - 132
Phosphorus (PHOS) (mg/dl)	2.5 - 6.2	2.9 - 7.7
Total Protein (TP) (g/dl)	5.8 - 7.9	6.1 - 8.8
Uric Acid (mg/dl)	0 - 0.6	0 - 0.2
Sodium (Na^+) (mEq/l)	146 - 156	151 - 161
Potassium (K^+) (mEq/l)	3.8 - 5.1	3.5 - 5.1
Chloride (Cl^-)	109 - 122	117 - 129
CO_2 Total (T CO_2) (mM/l)	17 - 27	13 - 25
Anion Gap	8 - 19	9 - 21
Osmolality (mOsm/l) -Calculated	289 - 313	299 - 327

Additional Serum Chemistries

Ammonia (μg/dl)	19 - 120	-
Ammonia Tolerance (μg/dl)	<200 @ 30 min.	<300
AST (SGOT) (IU/l)	<105	<51
Bilirubin, Direct	0 - 0.4	0 - 0.2
BSP retention at 30 minutes	0 - 5%	-
Cholesterol (mg/dl)	125 - 300	95 - 130
Gamma glutyltranspepdidase (GGT)	0 - 2.26	-
Lactate (mg/dl)	4 - 12	
Methemalbumin (mg/dl)	0 - 5	
Lipase (U/l)	0 - 600	0 - 600
Free Plasma Hgb (mg/dl)	<10	<10
Xylose toler. (mg/dl) @60-90 min.	70 - 90	
PABA tolerance (plasma) (μg/dl)	670 +/- 140	386 +/- 134

Additional Acid-Base/Electrolytes

pH	7.31 - 7.53	7.32 - 7.44
pO_2 (mm Hg) Arterial	85 - 95	-
Venous	35 - 40	35 - 40
pCO_2 (mm Hg) Arterial	29 - 36	-
Venous	35 - 44	38 - 46
Bicarb (HCO_3^-) (mEq/l)	25 - 35	24 - 34
Base Excess (mEq/l)	+6 to 0	+2 to -5
Magnesium (mg/dl)	1.7 - 2.9	2 - 3

Chemistry - Urinalysis

	DOG	CAT
Specific gravity	1.001 - 1.070	1.001 - 1.080
pH	5.5 - 7.5	5.5 - 7.5
Volume (ml/kg/day)	24 - 41	22 - 30
Osmolality	500 - 1200 50 min; 2400 max.	50 min; 3000 max.
Sediment leukocytes (per HPF) erythrocytes casts (per HPF)	 0 - 5 0 - 5 0	 0 - 5 0 - 5 0
Glucose/Ketones	0	0
Bilirubin	0 - trace	0
Calcium (mEq/l)	2 - 10	
Creatinine (mg/dl)	100 - 300	110 - 280
Chloride (mEq/l)	0 - 400	
Magnesium (mg/kg/24h)	1.7 - 3.0	3
Phosphorus (mEq/l)	50 - 180	
Potassium (mEq/l)	20 - 120	
Sodium (mEq/l)	20 - 165	
Urea Nitrogen (mg/kg/24h)	140 - 2302	374 - 1872

CSF Parameters

	DOG	CAT
Pressure (mm H_2O)	<170	<100
Specific gravity	1.005 - 1.007	1.005 - 1.007
lymphocytes/µl	<5	<5
Pandy's	neg. - trace	neg.
Protein (mg/dl)	<25	<25
CK (IU/l)	9 - 28	

Hormones

	DOG	CAT
Cortisol (ng/ml) -resting	Not-Detectable (ND) - 50	ND - 50
-3 hr post dexamethasone suppression test -2 hr post ACTH (@2.2mg/kg)	 ND 80 - 200	 ND 80 - 200
Estradiol (pg/ml) -follicular phase -anestrous/spayed females & males	 30 - 250 <35	 20 - 70 <20
Glucagon (pg/ml)	4 - 75	32 - 84
Insulin (µU/ml)	2 - 22	6 - 22
Parathormone, midmolecule (pMole/l)	72 - 220	
Progesterone (ng/ml) -luteal phase female -male, non-luteal phase female	 2 - 80 <2	 2 - 40 <2
Testosterone (ng/ml) -intact males	 0.5 - 9	 ND - 5
Thyroxine (T4) (mcg/dl) -resting -5 hr post TSH (5 IU IV) -6 hr post TSH (5 IU IV)	 2.0 - 4.0 >3.5 	 0.6 - 3.6 >4.0
Triiodothyronine (T3) (ng/ml) -resting -8 hour post TSH (5 IU IV)	 75 - 200 75 - 350	 60 - 200

Reference Laboratory Values: Cattle & Horses

The following reference values are those presently being used at the University of Minnesota, Veterinary Teaching Hospital. They should be used as a general reference only; refer to the laboratory normals from the lab you are using for specific reference values applicable to your practice situation.

HEMATOLOGY

	CATTLE	HORSES (adult)	(foals 1-16 hr's old)
PCV (%)	24 - 46	32 - 53	30 - 40
Hct		30.1 - 50.1	28.9 - 45.9
Hgb (g/dl)	8 - 15	10.7 - 18.1	10.7 - 16.3
RBC (X 10^6/µl)	5 - 10	6.27 - 11.06	7.33 - 11.27
WBC (X 10^3)	4 - 12	4.1 - 11.3	6 - 16
Total Protein (TPP) (g/dl)	7 - 8.5	6.1 - 7.9	3.8 - 6.6
MCV (fl)	40 - 60	38.7 - 54.4	37 - 43.7
MCH (pg)	11 - 17	14 - 19.4	13.2 - 15.8
MCHC (g/dl)	30 - 36	34.8 - 37	33.8 - 38.1
Reticulocytes (%)	0	0	
RBC diameter (microns)	4 - 8	5 - 6	
RBC life (days)	160	140 - 150	
M:E ratio	0.31 - 1.85:10	0.5-1.5:10	
Platelets (X 10^3/µl)	100 - 800	100 - 300	175 - 400
Icterus Index	2 - 15	7.5 - 20	
Fibrinogen (mg/dl)	300 - 700	100 - 400	100 - 300
RDW		16.5 - 24.8	15.7 - 27.9
PCT		.068 - .176	0.128 - 0.262
MPV		5.3 - 7.1	5.3 - 8.1
PDW		15.3 - 17.2	14.8 - 16.2

WBC Diff. - Absolute count/µl (% of total)

stabs	0-250 (0-2)	rare (0)	0-160 (0-1)
segs	600-5400 (15-45)	1350-8250 (33-73)	400-14700 (74-92)
lymphs	1800-9000 (45-75)	820-7350 (20-65)	300-3400 (5-21)
monos	80-850 (2-7)	40-700 (1-6)	60-1100 (1-7)
eos	80-2400 (2-20)	40-450 (1-4)	0-160 (0-1)
basos	0-250 (0-2) ·	40-80 (1-2)	rare

Coagulation (secs)

PT	6.8 - 8.4	8.7 - 10.5	9.5-12.7 (1-16 hr's old)
			8.1-12.3 (2 wk's old)
PTT	11.0 - 17.4	12.3 - 16.7	39.3-58.6 (1-16 hr's old)
			28.6-47 (2 wk's old)
TT	4.3 - 7.1	5.6 - 9.0	14.6-27.9 (1-16 hr's old)
			10.8-19.9 (2 wk's old)

CHEMISTRY - SERUM

	CATTLE (adult dairy)	HORSES
Blood Urea Nitro. (BUN) (mg/dl)	6 - 22	11 - 24
Sodium (Na^+) (mEq/l)	138 - 148	136 - 143
Potassium (K^+) (mEq/l)	3.8 - 5.1	2.6 - 4.9
Chloride (Cl^-)	96 - 109	97 - 105
CO_2 Total (TCO_2) (mM/l)	23 - 30	26 - 33
Glucose (g/dl)	54 - 79	72 - 132
Calcium, Total (mg/dl)	9.3 - 10.6	11 - 13.6
Creatinine (mg/dl)	0.8 - 1.4	0.9 - 1.8
Phosphorus (PHOS) (mg/dl)	5.1 - 9.3	2.4 - 4.8
Anion Gap - Calc.	10 - 20	6 - 12
Osmolality (mOsm/l) -Calc.	273 - 293	275 - 286
Albumin (ALB) (g/dl)	2.8 - 3.8	3 - 4.0
Alk. Phosphatase (ALP) (U/l)	10 - 77	56 - 140
AST (SGOT) (U/l)	39 - 79	170 - 345
Bilirubin Total (T Bili) (mg/dl)	0.1 - 0.4	0.2 - 3.1
Creatine Kinase (CK) (IU/l)	46 - 169	65 - 276
Gamma GT (U/l)	14 - 40	11 - 26
Total Protein (TP) (g/dl)	6.3 - 8.9	5.6 - 8.0
SDH (U/l)	9.3 - 22.5	0 - 12.1
Uric Acid (mg/dl)	0 - 0.9	
Ammonia (μg/dl)		11 - 74
D-Xylose (mg/dl)		17-25 @60-90 min.
Free plasma Hgb (mg/dl)	<10	<10

Reference Laboratory Values: Sheep, Goats & Swine

The following reference values are those presently being used at the University of Minnesota, Veterinary Teaching Hospital. They should be used as a general reference only; refer to the laboratory normals from the lab you are using for the specific reference values applicable to your practice situation.

HEMATOLOGY

	SHEEP	GOATS	SWINE
PCV (%)	27 - 45	22 - 38	32 - 50
Hgb (g/dl)	9 - 15	8 - 12	10 - 16
RBC (x 10^6/µl)	9 - 15	8 - 18	5 - 8
WBC (x 10^3)	4 - 12	4 - 13	11 - 22
Total Protein (TPP) (g/dl)	6.0 - 7.5	6 - 7.5	6 - 8
MCV (fl)	28 - 40	16 - 25	50 - 68
MCH (pg)	8 - 12	5.2 - 8	17 - 21
MCHC (g/dl)	31 - 34	30 - 36	30 - 34
Reticulocytes (%)	0	0	0 - 1.0
RBC diameter (microns)	3.2 - 6	2.5 - 3.9	4 - 8
RBC life (days)	140 - 150	125	75 - 98
M:E ratio	0.77 - 1.68:10	0.69:10	1.77 - 0.52:10
Platelets (x 10^3/µl)	250 - 750	300 - 600	325 - 715
Icterus Index		<5 Units	2 - 5
Fibrinogen (mg/dl)	100 - 500	100-400	1 - 500

WBC Diff. - Absolute count/µl (% of total)

	SHEEP	GOATS	SWINE
stabs	rare (0)	rare	0 - 900 (0-4)
segs	400 - 6000 (10-50)	1200 - 6250 (30-48)	3100 -10350 (28-47)
lymphs	1600 - 9000 (40-75)	2000 - 9100 (50-70)	1550 - 13650 (39-62)
monos	0 - 750 (0-6)	0 - 550 (0-4)	200 - 2200 (2-10)
eos	0 - 1200 (0 - 10)	50 - 1050 (1-8)	50 - 2400 (0.5-11)
basos	0 - 350 (0-3)	0 - 150 (0-1)	0 - 450 (0-2)

Coagulation (secs)

PT	13.5 - 15.9
PTT	27.9 - 40.7
TT	4.8 - 8.0

CHEMISTRY - SERUM

	SHEEP	GOATS	SWINE
Blood Urea Nitro. (BUN) (mg/dl)	8 - 20	13 - 28	8 - 24
Sodium (Na^+) (mEq/l)	139 - 152	135 - 154	135 - 150
Potassium (K^+) (mEq/l)	3.9 - 5.4	4.6 - 9.8	7.8 - 10.9
Chloride (Cl^-) (mEq/l)	95 - 103	105 - 120	94 - 106
Glucose (g/dl)	42 - 76	60 - 100	65 - 95
Calcium, Total (mg/dl)	11.5 - 12.8	8.6 - 10.6	10.2 - 11.9
Creatinine (mg/dl)	1 - 2.7	0.9 - 1.8	1 - 3
Phosphorus (PHOS) (mg/dl)	5 - 7.3	4.2 - 9.8	7.8 - 10.9
Alk. Phosphatase (ALP) (U/l)	68 - 387	9 - 131	9 - 20
Bilirubin Total (T Bili) (mg/dl)	0.14 - 0.32	0 - 0.9	0 - 0.7
Creatine Kinase (CK) (IU/l)	42 - 62	<38	
Gamma GT (U/l)	25 - 59	24 - 39	
Total Protein (TP) (g/dl)	6 - 7.9	6.4 - 7.8	7.4
Albumin (g/dl)	2.4 - 3	2 - 4.4	3.4
SDH (U/l)	5.8 - 27.9	14 - 23.6	

Phone Numbers
Product Failure and Adverse Reaction Reporting

Drugs, Devices, Animal Foods
Food and Drug Administration
(301) 443-4095 (collect)
After hours call (301) 443-1209 to leave a recorded message.

Biologics (including Vaccines, Bacterins, and Diagnostic Kits)
U.S. Department of Agriculture
(515) 232-5789 (collect).After hours leave a recorded message.

Food Animal Residue Avoidance Databank (FARAD)
1-888-USFARAD (1-888-873-2723)

(Due to inadequate funding, FARAD phone service has been temporarily discontinued. It will return to service once sufficient funding is received.)

Regional Centers:

Western Region	Eastern Region
Phone: (916) 752-7507	Phone: (919) 829-4431
FAX: (916) 752-0903	FAX: (919) 829-4358

Internet E-Mail: farad @ucdavis.edu or farad@ncsu.edu
The FARAD Web site is operational and has much useful information: http://www.farad.org/

Poison Centers

National Animal Poison Information Center (NAPIC)
1-900-680-0000 $30 per case. The charge will appear on your telephone bill.
or 1-800-548-2423 or 1-888-426-4435 $30/case - no extra charge for follow-up calls. You must use Visa, MasterCard, Discover, or American Express when you call.

Hennepin County Regional Poison Center
Pet Poisoning Information Service
(612) 337-7387

There are many regional poison centers that may be of assistance with animal poisonings; refer to your local poison center for more more information.

Additional Phone Numbers

Bibliography

Drug Information for the Health Care Professional - Volume 1 USP DI. Rockville: United States Pharmacopeial Convention, 1990-1997

Bennett, K. , ed. Compendium of Veterinary Products 2nd Edition. Port Huron. North American Compendiums 1993. 1152 pp.

Veterinary Pharmaceuticals and Biologicals: 1991/1992, 7th ed. Lenexa: Veterinary Medicine Publishing Company, 1991. 939 pp.

Booth, N.H., and L.E. McDonald, ed. Veterinary Pharmacology and Therapeutics. 6th ed. Ames: Iowa State University Press, 1988. 1227 pp.

Brander, C.G., D.M. Pugh, and R.J. Bywater. Veterinary Applied Pharmacology and Therapeutics. 4th ed. London: Baillière Tindall, 1982. 582 pp.

Davis, L.E., ed. Handbook of Small Animal Therapeutics. New York: Churchill Livingston, 1985. 718 pp.

Ettinger, S.J., ed. Textbook of Veterinary Internal Medicine. 3rd ed. Philadelphia: WB Saunders, 1989. 2399 pp.

Feldman, E.C., and R.W. Nelson. Canine and Feline Endocrinology and Reproduction. Philadelphia: WB Saunders, 1987. 564 pp.

Fox, P.R., ed. Canine and Feline Cardiology. New York: Churchill Livingstone, 1988. 676 pp.

Gilman, A.G. et al., ed. Goodman & Gilman's: The Pharmacological Basis of Therapeutics. 7th ed. New York: MacMillan, 1985. 1839 pp.

Greene, C.E. Infectious Diseases of the Dog and Cat. Philadelphia: WB Saunders, 1990. 971 pp.

Harrison, G.J., and L.R. Harrison, ed. Clinical Avian Medicine and Surgery. Philadelphia: Saunders, 1986. 717 pp.

Howard, J.L., ed. Current Veterinary Therapy 3, Food Animal Practice. Philadelphia: W.B. Saunders, 1993. 966 pp.

Kirk, R.W., ed. Current Veterinary Therapy X, Small Animal Practice. Philadelphia: W.B. Saunders, 1989. 1421 pp.

Kirk, R.W., Bonagura, J.D. eds. Current Veterinary Therapy XI, Small Animal Practice. Philadelphia: W.B. Saunders, 1992. 1348 pp.

McEvoy, G.K., ed. AHFS Drug Information. Bethesda: American Society of Hospital Pharmacists, 1990-1997.

Morgan, R.V., ed. Handbook of Small Animal Practice. New York: Churchill Livingstone, 1988. 1257 pp.

Morrow, D.A., ed. Current Therapy in Theriogenology 2: Diagnosis, Treatment and Prevention of Reproductive Diseases in Small and Large Animals. Philadelphia: WB Saunders, 1986. 1143 pp.

Olin, B.R., ed. Facts and Comparisons: Loose-leaf Drug Information Service. St. Louis: J.B. Lippincott, 1994-98.

Osol, A., ed. Remington's Pharmaceutical Sciences. 15th ed. Easton: Mack Publishing Co., 1975. 1961 pp.

Reynolds, J.E.F., ed. Martindale: The Extra Pharmacopoeia. 29th ed. London: The Pharmaceutical Press, 1989. 1896 pp.

Robinson, N.E., ed. Current Therapy in Equine Medicine-3. 3rd ed. Philadelphia: W.B. Saunders, 1992. 847 pp.

Sherding, R.G., ed. The Cat: Diseases and Clinical Management. New York: Churchill Livingstone, 1989. 1674 pp.

Sundlof, S.F., J.E. Riviere, and A.L. Craigmill. The Food Animal Residue Avoidance Databank: Trade Name File. 2nd ed. Gainesville: Institute of Food and Agricultural Sciences: University of Florida, 1988. 609 pp.

Trissel, L.A. Handbook on Injectable Drugs. 7th ed. Bethesda: American Society of Hospital Pharmacists, 1992. 1023 pp.

Upson, D.W. Handbook of Clinical Veterinary Pharmacology. 3rd ed. Manhattan: Upson Enterprises, 1988. 729 pp.

References

Adams, H.R. 1988a. Antianemic Drugs. In Veterinary Pharmacology and Therapeutics. Edited by N. H. Booth and L. E. McDonald. 469-481. Ames: Iowa State University Press.

Adams, H.R. 1988b. Hemostatic and Anticoagulant Drugs. In Veterinary Pharmacology and Therapeutics. Edited by N. H. Booth and L. E. McDonald. 481-494. Ames: Iowa State University Press.

Adams, S.B., C.H. Lamar, and J. Masty. 1984. Motility of the distal jejunem and pelvic flexure in ponies: Effects of six drugs. Am J Vet Res 45 : 795-799.

Alitalo, I. 1986. Clinical Experiences with Domesedan® in Horses and Cattle: A Review. Acta Vet Scand 82 : 193-196.

Allen, D., J. Pringle, D. Smith, P. Conlon and P. Burgmann. (1993). Handbook of Veterinary Drugs. Philadelphia, J.B. Lippincott Co. 678pp.

Allen, T.A. 1988. Mixed Infections. In Handbook of Small Animal Practice. Edited by R. V. Morgan. 1001-1004. New York: Churchill Livingstone.

Allen, T.A. 1989. Management of Advanced Chronic Renal Failure. In Current Veterinary Therapy X: Small Animal Practice. Edited by R. W. Kirk. 1195-1198. Philadelphia: W.B. Saunders.

Allen, W.M., and B.F. Sansom. 1986. Parturient Paresis (Milk fever) and Hypocalcemia (Cows, Ewes, and Goats). In Current Veterinary Therapy 2: Food Animal Practice. Edited by J.L. Howard. 311-317. Philadelphia: W.B. Saunders.

Amann, R.P. 1986. Reproductive Physiology and Endocrinology in the Dog. In Current Therapy in Theriogenology 2: Diagnosis, Treatment and Prevention of Reproductive Diseases in Small and Large Animals. Edited by D. A. Morrow. 532-538. Philadelphia: W.B. Saunders.

Ames, T. (1992). New equine therapeutic agents: Fact or fiction. Minnesota Veterinary Medicine Association: Annual Conference. Bloomington, 33-36

Anderson, N. (1994). Basic husbandry and medicine of pocket pets. Saunders Manual of Small Animal Practice. Edited by S. Birchard and R. Sherding; Philadelphia, W.B. Saunders Company. 1363-1389

Appel, M. and R. Jacobson. (1995). CVT Update: Canine Lyme Disease. Kirk's Current Veterinary Therapy:XII. Edited by J. Bonagura; Philadelphia, W.B. Saunders. 303-309

Armstrong, P.J., and M.S. Hand. 1989. Nutritional Disorders. In The Cat: Diseases and Clinical Management. Edited by R.G. Sherding. 141-161. New York: Churchill Livingstone.

Aronson, A.L., and D.P. Aucoin. 1989. Antimicrobial Drugs. In Textbook of Veterinary Internal Medicine. Edited by S. J. Ettinger. 383-412. Philadelphia: W.B. Saunders.

Auer, L.A., and K. Bell. 1986. Feline Blood Transfusion Reactions. In Current Veterinary Therapy (CVT) IX Small Animal Practice. Edited by R. W. Kirk. 515-521. Philadelphia: W.B. Saunders.

Baggot, J.D. 1983. Systemic Antimicrobial Therapy in Large Animals. In Pharmacological Basis of Large Animal Medicine. Edited by J. A. Bogan, P. Lees and A. T. Yoxall. 45-69. Oxford: Blackwell Scientific Publications.

Baggot, J.D., and J.F. Prescott. 1987. Antimicrobial Selection and Dosage in the Treatment of Equine Bacterial Infections. Equine Vet J 19 (2) : 92-96.

Baggot, J.D., G.V. Ling, and R.C. Chatfield. 1985. Clinical Pharmacokinetics of Amikacin in Dogs. Am Jnl of Vet Res 46 (8) : 1793-1796.

Baggot, J.D., W.D. Wilson, and S. Hietela. 1988. Clinical Pharmacokinetics of Metronidazole in Horses. J Vet Pharmacol Therap 11 : 417-420.

Bailey, E. and T. Garland. (1992a). Management of Toxicoses. Current Therapy in Equine Medicine 3. Edited by N. Robinson; Philadelphia, W.B. Saunders Co. 346-353

Bailey, E. M. and T. Garland. (1992b). Management of Toxicoses. Current Therapy in Equine Medicine 3. Edited by E. N. Robinson; Philadelphia, W.B. Saunders. 346-353

Bailey, E.M. 1986. Emergency and General Treatment of Poisonings. In Current Veterinary Therapy (CVT) IX Small Animal Practice. Edited by R. W. Kirk. 135-144. Philadelphia: W.B. Saunders.

Bailey, E.M. 1986. Management and Treatment of Toxicosis in Cattle. In Current Veterinary Therapy 2: Food Animal Practice. Edited by J. L. Howard. 341-354. Philadelphia: W.B. Saunders.

Bailey, E.M. 1989. Emergency and General Treatment of Poisonings. In Current Veterinary Therapy (CVT) X Small Animal Practice. Edited by R.W. Kirk. 116-125. Philadelphia: W.B. Saunders.

Ballard, S., T. Shults, A.A. Kownacki, J.W. Blake, and T. Tobin. 1982. The Pharmacokinetics, Pharmacological Responses and Behavioral Effects of Acepromazine in the Horse. J Vet Pharmacol Ther 5 (1) : 21-31.

Barr, S. and D. Bowman. (1994). "Giardiasis in Dogs and Cats." Comp CE. **16**(May): 603-610.

Barr, S., D. Bowman, R. Heller and H. Erb. Efficacy of albendazole against Giardia species in dogs and cats-Abstract. 38th Annual Meeting-AAVP. Edited by American Association of Veterinary Practitioners.

Barsanti, J.A. 1984. Opportunistic Fungal Infections. In Clinical Microbiology and Infectious Diseases of the Dog and Cat. Edited by C. E. Greene. 728-746. Philadelphia: W.B. Saunders.

Barsanti, J.A., and D.R. Finco. 1986. Feline Urinary Incontinence. In Current Veterinary Therap IX: Small Animal Practice. Edited by R. W. Kirk. 1159- 1163. Philadelphia: W.B. Saunders.

Barta, O. (1992ab). Immunoadjuvant therapy. Current Veterinary Therapy XI: Small Animal Practice. Edited by R. Kirk and J. Bonagura; Philadelphia, W.B. Saunders Company. 217-223

Barth, A.D. 1986. Induced Parturition in Cattle. In Current Therapy in Theriogenology 2: Diagnosis, Treatment and Prevention of Reproductive Diseases in Small and Large Animals. Edited by D. A. Morrow. 209-214. Philadelphia: W.B. Saunders.

Barton, C.L. 1988. Diseases of the Ovaries. In Handbook of Small Animal Practice. Edited by R. V. Morgan. 651-654. New York: Churchill Livingstone.

Barton, C.L., and A.M. Wolf. 1988. Disorders of Reproduction. In Handbook of Small Animal Practice. Edited by R. V. Morgan. 679-700. New York: Churchill Livingstone.

Batt, R.M. 1986. Wheat-Sensitive Enteropathy in Irish Setters. In Current Veterinary Therapy IX: Small Aniaml Practice. Edited by R. W. Kirk. 893-896. Philadelphia: W.B. Saunders.

Bauck, L. and H. Hoefer. (1993). "Avian antimicrobial therapy." Seminars in Avian & Exotic Med. 2(1): 17-22.

Bauer, T.G. 1988. Diseases of the Lower Airway. In Handbook of Small Animal Practice. Edited by R. V. Morgan. 185-193. New York: Churchill Livingstone.

Bauer, T.G. 1988. Pulmonary Parnechymal Disorders. In Handbook of Small Animal Practice. Edited by R. V. Morgan. 195-213. New York: Churchill Livingstone.

Baxter, J.G., C. Brass, J.J. Schentag, and R.L. Slaughter. 1986. Pharmacokinetics of Ketoconazole Administered Intravenously to Dogs and Orally as Tablet and Solution to Humans and Dogs. J Pharm Sci 75 (5) : 443-447.

Beasley, V.R., and D.C. Dorman. 1990. Management of Toxicoses. Vet Clin of North America: Sm Anim Pract 20 (2) : 307-337.

Beaver, B.V. 1989. Disorders of Behavior. In The Cat: Diseases and Clinical Management. Edited by R. G. Sherding. 163-184. New York: Churchill Livingstone.

Beck, D. (1992). "Effective long-term tratment of a suspected pituitary adenoma ina pony." Equine Vet Educ. 4(3): 119-122.

Bednarski, R. (1992). Recent advances in injectable chemical restraint. Current Veterinary Therapy XI: Small Animal Practice. Edited by R. Kirk and J. Bonagura; Philadelphia, W.B. Saunders Company. 27-31

Bednarski, R.M. 1989. Anesthesia and Pain Control. Vet Clin of North Amer: Small Anim Pract 19 (6) : 1223-1238.

Beech, J. 1987. Drug Therapy of Respiratory Disorders. Vet Clin North Am (Equine Practice) 3 (1) : 59-80.

Beech, J. 1987b. Respiratory Tract—Horse, Cow. In The Bristol Handbook of Antimicrobial Therapy. Edited by D. E. Johnston. 88-109. Evansville: Veterinary Learning Systems.

Beech, J. 1987b. Tumors of the Pituitary Gland (pars intermedia). In Current Therapy in Equine Medicine: 2. Edited by N. E. Robinson. 182-185. Philadelphia: W.B. Saunders.

Bell, F.W., and C.A. Osborne. 1986. Treatment of Hypokalemia. In Current Veterinary Therapy IX: Small Animal Practice. Edited by R. W. Kirk. 101-107. Philadelphia: W.B. Saunders.

Bellah, J.R. 1988. Acute Gastric Dilatation-Volvulus. In Handbook of Small Animal Practice. Edited by R. V. Morgan. 385-394. New York: Churchill Livingstone.

Bennett, D.G. 1986. Parasites of the Respiratory System. In Current Veterinary Therapy: Food Animal Practice 2. Edited by J. L. Howard. 684-687. Philadelphia: W.B. Saunders.

Berg, J.N. 1986. Aseptic Laminitis in Cattle. In Current Veterinary Therapy: Food Animal Practice 2. Edited by J. L. Howard. 896-898. Philadelphia: W.B. Saunders.

Bergman, P., E. MacEwen, I. Kurzman, C. Henry, A. Hammer and D. Knapp. (1996). "Amputation and carboplatin for treatment of dogs with osteosarcoma: 48 cases (1991 - 1993)." J Vet Intern Med. **10**((2)): 76-81.

Berkwitt, L., and J.L. Berzon. 1988. Pleural Cavity Diseases. In Handbook of Small Animal Practice. Edited by R.V. Morgan. 215-225. New York: Churchill Livingstone.

Bevier, D. (1990). "Long-term management of atopic disease in the dog." The Veterinary Clinics of North America; Small Animal Practice. 20(6: November): 1487-1507.

Black, L. 1986. Environmental Skin Conditions: Photosensitization with Gangrene. In Current Veterinary Therapy: Food Animal Practice 2. Edited by J. L. Howard. 932-933. Philadelphia: W.B. Saunders.

Blagburn, B.L., C.M. Hendrix, L.A. Hanrahan, D.S. Lindsay, R.G. Arther, and J.W. Drane. 1989. Controlled Dosage Titration of Febantel Paste in Naturally Parasitized Cattle. Am J Vet Res 50 (9) : 1574-1577.

Bloomberg, M. (1992). Pharmacokinetics of musculoskeletal drugs (Polysulfated Glycosaminoglycans, DMSO, Orgotein, and Hyaluronic Acid). Minnesota Veterinary Medicine Association: Annual Conference. Edited by Bloomington, 179-181

Bonagura, J. (1994). Bronchopulmonary disorders. Saunders Manual of Small Animal Practice. Edited by S. Birchard and R. Sherding; Philadelphia, W.B. Saunders Company. 561-573

Bonagura, J. and L. Lehmkuhl. (1994). Cardiomyopathy. Saunders Manual of Small Animal Practice. Edited by S. Birchard and R. Sherding; Philadelphia, W.B. Saunders Company. 464-480

Bonagura, J.D. 1989. Cardiovascular Diseases. In The Cat: Diseases and Clinical Management. Edited by R. G. Sherding. 649-686. New York: Churchill Livingstone.

Bonagura, J.D., and W. Muir. 1986. Vasodilator Therapy. In Current Veterinary Therapy (CVT) IX Small Animal Practice. Edited by R. W. Kirk. 329-334. Philadelphia: W.B. Saunders.

Booth, N.H. 1988. Inhalant Anesthetics. In Veterinary Pharmacology and Therapeutics - 6th Ed. Edited by N.H. Booth and L.E. McDonald. 181-211. Ames: Iowa State University Press.

Booth, N.H. 1988. Topical Agents. In Veterinary Pharmacology and Therapeutics. Edited by N. H. Booth and L. E. McDonald. 721-744. Ames: Iowa State University Press.

Booth, N.H. 1988a. Drugs Acting on the Central Nervous System. In Veterinary Pharmacology and Therapeutics - 6th Ed. Edited by N. H. Booth and L. E. McDonald. 153-408. Ames: Iowa State University Press.

Booth, N.H. 1988b. Topical Agents. In Veterinary Pharmacology and Therapeutics. Edited by N. H. Booth and L. E. McDonald. 721-744. Ames: Iowa State University Press.

Boothe, D. (1992). Control of pain in small animals. Proceedings of the Tenth Annual Veterinary Medical Forum. Edited by W. Morrison, San Diego, American College of Veterinary Internal Medicine. 240-242

Boothe, D.M. 1990. Drug Therapy in Cats: Recommended Dosing Regimens. JAVMA 196 (11) : 1845-1850.

Brander, C.G., D.M. Pugh, and R.J. Bywater. 1982. Veterinary Applied Pharmacology and Therapeutics. 4th ed. London: Baillière Tindall.

Brattan, G.R., and D.F. Kowalczyk. 1989. Lead Poisoning. In Current Veterinary Therapy (CVT) X Small Animal Practice. Edited by R.W. Kirk. 152-159. Philadelphia: W.B. Saunders.

Braun, R.K. 1986. Dairy Calf Health Management. In Current Veterinary Therapy 2: Food Animal Practice. Edited by J. L. Howard. 126-135. Philadelphia: W.B. Saunders.

Braun, W. (1995). Potbellied pigs: General medical care. Kirk's Current Veterinary Therapy:XII. Edited by J. Bonagura; Philadelphia, W.B. Saunders. 1388-1389

Breitschwerdt, E.B. 1988. Acute Renal Failure. In Handbook of Small Animal Practice. Edited by R. V. Morgan. 578-582. New York: Churchill Livingstone .

Bretzlaff, K. (1993). Production Medicine and Health Programs for Goats. Current Veterinary Therapy 3: Food Animal Practice. Edited by J. Howard; Philadelphia, W.B. Saunders Co. 162-167

Brewer, B.D. 1987. Disorders of Calcium Metabolism. In Current Therapy in Equine Medicine. Edited by N.E. Robinson. 189-192. Philadelphia: W.B. Saunders.

Brewer, B.D. 1987. Equine Protozoa Myeloencephalitis. In Current Therapy in Equine Medicine. Edited by N. E. Robinson. 359-363. Philadelphia: W.B. Saunders.

Brewer, G. J., R. D. Dick, W. Schall, V. Yuzbasiyan-Gurkan, T. P. Mullaney, C. Pace, J. Lindgren, M. Thomas and G. Padgett. (1992). "Use of zinc acetate to treat copper toxicosis in dogs." JAVMA. 201(August 15, 1992): 564-568.

Bright, J. (1992). Update: Diltiazem Therapy of Feline Hypertrophic Cardiomyopathy. Current Veterinary Therapy XI: Small Animal Practice. Edited by R. Kirk and J. Bonagura; Philadelphia, W.B. Saunders Company. 766-773

Bristol, F. 1986. Estrous Synchronization in Mares. In Current Therapy in Theriogenology 2: Diagnosis, Treatment and Prevention of Reproductive Diseases in Small and Large Animals. Edited by D. A. Morrow. 661-664. Philadelphia: W.B. Saunders.

Bristol, F. 1987. Synchronization of Estrus. In Current Therapy in Equine Medicine: 2. Edited by N. E. Robinson. 495-498. Philadelphia: W.B. Saunders.

Brooks, D.E. 1986. Canine and Feline Glaucomas. In Current Veterinary Therapy IX, Small Animal Practice. Edited by R. W. Kirk. 656-659. Philadelphia: W.B. Saunders.

Brooks, D.E. 1990. Glaucoma in the Dog and Cat. Vet Clin of North America: Small Anim Pract 20 (3) : 775-797.

Brooks, M. (1994). Coagulation disorders. Saunders Manual of Small Animal Practice. Edited by S. Birchard and R. Sherding; Philadelphia, W.B. Saunders Company. 164-170

Brown, S. (1997). Chronic Renal Failure. Handbook of Small Animal Practice 3rd Ed. Edited by R. Morgan; Philadelphia, WB Saunders. 512-516

Brown, S. and S. Forrester. (1989). "Serum disposition of oral clorazepate from regular-release and sustained-release tablets in dogs." J Vet Int Med. 3(2): 116.

Brown, S.A., and A.K. Prestwood. 1986. Parasites of the Urinary Tract. In Current Veterinary Therapy IX, Small Animal Practice. Edited by R. W. Kirk. 1153-1155. Philadelphia: W.B. Saunders.

Brown, S.A., and J.A. Barsanti. 1989. Diseases of the Bladder and Urethra. In Textbook of Veterinary Internal Medicine. Edited by S. J. Ettinger. 2108-2141. Philadelphia: W.B. Saunders.

Brumbaugh, G.W. 1987. Rational Selection of Antimicrobial Drugs for Treatment of Infections in Horses. Vet Clin North Am (Equine Practice) 3 (1) : 191-220.

Bruyette, D. (1991). Polyuria and polydipsia. Consultations in Feline Internal Medicine. Edited by J. August; Philadelphia, W.B. Saunders Company. 227-235

Bruyette, D.S., and E.C. Feldman. 1988. Ketoconazole and its use in the Management of Canine Cushing's Disease. Comp CE 10 (12) : 1379-1386.

Bucheler, J. and S. Cotter. (1995). Canine Immune-Mediated Hemolytic Anemia. Kirk's Current Veterinary Therapy:XII. Edited by J. Bonagura; Philadelphia, W.B. Saunders. 152-157

Buck, W. B. (1986). Copper-Molybdenum. Current Veterinary Therapy: Food Animal Practice 2. Edited by J. L. Howard; Philadelphia, W.B. Saunders. 437-439

Buerger, R. (1997). Congenital/Developmental Dermatoses. Handbook of Small Animal Practice 3rd Ed. Edited by R. Morgan; Philadelphia, Saunders. 871-877

Bufalari, A., S. Miller, C. Gionnoni and C. Short. (1998). "The use of propofol as an induction agent for halothane and isoflurane anesthesia in dogs." AAHA. 34: 83-91.

Bunch, S.E. 1986. Anticonvulsant Drug Therapy in Companion Animals. In Current Veterinary Therapy IX: Small Animal Practice. Edited by R. W. Kirk. 836-844. Philadelphia: W.B. Saunders.

Bunch, S.E. 1988. Diseases of the Exocrine Pancreas. In Handbook of Small Animal Practice. Edited by R.V. Morgan. 465-478. New York: Churchill Livingstone.

Burke, T.J. 1985. Reproductive Disorders. In Handbook of Small Animal Therapeutics. Edited by L. E. Davis. 605-616. New York: Churchill Livingstone.

Burke, T.J. 1986. Population Control in the Bitch. In Current Therapy in Theriogenology: 2. Edited by D. A. Morrow. 528-531. Philadelphia: W.B. Saunders.

Burke, T.J. 1986. Regurgitation in Snakes. In Current Veterinary Therapy (CVT) IX Small Animal Practice. Edited by R. W. Kirk. 749-750. Philadelphia: W.B. Saunders.

Burrows, C.F. 1983. Metoclopramide. JAVMA 183 (11) : 1341-1343.

Burrows, C.F. 1986. Constipation. In Current Veterinary Therapy IX: Small Animal Practice. Edited by R. W. Kirk. 904- 908. Philadelphia: W.B. Saunders.

Burrows, G.E. 1980. Systemic Antibacterial Drug Selection and Dosage. Bovine Practitioner 15 : 103-110.

Button, C., J.O. Errecalde, and M.S.G. Mulders. 1985. Loading and Maintenance Dosage Regimens for Theophylline in Horses. J Vet Pharm & Ther 8 (3) : 328-330.

Byars, T.D. 1987. Disseminated Intravascular Coagulation. In Current Therapy in Equine Medicine 2. Edited by N. E. Robinson. 306-309. Philadelphia: W.B. Saunders.

Calahan, P. 1987. Sand Colic. In Current Therapy in Equine Medicine 2. Edited by N. E. Robinson. 55-58. Philadelphia: W.B. Saunders.

Calvert, C. (1992). Update: Canine DIlated Cardiomyopathy. Current Veterinary Therapy XI: Small Animal Practice. Edited by R. Kirk and J. Bonagura; Philadelphia, W.B. Saunders Company. 773-779

Calvert, C. (1994). Heartworm Disease. Saunders Manual of Small Animal Practice. Edited by S. Birchard and R. Sherding; Philadelphia, W.B. Saunders Company. 487-493

Calvert, C. (1995). Diagnosis and management of ventricular tachyarrhythmias in Doberman pinschers with cardiomyopathy. Kirk's Current Veterinary Therapy:XII. Edited by J. Bonagura; Philadelphia, W.B. Saunders. 799-806

Calvert, C.A. 1987. Indications for the Use of Aspirin and Corticosteroid Hormones in the Treatment of Canine Heartworm Disease. Seminars Vet Med Surg (Small Animal) 2 (1) : 78-84.

Calvert, C.A. 1989. Feline Heartworm Disease. In The Cat: Diseases and Clinical Management. Edited by R. G. Sherding. 495-510. New York: Churchill Livingstone.

Calvert, C.A., and C.A. Rawlings. 1986. Therapy of Canine Heartworm Disease. In Current Veterinary Therapy IX: Small Animal Practice. Edited by R. W. Kirk. 406-419. Philadelphia: W.B. Saunders.

Caple, I, W. 1986. Downer Cow Syndrome. In Current Veterinary Therapy: Food Animal Practice 2. Edited by J. L. Howard. 327-328. Philadelphia: W.B. Saunders.

Caprile, K.A., and C.R. Short. 1987. Pharmacologic Considerations in Drug Therapy in Foals. Vet Clin North Am (Equine Practice) 3 (1) : 123-144.

Carleton, C.L., and W.R. Threlfall. 1986. Induction of Parturition in the Mare. In Current Therapy in Theriogenology 2: Diagnosis, Treatment and Prevention of Reproductive Diseases in Small and Large Animals. Edited by D. A. Morrow. 689-692. Philadelphia: W.B. Saunders.

Carothers, M., D. Chew and L. Nagode. (1994a). 25(OH)-Cholecalciferol Intoxication in Dogs. Proceedings of the Twelfth Annual Veterinary Medical Forum. Edited by R. DeNovo, San Francisco, American College of Veterinary Internal Medicine. 822-825

Carothers, M., D. Chew and T. Van Gundy. (1994b). Disorders of the parathyroid gland and calcium metabolism. Saunders Manual of Small Animal Practice. Edited by S. Birchard and R. Sherding; Philadelphia, W.B. Saunders Company. 229-237

Carro, T. (1994). L-forms and mycoplasmal infections. Consultations in Feline Internal Medicine: 2. Edited by J. August; Philadelphia, W.B. Saunders Company. 13-20

Carson, R.L. 1986. Synchronization of Estrus. In Current Veterinary Therapy: Food Animal Practice 2. Edited by J. L. Howard. 781-783. Philadelphia: W.B. Saunders.

Carson, T.L. 1986. Organophosphate and Carbamate Insecticide Poisoning. In Current Veterinary Therapy (CVT) IX Small Animal Practice. Edited by R. W. Kirk. 150-152. Philadelphia: W.B. Saunders.

Center, S. (1994). Hepatic lipidosis. Consultations in Feline Internal Medicine: 2. Edited by J. August; Philadelphia, W.B. Saunders Company. 87-101

Center, S.A., W.E. Hornbuckle, and T.D. Scavelli. 1986. Congenital Portosystemic Shunts in Cats. In Current Veterinary Therapy (CVT) IX Small Animal Practice. Edited by R. W. Kirk. 825-830. Philadelphia: W.B. Saunders.

Chastain, C.B. 1987. Aspirin: New Indications for an Old Drug. Comp CE 9 (2) : 165-169.

Chen, D.C.L., and O.W.I. Li 1987. Hypothyroidism. In Current Therapy in Equine Medicine 2. Edited by N. E. Robinson. 185-187. Philadelphia: W.B. Saunders.

Cheney, J.M., and G.T. Allen. 1989. Parasitism in Llamas. Vet Clin North America: Food Animal Practice 5 (1) : 217-232.

Chew, D.J., S.P. DiBartola, and W.F. Fenner. 1986. Pharmacologic Manipulation of Urination. In Current Veterinary Therapy IX: Small Animal Practice. Edited by R. V. Kirk. 1207-1212. Philadelphia: W.B. Saunders.

Chiapella, A. 1986. Diagnosis and Management of Chronic Colitis in the Dog and Cat. In Current Veterinary Therapy IX: Small Aniaml Practice. Edited by R. W. Kirk. 896-903. Philadelphia: W.B. Saunders.

Chiapella, A.M. 1988. Diseases of the Small Intestine. In Handbook of Small Animal Practice. Edited by R. V. Morgan. 395-420. New York: Churchill Livingstone.

Clark, D.R. 1986. Diseases of the General Circulation. In Current Veterinary Therapy: Food Animal Practice 2. Edited by J. L. Howard. 694-696. Philadelphia: W.B. Saunders.

Clark, D.R. 1988. Treatment of Circulatory Shock. In Veterinary Pharmacology and Therapeutics, 6th Ed. Edited by N. H. Booth and L. E. McDonald. 563- 570. Ames: Iowa State University Press.

Clark, E.S., and J.L. Becht. 1987. Clinical Pharmacology of the Gastrointestinal Tract. Vet Clin North Am (Equine Practice) 3 (1) : 101-122.

Clemmons, R. (1991). Therapeutic considerations for degenerative myelopathy of German Shepherds. Proceedings of the Ninth Annual Veterinary Medical Forum. Edited by W. Morrison, New Orleans, American College of Veterinary Internal Medicine. 773-779

Clubb, S.L. 1986. Therapeutics: Individual and Flock Treatment Regimens. In Clinical Avian Medicine and Surgery. Edited by G. J. Harrison and L. R. Harrison. 327-355. Philadelphia: W.B. Saunders.

Cohen, R. (1995). Systemic Anaphylaxis. Kirk's Current Veterinary Therapy:XII. Edited by J. Bonagura; Philadelphia, W.B. Saunders. 150-152

Concannon, P.W. 1986. Clinical and Endocrine Correlates of Canine and Ovarian Cycles and Pregnancy. In Current Veterinary Therapy IX, Small Animal Practice. Edited by R. W. Kirk. 1214-1224. Philadelphia: W.B. Saunders.

Constable, P. (1993). Diseases of the Digestive System: Introduction to the Ruminant Forestomach. Current Veterinary Therapy 3: Food Animal Practice. Edited by J. Howard; Philadelphia, W.B. Saunders Co. 706-

Coppoc, G.L. 1988. Chemotherapy of Neoplastic Diseases. In Veterinary Pharmacology and Therapeutics. Edited by N. H. Booth and L. E. McDonald. 861-876. Ames: Iowa State University Press.

Coppock, R.W., and M.S. Mostrom. 1986. Intoxication Due to Contaminated Garbage, Food, and Water. In Current Veterinary Therapy IX: Small Animal Practice. Edited by K. R.W. 221-225. Philadelphia: W.B. Saunders.

Cornelius, L.M., and D.E. Bjorling. 1988. Diseases of the Liver and Biliary System. In Handbook of Small Animal Practice. Edited by R. V. Morgan. 441-464. New York: Churchill Livingstone.

Cornelius, L.M., and E.L. Roberson. 1986. Treatment of gastrointestinal parasitism. In Current Veterinary Therapy IX: Small Animal Practice. Edited by K. R.W. 921-924. Philadelphia: W.B. Saunders.

Cornell Staff. 1985. Veterinary Drug Formulary: Cornell Research Foundation, Inc. Baltimore: Williams & Wilkins.

Cotter, S.M. 1988. Disorders of White Blood Cells. In Handbook of Small Animal Practice. Edited by R.V. Morgan. 749-760. New York: Churchill Livingstone.

Court, M.H., L.R. Engelking, N.H. Dodman, M.S. Anwer, D.C. Seeler, and M. Clark. 1987. Pharmacokinetics of Dantrolene Sodium in Horses. J Vet Pharmacol Ther 10 (3) : 218-226.

Couto, C. (1994). Lymphoma in the Horse. Proceedings of the Twelfth Annual Veterinary Medical Forum. Edited by R. DeNovo, San Francisco, American College of Veterinary Internal Medicine. 865

Couto, C.G. 1986. Canine Extranodal Lymphomas. In Current Veterinary Therapy IX: Small Animal Practice. Edited by R. W. Kirk. 473- 477. Philadelphia: W.B. Saunders.

Couto, C.G. 1989. Oncology. In The Cat: Diseases and Clinical Management. Edited by R. G. Sherding. 589-647. New York: Churchill Livingstone.

Couto, C.G. 1989a. Diseases of the Lymph Nodes and the Spleen. In Textbook of Veterinary Internal Medicine. Edited by S.J. Ettinger. 2225-2245. Philadelphia: W.B. Saunders.

Couto, C.G. 1989b. Oncology. In The Cat: Diseases and Clinical Management. Edited by R.G. Sherding. 589-647. New York: Churchill Livingstone.

Cowan, L. (1994). Diseases of the urinary bladder. Saunders Manual of Small Animal Practice. Edited by S. Birchard and R. Sherding; Philadelphia, W.B. Saunders Company. 826-836

Cowgill, L. (1992). Application of recombinant human erythropoietin in dogs and cats. Current Veterinary Therapy XI: Small Animal Practice. Edited by R. Kirk and J. Bonagura; Philadelphia, W.B. Saunders Company. 484-488

Cowgill, L.D., and A.J. Kallet. 1986. Systemic Hypertension. In Current Veterinary Therapy IX, Small Animal Practice. Edited by R. W. Kirk. 360-364. Philadelphia: W.B. Saunders.

Cox, V.S. 1986. Cryptorcidism in the Dog. In Current Therapy in Theriogenology 2: Diagnosis, Treatment and Prevention of Reproductive Diseases in Small and Large Animals. Edited by D. A. Morrow. 541-544. Philadelphia: W.B. Saunders.

Crowill-Davis, S. (1992). Tail chasing in dogs. Current Veterinary Therapy XI: Small Animal Practice. Edited by R. Kirk and J. Bonagura; Philadelphia, W.B. Saunders Company. 995-997

Cunningham, F., J. Fisher, C. Bevelle, M. Cwik and R. Jensen. (1992). "The pharmacokinetics of methocarbamol in the thoroughbred race horse." J Vet Pharmacol Therap. 15: 96-100.

Davenport, D. (1992). Hematemesis: diagnosis and treatment. Current Veterinary Therapy XI: Small Animal Practice. Edited by R. Kirk and J. Bonagura; Philadelphia, W.B. Saunders Company. 132-137

Davenport, D. (1994). Enteral/Parenteral nutrition for gastrointestinal disorders. Consultations in Feline Internal Medicine: 2. Edited by J. August; Philadelphia, W.B. Saunders Company. 107-118

Davis, L. (1993). Drugs Affecting the Digestive System. Current Veterinary Therapy 3: Food Animal Practice. Edited by J. Howard; Philadelphia, W.B. Saunders Co.

Davis, L.E. 1979. Fever. JAVMA 175 : 1210.

Davis, L.E. 1985. Handbook of Small Animal Therapeutics. New York: Churchill Livingstone.

Davis, L.E. 1985a. General Care of the Patient. In Handbook of Small Animal Therapeutics. Edited by L. E. Davis. 1-20. New York: Churchill Livingstone.

Davis, L.E. 1985b. Handbook of Small Animal Therapeutics. New York: Churchill Livingstone.

Davis, L.E. 1986. Drugs affecting the digestive system. In Curret Veterinary Therapy 2: Food Animal Practice. Edited by J. L. Howard. 760-763. Philadelphia: W.B. Saunders.

Day, K. (1993) Personal Communication

Debuf, Y. M. (1991). The Veterinary Formulary: Handbook of Medicines Used in Veterinary Practice. 448.

DeLellis, L. and M. Kittleson. (1992). Current uses and hazards of vasodilator therapy in heart failure. Current Veterinary Therapy XI: Small Animal Practice. Edited by R. Kirk and J. Bonagura; Philadelphia, W.B. Saunders Company. 700-708

DeNovo, R. and R. Bright. (1992). Chronic Feline Constipation/Obstruction. Current Veterinary Therapy XI: Small Animal Practice. Edited by R. Kirk and J. Bonagura; Philadelphia, W.B. Saunders Company. 619-626

DeNovo, R.C. 1988. Diseases of the Large Bowel. In Handbook of Small Animal Practice. Edited by R. V. Morgan. 421-439. New York: Churchill Livingstone.

DeNovo, R.C., Jr. 1986. Therapeutics of Gastrointestinal Diseases. In Current Veterinary Therapy (CVT) IX Small Animal Practice. Edited by R. W. Kirk. 862-871. Philadelphia: W.B. Saunders.

DeNovo, R.C., K.A. Potter, and J.M. Woolfson. 1988. Diseases of the Oral Cavity and Pharynx. In Handbook of Small Animal Practice. Edited by R. V. Morgan. 327-345. New York: Churchill Livingstone.

Derksen, F.J. 1987. Chronic Obstructive Pulmonary Disease. In Current Therapy in Equine Medicine. Edited by N. E. Robinson. 596-602. Philadelphia: W.B. Saunders.

Desiderio, J.V., and B.M. Rankin. 1986. Immunomodulators. In Current Veterinary Therapy IX: Small Animal Practice. Edited by R. W. Kirk. 1091-1096. Philadelphia: W.B. Saunders.

Dhupa, N. and N. Shaffron. (1995). Continuous Rate Infusion Formulas. Textbook of Veterinary Internal Medicine. Edited by S. Ettinger and E. Feldman; Philadelphia, W.B. Saunders. 2130-2145

Dial, S., M. Thrall and D. Hamar. (1989). "4-methylpyrazole as treatment for naturally acquired ethylene glycol intoxication in dogs." JAVMA. 195(1): 73-76.

Dill, S.G. 1986. Polioencephalomalacia in Ruminants. In Current Veterinary Therapy: Food Animal Practice 2. Edited by J. L. Howard. 868-869. Philadelphia: W.B. Saunders.

Dillon, R. 1986. Feline Heartworm Disease. In Current Veterinary Therapy IX: Small Animal Practice. Edited by R. W. Kirk. 420-425. Philadelphia: W.B. Saunders.

Dimski, D. (1995). Therapy of inflammatory bowel disease. Kirk's Current Veterinary Therapy:XII. Edited by J. Bonagura; Philadelphia, W.B. Saunders. 723-728

Dimski, D.S. 1989. Helminth and Noncoccidial Protozoan Parasites of the Gastrointestinal Tract. In The Cat: Diseases and Clinical Management. Edited by R. G. Sherding. 459-477. New York: Churchill Livingstone.

Dodds, W.J. 1988. Bleeding Disorders. In Handbook of Small Animal Practice. Edited by R. V. Morgan. 773-785. New York: Churchill Livingstone.

Dodman, N. (1992). "Advantages and guidelines for using antiprostaglandins." The Veterinary Clinics of North America; Small Animal Practice. 22(2: March): 367-369.

Donecker, J.M., R.A. Sams, and S.M. Ashcroft. 1986. Pharmacokinetics of Probenecid and the Effect of Oral Probenecid Administration on the Pharmacokinetics of Cefazolin in Mares. Am J Vet Res 47 (1) : 89-95.

Dougherty, S. (1994). Hemolytic anemia. Proceedings of the Twelfth Annual Veterinary Medical Forum. Edited by R. DeNovo, San Francisco, American College of Veterinary Internal Medicine. 152-154

Dow, S.W. 1989. Anaerobic Infections in Dogs and Cats. In Current Veterinary Therapy X: Small Animal Practice. Edited by R. W. Kirk. 1082-1085. Philadelphia: Saunders.

Drost, M. 1986. Elective Termination of Pregnancy. In Current Veterinary Therapy 2: Food Animal Practice. Edited by J. L. Howard. 797-798. Philadelphia: W.B. Saunders.

Duffee, N.E., J.M. Christensen, and A.M. Craig. 1989. The Pharmacokinetics of Cefadroxil in Foals. J Vet Pharmacol Therap 12 : 322-326.

Dumonceaux, G. (1995). Illicit drug intoxication in dogs. Kirk's Current Veterinary Therapy:XII. Edited by J. Bonagura; Philadelphia, W.B. Saunders. 250-252

Duran, S. (1992) Personal Communication

Duran, S. and W. Ravis. (1993). Comparative pharmacokinetics of H2 antagonists in horses. Proceedings of the Eleventh Annual Veterinary Medical Forum. Edited by R. DeNovo, Washington D.C., American College of Veterinary Internal Medicine. 687-690

Duran, S.H., W.R. Ravis, W.M. Pedersoli, and J. Schumacher. 1987. Pharmacokinetics of Phenobarbital in the Horse. Am Jnl Vet Res 48 (5) : 807-810.

Eastlake, P. and A. Snyder. (1998) Treatment of Shock: New Strategies

Edens, L. and J. Cargile. (1997). Medical Management of Colic. Current Therapy in Equine Medicine 4. Edited by N. Robinson; Philadelphia, Saunders. 182-191

Einarsson, S. 1986. Agalactia in Sows. In Current Therapy in Theriogenology 2: Diagnosis, Treatment and Prevention of Reproductive Diseases in Small and Large Animals. Edited by D. A. Morrow. 935-937. Philadelphia: W.B. Saunders.

Enos, L. R. (1993) Personal Communication

Enos, L.R. 1989. Personal Communication.

Enos, L.R., and K. Keiser. 1985. Formulary: Veterinary Medical Teaching Hospital; University of California at Davis. Davis:

Ettinger, S. and K. Barrett. (1995). Pain. Textbook of Veterinary Internal Medicine: Diseases of the Dog and Cat. Edited by S. Ettinger and E. Feldman; Philadelphia, WB Saunders. 57-60

Ettinger, S.J. 1989. Cardiac Arrythmias. In Textbook of Veterinary Internal Medicine. Edited by S. J. Ettinger. 1051-1096. Philadelphia: W.B. Saunders.

Evans, A. (1996). Hypersensitivity Reactions. Large Animal Internal Medicine, 2nd Ed. Edited by B. Smith; St Louis, Mosby. 1405-1411

Fadok, V. (1992). Appendicular Inflammatory Disorders. Current Therapy in Equine Medicine 3. Edited by N. Robinson; Philadelphia, W.B. Saunders Co. 161-165

Farnbach, G.C. 1985. Seizures in the Dog; Part II: Control. Comp CE 7 (6) : 505-510.

Farrow, B.R.H. 1986. Generalized Tremor Syndrome. In Current Veterinary Therapy IX: Small Animal Practice. Edited by R. W. Kirk. 800-801. Philadelphia: W.B. Saunders.

Feldman, B.F. 1985. Anemia and Bleeding Disorders. In Handbook of Small Animal Therapeutics. Edited by L. E. Davis. 189-216. New York: Churchill Livingstone.

Feldman, B.F. 1986. Thrombosis—Diagnosis and Treatment. In Current Veterinary Therapy IX: Small Animal Practice. Edited by R.W. Kirk. 505-509. Philadelphia: W.B. Saunders.

Feldman, B.F. 1989. Disorders of Platelets. In Current Veterinary Therapy X: Small Animal Practice. Edited by R.W. Kirk. 457-464. Philadelphia: W.B. Saunders.

Feldman, E., R. Nelson and R. Lynn. (1992). Desoxycorticosterone pivalate (DOCP) treatment of canine and feline hypoadrenocorticism. Current Veterinary Therapy XI: Small Animal Practice. Edited by R. Kirk and J. Bonagura; Philadelphia, W.B. Saunders Company. 353-355

Feldman, E.C. 1989. Adrenal Gland Disease. In Textbook of Veterinary Internal Medicine. Edited by S. J. Ettinger. 1721-1776. Philadelphia: W.B. Saunders.

Feldman, E.C., and M.E. Peterson. 1984. Hypoadrenocorticism. Vet Clin of North America: Small Anim Prac 14 (4) : 751-766.

Feldman, E.C., and R.W. Nelson. 1987a. Canine and Feline Endocrinology and Reproduction. Philadelphia: W.B. Saunders.

Feldman, E.C., and R.W. Nelson. 1987b. Hyperthyroidism and Thyroid Tumors. In Canine and Feline Endocrinology and Reproduction. 91-136. Philadelphia: WB Saunders.

Feldman, E.C., and R.W. Nelson. 1987c. Hypoglycemia. In Canine and Feline Endocrinology and Reproduction. 304-327. Philadelphia: WB Saunders.

Feldman, E.C., and R.W. Nelson. 1987d. Hypothyroidism. In Canine and Feline Endocrinology and Reproduction. 55-90. Philadelphia: WB Saunders.

Feldman, E.C., and R.W. Nelson. 1989. Diagnosis and Treatment Alternatives for Pyometra in Dogs and Cats. In Current Veterinary Therapy X: Small Animal Practice. Edited by R. W. Kirk. 1305-1310. Philadelphia: W.B. Saunders.

Feldman, E.C., L.A. Schrader, and D.C. Twedt. 1988. Diseases of the Adrenal Gland. In Handbook of Small Animal Practice. Edited by R. V. Morgan. 537-549. New York: Churchill Livingstone.

Felice, L. and M. Murphy. (1995). CVT Update: Anticoagulant rodenticides. Kirk's Current Veterinary Therapy:XII. Edited by J. Bonagura; Philadelphia, W.B. Saunders. 228-232

Fenner, W. (1994ab). Seizures, narcolepsy, and cataplexy. Saunders Manual of Small Animal Practice. Edited by S. Birchard and R. Sherding; Philadelphia, W.B. Saunders Company. 1147-1156

Fenner, W.R. 1986. Head Trauma and Nervous System Injury. In Current Veterinary Therapy IX: Small Animal Practice. Edited by R. W. Kirk. 830-836. Philadelphia: W.B. Saunders.

Fenner, W.R. 1986b. Meningitis. In Current Veterinary Therapy IX: Small Animal Practice. Edited by R. W. Kirk. 814-820. Philadelphia: W.B. Saunders.

Fenner, W.R. 1988. Diseases of the Brain. In Handbook of Small Animal Practice. Edited by R. V. Morgan. 247-268. New York: Churchill Livingstone.

Fenner, W.R. 1989. Neurologic Diseases. In The Cat: Diseases and Clinical Management. Edited by R.G. Sherding. 1163-1215. New York: Churchill Livingstone.

Ferguson, D.C. 1986. Thyroid Hormone Replacement Therapy. In Current Veterinary Therapy IX: Small Animal Practice. Edited by R. W. Kirk. 1018-1025. Philadelphia: W.B. Saunders.

Ferrante, P. and D. Kronfeld. (1992). Ergogenic Diets and Nutrients. Current Therapy in Equine Medicine 3. Edited by N. Robinson; Philadelphia, W.B. Saunders Co. 808-814

Fikes, J.D. 1990. Organophosphorous and Carbamate Insecticides. Vet Clinics of North Amer: Small Anim Pract 20 (2) : 353-367.

Fingeroth, J.M., and D.D. Smeak. 1988. Intravenous Methylene Blue Infusion for Intraoperative Identification of Pancreatic Islet-cell Tumors in Dogs. Part II: Clinical Trials and Results in Four Dogs. J Am Anim Hosp Assoc 24 (2) : 175-182.

Fingland, R.B. 1989. Tracheal Collapse. In Current Veterinary Therapy X: Small Animal Practice. Edited by R. W. Kirk. 353-360. Philadelphia: W.B. Saunders.

Fish, R. and C. Besch-Williford. (1992). Reproductive disorders in the rabbit and guinea pig. Current Veterinary

Therapy XI: Small Animal Practice. Edited by R. Kirk and J. Bonagura; Philadelphia, W.B. Saunders Company.

Flammer, K. (1992). An update on the diagnosis and treatment of avian chlamydiosis. Current Veterinary Therapy XI: Small Animal Practice. Edited by R. Kirk and J. Bonagura; Philadelphia, W.B. Saunders Company. 1150-1153

Flammer, K. 1986. Oropharyngeal Diseases in Caged Birds. In Current Veterinary Therapy IX: Small Animal Practice. Edited by R. W. Kirk. 699-702. Philadelphia: W.B. Saunders.

Foil, C.S. 1986. Antifungal Agents in Dermatology. In Current Veterinary Therapy IX: Small Animal Practice. Edited by R. W. Kirk. 560-565. Philadelphia: W.B. Saunders.

Ford, R. (1991). Gastrointestinal manifestations of viral diseases. Consultations in Feline Internal Medicine. Edited by J. August; Philadelphia, W.B. Saunders Company. 441-444

Ford, R.B., and A.L. Aronson. 1985. Antimicrobial Drugs and Infectious Diseases. In Handbook of Small Animal Therapeutics. Edited by L. E. Davis. 45-88. New York: Churchill Livingstone.

Forney, S. and R. Allen. (1992) Personal Communication

Forney, S., and R. Allen. 1984. Colorado State University, Veterinary Teaching Hospital Formulary. Fort Collins:

Forrester, S. and G. Lees. (1994). Disease of the Kidney and Ureter. Saunders Manual of Small Animal Practice. Edited by S. Birchard and R. Sherding; Philadelphia, W.B. Saunders Company. 799-820

Fowler, M.E. 1986. Zootoxins. In Current Veterinary Therapy: Food Animal Practice 2. Edited by J. L. Howard. 463-465. Philadelphia: W.B. Saunders.

Fowler, M.E. 1989. Medicine and Surgery of South American Camelids. Ames: Iowa State University Press.

Fox, J. (1995a). Desulfovibrio-associated proliferative colitis in ferrets. Kirk's Current Veterinary Therapy:XII. Edited by J. Bonagura; Philadelphia, W.B. Saunders. 1339-1341

Fox, L. (1995b). The paraneoplastic disorders. Kirk's Current Veterinary Therapy:XII. Edited by J. Bonagura; Philadelphia, W.B. Saunders. 530-542

Fox, P.R. 1989. Myocardial Diseases. In Textbook of Veterinary Internal Medicine. Edited by S.J. Ettinger. 1097-1131. Philadelphia: W.B. Saunders.

Franklin, J.S. 1986a. Dystocia and Obstetrics in Goats. In Current Therapy in Theriogenology 2: Diagnosis, Treatment and Prevention of Reproductive Diseases in Small and Large Animals. Edited by D. A. Morrow. 590-592. Philadelphia: W.B. Saunders.

Franklin, J.S. 1986b. Retained Placenta, Metritis and Pyometra. In Current Therapy in Theriogenology 2: Diagnosis, Treatment and Prevention of Reproductive Diseases in Small and Large Animals. Edited by D. A. Morrow. 595. Philadelphia: W.B. Saunders.

Frey, H.H., and B. Rieh. 1981. Pharmacokinetics of Naproxen in the Dog. AM J of Vet Res 42 (9) : 1615-1617.

Fulton, L. (1991). The use of lomustine in the treatment of brain masses. Proceedings of the Ninth Annual Veterinary Medical Forum. Edited by W. Morrison, New Orleans, American College of Veterinary Internal Medicine. 827-828

Furr, A., and W.B. Buck. 1986. Arsenic. In Current Veterinary Therapy: Food Animal Practice 2. Edited by J.L. Howard. 435-437. Philadelphia: W.B. Saunders.

Galey, F. (1993). Arsenic toxicosis. Current Veterinary Therapy 3: Food Animal Practice. Edited by J. Howard; Philadelphia, W.B. Saunders Co. 394-396

Gauvin, J. (1993). "Drug therapy in reptiles." Seminars in Avian & Exotic Med. 2(1): 48-59.

Geiser, D. (1992). Chemical restraint and anesthesia of the draft horse. Current Therapy in Equine Medicine 3. Edited by N. Robinson; Philadelphia, W.B. Saunders Co. 95-101

Geor, R. (1992). Equine gastroduodenal ulceration: Clinical syndromes, diagnosis and medical management. Minnesota Veterinary Medicine Association: Annual Conference. Edited by Bloomington, 27-32

Gershwin, L. (1992). Treatment of hypersensitivity: General guidelines. Current Veterinary Therapy XI: Small Animal Practice. Edited by R. Kirk and J. Bonagura; Philadelphia, W.B. Saunders Company. 54-59

Giger, U., and L.L. Werner. 1988. Immune-Mediated Diseases. In Handbook of Small Animal Practice. Edited by R. V. Morgan. 841-860. New York: Churchill Livingstone.

Gillespie, D. (1994). Reptiles. Saunders Manual of Small Animal Practice. Edited by S. Birchard and R. Sherding; Philadelphia, W.B. Saunders Company. 1390- 1411

Gilmour, M.A., and R. Walshaw. 1987. Naproxen-induced Toxicosis in a Dog. JAVMA 191 (11) : 1431-1432.

Gilson, S. and R. Page. (1994). Principles of Oncology. Saunders Manual of Small Animal Practice. Edited by S. Birchard and R. Sherding; Philadelphia, W.B. Saunders Company. 185-192

Golden, D.L., and V.C. Langston. 1988. Uses of Vincristine and Vinblastine in Dogs and Cats. JAVMA 193 (9) : 1114-1117.

Goodwin, J.K., and M. Schaer. 1989. Septic Shock. Vet Clin of North America—Small Anim Pract 19 (6) : 1239-1258.

Gorman, N.T., and L.L. Werner. 1989. Immune-mediated Diseases. In The Cat: Diseases and Clinical Management. Edited by R. G. Sherding. 511-527. New York: Churchill Livingstone.

Grandy, J.L., and R.B. Heath. 1987. Cardiopulmonary and Behavioral Effects of Fentanyl-droperidol in Cats. JAVMA 191 (1) : 59-61.

Grauer, G.F. , and J.J. Hjelle. 1988c. Pesticides. In Handbook of Small Animal Practice. Edited by R.V. Morgan. 1095-1100. New York: Churchill Livingstone.

Grauer, G.F., and J.J. Hjelle. 1988. Rodenticides. In Handbook of Small Animal Practice. Edited by R.V. Morgan. 1087-1093. New York: Churchill Livingstone.

Grauer, G.F., and J.J. Hjelle. 1988. Toxicology: Introduction. In Handbook of Small Animal Practice. Edited by R. V. Morgan. 1083-1086. New York: Churchill Livingstone.

Grauer, G.F., and J.J. Hjelle. 1988a. Household Drugs. In Handbook of Small Animal Practice. Edited by R.V. Morgan. 1115-1118. New York: Churchill Livingstone.

Grauer, G.F., and J.J. Hjelle. 1988b. Household Toxins. In Handbook of Small Animal Practice. Edited by R.V. Morgan. 1109-1114. New York: Churchill Livingstone.

Grauer, G.F., and J.J. Hjelle. 1988b. Toxicology: Introduction. In Handbook of Small Animal Practice. Edited by R. V. Morgan. 1083-1086. New York: Churchill Livingstone.

Grauer, G.F., and J.J. Hjelle. 1989a. Bacterial Toxins. In Handbook of Small Animal Practice. Edited by R. V. Morgan. 1105-1107. New York: Churchill Livingstone.

Grauer, G.F., and J.J. Hjelle. 1989b. Toxicology: Introduction. In Handbook of Small Animal Practice. Edited by R. V. Morgan. 1083-1086. New York: Churchill Livingstone.

Greco, D.S., and M.D. Peterson. 1989. Feline Hypoadrenocorticism. In Current Veterinary Therapy X: Small Animal Practice. Edited by R. W. Kirk. 1042-1045. Philadelphia: W.B. Saunders.

Green, R.A. 1989. Hemostatic Disorders: Coagulation and Thrombotic Disorders. In Textbook of Veterinary Internal Medicine. Edited by S.J. Ettinger. 2246-2264. Philadelphia: W.B. Saunders.

Greene, C.E. 1984. Clinical Microbiology and Infectious Diseases of the Dog and Cat. Philadelphia: W.B. Saunders.

Greene, C.E. 1986. Rocky Mountain Spotted Fever and Ehrlichiosis. In Current Veterinary Therapy IX: Small Animal Practice. Edited by R. W. Kirk. 1080-1084. Philadelphia: W.B. Saunders.

Greene, C.E., and K.G. Braund. 1989. Diseases of the Brain. In Textbook of Veterinary Internal Medicine. Edited by S.J. Ettinger. 578-623. Philadelphia: W.B. Saunders.

Greene, C.E., K.G. O'Neal, and J.A. Barsanti. 1984. Antimicrobial Chemotherapy. In Clinical Microbiology and Infectious Diseases of the Dog and Cat. Edited by C. E. Greene. 144-188. Philadelphia: W.B. Saunders.

Greene, R. (1995). Canine Ehrlichiosis: Clinical implications for humoral factors. Kirk's Current Veterinary Therapy:XII. Edited by J. Bonagura; Philadelphia, W.B. Saunders. 290-293

Greene, R.T. 1990. Lyme Borreliosis. In Infectious Diseases of the Dog and Cat. Edited by C. E. Greene. 508-514. Philadelphia: W.B. Saunders.

Greentree, W. and J. Hall. (1995). Iron Toxicosis. Kirk's Current Veterinary Therapy:XII. Edited by J. Bonagura; Philadelphia, W.B. Saunders. 240-242

Griffen, C. (1994). Flea allergy dermatitis. Saunders Manual of Small Animal Practice. Edited by S. Birchard and R. Sherding; Philadelphia, W.B. Saunders Company. 299-301

Grodsky, B. (1994) Personal Communication

Gross, M.E., and W.J. Tranquilli. 1989. Use of Alpha 2-Adrenergic Receptor Atagonists. JAVMA 195 (3) : 378-381.

Hackett, T. and D. Van pelt. (1995). Cardiopulmonary resuscitation. Kirk's Current Veterinary Therapy:XII. Edited by J. Bonagura; Philadelphia, W.B. Saunders. 167-175

Haddad, R.S., W.R. Ravis, W.M. Pedersoli, and R.L. Carson Jr. 1987. Pharmacokinetics and tissue Residues of Gentamicin in Lactating Cows after Multiple Intramuscular Doses are Administered. Am Jnl of Vet Res 48 (1) : 21-27.

Hall, I. and K. Campbell. (1994). Antibiotic-responsive dermatoses. Consultations in Feline Internal Medicine: 2. Edited by J. August; Philadelphia, W.B. Saunders Company. 233-239

Hall, J. (1994). Diagnosis and management of gastric motility disorders. Proceedings of the Twelfth Annual Veterinary Medical Forum. Edited by R. DeNovo, San Francisco, American College of Veterinary Internal Medicine. 180-182

Hall, J.A., and D.C. Twedt. 1988. Diseases of the Stomach. In Handbook of Small Animal Practice. Edited by R. V. Morgan. 371-384. New York: Churchill Livingstone.

Hall, L. W. and K. W. Clarke. (1983). Veterinary Anesthesia 8th Ed. London, Bailliere Tindall. 417pp.

Hameida, N.A., B.K. Gustafsson, and H.L. Whitmore. 1986. Therapy of Uterine Infections: Alternatives to Antibiotics. In Current Therapy in Theriogenology 2: Diagnosis, Treatment and Prevention of Reproductive Diseases in Small and Large Animals. Edited by D. A. Morrow. 45-47. Philadelphia: W.B. Saunders.

Hamlin, R. (1992). Current uses and hazards of ventricular antiarrhythmic therapy. Current Veterinary Therapy XI: Small Animal Practice. Edited by R. Kirk and J. Bonagura; Philadelphia, W.B. Saunders Company. 694-700

Handagama, P. 1986. Salicylate Toxicity. In Current Veterinary Therapy IX: Small Animal Practice. Edited by R. W. Kirk. 524-527. Philadelphia: W.B. Saunders.

Hansen, B. (1994). "Analgesic therapy." Comp on Cont Ed. 16(7): 868-875.

Hansen, S. (1995). Management of organophosphate and carbamate insecticide toxicoses. Kirk's Current Veterinary Therapy:XII. Edited by J. Bonagura; Philadelphia, W.B. Saunders. 245-248

Hardie, E.M. 1984. Actinomycosis and Nocardiosis. In Clinical Microbiology and Infectious Diseases of the Dog and

Cat. Edited by C. E. Greene. 663-674. Philadelphia: W.B. Saunders.

Hardy, R.M. 1985. Hepatic Diseases. In Handbook of Small Animal Therapeutics. Edited by L. E. Davis. 463- 484. New York: Churchill Livingstone.

Hardy, R.M. 1989. Diseases of the Liver and Their Treatment. In Textbook of Veterinary Internal Medicine. Edited by S.J. Ettinger. 1479-1527. Philadelphia: W.B. Saunders.

Hardy, R.M., and E.P. Robinson. 1986. Treatment of Alkalosis. In Current Veterinary Therapy IX, Small Animal Practice. Edited by R. W. Kirk. 67-75. Philadelpia: W.B. Saunders Co.

Hardy, R.M., and L.G. Adams. 1989. Hypophosphatemia. In Current Veterinary Therapy X: Small Animal Practice. Edited by R.W. Kirk. 43-47. Philadelphia: W.B. Saunders.

Harpster, N.K. 1986. Feline Myocardial Diseases. In Current Veterinary Therapy IX: Small Animal Practice. Edited by R. W. Kirk. 380- 398. Philadelphia: W.B. Saunders.

Harpster, N.K. 1988. Diseases of Peripheral Blood Vessels. In Handbook of Small Animal Practice. Edited by R.V. Morgan. 149-161. New York: Churchill LIvingstone.

Hartke, J., J. Rojko and L. Mathes. (1992). Cachexia associated with cancer and immunodeficiency in cats. Current Veterinary Therapy XI: Small Animal Practice. Edited by R. Kirk and J. Bonagura; Philadelphia, W.B. Saunders Company. 438-441

Harvey, J.W., T.W. French, and D.J. Meyer. 1982. Chronic Iron Deficiency in Dogs. JAAHA 18 : 946-960.

Haskins, S. (1992). Current concepts and techniques in small animal critical care. Minnesota Veterinary Association Annual Meeting. Edited by Bloomington, 199-254

Haskins, S.C. 1989. Cardiopulmonary Resuscitation. In Current Veterinary Therapy X: Small Animal Practice. Edited by R.W. Kirk. 330-336. Philadelphia: W.B. Saunders.

Hatch, R.C. 1988. Poisons Causing Abdominal Distress or Liver or Kidney damage. In Veterinary Pharmacology and Therapeutics. Edited by N. H. Booth and L. E. McDonald. 1102-1125. Ames: Iowa State Univ. Press.

Hatch, R.C. 1988b. Poisons Causing Respiratory Insufficiency. In Veterinary Pharmacology and Therapeutics. Edited by N.H. Booth and L.E. McDonald. 1007-1052. Ames: Iowa State Univ. Press.

Hatch, R.C., J.D. Clark, A.D. Jernigan, and C.H. Tracy. 1988. Searching for a Safe, Effective Antagonist to Telazol® Overdose. Vet Med (January) : 112-117.

Hawkins, E.C., S.J. Ettinger, and P.F. Suter. 1989. Diseases of the Lower Respiratory Tract (lung) and Pulmonary Edema. In Textbook of Veterinary Internal Medicine. Edited by S. J. Ettinger. 816-866. Philadelphia: W.B. Saunders.

Held, J.P. 1987. Retained Placenta. In Current Therapy in Equine Medicine, 2. Edited by N. E. Robinson. 547-550. Philadelphia: W.B. Saunders.

Helfand, S.C. 1989. Chemotherapy of Solid Tumors. In Current Veterinary Therapy X: Small Animal Practice. Edited by R.W. Kirk. 489-493. Philadelphia: W.B. Saunders.

Helton-Rhodes, K. (1994). Immune-mediated dermatoses. Saunders Manual of Small Animal Practice. Edited by S. Birchard and R. Sherding; Philadelphia, W.B. Saunders Company. 313-318

Henik, R., P. Snyder and L. Volk. (1997). "Treatment of systemic hypertension in cats with amlodipine besylate." J Am Anim Hosp Assoc. **33**(3): 226-234.

Henik, R.A., P.N. Olson, and R.A. Rosychuk. 1985. Progestagen Therapy in Cats. Comp CE 7 (2) : 132-141.

Herd, R.P. 1986a. Cestode Infections—Cattle, Sheep, Goats. In Current Veterinary Therapy: Food Animal Practice 2. Edited by J. L. Howard. 759-760. Philadelphia: W.B. Saunders.

Herd, R.P. 1986b. Trematode Infections—Cattle, Sheep, Goats. In Current Veterinary Therapy: Food Animal Practice 2. Edited by J. L. Howard. 756-759. Philadelphia: W.B. Saunders.

Herd, R.P. 1987. Chemotherapy of Migrating Strongyles. In Current Therapy in Equine Medicine, 2. Edited by N. E. Robinson. 331-332. Philadelphia: W.B. Saunders.

Herron, M.A. 1988. Disease of the External Genitalia. In Handbook of Small Animal Practice. Edited by R.V. Morgan. 673-678. New York: Churchill Livingstone.

Hillidge, C.J., and J-M.L. Zertuche. 1987. Corynebacterium equi Lung Abscesses in Foals. In Current Therapy in Equine Medicine, 2. Edited by N. E. Robinson. 230-232. Philadelphia: W.B. Saunders.

Hillman, R.B. 1987. Induction of Parturition. In Current Therapy in Equine Medicine, 2. Edited by N. E. Robinson. 533-537. Philadelphia: W.B. Saunders.

Hillyer, E. (1994). Avian dermatology. Saunders Manual of Small Animal Practice. Edited by S. Birchard and R. Sherding; Philadelphia, W.B. Saunders Company. 1271-1281

Hilwig, R.W. 1987. Cardiac Arrhythmias. In Current Therapy in Equine Medicine. Edited by N. E. Robinson. 154-164. Philadelphia: W.B. Saunders.

Hjerpe, C.A. 1986. The Bovine Respiratory Disease Complex. In Current Veterinary Therapy: Food Animal Practice 2. Edited by J. L. Howard. 670-681. Philadelphia: W.B. Saunders.

Hodgkins, E. and P. Franks. (1991). Nutritional requirements of the sick cat. Consultations in Feline Internal Medicine. Edited by J. August; Philadelphia, W.B. Saunders Company. 25-34

Hoeffer, H. (1995). Antimicrobials in pet birds. Kirk's Current Veterinary Therapy:XII. Edited by J. Bonagura; Philadelphia, W.B. Saunders. 1278-1283

Holland, M. and C. Chastain. (1995). Uses & misuses of aspirin. Kirk's Current Veterinary Therapy:XII. Edited by J. Bonagura; Philadelphia, W.B. Saunders. 70-73

Hooser, S.B., and V.R. Beasley. 1986. Methylxanthine Poisoning (Chocolate and Caffeine toxicosis). In Current Veterinary Therapy IX: Small Animal Practice. Edited by R. W. KIrk. 191-192. Philadelphia: W.B. Saunders.

Hopkins, S.M. 1987. Ovulation Management. In Current Therapy in Equine Medicine. Edited by N. E. Robinson. 498-500. Philadelphia: W.B. Saunders.

Hoskins, J.D. 1988. Juvenile Nutritional Disorders. In Handbook of Small Animal Practice. Edited by R.V. Morgan. 1061-1066. New York: Churchill Livingstone.

Hoskins, J.D. 1989. Thiacetarsemide and its Adverse Effects. In Current Veterinary Therapy X: Small Animal Practice. Edited by R. W. Kirk. 131-134. Philadelphia: W.B. Saunders.

Hoskins, J.D., J.B. Malone, and C.R. Root. 1981. Albendazole Therapy in Naturally-occurring Feline Paragonimiasis. AAHA 17 (2) : 265-269.

Howard, J. (1993). Table of Common Drugs: Approximate Doses. Current Veterinary Therapy 3: Food Animal Practice. Edited by J. Howard; Philadelphia, W.B. Saunders Co. 930-933

Howard, J.L. 1986. Current Veterinary Therapy 2, Food Animal Practice. Philadelphia: W.B. Saunders.

Hribernik, T.N. 1989. Canine and Feline Heartworm disease. In Current Veterinary Therapy X: Small Animal Practice. Edited by R. W. Kirk. 263-270. Philadelphia: W.B. Saunders.

Hubbell, J. (1994). PRactical methods of anesthesia. Saunders Manual of Small Animal Practice. Edited by S. Birchard and R. Sherding; Philadelphia, W.B. Saunders Company. 31-21

Hubbell, J. (1994). Practical methods of anesthesia. Saunders Manual of Small Animal Practice. Edited by S. Birchard and R. Sherding; Philadelphia, W.B. Saunders Company. 31-21

Hubbell, J.A.E., R.M. Bednarski, and W.W. Muir. 1989. Xylazine and Tiletamine-Zolazepam Anesthesia in Horses. Am J Vet Res 50 (5) : 737-742.

Huber, W.G. 1988a. Aminoglycosides, Macrolides, Lincosamides, Polymyxins, Chloramphenicol, and other Antibacterial Drugs. In Veterinary Pharmacology and Therapeutics. Edited by N. H. Booth and L. E. McDonald. 822-848. Ames: Iowa State University Press.

Huber, W.G. 1988b. Antifungal and Antiviral Agents. In Veterinary Pharmacology and Therapeutics. Edited by N. H. Booth and L. E. McDonald. 849-860. Ames: Iowa State University Press.

Huerkamp, M. (1995). Anesthesia and postoperative management of rabbits and pocket pets. Kirk's Current Veterinary Therapy:XII. Edited by J. Bonagura; Philadelphia, W.B. Saunders. 1322-1327

Hugnet, C., F. Buronrosse, X. Pineau, J. Cadore, G. Lorgue and P. Berny. (1996). "Toxicity and kinetics of amitraz in dogs." Am J Vet Res. **57**(10): 1506-10.

Hurvitz, A.I., and J. Johnessee. 1985. Immunologic Disorders. In Handbook of Small Animal Therapeutics. Edited by L. E. Davis. 149-174. New York: Churchill Livingstone.

Ihrke, P. and T. Gross. (1997). Ulcerative Dermatosis of Shetland Sheepdogs and Collies. Kirk's Current Veterinary Therapy XII: Small Animal Practice. Edited by J. Bonagura; Philadelphia, Saunders. 639-640

Ihrke, P.J. 1986. Antibacterial Therapy in Dermatology. In Current Veterinary Therapy IX: Small Animal Practice. Edited by R. W. Kirk. 566-571. Philadelphia: W.B. Saunders.

IJenkins, W.L. 1985. Pharmacologic Control of Inflammation. In Handbook of Small Animal Therapeutics. Edited by L. E. Davis. 127-148. New York: Churchill Livingstone.

Ilkiw, J. (1992). "Other potentially useful new injectable anesthetic agents." The Veterinary Clinics of North America; Small Animal Practice. 22(2: March): 281-293.

Jacobs, R., J. Lumsden and W. Vernau. (1992). Canine and Feline Reference Values. Current Veterinary Therapy XI: Small Animal Practice. Edited by R. Kirk and J. Bonagura; Philadelphia, W.B. Saunders Company. 1250-1277

Janssens, L. (1986). "Treatment of pseudopregnancy with bromocriptin, an ergot alkaloid." Vet Record. 119(8): 172-174.

Jenkins, T. (1993) Personal Communication

Jenkins, W.L. 1986. Antimicrobial Therapy. In Current Veterinary Therapy: Food Animal Practice 2. Edited by J. L. Howard. 8-23. Philadelphia: W.B. Saunders.

Jenkins, W.L. 1987. Pharmacologic Aspects of Analgesic Drugs in Animals: An overview. JAVMA 191 (10) : 1231-1240.

Jenkins, W.L. 1987a. Cephalosporins and Cephamycins. In The Bristol Handbook of Antimicrobial Therapy. Edited by D. E. Johnston. 249-256. Evansville: Veterinary Learning Systems.

Jenkins, W.L. 1987b. Chloramphenicol, Macrolides, Lincosamides,Vancomycin, Polymyxins, Rifamycins. In The Bristol Handbook of Antimicrobial Therapy. Edited by D. E. Johnston. 261-265. Evansville: Veterinary Learning Systems.

Jenkins, W.L. 1988. Drugs Affecting Gastrointestinal Functions. In Veterinary Pharmacology and Therapeutics 6th Ed. Edited by N. H. Booth and L. E. McDonald. 657- 671. Ames: Iowas Stae Univ. Press.

Jenkins, W.L., and D.M. Boothe. 1987. Amphotericin B, Nystatin, Flucytosine, Imidazoles, Griseofulvin. In The Bristol Handbook of Antimicrobial Therapy. Edited by D. E. Johnston. 270-271. Evansville: Veterinary Learning Systems.

Jergens, A. (1995). Acute diarrhea. Kirk's Current Veterinary Therapy:XII. Edited by J. Bonagura; Philadelphia, W.B. Saunders. 701-705

Jernigan, A.D., R.C. Wilson, and R.C. Hatch. 1988. Pharmacokinetics of Amikacin in Cats. Am Jnl of Vet Res 49 (3) : 355-358.

Jernigan, A.D., R.C. Wilson, N.D. Booth, R.C. Hatch, and A. Akbari. 1988. Comparative Pharmacokinetics of Yohimbine in Steers, Horses and Dogs. Can J Vet Res 52 : 172-176.

Jernigan, A.D., R.C. Wilson, R.C. Hatch, and D.T. Kemp. 1988. Pharmacokinetics of Gentamicin after Intravenous, Intramuscular and Subcutaneos Administration in Cats. Am Jnl of Vet Res 49 (1) : 32-35.

Johnessee, J.S., and A.I. Hurvitz. 1983. Thrombocytopenia. In Current Veterinary Therapy VII: Small Animal Practice. Edited by R. W. Kirk. 389-392. Philadelphia: W.B. Saunders.

Johnson, L. (1993). Llama Herd health management. Current Veterinary Therapy 3: Food Animal Practice. Edited by J. Howard; Philadelphia, W.B. Saunders Co. 172-177

Johnson, S. (1996). "Nonsteroidal antiinflammatory analgesics to manage acute pain in dogs and cats." Comp CE. (October 1996): 1117-1123.

Johnson, S. and R. Sherding. (1994). Diseases of the liver and biliary tract. Saunders Manual of Small Animal Practice. Edited by S. Birchard and R. Sherding; Philadelphia, W.B. Saunders Company. 722-760

Johnson, S., R. Sherding and R. Bright. (1994). Diseases of the stomach. Saunders Manual of Small Animal Practice. Edited by S. Birchard and R. Sherding; Philadelphia, W.B. Saunders Company. 655-675

Johnson, S.E. 1984. Clinical pharmacology of antiemetics and antidiarrheals. Columbus: Kal Kan Foods, Inc.

Johnson, S.E. 1986. Acute Hepatic Failure. In Current Veterinary Therapy (CVT) IX Small Animal Practice. Edited by R. W. Kirk. 945-952. Philadelphia: W.B. Saunders.

Johnston, J., and R.H. Whitlock. 1987. Botulism. In Current Therapy in Equine Medicine, 2. Edited by N. E. Robinson. 367-370. Philadelphia: W.B. Saunders.

Johnston, S. (1997). Skeletal Diseases. Practical Small Animal Internal Medicine. Edited by M. Leib and W. Monroe; Philadelphia, Saunders. 1189-1208

Johnston, S.D. 1986. Parturition and Dystocia in the Bitch. In Current Therapy in Theriogenology 2: Diagnosis, Treatment and Prevention of Reproductive Diseases in Small and Large Animals. Edited by D. A. Morrow. 500-501. Philadelphia: W.B. Saunders.

Jones, B.D. 1985. Gastrointestinal Disorders. In Handbook of Small Animal Therapeutics. Edited by L. E. Davis. 397-462. New York: Churchill Livingston.

Jones, R.S. 1985b. New Skeletal Muscle Relaxants in Dogs and Cats. JAVMA 187 (3) : 281-282.

Jones, R.S., and C.J. Seymour. 1985. Clinical Observations on the use of Vecuronium as a Muscle Relaxant in the Dog. J Small Anim Pract 26 (4) : 213-218.

Joseph, R., J. Carrillo and V. Lennon. (1988). "Myasthenia gravis in the cat." J Vet Int Med. 2(2): 75-79.

Juzwiak, J.S., M.P. Brown, R. Gronwall, and A.E. Houston. 1989. Effect of Probenecid Administration on Cephapirin Pharmacokinetics and Concentrations in Mares. Am J Vet Res 50 (10) : 1742-1747.

Karpinski, L.G., and S. L. Clubb. 1986. Clinical Aspects of Ophthalmology in Caged Birds. In Current Veterinary Therapy IX: Small Animal Practice. Edited by R. W. Kirk. 616-621. Philadelphia: W.B. Saunders.

Kaufmann, A.F. 1986. Anthrax. In Current Veterinary Therapy: Food Animal Practice 2. Edited by J. L. Howard. 566-567. Philadelphia: W.B. Saunders.

Kay, A.D., and K.P. Richter. 1988. Diseases of the Parathyroid Glands. In Handbook of Small Animal Practice. Edited by R.V. Morgan. 521-526. New York: Churchill Livingstone.

Kay, N.D., S. A. Kruth, and D.C. Twedt. 1988. Miscellaneous Endocrine Disorders. In Handbook of Small Animal Practice. Edited by R. V. Morgan. 551-559. New York: Churchill Livingstone.

Kay, W.J., and D.P. Aucoin. 1985. Seizure Disorders. In Handbook of Small Animal Therapeutics. Edited by L. E. Davis. 505-518. New York: Churchill Livingstone.

Keene, B. (1989). Canine Cardiomyopathy. Current Veterinary Therapy X, Small Animal Practice. Edited by R. Kirk; Philadelphia, W.B. Saunders. 240-251

Keene, B. (1992). L-Carnitine deficiency in canine dilated cardiomyopathy. Current Veterinary Therapy XI: Small Animal Practice. Edited by R. Kirk and J. Bonagura; Philadelphia, W.B. Saunders Company. 780-783

Keller, E. and S. Helfand. (1994). Clinical management of soft-tissue sarcomas. Consultations in Feline Internal Medicine: 2. Edited by J. August; Philadelphia, W.B. Saunders Company. 557-566

Kelly, M. (1995). Pain. Textbook of Veterinary Internal Medicine: Diseases of the Dog and Cat. Edited by S. Ettinger and E. Feldman; Philadelphia, WB Saunders. 21-25

Kemp, D. (1992) Personal Communication

Kemp, D. (1994) Personal Communication

Kemppainen, R.J. 1986. Principles of Glucocorticoid Therapy in Nonendocrine Disease. In Current Veterinary Therapy (CVT) IX Small Animal Practice. Edited by R. W. Kirk. 954-962. Philadelphia: W.B. Saunders.

Kemppainen, R.J., and C.A. Zerbe. 1989a/b. Common Endocrine Diagnostic Tests: Normal Values and Interpretation. In Current Veterinary Therapy X: Small Animal Practice. Edited by R. W. Kirk. 961-968. Philadelphia: W.B. Saunders.

Kern, T.J. 1986. Disorders of the Lacrimal System. In Current Veterinary Therapy IX: Small Animal Practice. Edited by R. W. Kirk. 634-641. Philadelphia: W.B. Saunders.

Kinosian, L. (1994) Personal Communication

Kintzer, P. and M. Peterson. (1995). Mitotane (o, p'-DDD) treatment of hyperadrenocorticism in dogs. Kirk's Current Veterinary Therapy:XII. Edited by J. Bonagura; Philadelphia, W.B. Saunders. 416-420

Kintzer, P.P., and M.E. Peterson. 1989. Mitotane (o,p'-DDD) Treatment of Cortisol-Secreting Adrenocortical Neoplasia. In Current Veterinary Therapy X: Small Animal Practice. Edited by R. W. Kirk. 1034-1037. Philadelphia: W.B. Saunders.

Kirk, R.W. 1986. Current Veterinary Therapy IX, Small Animal Practice. Philadelphia: W.B. Saunders.

Kirk, R.W. 1989. Current Veterinary Therapy X, Small Animal Practice. Philadelphia: W.B. Saunders.

Kirkpatrick, C.E., A.W. Knochenhauer, and S.L. Jacobsen. 1987. Use of Praziquantel for Treatment of Diphyllobothrium sp. in a Dog. JAVMA 190 (5) : 557-558.

Kirkpatrick, C.E., and E.A. Shelly. 1987. Paragonimiasis in a Dog: Treatment with Praziquantel. JAVMA 187 (1) : 75-76.

Kittleson, M.D. 1985. Cardiovascular Diseases. In Handbook of Small Animal Therapeutics. Edited by L. E. Davis. 217-265. New York: Churchill Livingstone.

Kittleson, M.D. 1985b. Pathophysiology and Treatment of Heart Failure. In Manual of Small Animal Cardiology. Edited by L. P. Tilley and J. M. Owens. 308-332. New York: Churchill Livingstone.

Kittleson, M.D., and G.G. Knowlen. 1986. Positive Inotropic Drugs in the Treatment of Heart Failure. In Current

Veterinary Therapy IX: Small Animal Practice. Edited by R. W. Kirk. 323- 328. Philadelphia: W.B. Saunders.

Klausner, J., F. Bell, D. Hayden, S. Johnston and E. Lund. (1994). Recent developments in the diagnosis and treatment of BPH and prostatic carcinoma. Proceedings of the Twelfth Annual Veterinary Medical Forum. Edited by R. DeNovo, San Francisco, American College of Veterinary Internal Medicine. 870-871

Klausner, J.S., and F.W. Bell. 1988. Personal Communication.

Knaack, K.E. 1988. Diseases of Muscle. In Handbook of Small Animal Practice. Edited by R. V. Morgan. 917-927. New York: Churchill Livingstone.

Knapp, D., R. Richardson, T. Chan, G. Bottoms, W. Widmer, D. DeNicola, R. Teclaw, P. Bonney and T. Kuczek. (1994). "Piroxicam therapy in 34 dogs with transitional cell carcinoma of the urinary bladder." J Vet Int Med. 8(4): 273-278.

Knapp, D.W., R.C. Richardson, P.L. Bonney, and K. Hahn. 1988. Cisplatin Therapy in 41 Dogs with Malignant Tumors. Jnl of Vet Int Med 2 : 41-46.

Knight, D. (1995). Guidelines for diagnosis and management of heartworm (Dirofilaria Immitis) infection. Kirk's Current Veterinary Therapy:XII. Edited by J. Bonagura; Philadelphia, W.B. Saunders. 879-887

Knight, D.H. 1987. Thiacetarsemide Treatment of Heartworm Infection in Dogs. Seminars in Vet Med (Small Animal) 2 (1) : 36-43.

Knight, D.H. 1988. Heartworm Disease. In Handbook of Small Animal Practice. Edited by R. V. Morgan. 139-148. New York: Churchill Livingstone.

Knowlen, G.G., and M.D. Kittleson. 1986. Captopril Therapy in Dogs with Heart Failure. In Current Veterinary Therapy (CVT) IX Small Animal Practice. Edited by R. W. Kirk. 334-339. Philadelphia: W.B. Saunders.

Kordick, D., M. Lappin and E. Breitschwerdt. (1995). Feline Rickettsial Diseases. Kirk's Current Veterinary Therapy:XII. Edited by J. Bonagura; Philadelphia, W.B. Saunders. 287-290

Koritz, G.D. 1986. Therapeutic Management of Inflammation. In Current Veterinary Therapy 2: Food Animal Practice. Edited by J. L. Howard. 23-27. Philadelphia: W.B. Saunders.

Koritz, G.D., C.A. Neff-Davis, and I.J. Munsiff. 1986. Bioavailability of Four Slow-release Theophylline Formulations in the Beagle Dog. J Vet Pharm & Ther 9 (3) : 293-302.

Kornegay, J.N. 1986. Diskospondylitis. In Current Veterinary Therapy IX: Small Animal Practice. Edited by R. W. Kirk. 810-814. Philadelphia: W.B. Saunders.

Kowalczyk, D.F., and J. Beech. 1983. Pharmacokinetics of Phenytoin in Horses. J Vet Pharmacol Ther 6 (2) : 133-140.

Kraemer, D.C., and M.J. Bowen. 1986. Embryo Transfer in Laboratory Animals. In Current Therapy in Theriogenology 2: Diagnosis, Treatment and Prevention of Reproductive Diseases in Small and Large Animals. Edited by D. A. Morrow. 73-78. Philadelphia: W.B. Saunders.

Krahwinkel, D.J. 1988. Disease of the Salivary Glands. In Handbook of Small Animal Practice. Edited by R. V. Morgan. 347-356. New York: Churchill Livingstone.

Kruger, J.M., C.A. Osborne, and D.J. Polzin. 1986. Treatment of Hypercalcemia. In Current Veterinary Therapy (CVT) IX Small Animal Practice. Edited by R. W. Kirk. 75-90. Philadelphia: W.B. Saunders.

Kummel, B. (1995). Medical treatment of canine pemphigus-pemphigoid. Kirk's Current Veterinary Therapy:XII. Edited by J. Bonagura; Philadelphia, W.B. Saunders. 636-638

Kunkle, G.A. 1986. Progestagens in Dermatology. In Current Veterinary Therapy IX: Small Animal Practice. Edited by R. W. Kirk. 601-605. Philadelphia: W.B. Saunders.

Kwochka, K. (1992). Treatment of seborrhea in the American cocker spaniel. Current Veterinary Therapy XI: Small Animal Practice. Edited by R. Kirk and J. Bonagura; Philadelphia, W.B. Saunders Company. 523-527

Kwochka, K. (1994). Keratinization Defects. Saunders Manual of Small Animal Practice. Edited by S. Birchard and R. Sherding; Philadelphia, W.B. Saunders Company. 318-325

Kwochka, K.W. 1986. Differential Diagnosis of Feline Miliary Dermatitis. In Current Veterinary Therapy (CVT) IX Small Animal Practice. Edited by R. W. Kirk. 538-544. Philadelphia: W.B. Saunders.

Labato, M. (1994). Micturition Disorders. Saunders Manual of Small Animal Practice. Edited by S. Birchard and R. Sherding; Philadelphia, W.B. Saunders Company. 857-864

Labato, M.A. 1988. Disorders of Micturation. In Handbook of Small Animal Practice. Edited by R. V. Morgan. 621-628. New York: Churchill Livingstone.

Lage, A.L., D. Polzin, and R.D. Zenoble. 1988. Diseases of the Bladder. In Handbook of Small Animal Practice. Edited by R. V. Morgan. 605-620. New York: Churchill Livingstone.

Laliberté, L. 1986. Pregnancy, Obstetrics, and Postpartum Management of the Queen. In Current Therapy in Theriogenology 2: Diagnosis, Treatment and Prevention of Reproductive Diseases in Small and Large Animals. Edited by D. A. Morrow. 812-821. Philadelphia: W.B. Saunders.

Lane, I. and J. Barsanti. (1994). Urinary incontinence. Consultations in Feline Internal Medicine: 2. Edited by J. August; Philadelphia, W.B. Saunders Company. 373-382

Lantz, G., S. Badylak, M. Hiles and T. Arkin. (1992). "Treatment of reperfusion injury in dogs with experimentally induced gastric dilatation volvulus." Am J Vet Res. 53(9): 1594-1598.

Lappin, M. (1995). CVT Update: Feline Toxoplasmosis. Kirk's Current Veterinary Therapy:XII. Edited by J. Bonagura; Philadelphia, W.B. Saunders. 309-314

Lappin, M. (1997). Rever, sepsis, and principles of antimicrobial therapy. Practical Small Animal Internal Medicine. Edited by M. Leib and M. WE; Philadelphia, Saunders. 829-836

Lappin, M.R. 1989. Feline Toxoplasmosis. In Current Veterinary Therapy X: Small Animal Practice. Edited by R. W. Kirk. 1112-1115. Philadelphia: W.B. Saunders.

Laratta, L.J. 1986. Ocular Infectious Diseases. In Current Veterinary Therapy IX: Small Animal Practice. Edited by R. W. Kirk. 673-678. Philadelphia: W.B. Saunders.

LeCouteur, R.A. 1988. Disorders of Peripheral Nerves. In Handbook of Small Animal Practice. Edited by R. V. Morgan. 299-318. New York: Churchill Livingstone.

LeCouteur, R.A., and J.M. Turrel. 1986. Brain Tumors in Dogs and Cats. In Current Veterinary Therapy IX: Small Animal Practice. Edited by R. W. Kirk. 820-825. Philadelphia: W.B. Saunders.

Legendre, A. (1993). Itraconazole: A new antifungal drug. Proceedings of the Eleventh Annual Veterinary Medical Forum. Edited by R. DeNovo, Washington D.C., American College of Veterinary Internal Medicine. 277-278

Legendre, A. (1995). Antimycotic Drug Therapy. Kirk's Current Veterinary Therapy:XII. Edited by J. Bonagura; Philadelphia, W.B. Saunders. 327-331

Legendre, A.M. 1989. Systemic Mycotic Infections. In The Cat: Diseases and Clinical Management. Edited by R. G. Sherding. 427-457. New York: Churchill Livingstone.

Leib, M.S., W.H. Hay, and L. Roth. 1989. Plasmacytic-Lymphocytic Colitis in Dogs. In Current Veterinary Therapy X: Small Animal Practice. Edited by R. W. Kirk. 939-944. Philadelphia: W.B. Saunders.

Leifer, C.E. 1986. Hypoglycemia. In Current Veterinary Therapy IX: Small Animal Practice. Edited by R. W. Kirk. 982-983. Philadelphia: W.B. Saunders.

Lein, D.H. 1986. Prostaglandins in Therapy in Small Animal Reproduction. In Current Veterinary Therapy IX: Small Animal Practice. Edited by R. W. Kirk. 1233-1236. Philadelphia: W.B. Saunders.

Lein, D.H. 1989. Female Reproduction. In The Cat: Diseases and Clinical Management. Edited by R. G. Sherding. 1479-1497. New York: Churchill Livingstone.

Leveille-Webster, C. and S. Center. (1995). Chronic hepatitis: Therapeutic considerations. Kirk's Current Veterinary Therapy:XII. Edited by J. Bonagura; Philadelphia, W.B. Saunders. 749-756

Lewis, L.D., M.L. Morris Jr., and M.S. Hand. 1987. Feline Urological Syndrome. In Small Animal Clinician Nutrition III. Topeka: Mark Morris Assoc.

Line, S. (1998) Personal Communication

Lissman, B.A. 1986. Lyme Disease. In Current Veterinary Therapy IX: Small Animal Practice. Edited by R. W. Kirk. 1100. Philadelphia: W.B. Saunders.

Lissman, B.A. 1988. Rickettsial Diseases. In Handbook of Small Animal Practice. Edited by R. V. Morgan. 1005-1008. New York: Churchill Livingstone.

Littman, M. (1992). Update: Treatment of hypertension in dogs and cats. Current Veterinary Therapy XI: Small Animal Practice. Edited by R. Kirk and J. Bonagura; Philadelphia, W.B. Saunders Company. 838-839

Livesay, M. (1996). Navicular disease. Large Animal Internal Medicine. Edited by B. Smith; St Louis, Mosby. 1291-1297

Loar, A. (1994). Anemia: Diagnosis and treatment. Consultations in Feline Internal Medicine: 2. Edited by J. August; Philadelphia, W.B. Saunders Company. 469-487

Loar, A.S. 1988. Diseases of the Mammary Glands. In Handbook of Small Animal Practice. Edited by R. V. Morgan. 707-717. New York: Churchill Livingstone.

Lofstedt, R.M. 1986. Termination of Unwanted Pregnancy in the Mare. In Current Therapy in Theriogenology 2: Diagnosis, Treatment and Prevention of Reproductive Diseases in Small and Large Animals. Edited by D. A. Morrow. 715-718. Philadelphia: W.B. Saunders.

London, C. and A. Frimberger. (1997). Principles of Oncology. Handbook or Small Animal Practice, 3rd Ed. Edited by R. Morgan; Philadelphia, Saunders. 745-760

Long, R.E. 1986. Potential of Chrysotherapy in Veterinary Medicine. JAVMA 188 (5) : 539-542.

Longhofer, S.L. 1988. Chemotherapy of Rickettsial, Protozoal, and Chlamydial Diseases. Vet Clin of North America: Sm Anim Pract 18 (6) : 1183-1196.

Lorenz, M.D. 1984. Integumentary Infections. In Clinical Microbiology and Infectious Diseases of the Dog and Cat. Edited by C. E. Greene. 189-207. Philadelphia: W.B. Saunders.

Lothrop, C.D. 1989. Medical Treatment of Neuroendocrine Tumors of the Gastroenteropancreatic System with Somatostatin. In Current Veterinary Therapy X: Small Animal Practice. Edited by R. W. Kirk. 1020-1024. Philadelphia: W.B. Saunders.

Lothrop, C.D., and G.J. Harrison. 1986. Miscellaneous Diagnostic Tests. In Clinical Avian Medicine and Surgery. Edited by G. J. Harrison and L. R. Harrison. 293-297. Philadelphia: W.B. Saunders.

Lothrop, C.D., G.J. Harrison, D. Schultz, and T. Utteridge. 1986. Miscellaneous Diseases. In Clinical Avian Medicine and Surgery. Edited by G. J. Harrison and L. R. Harrison. 535-536. Philadelphia: W.B. Saunders.

Love, D.N., R.J. Rose, C.A. Martin, and M. Bailey. 1983. Serum Concentrations of Penicillin in the Horse After Administration of a Variety of Penicillin Preparations. Equine Vet J 15 (1) : 43-48.

Ludders, J. (1992). "Advantages and guidelines for using isoflurane." The Veterinary Clinics of North America; Small Animal Practice. 22(2: March): 328-331.

Lulich, J., C. Osborne and C. Smith. (1992). Canine calcium oxalate urolithiasis: Risk factor management. Current Veterinary Therapy XI: Small Animal Practice. Edited by R. Kirk and J. Bonagura; Philadelphia, W.B. Saunders Company. 892-899

Lumb, W.V., and E.W. Jones. 1984. Veterinary Anesthesia, 2nd Ed. Philadelphia: Lea & Febiger.

Lunney, J. and S. Ettinger. (1991). "Mexiletine administration for management of ventricular arrhythmia in 22 dogs." AAHA. 27(6): 597-600.

MacEwen, E.G., and R.C. Rosenthal. 1989. Approach to Treatment of Cancer Patients. In Textbook of Veterinary Internal Medicine. Edited by S.J. Ettinger. 527-546. Philadelphia: W.B. Saunders.

Mack, R. (1993). Chronic hepatitis in dogs. Proceedings of the Eleventh Annual Veterinary Medical Forum. Edited by R. DeNovo, Washington D.C., American College of Veterinary Internal Medicine. 206-207

Macy, D.W. 1986. Chemotherapeutic Agents Available for Cancer Treatment. In Current Veterinary Therapy IX: Small Animal Practice. Edited by R.W. Kirk. 467-470. Philadelphia: W.B. Saunders.

Macy, D.W. 1987. Fungal Diseases—Dog, Cat. In The Bristol Handbook of Antimicrobial Therapy. Edited by D. E. Johnston. 152-157. Evansville: Veterinary Learning Systems.

Macy, D.W. 1988. Systemic Mycoses. In Handbook of Small Animal Practice. Edited by R. V. Morgan. 963-973. New York: Churchill Livingstone.

Macy, D.W., and S.L. Ralston. 1989. Cause and Control of Decreased Appetite. In Current Veterinary Therapy X: Small Animal Practice. Edited by R. W. Kirk. 18-24. Philadelphia: W.B. Saunders.

Mader, D.R., G.M. Conzelman, and J.D. Baggot. 1985. Effects of Ambient Temperature on the Half-life and Dosage Regimen of Amikacin in the Gopher Snake. JAVMA 187 (11) : 1134-1136.

Maggio-Price, L. 1988. Disorders of Red Blood Cells. In Handbook of Small Animal Practice. Edited by R. V. Morgan. 725-748. New York: Churchill Livingstone.

Magne, M.L. 1986. Acute Metritis in the Bitch. In Current Therapy in Theriogenology 2: Diagnosis, Treatment and Prevention of Reproductive Diseases in Small and Large Animals. Edited by D. A. Morrow. 500-501. Philadelphia: W.B. Saunders.

Magne, M.L. 1989. Canine Plasmacytic-Lymphocytic Enteritis. In Current Veterinary Therapy X: Small Animal Practice. Edited by R. W. Kirk. 922-926. Philadelphia: W.B. Saunders.

Mandsager, R.E. 1988. Personal Communication.

Manning, T.O., and V.J. Scheidt. 1986. Bovine Hypersensitivity Skin Disease. In Current Veterinary Therapy 2 : Food Animal Practice. Edited by J. L. Howard. 934-936. Philadelphia: W.B. Saunders.

Mapletoff, R.J. 1986. Bovine Embryo Transfer. In Current Therapy in Theriogenology 2: Diagnosis, Treatment and Prevention of Reproductive Diseases in Small and Large Animals. Edited by D. A. Morrow. 54-58. Philadelphia: W.B. Saunders.

Marder, A. (1991). "Psychotropic drugs and behavioral therapy." Veterinary Clinics of North America: Small Animal Practice. 21(2): 329-342.

Marks, S., C. Mannella and M. Schaer. (1990). "Coral snake enevenomation in the dog: Report of four cases and review of the literature." AAHA. 26(6): 629-634.

Marshall, R. (1993). "Avian anthelmintics and antiprotozoals." Seminars in Avian & Exotic Med. 2(1): 33-41.

Martens, R.J., and W.L. Scrutchfield. 1982. Foal Diarrhea: Pathogenesis, Etiology, and Therapy. Comp Cont Ed 4 (4) : S175-S186.

Mathews, N.S., et al 1986. Cardiovascular and Pharmacokinetic Effects of Isoxsuprine in the Horse. Am J Vet Res 47 (10) : 2120-2133.

Matus, R.E. 1989. Chemotherapy of Lymphoma and Leukemia. In Current Veterinary Therapy X: Small Animal Practice. Edited by R.W. Kirk. 482-488. Philadelphia: W.B. Saunders.

Matz, M. (1995). Gastrointestinal ulcer therapy. <u>Kirk's Current Veterinary Therapy:XII</u>. Edited by J. Bonagura; Philadelphia, W.B. Saunders. 706-710

McCaw, D. (1994). Advances in therapy for retroviral infections. Consultations in Feline Internal Medicine: 2. Edited by J. August; Philadelphia, W.B. Saunders Company. 21-25

McClary, D. 1986. Retained Placenta. In Current Veterinary Therapy: Food Animal Practice 2. Edited by J. L. Howard. 773-775. Philadelphia: W.B. Saunders.

McConnell, V. C. and T. Hughey. (1992) Formulary 1989: Update, The University of Georgia, Veterinary Medical Teaching Hospital

McConnell, V.C., and T Hughey. 1987. Formulary, The University of Georgia, Veterinary Medical Teaching Hospital. Athens, GA:

McCormack, J. 1986. Pyometra in Cattle. In Current Veterinary Therapy: Food Animal Practice 2. Edited by J. L. Howard. 777-778. Philadelphia: W.B. Saunders.

McDonald, L.E. 1988. Hormones of the Pituitary Gland. In Veterinary Pharmacology and Therapeutics - 6th Ed. Edited by N. H. Booth and L. E. McDonald. 581-592. Ames: Iowa State University Press.

McDonald, S.E. 1986. Lead Poisoning in Psittacine Birds. In Current Veterinary Therapy IX: Small Animal Practice. Edited by R. W. Kirk. 713-718. Philadelphia: W.B. Saunders.

McDonald, S.E. 1989. Summary of Medications for Use in Psittacine Birds. JAAV 3 (3) : 120-127.

McDougald, L. and E. Roberson. (1988). Antiprotazoan Drugs. Veterinary Pharmacology and Therapeutics. Edited by N. H. Booth and L. E. McDonald; Ames, Iowa State University Press. 950-968

McGrath, C. and J. Ko. (1997a). <u>How to use medetomidine (Domitor®) in dogs</u>. Virgina Veterinary Notes, Veterinary Teaching Hospital.

McGrath, C. and J. Ko. (1997b). <u>How to use the new alpha-2 antagonist, Atipamezole (Antisedan®) to reverse medetomidine (Domitor®) in the dog</u>. Virgina Veterinary Notes, Veterinary Teaching Hospital.

McHardy, N., R. Woolon and R. Clampitt. (1986). "Efficacy, toxicity and metabolism of imidocarb dipropionate in the treatment of Babesia ovis infection in sheep." Res Vet Sci. **41**((1)): 14-20.

McKeever, P.J. 1986. Stomatitis. In Current Veterinary Therapy IX: Small Animal Practice. Edited by R. W. Kirk. 846-848. Philadelphia: W.B. Saunders.

McKiernan, B. (1992). Current uses and hazards of bronchodilator therapy. Current Veterinary Therapy XI: Small Animal Practice. Edited by R. Kirk and J. Bonagura; Philadelphia, W.B. Saunders Company. 515-518

McKiernan, B.C., G.D. Koritz, L.E. Davis, C.A. Neff-Davis, and D.R. Pheris. 1983. Pharmacokinetic studies of theophylline in cats. J Vet Pharm & Ther 6 (2) : 99-104.

Medleau, L. and K. Moriello. (1992). Feline Dermatophytosis. Current Veterinary Therapy XI: Small Animal Practice. Edited by R. Kirk and J. Bonagura; Philadelphia, W.B. Saunders Company. 547-551

Meredith, M.J. 1986. Bacterial Endometritis. In Current Therapy in Theriogenology 2: Diagnosis, Treatment and Prevention of Reproductive Diseases in Small and Large Animals. Edited by D. A. Morrow. 953-956. Philadelphia: W.B. Saunders.

Meric, S.M. 1989. Diagnosis and Management of Feline Hyperthyroidism. Comp Cont Educ 11 (9) : 1053-1062.

Merkt, H., A. Graser, H. Sackman, and A.-R. Gunzel. 1979. [Perforation of the rectum in the horse. Trials on temporary inhibition of peristalsis by drugs.] Mastdarmperforation beim pferd. Versuche zur temporaren medikamentosen Peristaltikhemmung. Abstract. Praktische Tierarzt 60 (3) : 189-190.

Merrall, M., and D.M. West. 1986. Rumiant Hypomagnesemic Tetanies. In Current Veterinary Therapy: Food Animal Practice 2. Edited by J.L. Howard. 328-332. Philadelphia: W.B. Saunders.

Merritt, A.M. 1987. Diabetes Mellitus. In Current Therapy in Equine Medicine, 2. Edited by N. E. Robinson. 181-182. Philadelphia: W.B. Saunders.

Meurs, K. and E. Breitschwerdt. (1995). CVT Update: Zinc Toxicity. Kirk's Current Veterinary Therapy:XII. Edited by J. Bonagura; Philadelphia, W.B. Saunders. 238-239

Meuten, D.J., and P.J. Armstrong. 1989. Parathyroid Disease and Calcium Metabolism. In Textbook of Veterinary Internal Medicine. Edited by S.J. Ettinger. 1610-1631. Philadelphia: W.B. Saunders.

Miller, M. (1994). Diagnosis and management of dirofilariasis. Consultations in Feline Internal Medicine: 2. Edited by J. August; Philadelphia, W.B. Saunders Company. 267-271

Miller, M. and L. Tilley. (1995). Manual of Canine and Feline Cardiology, 2nd Ed. 562pp.

Miller, M., L. Tilley and F. Smith. (1994). Disorders of cardiac rhythm. Saunders Manual of Small Animal Practice. Edited by S. Birchard and R. Sherding; Philadelphia, W.B. Saunders Company. 421-435

Miller, M.S. 1985. Treatment of Cardiac Arrhythmias and Conduction Disturbances. In Handbook of Small Animal Cardiology. Edited by L. P. Tilley and J. M. Owens. 333-386. New York: Churchill Livingstone.

Miller, W. (1989). Nonsteroidal anti-inflammatory agents in the management of canine and feline pruritis. Current Veterinary Therapy X, Small Animal Practice. Edited by R. Kirk; Philadelphia, W.B. Saunders. 566-569

Miller, W. (1992). Follicular Disorders of the Doberman Pinscher. Current Veterinary Therapy XI: Small Animal Practice. Edited by R. Kirk and J. Bonagura; Philadelphia, W.B. Saunders Company. 515-518

Miller, W. (1993). Nutritional, Endocrine, and Keratinization Abnormalities. Current Veterinary Therapy 3: Food Animal Practice. Edited by J. Howard; Philadelphia, W.B. Saunders Co. 911-913

Moreau, P.M., and M.R. Lappin. 1989. Pharmacologic Management of Urinary Incontinence. In Current Veterinary Therapy X: Small Animal Practice. Edited by R. W. Kirk. 1214-1222. Philadelphia: Saunders.

Moreland, K.J. 1988. Ulcer disease of the upper gastrointestinal tract in small animals: Pathophysiology, diagnosis, and management. Comp CE 10 (11) : 1265-1280.

Morgan, R. (1997). Appendix IV: Recommended Drug Dosages. Handbook of Small Animal Practice 3rd Ed. Edited by R. Morgan; Philadelphia, Saunders. 1339-1375

Morgan, R.V. 1988. Burns. In Handbook of Small Animal Practice. Edited by R.V. Morgan. 1135-1142. New York: Churchill Livingstone.

Morgan, R.V. 1988. Collection and Interpretation of Laboratory Data. In Handbook of Small Animal Practice. Edited by R. V. Morgan. 13-22. New York: Churchill Livingstone.

Morgan, R.V. 1988. Handbook of Small Animal Practice. New York: Churchill Livingstone.

Moriello, K. (1992). Treatment of Sarcoptes and Cheyletiella infestations. Current Veterinary Therapy XI: Small Animal Practice. Edited by R. Kirk and J. Bonagura; Philadelphia, W.B. Saunders Company.

Moses, B.L. 1988. Cardiac Arrhythmias and Cardiac Arrest. In Handbook of Small Animal Practice. Edited by R. V. Morgan. 71-90. New York: Churchill Livingstone.

Mount, M.E. 1989. Toxicology. In Textbook of Veterinary Internal Medicine. Edited by S.J. Ettinger. 456-483. Philadelphia: W.B. Saunders.

Mount, M.E., B.J. Woody, and M.J. Murphy. 1986. The Anticoagulant Rodenticides. In Current Veterinary Therapy IX: Small Animal Practice. Edited by R.W. Kirk. 156-165. Philadelphia: W.B. Saunders.

Muir, W. (1994). Cardiopulmonary cerebral resuscitation. Saunders Manual of Small Animal Practice. Edited by S. Birchard and R. Sherding; Philadelphia, W.B. Saunders Company. 513-524

Muir, W. and J. Bonagura. (1994). Drugs for the treatment of cardiovascular disease. Saunders Manual of Small Animal Practice. Edited by S. Birchard and R. Sherding; Philadelphia, W.B. Saunders Company. 436-443

Muir, W.W., and C.R. Swanson. 1989. Principles, Techniques, and Complications of Feline Anesthesia and Chemical Restraint. In The Cat: Diseases and Clinical Management. Edited by R.G. Sherding. 81-116. New York: Churchill Livingstone.

Muir, W.W., and S. McGuirk. 1987. Cardiovascular Drugs: Their Pharmacology and Use in Horses. Vet Clin of North America, Equine Prac 3 (1) : 37- 57.

Muir, W.W., III. 1987. Analgesics in the Treatment of Colic. In Current Therapy in Equine Medicine. Edited by N. E. Robinson. 27-29. Philadelphia: W.B. Saunders.

Muir, W.W., III. An Outline of Veterinary Anesthesia. Columbus: Anesthesia Dept., Dept. of Veterinary Clinical Sciences, Ohio State University.

Muir, W.W., R.A. Sams, and S. Ashcraft. 1984. Pharmacologic and Pharmacokinetic Properties of Methocarbamol in the Horse. Am J Vet Res 45 (11) : 2256-2260.

Mullowney, P.C. 1986. Bovine Mange. In Current Veterinary Therapy: Food Animal Practice 2. Edited by J. L. Howard. 920-924. Philadelphia: W.B. Saunders.

Mulnix, J.A. 1985. Endocrine Disorders. In Handbook of Small Animal Therapeutics. Edited by L. E. Davis. 577-603. New York: Churchill Livingstone.

Mundell, A. (1994). Demodicosis. Saunders Manual of Small Animal Practice. Edited by S. Birchard and R. Sherding; Philadelphia, W.B. Saunders Company. 290-294

Murtaugh, R.J. 1988. Protozoal Diseases. In Handbook of Small Animal Practice. Edited by R. V. Morgan. 1009-1028. New York: Churchill Livingstone.

Murtaugh, R.J., and J.N. Ross. 1988. Cardiac Arrhythmias: Pathogenesis and Treatment in the Trauma Patient, Comp CE 10 (2) : 332-339.

Neer, T. (1994). Seizures (Part I & II). Proceedings of the Twelfth Annual Veterinary Medical Forum. Edited by R.

DeNovo, San Francisco, American College of Veterinary Internal Medicine. 463-471

Neer, T.M. 1988. Clinical Pharmacologic Features of Fluoroquinolone Antimicrobial Agents. JAVMA 193 (5) : 577-580.

Neer, T.M. 1988. Diseases of the Middle Ear and Inner Ear. In Handbook of Small Animal Practice. Edited by R. V. Morgan. 945-952. New York: Churchill Livingstone.

Neff-Davis, C.A. 1985. Clinical Monitoring of Drug Concentrations. In Handbook of Small Animal Therapeutics. Edited by L. E. Davis. 633-655. New York: Churchill Livingstone.

Neiger, R. D. 1989. Arsenic Poisoning. In Current Veterinary Therapy X: Small Animal Practice. Edited by R.W. Kirk. 159-161. Philadelphia: W.B. Saunders.

Nelson, D.L. 1986. Diseases of the Cornea. In Current Veterinary Therapy IX: Small Animal Practice. Edited by R. W. Kirk. 642-649. Philadelphia: W.B. Saunders.

Nelson, R. (1994). Diabetes Mellitus. Saunders Manual of Small Animal Practice. Edited by S. Birchard and R. Sherding; Philadelphia, W.B. Saunders Company. 249-256

Nelson, R. and E. Feldman. (1992). Treatment of feline diabetes mellitus. Current Veterinary Therapy XI: Small Animal Practice. Edited by R. Kirk and J. Bonagura; Philadelphia, W.B. Saunders Company. 364-367

Nelson, R. and E. Feldman. (1995). Treatment of feline diabetes mellitus with the oral sulfonylurea, glipizide. Kirk's Current Veterinary Therapy:XII. Edited by J. Bonagura; Philadelphia, W.B. Saunders. 401-403

Nelson, R.W. 1988a. Diseases of the Uterus. In Handbook of Small Animal Practice. Edited by R. V. Morgan. 661-666. New York: Churchill Livingstone.

Nelson, R.W. 1989b. Treatment of Canine Hypothyroidism. In Current Veterinary Therapy X: Small Animal Practice. Edited by R. W. Kirk. 993-997. Philadelphia: W.B. Saunders.

Nelson, R.W., and E.C. Feldman. 1986. Canine Diabetes Mellitus. In Current Veterinary Therapy IX: Small Animal Practice. Edited by R. W. Kirk. 991-999. Philadelphia: W.B. Saunders.

Nelson, R.W., and E.C. Feldman. 1988. Diseases of the Endocrine Pancreas. In Handbook of Small Animal Practice. Edited by R. V. Morgan. 527-535. New York: Churchill Livingstone.

Nichols, C. (1992). Endocrine and metabolic causes of polyuria and polydipsia. Current Veterinary Therapy XI: Small Animal Practice. Edited by R. Kirk and J. Bonagura; Philadelphia, W.B. Saunders Company. 293-301

Nichols, C.E., and J.B. Miller. 1988. Diseases of the Pituitary Gland. In Handbook of Small Animal Practice. Edited by R. V. Morgan. 501-506. New York: Churchill Livingstone.

Nichols, R. 1989. Diabetes Insipidus. In Current Veterinary Therapy X: Small Animal Practice. Edited by R. W. Kirk. 973-978. Philadelphia: W.B. Saunders.

Nichols, R., M Peterson and H. Mullen. (1994). Adrenal gland. Saunders Manual of Small Animal Practice. Edited by S. Birchard and R. Sherding; Philadelphia, W.B. Saunders Company. 238-248

Nicholson, S. (1993). Cyanogenic Plants. Current Veterinary Therapy 3: Food Animal Practice. Edited by J. Howard; Philadelphia, W.B. Saunders Co. 367-368

Nixon, A. (1992). Intra-articular medication. Current Therapy in Equine Medicine 3. Edited by N. Robinson; Philadelphia, W.B. Saunders Co. 127-131

Nixon, M. (1994). "Cisapride-The newest gastrointestinal prokinetic drug." Academy of Feline Practitioners Newsletter. : 6.

Noone, K.E. 1986. Pulmonary Hypersensitivities. In Current Veterinary Therapy (CVT) IX Small Animal Practice. Edited by R. W. Kirk. 285-292. Philadelphia: W.B. Saunders.

Nouws, J.F.M., D.J. Mevius, T.B. Vree, A.M. Baars, and J. Laurensen. 1988. Pharmacokinetics, Renal Clearance and Metabolism of Ciprofloxacin Following Intravenous and Oral Administration to Calves andPiigs. Vet Quarterly 10 (3): 156-163.

Novotney, M.J., and H.R. Adams. 1986. New Perspectives in Cardiology; Recent Advances in Antiarrhythmic Drug Therapy. JAVMA 189 (5) : 533-539.

Noxon, J. (1997). Bacterial and Fungal Diseases of the Skin. Practical Small Animal Internal Medicine. Edited by M. Leib and M. WE; Philadelphia, Saunders. 33-48

Noxon, J.O. 1989. Systemic Antifungal Therapy. In Current Veterinary Therapy X: Small Animal Practice. Edited by R. W. Kirk. 1101-1108. Philadelphia: W.B. Saunders.

Nye, R.R. 1986. Dealing with the Egg-bound Bird. In Current Veterinary Therapy (CVT) IX Small Animal Practice. Edited by R.W. Kirk. 746-747. Philadelphia: W.B. Saunders.

O'Brien, J.A. 1986. Laryngeal Paralysis in Dogs. In Current Veterinary Therapy IX: Small Animal Practice. Edited by R. W. Kirk. 789-792. Philadelphia: W.B. Saunders.

O'Keefe, D.A., and C.L. Harris. 1990. Toxicology of Oncologic Drugs. Vet Clinics of North America: Small Animal Pract 20 (2) : 483-504.

Oehme, F.W. 1986a. Aspirin and Acetominophen. In Current Veterinary Therapy IX: Small Animal Practice. Edited by R. W. Kirk. 188-190. Phialdelphia: W.B. Saunders.

Oehme, F.W. 1986b. Cyanogenic Plants. In Current Veterinary Therapy: Food Animal Practice 2. Edited by J.L. Howard. 390-392. Philadelphia: W.B. Saunders.

Oehme, F.W. 1987. General Principles in Treatment of Poisoning. In Current Therapy in Equine Medicine 2. Edited by N. E. Robinson. 653-656. Philadelphia: W.B. Saunders.

Oehme, F.W. 1987. Insecticides. In Current Therapy in Equine Medicine. Edited by N. E. Robinson. 658-660. Philadelphia: W.B. Saunders.

Oehme, F.W. 1987a. Arsenic. In Current Therapy in Equine Medicine. Edited by N.E. Robinson. 668-670. Philadelphia: W.B. Saunders.

Oehme, F.W. 1987b. General Principles in Treatment of Poisoning. In Current Therapy in Equine Medicine 2. Edited by N.E. Robinson. 653-656. Philadelphia: W.B. Saunders.

Oehme, F.W. 1987c. Insecticides. In Current Therapy in Equine Medicine. Edited by N.E. Robinson. 658-660. Philadelphia: W.B. Saunders.

Oehme, F.W. 1987d. Lead. In Current Therapy in Equine Medicine. Edited by N.E. Robinson. 667-668. Philadelphia: W.B. Saunders.

Ogburn, P.N. 1988. Myocardial Diseases. In Handbook of Small Animal Practice. Edited by R. V. Morgan. 109-128. New York: Churchill Livingstone.

Ogilvie, G.K. 1988. Principles of Oncology. In Handbook of Small Animal Practice. Edited by R.V. Morgan. 805-817. New York: Churchill Livingstone.

Oglesbee, B. (1995). Emergency medicine for pocket pets. Kirk's Current Veterinary Therapy:XII. Edited by J. Bonagura; Philadelphia, W.B. Saunders. 1328-1331

Oglesbee, B. and C. Bishop. (1994a). Avian Infectious disease. Saunders Manual of Small Animal Practice. Edited by S. Birchard and R. Sherding; Philadelphia, W.B. Saunders Company. 1257-1270

Oglesbee, B. and C. Bishop. (1994b). Avian Infectious Diseases. Saunders Manual of Small Animal Practice. Edited by S. Birchard and R. Sherding; Philadelphia, W.B. Saunders Company. 1257-1270

Olson, J.D., and P.N. Olson. 1986. Disorders of the Canine Mammary Gland. In Current Therapy in Theriogenology 2: Diagnosis, Treatment and Prevention of Reproductive Diseases in Small and Large Animals. Edited by D. A. Morrow. 506-509. Philadelphia: W.B. Saunders.

Olson, P.N., R.A. Bowen, P.W. Husted, and T.M. Nett. 1986. Terminating Canine and Feline Pregnancies. In Current Veterinary Therapy IX: Small Animal Practice. Edited by R. W. Kirk. 1236-1240. Philadelphia: W.B. Saunders.

Orsini, J.A. 1988. Butorphanol tartrate: Pharmacology and Clinical Indications. Comp CE 10 (7) : 849-854.

Orsini, J.A., L.R. Soma, J.E. Rourke, and M. Park. 1985. Pharmacokinetics of Amikacin in the Horse Following Intravenous and Intramuscular Administration. Jnl of Vet Pharm & Ther 8 (2) : 194-201.

Orton, C.E. 1986. Gastric Dilatation-volvulus. In Current Veterinary Therapy (CVT) IX Small Animal Practice. Edited by R. W. Kirk. 856-862. Philadelphia: W.B. Saunders.

Osborne, C., J. Lulich, L. Unger, J. Bartges and L. Felice. (1993). Canine and feline urolithiasis: Relationship and etiopathogenesis with treatment and prevention. Disease mechanisms in small animal surgery. Edited by M. Bojrab; Philadelphia, Lea & Febiger. 464-511

Osborne, C.A., A. Hoppe, and T.D. O'Brien. 1989. Medical Dissolution and Prevention of Cystine Urolithiasis. In Current Veterinary Therapy X: Small Animal Practice. Edited by R.W. Kirk. 1189-1193. Philadelphia: W.B. Saunders.

Osborne, C.A., and J.P. Lulich. 1987. Urinary Tract and Prostate Gland. In The Bristol Handbook of Antimicrobial Therapy. Edited by D. E. Johnston. 74-87. Evansville: Veterinary Learning Systems.

Osborne, C.A., D.J. Polzin, G.R. Johnston, and T.D. O'Brien. 1989. Canine Urolithiasis. In Textbook of Veterinary Internal Medicine. Edited by S.J. Ettinger. 2083-2107. Philadelphia: W.B. Saunders.

Osweiler, G.D. 1986. Nephrotoxic Plants. In Current Veterinary Therapy: Food Animal Practice 2. Edited by J. L. Howard. 401-404. Philadelphia: W.B. Saunders.

Osweiler, G.D., and B.S. Hook. 1986. Mercury. In Current Veterinary Therapy: Food Animal Practice 2. Edited by J.L. Howard. 440-442. Philadelphia: W.B. Saunders.

Osweiler, G.D., and L.P. Ruhr. 1986. Plants Affecting Blood Coagulation. In Current Veterinary Therapy: Food Animal Practice 2. Edited by J. L. Howard. 404-406. Philadelphia: W.B. Saunders.

Ott, R.S. 1986a. Breeding Management Problems in Sheep and Goats. In Current Veterinary Therapy: Food Animal Practice 2. Edited by J. L. Howard. 811-813. Philadelphia: W.B. Saunders.

Ott, R.S. 1986b. Prostaglandins for Induction of Estrous, Estrous Synchronization, Abortion and Induction of Parturition. In Current Therapy in Theriogenology 2: Diagnosis, Treatment and Prevention of Reproductive Diseases in Small and Large Animals. Edited by D. A. Morrow. 583-585. Philadelphia: W.B. Saunders.

Overall, K. (1997). Clinical behavioral medicine for small animals. St Louis, Mosby. 544pp.

Papich, M. (1992). Table of Common Drugs: Approximate Dosages. Current Veterinary Therapy XI: Small Animal Practice. Edited by R. Kirk and J. Bonagura; Philadelphia, W.B. Saunders Company. 1233-1249

Papich, M. (1995). Table of Common Drugs: Approximate Dosages. Current Veterinary Therapy XII: Small Animal Practice. Edited by J. Bonagura; Philadelphia, W.B. Saunders Company. 1429-1446

Papich, M.G. 1986. Bronchdilator Therapy. In Current Veterinary Therapy IX, Small Animal Practice. Edited by R. W. Kirk. 278-284. Philadelphia: W.B. Saunders.

Papich, M.G. 1990. Toxicoses from Over-the-Counter Human Drugs. Vet Clin of North Amer: Sm Anim Prac 20 (2) : 431-451.

Papich, M.G., L.E. Davis, C.A. Davis, B.C. McKiernan, and S.A. Brown. 1986. Pharmacokinetics of Procainamide Hydrochloride in Dogs. Am J Vet Res 47 (11) : 2351-2357.

Paradis, M. 1989. Ivermectin in Small Animal Dermatology. In Current Veterinary Therapy X: Small Animal Practice. Edited by R. W. Kirk. 560-563. Philadelphia: W.B. Saunders.

Paradis, M. and D. Scott. (1992). Nonsteroidal therapy for canine and feline pruritis. Current Veterinary Therapy XI: Small Animal Practice. Edited by R. Kirk and J. Bonagura; Philadelphia, W.B. Saunders Company. 563-566

Pascoe, P.J. 1986. Short-term Ventilatory Support. In Current Veterinary Therapy IX: Small Animal Practice. Edited by R. V. Kirk. 269-277. Philadelphia: W.B. Saunders.

Paul, J.W. 1986. Anthelmintic Therapy. In Current Veterinary Therapy: Food Animal Practice 2. Edited by J. L. Howard. 39-44. Philadelphia: W.B. Saunders.

Pechman, R.D. 1989. Respiratory Parasites. In The Cat: Diseases and Clinical Management. Edited by R. G. Sherding. 485-494. New York: Churchill Livingstone.

Pedroia, V. 1989. Disorders of the Skeletal Muscles. In Textbook of Veterinary Internal Medicine. Edited by S.J. Ettinger. 733-744. Philadelphia: W.B. Saunders.

Penzhorn, B. and G. Swan. (1993). Coccidiosis. Current Veterinary Therapy 3: Food Animal Practice. Edited by J. Howard; Philadelphia, W.B. Saunders Co. 599-604

Peterson, J. and C. Couto. (1994a). Lymphoid leukemias. Peterson, J. and C. Couto. (1994a). Lymphoid leukemias. Consultations in Feline Internal Medicine: 2. Edited by J. August; Philadelphia, W.B. Saunders Company. 509-513

Peterson, J. and C. Couto. (1994b). Tumors of the skin and subcutaneous tissues. Saunders Manual of Small Animal Practice. Edited by S. Birchard and R. Sherding; Philadelphia, W.B. Saunders Company. 211-217

Peterson, M.E. 1986. Canine Hyperadrenocorticism. In Current Veterinary Therapy IX: Small Animal Practice. Edited by R. W. Kirk. 963-972. Philadelphia: W.B. Saunders.

Peterson, M.E. 1986. Hypoparathyroidism. In Current Veterinary Therapy IX: Small Animal Practice. Edited by R.W. Kirk. 1039-1045. Philadelphia: W.B. Saunders.

Peterson, M.E., and D.C. Ferguson. 1989. Thyroid Diseases. In Textbook of Veterinary Internal Medicine. Edited by S. J. Ettinger. 1632-1675. Philadelphia: W.B. Saunders.

Peterson, M.E., and J.F. Randolph. 1989. Endocrine Diseases. In The Cat: Diseases and Clinical Management. Edited by R. G. Sherding. 1095-1161. New York: Churchill Livingstone.

Peterson, M.E., P.P. Kintzer, and A.I. Hurvitz. 1988. Methimazole Treatment of 262 Cats With Hyperthyroidism. Jnl of Vet Int Med 2 (3) : 150-157.

Phillips, R.W. 1988a. Trace Elements. In Veterinary Pharmacology and Therapeutics - 6th Ed. Edited by N.H. Booth and L.E. McDonald. 708-719. Ames: Iowa State University Press.

Phillips, R.W. 1988b. Water-soluble Vitamins. In Veterinary Pharmacology and Therapeutics - 6th Ed. Edited by N. H. Booth and L. E. McDonald. 698-702. Ames: Iowa State University Press.

Pier, A.C. 1986. Dermatophytosis. In Current Veterinary Therapy: Food Animal Practice 2. Edited by J. L. Howard. 924-927. Philadelphia: W.B. Saunders.

Pion, P. (1992). Current uses and hazards of calcium channel blocking agents. Current Veterinary Therapy XI: Small Animal Practice. Edited by R. Kirk and J. Bonagura; Philadelphia, W.B. Saunders Company. 684-688

Pion, P.D., and M.D. Kittleson. 1989. Therapy for Feline Aortic Thromboembolism. In Current Veterinary Therapy X:

Small Animal Practice. Edited by R.W. Kirk. 295-302. Philadelphia: W.B. Saunders.

Plumb, D.C. 1988. Veterinary Pharmacy Formulary. 2nd ed. St. Paul: Minnesota Veterinary Teaching Hosp.

Polzin, D.J., and C.A. Osborne. 1985. Diseases of the Urinary Tract. In Handbook of Small Animal Therapeutics. Edited by L. E. Davis. 333-395. New York: Churchill Livingstone.

Powe, T.A. 1986. Lactation Failure: Dysglactia, Agalactia, Hypogalactia. In Current Veterinary Therapy: Food Animal Practice 2. Edited by J. L. Howard. 771-773. Philadelphia: W.B. Saunders.

Power, H. and P. Ihrke. (1995). The use of synthetic retinoids in veterinary medicine. Kirk's Current Veterinary Therapy:XII. Edited by J. Bonagura; Philadelphia, W.B. Saunders. 585- 590

Powers, J.F. 1985. Butorphanol Analgesia in the Bovine. From a lecture. AABP Conference. Buffalo:

Prescott, J.F., D.J. Hoover, and I.R. Dohoo. 1983. Pharmacokinetics of Erythromycin in Foals and in Adult Horses. J Vet Pharmacol Therap 6 : 67-74.

Prueter, J.C. 1988. Diseases of the Larynx. In Handbook of Small Animal Practice. Edited by R. V. Morgan. 173-178. New York: Churchill Livingstone.

Prueter, J.C. 1988. Diseases of the Nasal Cavity and Sinus. In Handbook of Small Animal Practice. Edited by R. V. Morgan. 167-172. New York: Churchill Livingstone.

Prueter, J.C. 1988. Diseases of the Nasal cavity and Sinus. In Handbook of Small Animal Practice. Edited by R. V. Morgan. 167-172. New York: Churchill Livingstone.

Prueter, J.C. 1988b. Diseases of the Trachea. In Handbook of Small Animal Practice. Edited by R. V. Morgan. 179-184. New York: Churchill Livingstone.

Pugh, D.M. 1982. The Hormones II: Control of Reprductive Function. In Veterinary Applied Pharmacolgy and Therapeutics. 181-201. London: Baillière Tindall.

Rackear, D, B Feldman, T Farver, and L Lelong. 1988. The Effect of Three Different Dosages of Acetylsalicylic Acid on Canine Platelet Aggregation. AAHA 24 (1) : 23-26.

Radostits, O.M. 1986. Neonatal Diarrhea in Ruminants (Calves, Lambs and Kids). In Current Veterinary Therapy 2: Food Animal Practice. Edited by J.L. Howard. 105-113. Philadelphia: W.B. Saunders.

Raffe, M.R. 1986. Personal communication.

Ralston, S.L. 1987. Feeding Problems. In Current Therapy in Equine Medicine. Edited by N. E. Robinson. 123-126. Philadelphia: W.B. Saunders.

Randolph, J. and M. Peterson. (1994). Hypothalamus and pituitary gland. Saunders Manual of Small Animal Practice. Edited by S. Birchard and R. Sherding; Philadelphia, W.B. Saunders Company. 263-271

Randolph, R.W. 1986. Preventive Medical Care for the Pet Ferret. In Current Veterinary Therapy IX: Small Animal Practice. Edited by R. W. Kirk. 772-774. Philadelphia: W.B. Saunders.

Raskin, R. (1994). Erythrocytes, leukocytes and platelets. Saunders Manual of Small Animal Practice. Edited by S. Birchard and R. Sherding; Philadelphia, W.B. Saunders Company. 147-163

Ravis, W.R., R.F. Nachreiner, W. Pedersoli, and N.S. Houghton. 1987. A Pharmacokinetic Study of Phenobarbital in Mature Horses after Oral Dosing. J Vet Pharmacol Ther 4 : 283-289.

Rawlings, C.A., and C.A. Calvert. 1989. Heartworm Disease. In Textbook of Veterinary Internal Medicine. Edited by S. J. Ettinger. 1163-1184. Philadelphia: W.B. Saunders.

Rebhun, W.C. 1986. Diseases of the Peripheral Nerves. In Current Veterinary Therapy 2: Food Animal Practice. Edited by J. L. Howard. 874-876. Philadelphia: W.B. Saunders.

Refsal, K. and R. Nachreiner. (1995). Monitoring thyroid hormone replacement therapy. Kirk's Current Veterinary Therapy:XII. Edited by J. Bonagura; Philadelphia, W.B. Saunders. 364-368

Reid, F.M., and F.W. Oehme. 1989. Toxicoses. In The Cat: Diseases and Clinical Management. Edited by R.G. Sherding. 185-215. New York: Churchill Livingstone.

Reidesel, D.H. 1986 Opioids in Small Animal Practice. From a lecture.

Reinemeyer, C. (1992). Feline Gastrointestinal Parasites. Current Veterinary Therapy XI: Small Animal Practice. Edited by R. Kirk and J. Bonagura; Philadelphia, W.B. Saunders Company. 626-630

Reinemeyer, C. (1995). Parasites of the respiratory system. Kirk's Current Veterinary Therapy:XII. Edited by J. Bonagura; Philadelphia, W.B. Saunders. 895-898

Reinemeyer, C.R. 1985. Strategies for Management of Gastrointestinal Parasitism of Small Animals. In Eith Annual Kal Kan Symposium for the Treatment of Small Animal Diseases. 25-32. Vernon: Kal Kan Foods, Inc.

Richey, E.J. 1986. Bovine Anaplasmosis. In Current Veterinary Therapy: Food Animal Practice 2. Edited by J. L. Howard. 622-626. Philadelphia: W.B. Saunders.

Richter, K.P. 1989. Diseases of the Large Bowel. In Textbook of Veterinary Internal Medicine. Edited by S. J. Ettinger. 1397-1420. Philadelphia: W.B. Saunders.

Riis, R.C. 1986. Tumors of the Eye and Adnexa. In Current Veterinary Therapy (CVT) IX Small Animal Practice. Edited by R. W. Kirk. 679-684. Philadelphia: W.B. Saunders.

Rikihisa, Y. and G. Zimmerman. (1995). Salmon Poisoning Disease. Kirk's Current Veterinary Therapy:XII. Edited by J. Bonagura; Philadelphia, W.B. Saunders. 297-300

Riviere, J.E. 1985. Clinical Management of Toxicoses and Adverse Drug Reactions. In Handbook of Small Animal Therapeutics. Edited by L. E. Davis. 657-683. New York: Churchill Livingstone.

Riviere, J.E. 1989. Cephalosporins. In Current Veterinary Therapy X: Small Animal Practice. Edited by R. W. Kirk. 74-77. Philadelphia: W.B. Saunders.

Roberson, E.L. 1988a. Anticestodal and Antitrematodal drugs. In Veterinary Pharmacology and Therapeutics. Edited by N. H. Booth and L. E. McDonald. 928-949. Ames: Iowa State University Press.

Roberson, E.L. 1988b. Antinematodal Agents. In Veterinary Pharmacology and Therapeutics. Edited by N. H. Booth and L. E. McDonald. 882-927. Ames: Iowa State University Press.

Roberts, S.E. 1985. Assessment and Management of the Ophthalmic Emergency. Comp CE 7 (9) : 739-752.

Roberts, S.J. 1986a. Abortion and Other Gestational Diseases in Mares. In Current Therapy in Theriogenology 2: Diagnosis, Treatment and Prevention of Reproductive Diseases in Small and Large Animals. Edited by D. A. Morrow. 705-710. Philadelphia: W.B. Saunders.

Roberts, S.J. 1986b. Gestation and Pregnancy Diagnosis in the Mare. In Current Therapy in Theriogenology 2: Diagnosis, Treatment and Prevention of Reproductive Diseases in Small and Large Animals. Edited by D. A. Morrow. 670-678. Philadelphia: W.B. Saunders.

Robinson, E., S. Sanderson and R. Machon. (1993) Personal Communication

Robinson, N. (1992). Table of Drugs: Approximate Doses. Current Therapy in Equine Medicine 3. Edited by N. Robinson; Philadelphia, W.B. Saunders Co. 815-821

Robinson, N.E. 1987. Table of Common Drugs: Approximate Doses. In Current Therapy in Equine Medicine, 2. Edited by N. E. Robinson. 761. Philadelphia: W.B. Saunders.

Rogers, K.S., and G.E. Lees. 1989. Management of Urinary Tract Infections. In Current Veterinary Therapy X: Small Animal Practice. Edited by R. W. Kirk. 1204-1209. Philadelphia: W.B. Saunders.

Romatowski, J. 1989. Use of Megestrol Acetate in Cats. JAVMA 194 (5) : 700-702.

Root, M. and S. Johnston. (1995). Pregnancy termination in the bitch using prostaglandin F2-alpha. Kirk's Current Veterinary Therapy:XII. Edited by J. Bonagura; Philadelphia, W.B. Saunders. 1079-1080

Rosenkrantz, W. (1989). Immunomodulating drugs in dermatology. Current Veterinary Therapy X: Small Animal Practice. Edited by R. W. Kirk; Philadelphia, WB Saunders. 570-577

Rosenkrantz, W. 1989. Immunomodulating Drugs in Dermatology. In Current Veterinary Therapy X: Small Animal Practice. Edited by R. W. Kirk. 570-577. Philadelphia: W.B. Saunders.

Rosenthal, R.C. 1985. Chemotherapy of Neoplastic Diseases. In Handbook of Small Animal Therapeutics. Edited by L. E. Davis. 175- 188. New York: Churchill Livingstone.

Rosin, E., T.S. Uphoff, C. Santulus, and M.T. Collins. 1988. Surgical Wound Conncentrations of Cephalothin, Cefazolin, Ampicillin, and Gentamicin in the Dog (Abstract). Veterinary Surgery Scientific Meeting Abstracts-American College of Veterinary Surgery 1988 : 39.

Ross, L.A., E.B. Breitschwerdt, T.A. Allen, D.J. Polzin, and R.D. Zenoble. 1988. Diseases of the Kidney. In Handbook of Small Animal Practice. Edited by R. V. Morgan. 567-593. New York: Churchill Livingstone.

Rossdale, P.D. 1987. Exogenous Control of the Breeding Season. In Current Therapy in Equine Medicine, 2. Edited by N. E. Robinson. 493-494. Philadelphia: W.B. Saunders.

Rosser, E. (1992). Sebaceous adenitis. Current Veterinary Therapy XI: Small Animal Practice. Edited by R. Kirk and J. Bonagura; Philadelphia, W.B. Saunders Company. 534-539

Rosser, E. (1993). Parasitic Dermatoses. Current Veterinary Therapy 3: Food Animal Practice. Edited by J. Howard; Philadelphia, W.B. Saunders Co. 882-890

Rosskopf, W.J. 1986. Shell Diseases in Turtles and Tortoises. In Current Veterinary Therapy (CVT) IX Small Animal Practice. Edited by R. W. Kirk. 751-759. Philadelphia: W.B. Saunders.

Rossoff, I.S. 1974. Handbook of Veterinary Drugs. New York: Springer Publishing.

Rosychuck, R. (1991). Newer therapies in veterinary dermatology. Proceedings of the Ninth Annual Veterinary Medical Forum. Edited by W. Morrison, New Orleans, American College of Veterinary Internal Medicine. 101-104

Rosychuck, R. and M. Swartout. (1997). Endocrine/Metabolic Skin Diseases. Handbook of Small Animal Practice 3rd Ed. Edited by R. Morgan; Philadelphia, Saunders. 928-940

Rosychuk, R.A.W. 1989. Llama Dermatology. Vet Clin of North Amer: Food Anim Prac 5 (1) : 203-215.

Roudebush, P. 1985. Respiratory Diseases. In Handbook of Small Animal Therapeutics. Edited by L. E. Davis. 287-332. New York: Churchill Livingstone.

Roussel, A. (1992). Motility-Modifying Drugs in Large Animals. Proceedings of the Tenth Annual Veterinary Medical Forum. Edited by W. Morrison, San Diego, American College of Veterinary Internal Medicine. 515-517

Rubin, S.I., D.R. Krawiec, Gelberg. H., and R.D. Shanks. 1989. Nephrotoxicity of Amphotericin B in Dogs: A comparison of Two Methods of Administration. Cna J Vet Res 53 : 23-28.

Ruhr, L.P., and G.D. Osweiler. 1986. Nitrate Accumulators. In Current Veterinary Therapy 2: Food Animal Practice. Edited by J. L. Howard. 392-394. Philadelphia: W.B. Saunders.

Russell, L. and J. Rush. (1995). Cardiac Arrhythmias in Systemic Disease. Kirk's Current Veterinary Therapy:XII. Edited by J. Bonagura; Philadelphia, W.B. Saunders. 161-166

Russo, E.A., and G.E. Lees. 1986. Treatment of Hypocalcemia. In Current Veterinary Therapy (CVT) IX Small Animal Practice. Edited by R. W. Kirk. 91-94. Philadelphia: W.B. Saunders.

Rutgers, H. (1994). Primary hepatic fibrosis in the dog. Proceedings of the Twelfth Annual Veterinary Medical Forum. Edited by R. DeNovo, San Francisco, American College of Veterinary Internal Medicine. 772-773

Schaer, M. 1986. The Diagnosis and Treatment of Metabolic and Respiratory Acidosis. In Current Veterinary Therapy (CVT) IX Small Animal Practice. Edited by R.W. Kirk. 59-66. Philadelphia: W.B. Saunders.

Schall, W.D. 1985. Pancreatic Diseases. In Handbook of Small Animal Therapeutics. Edited by L.E. Davis. 485-504. New York: Churchill Livingstone.

Schmitz, D.G., and J.C. Reagor. 1987. Cantharidin (Blister Beetle) Toxicity. In Current Therapy in Equine Medicine. Edited by N. E. Robinson. 120-122. Philadelphia: W.B. Saunders.

Schrader, L.A. 1986. Hypoadrenocorticism. In Current Veterinary Therapy (CVT) IX Small Animal Practice. Edited by R. W. Kirk. 972-977. Philadelphia: W.B. Saunders.

Schultz, C.S. 1986. Formulary, Veterinary Hospital Pharmacy, Washington State University. Pullman, Washington: Washington State University Press.

Schunk, K.L. 1988. Disorders of the Spinal Cord. In Handbook of Small Animal Practice. Edited by R. V. Morgan. 269-297. Nw York: Churchill Livingstone.

Schunk, K.L. 1988. Seizure disorders. In Handbook of Small Animal Practice. Edited by R. V. Morgan. 239-246. New York: Churchill Livingstone.

Schunk, K.L. 1988a. Disorders of the Spinal Cord. In Handbook of Small Animal Practice. Edited by R. V. Morgan. 269-297. Nw York: Churchill Livingstone.

Schunk, K.L. 1988b. Seizure Disorders. In Handbook of Small Animal Practice. Edited by R. V. Morgan. 239-246. New York: Churchill Livingstone.

Schwark, W.S., N.G. Ducharme, S.J. Shin, W.T. Beilman, and J.T. Elwell. 1983. Absorption and Distribution Patterns of Oral Phenoxymethyl Penicillin (penicillin V) in the Horse. Cornell Vet 73 : 314-322.

Schwartz-Porsche, D. (1992). Management of Refractory Seizures. Current Veterinary Therapy XI: Small Animal Practice. Edited by R. Kirk and J. Bonagura; Philadelphia, W.B. Saunders Company. 986-991

Schwartz-Porsche, D. 1986. Epidemiological, Clinical, and Pharmacokinetic Studies in Spontaneously Epileptic Dogs and Cats. Proceedings. ACVIM.

Scott, D.W. 1982. Dermatologic Use of Glucocorticoids: Systemic and Topical. Vet Clin of North America: Small Anim Prac 12 (1) : 19-32.

Seeler, D.C., and J.C. Thurmon. 1985. Fluid and Electrolyte Disorders. In Handbook of Small Animal Therapeutics. Edited by L. E. Davis. 21-44. New York: Churchill Livingstone.

Sellers, A.F., and J.E. Lowe. 1987. Large Colon Impaction. In Current Therapy in Equine Medicine 2. Edited by N. E. Robinson. 53-55. Phialdelphia: W.B. Saunders.

Sellon, R. and E. Breitschwerdt. (1995). CVT Update: Rocky Mountain Spotted Fever. Kirk's Current Veterinary Therapy:XII. Edited by J. Bonagura; Philadelphia, W.B. Saunders. 293-297

Semrad, S.D., and J.N. Moore. 1987. Endotoxemia. In Current Therapy in Equine Medicine 2. Edited by N. E. Robinson. 81-87. Philadelphia: W.B. Saunders.

Senior, D.F. 1989. Fluid Therapy, Electrolyte and Acid-base Control. In Textbook of Veterinary Internal Medicine. Edited by S. J. Ettinger. 429-449. Philadelphia: W.B. Saunders.

Senior, D.F. 1989. Medical Management of Urate Uroliths. In Current Veterinary Therapy X: Small Animal Practice. Edited by R. W. Kirk. 1178-1181. Philadelphia: W.B. Saunders.

Sexton, J.W., and W.B. Buck. 1986. Lead. In Current Veterinary Therapy: Food Animal Practice 2. Edited by J. L. Howard. 439-440. Philadelphia: W.B. Saunders.

Shanley, K. and K. Overall. (1992). Psychogenic dermatoses. Current Veterinary Therapy XI: Small Animal Practice. Edited by R. Kirk and J. Bonagura; Philadelphia, W.B. Saunders Company. 552-558

Shapiro, W. 1989. Cisplatin Chemotherapy. In Current Veterinary Therapy X: Small Animal Practice. Edited by R.W. Kirk. 497-502. Philadelphia: W.B. Saunders.

Sharp, N. 1989. Nasal Aspergillosis. In Current Veterinary Therapy X: Small Animal Practice. Edited by R. W. Kirk. 1106-1109. Philadelphia: W.B. Saunders.

Shaw, K, C.M. Trim, A Palminteri, D.C. Sawyer, J.A.E. Hubbell, and D.J. Krahwinkel Jr. 1986. The Use of Oxymorphone in Veterinary Medicine. Proceedings. University of Pennsylvania, Philadelphia:

Shelton, G. (1992). Canine Myasthenia Gravis. Current Veterinary Therapy XI: Small Animal Practice. Edited by R. Kirk and J. Bonagura; Philadelphia, W.B. Saunders Company. 1039-1042

Sherding, R. (1994). Anorectal diseases. Saunders Manual of Small Animal Practice. Edited by S. Birchard and R. Sherding; Philadelphia, W.B. Saunders Company. 777-792

intestines. Saunders Manual of Small Animal Practice. Edited by S. Birchard and R. Sherding; Philadelphia, W.B. Saunders Company. 687-714

Sherding, R. and S. Johnson. (1994b). Systemic mycoses. Saunders Manual of Small Animal Practice. Edited by S. Birchard and R. Sherding; Philadelphia, W.B. Saunders Company. 133-140

Sherding, R. G. (1986). Intestinal Lymphangiectasia. Current Veterinary Therap IX: Small Animal Practice. Edited by R. W. Kirk; Philadelphia, W.B. Saunders. 885-888

Sherding, R.G. 1989. Diseases of the Intestines. In The Cat: Diseases and Clinical Management. Edited by R. G. Sherding. 955-1006. New York: Churchill Livingstone.

Sherding, R.G. 1989. Diseases of the Small Bowel. In Textbook of Veterinary Internal Medicine. Edited by S. J. Ettinger. 1323-1396. Philadelphia: W.B. Saunders.

Shewen, P. and K. Bateman. (1993). Pasteurellosis in Cattle. Current Veterinary Therapy 3: Food Animal Practice. Edited by J. Howard; Philadelphia, W.B. Saunders Co. 555-559

Shideler, R.K., J.L. Voss, W.M. Aufderheide, C.P. Hessemann, and E.L. Squires. 1983. The Effect of Altrenogest, an Oral Progestin, on Hematologic and Biochemical Parameters in Mares. Vet Hum Tox 25 (4) : 250-252.

Shille, V.M. 1986. Management of Reproductive Disorders in the Bitch and Queen. In Current Veterinary Therapy (CVT) IX Small Animal Practice. Edited by R. W. Kirk. 1225-1229. Philadelphia: W.B. Saunders.

Shille, V.M., and P.N. Olson. 1989. Dynamic Testing in Reproductive Endocrinology. In Current Veterinary Therapy X: Small Animal Practice. Edited by R. W. Kirk. 1282-1291. Philadelphia: W.B. Saunders.

Shores, A. 1989. Craniocerebral Trauma. In Current Veterinary Therapy X: Small Animal Practice. Edited by R. W. Kirk. 847-853. Philadelphia: W.B. Saunders.

Shull-Selcer, E. and W. Stagg. (1991). "Advances in the understanding and treatment of noise phobias." Veterinary Clinics of North America: Small Animal Practice. 21(2): 353-367.

Sikarskie, J.G. 1986. The Use of Ivermectin in Birds, Reptiles, and Small Mammals. In Current Veterinary Therapy (CVT) IX Small Animal Practice. Edited by R. W. Kirk. 743-745. Philadelphia: W.B. Saunders.

Silley, P., A.P. Rudd, W.M. Symington, and A.J. Tait. 1988. Pharmacokientics of Cephalexin in Dogs and Cats after Oral, Subcutaneous, and Intramuscular Administration. Vet Record (Jan 2 1988) : 15-17.

Simpson, S.T. 1989. Hydrocephalus. In Current Veterinary Therapy X: Small Animal Practice. Edited by R. W. Kirk. 842-847. Philadelphia: W.B. Saunders.

Sisson, D., and W.P. Thomas. 1986. Bacterial Endocarditis. In Current Veterinary Therapy (CVT) IX Small Animal Practice. Edited by R. W. Kirk. 402-406. Philadelphia: W.B. Saunders.

Slappendel, R.J. 1989. Disseminated Intravascular Coagulation. In Current Veterinary Therapy X: Small Animal Practice. Edited by R.W. Kirk. 451-457. Philadelphia: W.B. Saunders.

Smith, B. (1996a). Actinobacillosis. Large Animal Internal Medicine 2nd Ed. Edited by B. Smith; St Louis, Mosby. 794-796

Smith, B. (1996b). Actinomycosis. Large Animal Internal Medicine 2nd Ed. Edited by B. Smith; St Louis, Mosby. 796-797

Smith, J.A. 1986. Toxic Encephalopathies in Cattle. In Current Veterinary Therapy 2: Food Animal Practice. Edited by J. L. Howard. 855-863. Philadelphia: W.B. Saunders.

Smith, J.A. 1989. Noninfectious Diseases, Metabolic Diseases, Toxicities, and Neoplastic Diseases of South American Camelids. Vet Clin of North Amer: Food Anim Pract 5 (1) : 101-143.

Smith, M.C. 1986a. Anestrus, Pseudopregnancy and Cystic Follicles. In Current Therapy in Theriogenology 2: Diagnosis, Treatment and Prevention of Reproductive Diseases in Small and Large Animals. Edited by D. A. Morrow. 585-586. Philadelphia: W.B. Saunders.

Smith, M.C. 1986b. Synchronization of Estrus and the Use of Implants and Vaginal Sponges. In Current Therapy in Theriogenology 2: Diagnosis, Treatment and Prevention of Reproductive Diseases in Small and Large Animals. Edited by D. A. Morrow. 582-583. Philadelphia: W.B. Saunders.

Snyder, P. (1998). "Amlodipine: a randomized, blinded clinical trial in 9 cats with systemic hypertension." J Vet Intern Med. 12(May (3)): 157-162.

Sojka, N.J. 1986. Management of Artificial Breeding in Cats. In Current Therapy in Theriogenology 2: Diagnosis, Treatment and Prevention of Reproductive Diseases in Small and Large Animals. Edited by D. A. Morrow. 805-808. Philadelphia: W.B. Saunders.

Spehar, A.M. , M.R. Hill, I.G. Mayhew, and L. Hendeles. 1984. Preliminary Study on the Pharmacokinetics of Phenobarbital in the Neonatal Foal. Eq Vet Jnl 16 (4) : 368-371.

Spink, R.R. 1986. Aerosol Therapy. In Clinical Avian Medicine and Surgery. Edited by G. J. Harrison and L. R. Harrison. 376-379. Philadelphia: W.B. Saunders.

Squires, E.L., and A.O. McKinnon. 1987. Hormone therapy for control of reproduction in mares and stallions. Vet Clin North Am (Equine Practice) 3 (1) : 81-100.

Squires, E.L., R.K. Shideler, J.L. Voss, and S.K. Webel. 1983. Clinical Applications of Progestins in Mares. Comp CE 5 (1) : S16-S22.

Stann, S.E. 1988a. Diseases of Lymph Nodes and the Lymphatics. In Handbook of Small Animal Practice. Edited by R.V. Morgan. 787-797. New York: Churchill Livingstone.

Stann, S.E. 1988b. Disorders of the Spleen. In Handbook of Small Animal Practice. Edited by R.V. Morgan. 799-804. New York: Churchill Livingstone.

Stover, S.M. 1987. Pre- and Postoperative Management of the Colic Patient. In Current Therapy in Equine Medicine: 2. Edited by N. E. Robinson. 33- 38. Philadelphia: W.B. Saunders.

Stunkard, J.M. 1984. Diagnosis, Treatment and Husbandry of Pet Birds. Edgewater, MD: Stunkard Publishing.

Suter, P.F. 1989. Peripheral Vascular Disease. In Textbook of Veterinary Internal Medicine. Edited by S.J. Ettinger. 1185-1199. Philadelphia: W.B. Saunders.

Swango, L.J., K.W. Bankemper, and L.I. Kong. 1989. Bacterial, Rickettsial, Protozoal, and Miscellaneous Infections. In Textbook of Veterinary Internal Medicine. Edited by S. J. Ettinger. 265-297. Philadelphia: W.B. Saunders.

Swanson, J.F. 1989. Uveitis. In Current Veterinary Therapy X: Small Animal Practice. Edited by R. W. Kirk. 652-656. Philadelphia: W.B. Saunders.

Sweeney, C.R., and T.O. Hansen. 1987. Narcolepsy and Epilepsy. In Current Therapy in Equine Medicine. Edited by N. E. Robinson. 349-353. Philadelphia: W.B. Saunders.

Sweeney, R.W., L.R. Soma, C.B. Woodward, and C.B. Charlton. 1986. Pharmacokinetics of Metronidazole Given to Horses by Intravenous and Oral Routes. JAVMA 47 (8) : 1726-1729.

Sweeney, R.W., M. MacDonald, J. Hall, T.J. Divers, and C.R. Sweeney. 1988. Kinetics of gentamicin Elimination in Two Horses with Acute Renal Failure. Equine Vet J 20 (3) : 182-184.

Swindle, M.M. 1985. Anesthesia in Swine. Charles River Tech Bul 3 (3)

Swinyard, E.A. 1975. Diuretic Drugs. In Remington's Pharmaceutical Sciences. Edited by A. Osol. 861-873. Easton: Mack Publishing.

Swinyard, E.A. 1975. Histamine and Antihistamines. In Remington's Pharmaceutical Sciences. Edited by A. Osol. 1055-1066. Easton: Mack Publishing Co.

Tams, T. (1994). Cisapride: Clinical experience with the newest GI prokinetic drug. Proceedings of the Twelfth Annual Veterinary Medical Forum. Edited by R. DeNovo, San Francisco, American College of Veterinary Internal Medicine. 101-102

Tams, T.R. 1986. Feline Inflammatory Bowel Disease. In Current Veterinary Therapy IX, Small Animal Practice. Edited by R. W. Kirk. 881-885. Philadelpia: W.B. Saunders Co.

Tangner, C.H., and D.A. Hulse. 1988. Joint Diseases. In Handbook of Small Animal Practice. Edited by R.V. Morgan. 873-891. New York: Churchill Livingstone.

Taylor, J.B., J.H. Verrall, N. Chandler, R.D. Jones, and J. Parker. 1983. Clinical Efficacy of a Revised Dosage Schedule of Phenylbutazone in Horses. Vet Rec 113 (8) : 183-184.

Teske, E. 1986. Estrogen-Induced Bone Marrow Toxicity. In Current Veterinary Therapy IX, Small Animal Practice. Edited by R. W. Kirk. 495-498. Philadelpia: W.B. Saunders

Thoday, K.L. 1986. Differential Diagnosis of Ayrmetric Alopecia in the Cat. In Current Veterinary Therapy IX: Small

Animal Practice. Edited by R. W. Kirk. 545-553. Philadelphia: W.B. Saunders.

Thompson, J. (1994). Systemic immune-mediated disease. Saunders Manual of Small Animal Practice. Edited by S. Birchard and R. Sherding; Philadelphia, W.B. Saunders Company. 171-178

Thompson, J. A. (1992). Formulary: University of Florida Veterinary Medical Teaching Hospital. Gainesville, 207pp.

Thompson, J. R. and W. B. Buck. (1993a). Copper-Molybdenum Toxicosis. Current Veterinary Therapy 3: Food Animal Practice. Edited by J. L. Howard; Philadelphia, W.B. Saunders. 396-398

Thompson, J.P. 1989. Antineoplastic Agents in Cancer Therapy. In Current Veterinary Therapy X: Small Animal Practice. Edited by R. W. Kirk. 1367-1369. Philadelphia: W.B. Saunders.

Thompson, J.P. 1989b. Immunologic Diseases. In Textbook of Veterinary Internal Medicine. Edited by S.J. Ettinger. 2297-2328. Philadelphia: W.B. Saunders.

Thompson, L. and W. Buck. (1993b). Copper-Molybdenum Toxicosis. Current Veterinary Therapy 3: Food Animal Practice. Edited by J. Howard; Philadelphia, W.B. Saunders Co. 396-398

Thurmon, J.C., and G.J. Benson. 1986. Anesthesia in Ruminants and Swine. In Current Veterinary Therapy 2: Food Animal Practice. Edited by J. L. Howard. 51-71. Philadelphia: W.B. Saunders.

Thurmon, J.C., and G.J. Benson. 1987. Injectable Anesthetics and Anesthetic Adjuncts. Vet Clin North Am (Equine Practice) 3 (1) : 15-36.

Tilley, L.P. , and M.S. Miller. 1986. Antiarrhythmic drugs and management of cardiac arrhythmias. In Current Veterinary Therapy IX: Small Animal Practice. Edited by R. V. Kirk. 346-360. Philadelphia: W.B. Saunders.

Tilley, L.P., and J.M. Owens. 1985. Manual of Small Animal Cardiology. New York: Churchill Livingstone.

Tilley, L.P., and M.S. Miller. 1986. Antiarrhythmic Drugs and Management of Cardiac Arrhythmias. In Current Veterinary Therapy IX: Small Animal Practice. Edited by R. V. Kirk. 346-360. Philadelphia: W.B. Saunders.

Todd, K.S., A.J. Paul, and J.A. DiPietro. 1985. Parasitic Diseases. In Handbook of Small Animal Therapeutics. Edited by L. E. Davis. 89-126. New York: Churchill Livingstone.

Todd, K.S., J.A. Dipietro, and W.M. Guterbock. 1986. Coccidiosis. In Current Veterinary Therapy 2: Food Animal Practice. Edited by J. L. Howard. 632-636. Philadelphia: W.B. Saunders.

Tomlinson, R.V., H.R. Spires, and J.L. Bowen. 1985. Absorption and Elimination of a Prostaglandin F Analog, Fenprostalene, in Lactating Dairy Cows. Jnl Dairy Sci 68 (8) : 2072-2077.

Trepanier, L.A., M.E. Peterson, and D.A. Aucoin. 1989. Methimazole Pharmacokinetics in the Normal Cat. Abstract. ACVIM

Trotter, E.J. 1986. Canine Wobbler Syndrome. In Current Veterinary Therapy IX: Small Aniaml Practice. Edited by R. W. Kirk. 806-810. Philadelphia: W.B. Saunders.

Twedt, D.C., and E.L. Whitney. 1989. Management of Hepatioc Copper Toxicosis in Dogs. In Current Veterinary Therapy X: Small Animal Practice. Edited by R. W. Kirk. 891-893. Philadelphia: W.B. Saunders.

Twedt, D.C., and M.L. Magne. 1986. Chronic Gastritis. In Current Veterinary Therapy IX: Small Animal Practice. Edited by R. V. Kirk. 852-856. Philadelphia: W.B. Saunders.

Upson, D.W. 1988. Handbook of Clinical Veterinary Pharmacology. 3rd ed. Manhattan: Dan Upson Enterprises.

USPC. 1989. Veterinary Information- Appendix V. In Drug Information for the Health Professional. 2523-2565. Rockville: United States Pharmacopeial Convention.

USPC. 1990. Veterinary Information- Appendix III. In Drug Information for the Health Professional. 2811- 2860. Rockville: United States Pharmacopeial Convention.

Vaden, S. and G. Grauer. (1992). Medical management of canine glomerulonephritis. Current Veterinary Therapy XI: Small Animal Practice. Edited by R. Kirk and J. Bonagura; Philadelphia, W.B. Saunders Company. 861-864

Vaden, S. and L. Cohn. (1994). Immunosuppressive Drugs: Corticosteroids and Beyond. Proceedings of the Twelfth Annual Veterinary Medical Forum. Edited by R. DeNovo, San Francisco, American College of Veterinary Internal Medicine. 264-266

Vaden, S. and M. Papich. (1995). Empiric Antibiotic Therapy. Kirk's Current Veterinary Therapy:XII. Edited by J. Bonagura; Philadelphia, W.B. Saunders. 276-280

Vail, D. and G. Ogilvie. (1994). Lymphoid neoplasia. Saunders Manual of Small Animal Practice. Edited by S. Birchard and R. Sherding; Philadelphia, W.B. Saunders Company. 193-199

Van Camp, S.D. 1986. Breeding Soundness Examination of the Mare and Common Genital Abnormalities Encountered. In Current Therapy in Theriogenology 2: Diagnosis, Treatment and Prevention of Reproductive Diseases in Small and Large Animals. Edited by D. A. Morrow. 654-661. Philadelphia: W.B. Saunders.

Vestre, W.A. 1985. Ophthalmic Diseases. In Handbook of Small Animal Therapeutics. Edited by L. E. Davis. 549-575. New York: Chirchill Livingstone.

Voith, V.L., and A.R. Marder. 1988a. Canine Behavioral Disorders. In Handbook of Small Animal Practice. Edited by R. V. Morgan. 1033-1043. New York: Churchill Livingstone.

Voith, V.L., and A.R. Marder. 1988b. Feline Behavioral Disorders. In Handbook of Small Animal Practice. Edited by R. V. Morgan. 1045-1051. New York: Churchill Livingstone.

Vrins, A., G. Carlson, and B. Feldman. 1983. Warfarin: A Review with Emphasis on its Use in the Horse. Can Vet Jnl 24 : 211-213.

Walker, R. (1992). Antimicrobial Chemotherapy. Current Therapy in Equine Medicine 3. Edited by N. Robinson; Philadelphia, W.B. Saunders Co. 1-13

Wallace, L.J. 1988. Personal Communication.

Walter, P. A., D.A. Feeney, and G.R. Johnston. 1986. Diagnosis and Treatment of Adverse Reactions to Radiopaque Contrast Agents. In Current Veterinary Therapy IX: Small Animal Practice. Edited by R. W. Kirk. 47-52. Philadelphia: W.B. Saunders.

Walton, D.K. 1986. Psychodermatoses. In Current Veterinary Therapy IX: Small Animal Practice. Edited by R. W. Kirk. 557-559. Philadelphia: W.B. Saunders.

Ware, W. (1992). Current Uses and Hazards of Beta-Blockers. Current Veterinary Therapy XI: Small Animal Practice. Edited by R. Kirk and J. Bonagura; Philadelphia, W.B. Saunders Company. 676-684

Ware, W. (1997). Acquired Valvular Diseases. Handbook of Small Animal Practice 3rd Ed. Edited by R. Morgan; Philadelphia, WB Saunders. 91-97

Ware, W.A., and J.D. Bonagura. 1986. Canine Myocardial Diseases. In Current Veterinary Therapy IX: Small Animal Practice. Edited by R. V. Kirk. 370-380. Philadelphia: W.B. Saunders.

Washabau, R. and M. Elie. (1995). Antiemetic therapy. Kirk's Current Veterinary Therapy:XII. Edited by J. Bonagura; Philadelphia, W.B. Saunders. 679-684

Wass, W.M., J.R. Thompson, E.W. Moss, J.P. Kunesh, P.G. Eness, and L.S. Thompson. 1986a. Diseases of the ruminat

forestomach. In Current Veterinary Therapy 2: Food Animal Practice. Edited by J. L. Howard. 715-723. Philadelphia: WB Suanders.

Wass, W.M., J.R. Thompson, E.W. Moss, J.P. Kunesh, P.G. Eness, and L.S. Thompson. 1986b. Gastric ulcer syndrome in swine. In Current Veterinary Therapy 2: Food Animal Practice. Edited by J. L. Howard. 723-724. Philadelphia: W.B. Saunders.

Watrous, B.J. 1989. Diseases of the esophogus. In Handbook of Small Animal Practice. Edited by R. V. Morgan. 357-370. New York: Churchill LIvingstone .

Weiser, M.G. 1989a. Erythrocytes and Associated Disorders. In The Cat: Diseases and Clinical Management. Edited by R.G. Sherding. 529-556. New York: Churchill Livingstone.

Weiser, M.G. 1989b. Erythrocytes and Associated Disorders. In Textbook of Veterinary Internal Medicine. Edited by S.J. Ettinger. 2145-2180. Philadelphia: W.B. Saunders.

Weiss, D.J. 1986. Therapy for Disorders of Erythropoiesis. In Current Veterinary Therapy IX: Small Animal Practice. Edited by R. W. Kirk. 490-495. Philadelphia: W.B. Saunders.

Weiss, R. (1994). Feline infectious peritonitis virus: Advances in therapy and control. Consultations in Feline Internal Medicine: 2. Edited by J. August; Philadelphia, W.B. Saunders Company. 3-12

Weller, R.E. 1988. Paraneoplastic Syndromes. In Handbook of Small Animal Practice. Edited by R. V. Morgan. 819-827. New York: Churchill Livingstone.

Weller, R.E. 1988. Paraneoplastic Syndromes. In Handbook of Small Animal Practice. Edited by R. V. Morgan. 819-827. New York: Churchill Livingstone.

Wertz, E.M., G.J. Benson, J.C. Thurmon, W.J. Tranquilli, L.E. Davis, and G.D. Koritz. 1988. Pharmaco-kinetics of Thiamylal in Cats. Am J Vet Res 49 (7) : 1079-1083.

Wheaton, L.G. 1989. Drugs that Affect Uterine Motility. In Current Veterinary Therapy X: Small Animal Practice. Edited by R. W. Kirk. 1299-1302. Philadelphia: W.B. Saunders.

Wheeler, S.L. 1986. Canine Pheochromocytoma. In Current Veterinary Therapy IX: Small Animal Practice. Edited by R. W. Kirk. 977-981. Phialdelphia: W.B. Saunders.

Wheler, C. (1993). "Avian anesthetics, analgesics, and tranquilizers." Seminars in Avian & Exotic Med. 2(1): 7-12.

White, P. (1994). Atopy. Saunders Manual of Small Animal Practice. Edited by S. Birchard and R. Sherding; Philadelphia, W.B. Saunders Company. 302-312

White, S.D., L.J. Stewart, and M. Bernstein. 1987. Corticosteroid (Methylprednisolone Sodium Succinate) Pulce Therapy in 5 Dogs with Autoimmune Skin Disease. JAVMA 191 (9) : 1121-1124.

Whitlock, R.H. 1986a. Abomasal Ulcers. In Current Veterinary Therapy 2: Food Animal Practice. Edited by J. L. Howard. 740-741. Philadelphia: W.B. Saunders.

Whitlock, R.H. 1986b. Constipation. In Current Veterinary Therapy 2: Food Animal Practice. Edited by J. L. Howard. 711. Philadelphia: W.B. Saunders.

Whittem, T. (1993) Personal Communication

Wilcke, J.R. 1985. Cardiac Dysrhythmias. In Handbook of Small Animal Therapeutics. Edited by L. E. Davis. 267-286. New York: Churchill Livingstone.

Wilcke, J.R. 1986. Allergic Drug Reactions. In Current Veterinary Therapy IX: Small Animal Practice. Edited by R. W. Kirk. 444-448. Phialdelphai: W.B. Saunders.

Wildt, D.E. 1986. Estrous Cycle Control—Induction and Prevention in Cats. In Current Therapy in Theriogenology: 2. Edited by D. A. Morrow. 808-812. Philadelphia: W.B. Saunders.

Willard, M. D. (1986). Treatment of hyperkalemia. Current Veterinary Therapy IX: Small Animal Practice. Edited by R. W. Kirk; Phialdelphai, W.B. Saunders. 94-101

Willard, M.D. 1986. Treatment of Hyperkalemia. In Current Veterinary Therapy IX: Small Animal Practice. Edited by R.W. Kirk. 94-101. Philadelphia: W.B. Saunders.

Willemse, T. (1992). Zinc-related cutaneous dosrders of dogs. Current Veterinary Therapy XI: Small Animal Practice. Edited by R. Kirk and J. Bonagura; Philadelphia, W.B. Saunders Company. 532-534

Williams, C.S.F. 1986. Practical Management of Induced Parturition. In Current Therapy in Theriogenology 2: Diagnosis, Treatment and Prevention of Reproductive Diseases in Small and Large Animals. Edited by D. A. Morrow. 588-589. Philadelphia: W.B. Saunders.

Williams, D.A. 1989. Exocrine pancreatic insufficiency. In Current Veterinary Therapy X: Small Animal Practice. Edited by R. W. Kirk. 927-932. Philadelphia: W.B. Saunders.

Wilson, J.H. 1987. Eastern Equine Encephalitis. In Current Therapy in Equine Medicine. Edited by N. E. Robinson. 345-347. Philadelphia: W.B. Saunders.

Wilson, J.H. 1987. Gastrointestinal Problems in Foals. In Current Therapy in Equine Medicine. Edited by N. E. Robinson. 232-241. Phialdelphia: W.B. Saunders.

Wingfield, W.E. 1985. Cardiopulmonary Arrest and Resuscitation. In Manual of Small Animal Cardiology. Edited by L. P. Tilley and J. M. Owens. 387-414. New York: Churchill Livingstone.

Wingfield, W.E., and D. Van Pelt. 1989. Abnormal Bleeding. Vet Clin of North Amer: Sm Anim Pract: Critical Care 19 (6)

Wolf, A. (1994). Antifungal agents. Consultations in Feline Internal Medicine: 2. Edited by J. August; Philadelphia, W.B. Saunders Company. 53-57

Wolfe, D.F. 1986. Surgical Procedures of the Reproductive System of the Bull. In Current Therapy in Theriogenology 2: Diagnosis, treatment and prevention of reproductive diseases in small and large animals. Edited by D. A. Morrow. 353-379. Philadelphia: W.B. Saunders.

Wood, R.L. 1986. Swine Erysipelas. In Current Veterinary Therapy 2: Food Animal Practice. Edited by J. L. Howard. 561-562. Philadelphia: W.B. Saunders.

Woody, B.J. 1988. Prevention of Estrus and Pregnancy. In Handbook of Small Animal Practice. Edited by R. V. Morgan. 701-705. New York: Churchill Livingstone.

Wykes, P.M. 1986. Diseases of the Vagina and Vulva in the Bitch. In Current Therapy in Theriogenology 2: Diagnosis, Treatment and Prevention of Reproductive Diseases in Small and Large Animals. Edited by D. A. Morrow. 476-481. Philadelphia: W.B. Saunders.

Wyman, M. 1986. Contemporary Ocular Therapeutics. In Current Veterinary Therapy IX, Small Animal Practice. Edited by R. W. Kirk. 684-696. Philadelphia: W.B. Saunders.

Yeary, R.A. 1980. Serum Concentrations of Primidone and its Metabolites, Phenylethylmalonamide and Phenobarbital in the Dog. Am J Vet Res 41 (10) : 1643-1645.

Young, K.M. 1988. Disorders of Platelets. In Handbook of Small Animal Practice. Edited by R.V. Morgan. 765-772. New York: Churchill Livingstone.

Zerbe, C.A. 1989. Feline Hyperadrenocorticism. In Current Veterinary Therapy X: Small Animal Practice. Edited by R. W. Kirk. 1038-1045. Philadelphia: W.B. Saunders.

Zimmer, J. (1986). Nutritional management of gastrointestinal diseases. Current Veterinary Therap IX: Small Animal Practice. Edited by R. W. Kirk; Philadelphia, W.B. Saunders. 909-916

DRUGS SORTED BY THERAPEUTIC CLASS/MAJOR INDICATION

Where dosages are available for a given species, the following code is used in parentheses after the drug name:

A=Avian; Pet Bird
B=Bovine, Cattle
C=Cat, Feline
D=Dog, Canine
H=Horse, Equine
L=Llama, Camelid

O=Ostrich, Rattite
Po=Pocket Pets/Rabbits/Small Lab Animals
R=Reptiles/Amphibians
Sw=Swine, Pigs
Sh=Sheep/Goats; Ovine/Caprine
Z=Wildlife/Zoo Animals

Note: As some drugs have multiple indications, there may not be a specific dosage listed for that indication for every species noted.

Central Nervous System Drugs

(including antiinflammatories, analgesics, muscle relaxants)

CNS/Respiratory Stimulants
Doxapram (D,C,B,SW,H) 224

Analgesics
Narcotic Agonists
Codeine (D) 156
Fentanyl (D,C) 272
Meperidine (D,C,B,H) 403
Morphine (D,C,H,Sw,Sh) 440
Oxymorphone (D,C,H,Sw,P) 473
Narcotic agonist/antagonists
Buprenorphine (H) 85
Butorphanol (D,C,B,H,A) 89
Pentazocine (D,C,H,Sw) 494

Micellaneous Analgesics
Acetaminophen (D) 3

Nonsteroidal Anti-inflammatory/ Analgesic Agents
Aspirin (D,C,B,H,Sw,A) 56
Carprofen (D) 102
DMSO (D,H) 208
Etodolac (D) 260
Flunixin (D,B,H,A) 288
Ketoprofen (H) 370
Meclofenamic Acid (D,H) 392
Naproxen (D,H) 449
Phenylbutazone (D,B,H,Sw) 504
Piroxicam (D) 518

Gold Compounds
Aurothioglucose (D,C,H) 68
Auranofin (D) 67

Behavior-Modifying Agents
Amitriptyline (D,C) 30
Buspirone (D,C) 87
Clomipramine (D,C) 148
Clorazepate (D) 152
Imipramine (D,C) 338

Tranquilizers/Sedatives
Acepromazine (D,C,P,B,H,Sw,Sh) 1
Azaperone (Sw) 70
Detomidine (H,B) 177
Diazepam (D,C,B,H,Sw,Sh) 184
Doxepin (D,C,B,Sw,H) 225
Medetomidine (D,C) 394
Midazolam (D,C,H) 429
Promazine (D,C,B,H,Sw) 541
Tiletamine/Zolazepam (D,C,H,Z) 617
Xylazine (D,C,B,H,Sh,Z) 648

Anesthetic Agents
Barbiturates
Pentobarbital (D,C,B,H) 496
Thiamylal (D,C,B,H,Sw,Sh) 607
Thiopental (D,C,B,H,Sw,Sh) 610
Inhalants
Isoflurane (D,C,P,R,A) 348
Halothane (D,C,P,H) 316
Methoxyflurane (D,C,B,Sh,Sw) 416
Miscellaneous
Fentanyl/Droperidol (D,C) 274
Ketamine (D,C,B,H,Sw,Sh,R,A,Z) 362
Propofol (D,C) 545
Xylazine (D,C,B,H,Sh,Z) 649
Tiletamine/Zolazepam (D,C,H,Z) 617

Reversal Agents
Atipamezole (D) 62
Flumazenil (D,C) 287
Naloxone (D,C,H) 445
Naltrexone (D) 446
Neostigmine (D,B,H,Sw,Sh) 454
Tolazoline (D,C,H,Sh,B,Z) 625
Yohimbine (D,C,H,L,Z) 651

Anticonvulsants
Bromides (D) 82
Clonazepam (D) 150
Clorazepate (D) 152
Diazepam (D,C,B,H,Sw,Sh) 184
Mephenytoin (D) 406
Phenobarbital (D,C,B,H) 500
Phenytoin (D,C,H) 509
Primidone (D,C) 535
Valproic Acid (D) 634

Oxybutynin (D,C) 472
Phenoxybenzamine (D,C,H) 503
Phenylpropanolamine (D,C) 508

Urinary Alkalinizers
Sodium Bicarbonate (D,C,H,B,Sh,A) 569

Urinary Acidifiers
Methionine (D,C,B,H) 411
Ammonium Chloride (D,C,H,B,Sh) 32

Cholinergic Stimulants
Bethanechol (D,C,H,R) 76

Agents for Urolithiasis
Acetohydroxamic Acid (D) 7
Allopurinol (D,C,A) 14
Ammonium Chloride (D,C,H,B,Sh) 32
Citrate Salts (D) 142
Methionine (D,C,B,H) 411
Tiopronin (D) 620

Gastrointestinal Agents
Antiemetic Agents
Chlorpromazine (D,C,B,H,Sw,Sh) 129
Dimenhydrinate (D,C) 205
Diphenhydramine (D,C,B) 214
Meclizine (D,C) 391
Metoclopramide (D,C,H) 421
Prochlorperazine (D,C) 539

Antiulcer Medications
  Antacids
Aluminum Gels (D,C) 48
Calcium Salts, Oral (D,C,B,H,Sh,Sw,A,R) 92
Na Bicarbonate (D,C,H,B,Sh,A) 569
  H2 Antagonists
Cimetidine (D,C,B,H,Sw,R) 134
Famotidine (D,H) 264
Ranitidine (D,H) 562
  Gastromucosal Protectants
Sucralfate (D,C,H,R) 583
  Protaglandin E1 Analogs
Misoprostol (D) 434
  Proton Pump Inhibitors
Omeprazole (D,H) 462

Appetite Stimulants
Cyproheptadine (D,C) 164
Diazepam (D,C,B,H,Sw,Sh) 184
Oxazepam (D,C,H) 469

GI Antispasmodics-Anticholinergics
Aminopentamide (D,C) 22
Isopropamide (D,C) 349
Propantheline (D,C,H) 542

GI Stimulants
Cisapride (D,C,H) 139
Dexpanthenol (D,C,H) 182
Metoclopramide (D,C,H) 421
Neostigmine (D,B,H,Sw,Sh) 454

Digestive Enzymes
Pancrelipase (D,C,A) 483

Laxatives
  Saline
Oral Colonic Lavage (OCL) (D) 567
Saline Hyperosmotics (D,C,B,H,Sw,A) 567
  Magnesium Salts
  Sodium Salts
  Irritant
Bisacodyl (D,C) 78
  Bulk producing
Psyllium (D,C,H) 551
  Lubricant
Mineral Oil (D,C,B,H,Sw,Sh,A) 432
  Surfactant
Docusate (D,C,H) 219
  Misc.
Lactulose (D,C,A) 371

Antidiarrheals
Diphenoxalate/Atropine (D,C) 216
Kaolin/Pectin (D,C,B,H,Sw,Sh,A) 361
Bismuth Subsalicylate (D,B,H,Sw) 78
Clioquinol (H) 148

Misc. GI Drugs
Bismuth Subsalicylate (D,B,H,Sw) 78
Pancrelipase (D,C,A) 483
Sulfasalazine (D,C) 592
Ursodiol (D) 633

Hormones/Endocrine/Reproductive Agents
Sex Hormones
  Estrogens
Estradiol (D,C,B,H) 253
DES (D) 193

  Progestins
Altrenogest (H) 16
Medroxyprogesterone (D,C,A) 396
Megesterol (D,C) 398

  Androgens
Danazol (D,C) 170
Mibolerone (D,C,H) 428
Testosterone (D,C,B) 595

  Anabolic steroids
Boldenone (H) 81
Stanozolol (D,C,H,Sh,A,R) 579
Nandrolone (D,C) 447

Posterior Pituitary Hormones
  Vasopressin Derivatives
Desmopressin (D,C) 175
Vasopressin (D,C) 636

  Oxytocics
Oxytocin (D,C,B,H,Sw,Sh,A,R) 479

Adrenal Cortical Steroids
Corticotropin-ACTH (D,C,B,H,A) 159
  Mineralocorticoids
Desoxycorticosterone Piv. (D) 176
Fludrocortisone (D,C) 286

Glucocorticoids
Betamethasone (D) 75
Dexamethasone (D,C,B,H,Sw,L,A,R) 178
Fludrocortisone (D,C) 286
Flumethasone (D,C,H) 288
Hydrocortisone (D,C,B,H) 330
Methylprednisolone (D,C,H) 418
Prednisolone (D, C,B,H,L,Sw,A,R) 528
Prednisone (D,C,B,H,L,Sw,A,R) 528
Triamcinolone (D,C,B,H) 627

Adrenal Steroid Inhibitors
Mitotane (D)435
Selegiline (D) 567

Antidiabetic Agents
Insulin (D,C,B,H,A) 339
Chlorpropamide (D,C,A,B,Sw) 131
Glipizide (C) 304

Glucose elevating agents
Diazoxide (D) 187
Glucose/Dextrose

Thyroid Drugs
Thyroid Hormones
Levothyroxine (D,C,H,B,R) 377
Liothyronine (D,C) 384
TSH (D,C,H) 614
Antithyroid Drugs
Methimazole (C) 409

Misc. Endocrine/Reproductive Drugs
Bromocriptine (D,H) 84
Chorionic Gonadotropin-HCG
    (D,C,B,H,Sh) 132
Follicle Stimulating Hormone
    (D,C,B,H,Sw,Sh,P) 293
Gonadorelin (D,C,B,Sh) 311
Mibolerone (D) 428
Prostaglandins
Cloprostenol (B,H,Sw,Sh) 151
Dinoprost (D,C,B,H,Sw,Sh) 210
Fenprostalene (B) 271
Fluprostenol (H) 292

Antiinfective Drugs
Antiparasitics
Amitraz (D,Sh) 28
Albendazole (D,C,B,Sw,Sh) 11
Clorsulon (B,Sh,L) 154
Cythioate (D) 167
Dichlorvos (D,C,P,B,H) 189
Diethylcarbamazine (D,C) 191
Doramectin (B) 223
Eprinomectin (B) 246
Epsiprantel (D,C) 247
Ethylisobutrazine (D) 258
Febantel (D,C,B,Sh,H) 266
Fenbendazole (D,C,B,H,Sw,Sh,L,A,R) 268
Fenthion (D) 276
Fipronil (D,C) 280
Furazolidone (D,C) 296

Imidocarb (D,Sh) 335
Imidacloprid (D,C) 334
Ivermectin (D,B,H,Sw,Sh,L,A,R) 357
Levamisole (D,C,B,L,Sw,Sh,A) 373
Lufenuron (D,C) 385
Melarsomine (D) 401
Metronidazole (D,C,H,A,R) 424
Milbemycin (D,C) 431
Morantel (B,Sh) 439
Moxidectin (D,H,B) 443
Oxfendazole (H,B,Sw,Sh) 470
Oxibendazole (H,B,Sw,Sh) 471
Piperazine (D,C,H,B,Sw,A) 516
Praziquantal (D,C,Sh,L,A,R) 527
Pyrantal (D,C,H,Sw,B,Sh,L,A) 552
Pyrimethamine (D,C,H) 556
Quinacrine (D,C) 558
Thiabendazole (D,B,H,Sw,Sh,L,A) 600
Thiacetarsemide (D,C) 602

Anticoccidial Agents
Amprolium (D,B,Sw,Sh,A) 45
Decoquinate (B,Sh,L) 173

Antibiotics
Aminocyclitols
Amikacin (D,C,B,H,A,R) 17
Apramycin (Sw,B) 53
Gentamicin (D,C,B,H,Sw,A,R) 299
Neomycin (D,C,B,H,Sw,Sh,A,R) 451
Spectinomycin (D,C,B,H,Sw,A) 575
Tobramycin (D,C,H,A,R) 621
Cephalosporins
Cefadroxil (D,C) 103
Cefazolin (D,C,H) 104
Cefoperazone (H) 106
Cefotaxime (D,C,H,A,R) 107
Cefoxitin (D,C,H) 109
Ceftiofur (B,H,R) 110
Ceftriaxone (D,C,H)111
Cephalexin (D,C,H,A) 112
Cephalothin (D,C,B,H,A,R) 116
Cephapirin (D,C,B,H) 117
Macrolides
Erythromycins (D,C,B,H,Sw,Sh) 248
Tylosin (D,C,B,Sw,Sh,A,R) 631
Penicillins
Amoxicillin (D,C,B,H,A,R) 34
Amoxicillin/Clavulanate (D,C) 36
Ampicillin (D,C,B,H,Sw,P,A,R) 42
Carbenicillin (D,C,H,A,R) 98
Cloxacillin (D,C,B) 155
Dicloxacillin (D,C) 191
Hetacillin (D,C,B) 323
Oxacillin (D,C,H) 467
Penicillin G (D,C,B,H,Sw,A) 489
Penicillin V (D,C,H) 493
Ticarcillin (D,C,B,H,L,Sw,A,R) 616

Miscellaneous Agents

Antidotes
Acetylcysteine (D,C) 8
Ammonium Molybdate (Sh) 34
Antivenin Polyvalent/Coral Snake (D,H) 50
Atipamezole (D) 62
Deferoxamine (D,C) 174
Dimercaprol (D,C,H,B) 206
Edetate Calcium Disodium (D,C,H,A,B) 233
Ethanol (D,C) 257
Fomepizole--4-MP(D) 295
Methylene Blue (D,B,Sh) 417
Naloxone (D,C,H) 445
Penicillamine (D,C) 485
Phytonadione (D,C,B,H,Sw,Sh,A) 513
Pralidoxime (D,C,B,H) 523
Protamine Sulfate (D,C,B) 550
Sodium Polystyrene Sulfonate (D) 573
Sodium Sulfate (B,Sh,Sw) 574
Sodium Thiosulfate (H,B,Sh) 574
Thiamine (D,C,B,H,Sw,Sh) 605
Zinc Acetate/Sulfate (D,C) 652
Activated charcoal (D,C,B,Sh,H) 119

Bone/Joint Agents
Allopurinol (D,C,A) 14
Hyaluronate (D) 325
Etidronate (D,C) 259
Polysulfated Glycosaminoglycan (H,D) 520

Dermatologic Agents (Systemic)
Fatty Acids, Essential (D,C) 265
Etretinate (D) 261
Isotretinoin (D,C) 353
Pentoxifylline (D,H) 499

Emetics
Apomorphine (D,C) 51
Ipecac (D,C) 345

Vitamins and Minerals/Nutrients
Ascorbic Acid/Vit. C (D,C,P,H,B) 53
Carnitine (D,C) 101
Fatty Acids, Essential (D,C) 265
MCT Oil (D) 396
Thiamine (D,C,B,H,Sw,Sh) 605
Vitamin E/Selenium (B,Sw,Sh,H) 644
Zinc Acetate/Sulfate (D,C) 652

Immune Stimulants
Propionibacterium Acnes Inj. (D,C) 544

Cholinergic Muscle Stimulants
Pyridostigmine (D,C) 554

Systemic Acidifiers
Acetazolamide (D,C,B,Sh,Sw) 5
Acetic Acid (B,Sh,H) 6

Systemic Alkalinizers
Sodium Bicarbonate (D,C,H,B,Sh,A) 569

Unclassified
Aminocaproic Acid (D) 21
Colchicine (D) 158

Edrophonium (D,C) 235
Methylene Blue (D,B,Sh) 417
Pyridostigmine (D,C) 554

Index

Notes:

Notes:

Notes:

ISBN 0-8138-2444-3

9 780813 824444   90000